RESPIRATORY
DISEASES

RESPIRATORY
DISEASE

RESPIRATORY DISEASES

JOHN CROFTON

M.A., M.D.(Camb.), F.R.C.P.(Edin. & Lond.)

Professor of Respiratory Diseases and Tuberculosis
University of Edinburgh,
Honorary Consultant Physician
South-Eastern Regional Hospital Board, Scotland

AND

ANDREW DOUGLAS

M.B., Ch.B., F.R.C.P.(Edin.)

Senior Lecturer, Department of Respiratory Diseases and Tuberculosis
University of Edinburgh,
Honorary Consultant Physician
South-Eastern Regional Hospital Board, Scotland

SECOND PRINTING

BLACKWELL SCIENTIFIC PUBLICATIONS

OXFORD AND EDINBURGH

First published 1969
Reprinted 1971

ISBN 0 632 05480 8

Distributed in the U.S.A. by

F. A. DAVIS COMPANY, 1915 ARCH STREET
PHILADELPHIA, PENNSYLVANIA

Printed and bound in Great Britain by

WILLIAM CLOWES AND SONS LIMITED, LONDON,
BECCLES AND COLCHESTER

Contents

11   Primary Pulmonary Tuberculosis   196

12   Miliary Tuberculosis   207

13   Postprimary Pulmonary Tuberculosis   215

14   Treatment of Pulmonary Tuberculosis   234

15   Pulmonary Disease due to 'Atypical' Mycobacteria   259

16   Pleurisy and Pleural Effusion   263

29 Tumours of the Lung 517

30 Other Pulmonary Tumours 552

31 Diffuse Fibrosing Alveolitis and Honeycomb Lung 565

32 Respiratory Manifestations of Systemic Diseases 577

Preface

This book is designed principally for postgraduates wishing to learn something of chest disease and as a modest reference book for general physicians or others. It is not primarily an undergraduate book but we hope the occasional enthusiastic undergraduate may dip into it in search of more detail on a particular theme.

We are well aware that no one, certainly not ourselves, can know all about respiratory disease. The book is founded on our own clinical practice, on many years' experience of teaching undergraduates and postgraduates and on an inevitably limited study of the literature. As the book purports to be in English we have mainly confined ourselves to references in that language. On the more important themes we have given only a few key foreign references, if any at all, but we have been a little more ecumenical in the case of some of the more exotic diseases.

In order to enable us to deal with certain important subjects more fully, and yet to keep the book within a reasonable compass and within a reasonable price, we have severely curtailed the number of x-rays included, though in places we have thought it useful to elaborate the text with diagrams or drawings. The reader in search of illustrative x-rays is recommended to consult radiological textbooks, such as Le Roux B. T. and Dodds T. C. (1964) *A Portfolio of Chest Radiographs*, Edinburgh: Livingstone; Le Roux B. T. and Dodds T. C. (1968) *A Second Portfolio of Chest Radiographs*, Edinburgh: Livingstone; Simon G. (1962) *The Principles of Chest X-ray Diagnosis*, 2nd Edition, London: Butterworth or Shanks S. C. and Kerley P. eds (1962) *A Textbook of X-ray Diagnosis by British Authors*, vol. 2, 3rd Edition, London: Lewis.

A number of colleagues have been kind enough to read individual chapters. Their constructive criticism has been of great value to us, although of course we alone are responsible for any residual errors. For this help our sincere thanks are due to Professor A. L. Cochrane, Dr. Charles Fletcher, Dr. Wallace Fox, Professor L. P. Garrod, Dr. I. W. B. Grant, Dr. N. W. Horne, Mr. R. J. M. McCormack, Dr. G. J. R. McHardy, Dr. A. T. Wallace and Dr. F. J. Wright. We are most grateful to Dr. Eileen Crofton for providing much epidemiological information and for reading the proofs, and to both our wives for tolerating the distortions of family life implicit in authorship. We would also like to thank our junior colleagues not only for all they have taught us but also for inevitably taking an increased share of the routine work while we have been engaged in writing the book.

We cannot too greatly praise Miss May Corkey and Miss Margaret Ballantine for their skill in typing, for their disciplined marshalling of our disordered references into orderly ranks, for their brilliant interpretation of scribbled drafts which must sometimes have been as challenging as Etruscan, and for facing all these exacting tasks with unfailing intelligence and good humour.

We would also like to thank Mr. Per Saugman, Managing Director of Blackwell Scientific Publications, who cajoled us into writing this book in the first place and Mr. Nigel Palmer, Manager of their Edinburgh office, for patiently nursing a pair of tyros through the vicissitudes of publication.

Some Symbols used in Respiratory Physiology

PRIMARY SYMBOLS

V	Volume of gas
$\dot{V}$	Volume of gas per unit time
Q	Volume of blood
$\dot{Q}$	Volume of blood per unit time
P	Pressure
S	Saturation
RQ	Respiratory quotient
R	Respiratory exchange ratio (under steady state conditions $=$ RQ)
D	Diffusing capacity
T	Transfer factor

SUFFIXES

E	Expired gas
A	Alveolar gas
T	Tidal gas
D	Deadspace
a	Arterial blood
v	Venous blood
c	Capillary blood
L	Lung

Examples of use of symbols and suffixes

Pa,O_2	Partial pressure of oxygen in arterial blood
PA,O_2	Partial pressure of oxygen in alveolar gas
$\dot{V}A$	Alveolar ventilation per unit time
VD	Volume of deadspace gas
VT	Tidal volume
DL	Diffusing capacity of the lung

CHAPTER 1

The Structure and Function
of the Respiratory Tract

The respiratory system brings air into contact with the mixed venous blood, so that appropriate gas exchange ensures an adequate content of oxygen in the systemic circulation to the tissues and the gaseous product of metabolism, carbon dioxide, is eliminated. In land animals the lungs not only provide an enormous interface for oxygen and carbon dioxide transfer between blood and environment but have the secondary function of an air pump. Atmospheric air undergoes purification, warming and humidification within the upper respiratory tract before onward transmission through the conducting passages (bronchi and bronchioles) to the alveoli where it comes into intimate contact with the mixed venous blood. The structure of each part of the respiratory system reflects its function.

The respiratory tract is arbitrarily divided at the level of the lower border of the cricoid cartilage into upper and lower parts. Whereas the lower respiratory tract is primarily concerned with conduction of air to and from the alveoli, the upper respiratory tract has several physiological functions in addition to air conduction. Among these are swallowing, conditioning of air before its passage into the trachea, smell and speech. A list of the symbols used in respiratory physiology, and their meaning, is given on p. xiv.

THE UPPER RESPIRATORY TRACT

THE NOSE

The nose has 4 important respiratory functions.

Air conduction

Unless there is obstruction, e.g. nasal polypi or mucosal congestion, the adult breathes through the nose. In normal subjects the resistance to air flow is 50% greater with nose breathing than with mouth breathing.

Defence mechanism

The hairs in the anterior part of the nose, the vascular mucous membrane, the ciliated epithelium, the watery secretions with their bactericidal properties and the extensive lymph drainage all combine to provide an important defence against noxious elements in the inspired air.

Warming and humidification of inspired air

These are probably the most important functions of the nose. Inspired air is heated to approximately body temperature (37°C) by the highly vascular mucous membrane of the nose, and the relative humidity of the inspired air is raised to the 95% which the bronchi and alveoli require for adequate function. The moisture is obtained from transudation through the mucosal epithelium, to a less extent from the secretions of mucous glands and goblet cells and also from the inspired air. 10,000 l (litres) of air pass through the nose every 24 hours and require about 0·75 l of nasal secretion for appropriate humidification. The vascularity of the nasal mucous membrane and the activity of the numerous mucous glands is under control of the autonomic nervous system.

When inspired air bypasses the nose, e.g. after endotracheal intubation or tracheostomy, the lower respiratory mucosa becomes dry and cessation of ciliary activity rapidly follows, predisposing to infection. It is important, therefore, to ensure that inspired air is adequately humidified. Even the nasal inhalation of dry gas can be harmful if prolonged. The importance of the warming and humidifying function is readily appreciated after strenuous exercise in a cold atmosphere when rapid mouth breathing leads to drying of the tracheal mucous membrane and retrosternal soreness.

There is no doubt, however, that the tracheobronchial mucosa can adapt itself to those situations in which the warming and humidifying functions of the nose are no longer effective. Patients with total laryngectomy breathe directly in and out of the trachea and, although there is initially a period of adjustment, there appears to be little final inconvenience from excluding the nose from the airways [35, 74 & 127].

THE PARANASAL SINUSES

There is no general agreement regarding the functions of the accessory air sinuses but among those more frequently mentioned are temperature insulation, voice resonance and protection combined with lightness. They are lined by ciliated columnar epithelium and communicate with the nasal cavity by narrow openings which may become occluded if the sinuses are infected. Impaired drainage results in infection persisting chronically in the sinuses, providing a potential source for aspiration of infected material into the lower respiratory tract.

THE EUSTACHIAN TUBE

At rest the walls are normally in apposition, acting as a valve, but during yawning, eating and swallowing they separate through the action of the tensor veli palatini [152]. Blowing against the closed lips and nose can raise the pressure in the nasopharynx sufficiently to open the tube. Pressures of 25–35 mm Hg are required for this [45, 129, 130 & 162]. Mucosal oedema, tenacious secretions and excessive adenoid tissue may occlude the tube so that a negative pressure develops in the middle ear and mastoid air cells, drawing the tympanic membrane inwards.

THE PHARYNX

The pharynx is divided by the soft palate into an upper nasopharyngeal portion and a lower orolaryngeal portion. The nasopharyngeal part has numerous lymph glands including the nasopharyngeal tonsil (or adenoids) and the Eustachian, lingual and palatine tonsils which are arranged in a circular fashion around the nasopharynx. Swelling of the lymphoid tissue can result in partial obstruction of the airway. Infection of lymph glands in the posterior wall of the pharynx may result in a retropharyngeal abscess, most commonly associated with extension of infection from a peritonsillar abscess but sometimes from sepsis of cervical vertebrae. A large retropharyngeal abscess presents difficulties for the anaesthetist if nasal intubation is necessary.

In the unconscious patient the tongue tends to fall back and obstruct the laryngeal opening. This may be prevented by bringing the lower jaw forwards and upwards so that the lower incisors lie in front of the upper teeth, and by hyperextending the head so that the tongue is carried upwards and forwards. If there are no contra-indications the unconscious patient, e.g. after anaesthesia, should be nursed on his side for in this position the tongue falls away from the posterior pharyngeal wall and aspiration into the larynx is less likely.

THE LARYNX

The larynx comprises a number of articulated cartilages, the vocal cords and the various laryngeal muscles and ligaments. The nerve supply of the mucous membrane is from both the superior and the recurrent laryngeal nerves. The principal motor nerve to the larynx is the recurrent laryngeal. The only other motor nerve is the external branch of the *superior laryngeal nerve*. This supplies the cricothyroid muscle, which is the principal tensor of the vocal cords. Paralysis of this nerve results in reduction in the antero-posterior diameter of the glottis and laxity of the vocal cords. Local anaesthesia of the throat and larynx as well as blocking the sensory nerve endings of the superior and recurrent laryngeal nerves may block the external branch of the superior laryngeal nerve and result in alteration of the shape of

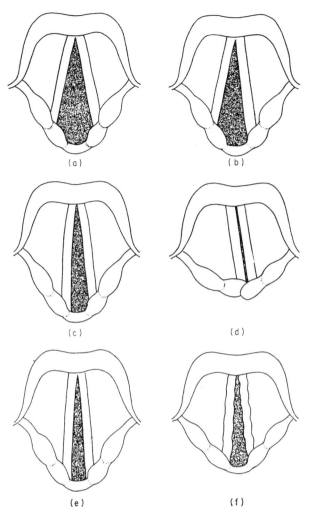

FIG. 1.1. Normal and some abnormal appearances of the vocal cords; all drawn as seen in the mirror, i.e. patient's left to observer's right. (a) Normal larynx during inspiration. (b) Left recurrent laryngeal nerve paralysis during inspiration. (c) Uncompensated left recurrent laryngeal nerve paralysis during phonation. (d) Compensated left recurrent laryngeal nerve paralysis during phonation. (e) Bilateral recurrent laryngeal nerve paralysis during inspiration. (f) Superior laryngeal nerve paralysis resulting in foreshortened larynx and lax vocal cords.

the glottis and the vocal cords (fig. 1.1.). It is important to remember this when local anaesthesia is employed for diagnostic laryngoscopy (p. 77). The superior laryngeal nerve may be injured at thyroidectomy. The functional effect of injury to the superior laryngeal nerve is that the voice is weak, rough and easily fatigued, and the pitch is lower so that the singing voice is lost.

The left *recurrent laryngeal nerve* leaves the vagus at the level of the aortic arch and after hooking round the arch runs upward through the mediastinum, between the trachea and the oesophagus and then deep to the thyroid to reach the larynx beneath the lower edge of the inferior constrictor muscle. The course of the right recurrent laryngeal nerve differs in the lower part, the origin being at the level of the subclavian artery, which it hooks round before passing upwards into the neck. Apart from the sensory fibres to the mucous membrane of the larynx below the level of the vocal cords, the recurrent laryngeal nerve supplies all the muscles of the larynx with the exception of the cricothyroid muscle.

As well as being the site of some of the most important protective mechanisms in the respiratory tract, e.g. cough reflex, the larynx is also the organ of voice production. Disease affecting the larynx is usually associated with some disturbance of phonation, commonly hoarseness or huskiness and sometimes complete loss of voice. The extent of the loss of voice may not match the seriousness of the lesion, e.g. a simple laryngitis may permit only a toneless whisper for several days.

The symptoms of vocal cord paralysis, which vary from practically none to almost complete loss of voice, depend on whether the condition is unilateral or bilateral, the position of the paralysed cord and the amount of compensation which the normal cord can achieve. In unilateral paralysis of the recurrent laryngeal nerve (fig. 1.1), abduction of the normal cord can provide an adequate airway so dyspnoea due to obstruction is not a feature. Bilateral palsy resulting in approximation of both cords to the midline may cause distressing dyspnoea.

Unilateral recurrent laryngeal nerve palsy leaves the affected cord close to the midline but since the glottis cannot be completely closed phonation is imperfect leading to hoarseness, loss of the singing voice and the ability to modulate. In time the voice may improve through the compensatory action of the normal cord which crosses the midline to meet the paralysed cord. The paralysed cord may become fixed in the paramedian position and the patient become unaware of the paralysis in ordinary conversation although the ability to sing remains impaired.

Bilateral recurrent laryngeal nerve palsy results in adduction of the cords so that the glottic opening becomes only a 2–3 mm chink. The voice is, therefore, weak but the main disability relates to obstruction of the airway so that any exertion may provoke dyspnoea and stridor.

The phenomenon of cough requires closure of the glottis, increase in the intrathoracic pressure and its sudden release when the glottis relaxes. When *vocal cord paralysis* occurs the explosive element of cough is lost (bovine cough). Motor paralysis of the larynx is usually due to involvement of the left recurrent laryngeal nerve by a bronchial carcinoma in the left hilar region. Syphilitic aortic aneurysm was once a frequent cause but is now rare. Other causes are oesophageal carcinoma, thyroid carcinoma and mediastinal swellings such as malignant glands, a dilated left auricle or a pericardial effusion. Paralysis of the right vocal cord is rare and is most commonly due to aneurysm of the right subclavian artery or thyroid carcinoma. The recurrent laryngeal nerve carries motor fibres to both the abductor and adductor muscles of the vocal cord. The abductor fibres are more vulnerable so that moderate trauma usually results in pure abductor paralysis while severe trauma or section of the nerve causes both abductor and adductor paralysis. Pure adductor paralysis does not occur except as a functional disorder. In hysterical aphonia the ability to cough normally is preserved. Commonly the condition is transient and self-limiting.

THE LOWER RESPIRATORY TRACT

CONDUCTING AIRWAYS

GROSS ANATOMY

THE TRACHEA [70]

The trachea extends from the larynx to the bifurcation in the mediastinum. It is fixed above to the larynx and so to the skull.

Below it is anchored to the mediastinum by means of the main bronchi and oblique connective tissue fibres running to the dorsal surface of the pericardium. The bifurcation is normally displaced slightly to the right, possibly because of the greater elastic pull of the right lung. As both ends can move independently the length is variable, averaging 10–12 cm. The transverse diameter is approximately 25% greater than the sagittal. About half the trachea lies in the cervical region and half is intrathoracic. The calibre of the intrathoracic portion is affected by intrathoracic pressure changes, while that of the cervical portion is not (p. 12). *Position and movements of the body* affect the position and length of the trachea. With flexion of the head the cricoid cartilage at the upper end of the trachea may be only 1 cm above the manubrium, whereas with full extension it may be 7 cm higher. There is up to 3 cm movement of the upper trachea with swallowing, while the bifurcation may move 1 cm. In the supine position and in expiration the bifurcation lies at the cranial end of the 5th thoracic vertebra, separated from it only by the oesophagus. In the prone position it moves forward about 2 cm. On inspiration the bifurcation moves caudally by about 1 vertebral level and away from the vertebrae by about 3 cm. The angle of bifurcation narrows on deep inspiration but the amount probably varies with the relation between diaphragmatic and costal breathing.

THE BRONCHI

The trachea divides into the right and left main bronchi, the left running somewhat more horizontally than the right. The angle between the bronchi varies from 50 to 100°. The right main bronchus gives rise to 3 *lobar bronchi*, the left to 2. The *right main bronchus* is only 1–2·5 cm in length before it gives off the *right upper lobe bronchus* (fig. 1.2). The intermediate bronchus then passes down to divide into the *middle* and *lower lobe bronchi*. The *left main bronchus* is approximately 5 cm in length before it divides into the *left upper lobe* and *lower lobe bronchi*. Each lobar bronchus divides in turn into *segmental divisions* which are shown in fig. 1.2. These are important clinically as pathological processes are often confined to segments. The precise anatomy of divisions below segmental are in general not important to the clinician, with the exception of the axillary subdivisions of the anterior and posterior segmental bronchi

of the right upper lobe. As individuals often lie on their side in sleep, aspirated material from the upper respiratory tract may gravitate into these divisions and give rise to pneumonia or lung abscess. It may also be noted that the apical bronchus of the right

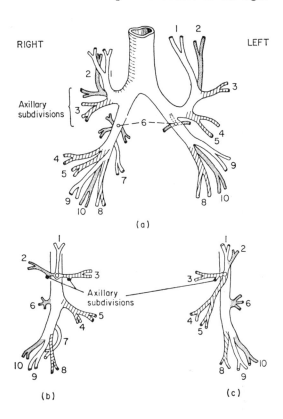

FIG. 1.2. Segmental bronchi; (a) anterior, (b) right lateral and (c) left lateral. Upper lobes: 1 apical, 2 posterior, 3 anterior; 4 and 5 superior and inferior lingular branches (left only). Middle lobe: 4 lateral, and 5 medial, branches. Lower lobes: 6 apical lower, 7 medial (right only), 8 anterior, 9 lateral, and 10 posterior, branches. After Brock [16] and Foster-Carter [57].

lower lobe usually comes off the lower lobe bronchus almost opposite the origin of the middle lobe bronchus. A lower subapical bronchus is not uncommon. Another relatively frequent variation is that the anterior segmental bronchus of the left upper lobe comes directly off the left upper lobe bronchus, thus forming a trifurcation with the apicoposterior and lingular bronchi. Very occasionally a separate bronchus comes directly off the trachea to the apex of the right upper lobe. Variations in bronchial segmental anatomy are common and are given in detail by Boyden [14].

Number of divisions in the bronchial tree. The lower airways are known as bronchi down to the smallest divisions containing cartilage, however sparse, in their walls. Thereafter they become *bronchioles*, which remain purely conducting airways. The final branch of this type of airway is known as the *terminal bronchiole* which gives off the *respiratory bronchioles*, so named because alveoli occur in their walls. From the tracheal bifurcation the smallest bronchi are reached after some 8–13 divisions, depending on the area of lung supplied [70]. There is a good deal of variation according to the size and shape of the segments. For instance, in the apical lower segment, where the bronchi run a relatively short course, the terminal bronchioles may be reached after some 15 generations from the origin of the segmental bronchus, whereas in the lingula it may be 25. There tend to be fewer generations in lateral branches than in axial [138].

From the smallest bronchi, which are about 1 mm in diameter, there are usually 3–4 further subdivisions of bronchioli before the terminal bronchiole is reached. There are therefore about 20 terminal bronchioles for each small bronchus [70]. There may be up to 50 respiratory bronchioles per terminal bronchiole. It has been estimated that some 200 alveoli are supplied by each respiratory bronchiole.

Diameters of branches of the airways. In most cases branching is by bifurcation. Although the cross section of each individual branch is smaller than that of the stem from which it arises the total cross section of both branches is greater than that of the stem. Therefore the total cross section of all the branches of the airways tends to increase peripherally. The total cross section of the respiratory bron-

chioles has an area some 10 times that of the trachea [70]. It is stated that the changes in diameter with respiration are relatively greater in the peripheral bronchi, perhaps because of their less rigid walls.

The pattern of terminal branching as seen in the bronchogram has been described by Reid [138]. After about the 8th to 10th division from the segmental bronchus the small bronchi and bronchioles show as parallel-walled line shadows, mostly consisting of bronchioli but including some small bronchi. These at first divide every 0·5–1 cm until near their termination when the branches occur every 2–3 mm and are only 2–3 mm long; these represent the terminal bronchioli.

The lung of the newborn child is not merely a miniature of the adult lung in that development continues after birth, particularly in relation to a number of branches of the airways. From about the 6th month of gestation until birth the human lung has 17 divisions of branching airways [125]. There is a resumption of lung growth after birth when additional branches are added, bringing the total number of divisions to about 25 in the adult lung.

Segmental anatomy. The lobes of the lung are divided into segments corresponding to the segmental bronchi. The distribution of these segments is shown in figs. 1.3, & 1.4, but

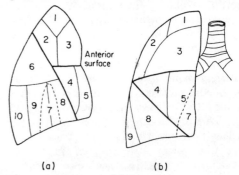

FIG. 1.3. Segmental anatomy of the right lung, (a) lateral and (b) anterior aspects. For key see fig. 1.2. After Foster-Carter [57].

there are frequent variations in the sizes of the segments and sometimes in their distribution [14]. It should be noted that the division between the segments is incomplete. There are only partial divisions by fibrous septa, mainly peripheral, and collateral airdrift can occur between the segments (p. 10). Frequently the divisions between segments can only be identified by the branches of the pulmonary

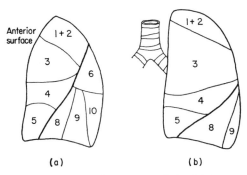

FIG. 1.4. Segmental anatomy of the left lung; (a) lateral and (b) anterior aspects. For key see fig. 1.2. After Foster-Carter [57].

vein which run between them. On the other hand sometimes partial fissures occur between segments, with infoldings of the pleura which may be visible radiologically, especially if thickened by pleurisy. Segmental anatomy is important clinically as pathological processes are often localized to individual segments and segmental pneumonia or collapse is common. Radiologically, segmental anatomy is most readily recognized on a lateral film.

Important abnormalities of segmental anatomy. Variations in segmental anatomy are common. (For details see Boyden [14]). Most of these are not of great importance to the physician, although they may be to the surgeon. Radiologically the so-called *azygos lobe* occurs in about 0·1% of right lungs [57]. This is a developmental abnormality caused by the azygos vein looping over a portion of the apical segment of the upper lobe rather than directly over the right main bronchus. This causes an infolding of both layers of the pleura, showing as a thin outwardly convex line ending in a rounded or oval shadow below, the latter representing the azygos vein. There is no abnormality of bronchial anatomy.

The azygos lobe is only very rarely the site of a localized pathological process. The so-so-called *sequestration* of part of the lung [13 & 57] is another congenital abnormality by which a portion, usually of a lower lobe, becomes isolated from the rest of the lung during development. The isolated segment is most often included within the lower lobe, although the bronchi, which are usually dilated and cystic, do not connect with the rest of the bronchial tree. There is almost always an abnormal blood supply to the sequestrated area, usually from the thoracic aorta, but sometimes from the abdominal aorta with a branch running up through the diaphragm. The abnormality is slightly commoner on the left than the right and usually comes to attention after becoming infected and suppurating. Radiologically it may show as a somewhat rounded opacity which may be mistaken for a tumour. Occasionally the sequestration is not included in the lung (*extralobar sequestration*). Although some of these are pulmonary in origin, others may develop embryonically from separate diverticula from the foregut and have a connection with the oesophagus [13].

STRUCTURE OF THE WALLS OF THE AIRWAYS (mainly from von Hayek [70]) The walls of the trachea and bronchi contain 3 important layers:

(1) the mucosa,
(2) the submucosa and
(3) the fibrocartilaginous layer which also includes the plain muscle.

The arrangement for a large bronchus is shown diagrammatically in fig. 1.5.

The *mucosa* is a *pseudostratified ciliated epithelium*. Most of the superficial layer consists of ciliated cells (p. 10). Scattered among the ciliated cells are the goblet cells which are mucus-secreting. The majority of goblet cells are surrounded by ciliated cells and they decrease in numbers in the smaller bronchi. Beneath the superficial cells in the large bronchi are 2 or 3 further rows of more cuboidal transitional cells, gradually decreasing in numbers peripherally until there is only

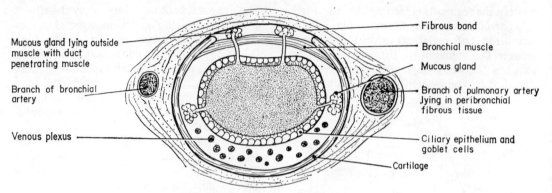

Fig. 1.5. Diagrammatic cross-section of a large bronchus.

a single row of ciliated cells, with occasional goblet cells, in the bronchioli. The mucosa is limited externally by the basement membrane which consists of strands of interweaving fibrils. Over the carina of the tracheal bifurcation, and frequently in the region of lower bifurcations, ciliated epithelium is replaced by *squamous*. There are intercellular clefts in the mucosa which may contain lymphocytes, leucocytes and mast cells, and also large rounded faintly staining cells, especially near bifurcations, which are probably sensory receptors [70 & 178]. The mucosa is often disposed in longitudinal folds, the thickness of which perhaps partially depends on the tone of the bronchial muscle.

The *submucosa* is thicker beneath the folds of mucosa and, in the trachea and larger bronchi, posteriorly between the ends of the cartilaginous rings. In the submucosa a capillary network lies directly on the basement membrane, with pre- and postcapillary vessels lying in the deeper layers between the elastic fibres. The *elastic fibres* are mainly disposed longitudinally in bundles along the folds of the mucous membrane with thin intervening layers, but are also connected with the mucous membrane, with the cartilage and with circular elastic fibres in the fibro-cartilaginous layer. In the bronchioli elastic fibres pass outwards and connect with the alveolar elastic tissue.

Mucous glands occur from the trachea to the smallest bronchi and are most numerous in medium sized bronchi. In the large bronchi

they are situated in the submucosa between the mucous membrane and the cartilage, often extending outwards between gaps in the cartilage. They may lie external to the muscle with their ducts penetrating the latter and may even protrude outwards through the fibrous layer into the peribronchial connective tissue. They are mostly sausage shaped with the duct opening at one end and running transversely to the long axis of the bronchus to discharge on the surface of the bronchial mucous membrane. The size of the glands is very variable, the largest being up to 1 mm in length. They greatly increase in number and size in chronic bronchitis (p. 310). The epithelium of the mucous glands is ciliated with a variable number of goblet cells. External to the bronchial muscle the ducts may be ampullary and surrounded by lymphoid tissue. Some of the cells of the mucous glands seem granular and have been thought to secrete a serous fluid, although Florey et al. consider on histochemical grounds that this appearance may be deceptive and that most may be mucus-secreting [55]. The mucus and its function are discussed on p. 15.

In the trachea and larger bronchi, down to the 4th or 5th generation of the segmental bronchi, the *cartilages* are semicircular, somewhat horseshoe shaped and with a posterior gap. This posterior 'membranous' portion of the bronchus is limited externally by a fibrous membrane joining the tips of the cartilages and continuous longitudinally between successive cartilages.

The bifurcations of the bronchi, and of the trachea, are marked by cartilaginous spurs with a ridge concave towards the trachea. In the smaller bronchi the cartilage breaks up into irregular plates which become more and more sparse as the bronchial tree is descended, the airways becoming known as bronchioles when cartilage can no longer be found in their walls.

In the trachea the *plain muscle* connects the tips of the cartilages and lies internal to the fibrous membrane. Contraction of the muscle brings the tips of the cartilages together and results in invagination of the posterior mucous membrane into the tracheal lumen. As the bronchial tree is descended the muscle is inserted further and further forward on the inner surface of the cartilages until it comes to form a ring. As the cartilages cease to be circumferential the bronchial muscle becomes disposed more longitudinally in a spiral manner and its contraction both narrows and shortens the bronchi. In the smaller bronchi the muscle is separated from the cartilage by a loose vascular layer with numerous bronchovenous vessels and lymphatics. In the bronchioles the muscle tends to merge with the surrounding lung tissue. Relative to the thickness of the wall the muscle is largest in the bronchioles. The extramuscular venous network terminates at the bronchioles where the fibrous layer and the mucous membrane become united.

The bronchi are surrounded by *peribronchial tissue* mostly consisting of loose connective tissue which allows the bronchi to move within it and which is continuous with the periarterial tissue of the pulmonary arteries and the large veins. This tissue also contains bronchial arteries and veins, nerves, lymph vessels, lymphoid and adipose tissue. Dust is often deposited in the peribronchial tissue especially in areas where lymphoid tissue surrounds dust-containing macrophages in the region of the dividing angles of the bronchi [70].

The *bronchioli* contain no cartilage or mucous glands. They consist of a single layer of ciliated epithelium with very occasional goblet cells. The terminal bronchiole is the most distant bronchiole with complete epithelial lining. The *respiratory bronchiole* is partly lined by alveoli opening off it.

BLOOD SUPPLY OF THE BRONCHI

The bronchi are primarily supplied by the *bronchial arteries* derived from the aorta but *anastomoses with the pulmonary artery* make it possible for the latter also to convey blood to the distal portions of the medium and small bronchi, and it is probable that the bronchioles are mainly supplied by the pulmonary artery. The bronchi drain both into the pulmonary veins and into the vena cava. The smaller bronchi drain into the pulmonary veins of the segments while the larger bronchi drain by small venous bundles into the pulmonary veins at the hilum. They connect also by a plexus with the venous network of the posterior mediastinum and so with the azygos and hemiazygos veins.

THE TERMINAL AIR UNITS

The terminal bronchiole is the last purely conducting structure in the respiratory tract, and it is the last part of the bronchial tree which has a continuous lining of cuboidal epithelial cells [70]. Distal to this is the acinus

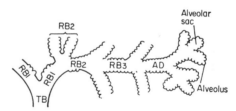

FIG. 1.6. A diagrammatic view of the acinus and its components showing the terminal bronchiole (TB), respiratory bronchioles (RB 1st, 2nd & 3rd orders) and the alveolar duct (AD). By permission of Professor A.D. Heppleston.

(fig. 1.6), which is the part of the lung concerned with gas exchange and which consists of three orders of respiratory bronchioles with their distal connections [170]. These bronchioles, as their name suggests, bear alveoli which increase in number from the 1st to the 3rd order of respiratory bronchioles. The alveoli are shallow and are separated by smooth portions of the wall in which a continuous cuboidal epithelium is no longer present. Each 3rd order of respiratory bronchiole leads into 2 or 3 alveolar ducts. An alveolar duct can scarcely be said to possess walls for the alveolar entrances are so close together but between the alveoli wisps of smooth muscle, collagen and elastic fibres can be identified. This is the last part of the bronchial tree with continuous muscle fibres and closure of terminal air units may occur through contraction of these fibres [157]. An alveolar duct and its distal connections constitute a *primary lobule*. The last in a short series of alveolar ducts terminates in one or more alveolar sacs which, in turn, bear a small and variable number of terminal alveoli. The alveolar sacs, like the alveolar ducts, have no proper walls but open out on all sides into alveoli. The term 'atrium' was applied by Miller to an irregularly shaped space intervening between the alveolar duct and the alveolar sacs [113]. Further studies have shown, however, that the atria may have their basis in shrinkage artefacts. On this account and because the term does not have a precise meaning Krahl has suggested that it should no longer be used [92].

The diameter of an alveolus varies with the depth of respiration but an average is about 0·25 mm. It is estimated that there are about 300 million alveoli in each lung and in the normal subject the internal surface area of the lungs varies from 40.to 80 m² [168, 169 & 170]. The term *secondary lobule* [113] is applied to the smallest division of the lung parenchyma which is bounded by connective tissue septa. It is variable in size because the lobular septa vary in size but, because it is easily recognized, it is a useful unit for descriptive purposes.

THE RESPIRATORY EPITHELIUM

From the trachea to the beginning of the respiratory bronchioles the respiratory tract is lined by ciliated columnar epithelium interspersed with variable numbers of goblet cells. At the beginning of the respiratory bronchiole the lining cell becomes cuboidal and has no cilia. Electron microscopy studies by Low

and many others have given conclusive proof that there is a complete epithelial covering of each alveolar surface [102, 103 & 104]. The alveolar wall consists of a layer of flattened epithelium comprising two types of cell (large and small) on a basement membrane. Some of the alveolar epithelial cells have phagocytic properties and can readily ingest carbon particles, red blood cells, etc. when these are instilled intratracheally. Between adjacent alveoli the interalveolar septa contain the pulmonary capillaries, reticulum and elastic fibres and phagocytes of mesodermal origin. Electron microscopy studies have shown that the distance from alveolar air to the capillary blood is from 0·36 to 2·5 μ [145].

The alveolar epithelium is covered by a mucoid film which is probably derived from septal cells in the alveolar wall. This contains a surface acting agent (p. 11) which appears to be secreted by the larger of the alveolar epithelial cells. The functions of this mucoid layer are said to include removal of fine particulate matter, protection of the underlying tissue from drying, facilitation of gas exchange and the maintenance of a near constant alveolar surface tension [108] (p. 11).

ALVEOLAR PORES

Collateral drift of alveolar gas may occur through the pores of Kohn which are openings in the alveolar wall 10–15 μ in diameter [91]. These allow communication between alveoli, even between adjoining segments. They may prevent collapse of lobules when the supplying bronchiole is occluded.

BRONCHIOLE–ALVEOLAR COMMUNICATIONS

Lambert has described short epithelium-lined communications between distal bronchioles and some of the neighbouring alveoli [93 & 94]. They are approximately 30 μ in diameter and therefore 2 or 3 times the diameter of most interalveolar pores. Apparently these tubular communications are able to remain open regardless of the degree of contraction of bronchiolar smooth muscle and probably play an important part in collateral ventilation in health and in disease. Interalveolar pores permit collateral ventilation between adjacent alveoli only whereas the bronchiole-alveolar communication provides a means of aerating many alveoli.

ALVEOLAR MUSCLE FIBRES

Isolated or interlacing smooth muscle fibres have been described throughout the interstitium of the lung and in the alveolar walls [8 & 34]. The precise physiological significance of these fibres is not known. Corssen found that these smooth muscle fibres occurred mainly in diseased tissue [34], for example in bronchitis and emphysema and particularly in pulmonary hypertension. He suggests that the lung parenchyma may be capable of active contraction which might explain some cases of atelectasis in which no bronchial obstruction can be demonstrated.

PULMONARY SURFACTANT
(Surface acting agent)

As early as 1929 von Neergaard suggested that retraction of the lungs during passive expiration was not due entirely to elastic tissue recoil and that surface tension forces were likely to be important [120]. After Macklin's demonstration of the mucoid film lining the alveoli [108], interest was stimulated in its nature by two observations. Radford showed by a study of pressure–volume loops (p. 43) that hysteresis was much less in a saline filled lung compared with an air filled lung [134 & 160], suggesting that surface forces are reduced when the gas–tissue interface is eliminated. Pattle demonstrated that pulmonary oedema fluid had much less surface tension than plasma [128]. Subsequent work by Clements and his colleagues showed that the retractive forces due to surface tension were as important as those due to the elastic tissues of the lung itself [29]. The surface acting forces became much less as the alveolar surface contracted during expiration. The effect of this is to enable alveoli to remain open for a longer period during expiration.

The surface tension of the mucoid layer lining the alveoli is regulated by a surface acting material secreted by the mitochondria of certain cells within the alveolar walls. Due to this pulmonary surfactant the surface tension of the alveolar wall decreases as surface area decreases (expiration) and increases as the area increases (inspiration). This stabilizes the alveolar spaces by equalizing pressure within them as they expand and contract and by distributing pressure evenly between small and large alveoli. Without surface acting agent alveoli would collapse and enormous forces would be required to expand them. It is also thought that surface acting agent assists osmotic forces acting across the alveolar capillary membrane and prevents the alveolar lining fluid from drawing further fluid into the alveoli. Pulmonary surfactant is a lipoprotein based on lecithin and sphyngomyelin radicles and appears at about the 30th week of intra-uterine life.

Absence of surface acting agent in the premature infant results in the *respiratory distress syndrome (hyaline membrane disease)* (p. 591). The surface tension in the lungs is increased and very high pressures are required to distend them. Osmotic pressure relationships are disturbed and fluid passes into the alveolar lumen. This fluid, which lacks surface acting material, does not foam as does ordinary pulmonary oedema fluid, and it is rich in eosinophilic material and in fibrin. The histopathological appearances due to this highly proteinous fluid give rise to the term 'hyaline membrane disease'. The child has all the features of respiratory distress including chest retraction, expiratory grunting and gross cyanosis. Paradoxical in-drawing of the ribs occurs with inspiration. The chest radiograph usually shows fine mottling throughout the lung fields. The outlook is poor but assisted respiration may be successful in some cases [12 & 159]. In a severe case hypoxia may not be relieved by oxygen therapy because of atelectasis resulting in blood flowing through unventilated lung (p. 37). To a pure respiratory acidosis (p. 47) a metabolic acidosis is added due to progressive anoxia and the accumulation of lactic acid. The giving of intravenous glucose and sodium bicarbonate after birth may improve the metabolic disorder [167].

Early delivery because of maternal diabetes or toxaemia of pregnancy may also result in the respiratory distress syndrome.

Surface acting agent is temporarily not produced or is inactivated after bronchial occlusion or the use of cardiac bypass, with consequent development of atelectasis [97]. Ozone [112], prolonged inhalation of 100% oxygen [27 & 133] and x-rays may also inactivate the surface film.

THE CALIBRE OF THE AIRWAYS AND ITS REGULATION

Adequate calibre of the airways is obviously crucial to efficient respiration. Flow in a tube varies inversely as the 4th power of its radius, so that slight changes in calibre have a major effect on flow. Airways obstruction is an important factor in causing disability in respiratory diseases such as chronic bronchitis and asthma. The available evidence regarding control of calibre, derived from the study of normal man and of experimental animals, has been reviewed by Widdicombe [175 & 178].

Factors affecting bronchial calibre may be classified as follows.

In the normal respiratory tract,

(1) mechanical factors,
    (a) the tension of the elastic tissues of the lung on the bronchial wall,
    (b) the relation between the extrabronchial pressure (alveolar pressure) and the pressure in the alveolar lumen, i.e. the transmural bronchial pressure.
(2) bronchial muscular tone.

In disease the following additional factors may be important,

(3) swelling of the bronchial mucous membrane due to inflammation, oedema, congestion or enlargement of the mucous glands,
(4) excessive mucus,
(5) distortion of the airways by fibrosis, emphysema, etc.

Only the first 2 factors will be considered here. Changes in disease are reviewed in the appropriate chapters.

The bronchi become longer and wider on inspiration, shorter and narrower on expiration. This has been shown both by radiological studies with the bronchi outlined by radioopaque material (bronchography), and by studying changes in anatomical dead space (p. 28). Various published studies indicate that on inflating the lungs 2–4% of the increased volume represents increased anatomical deadspace. Although some of this increase is in the larynx Widdicombe concludes that the volume of the airways increases in parallel with that of the lungs [178].

MECHANICAL FACTORS
AFFECTING AIRWAYS CALIBRE

It has been shown, as might be expected, that the resistance of the airways diminishes as the *lung volume* becomes greater and the bronchi dilate [38 & 178]. In fact resistance varies inversely as the lung volume under normal circumstances. It seems that the most important factor in reducing resistance is the *elastic pull of the lungs* on the airways (transpulmonary pressure), for if the chest wall of a healthy subject is appropriately strapped the relationship between airways resistance and transpulmonary pressure is maintained but the relationship with lung volume is not, probably due to the closure of lung units [19 & 26]. *Bronchial transmural pressure* is also a factor. During inspiration when the air is flowing into the alveoli the intraluminal pressure in the airways will clearly be above that of the alveoli, tending to push the walls of the airways outwards. During expiration the reverse holds. Intraluminal pressure in a gas flowing through a tube depends on the rate of flow and the resistance of the tube. On expiration, as the flow is occurring outwards, there is clearly a progressive fall of intraluminal pressure from the alveoli to the mouth. On the other hand the pressure in the alveoli surrounding the bronchi will be relatively constant. The inward pressure on the walls of the bronchi will therefore be greater in the proximal bronchi than in the distal. In addition, at constant volume flow, the intraluminal pressure decreases as the velocity increases (Bernoulli's theorem). The total cross-section of the larger bronchi is smaller than that of the smaller bronchi (p. 6). Therefore the velocity of the gas is increased in the larger bronchi, resulting in an even larger transmural pressure difference than in the smaller bronchi. With their more rigid walls the larger bronchi are more able to remain patent with this larger transmural pressure difference but with forced expiration the difference may be sufficient to invaginate the softer posterior walls between the gaps in the semicircular cartilage and cause air trapping. This only occurs at volumes between 75 and 20% of vital capacity [107]. It is possible that under these circumstances changes in smooth muscle tone may also contribute.

By measuring intrabronchial and transpulmonary pressure Macklem and Wilson conclude that in normal man lung volume is the major factor affecting the calibre of the airways peripheral to the segmental bronchi [107]. The proximal bronchi are affected both by the lung volume and expiratory pleural pressure, while the intrathoracic trachea is mainly affected by the pleural pressure. In quiet breathing the main resistance lies in the peripheral airways, in forced expiration in the proximal.

BRONCHIAL MUSCLE

Contraction of bronchial smooth muscle narrows the airways. In the trachea and larger bronchi, where the muscle is largely posterior and attached to the semicircular cartilages, contraction approximates the posterior ends of the cartilages, narrowing the bronchus both by reducing its diameter and by rendering the posterior mucous membrane redundant, the shape of the lumen becoming somewhat crescentic. Further down the bronchial tree the muscle fibres become more nearly circular and contraction of the lumen more symmetrical. More peripherally the fibres run spirally and contraction both narrows the lumen and shortens the bronchi. Contraction of circular muscle not only diminishes the overall diameter but renders the mucous membrane redundant so that it becomes

puckered and folded, further narrowing the lumen.

The *nerve supply* of the trachea and bronchi is derived from the vagus and sympathetic. These two groups of nerves are closely interrelated anatomically, with connecting branches and contributions to common plexuses, so that it is difficult to define the precise anatomy [70]. There is apparently a good deal of variation between individuals. The trachea is mainly supplied by the *recurrent laryngeal* nerves containing both vagal and sympathetic fibres. The bronchi are supplied by means of a smaller anterior and a larger posterior plexus to which both groups of nerves contribute. Most ganglia occur external to the cartilage and in the nonfibrous layer between the posterior ends of cartilages in the larger bronchi. They tend to be particularly related to the mucous glands. They are also found in the submucosa at the bronchial divisions.

With the interweaving of the sympathetic and parasympathetic fibres and the large number of variables which have been shown to affect bronchial calibre the precise definition of the influence of individual factors on bronchial calibre is a difficult task. A good deal of the experimental work is contradictory, probably because of differences in experimental conditions. Much still remains to be learned and the outline given below is inevitably oversimplified and provisional. For fuller details see the reviews by Widdicombe [175 & 178].

In general the vagal nerves are constrictor and the sympathetic dilator. There is apparently some nervous control of bronchial tone from the medulla independent of the control of respiratory movement, but its precise significance is still undefined [178]. Tone is probably controlled by reflexes affected by a large number of potential factors, some of which are mentioned below.

STATIC AND DYNAMIC TONE OF BRONCHIAL MUSCLE

We have used the word 'static' tone to indicate tone of the bronchial muscle which does not change throughout the respiratory cycle and 'dynamic' tone to indicate tone which may change during the respiratory cycle, increasing on expiration as the bronchi narrow and decreasing on inspiration [47 & 48]. Dynamic tone might also increase in cough. The existence of static tone in healthy normal subjects has been frequently shown by the increase of anatomical deadspace and decrease of airways resistance following the injection of atropine or inhalation of isoprenaline [178]. The effect of these drugs, and of vagotomy, on anaesthetized animals is the same [175]. Whether any change of tone occurs in normal respiration is uncertain; most of the changes in calibre are due to the mechanical factors outlined above. Any additional contribution from changes in tone, if it exists, must be small [178]. Major changes in lung inflation can probably affect bronchial muscular tone. Experimentally artificial inflation of lungs, isolated from the cervical trachea, has been shown to relax tracheal muscle while deflation contracts it, though the degree of inflation and the speed of the reaction were different from those of normal breathing [86, 101 & 176]. It is rational to suppose that inflation reflexes also affect bronchial muscle and there is some indirect evidence for this [178]. We have found that certain wheezy patients with bronchitis or asthma have greater endo-bronchial pressure changes than can be accounted for by mechanical influences. This suggests an increase in bronchomotor tone on expiration which may possibly be a pathological exaggeration of a small normal variation with breathing [47].

FACTORS AFFECTING
BRONCHIAL MUSCULAR TONE
These are by no means well defined in health and disease. Moreover, many experimental results are conflicting, probably because of the number of variables involved.

CO_2. In experimental animals there is good evidence that high concentrations of CO_2 produce constriction [101 & 176]. This appears to be nervously mediated, possibly by a reflex via the medulla. On the other hand Severinghaus et al., using bronchospirometry in dogs, showed that occlusion of a pulmonary artery to one lung, and consequent decrease of CO_2 excretion, diminished ventilation to that lung, probably by contraction of bronchial muscle, the effect being abolished by 2% CO_2 [147]. Similar results have been obtained in man and were reversed by 6% CO_2 [158]. In dogs the effect did not appear to be nervously mediated as it was blocked by isoprenaline but not by vagotomy or atropine. In man the breathing of 4–10% CO_2 does not consistently change airways resistance [19], but an actual effect may be masked by the resulting hyperpnoea. On the other hand voluntary overbreathing, which decreases CO_2, increases total lung resistance and this may be abolished by adding CO_2 [122]. In summary, it seems likely that CO_2 concentration has a direct effect on bronchial muscle, though possibly not within the normal physiological range, and that this effect may be of importance in reducing the ventilation to areas of the lung which are underperfused with blood. Conclusive evidence for this attractive theory is not at present available.

O_2. Although this has been less studied, there is good evidence that breathing 10% O_2, both in animals and man, can lead to increased airways resistance and this can be abolished by high concentrations [118 & 178].

Endocrine and metabolic factors.
(1) Isoprenaline, adrenaline and noradrenaline relax bronchial muscular tone and cause dilatation of the airways but the quantities likely to be present in the blood in physiological conditions are probably insufficient to have an effect [69 & 178].
(2) Histamine and 5-hydroxytryptamine (5-HT) produce constriction and may be important in anaphylaxis and in the bronchoconstriction of pulmonary embolism (p. 23). 'Slow reacting substance' may be important in asthma in man (p. 401).

Lung inflation and deflation. Lung inflation relaxes bronchial and tracheal muscle, probably through the pulmonary stretch receptors (Hering–Breuer reflex) [86, 101 & 176]. Deflation has the opposite effect. On the other

hand very large inflations may have a bronchoconstrictor effect [99] although, if there is
initial bronchoconstriction, the immediate
effect may be relaxation [117]. The previous
state of the muscle, the degree of inflation and
the exact time at which measurements are
made may all be relevant.

Painful stimuli have frequently been shown to
cause bronchodilatation.

Irritation of the airways mucosa. Irritation of
the respiratory epithelium, for instance by
inhalation of dusts or irritant gases, has often
been shown to produce reflex bronchoconstriction. In some instances irritation of
the upper airways causes dilatation instead of
constriction [178].

THE PHYSIOLOGICAL INFLUENCE OF CHANGES IN AIRWAYS CALIBRE

The larger the airways the larger the anatomical deadspace and therefore the greater the
respiratory work necessary to maintain a
given alveolar ventilation rate. On the other
hand, constriction of the airways, though
diminishing the deadspace, increases the
resistance of the airways and therefore increases respiratory work. One can imagine,
therefore, that, for any given alveolar ventilation rate, there is an optimum calibre for the
airways. Widdicombe calculates that the
optimum anatomical deadspace may be
about 125 ml [178]. It is not yet known
whether the calibres are at their optimum in
different physiological or pathological conditions or whether there is any appropriate
alteration in bronchial muscular tone. Calibre,
of course, is also increased by increasing lung
inflation (p. 12). It is thought that the increased lung inflation in patients with airways
obstruction may be partly a compensatory
response, attempting to widen the airways
by increasing the elastic tension of the lung

on their walls. Such inflation may also decrease bronchial muscular tone, at least when
there is prior bronchoconstriction [117].

UNIFORMITY OF CALIBRE CHANGES IN THE AIRWAYS

Widdicombe concludes that at present there
is no evidence that nervous control applies
differentially in different parts of the bronchial
tree [178], but little direct testing has been
carried out. Although it is often assumed that
most of the resistance is in the bronchioli in
fact most of the anatomical deadspace of the
bronchial tree is in the terminal and respiratory bronchioles and most of the resistance in
the lobar and segmental bronchi. That is to
say, decrease in bronchiolar calibre has a
more important effect in decreasing anatomical deadspace than in increasing resistance,
whereas the reverse is true for lobar and segmental bronchi. This is still controversial
and relative resistance in the airways may be
influenced by the type of breathing (see
Macklem and Wilson's findings [107] summarized on p. 13). In pathological conditions
there may be differential effects on the calibre
in different parts of the bronchial tree. For
instance, the peripheral parts, with thinner
and softer walls, are more likely to be distorted by fibrosis or emphysema or to be
obstructed by mucus, though these factors
will have to affect a very large number of the
small branches to have a major overall effect.
It is also possible that changes in CO_2 content
of the gas within the airways may have a
direct local effect on muscle tone (p. 14). It
has been shown (p. 13) that forced expiration,
with an intrathoracic pressure above atmospheric, tends particularly to obstruct the
intrathoracic trachea and larger bronchi by
invagination of their posterior walls. It is
possible that this may be of some clinical
importance in grossly dyspnoeic patients with
airways obstruction, at least during exercise.

THE SECRETIONS OF THE RESPIRATORY AIRWAYS

NATURE OF THE SECRETIONS

We are far from having a complete knowledge
of the secretions of the respiratory tract. The

mucous secretion consists mainly of acid and
neutral polysaccharides, the acid arising
partly from the presence of sialic acid or

sulphate [139]. Albumin and globulins are also present. The pH is usually neutral and the concentration of sodium and potassium midway between that in the blood serum and that within the cells [60]. Specific antibodies to such substances as tetanus toxoid and streptococcal antigens have been shown to be present in nasal secretions; reaginic antibodies have been found in allergic subjects [140]. The relative concentrations of the different types of globulins in tracheobronchial secretions are different from those in blood serum, and it has been suggested that a contribution is made by the lymphoid tissue of the respiratory tract [68 & 87]. In addition substances such as lysozyme and transferrin are present which may have a nonspecific, anti-infective function [60 & 61].

SOURCE

Mucus is derived from the goblet cells and the mucous glands. In the latter there are two types of cell, one distended with mucous globules and the other serous and with a granular appearance. In addition there is a transudation through the other cells in potentially quite large quantities [55]; some transudate may also be derived from the alveoli [60].

CONTROL

Secretion from the goblet cells is initiated by direct irritation of the cells, whereas the mucous glands secrete via a vagal reflex, though probably also by direct irritation [55 & 139]. Acetylcholine empties both types of cell in mucous glands but does not affect goblet cells. Atropine decreases secretion of the mucous glands.

FUNCTIONS

Knowledge of the functions of the respiratory secretions is incomplete but the following are probable.

(1) A 'waterproofing' effect which diminishes water loss in the respiratory tract as has been shown in the case of skin mucus in lower animals [121].

(2) A physical barrier is formed between inhaled irritants and the delicate cells of the mucous membrane. This barrier may be effective partly by its resistance to the passage

of water but mucoproteins also have a buffering effect which will tend to keep the hydrogen ion concentration constant.

(3) The secretions form the 'mucous blanket' which, by ciliary action, conveys trapped particles, etc. upwards and out of the respiratory tract (p. 17).

(4) They have an anti-infective action on inhaled pathogens by means of antibodies and nonspecific, anti-infective substances, as mentioned above.

IMPORTANCE IN DISEASE

Increased secretion of mucus, and perhaps increased transudation, probably form part of the response to infection and irritation and may have some of the protective effects already outlined. It has been shown experimentally that chronic irritation causes increase in the numbers of goblet cells [55 & 139]. The most important chronic condition leading to excessive mucus secretion is *chronic bronchitis* (p. 310). in which excess mucus floods the cilia so that they beat ineffectively and there is no thin mucous blanket to be passed upwards. The excess mucus is liable to obstruct small bronchi and sometimes even quite large ones. This mechanical effect reduces the drainage of the respiratory tract and renders it liable to infection. It has been shown also that mucus may coat bacteria and protect them from the body's defences [123]. On the other hand insufficient mucus or excessive drying of it, as may happen in tracheostomy, dries up the mucous blanket and prevents the effective action of the cilia. In *mucoviscidosis* (p. 592) the basic defect is probably a congenital abnormality of mucus, and it is possible that there are other qualitative abnormalities in disease which are as yet undefined. A rare disorder of mucous secretion occurs, known as *pituitous catarrh*, in which there is grossly excessive secretion of watery mucus, up to 500 ml/day. Histologically there is no hypertrophy of the mucous glands, and it seems possible that the fluid is derived from transudation. The excessive secretion is prevented by corticosteroid drugs which have little effect in other disorders of secretion such as chronic bronchitis [139].

THE CILIA OF THE RESPIRATORY TRACT

DISTRIBUTION AND FUNCTION

Cilia are distributed throughout the respiratory tract except in the anterior nares, in the back of the pharynx and over the vocal cords, though they extend between the cords posteriorly. Their general function is to cleanse the tract of particulate and other material by moving upwards a blanket of mucus about 5 μ in thickness. The blanket rests on the tips of the cilia which beat in less viscid fluid, possibly derived from transudation from the cells (p. 16). In the nasal sinuses the *direction of flow* is towards the ostia; in the nose backwards towards the posterior nares; in the bronchi upwards; in the trachea upwards, backwards between the vocal cords posteriorly and again upwards, until finally the mucous blanket tips over into the oesophagus. For correct functioning the mechanism requires:

(1) properly functioning cilia,
(2) the correct fluid in which to beat,
(3) a mucous blanket of the correct thickness and viscosity.

CILIARY MORPHOLOGY

The cilia are carried on the ciliary cells of the mucous membrane, about 200 cilia per cell, with some 1500 to 2000 million cilia/cm². The length of the cilia is some 6–7 μ in man, about the same as the thickness of the mucous blanket. Electron microscopy has shown that each individual cilium has a well organized structure [142].

ACTION OF THE CILIA

CILIARY MOVEMENT

Cilia act by a rapid forward movement with a rigid cilium followed by a slower recovery movement with a limp cilium. There is presumably contractile material within the cilium but this has not yet been precisely defined. The rate of ciliary beat varies; it is approximately 21 beats/sec in rats [39]. The cilia beat successively to produce a *wave motion* with waves about 20 μ in length. Such sequential movement is known as 'metachronal'. Apparently in mammals the movement of the waves is in the opposite direction to the effective beat of the cilia (antiplectic metachronism), an action which is said to be more effective in moving mucus [153]. The *factors controlling* ciliary movement are still incompletely defined. The metachronal action is said to depend on a principle of 'least interference' between the movement of individual cilia [153]. There is some evidence of nerve endings in close approximation to the cilia [142]. Although parasympathetic stimulation in the frog stimulates ciliary activity [105], and there is evidence that acetylcholine in large doses stimulates ciliary mucous membrane removed from man [33], it is uncertain whether such control is relevant to physiological conditions [62].

Rate of movement of the mucous blanket
Estimates in different animals with different techniques vary from 2·5 to 35 mm/min Smaller particles carried on the blanket usually move faster than do larger.

Factors affecting ciliary movement and movement of the mucous blanket
The rate of movement is unaffected by sleep or by gravity. *Drying* of the mucous blanket has a marked effect, the blanket tending to break. Ordinarily, when breathing through the nose, the tracheal air is more than 80% saturated with water vapour but with continuous mouth breathing this decreases. When a patient is breathing ordinary air through a tracheostomy the tracheal air may be only 50% saturated; humidification is therefore important. In experimental animals internal dehydration also affects the mucous blanket [9]. *Excess* mucus renders the action of the cilia ineffective as they are unable to move the large amount of mucus and the mucous blanket disappears. There is much evidence that *cigarette smoking* adversely affects ciliary action and the movement of the mucous blanket [40]. The cilia in cigarette smokers are alleged to be shorter than in nonsmokers [84]. Islands of squamous epithelium are said to occur in most subjects,

particularly in the region of bronchial divisions. Hilding has produced some evidence to indicate that cigarette tar may accumulate round the distal margins of such islands and suggests that these form the foci for the carcinogenetic effect of tobacco [75]. *Alcohol* has a major effect in diminishing the movement of the mucous blanket in mice, although the more important factor in increasing the susceptibility to infection may be the inhibition of the mobilization of alveolar macrophages [96] (p. 24). Certain *drugs* affect ciliary action. 10% cocaine inhibits the action, although some other local anaesthetics, such as xylocaine, do not [9]. Atropine inhibits the action by causing drying and increased viscosity of the mucous blanket.

IMPORTANCE IN DISEASE

The importance of the ciliary mechanism in disease will be obvious from what has been said. The effect of smoking is probably a factor in the development of *chronic bronchitis* and *carcinoma of the bronchus*. In *bronchitis* and *bronchiectasis* the cilia may be diminished in number and the excessive mucus renders their action ineffective. The effect of alcohol on the mechanism may predispose to *pneumonia* and *lung abscess*, although alcohol probably also depresses other defence mechanisms (p. 24). The influenza virus causes destruction of ciliary cells [73], and certain other viruses affecting the upper respiratory tract may also cause damage to cilia [78].

BLOOD VESSELS OF THE LUNG

The lungs have a dual blood supply. The bronchial arteries are derived usually from the thoracic aorta but sometimes from the intercostal, subclavian or internal mammary arteries and supply the bronchi and pulmonary tissue down to the level of the respiratory bronchioles. Distal to this the lung lobules are supplied by the pulmonary artery which conveys nearly the whole of the output of the right ventricle to the alveolar capillaries.

The bronchial arteries incorporated in the connective tissue surrounding the bronchi follow the airways and divide with them until the distal end of the terminal bronchiole is reached. Branches of the bronchial artery form an arterial plexus in the adventitia of the bronchial wall and from this plexus branches pierce the muscle layer to enter the submucosa where they break up into a fine capillary plexus which supplies the mucous membrane. Venous radicles arising from the capillary network pierce the muscle layer to reach the adventitia where a venous plexus is formed. Veins arising from this plexus form one of the sources of the pulmonary vein. There is therefore an arterial and venous plexus on the outside of the muscle layer and a capillary plexus on the inside. Blood flow between the various plexuses involves passage through the muscle layer. When the muscle contracts the arterial plexus which is supplied at systemic pressure is likely to maintain a flow to the capillary plexus which, however, may not be able to pass the blood to the venous plexus. This is likely to result in oedema of the mucous membrane and narrowing of the lumen. This may partly explain the redundant, oedematous mucous membrane sometimes seen at bronchoscopy in the chronic asthmatic. Beyond the terminal bronchiole the bronchial arteries cease as distinct vessels and the internal capillary plexus merges with the pulmonary capillaries.

The pulmonary artery divides into right and left main branches and these divide and subdivide into branches corresponding with divisions of the bronchial tree to end in the terminal arterioles which supply the acini. The terminal arterioles, which are end arteries, break up into pulmonary capillaries which form networks in the interalveolar septa.

The pulmonary venous system arises from venules draining the capillary bed. These unite to form veins which drain into the interlobular septa and, therefore, do not follow the bronchial tree. The main pulmonary veins end in the left atrium.

In addition to the alveolar capillary bed the pulmonary veins drain the larger bronchi and the tracheal bifurcation by channels (the bronchial veins) which enter the pulmonary veins near the hilum. The pulmonary veins also drain the visceral pleura (p. 21). The bronchial veins anastomose with the pulmonary veins.

It is possible but not conclusively proved that the terminal arterioles, although they do not anastomose with each other, may communicate with the pulmonary veins through relatively large arteriovenous anastomoses [97 & 166]. Normally the volume of blood which bypasses the alveolar capillaries is small but this may be increased in disease by precapillary anastomoses between pulmonary arteries and veins and between bronchial and pulmonary arteries. These anastomoses are present particularly in pulmonary fibrosis, bronchiectasis and bronchial carcinoma. Pulmonary arteriovenous anastomoses occur in cirrhosis of the liver. Their development is thought to be due to the presence in the circulation of some substance normally inactivated by the liver. In fibrotic areas the bronchial arteries are often markedly dilated. The severe haemoptysis which may be associated with bronchiectasis commonly occurs from dilated bronchial arteries supplied at systemic pressure (p. 351).

THE PULMONARY LYMPHATICS

The pleura and all of the lung substance with the possible exception of the alveoli [163 & 164] are richly supplied with lymphatic vessels which are located beneath the pulmonary pleura, around the vessels and bronchi and also within the bronchial wall. The constant movement of the structures with which the lymphatic vessels are intimately related promotes the flow of lymph into the draining glands alongside the bronchi and at the hila. Simple valves direct flow proximally. Lymph drains finally into the systemic venous system at the junctions of the subclavian and internal jugular veins via the thoracic duct for the left lung and the right lymphatic duct for the right.

Aggregations of lymphoid tissue are found in the angles of bronchial branches from the periphery inwards. The most distal of these aggregations surround the division of the last respiratory bronchiole into alveolar ducts. True lymph glands (the bronchopulmonary glands) are not found until the first division of the lobar bronchi [70]. The 'hilar' glands around the main lobar bronchi form part of a large group which are clustered about the lung root. The glands lying lateral and inferior to the tracheal bifurcation are the upper and lower tracheobronchial groups. The lower group lies in the angle of bifurcation and unites the tracheobronchial groups of the two sides. Usually the upper tracheobronchial glands are larger on the right. On the left side one or more glands (para-aortic) are separated from the upper tracheobronchial group by the course of the aorta and the left pulmonary artery and these are closely related to the ligamentum arteriosum, the recurrent laryngeal nerve and the vagal fibres to the pulmonary plexus. Paratracheal glands on either side of the trachea are closely related to the recurrent laryngeal nerves. Efferent vessels from the paratracheal glands pass to the lower deep cervical glands. Other intrathoracic lymphatic gland groups are those on the inner surface of the anterior chest wall along the distribution of the internal mammary arteries (sternal glands), the internal intercostal glands near the heads of the ribs and the anterior and posterior mediastinal lymph glands.

Von Hayek has described the pulmonary lymph drainage as follows [70].

(1) Upper $\frac{2}{3}$ right upper lobe: right tracheobronchial glands,

(2) lower $\frac{1}{3}$ right upper lobe: dorsolateral hilar glands,

(3) right middle lobe: hilar glands around origin of middle lobe bronchus,

(4) dorsolateral parts of right lower lobe: dorsolateral hilar glands,

(5) venteromedial parts of right lower lobe: venteromedial hilar glands and glands in tracheal bifurcation,

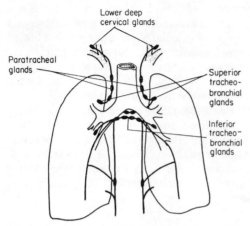

FIG. 1.7. The pulmonary lymph glands. Note connections with neck and abdominal glands. From von Hayek.

(6) apex of left upper lobe: para-aortic glands,

(7) left upper lobe excluding apex: anterior and posterior hilar glands and glands in tracheal bifurcation,

(8) left lower lobe: drainage similar to right lower lobe.

The lower lobe also drains to glands in the posterior mediastinum and, through the diaphragm, to the retroperitoneal lymph glands (fig. 1.7).

The abundance of pulmonary lymphatics is clearly seen when they are distended due to lymphatic carcinomatosis or pulmonary oedema. The dilated lymphatic vessels and anastomotic channels between them may then be visible in the chest radiograph.

INNERVATION OF THE LUNGS

While much remains to be learned about the innervation of the lung [70], it is generally agreed that the lung is supplied from the vagi and the fibres of the upper 6 thoracic sympathetic ganglia. The phrenic nerve may also be involved, possibly in relation to vascular control, but its distribution in the lung and its role are poorly understood.

The vagal and thoracic sympathetic fibres form a pulmonary plexus which ensheathes the bronchi and bronchioles and in which the parasympathetic ganglia are embedded. The motor supply to the bronchial muscle (p. 13) and probably also dilator fibres to the pulmonary blood vessels are derived from vagal efferents, which also control the activity of bronchial mucous glands. Most of the vagal afferent fibres convey impulses from stretch receptors, but the vagus is also stated to contain pain and other sensory fibres and unilateral section abolishes pain of pulmonary origin as well as cough reflexes [89]. The sympathetic nerves carry bronchodilator fibres. The sympathetic contribution to vascular control is not fully known.

THE PLEURA

The pleura is a serous membrane of mesodermal origin consisting of a layer of connective tissue covered by a simple squamous epithelium. The *visceral* pleura which covers the surface of the lung and lines the interlobar fissures is continuous at the hilum with the *parietal* pleura which lines the hemithorax. A thin, double fold of pleura below the pulmonary hilum and extending almost to the diaphragm is called the pulmonary ligament.

The pleural cavity is only a potential space for under normal conditions the visceral and parietal pleura are in apposition save for a small quantity of lubricating fluid. The volume of this fluid remains constant due to a balance between filtration from surrounding tissues and absorption into the pleural lymphatics.

The parietal pleura is divided for descriptive purposes into costal, mediastinal and diaphragmatic portions. There is no basement membrane and the epithelium lies directly on the connective tissue layer. The nuclei of the surface cells are ovoid and have deeply staining nucleoli. The connective tissue layer varies in composition and thickness in different parts. Over the pericardium it is almost entirely collagenous; over the diaphragm and central tendon elastic fibres predominate. Normally the diaphragmatic and costal pleura come into contact in the costophrenic angle during expiration.

Deep to the epithelium of the visceral pleura there is, successively, a fine layer of connective tissue (collagenous and elastic fibres), a strong fibrous layer and a layer of highly vascular connective tissue continuous with the underlying interlobular septa.

BLOOD SUPPLY OF THE PLEURA

VISCERAL PLEURA

Branches of the bronchial artery which reach the pleura in the interlobular septa provide the main blood supply, but a few branches of the pulmonary artery supply the deepest part of the visceral pleura. The terminal branches of the arteries supplying the pleura ramify in a loose network of capillaries which are about 10 times the width of alveolar capillaries and have been termed by Von Hayek 'giant capillaries' [70].

PARIETAL PLEURA

The blood supply of the costal part of the parietal pleura is from the intercostal arteries. The mediastinal and diaphragmatic pleura is supplied by the pericardiacophrenic branch of the internal mammary artery.

THE PLEURAL LYMPHATICS

VISCERAL PLEURA

A subpleural network of lymphatics drains into the hilar glands.

PARIETAL PLEURA

The costal lymphatics drain into glands along the internal mammary artery (sternal glands) and to the internal intercostal glands near the heads of the ribs. Lymph vessels are especially numerous over the muscular part of the diaphragm. These drain to the sternal and to the anterior and posterior mediastinal lymph glands. Lymphatics are sparse beneath the mediastinal pleura and are found only where fatty tissue is present. They accompany the pericardiacophrenic artery and drain to the posterior mediastinal glands.

INNERVATION OF THE PLEURA

The visceral pleura is supplied by autonomic fibres only. The parietal pleura overlying the central part of the diaphragm is innervated by the phrenic nerve and the peripheral diaphragmatic pleura is supplied from adjacent intercostal nerves. Spinal nerves supply the costal parietal pleura.

INTRAPLEURAL PRESSURE

The mean pressure within the pleural cavity is subatmospheric. This is because of the retractive force of the lung which consists of:

(1) the elastic tissue throughout the interstitium of the lung and in the bronchial wall,
(2) the 'geodesic' pattern of bronchial muscle (p. 9) which tends to shorten the airways and
(3) the surface tension of the alveolar lining film (p. 11).

The intrapleural pressure is different in different parts of the pleura and may vary by as much as 5 cm H_2O between the apex and the base due to the weight of the thoracic viscera. There are, therefore, many intrapleural pressures. A representative pressure can be recorded by the induction of a small pneumothorax, but this potentially dangerous procedure is not feasible for routine investigation and is unnecessary since it has been shown in many studies that there is a close correspondence between the intraoesophageal and the intrathoracic pressure. The relationship is most accurate when the intraoesophageal pressure is measured in the upright position by means of a polythene tube of 1 mm internal diameter with lateral apertures at its end which are covered by a latex balloon 10 cm long and 1 cm in diameter containing 0·2 ml of air. The lubricated balloon is passed through the nose and guided into the oesophagus by having the subject suck water through a straw. The tube is passed until positive deflections on inspiration are noted on the manometer or gauge indicating that the balloon is in the stomach. The tube is then withdrawn slowly until inspiration records negative deflections. The balloon is finally sited in the oesophagus at a point where transmitted cardiac pulsations least interfere with the recording.

Average intraoesophageal amplitudes on quiet breathing in the upright subject are from -6 cm H_2O on inspiration to -2.5 cm H_2O on expiration [36]. The amplitude varies with the depth of breathing and with the effort required to move air. The intraoesophageal pressure amplitude can be used to measure the work performed in stretching the lungs. Almost all patients with dyspnoea have increased negative intraoesophageal pressures on inspiration, i.e. a greater oesophageal pressure amplitude, showing that the work of breathing is increased. When obstructive airways disease is present the end-expiratory pressure becomes more positive the greater the obstruction (p. 406) and may exceed atmospheric pressure when active efforts have to be made to drive air out of the thorax. High intrathoracic pressures impede the venous return to the heart and tachycardia results. A fall in the pulse rate accompanies relief of airways obstruction in an asthmatic attack (p. 406). An increase in the pulse rate is an ominous sign in asthma; death in status asthmaticus often occurs with an almost empty heart.

PASSAGE OF FLUID THROUGH THE VISCERAL PLEURA

Although the precise mechanism is not understood it is believed that there is a constant movement of fluid through the pleural cavity from the visceral pleura to the parietal pleura where resorption occurs mainly by lymphatics but also by way of the blood stream [64 & 100]. The uptake by the parietal lymphatics is increased by respiratory movements. Studies with dyes have shown that resorption from the pleural cavity also occurs through the adipose tissue of the intercostal spaces [54, 100 & 146], at least in the first instance, although further removal may be via blood or lymph vessels.

RESPIRATORY REFLEXES

It is now appreciated that stimulation of any visceral or somatic nerve may influence breathing and that a multiplicity of afferent pathways are concerned in respiratory reflexes. At least 9 respiratory nervous reflexes originate in the thoracic viscera, and 5 of these are sufficiently well evaluated to be given specific designation.

THE INFLATION REFLEX
(Hering–Breuer)

Hering [72] and Breuer [15] in 1868 showed that maintained inflation of the lungs decreased the frequency of inspiratory efforts in anaesthetized animals and that maintained collapse had the reverse effect. Vagotomy prevents these responses, proving that they are reflex, and Adrian in 1933 showed that the reflex was mediated through pulmonary stretch receptors which are unencapsulated and are believed to be smooth muscle endings [2], found mainly in the walls of the bronchi and bronchioles [49, 113 & 174]. The inflation reflex is present in the newborn but becomes weaker in later life. Its significance was overshadowed when the importance of the chemical control of respiration (p. 25) was established. It is now regarded as only one of a number of chemical and nervous mechanisms which regulate the pattern of breathing. It is probable that it affects bronchial muscle tone (p. 14).

THE DEFLATION REFLEX

Deflation of the lungs stimulates breathing by activating a group of receptors which are believed to lie in the respiratory bronchioles or distal to them [124]. The precise significance of the deflation reflex is difficult to determine because deflation of the lungs alters breathing through several other mechanisms as well. Although it is uncertain whether the deflation reflex is active in ordinary breathing, it is probably important in forced deflation of the lungs and in atelectasis, the rate and force of the inspiratory effort being increased through its action in these circumstances. Vagotomy usually abolishes the deflation reflex in animals.

THE PARADOXICAL REFLEX

Head in 1889 showed that inflation of the lungs of rabbits when the vagus nerve was partially blocked (during recovery from freezing) gave no inflation reflex but instead resulted in a prolonged and vigorous contraction of the diaphragm [71]. The response was abolished by section of the vagus and because the effect is the opposite to that obtained by the normal inflation reflex it was termed 'paradoxical'. Two observations have suggested possible physiological roles for the paradoxical reflex. The occasional deep breaths which punctuate ordinary quiet breathing [106], and which are believed to prevent the microatelectasis that would otherwise occur, disappear after vagotomy and it has been suggested that they may be due to the paradoxical reflex [95]. Cross and his colleagues observed gasps when the lungs of newborn babies were inflated during the first 5 days [37]. They have suggested that the mechanism is analogous to the paradoxical reflex and that it may promote aeration of the neonatal lung.

IRRITANT REFLEXES

Subepithelial receptors in the trachea and bronchi are responsible for the cough reflex [49, 59, 77, 113 & 174]. These receptors are mainly congregated in the posterior wall of the trachea and at the bronchial bifurcations (as far as the proximal end of the respiratory bronchioles) and are most numerous at the main carina. Adequate anaesthesia of the tracheal bifurcation is essential for good bronchoscopy under local anaesthesia (p. 77).

The inhalation of mechanical or chemical irritants results in reflex closure of the glottis and bronchoconstriction. There is probably a peripheral intrinsic reflex arc within the bronchial wall as well as a central component acting through the vagus [30].

PULMONARY VASCULAR REFLEXES

Raising of the vascular pressure in the lungs of cats and dogs results in apnoea followed by rapid, shallow breathing associated with hypotension [28, 41 & 113]. These effects are prevented by vagotomy and are more in evidence when the venous rather than the arterial side of the circulation is distended. The precise site of the receptors has not yet been identified although present evidence suggests they are in the pulmonary veins or capillaries.

Multiple pulmonary embolism results in prolonged, rapid, shallow breathing in animals [110 & 111] and in man [143]. These effects are abolished by vagotomy in animals. As well as this respiratory reflex to embolization many other changes occur which affect respiration. These include fall in blood pressure and pulse rate, generalized pulmonary vasoconstriction and possibly oedema, decrease in lung compliance (p. 42) and increased resistance to air flow [20 & 66]. Because injections of 5-hydroxytryptamine can closely simulate the effects of embolism it has been suggested that this substance is liberated during the formation of vascular thrombi, possibly from platelets [161]. That this is not a complete explanation is shown by the fact that anti-5-hydroxytryptamine drugs are only partially successful in blocking the effects of embolism [66 & 85].

REFLEXES IN THE UPPER AIRWAYS

These are primarily protective. Sneezing and coughing are both reflex vigorous efforts. Sneezing is a response to irritation within the nose, but it may also occur on sudden exposure of the retina to bright light [17]. Coughing is a response to any irritating stimulus from the level of the pharynx down. The gag reflex prevents the entrance of unwanted material into the oesophagus but also results in closure of the glottis. Broncho-constrictor (p. 15), cardioinhibitory and vasomotor reflexes have been reported as the result of stimulation of the nose or throat [50, 67, 88 & 136].

OTHER RESPIRATORY REFLEXES

Reflexes from respiratory muscles, tendons and joints, from the heart and systemic circulation, from alimentary viscera, pain and temperature receptors, and also certain postural reflexes can all influence breathing. A well known example is the gasping which follows sudden application of cold to the skin.

For detailed descriptions of the respiratory reflexes the reader is referred to Widdicombe's review [177].

THE DEFENCES OF THE RESPIRATORY TRACT

We will now briefly summarize some of the defence mechanisms of the respiratory tract, concerned with protecting it not only against infection but also against dusts, noxious gases, etc. These may be listed as follows:

The gag reflex (p. 23).

The cough reflex (p. 23).

The normal movement of the bronchi with respiration. The shortening and narrowing of the bronchi on expiration will tend to 'milk' material from the lower respiratory tract towards the upper. Whether in addition there is any 'peristaltic' form of bronchial muscular contraction is at present uncertain although there are a few findings in the literature which suggest this possibility [178].

Ciliary action and the mucous blanket, concerned with carrying away particulate material, bacteria, etc. The action of mucus in protecting the mucous membrane and perhaps combating infection has been outlined on p. 16.

The alveolar macrophages. These appear to play an important part in dealing with relatively nonpathogenic bacteria which may reach the lower respiratory tract. The alveolar macrophage is said to be a specialized cell and seems to differ in metabolic and enzyme characteristic from other macrophages and polymorphs [96]. The lungs of mice which have inhaled aerosols of staphylococci are cleared of bacteria with astonishing speed. It has been shown that the alveolar macro-phages are mainly responsible for this. Bacteria which have been labelled with radioactive material can no longer be cultured from the lungs after quite a brief period, although most of the radioactive material remains in the lungs and antigens derived from the bacteria can be demonstrated within the macrophages [63]. This process is accompanied by no obvious inflammatory reaction, although of course the latter, with neutrophils, occurs with pathogenic infections. Alveolar macrophages also take part in clearing dust particles and are important in the pathogenesis of pneumoconiosis (p. 472). It had been found many years ago that alcohol decreased the rate at which pneumococci, haemolytic streptococci and *H. influenzae* were cleared from the lungs of mice [156]. It seems that this is due to inadequate mobilization of macrophages [96]. With infection by pathogenic bacteria alcohol also inhibits the capillary dilatation and leucocyte response of the inflammatory reaction [131].

THE CONTROL OF RESPIRATION

NERVOUS CONTROL

Respiration is influenced by many factors. The automatic rhythm of respiration is, however, under the control of nerve cells in the reticular formation of the medulla. These are usually referred to as *the respiratory centre*, which comprises inspiratory and expiratory components, functioning reciprocally. Impulses from the inspiratory centre stimulate the respiratory muscles, the thoracic cage expands and the lungs inflate. Afferent impulses from the distended lungs then pass to the expiratory centre which inhibits the inspiratory centre so that the lungs deflate. The activity of the respiratory centre is related to the general level of activity of the brain stem. Thus wakefulness has a stimulant effect on respiration and depression of brain activity by sleep, hypnotics and anaesthesia reduces ventilation.

Many of the higher centres can influence respiration. Swallowing, speaking, laughing and crying all influence the respiratory pattern. Pyrexia, acting via a temperature regulating centre in the hypothalamic region, stimulates breathing.

The nervous control of breathing is especially important in exercise. Currently there are no theories based on the chemical control of respiration which can fully explain ventilation on exercise.

CHEMICAL CONTROL

In the normal subject the volume of ventilation is adjusted principally by the partial pressure of CO_2 (P_{CO_2}), the pH of arterial blood and, to a much lesser extent, by the partial pressure of oxygen (P_{O_2}). Recently a *central chemosensitive area* has been discovered within the pial membrane overlying the anterolateral medulla of cats and dogs [113]. This responds to the hydrogen ion activity (H^+) in the cerebrospinal fluid (CSF) and indirectly to changes of P_{CO_2} in the blood. It is not certain whether CO_2 exerts its effect directly on the respiratory centre or through the medium of this chemosensitive area [18, 115 & 126].

The pH of the CSF remains remarkably constant despite marked changes in blood pH. Thus a fairly constant environment is ensured for the nerve cells. The blood–brain barrier appears to be capable of actively transporting ions in such a way as to regulate the pH of the CSF [148 & 150]. There are virtually no buffer systems in the CSF and the homeostasis is probably effected by a 'pump' action of the choroid plexus and ependyma driving H^+ ions, when necessary, from the blood into the CSF where they react with HCO_3^- ions. CO_2 is liberated and this diffuses out again. Thus each H^+ ion pumped in destroys one HCO_3^- ion.

The principal chemical stimuli to breathing are a rise in P_{CO_2} and a fall in pH. Because of the reciprocal relationship between these factors it has been difficult to study the effect of each separately. However, the ability of each to stimulate breathing is unquestioned although the precise mechanism is not known.

Whenever the P_{CO_2} rises above the level of about 40 mm Hg breathing is stimulated so that the excess is blown off. There is, therefore, a very sensitive feedback mechanism based on the level of the P_{CO_2} and hydrogen ion activity in the blood which ensures an appropriate depth of respiration for particular metabolic and environmental situations. The level of P_{CO_2} to which the respiratory centre responds by initiating hyperventilation may vary in certain abnormal conditions. In the relatively reduced environmental oxygen pressure at high altitudes the initial acclimatization of normal subjects includes a ventilatory response which reduces the P_{CO_2} to a new lower level to which the respiratory centre becomes accustomed. Any important increase in P_{CO_2} above this level, although still perhaps below 40 mm Hg, may for a time result in dyspnoea. After 8 hours at high altitudes the CSF bicarbonate begins to fall and the hydrogen ion activity in the CSF is thus restored to normal at the lower P_{CO_2} dictated by the low Pa_{O_2}. It takes several days for the processes of readjustment to be complete, largely due to the need to change the HCO_3^- concentration in the large amount of CSF already formed.

A situation similar to that at high altitudes develops in the patient with respiratory failure who has been overventilated by a respirator for long periods [154].

Peripheral chemoreceptors in the carotid and aortic bodies sense changes in the P_{O_2} and pH of the blood and relay these reflexly to the respiratory centre via the glossopharyngeal and vagus nerves. The carotid body is situated at the bifurcation of the carotid artery, and the aortic body is on the ascending aorta close to the pulmonary artery. These chemoreceptors are formed of a mass of glandular looking epithelioid cells which are very active metabolically and are richly supplied with sinusoidal blood vessels and nerve endings. Decrease in P_{O_2} and decrease in the pH of arterial blood, from whatever cause, stimulate breathing via the aortic and carotid chemoreceptors. Increase in P_{CO_2} is also effective, acting via a rise in (H^+). The anoxic stimulus is the most effective and applies when the arterial P_{O_2} is low or the blood flow to the chemoreceptors is reduced, as in hypotension. In man the peripheral chemoreceptors are not highly sensitive to small variations in Po_2 and the oxygen content of inspired gas has to fall to 16% before stimulation results in increase in the tidal volume and slight increase in the respiratory rate. Anoxic stimulation of ventilation in the normal subject is small compared with the effect of CO_2 increase and is unimportant at rest. It is estimated that about 20% of the resting ventilatory drive originates in the peripheral chemoreceptors [150]. The anoxic drive to respiration becomes important in the alveolar hypoventilation states due to such varied pathology as brain stem lesions, the Pickwickian syndrome (characterized by somnolence, obesity, polycythaemia and evidence of pituitary hypofunction), depression of the respiratory centre by drugs and, most common of all, chronic obstructive airways disease due to chronic bronchitis. Alveolar hypoventilation leads to rise in the Pco_2, fall in the blood and urine pH, increased renal excretion of ammonium salts and retention of sodium. Bicarbonate is reabsorbed by the kidneys and the buffering capacity of the body is raised so that subsequent increases in Pco_2 result in a proportionately smaller increase in $[H^+]$ and a smaller stimulus to ventilation than in the normal. The hypercapnic drive to respiration is reduced and CO_2 retention no longer protects the body from further hypercapnia. Levels of Pco_2 above 70 mm Hg also have a direct depressive effect on the respiratory centre. Ventilation may then largely depend on anoxia and the giving of high concentrations of oxygen may deprive the patient of the principal remaining ventilatory drive. Ventilation will, therefore, progressively fall and Pco_2 progressively rise (p. 324).

PERIODIC RESPIRATION

Periodic respiration, described by Cheyne in 1818 and commonly termed Cheyne–Stokes respiration, is usually ascribed to increased chemoreceptor drive resulting in hyperventilation with excretion of excessive quantities of CO_2. This is followed by reduction in the central drive to respiration so that ventilation decreases until the CO_2 builds up sufficiently to initiate the next cycle. Periodic breathing is common in the elderly during sleep, in cardiac failure, in cerebral lesions, particularly those associated with increased intracranial pressure, and in states of metabolic acidosis such as those produced by diabetes mellitus and uraemia.

Studies by Guyton and his colleagues have shown that periodic breathing can be produced by imposing a circulatory delay between the thorax and the respiratory centre through the insertion of plastic tubes between proximal carotid arteries and distal carotid or vertebral arteries in dogs [65]. This supports the concept that one of the basic mechanisms is the prolongation of the circulation time from lung to brain, such as may occur in cardiac failure. Bates and Christie have demonstrated that the patient with periodic breathing is capable of taking as deep a breath during the period of apnoea as during the hyperventilation phase [10], indicating that there can be no significant cyclical change in the distensibility of the lungs. They have further shown the unexpected finding that the arterial oxygen saturation measured by oximetry (p. 45) is normal during apnoea and low during hyperpnoea, i.e. 90° out of phase with the oxygen saturation in the pulmonary vein. Also the level of mean arterial Pco_2 is usually low in periodic breathing showing that the cyclical ventilatory control actually results in a higher level of alveolar ventilation than is necessary for CO_2 elimination.

POSTHYPERVENTILATION APNOEA

Although described by Haldane, posthyperventilation apnoea is not universal and is most frequently demonstrated in medical students, who, having read the text books, think they know what pattern of breathing they should adopt. If it is demonstrated in an unsophisticated subject it may be a sign of supramedullary brain damage [132]. Normal subjects after hyperventilation have only a few seconds of apnoea or continue to breathe rhythmically with a reduced tidal volume until the arterial Pco_2 reaches the resting level [52]. Patients with bilateral cerebral injury or mild metabolic disease involving the brain [116], stop breathing after hyperventilation until the P_{CO_2} reaccumulates. It seems probable, therefore, that the normal brain provides a stimulus, originating either in the cerebral hemispheres or in connections between these and the reticular formation, which can maintain the rhythm of respiration even when chemical stimuli are no longer effective.

RESPIRATORY FUNCTION

The term *respiration* includes the processes by which cells utilize oxygen, produce carbon dioxide and exchange these gases with the atmosphere. Normal respiration requires the interdependence and integration of many functions of the lungs and of the cardiovascular and nervous systems.

GENERAL DESCRIPTION OF LUNG FUNCTION

NORMAL LUNG FUNCTION

The lungs maintain normal and nearly constant oxygen and carbon dioxide pressures and content in the arterial blood in all physiological circumstances. In normality this is achieved without ventilatory discomfort or adverse effect on the heart or other organs. Constancy of the arterial blood gases is maintained by the efficient transfer of gas between the alveolar air and the blood passing through the alveolar capillaries. Gas exchange is achieved by bringing the mixed venous blood into intimate contact with alveolar gas over the very large surface area provided by the alveolar membrane. On one side of the interface blood is brought to the pulmonary capillaries by the action of the right ventricle and on the other side inspired air is brought by the bellows action of the lung. Thus there are 3 components of pulmonary gas exchange:

(1) *ventilation* which must not only be adequate in total quantity but be efficiently distributed to all perfused alveoli

(2) *pulmonary capillary blood flow* which in the healthy lung is delivered in adequate volume and distributed efficiently to all the ventilated alveoli;

(3) *diffusion* across the alveolar capillary membrane, the transfer of gas between alveolar air and pulmonary capillary blood being determined by the gas tension gradients between them.

Ventilation ($\dot{V}$) and perfusion ($\dot{Q}$) are remarkably integrated in health and the whole process of pulmonary gas exchange is achieved with the minimum expenditure of energy by the respiratory and cardiovascular systems. Any imbalance between the ventilation and the circulation of the lungs in the form of ventilation of underperfused alveoli or perfusion of underventilated alveoli will result in a reduction in the effective blood–gas interface. Ventilatory effort may be wasted or there may be imperfect oxygenation of the blood (fig. 1.19, p. 39).

VENTILATION

MECHANISM

Pulmonary ventilation, or the mass movement of air up and down the respiratory passages, depends on the rhythmic expansion and contraction of the lung. Contraction of the intercostal muscles and of the diaphragm causes an upward and outward movement of the ribs and flattening of the diaphragm during normal quiet inspiration. During vigorous breathing the accessory muscles of respiration (the sternomastoids, the scaleni, the pectorals and the latissimus dorsi) also come into play. Expiration is essentially passive but may be assisted during vigorous breathing by contraction of the abdominal muscles. Contraction of the inspiratory muscles lowers the intrathoracic and alveolar pressures so that air flowing from a higher to a lower pressure enters the lungs. During expiration the elastic recoil of the lungs and chest wall raises the intrathoracic and alveolar pressures so that the air flow is reversed. The rhythmicity, rate and depth of respiration are controlled by the respiratory centre which ensures that alveolar ventilation is at the appropriate level and is achieved with a minimum energy cost.

THE LUNG VOLUMES AND CAPACITIES

There are 4 primary lung volumes and 4 lung capacities. Each capacity includes 2 or more of the primary volumes (fig. 1.8).

The volume of gas inspired or expired with each breath is called the *tidal volume* (V_T). On quiet breathing this measures about 500 ml in adults. About 150 ml of this fills the conducting airways from the nose and mouth

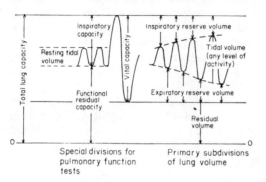

FIG. 1.8. Subdivisions of the lung volume. Pappenheimer (1950).

down to the respiratory bronchioles and does not take part in gas exchange; this is the *anatomical deadspace* (V_D). The other 350 ml is available for alveolar ventilation (V_A). This mixes with the volume of gas remaining in the lung after a quiet expiration (the *functional residual capacity*, FRC) which ranges from 1800 ml in small females to 3500 ml in large males. At a respiratory rate of 12/min V_A will be about 12×350 ml, or 4·2 l/min. Calculation of alveolar ventilation in this way is an oversimplification which assumes that inspired gas moves with a square front (fig. 1.9), whereas, in fact, it has a cone front (fig. 1.9). Square front flow would mean that if V_T were reduced to the value of V_D alveolar ventilation would be nil. Because of the cone front some alveolar ventilation (but very little) can occur even when V_T is less than V_D. Thus the above method of calculating alveolar ventilation is not accurate when V_T is greatly reduced.

Expiration ends and air flow ceases when the alveolar pressure (P_A) becomes equal to atmospheric pressure. At this point there is a balance between the elastic recoil of the lung and the tendency of the chest wall to spring outwards. By contraction of the muscles of expiration, principally the abdominal muscles, a further volume of gas can be expired. This is the *expiratory reserve volume* (ERV) which varies according to the size of the tidal volume. The amount of gas remaining in the lungs after this voluntary expiration is the *residual*

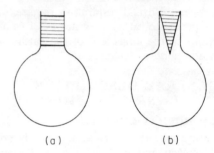

FIG. 1.9. Diagrammatic representations of (a) square and (b) cone front flow.

volume (RV) which is usually about 1200 ml. The residual volume is less than 30% of the *total lung capacity* (TLC), which is the volume of gas contained in the lungs at the end of a full inspiration. The *vital capacity* (VC) is the maximum volume of gas which can be expired after a maximum inspiration. In a young healthy person the vital capacity is about 80% of the total lung capacity. During the performance of the vital capacity manoeuvre expiratory muscle effort causes the air to flow until the pressure in the surrounding lungs exceeds that within the lumen of the small airways which then collapse, trapping the residual volume which can never be expelled in life. The *inspiratory capacity* (IC) is the maximum volume of air which can be inspired from the resting expiratory level. It is about 75% of the VC. The *inspiratory reserve volume* is the maximum volume which can be inspired from the end tidal inspiratory position.

METHODS OF MEASURING LUNG VOLUMES

The vital capacity and its subdivisions (IRV, ERV and TV) are measured directly by simple spirometry. The residual volume or the functional residual capacity can be measured by the degree of dilution of a measured volume of inert gas (usually helium) when the patient is breathing into a spirometer of known volume. The volume is kept constant by adding O_2 at the same rate as the expired CO_2 is removed by the absorber. The TLC can also be measured by this method but is usually calculated by adding FRC to IC or RV to VC. Switching the patient into the circuit after a maximum expiration, at the end of a normal expiration and at full inspiration will measure the RV, FRC and TLC respectively. The following calculation is used.

$$a \times V = b\,(V + RV^*)$$

$$RV^* = \frac{(a-b) \times V}{b}$$

V, spirometer volume; a, initial concentration of helium in %; b, concentration of helium in % at end of equilibration; *, or FRC or TLC.

The RV, FRC and TLC can also be measured by the technique of open circuit nitrogen clearance [42 & 43]. Nitrogen is displaced from the lungs by oxygen breathing and the volume of nitrogen expired is calculated by analysis of the nitrogen content of the expired air by a nitrogen meter. The formula employed is:

$$RV^* = \frac{V \times b}{a-b}$$

V, spirometer volume; a, initial concentration of nitrogen in the lung; b, end concentration of nitrogen in the spirometer–lung system; *, or FRC or TLC.

It will be seen that

$$IC = TLC - FRC;$$
$$RV = FRC - ERV;$$
$$TLC = RV + VC = FRC + IC.$$

CLINICAL SIGNIFICANCE OF VARIATION IN LUNG VOLUMES AND CAPACITIES

The static lung volumes are essentially anatomical measurements and do not evaluate function. Nevertheless alteration in the lung volumes may be associated with disease processes affecting function.

Each degree centigrade makes a difference of about 0·5% in the lung volumes, and these should be corrected to body temperature and ambient pressure saturated with water vapour (BTPS) [31].

John Hutchinson, a surgeon, in 1844 was aware that the vital capacity was greater in summer than in winter and corrected volumes to 15°C, the average indoor temperature at the time [79, 80, 81, 82 & 83]. In 1954 Needham and his colleagues corrected to 20°C and nowadays with central heating a common indoor temperature is 25°C [119].

VITAL CAPACITY

The vital capacity in the healthy subject varies with posture, age, sex, body type and state of physical training. Sometimes performance of the test improves with repeated examinations. A reduction of more than 20% of the predicted normal value on repeated testing may be considered abnormal. There are so many disease processes which can lower the vital capacity that it cannot be used for specific diagnosis as an isolated test. Indeed reduction in VC need not signify pulmonary disease at all. The vital capacity is reduced where there is:

(1) reduction in functioning lung tissue due to pulmonary resection, tumours, pneumonia, collapse, oedema and fibrosis,

(2) limitation of expansion of normal lung due to pain, chest deformity, neuromuscular disease, ascites, pneumothorax, pleural thickening or effusion and the later stages of pregnancy.

Serial estimations of the VC may be helpful in assessing progress in the course of a disease with a restrictive pattern of ventilatory abnormality. Restrictive ventilatory impairment is due to conditions which encroach upon the lung volume, e.g. pleural fibrosis, or which reduce the ability of the thoracic cage or lungs to expand, e.g. ankylosing spondylitis or diffuse interstitial pulmonary fibrosis.

FUNCTIONAL RESIDUAL CAPACITY AND RESIDUAL VOLUME

FRC and RV usually vary together. Increase in FRC indicates hyperinflation during quiet breathing. Increase in RV indicates hyperinflation even after the patient has made a maximal voluntary effort to force the lungs back to their normal size. Increase in FRC and RV may be reversible as in asthma or irreversible as in emphysema.

TOTAL LUNG CAPACITY

This is reduced in restrictive pulmonary disease such as diffuse interstitial pulmonary fibrosis, in extensive pulmonary lesions such as massive pneumonia, in atelectasis and when there is compression of pulmonary tissue as in pneumothorax. In emphysema it may be unaltered or increased.

In *chronic obstructive airways disease* (asthma or bronchitis with varying degrees of emphysema) the total lung capacity is unaltered or increased. The FRC is increased owing to reduced elastic lung recoil, increased resistance to expiration and collapse or narrowing of bronchioles. Also because of these factors the VC is reduced below the normal 80% of the total lung capacity and the RV is increased. If there is a reversible component in the airways obstruction these changes are not permanent. Similar changes in the lung volumes may occur with increasing age. In uncomplicated diffuse lung fibrosis and in heart disease with pulmonary congestion the TLC and VC are reduced and the RV is commonly normal.

THORACIC GAS VOLUME

In severe obstructive airways disease and in some pulmonary bullae air may be trapped in the alveoli so that it only very slowly mixes with the inspired gas. In such cases the helium dilution and nitrogen washout techniques cannot assess the residual volume accurately. The body plethysmograph can, however, measure the total gas volume in the thorax whether it is communicating with the airways or not and the amount of air trapping can be calculated when the RV as determined by the nitrogen or helium methods is known.

The principle of the measurement of the thoracic gas volume is based on Boyle's Law, $PV = P^1V^1$ (fig. 1.10). The patient is enclosed in the body plethysmograph and breathes freely within the box. Alveolar pressure (P) equals atmospheric pressure at end-expiration when there is no gas flow. The thoracic gas volume (V) is unknown. At the appropriate point in the respiratory cycle a shutter mechanism suddenly occludes the airway.

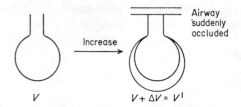

FIG. 1.10. Plethysmograph technique of measuring thoracic gas volume.

Inspiration against the obstruction results in a fall in intrathoracic pressure (to P^1), decompression of the thoracic gas which is now $V + \Delta V$ (or V^1) and a rise in pressure in the plethysmograph due to ΔV. ΔV is derived from the pressure change it causes.

$$PV = P^1V^1 = P^1 (V + \Delta V)$$

P, P^1 and ΔV are known; V, the thoracic gas volume can now be calculated.

Attempts have been made to determine the lung volume by various radiological procedures. None has been shown to be as sufficiently reliable or as easily performed as the standard physiological test.

DEADSPACE

The term *physiological deadspace* is used to describe *all* the air in the respiratory tract which does not take part in gas exchange. It comprises the anatomical deadspace (p. 28) plus the volume of alveoli in which the blood flow fails to match the ventilation. Thus those alveoli which have an imperfect capillary blood flow, e.g. pulmonary artery thrombosis, and those which are distended and, therefore, contain excess air, e.g. emphysema, contribute to the physiological deadspace, provided they receive ventilation in excess of perfusion. It should be noted that bullae are often *under-ventilated*.

The *anatomical deadspace* (p. 28) is measured by continuous analysis of the nitrogen concentration in the expired breath and simultaneous measurement of expired volume flow rate. Nitrogen is used because it does not take part in gas exchange. By means of a nitrogen meter a single expiration is monitored following a deep breath of oxygen (fig.

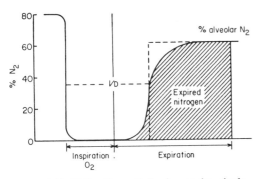

FIG. 1.11. Estimation of deadspace by single breath analysis. Modified from Comroe *et al.* [32] *The Lung.* Chicago, Yearbook Medical Publishers.

1.11). The first part of the record at the beginning of expiration represents pure deadspace gas in which no nitrogen is present. This is followed by a short phase of rapidly rising nitrogen concentration when mixed deadspace and alveolar air is recorded, and finally the pure alveolar sample which will reflect the degree of dilution of alveolar nitrogen by the oxygen. If no mixing occurred in the airways the rise in nitrogen concentration would occur abruptly as a square front and the anatomical deadspace would be the amount expired up to this point. The theo-

retical situation of a square front can be determined by the method of Fowler which divides the rising phase of the curve into two equal parts. This gives the anatomical dead space.

The *physiological deadspace* can be calculated by the Bohr equation which is based on the fact that expired gas comprises gas from the anatomical deadspace plus gas from alveoli. The alveolar gas may be from alveoli with appropriate ventilation and perfusion and/or from alveoli whose ventilation–perfusion ratio is abnormal (p. 37).

$$V_D = \frac{(P_{a,CO_2} - P_{E,CO_2})\, V_T}{P_{a,CO_2}}$$

P_{a,CO_2}, CO_2 partial pressure in arterial blood (assumed to be equal to 'ideal' alveolar CO_2 pressure); P_{E,CO_2}, pressure of CO_2 in mixed expired air; V_T, tidal volume. This method simply requires analysis of expired air and of a sample of arterial blood. It expresses the ratio of deadspace (V_D) to tidal volume (V_T) as if the lung were in two parts physiologically, one normal as regards ventilation and perfusion and the other infinitely ventilated but not perfused.

ALVEOLAR VENTILATION (USEFUL VENTILATION)

It is the *alveolar* ventilation which is all important in the maintenance of normal blood gases. It may be normal in amount or even increased but still inadequate to oxygenate the blood fully if:

(1) ventilation is not uniformly distributed,
(2) pulmonary capillary blood flow is not uniform or
(3) diffusing capacity is decreased.

Hypoventilation (alveolar underventilation) occurs when the volume of air entering the alveoli and taking part in gas exchange each minute is insufficient for the metabolic needs of the body. When the patient is breathing air alveolar hypoventilation leads to retention of carbon dioxide with consequent respiratory acidosis and anoxaemia. The carbon dioxide added to the alveoli from pulmonary capillary blood is not adequately removed in hypoventilation so that the arterial P_{CO_2}, which is in equilibrium with alveolar P_{CO_2}, rises. The alveolar P_{O_2} must fall and arterial P_{O_2} and oxygen saturation (S_{O_2}) decrease. Rise in P_{CO_2} leads to a fall in pH (respiratory acidosis) (p. 47).

The relationship between the mean alveolar P_{CO_2} and the mean alveolar P_{O_2} can be determined by the *alveolar gas equation* which states that the sum of the partial pressures of each of the alveolar gases, O_2, CO_2, N_2 and water vapour, equals atmospheric pressure (760 mm Hg). Thus if any 3 are known the 4th can be calculated. If the volume of gas entering and leaving the alveoli were constant (V) the respiratory quotient (RQ) would be

$$\frac{CO_2 \text{ produced}}{O_2 \text{ taken up}}$$

$$= \frac{P_{CO_2} \text{ gradient between} \atop \text{alveolar and inspired air} \times V}{P_{O_2} \text{ gradient between} \atop \text{inspired and alveolar air} \times V}$$

Normally the inspired $P_{CO_2}=0$ but not in every situation, e.g. anaesthesia; use of masks and valve boxes which have a deadspace of their own.

$$= \frac{\text{alveolar } P_{CO_2}}{\text{inspired } P_{O_2} - \text{alveolar } P_{O_2}}$$

i.e.

$$\text{alveolar } P_{O_2} = \text{inspired } P_{O_2} - \frac{\text{arterial } P_{CO_2}}{RQ}$$

But RQ is not unity since in most cases more O_2 is taken up per minute than CO_2 is added. The resting RQ is usually about 0·8. As N_2 is not absorbed or excreted in the lung the amount of N_2 is unchanged so this results in N_2 being slightly more concentrated. In turn this alters the volume and pressure of O_2 and CO_2. Taking this into account the equation now reads:

$$\text{alveolar } P_{O_2} = \text{inspired } P_{O_2} - \frac{\text{arterial } P_{CO_2}}{RQ} \times [RQ + 0.79 \, (1 - RQ)]$$

0·79, fraction of N_2 in inspired air.

When the alveolar gas equation is used the assumption is made that $\dot{V}_A/\dot{Q}$ (p. 37) is even throughout the lung. Oxygen equilibration between alveolus and capillary is assumed so that arterial blood P_{O_2} should be the same as the calculated alveolar P_{O_2} (or 'ideal alveolar P_{O_2}') point 0 in fig. 1.12. Thus we have a measure of what the arterial P_{O_2} (point 0 in fig. 1.12) should be in the perfect lung. The

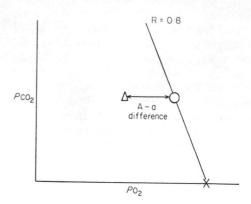

FIG. 1.12. The O_2–CO_2 diagram. The effect of RQ is represented by a fan of lines of which the normal (0·8) is shown. The line describes the composition of alveolar gas in a normal resting patient with an RQ of 0·8. To determine the alveolar P_{O_2} read across from the measured P_{CO_2} to the line. The difference between the measured arterial P_{O_2} and the ideal alveolar P_{O_2} is the A–a difference. ×, inspired air point (P_{O_2} 150, P_{CO_2} 0); ○, ideal alveolar point (P_{O_2} 100, P_{CO_2} 40); △, arterial point (P_{O_2} 80, P_{CO_2} 40). This is an example of an abnormal reading.

difference between the measured arterial P_{O_2} (point Δ in fig. 1.12 as an example of the abnormal) and the ideal alveolar figure (point 0) i.e. ideal alveolar–arterial P_{O_2} or A−a difference, is a measure of underventilation of perfused alveoli or physiological shunting (venous admixture effect).

The interrelationships between the pressures of alveolar gases can be depicted graphically in the O_2–CO_2 diagram of Rahn and Fenn (fig. 1.13) [135]. The alveolar gas equation can be readily solved by use of the diagram and additional information may be obtained by modification of the diagram.

The only worthwhile index of alveolar

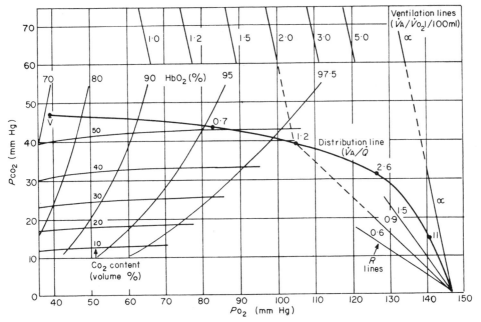

FIG. 1.13. O_2–CO_2 diagram of Rahn and Fenn with alveolar ventilation and "R" lines.

On a grid formed of the coordinates PO_2 and PCO_2 on equal scales are superimposed isopleths for SO_2 and CO_2 content. The SO_2 and CO_2 content isopleths are curved because of the effect of changing PCO_2 and PO_2. This is another way of depicting the dissociation curves of O_2 and CO_2. When any two of the variables (PO_2 PCO_2, SO_2 and CO_2 content) are known the other two may be predicted. The diagram is made more complex but much more useful by superimposition of coordinates for the respiratory exchange ratio (R—ratio of rate of appearance of CO_2 in the lung to rate of disappearance of O_2) and alveolar ventilation, and a curved distri- bution line of the PO_2 and PCO_2 combinations which may occur for different $\dot{V}A/\dot{Q}$ ratios in a particular subject. The use of the diagram assumes that there is no difference between PCO_2 in alveolar gas and arterial blood.

A patient with a PA,O_2 of 104 mm Hg and a value for R of 0·9 (calculated from analysis of expired gas) will have a $\dot{V}A/\dot{Q}$ ratio of 1·2, an alveolar ventilation of 2·0 1/min for each 100 ml of O_2 consumed and a Pa,CO_2 of 39 mm Hg. The values for SO_2 and CO_2 content can also be read off.

Alveolar ventilation can, therefore, be determined from the diagram by knowledge of (a) PA,O_2 and Pa,CO_2, (b) PA,O_2 and R, (c) Pa,CO_2 and R.

From Cotes J.E. (1965) *Lung Function*. Oxford, Blackwell Scientific Publications.

ventilation is the PCO_2. Because of the S-shape of the oxygen dissocation curve (fig. 1.14) the oxygen saturation is relatively uninfluenced until the partial pressure of oxygen in alveolar gas falls to relatively low levels. Oxygen saturation, therefore, is no guide to the degree of alveolar hypoventilation. The arterial PO_2 is fallacious as an index of alveolar hypo- ventilation for it is also influenced importantly by impairment in alveolar–capillary diffusion and by low $\dot{V}A/\dot{Q}$ ratios whereas the arterial PCO_2 is not, to all intents and purposes be- cause of the shape of the CO_2 dissociation curve.

The amount of CO_2 contained in the blood varies with the CO_2 pressure to which the blood is subjected, and it is possible to con- struct a dissociation curve (fig. 1.15). The curve is virtually linear over the resting physiological range. The curve is influenced by the degree of oxygenation since the more the Hb is saturated the less CO_2 it can carry, and vice versa. There is, therefore, a different curve for each degree of oxygenation. In the tissues where the percentage oxygenation is low more CO_2 is taken up; the reverse applies in the pulmonary capillaries so that the CO_2 held in the blood tends to fall.

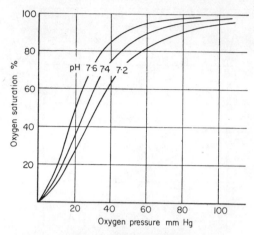

FIG. 1.14. Oxyhaemoglobin dissociation curve relating partial pressure of O_2 to percentage saturation (O_2 content). In the upper ranges large changes of Po_2 cause little change in So_2. In the lower ranges small changes in Po_2 cause large changes in So_2. Note that a falling pH moves the curve to the right.

The commonest causes of *alveolar hypoventilation* are:

(1) conditions associated with uneven distribution of inspired air, e.g. chronic bronchitis,

(2) neuromuscular or skeletal disease affecting the thorax, e.g. poliomyelitis, myasthenia, thoracic deformities,

(3) depression of responsiveness of the respiratory centre to CO_2, e.g. chronic bronchitis, effect of morphine, barbiturates, etc. and

(4) severe reduction of functioning lung tissue, e.g. atelectasis, emphysema, massive pleural effusion.

In recent years the syndrome of *primary alveolar hypoventilation* has been recognized in which the lungs are normal but control of breathing is not. In this syndrome ventilatory capacity may be normal and diffusion and $\dot{V}_A/\dot{Q}$ balance unimpaired yet the resting level of ventilation may be so low as to cause hypoxia and hypercapnia with consequent polycythaemia and an increased but reversible (at least initially) pulmonary vascular resistance (p. 36). Commonly this syndrome is

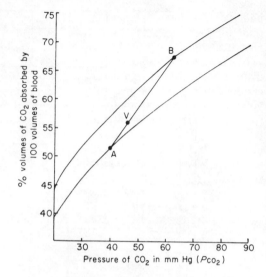

FIG. 1.15. Carbon dioxide dissociation curve. Upper line fully reduced human blood, lower line, fully oxygenated human blood; A, volume and tension of CO_2 in arterial blood; V, volume and tension of CO_2 in venous blood; B, contents in fully reduced blood.

Line AV is the dissociation of CO_2 in human blood. A rise in the respiratory quotient moves it to the right; a fall in the respiratory quotient moves it to the left. From Wylie W.D. & Churchill-Davidson H.C. (1966) *A Practice in Anaesthesia*. London, Lloyd-Luke.

seen in obese patients [5, 137 & 151], but rarely it has been recorded in patients of normal weight. Of course not all obese patients underventilate.

Oxygen therapy will increase the oxygen saturation to normal in alveolar hypoventilation but will not rid the blood of excess carbon dioxide, which can only be removed by increasing alveolar ventilation, if necessary by assisted respiration.

Hyperventilation, which occurs with major pulmonary embolism and recurrent pulmonary microembolism, anxiety, lesions in the region of the pons, hyperthyroidism, fever, etc., blows off CO_2 and produces respiratory alkalosis but because of the shape of the oxygen dissociation curve can add little to the oxygenation of the blood unless there has been preceding alveolar hypoventilation. The changes in Pco_2 due to overventilation and underventilation are related to blood pH and total blood bicarbonate by the Henderson–Hasselbalch equation (p. 45).

In the normal subject with uniform gas distribution alveolar ventilation per minute can be calculated from respiratory rate, tidal volume and predicted anatomical deadspace (p. 28). If, as is usual in disease, gas distribution is not uniform this method of calculating effective alveolar ventilation does not apply and methods based on CO_2 elimination must be used.

less marked. Distributional efficiency can be assessed by the rate of washing out of nitrogen from the alveoli during oxygen breathing in an open circuit, or the rate of mixing of helium in a closed circuit. Rapid analysis of tidal air with or without a previous breath of oxygen or helium also gives valuable information regarding gas distribution and the equality of alveolar ventilation. Inequality of alveolar ventilation may be spatial when ventilation is uneven with respect to volume or temporal when it is uneven with respect to time. If

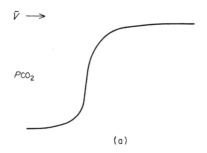
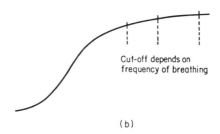

FIG. 1.16. Analysis of P_{CO_2} in expired gas. (a) In a normal subject (fairly square front trace), (b) in a patient with obstructive airways disease (slower rise in P_{CO_2} and end-point reached much later).

Uneven distribution of inspired air occurs when there are areas of the lung with altered elasticity, e.g. emphysema, altered expansion, e.g. interstitial lung disease, pulmonary congestion, atelectasis, tumour, regional obstruction, e.g. asthma, or regional 'check valves', e.g. obstructive emphysema. This results in some alveoli being underventilated and some perhaps overventilated. Anoxaemia occurs but not necessarily CO_2 retention because hyperventilation in relation to blood flow in some areas can blow off CO_2 and compensate for the effect of hypoventilated areas.

The efficiency of distribution of inspired air in the normal subject is disturbed by anaesthesia, restriction of chest wall movement, deliberate changes in the pattern of breathing in relation to depth or rhythm and probably also by extreme exercise. In patients with chronic obstructive airways disease there is usually marked disturbance of gas distribution whereas in those with lung fibrosis without obstructive airways diseases the evidence of impaired gas distribution is much

distribution is imperfect the less well ventilated alveoli empty later in expiration. Carbon dioxide pressure in expired gas will then be higher and oxygen pressure lower towards the end of expiration (fig. 1.16).

THE PULMONARY CIRCULATION

At rest the right ventricle pumps about 5 l of blood per min through the pulmonary circulation. The mean pulmonary arterial pressure is only about 15 mm Hg and since

$$\text{blood flow} = \frac{\text{driving pressure}}{\text{resistance}}$$

the resistance in the pulmonary circulation is only about $\frac{1}{10}$ that of the systemic circulation. The pulmonary circulation has a remarkable reserve capacity and in the young subject blood flow can be doubled to both lungs in exercise and to one lung after pneumonectomy (provided the vascular bed in the remaining lung is normal) with scarcely any rise in the pulmonary artery pressure. This reserve is apparently due to the great distensibility of the pulmonary vasculature and also to the fact that all available vessels are not in use at rest. Vascular distensibility lessens with age.

CONTROL OF PULMONARY CIRCULATION

So far as is known there is no effective nervous control over pulmonary vascular resistance. There is, however, an efficient regulating mechanism in the normal lung based on the pressure of O_2 and CO_2 in the blood. Anoxia increases pulmonary vascular resistance, an important point to remember in the management of respiratory failure (p. 339). A fall in Pa,CO_2 after obstruction of a pulmonary artery results in a 25% reduction in local ventilation [147]. It may be that there is a homeostatic mechanism mediated by Po_2 or Pco_2 correlating pulmonary blood flow and local ventilation.

VARIATIONS IN PULMONARY CIRCULATION

The amount of the pulmonary circulation varies with the right heart output. Thus it is increased in exercise, thyrotoxicosis, fever, anaemia and left to right shunts associated with septal defects and patent ductus arteriosus, and decreased in congestive cardiac failure and right to left shunts. The fact that the pulmonary circulation may be doubled without rise in the pulmonary vascular pressure only holds true if the resistance is not increased. Pulmonary vascular resistance increases when there is a reduction in the number or calibre of the pulmonary vessels, such as may occur in diffuse pulmonary fibrosis, extensive lung resection, multiple embolism, 'primary' pulmonary hypertension and, most common of all, the pulmonary attrition associated with chronic bronchitis and emphysema. All of these can result in a rise in pulmonary arterial pressure. Pulmonary vasoconstriction due to anoxia can result in a temporary rise in pulmonary vascular pressure.

PULMONARY OEDEMA

Because the pressure in the pulmonary capillaries is low and less than the colloid osmotic pressure fluid tends to be drawn into the capillaries (fig. 1.17). In disease such as mitral stenosis and left ventricular failure there is a rise in pressure in the pulmonary capillaries which may now exceed the osmotic pressure so that fluid passes across the capillary membrane into the interstitium of the lung and into the alveoli, resulting in pulmonary oedema. Not all cases of mitral

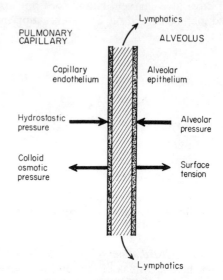

FIG. 1.17. Forces acting across an alveolar-capillary membrane.

stenosis with a raised pulmonary arterial pressure have pulmonary oedema, and it is thought that this may be due to a compensating rise in pressure of the interstitial fluid preventing transudation from the pulmonary capillaries [32].

MEASUREMENT OF PULMONARY BLOOD FLOW

Pulmonary blood flow can be measured by

(1) the direct Fick method, using the equation

blood flow (l/min)
$$= \frac{O_2 \text{ uptake ml/min}}{(\text{arterial}-\text{venous}) \ O_2 \text{ difference (ml/l)}},$$

(2) the indirect Fick method using nitrous oxide [25],

(3) dye dilution methods,

(4) a plethysmographic method based on the uptake of nitrous oxide from a mixture containing 80% nitrous oxide and 20% oxygen and calculated from knowledge of the alveolar volume, the partial pressure of nitrous oxide in the alveoli and its solubility in the blood,

(5) the technique of lung scanning after the inhalation of radio-oxygen ($^{15}O_2$) or the intravenous injection of radio-Xenon (^{133}Xe) [7, 171 & 172] p. 49).

VENTILATION–PERFUSION RATIO

Despite its apparent anatomical homogeneity the lung is physiologically nonhomogeneous and the most important disorders of function affect it differentially. The commonest cause of failure to oxygenate adequately the mixed venous blood is an imbalance between alveolar ventilation ($\dot{V}A$) and pulmonary capillary blood flow ($\dot{Q}$) [171 & 172].

Even in the normal lung *air* is not distributed evenly. In the erect position resting ventilation per unit volume of lung is greater at the bases than at the apices. The difference becomes less on lying down and on exercise. In the abnormal lung airways obstruction due to distortion and narrowing of the smaller bronchi and bronchioles, extensive destructive lesions and conditions associated with altered distensibility of parts of the lung all result in maldistribution of inspired air (p. 35).

There are also regional differences in *blood flow* in the normal lung and these are largely determined by posture. It had for long been postulated that the upper parts of the lung would receive less blood than the bases simply on account of the weight of the column of blood in the lung. This has been shown to be the case and it has been demonstrated that between the 1st and the 5th intercostal spaces the blood flow is increased 9 fold [173]. The regional differences in ventilation are much less marked than the variation in blood flow. It is estimated that about $\frac{1}{7}$ of the ventilated lung is not perfused.

In health the $\dot{V}A/\dot{Q}$ ratio varies from alveolus to alveolus and at different times in

the same alveolus, but the overall effect maintains a P_{O_2} of approximately 96 mm Hg and a P_{CO_2} of about 40 mm Hg. Since alveolar ventilation ($\dot{V}A$) at rest is about 4 l/min and pulmonary blood flow ($\dot{Q}$) is about 5 l/min the $\dot{V}A/\dot{Q}$ ratio is 0·8.

The *functional effect* of uneven gas distribution depends on the corresponding blood distribution. If disease were to cause uneven ventilation and correspondingly uneven perfusion the blood gases would remain normal. The parallel reduction in blood flow to preserve the $\dot{V}A/\dot{Q}$ ratio could be effected by capillary vasoconstriction in response to reduced alveolar oxygen pressure. If, as is usual in disease, gas distribution is uneven and perfusion is either even or uneven, but disproportionate to ventilation, the blood gases cannot be maintained normal.

Those parts of the lung with a raised $\dot{V}A/\dot{Q}$ ratio resemble *deadspace*. When blood flow is increased in relation to ventilation and the $\dot{V}A/\dot{Q}$ ratio is reduced, e.g. in atelectasis, venous blood is bypassing the lung so far as the process of arterialization is concerned and this is referred to as a *shunt* or venous admixture. Extensive shunting results in reduced oxygen saturation of arterial blood. The $\dot{V}A/\dot{Q}$ ratio is reduced at the lung bases because blood flow is proportionately greater than ventilation. The effect of this is small, however, resulting only in a reduction of about 4 mm in the Pa,O_2 and not materially affecting arterial oxygen saturation (Sa,O_2).

Alterations in $\dot{V}A/\dot{Q}$ ratios affect Pa,O_2 far more than P_{CO_2}. The blood leaving well ventilated alveoli is already almost fully oxygenated and increased ventilation of these cannot compensate for the underoxygenation arising from underventilated areas. Increased ventilation will, however, increase the elimination of CO_2 from well ventilated areas and so partially compensates for reduced or absent transfer of CO_2 in underventilated parts (p. 35).

The raised $\dot{V}A/\dot{Q}$ or deadspace effect can be estimated by the Bohr Equation (p. 31) which states that expired gas may be treated as a mixture of dead space gas and alveolar gas and that increase in one fraction of the mixture must imply a decrease in the other. Alveolar CO_2 will be low in those parts of the lung acting as *deadspace* resulting in higher values for the physiological deadspace than for the anatomical deadspace. Major pulmonary embolism with resulting impairment or total lack of perfusion of large areas of ventilated lung will show a marked difference between the arterial and alveolar CO_2 pressures indicating a large deadspace.

The *shunting effect* can be estimated by the difference in oxygen tension between alveolar gas and arterial blood (A−aPo_2 difference*) [51] if no major diffusion defect or anatomical shunt is present (p. 32). The ideal PA,O_2 and Pa,O_2 can be calculated from analysis of respired gas and arterial blood. The normal A−aPo_2 difference is about 9 mm Hg, 4 mm of which is due to those parts of the lung with a low $\dot{V}A/\dot{Q}$ ratio and the remainder to the effect of diffusion and anatomical shunts (bronchial to pulmonary veins, coronary veins to left heart).

Normally 1–4% of the cardiac output is involved in right to left shunts; in anaesthesia this may be raised to 10–15% due to micro-atelectasis. Just as it is important to have intermittent sighs (or yawns) in normal respiration so it is important for the anaesthetist to inflate the lungs fully from time to time [11].

Reduction in the $\dot{V}A/\dot{Q}$ ratio increases the A−aPo_2 difference. In a patient with severe bronchitis it may be as high as 50 mm Hg.

Regional defects in ventilation and pulmonary blood flow can now be studied by means of gas isotopes (p. 49) and by differential lobar sampling and gas analysis (p. 48).

DIFFUSION

The 3rd component in pulmonary gas exchange is *diffusion*. Its importance was recognized at the beginning of this century, but only in the last 20 years has it been clearly understood and studied precisely. More

recently what had been intellectually satisfying concepts of diffusion have been seriously questioned and many problems relating to diffusion remain unsolved.

Diffusion is concerned with the volume of gas transferred from alveolus to capillary or from capillary to alveolus. The volume of gas transferred to or from a single alveolus depends on

(1) the area for diffusion,
(2) time,
(3) the pressure difference between alveolar and capillary gas,
(4) the thickness of the alveolar capillary membrane,
(5) a diffusion coefficient for the membrane.

When the volume of gas transferred is expressed in terms of time and unit difference in partial pressure between the gas in the alveoli and in the mean capillary blood (ml/min/mm Hg) this is known as the *diffusing capacity of the lung* (DL). Every gas has a diffusing capacity but in practice the soluble gases CO or O_2 are used to determine DL.

Oxygen has to cross the alveolar membrane, the interstitial fluid, the capillary membrane, the blood plasma and the membrane of the RBC before combination with haemoglobin occurs (fig. 1.18). Thus theoretically diffusion may be influenced by intra-alveolar oedema or exudate, interstitial oedema, exudate or fibrosis, thickening of the alveolar wall, thickening of the capillary membrane, or increase in the intracapillary path for oxygen due to capillary dilatation. Pulmonary diffusing capacity measures the impediment produced by *all* the factors involved in transfer of oxygen to the RBC, and for the whole lung the influence of the $\dot{V}A/\dot{Q}$ ratio is important.

Any membrane must cause some impediment to gas diffusion through it. If the membrane has a uniform structure the defect in diffusion depends on the thickness of the membrane. The total amount of diffusion is also limited by the surface area available. It is now agreed that the normal alveolar membrane causes no appreciable impediment to oxygen diffusion from alveolus to blood [10

* A−a Po_2 difference is an overall indication of the efficacy of the lung as a gas exchanger. Certain assumptions are necessary in its calculation and in expressing it as 'shunt'.

& 56]. A number of conditions have been recognized in which there is desaturation of arterial blood associated with pathological evidence of thickening of the alveolar lining membrane. Among these are included interstitial lung disease of the type described by

gas and perfusion (e.g. relative overperfusion of poorly ventilated areas) underoxygenation may occur although Pa,CO_2 may be normal (p. 37). In those conditions associated with alteration in the alveolar wall the abnormality is usually uneven; so also is ventilation and

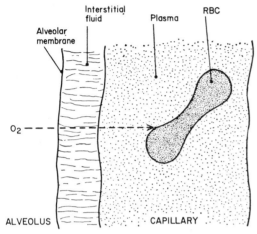

FIG. 1.18. Pathway for O_2 from alveolus to red blood cell.

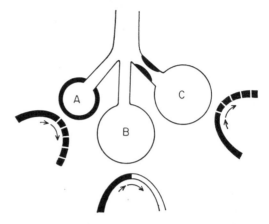

FIG. 1.19. Diagrammatic representation of effects of diffusion impediment and $\dot{V}/\dot{Q}$ imbalance.

A, Alveolus with diffusion impediment; B, normal alveolus with appropriate perfusion and ventilation; C, Alveolus with hypoventilation relative to blood flow ($\dot{V}/\dot{Q}$ imbalance).

Blood leaving alveolus A and alveolus C has low Po_2. Present techniques cannot distinguish which of the two processes causes the hypoxia.

Hamman and Rich and the more chronic varieties of 'fibrosing alveolitis' (p. 565), sarcoidosis (p. 371), pulmonary berylliosis (p. 498) asbestosis (p. 482), Farmer's lung (p. 506), pulmonary scleroderma (p. 585), polyarteritis nodosa (p. 434) and lymphatic carcinomatosis (p. 529). The clinical picture of these conditions includes dyspnoea, overventilation, decreased VC and TLC, cyanosis and decreased So_2 (if not at rest then induced by exercise), normal or decreased Pa,CO_2 and diffuse radiographic abnormality. In the conditions mentioned it was initially believed that the thickened membrane was responsible for the hypoxaemia since it could be corrected by increasing the oxygen content of inspired air. The normal or decreased Pa,CO_2 was explainable by the greater diffusibility of CO_2 (20 times more diffusible than O_2). But oxygen has a high rate of diffusion so that this aspect of gas exchange is unlikely to be impaired. Also, precisely the same functional abnormality may be caused by $\dot{V}A/\dot{Q}$ inequality (fig. 1.19). If there is mismatching of alveolar

perfusion. There are no methods at present available which can distinguish between $\dot{V}A/\dot{Q}$ abnormality and impaired diffusing capacity [144] but the general consensus of opinion is that $\dot{V}A/\dot{Q}$ disturbances are far more important than thickening of the alveolar membrane [53].

Despite the above reservations the measurement of the diffusing capacity (or transfer factor) for CO or O_2 is a useful index of the severity of the conditions listed above in which the fine structure of the lung is affected. DL may also be of value in diagnosis and prognosis and in assessing response to treatment. In some conditions, e.g. sarcoidosis (p. 380) DL is a more sensitive measure of the extent of disease than the x-ray appearances. The test is readily tolerated by the patient.

Ideally the gas used for DL estimations

should be oxygen and DL,O_2 can, in fact, be measured, though with difficulty.

$$DL,O_2 = \frac{\dot{V}O_2}{PA,O_2 - P\bar{C}_{O2}}$$

$\dot{V}O_2 = O_2$ consumption/min; PA,O_2, mean alveolar O_2 pressure; $P\bar{C}_{O2}$, mean pulmonary capillary O_2 pressure.

Because of the difficulty in measuring PA,O_2 and $P\bar{C}_{O2}$ the O_2 method for measuring diffusing capacity is not used routinely. DL,O_2 is normally more than 15 ml O_2/min/mm Hg.

In routine practice the diffusing capacity for CO (DL,CO) is used. CO has a great affinity for Hb (200 times that of O_2) so that any CO near a Hb molecule becomes bound to it. At low alveolar pressures of CO only a small fraction of the Hb is saturated with CO during the passage of the RBC through the pulmonary capillaries so that the pressure of CO in the blood is small relative to the CO pressure in the alveoli. The relatively large difference between PA,CO and $P\bar{C}_{CO}$ (or Pa,CO) makes the CO method for measuring diffusion capacity more accurate than the O_2 method. In all of the several ways of estimating DL,CO the plasma level of CO (Pa,CO) is kept very low so that the only limiting factor in CO uptake is diffusion. In essential the techniques employed require measurement of the uptake of CO ($\dot{V}CO$) and the pressure of CO in the alveolar gas by means of an infra-red analyser. Pa,CO is assumed to be zero.

$$DL,CO = \frac{\dot{V}CO}{PA,CO - Pa,CO} = \frac{\dot{V}CO}{PA,CO}$$

The difficulty with DL,CO measurements is in determining representative values for PA,CO because of uneven ventilation [56]. The value for DL,CO varies with the technique. With the commonly used single breath method the DL,CO is about 25 ml CO/min/mm Hg. Usually 50% of inspired CO is extracted; values less than 25% indicate $\dot{V}A/\dot{Q}$ inequality and/or diffusion abnormality. Other techniques may indicate whether $\dot{V}A/\dot{Q}$ imbalance is present. (For details of DL measurements the reader is referred to textbooks of respiratory physiology.)

AIRWAYS RESISTANCE AND ITS MEASUREMENT

The resistance of the flow of gas in the bronchi is proportional to the driving pressure and inversely proportional to the rate of flow, i.e.

$$\text{resistance} = \frac{\text{driving pressure}}{\text{rate of flow}}$$

The driving pressure in the airways on inspiration is the pressure at the mouth (atmospheric) *minus* alveolar pressure, and on expiration is the reverse. Factors influencing airway resistance include the calibre of the bronchi, whether flow is *laminar* (streamlined) or *turbulent* (eddy formation) and the density and viscosity of the gas. Flow is mainly laminar in quiet breathing; in rapid breathing turbulence becomes more important. In quiet breathing airway resistance depends more on the viscosity of the gas; in rapid breathing it depends more on the density. If the bronchial lumen is irregular turbulence may become important at low flow rates. This occurs in bronchitis (distortion, excess mucus, etc.), bronchial tumour or foreign body.

Airways resistance can be calculated accurately (and is expressed in cm H_2O/l/sec) by measuring atmospheric and alveolar pressure and rate of air flow. Air flow is measured by a pneumotachograph and alveolar pressure by the body plethysmograph using an interrupter technique [58]. Normal values for airway resistance are around 1·5–3·0 cm H_2O/l/sec with average flow rates. In chronic obstructive airways disease it may exceed 10 cm H_2O/l/sec.

For routine clinical use a reliable estimate of airways resistance may be made much more easily by determining the maximal flow rates on inspiration and expiration by simple spirometry. Even simpler is the measurement of the volume of gas expired by maximal effort in unit time after a maximal inspiration (V/t = flow rate) which is the *forced expiratory volume* (FEV). The usual unit of time employed is 1 sec (FEV_1). The total volume expired with the greatest force and speed after a maximal inspiration is the *forced vital capacity* (FVC) which differs very little from the VC in the normal subject but is proportionately more reduced when there is airways obstruction with air trapping. In young people the FEV is normally about 80% of the FVC; lesser values signify obstruction to air flow. Generalized airways obstruction is the commonest disorder of respiratory function and the FEV is the most useful single test available to the clinician.

In restrictive lung disease the FVC is reduced but if there is no obstructive component the FEV will be the normal proportion of the FVC and the FEV/FVC ratio will be around 80%.

Previously the *maximum breathing capacity* (MBC) or the *maximum voluntary ventilation* (MVV) (equivalent terms for the maximum volume of gas which can be breathed per minute), was calculated from the FEV by a multiplication factor (35 for FEV_1, 40 for $FEV_{0.75}$) and it was customary to use the MBC or MVV when referring to ventilatory reserve. The MVV is estimated directly by having the patient breathe as rapidly and deeply as possible for 15 sec and collecting the expired gas in a Douglas Bag. This volume is multiplied by 4 and the MVV is then expressed in l/min. Low values for MVV correlate well with subjective dyspnoea but with a few exceptions it gives no more information than the FEV. The direct MVV is is still of value when a repetitive test of function is necessary to assess the effect of tiring of the respiratory muscles as in myasthenia gravis.

Just as the VC is the most useful monitor for the progress of restrictive lung disease so the FEV is the most useful monitor for the progress of obstructive lung disease (fig. 1.20). In reversible generalized airways obstruction the FEV is recorded before and after a bronchodilator (usually the inhalation of 1% isoprenaline aerosol given for 2 min or 0·5 ml. of 1:1000 adrenaline given subcutaneously) Improvement must be assessed on the abso-

lute readings of the FEV and not on the FEV/FVC ratio, since the FVC is also reduced in obstructive airways disease (though proportionately less).

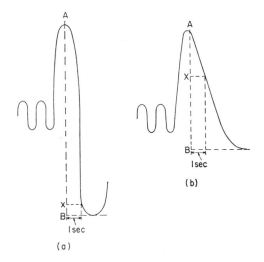

FIG. 1.20. (a) Normal spirogram during FVC manoeuvre. AB, FVC; AX, FEV, greater than 80% FVC. (b) Spirogram in obstructive airways disease. AB, FVC; AX, FEV, less than 80% FVC.

MEASUREMENT OF AIRWAYS RESISTANCE

The FVC and FEV are usually recorded on a spirometer with an electronic timing attachment. 'Dry' spirometers which are portable are now available and also portable machines which give a spirogram trace (Vitalograph; Vitalor). The spirogram may give useful information, e.g. in air trapping (fig. 1.21). Changes in airways resistance may also be measured by the *peak expiratory flow meter* [179]. This measures maximum flow over 10 milli-secs at the beginning of expiration (peak expiratory flow rate = PEFR). The peak flow meter is a robust machine, particularly useful for field studies and reliable as a means of serial assessment of generalized airways obstruction treated with bronchodilator drugs.

The *Snider match test* provides a crude assessment of airways resistance which is useful as a screening test for fitness for surgery. A lighted match is held 6 in. (15 cm) from the open mouth and the patient tries to blow it out. Failure to extinguish the match equates with an FEV_1 of less than 1000 ml, and quantitative measurements are then indicated to determine the FEV precisely.

Clinical assessment of obstructive limitation of respiration includes estimation of wheezing and rhonchi and the measurement

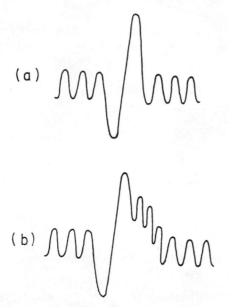

FIG. 1.21. (a) Normal spirogram during measurement of inspiratory capacity. Note immediate return of trace to previous level. (b) Spirogram during same manoeuvre as in (a) but demonstrating air trapping. Previous trace level reached only after several breaths.

of the *forced expiratory time* (FET). The latter is performed by asking the patient to expire forcibly with the mouth wide open, after a maximum inspiration, and listening with a stethoscope over the trachea. Normally the VC is expired in 3–4 sec and air flow stops. A value of 6 sec or over for the FET indicates airways obstruction and a FEV/FVC% below 65.

THE WORK OF BREATHING

The work of breathing refers to the energy expended in moving air into the lungs against the combined resistance of the abdominal contents, the chest wall and the lung. Thoracic resistance is both *elastic* and *nonelastic* (or viscous); when increased it may result in dyspnoea [109].

Active muscular contraction during inspiration must overcome (a) the elastic recoil of the lungs and thorax (elastic resistance) and (b) frictional resistance to movement of the tissues of the lung and chest wall along with the resistance to air flow in the airways due to friction and turbulence (nonelastic resistance).

ELASTIC RESISTANCE

This comprises the elastic recoil of the lung and also of the chest wall. The elastic properties of the lungs are due to elastic fibres but also to collagen, the reticulum of the lungs, pleura, bronchi and blood vessels, the surface tension of gas–liquid interfaces (p. 11), the smooth muscle of the bronchi, the pulmonary blood volume and probably also bronchial mucus. Elasticity ensures that the normal lung returns to its original size after inspiration.

Work done = force × distance. The force required for inspiration is equivalent to the change of intrathoracic or intrapleural pressure (p. 21). The distance over which this force acts is proportional to the resulting change in lung volume. When change in lung volume is related to unit change in intrapleural (in practice intraoesophageal) pressure this measures the distensibility or *compliance* of the lung which is simply a way of expressing the elastic properties of the lung.

$$\text{Compliance} = \frac{\text{change in lung volume (in l)}}{\begin{array}{c}\text{change in intraoesophageal}\\\text{pressure (in cm } H_2O)\end{array}}$$

Compliance can be measured by recording the variation in intraoesophageal pressure (p. 21) which occurs when the patient inspires a measured volume of air then holds his breath while keeping the glottis open. Many patients find this difficult. Transpulmonary pressure is then being measured under static conditions with no gas flow. It is possible to train the patient to fractionate inspiration into 2 or 3

Compliance = vol. change needed to produce 1cm.H₂O change
— in intrapleural or intra-oesophageal pressure.

parts so that the oesophageal pressure variation can be measured for each of the steps (fig. 1.22). From the data a pressure-volume line can be calculated (e.g. AB in fig. 1.23). The lung compliance is reflected in the slope of the curve. The normal value is about 0·2 l/cm

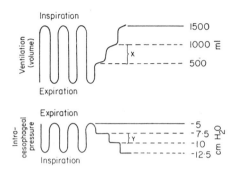

FIG. 1.22. Measurement of pulmonary compliance by fractionation of inspiration with glottis kept open. Taking measurements for middle part of recording (X and Y), compliance=
$$\frac{X}{Y} = \frac{0·5 \; 1}{2·5 \; cm} = 0·2 \; 1/cm \; H_2O.$$

H_2O (e.g. 0·5 l/2·5 cm H_2O). The compliance for each lung can be measured by bronchospirometry.

Compliance may also be measured with the patient breathing continuously, measuring end-inspiratory and end-expiratory levels of oesophageal pressure and relating these to the tidal volume (fig. 1.23). In the normal subject the results with the interrupted ('static') and continuous ('dynamic') breathing methods are virtually the same but when the lungs are diseased the values for compliance measured with continuous breathing are much lower, especially at fast respiratory rates, than those obtained by the interrupted method. This is because complete filling of the lung units cannot occur during the relatively short inspiratory phases. This discrepancy may be one of the first signs of chronic bronchitis.

Whenever pathological changes in the lungs cause increased tissue density the lungs become 'stiffer' and compliance is reduced. The increase in work to stretch the lungs can be kept to a minimum by breathing with a smaller

tidal volume, but more rapidly. This, however, increases the physiological deadspace.

Pulmonary compliance is reduced in pulmonary congestion and oedema, restrictive lung disease (due to pleural, interstitial or pulmonary fibrosis), respiratory disease of the

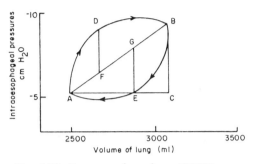

FIG. 1.23. Pressure–volume loop ADBEA constructed by relating intraoesophageal pressure and lung volume during one respiratory cycle. Line AB represents pressure necessary to inflate lung and elastic work expended is represented by triangle ABC. If lung were fully compliant the loop and line AB would be horizontal. Extra negative pressure to move air through airways (nonelastic resistance) on inspiration is represented by vertical line DF and work done to overcome nonelastic resistance on inspiration is equivalent to area ADBA. Area ABEA represents work done on expiration. Normally this is simply energy stored on inspiration when lung is stretched but extra work is necessary on expiration if chronic obstructive airways disease is present.

newborn, atelectasis, pneumonia, pleural effusion, pulmonary resection and sometimes in anaesthesia (probably due to microatelectasis). Compliance in emphysema varies with the rate of breathing. Measured by the static method the compliance is increased; measured by the dynamic method it is reduced because the easily ventilated areas are disproportionately stretched, thus increasing the elastic resistance to distension.

Although compliance studies have made important contributions to the understanding of pulmonary mechanics the test is not very discriminating, the details of the technique are extremely important if repeatable results are to be obtained and the range of 'normality' is wide. Tests of compliance do not distinguish between diffuse pulmonary disease causing stiffening of the lung and simple loss of functioning lung tissue even when this is due to extrapulmonary causes.

Thoracic cage compliance is reduced in a number of conditions affecting the chest wall including kyphoscoliosis, pectus excavatum, thoracoplasty, spastic conditions of the skeletal muscles and in patients with marked obesity. The compliance of chest wall and lung can be estimated using a Drinker respirator and measuring the change in tidal volume with the pressure variation. If the lung compliance is known the chest wall compliance can be calculated. The two are of the same order in the normal subject.

EFFECTS OF DECREASED COMPLIANCE

The less compliant the lungs the greater the work necessary to move air. In the 'stiff' lung of diffuse interstitial pulmonary fibrosis a tidal volume of 500 ml may only be achieved by intrapleural (intraoesophageal) pressure amplitudes of 50 cm H_2O, i.e. the pulmonary compliance is only 0·5 1/50 cm $H_2O = 0·01$ l/cm H_2O. The increased work needed to move poorly compliant lungs is particularly marked when the tidal volume is large; on this account the patient usually breathes less deeply and more rapidly.

Altered compliance, like most disturbances of lung function, usually affects the lung unevenly. This results in uneven ventilation and $\dot{V}A/\dot{Q}$ imbalance.

NONELASTIC RESISTANCE

As mentioned already, the elastic work needed to stretch the lungs is measured by relating the volume inspired to the increase of pressure gradient from the beginning to the end of inspiration when there is no air flow. The pressure–volume relationships are almost linear in the middle ranges of breathing (fig. 1.23). If the added pressure gradient required to maintain air flow during inspiration and expiration is related to the simultaneous volume change it will be seen that the changes are not linear but form a loop (AEB in fig. 1.23). The deviation from the line between the points of no flow (which represents compli-

ance) measures the total nonelastic resistance. At end inspiration and end expiration when there is no air flow the nonelastic resistance is nil. The deviation from the line joining the points of no flow will be greater with greater nonelastic resistance, i.e. the loop will be fatter.

Because obstructive airways disease is the commonest form of disordered lung function increase in nonelastic work is the most important disturbance in lung disease. It is greatly increased in asthma, bronchitis and emphysema. The factors of bronchospasm, mucosal oedema, excess mucoid secretion and distortion of the airways play a variable role. There is greater delay of flow in expiration than in inspiration. If the elastic recoil is impaired expiratory muscle effort may be required to empty the lungs. This may mean that positive pressures generated outside the lung are transmitted to the alveoli around the bronchioles which become compressed causing air trapping (p. 13).

To some extent the increase in nonelastic work due to chronic obstructive airways disease can be minimized by slow, deep breathing since the resistance to air flow rises rapidly with increase in velocity of air flow.

THE BLOOD GASES

Normal respiration maintains the Pa,O_2 around 96 mm Hg and the Pa,CO_2 around 40 mm Hg even though oxygen requirement varies from as little as 100 ml/min in sleep to 2–3 l/min in strenuous exercise. About 80% of these amounts of CO_2 are eliminated.

Clinical estimation of oxygen undersaturation by cyanosis is rarely accurate and saturation has to fall below 85% before it can be appreciated. Accurate measurement of So_2 can be made by the *Van Slyke manometric method* or by *spectrophotometry* (e.g. Brinkman haemoreflector). The Van Slyke method which measures both O_2 and CO_2 content of blood samples is the standard by which all other methods for measuring So_2 are compared. It is based on the absorption of O_2 by sodium hydrosulphite and CO_2 by sodium hydroxide. In the technique the volume and temperature are kept constant and variations in pressure are measured. Spectrophotometry will give an answer more quickly but it is important to remember that with some instruments abnormal pigment such as methaemoglobin can lead to inaccuracies. The *ear oximeter* is useful for measuring variations in So_2 although it is not reliable for measuring absolute levels.

The arterial Po_2 is replacing So_2 as the standard measurement for arterial oxygenation in most laboratories since the development of reliable *oxygen electrodes* which function on the polarigraphic principle [149]. The oxygen electrode can be accurately calibrated by tonometry to the highest levels of Po_2 needed for gas studies (600 mm Hg). The electrode functions on the principle that an electrical current can flow from a silver reference electrode to a platinum electrode in the presence of oxygen.

The arterial Pco_2 is now also most commonly measured by an electrode system using a sample of arterial blood [149]. The electrode is a glass one covered by teflon membrane through which CO_2 diffuses and forms H_2CO_3 in a watery film. The H_2CO_3 dissociates into H^+ and HCO_3^- ions and the former are measured. The *Astrup interpolation micro method* is also used and has the advantage of being applicable to capillary blood [4]. It is based on the principle that the relation between the logarithm of Pco_2 and the pH is a straight line. This line is constructed by recording the pH of arterial blood at 37°C without contact with air and after equilibration with two known concentrations of CO_2. Knowing the actual pH of the blood the corresponding Pco_2 can be determined. End tidal sampling of expired air can also be used to measure the Pa,co_2 but is applicable only when the lungs are healthy. This involves monitoring the CO_2 concentration during the whole of expiration, the last part giving a fair measure of alveolar Pco_2 which approximates to arterial Pco_2. The method is invalid if there is uneven distribution of ventilation. Another method is the use of the *Henderson–Hasselbalch equation* which requires knowledge of the pH and the plasma bicarbonate.

$$pH = pK^1 + \log \frac{(HCO_3^-)}{(H_2CO_3)}$$

(pK^1 is a constant,* 6·10 at a plasma temperature of 37°C). H_2CO_3 is in equilibrium with dissolved CO_2 and this in turn is a function of the Pa,co_2. Hence

$$pH = 6·1 + \log \frac{(HCO_3^-)}{0·03\ Pa,co_2}$$

The Pa,co_2 can, therefore, be calculated.

A bloodless technique which is applicable to conditions of uneven ventilation and which measures mixed venous Pco_2 by equilibration and is known as the *rebreathing method*, has been devised by Campbell and Howell [21 & 22]. The patient respires from a 1·5 l oxygen filled bag for 1½ min then rests. During this period the CO_2 content gradually rises until the Pco_2 in the bag is slightly higher than the Pa,co_2 After 2 or more min during which the Pa,co_2 reaches its previous level the patient then rebreathes into the bag for 20 sec or 5 breaths, whichever takes the longest. The gas in the bag, which is now in equilibrium with alveolar gas and mixed venous blood is then analysed by the modified Haldane or other gas analyser and the percentage of CO_2 found. The partial pressure of CO_2 is obtained by multiplying this percentage by the barometric pressure, corrected for vapour pressure, say $6\% \times 700$ mm Hg. This gives 42 mm Hg which is the Pco_2 of *mixed venous blood*. The Pco_2 of mixed venous blood is estimated to be 6 mm Hg higher than arterial Pco_2 so the arterial Pco_2 is $42 - 6 = 36$ mm Hg. The rebreathing method of assessing Pco_2 has become a standard side room test in most centres dealing with respiratory failure. The principal source of error is leakage around the mouth piece during rebreathing.

The *arterial blood pH* is usually measured by an electrode but it may be calculated by the Henderson–Hasselbalch equation if plasma CO_2 content and pressure are known.

* It has been found that this is not always the case if there has been an acute change in the patient's condition [165]. When the condition is stable the K^1 may be assumed to be constant.

ALTERATION IN THE BLOOD GASES

OXYGEN

Deficient oxygenation of arterial blood at sea level due to pulmonary causes results from one or more of the following:

(1) General inadequacy of alveolar ventilation.
(2) Intrapulmonary shunts.
(3) Impaired diffusion.
(4) Mismatching of ventilation and blood flow—$\dot{V}_A/\dot{Q}$ imbalance.

Of these the last is the most important. About one third of the mixed venous blood has to pass through underventilated alveoli before the So_2 is reduced below 90%. Under these circumstances exercise which reduces the oxygen saturation of mixed venous blood also reduces the Pa,o_2 and cyanosis may then become evident or, if present, is worsened. If desaturation is not worsened by exercise there is a disorder of ventilation which is not due to lung disease (e.g. primary hypoventilation). When arterial desaturation is due to a pulmonary cause the breathing of 100% O_2 results in a rapid rise of So_2 to 100%. 30% O_2 is almost as effective. If there is a major right to left shunt of blood bypassing the lung the breathing of 100% oxygen results in a slow slight rise (usually less than 10%) of So_2 due to an increased amount of dissolved oxygen in the plasma mixing with the shunted blood. The only cause of anoxaemia in which inhalation of 100% O_2 will not eventually increase the Pa,o_2 to maximum values (over 600 mm Hg) is a major right to left shunt.

CARBON DIOXIDE

The Pa,co_2 reflects the adequacy or otherwise of the volume of ventilation. Underventilation results in a rise in Pa,co_2 and if this is marked it may be accompanied by the clinical features of CO_2 retention which include tachycardia, rise in blood pressure with a bounding pulse, sweating and warm extremities, muscle twitching, coarse tremor, confusion and coma. Cerebral blood flow is highly sensitive to changes in Pa,co_2. Rise in Pa,co_2 causes a rise in intracranial pressure and headache

and papilloedema may result. When the clinical features of CO_2 retention are evident it usually means a rise in Pa,co_2 above 80 mm Hg. More moderate rises of Pa,co_2 have no associated specific features and are recognizable only when measured by the techniques already mentioned. For example reduction in alveolar ventilation by 20% results in a rise in Pa,co_2 to about 50 mm Hg which does not usually cause any symptoms, and a fall in Pa,o_2 to 76 mm Hg, which is still sufficient to maintain So_2 near normal so that cyanosis does not occur.

Hyperventilation reduces the Pa,co_2 but unless severe this results in no ill effects. Marked reduction in Pa,co_2 (e.g. overventilation during assisted respiration) leads to increase in pH and a low bicarbonate (respiratory alkalosis). Tetany may result. Cerebral blood flow may be greatly reduced.

The features associated with increase or decrease in Pa,co_2 are much less in evidence when the hypoventilation or hyperventilation is a chronic phenomenon.

Estimation of the Pa,co_2 is most commonly employed for evaluation of the severity and progress of hypoventilation due to chronic obstructive airways disease. It may be of diagnostic value in the older patient with congestive cardiac failure who may have a history of chronic bronchitis and in whom it is difficult to determine if the heart failure is right sided due to *cor pulmonale* or principally left sided due to ischaemic heart disease. In the latter the Pa,co_2 is normal or low due to hyperventilation. Cor pulmonale due to obstructive airways disease is always associated with a raised Pa,co_2.

Acid–base balance [44]
The principal organs concerned with acid–base regulation are the kidneys and the lungs. The lungs are much the more important. CO_2 is a rapidly effective regulator of the blood pH.

$$CO_2 + H_2O = H_2CO_3 = H^+ + HCO_3^-$$

(i.e. each CO_2 molecule excreted means one H^+ less).

Although strictly the CO_2–HCO_3^- system

is not a buffer chemically, it is physiologically vitally important in maintaining a stable hydrogen ion activity. CO_2 is regulated by the lungs (p. 44), HCO_3^- by the kidneys. Pulmonary compensation for variation in Pa,CO_2 is rapid in the normal subject. Renal compensation is usually slow.

Normally at rest the PCO_2 of mixed venous blood is 46 mm Hg. The PA,CO_2 is 40 mm Hg so that there is a pressure gradient of 6 mm across the alveolar–capillary membrane. CO_2 is carried in the blood in 3 forms, in solution (6%), as bicarbonate (70%) and as a carbamino compound (24%).

CO_2 as bicarbonate

Carbonic anhydrase in the red cell speeds the union of CO_2 with H_2O to form H_2CO_3; in the pulmonary capillaries this enzyme speeds the reverse process. The take up of CO_2 in the red cell is actually facilitated by the liberation of O_2 as follows:

$$HbO_2 \rightarrow Hb + O_2$$

Hb provides the base with which H^+, provided by dissociation of H_2CO_3, combines and HCO_3^- accumulates in the red cell. The red cell membrane is permeable only to anions e.g. Cl^- and HCO_3^- and to positively charged H ions. When HCO_3^- reaches a certain concentration within the cell there is ionic imbalance and HCO_3 ions pass out of the red cell and Cl ions pass in. The process is known as the *Hamburger phenomenon* or the *chloride shift*. In the pulmonary capillaries the process occurs in reverse. Hydrogen ions are liberated as Hb becomes HbO_2 and combines with HCO_3 ions to form H_2CO_3. Under the influence of carbonic anhydrase H_2CO_3 breaks down to CO_2 and H_2O. CO_2 then leaves the cell, HCO_3 ions enter and Cl ions move out into the plasma. The extracellular fluid bicarbonate thus forms a major part of the store of CO_2 in the body and plays an important part in maintaining a normal acid–base balance and a normal pH. From the Henderson–Hasselbalch equation it will be seen that the pH depends on the *ratio* of HCO_3^- to H_2CO_3 (normally 20 : 1 in the plasma) and not the absolute amounts.

CO_2 as a carbamino compound

CO_2 is combined with the amino group of Hb and to a very much lesser extent with plasma proteins.

Hb plays an important role as a buffer in acid–base balance. The plasma proteins by holding sodium ions which can be replaced by hydrogen ions also help.

Compensation for raised Pa,CO_2

Rapid increase in Pa,CO_2 evokes an immediate response by hyperventilation to restore normality. The response is dependent on normal sensitivity of the medullary chemosensitive centre, normal nervous pathways from the respiratory centre to the respiratory muscles, normal respiratory muscles and relatively normal lungs. A more gradual increase in Pa,CO_2 allows renal compensation to occur. Sodium ions are retained and H^+ excreted as NaH_2PO_4 or NH_4Cl while HCO_3^- is reabsorbed. The HCO_3^- combines with retained sodium so that in compensated respiratory acidosis the sodium concentration in the plasma does not decrease but the chloride concentration does. The ammonia (NH_3) which eliminates excess of H^+ in the urine is synthesized by the tubular cells from glutamine. The relation between the daily excretion of ammonia and the Pa,CO_2 is roughly linear [1]. Usually renal compensation is not fully effective and increase in Pa,CO_2, especially if rapid, results in some fall in pH (respiratory acidosis).

Assessment of the metabolic and respiratory contributions to alteration in acid–base balance requires knowledge of the arterial pH and bicarbonate. The interrelation of bicarbonate (HCO_3^-), pH and PCO_2 can be represented graphically in a fashion which demonstrates the effects of metabolic as well as respiratory acidosis and alkalosis (fig. 1.24). Single readings may be difficult to interpret but the position usually becomes clearer if the previous course of the illness is known. A rise in Pa,CO_2 due to respiratory acidosis must be associated with a rise in total blood CO_2 (bicarbonate). The latter also occurs in metabolic alkalosis. The distinction is made by simultaneous measurements of pH and Pa,CO_2. In respiratory acidosis there is a raised Pa,CO_2 and a high plasma bicarbonate. The combination of a raised pH, a low Pa,CO_2 and a low plasma bicarbonate indicates respiratory alkalosis.

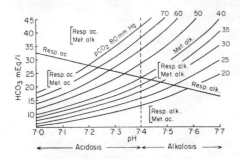

Fig. 1.24. Interrelation of bicarbonate (HCO_3), pH and PCO_2 in blood plasma. The values of these components which are associated with acidosis (AC) or alkalosis (ALK) of respiratory (RESP) or metabolic (MET) origin are shown. Thus at an (HCO_3) of 15 mEq/1 a pH of 7·15 is associated with a PCO_2 of 50 mm Hg and this occurs in metabolic acidosis. Reproduced from Beaumont & Dodds (1965) *Recent Advances in Medicine*. London, Churchill.

In the common form of respiratory failure where an acute is superimposed on a chronic hypercapnia repeated monitoring during the first few days of recovery shows a fall of Pa,CO_2 (say from 80 to 50 mm Hg), a rise in arterial blood pH (say from 7·28 to 7·35), and a fairly sustained high level of blood bicarbonate with an increased urine excretion of bicarbonate. The blood bicarbonate falls gradually during the second week and the urine bicarbonate correspondingly falls and finally reaches the normal negligible levels [1].

ASSESSMENT OF REGIONAL LUNG FUNCTION

Most commonly the evaluation of the function of each lung separately, of or subdivisions of the lungs, is required in the assessment for resectional surgery of patients with border line respiratory reserve. In general, ventilation, pulmonary blood flow and gas exchange are proportional to each other so that an estimate of one (usually ventilation) is commonly a reliable guide to all. Important exceptions are avascular bullous areas, areas with pulmonary artery occlusion which may still be well ventilated, or areas of atelectasis which may be well perfused.

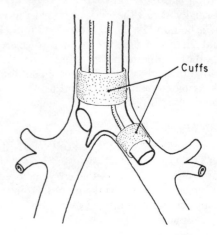

Fig. 1.25. Carlens catheter in position.

Normally the right lung accounts for 55% of the total ventilation and oxygen uptake and the left lung for 45%. The contribution of each lung to the overall respiratory function can be measured by *differential bronchospirometry*. A double channelled Carlens catheter (fig. 1.25) is inserted into the trachea after local anaesthesia and positioned so that the tip of the catheter enters the left main bronchus. The channel for the right lung ends in the trachea. Inflatable cuffs around the catheter, in the left main bronchus and in the trachea proximal to the aperture for the right lung channel, ensure that the ventilation to each lung can be recorded on separate spirometers. It is possible by this technique to measure the ventilation, minute volume, lung volume, pulmonary blood flow, exchanges of oxygen, carbon dioxide and carbon monoxide and ventilation–perfusion ratios for each lung. Commonly only the ventilation and oxygen uptake are required (fig. 1.26) and these are the easiest to measure.

Lobar or segmental analysis of lung function is now possible using techniques developed at the Postgraduate Medical School in London for measuring gas concentration and gas flow [46]. The composition of gas respired by the individual lobe or some segments is sampled through a hollow probe inserted under direct vision through a bronchoscope. The gas flow is measured by a device consisting essentially of a jet of argon passing transversely from a point of emission to a sampling

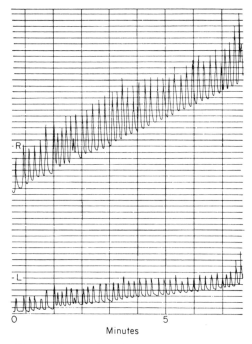

FIG. 1.26. Bronchospirometry trace in patient with large bulla in the left lung. Ventilation is indicated by excursion of trace and oxygen uptake by slope.

point, the whole being enclosed in a wire cage 6 mm in diameter which can be inserted into a bronchus until it is wedged. The argon is sampled by a mass spectrometer and when no gas flow occurs in the bronchus the concentration of argon is high. When there is gas flow in the bronchus the jet is deflected and the concentration sampled is less. By means of a calibration factor derived from *in vitro* measurements the actual flow of gas can be calculated. The results from these studies can indicate the *anatomical* location of areas of

lung with impaired function (e.g. pulmonary bullae) and can give valuable information when it is imperative that pulmonary resection should be as conservative as possible.

Topographical function can be studied by techniques using *radioactive gases* which can measure regional ventilation and blood flow [7, 171 & 172]. After a single breath of oxygen-15 (half life 2 min) or Xenon-133 (half life 5·3 days) the level of radioactivity is measured by multiple counters over the chest wall. This records regional ventilation. Regional perfusion can be assessed either by the patient inhaling oxygen-15 and holding the breath while the rate of removal is recorded by the counters, or by the intravenous injection of the relatively insoluble Xenon-133 which is excreted into the alveoli whenever it reaches the pulmonary capillaries. Radioactive gas studies express regional ventilation and perfusion quantitatively. Qualitative estimation of pulmonary blood flow can be obtained by intravenous injection of macro-aggregated *radio-iodinated human serum albumin* and recording radioactivity over the lungs by a scintillation scanner. This technique, which is entirely safe, may replace pulmonary angiography in the detection of pulmonary embolism (p. 459). It is, however, less discriminative.

These methods of assessment of regional lung function are not generally available. Lobar analysis and the radioactive gas techniques require costly apparatus and skilled technical assistance. Even the relatively crude assessment of bronchospirometry requires a degree of expertise and some technical help. But it is possible to learn a lot about regional function by the simple methods of clinical examination and standard radiographic procedures. Inspection, palpation and auscultation can give some indication of the degree of ventilation of the lung and PA and lateral radiographs can give reasonably reliable estimates of the relative aeration of different parts of the lungs. The most valuable of the simple procedures is *fluoroscopy*. The relative density of the lungs and the movement of the ribs, diaphragm and mediastinum give important indications of the relative ventilation in the various lobes, and lag in movement of the diaphragm or mediastinum may indicate some inequality of airways obstruction. Screening may determine the degree of ventilation of cysts and their contribution to air-trapping in the adjacent lung, particularly when a forced expiration is observed. The technique of *fluorodensitometry* is still in the experimental stage so far as assessment of regional lung function is concerned [153].

PULMONARY FUNCTION DURING EXERCISE

Valuable information regarding the cardiac, pulmonary, metabolic and psychological state of the patient can be obtained by observing the response to exercise. The effects of quantitated exercise can be studied by means of step tests, the bicycle ergometer and the treadmill. The bicycle ergometer has many advantages [3, 76 & 98] and is being used increasingly. Measurements which can be made before, during and after exercise include the pulse rate and the blood pressure, the respiratory rate, tidal volume, minute volume, alveolar ventilation and oxygen consumption. Precise evaluation of the results of these observations is dependent on having normal data for comparison. There can be quite wide ranges of 'normality' for these in the absence of pulmonary disease because of such factors as general fitness, state of training, age, etc. Estimations of So_2, Po_2, Pco_2, pH and diffusing capacity during exercise can be interpreted more accurately.

The ratio of the minute volume of ventilation to the oxygen uptake (l/ml O_2) has been termed the *ventilation equivalent* [90]. It is fairly constant in normal subjects (between 2 and 3 l/100 ml) but is increased in any condition resulting in hyperventilation in relation to the oxygen uptake including nervousness, thyrotoxicosis, anaemia, mitral stenosis, left ventricular failure, diffuse interstitial pulmonary fibrosis and pulmonary thrombo-embolism (p. 458).

The *maximal oxygen uptake* (measured when a pulse rate of 180/min is reached on moderate exercise) has been shown to be a reliable measure of working capacity in normal subjects and in patients with heart or lung disease [3, 98 & 114].

The *pulse–work relationship* is linear for most practical purposes since the heart rate is a linear function of O_2 consumption up to a maximum value which varies with age. Because of this it is possible to extrapolate from lower work levels once the pulse–work relationship has been determined for an individual during submaximal exercise. This is the most useful and one of the simplest and most easily tolerated of laboratory exercise tests. The O_2 consumption (or rate of work) corresponding to a pulse rate of 170 is commonly calculated and is referred to as the *physical working capacity* [172].

CLINICAL VALUE OF LUNG FUNCTION TESTS

Few branches of medicine have been affected more by the rapidly advancing technology of recent years than the study of respiratory physiology. The physician is now faced with a bewildering complexity of tests and techniques from which it is often difficult to distinguish what is valuable and what superfluous in the elucidation of problems relating to pulmonary function. The stage has been reached where an abundance of laboratory tests has made it imperative for critical appraisal to be made of their respective merits so that only the most useful and most easily performed tests can be selected for a particular problem. The aim, therefore, is towards increasing simplification so that only the simplest and most meaningful tests will be retained for general use. It cannot be overemphasized that the details of the history and the physical examination can, in most cases, be much more valuable than lung function tests in the aetiological sense and tests are frequently only necessary to quantitate the severity of a disorder. This is particularly true in conditions such as chronic bronchitis and asthma in which the history is the most important part of the whole assessment.

Lung function tests only show the effect of disease on function and cannot be used to give diagnosis on the basis of pathological change.

Some diseases do have a characteristic pattern of disordered function, however, and it is possible to distinguish an obstructive pattern of ventilatory abnormality (e.g. chronic bronchitis and emphysema) from a restrictive one (e.g. diffuse interstitial pulmonary fibrosis) (table 1.1).

TABLE 1.1. Characteristic patterns of disordered respiratory function.

OBSTRUCTIVE PATTERN (e.g. chronic bronchitis with emphysema)

(1) Reduced FVC, FEV, MVV and PEFR.
(2) Relatively greater reduction in FEV than in FVC.
(3) Increased RV.
(4) Uneven distribution of inspired gas.
(5) Increased nonelastic (viscous) work of breathing.
(6) Reduced Po_2 and So_2.
(7) Increased Pco_2 of arterial blood.
(8) Lowered arterial pH in exacerbations. In the chronic state the pH is usually normal.

RESTRICTIVE PATTERN (e.g. diffuse interstitial pulmonary fibrosis)

(1) Reduced FVC. (But MVV reasonably good because of ability to breathe rapidly, though shallowly. High frequency breathing can, however, compensate only up to a point.)
(2) FEV reduced proportionately with FVC; therefore FEV/FVC normal.
(3) Evidence of impaired gas distribution usually slight.
(4) Decreased lung compliance (increased elastic work of breathing).
(5) Decreased values for CO transfer factor.
(6) Reduced Po_2 and So_2 (at first on exertion only, later at rest).
(7) Normal Pco_2 of arterial blood (may even be low from overventilation).
(8) Normal or high arterial pH.

Broadly speaking there are 3 main values of lung function tests:

(1) They may assist in the diagnosis of some disease states which produce a characteristic pattern of altered function e.g. asthma, emphysema and interstitial fibrosis.
(2) They may explain why a patient is breathless or cyanosed although the diagnosis of functional abnormality, e.g. decreased compliance associated with 'stiff' lungs, may be pathologically nonspecific.

3—R.D.

(3) Lung function tests are of the first importance in the assessment of patients:

(a) Assessing the results of treatment, e.g. corticosteroid therapy in asthma, irradiation pneumonia, diffuse interstitial fibrosis, surgical treatment of heart disease, pleural fibrosis, etc.

(b) Assessing fitness for operation. Lung function tests can determine whether a patient can tolerate lung resection and may indicate the likelihood of postoperative trouble in other types of surgery. The dyspnoea of postoperative respiratory failure can nearly always be anticipated by performing simple tests of ventilatory capacity before operation. Commonly those patients with only moderately reduced ventilatory capacity are at greatest risk since the danger of the increased metabolic demands of the first few postoperative days is not appreciated. In general the FEV_1 should be above 1 litre (preferably above 1·5 l) in an average sized patient if operation requires resection of functioning lung. From the point of view of gas studies it is preferable for the So_2 to be above 90% and the Pco_2 to be less than 50 mm Hg.

(c) Lung function tests can give an objective quantitative measurement of lung damage due to industrial or other injury and assist in the assessment of compensation.

For clinical purposes the following are the most useful tests of respiratory function

(1) FEV_1 or peak flow, and FVC.
(2) Pa,o_2 (sometimes before and after exercise).
(3) Pa,co_2
(4) Dco (Tco).

DYSPNOEA

Dyspnoea is the commonest complaint for which the help of the pulmonary function laboratory is sought. First it is important to recognize what dyspnoea is not. It is not *tachypnoea*, which means rapid breathing, *hyperpnoea*, which means an increase in ventilation in proportion to increase in metabolism, or *hyperventilation* where increased ventilation is proportionately in excess of metabolic needs. Dyspnoea is a *subjective phenomenon* and is related to an awareness of the need for increased respiratory effort. Breathing involves the use of voluntary muscles and must, therefore, share many nervous mechanisms with voluntary movement. It is not surprising, therefore, that one can be aware of many facets of the act of normal breathing simply by focusing attention on it. Dyspnoea need not imply disease affecting the respiratory mechanism though most commonly it does. It occurs when the *demands* made on the lungs are out of proportion to their *capacity* to respond so that breathing is difficult, laboured and uncomfortable. There are, at least, 3 possible mechanisms, functioning singly or in combination, which can result in dyspnoea— increased work of breathing, reduction in ventilatory capacity and an undue awareness by the subject of the act of breathing. In most lung conditions it is possible to have some objective assessment of the abnormality which results in a greater expenditure of energy to move air in and out of the lungs. Also the degree of dyspnoea is usually related to the severity of the disorder of function and this correlation can be measured when studies are made during exercise as well as at rest. This is not absolute, however, and no single test or combination of tests has yet been devised which will, in all cases, correlate with dyspnoea or the absence of it since dyspnoea not only involves perception of respiratory discomfort but also the patient's individual reaction to it.

Numerous theories have been propounded over the years, some of them not capable of being readily proved or disproved because of the complex technology which testing would involve. Although no current theory explains every case of dyspnoea the most acceptable is the concept of *length–tension appropriateness* [23]. This theory suggests that the sensation of dyspnoea results when there is disturbance in the relationship between the force applied to the lung and the movement to which it gives rise so that the actual ventilation produced does not equate with the demand of the respiratory centres for ventilation. Campbell and Howell [24] have suggested that comparison is being made continuously, but unconsciously, of one or more of the following:

(1) Ventilation with activity,
(2) ventilation demanded with ventilation achieved,
(3) muscle tension exerted with change in muscle length achieved (or length demanded with length achieved).

If inappropriateness between these relations occurs beyond a certain degree this reaches consciousness as an awareness of respiratory distress, i.e. dyspnoea. For example, these workers postulate that the dyspnoea due to bronchial asthma or pulmonary oedema which awakes a sleeping patient results from the increased resistance to air flow or reduced compliance changing the relative signals of the chest wall length and tension receptors. The altered pulmonary mechanics may cause a chemical drive to respiration through underventilation and may also result in a drive mediated through the vagus nerves. It is possible that the summated information from *several* sources—somatic (principally the respiratory muscles), chemoreceptor, pulmonary and medullary reticular—results in awakening when a certain threshold is reached. On awakening the patient is aware of the summated distress in the subcortical region and also its origin in the mechanical difficulty of breathing (length–tension inappropriateness).

It should be stressed that much may be learned about the probable mechanism involved in dyspnoea by *clinical observation* with particular reference to:

(1) the rate and depth of breathing (e.g. abnormally rapid or deep),
(2) the apparent effort necessary for each breath,
(3) the congruity or otherwise of the volume of air moved and the effort expended.

Each of these gives information relating

ventilatory demands to ventilatory capacity. In most cases the appropriate tests of disordered function for any particular patient can be selected on the basis of the history and the clinical examination. Sometimes, for example, when patients are referred for compensation purposes and have insubstantial radiographic or clinical evidence of disease, it may be necessary to perform a battery of tests aiming at assessing the various components of lung function before pronouncing on the normality of the ventilatory processes. It is important in these circumstances to include tests requiring the full cooperation of the patient for these may indicate a lack of maximum effort, e.g. MVV. If normal values are obtained for the lung volumes, the VC, tests for distribution of inspired gas, pulmonary compliance, exercise ventilation, oxygen uptake, CO transfer factor and blood gas analysis a pulmonary cause for dyspnoea can fairly confidently be excluded. These tests cannot, however, exclude pulmonary pathology, e.g. pulmonary tuberculosis, small pulmonary neoplasm, etc. Nor may they discover ill recognized but possible factors which may cause dyspnoea such as chronic irritation of nerve endings in the respiratory tract or the presence of some poorly compliant and therefore poorly ventilated alveoli.

Psychogenic dyspnoea is often an uncomfortable diagnosis for the physician and regular follow up may be necessary to substantiate it. The aim should be to diagnose positively rather than by exclusion whenever possible.

The effect of individual abnormalities of function is not the same in different types of disease and this fact must modify the statement that dyspnoea and the measure of disturbance of function commonly correlate. For example a patient with an FEV_1 of 1200 ml with restrictive lung disease may be severely crippled whereas a patient with obstructive airways disease with a similar FEV_1 may have little or no complaint of dyspnoea. Thus the relation between measurable disorder of function and dyspnoea is only close within particular patterns of functional abnormality.

In the absence of a holistic theory of breathlessness attempts at *classification* of the symptom on a clinical or physiological basis always leave an embarrassingly large group headed 'Miscellaneous'. One or more of the following classifications may be applied in any particular case.

I. Classification may be made purely of *severity* as expressed by the patient or observed by the doctor and provided this classification is applied to the commonest cause of dyspnoea, namely chronic obstructive airways disease, the different grades can be quantitated very approximately, bearing in mind the subjective nature of the symptom.

Grade 1. Normal.

Grade 2. The patient is able to walk with normal persons of his own age, sex and build, on the level but cannot keep up on hills or stairs.

Grade 3. The patient is unable to keep up with normal persons on the level but can walk long distances at his own speed.

Grade 4. The patient is unable to walk more than about 100 yards on the level before dyspnoea makes him stop.

Grade 5. The patient is unable to walk more than a few steps without dyspnoea and becomes breathless even when washing or dressing.

Grade 1 usually equates with an FEV_1 of 3 l or over and Grade 5 with 0·6 l or less.

II. Dyspnoea may be classified according to *aetiology*, e.g. respiratory, cardiac, metabolic causes, etc., although, as stated, the number of conditions in the 'Miscellaneous Group' limits its usefulness as a working classification.

III. Dyspnoea may be classified according to whether it occurs on *exertion or at rest*.

Exertional dyspnoea

(1) Simple hyperventilation, e.g. anaemia or pregnancy; certain cases of pulmonary thromboembolism (p. 458).

(2) Early heart disease, e.g. the simple

hyperventilation of mitral stenosis in the absence of evidence of pulmonary disease.

(3) Obstructive airways disease, e.g. chronic bronchitis, bronchial asthma.

(4) Restrictive pulmonary disease, e.g. kyphoscoliosis, pulmonary fibrosis.

It is usually easy to distinguish those conditions associated with exertional breathlessness which are due to lung disease and those in which the lungs are normal.

Dyspnoea at rest

(1) Acute mechanical or infective conditions, e.g. pneumothorax, pleural effusion, pulmonary infarction, pneumonia.

(2) Paroxysmal dyspnoea, e.g. bronchial asthma, pulmonary oedema.

(3) Psychogenic dyspnoea, e.g. hyperventilation syndrome.

(4) Metabolic causes of dyspnoea (really hyperpnoea), e.g. acidosis from uraemia, diabetes.

(5) Cheyne–Stokes respiration (hyperpnoea and apnoea), e.g. in cerebrovascular disease.

IV. A classification which is strictly concerned with *ventilatory discomfort* and no other sensation is one based on the patient's awareness of 1 of 3 principal ventilatory abnormalities.

Awareness of increased ventilation

(1) Normal increase as in exercise, and proportional to O_2 uptake.

(2) Abnormal increase disproportionate to O_2 uptake, e.g. hyperventilation due to organic or psychogenic causes.

Awareness of ventilatory difficulty

(1) Obstructive abnormality, associated with increased viscous work.

(2) Restrictive abnormality, associated with increased elastic work. (The theory of length–tension inappropriateness explains this group.)

Awareness of need for increased ventilation
Neurological paralysis, where the discomfort is relieved by increasing ventilation by whatever means. Often the paralysis has to be very severe before dyspnoea occurs (VC less than normal V_T).

V. A classification which adds little to the understanding of dyspnoea but which is clinically useful is one in which the symptom is classified according to *mode of onset and progression:*

(1) *Dyspnoea of sudden onset*, e.g. pneumothorax, pulmonary embolism, pulmonary oedema from whatever cause, bronchial asthma, sudden occlusion of a major airway as by foreign body, inhalation of noxious gases or fumes, Farmer's lung, etc.

(2) *Dyspnoea subacutely progressive over weeks or months*, e.g. congestive cardiac failure, anaemia, obesity, pregnancy, pleural effusion, subacute occlusion of a major airway as by tumour, diffuse interstitial lung disease of the Hamman–Rich variety, etc.

(3) *Dyspnoea progressive over months or years*, e.g. chronic bronchitis and emphysema, pneumoconiosis, the pulmonary fibroses, etc.

REFERENCES

[1] ABER G.M. & BISHOP J.M. (1965) Serial changes in renal function, arterial gas tensions and the acid-base state in patients with chronic bronchitis and oedema. *Clin. Sci.* **28**, 511.

[2] ADRIAN E.D. (1933) Afferent impulses in the vagus and their effects on respiration. *J. Physiol (Lond.)*, **79**, 332.

[3] ASTRAND P.O. & SALTIN B. (1961) Oxygen uptake during the first minutes of heavy muscular exercise. *J. appl. Physiol.* **16**, 971.

[4] ASTRUP P., JØRGENSEN K., SIGGAARD-ANDERSEN O. & ENGEL K. (1960) Acid-base metabolism. A new approach. *Lancet*, **i**, 1035.

[5] AUCHINCLOSS J.H.JR., COOK E. & RENZETTI A.D. (1955) Clinical and physiological aspects of a case of obesity, polycythaemia and alveolar hypoventilation. *J. clin. Invest.* **34**, 1537.

[6] AVIADO D.M., LI T.H., KALOW W., SCHMIDT C.F. TURNBULL G.L., PESKIN G.W., HESS M.E. & WEISS A.J. (1951) Respiratory and circulatory reflexes from the perfused heart and pulmonary circulation of the dog. *Am. J. Physiol.* **165**, 267.

[7] BALL W.C., STEWART P.B., NEWSHAM L.G.S. & BATES D.V. (1962) Regional pulmonary function studies with Xenon[133] *J. clin. Invest.* **41**, 519.

[8] BALTISBERGER W. (1921) Ueber die glatte Muskulatur der meschlichen Lunge. *Z. Anat. EntwGesch.* **61**, 249.

[9] BANG F.B., BANG B.G. & FOARD M.A. (1966) Responses of upper respiratory mucosa to drugs and viral infections. *Am. Rev. resp. Dis.* **93**, Suppl. 142.

[10] BATES D.V. & CHRISTIE R.V. (1964) *Respiratory Function in Disease.* Philadelphia: Saunders.

[11] BENDIXEN H.H., HEDLEY-WHITE J. & LAVER M.B. (1963) Impaired oxygenation in surgical patients during general anaesthesia with controlled ventilation: A concept of atelectasis. *New Engl. J. Med.* **269**, 991.

[12] BENSON F., CELANDER O., HAGLUND G., NILSSON L., PAULSEN L., & RENCK L. (1958) Positive-pressure respiratory treatment of severe pulmonary insufficiency in the newborn infant: a clinical report. *Acta anaesth. scand.* **2**, 37.

[13] BLESOVSKY A. (1967) Pulmonary sequestration. A report of an unusual case and a review of the literature. *Thorax* **22**, 351.

[14] BOYDEN E.A. (1955) *Segmental Anatomy of the Lungs.* New York, McGraw-Hill.

[15] BREUER J. (1868) Die Selbststeuerung der Atmung durch den Nervus vagus. *Sber. Akad. Wiss. Wien.* **58** (ii), 909.

[16] BROCK R.C. (1954) *The Anatomy of the Bronchial Tree*, 2nd Edition, London, Oxford University Press.

[17] BRUBACKER A.P. (1919) The physiology of sneezing. *J. Am. med. Ass.* **23**, 585.

[18] BURNS B.D. (1963) The central control of respiratory movements. *Br. med. Bull.* **19**, 7.

[19] BUTLER J., CARO C.G., ALCALA R. & DUBOIS A.B. (1960) Physiological factors affecting airways resistance in normal subjects and in patients with obstructive respiratory disease. *J. clin. Invest.* **39**, 584.

[20] CAHILL J.M., ATTINGER E.O. & BYRNE J.J. (1961) Ventilatory responses to embolization of lung. *J. appl. Physiol.* **16**, 469.

[21] CAMPBELL E.J.M. & HOWELL J.B.L. (1960) Simple rapid methods of estimating arterial and mixed venous P_{CO_2}. *Br. med. J.* **i**, 458.

[22] CAMPBELL E.J.M. & HOWELL J.B.L. (1962) Rebreathing method for measurement of mixed venous P_{CO_2}. *Brit. med. J.* **ii**, 630

[23] CAMPBELL E.J.M. & HOWELL J.B.L. (1963a) The sensation of breathlessness. *Br. med. Bull.* **19**, 36.

[24] CAMPBELL E.J.M. & HOWELL J.B.L. (1963b) The sensation of dyspnoea. *Br. med. J.*, **ii**, 868.

[25] CANDER L. & FORSTER R.E. (1959) Determination of pulmonary parenchymal tissue volume and pulmonary capillary blood flow in man. *J. appl. Physiol.* **14**, 541.

[26] CARO C.G., BUTLER J. & DUBOIS A.B. (1960) Some effects of restriction of chest cage expansion on pulmonary function in man; an experimental study. *J. clin. Invest.* **39**, 573.

[27] CEDERGREN B., GYLLENSTEN L. & WERSALL J. (1959) Pulmonary damage caused by oxygen poisoning: an electronmicroscopic study in mice. *Acta paediat.* **48**, 477.

[28] CHURCHILL E.D. & COPE O. (1929) The rapid shallow breathing resulting from pulmonary congestion and edema. *J. exp. Med.* **49**, 531.

[29] CLEMENTS J.A., HUSTEAD R.F., JOHNSON R.P. & GRIBETZ I. (1961) Pulmonary surface tension and alveolar stability. *J. appl. Physiol* **16**, 444.

[30] COLEBATCH H.J.H. & HALMAGYI D.F.J. (1962) Reflex airway reaction to fluid aspiration. *J. appl. Physiol.* **17**, 787.

[31] COMROE, J.H., COURNAND A., FERGUSON J.K., FILLEY, G.F., FOWLER W.S., GRAY J.S., HELMHOLZ H.F.Jr., OTIS A.B., PAPPENHEIMER J.R., RAHN H. & RILEY R.L. (1950) Standardization of definitions and symbols in respiratory physiology. *Fed. Proc.* **9**, 602.

[32] COMROE J.H., FORSTER R.E., DUBOIS A.B., BRISCOE W.A. & CARLSEN E. (1962) *The Lung. Clinical Physiology and Pulmonary Function Tests*, 2nd Edition, p. 103. Chicago, Year Book.

[33] CORSSEN G. & ALLEN C.R. (1959) Acetylcholine: its significance in controlling ciliary activity of human respiratory epithelium *in vitro. J. appl. Physiol.* **14**, 901.

[34] CORSSEN G. (1963) Pulmonary atelectasis. *J. Am. med. Ass.* **183**, 314.

[35] CRAMER I.I. (1957) Heat and moisture exchange of respiratory mucous membrane. *Ann. Otol. Rhinol. Lar.* **66**, 327.

[36] CROMPTON G.K., MERCHANT SYLVIA & SCHONELL M.E. (1966) The effect of epinephrine and of the supine position on esophageal pressure recordings. *Amer. Rev. resp. Dis.* **93**, 716.

[37] CROSS K.W., KLAUS M., TOOLEY W.H. & WEISSER K. (1960) The response of the newborn baby to inflation of the lungs. *J. Physiol. (Lond.)* **151**, 551.

[38] CROTEAU J.R. & COOK C.D. (1961) Volume-pressure and length-tension measurement in human tracheal and bronchial segments. *J. appl. Physiol.* **16**, 170.

[39] DALHAMN T. (1956) Mucous flow and ciliary activity in the tracheas of healthy rats and rats exposed to respiratory irritant gases (SO_2, NH_3, $HCHO$). *Acta physiol. scand.* **36**, Suppl. 123.

[40] DALHAMN T. (1966) Effect of cigarette smoke on ciliary epithelium. *Am. Rev. resp. Dis.* **93**, Suppl. 108.

[41] DALY I. DE B., LUDANY G., TODD A. & VERNEY E.B. (1937) Sensory receptors in the pulmonary vascular bed. *Quart. J. exp. Physiol.* **27**, 123.

[42] DARLING R.C., COURNAND A., MANSFIELD J.S., & Richards D.W.Jr. (1940) Studies on the intrapulmonary mixture of gases. I. Nitrogen elimination from blood and body tissues during high oxygen breathing. *J. clin. Invest.* **19**, 591.

[43] DARLING R.C., COURNAND A. & RICHARDS D.W.Jr. (1940) Studies on the intrapulmonary mixture of gases. III. An open circuit method for measuring residual air. *J. clin. Invest.* **19**, 609.

[44] DAVENPORT H.W. (1958) *The ABC of Acid-base Chemistry*, 4th Edition. Chicago, University of Chicago Press.

[45] DISHOECK H.A.E. VAN (1941) Measurement of the tension of the tympanic membrane and of the resistance of the Eustachian tube. *Arch. Otolar.* **34**, 596.

[46] DOLLERY C.T. & HUGH-JONES P. (1963) Distribution of gas and blood in the lungs in disease. *Br. med. Bull.* **19**, 59.

[47] DOUGLAS A., SIMPSON D., MERCHANT SYLVIA, CROMPTON G. & CROFTON J. (1966a) The measurement of endomural bronchial (or 'squeeze') pressures in bronchitis and asthma. *Am. Rev. resp. Dis.* **93**, 693.

[48] DOUGLAS A., SIMPSON D., MERCHANT SYLVIA, CROMPTON G. & CROFTON J. (1966b) The effect of antispasmodic drugs on the endomural bronchial (or 'squeeze') pressures in bronchitis and asthma. *Am. Rev. resp. Dis.* **93**, 703.

[49] ELFTMAN A.G. (1943) The afferent and parasympathetic innervation of the lungs and trachea of the dog. *Amer. J. Anat.* **72**, 1.

[50] ELLIS M. (1936) The mechanism of the bronchial movements and the nasal-pulmonary reflex. *J. Lar. Otol.* **51**, 399.

[51] FAHRI L.E. (1966) Ventilation-perfusion relationship and its role in alveolar gas exchange, in *Advances of Respiratory Function*, ed. Caro C.O. London, Arnold.

[52] FINK B.R. (1961) Influence of cerebral activity in wakefulness on regulation of breathing. *J. appl. Physiol.* **16**, 15.

[53] FINLEY T.N., SWENSON E.W. & COMROE J.H. (1962) The cause of arterial hypoxaemia at rest in patients with 'alveolar-capillary block syndrome'. *J. clin. Invest.* **41**, 618.

[54] FLEINER W. (1888) Über die Resorption corpusculärer Elemente durch Lunge und Pleura. *Virchows Arch. path. Anat.* **112**, 97, 282

[55] FLOREY H., CARLETON H.M. & WELLS A.Q. (1932) Mucus secretion in the trachea. *Br. J. exp. Path.* **13**, 269.

[56] FORSTER R.E. (1964) Rate of gas uptake by red cells, in *Handbook of Physiology*, ed. Fenn W.O. & Rahn H. p. 839. *Am. Physiol. Soc.*, Washington.

[57] FOSTER-CARTER A.F. (1963) Broncho-pulmonary anatomy, in *Chest Diseases*, ed. Perry K.M.A. & Sellors T.H., London, Butterworths.

[58] GAENSLER E.A. (1961) Evaluation of pulmonary function: methods. *Annu. Rev. Med.* **12**, 385.

[59] GAYLOR J.B. (1934) The intrinsic nervous mechanism of the human lung. *Brain* **57**, 143.

[60] GERNEZ-RIEUX C., BISERTE G., HAVEZ R., VIOSIN C. & CUVELIER R. (1963) Etude biochemique de l'expectoration bronchique. *Sem. Hôp. Paris* **11**, 729.

[61] GERNEZ-RIEUX C., VIOSIN C., HAVEZ R., WATTEL F. & AERTS C. (1967) The factors favouring bronchial infection in chronic bronchitis. *Royal Netherlands Tuberculosis Association: Selected Papers* **10**, 21.

[62] GOSSELIN R.E. (1966) Physiologic regulations of ciliary motion. *Am. Rev. resp. Dis.* **93**, Suppl. 41.

[63] GREEN G.M. & KASS E.H. (1964) The role of the alveolar macrophage in the clearance of bacteria from the lung. *J. exp. Med.* **119**, 167.

[64] GROBER J. (1901) Die Resorptionskraft der Pleura. *Beitr. path. Anat.* **30**, 265.

[65] GUYTON A.C., CROWELL J.W. & MOORE J.W. (1956) Basic oscillating mechanism of Cheyne-Stokes breathing. *Am. J. Physiol.* **187**, 395.

[66] HALMAGYI D.F.J. & COLEBATCH H.J.H. (1961) Cardio-respiratory effects of experimental lung embolism. *J. clin. Invest.* **40**, 1785.

[67] HARRIS A.S. (1939) Cardio-inhibitory and vasomotor reflexes from the nose and throat *Ann. Otol. Rhinol. Lar.* **48**, 311.

[68] HAVEZ R., ROUSSEL P., MOSCHETTO Y., DEGAND P. & BISERTE G. (1965) Caractérisation électrophorétique des composants du mucus bronchique. *C. R. Hebd. Séanc. Acad. Sci. Paris* **260**, 4853.

[69] HAWKINS D.F. & SCHILD H.O. (1951) The action of drugs on isolated human bronchial chains. *Br. J. Pharmacol.* **6**, 682.

[70] HAYEK H. VON (1960) *The Human Lung* (translated by Krahl V.E.) New York, Hafner.

[71] HEAD H. (1889) On the regulation of respiration. *J. Physiol. (Lond.)* **10**, 1 & 279.

[72] HERING E. & BREUER J. (1868) Die Selbststeuerung der Atmung durch den Nervus vagus. *Sber. Akad. Wiss. Wien.* **57**, (ii), 672.

[73] HERS J.F.Ph. (1966) Disturbances of the ciliated epithelium due to influenza virus. *Am. Rev. resp. Dis.* **93**, Suppl. 162.

[74] HEYDEN R. (1950) Respiratory function in laryngectomized patients. *Acta Oto-Lar. Suppl.* **85**, 1.

[75] HILDING A.C. (1956) On cigarette-smoking, bronchial carcinoma and ciliary action: III. Accumulation of cigarette tar upon artificially produced deciliated islands in the respiratory epithelium. *Ann. Otol. Rhinol. Lar.* **65**, 116.

[76] HOLMGREN A., JONSSON B. & SJÖSTRAND T. (1960) Circulatory data in normal subjects at

rest and during exercise in recumbent position, with special reference to the stroke volume at different work intensities. *Acta physiol. scand.* **49**, 343.

[77] HONJIN R. (1956) On the nerve supply of the lung of the mouse, with special reference to the structure of the peripheral vegetative nervous system. *J. Comp. Neurol.* **105**, 587.

[78] HOORN B. & TYRRELL D.A.J. (1966) Effects of some viruses on ciliated cells. *Am. Rev. resp. Dis.* **93**, *Suppl.* 156.

[79] HUTCHINSON J. (1844a) Pneumatic apparatus for valuing the respiratory powers. *Lancet* **i**, 390.

[80] HUTCHINSON J. (1844b) Lecture on vital statistics, embracing an account of a new instrument for detecting the presence of disease in the system. *Lancet* **i**, 567.

[81] HUTCHINSON J. (1844c) Lecture on vital statistics, concluded. *Lancet* **i**, 594.

[82] HUTCHINSON J. (1846a) On the capacity of the lungs and on the respiratory function: with a view of establishing a precise and easy method of detecting disease by the spirometer. *Trans. Med.-Chir. Soc. London* **29**, 137.

[83] HUTCHINSON J. (1846b) On the capacity of the lungs and on the respiratory movements with the view of establishing a precise and easy method of detecting disease by the spirometer. *Lancet* **i**, 630.

[84] IDE G., SUNTZEFF VALENTINA & COWDRY E.V. (1959) A comparison of the histopathology of tracheal and bronchial epithelium of smokers and non-smokers. *Cancer (Philad.)* **12**, 473.

[85] KABINS S.A., FRIDMAN J., NEUSTADT J., ESPINOSA G. & KATZ L.N. (1960) Mechanisms leading to lung oedema in pulmonary embolism. *Am. J. Physiol.* **198**, 543.

[86] KAHN R.H. (1907) Zur Physiologie der Trachea. *Arch. Anat. Physiol.* p. 398.

[87] KEIMOWITZ R.I. (1964) Immunoglobulins in normal human tracheobronchial washings. *J. Lab. clin. Med.* **63**, 54.

[88] KING B., ELDER J., PROCTOR D.F. & DRIPPS R.D. (1954) Reflex circulatory responses to tracheal intubation performed under topical anaesthesia. *Anaesthesiology* **15**, 231.

[89] KLASSEN K.P., MORTON D.R. & CURTIS G.M. (1951) The clinical physiology of the human bronchi. III. The effect of vagus section on the cough reflex, bronchial caliber and clearance of bronchial secretions. *Surgery* **29**, 483.

[90] KNIPPING H.W. & MONCRIEFF A. (1932) The ventilation equivalent for oxygen. *Quart. J. Med. (n.s.)* **1**, 17.

[91] KOHN H.N. (1893) Zur Histologie des indurirenden fibrinösen Pneumonie. *Muench. med. Wschr.* **40**, 42.

[92] KRAHL V.E. (1963) Microstructure of the lung. *Arch. environ. Hlth.* **6**, 37.

[93] LAMBERT M.W. (1955) Accessory bronchiole-alveolar communications. *J. Path. Bact.* **70**, 311.

[94] LAMBERT M W (1957) Accessory bronchiole-alveolar channels. *Anat. Rec.* **127**, 472.

[95] LARRABEE M.G. & KNOWLTON G.C. (1946) Excitation and inhibition of phrenic motoneurones by inflation of the lungs. *Am. J. Physiol.* **147**, 90.

[96] LAURENZI G.A. & GUARNERI J.J. (1966) A study of the mechanisms of pulmonary resistance to infection: the relationship of bacterial clearance to ciliary and alveolar macrophage function. *Am. Rev. resp. Dis.* **93**, *Suppl.* 134.

[97] LIEBOW A.A. (1962) In Ciba Foundation *Symposium on Pulmonary Structure and Function*, ed. de Reuck and O'Connor. London, Churchill.

[98] LINROTH K. (1957) Physical working capacity in conscripts during military service: its relation to some anthropometric data; methods to assess individual physical capabilities. *Acta. med. scand.* **157**, *Suppl.* 324.

[99] LLOYD T.C. (1963) Bronchoconstriction in man following single deep inspirations. *J. appl. Physiol.* **18**, 114.

[100] LOESCHCKE, H. (1934) Experimentelle Untersuchungen über Saftstrom- und Resorptionswege. *Virchows Arch. path. Anat.* **292**, 281.

[101] LOOFBOURROW, G.N., WOOD W.B. & BAIRD I.L. (1957) Tracheal constriction in the dog. *Am. J. Physiol.* **191**, 411.

[102] LOW F.N. (1952) Electron microscopy of the rat lung. *Anat. Rec.* **113**, 437.

[103] LOW F.N. (1953) The pulmonary alveolar epithelium of laboratory mammals and man. *Anat. Rec.* **117**, 241.

[104] LOW F.N. (1954) Electron microscopy of sectioned lung tissue after varied duration of fixation in buffered osmium tetroxide. *Anat. Rec.* **120**, 827.

[105] LUCAS A.M. (1935) Neurogenous activation of ciliated epithelium. *Am. J. Physiol.* **112**, 468.

[106] MCCUTCHEON F.J. (1953) Atmospheric respiration and the complex cycles in mammalian breathing patterns. *J. Cellular Comp. Physiol.* **41**, 291.

[107] MACKLEM P.T. & WILSON N.J. (1965) Measurement of intrabronchial pressure in man. *J. appl. Physiol.* **20**, 653.

[108] MACKLIN C.C. (1954) The pulmonary alveolar mucoid film and pneumonocytes. *Lancet* **i**, 1099.

[109] MEAD J. (1961) Mechanical properties of lungs. *Physiol. Rev.* **41**, 281.

[110] MEGIBOW R.S., KATZ L.N. & STEINITZ F.S. (1942) Dynamic changes in experimental pulmonary embolism. *Surgery* **11**, 19.

[111] MEGIBOW R.S., KATZ L.N. & FERNSTEIN M. (1943) Kinetics of respiration in experimental pulmonary embolism. *Arch. intern. Med.* **71**, 536.

[112] MENDENHALL R.M. & STOKINGER H.E. (1962) Films from lung washings as a mechanism model for lung injury by Ozone. *J. appl. Physiol.* **17**, 28.

[113] MILLER W. S. (1947) *The Lung*, 2nd Edition. Springfield, Thomas.

[114] MITCHELL J.H., SPROULE B.J. & CHAPMAN C.B. (1958) The physiological meaning of the maximal oxygen intake test. *J. clin. Invest.* **37**, 538.

[115] MITCHELL R.A., LOESCHCKE H.H., MASSION W.H. & SEVERINGHAUS J.W. (1963) Respiratory responses mediated through superficial chemosensitive areas on the medulla. *J. appl. Physiol.* **18**, 523.

[116] MOSER K.M., RHODES P.G. & KWAAN P.L. (1965) Posthyperventilation apnoea. *Fed. Proc.* **24**, 273.

[117] NADEL J.A. & TIERNEY D.F. (1961) Effect of a previous deep inspiration on airway resistance in man. *J. appl. Physiol.* **16**, 717.

[118] NADEL J.A. & WIDDICOMBE J.G. (1962) Effect of changes in blood gas tensions and carotid sinus pressure on tracheal volume and total lung resistance to airflow. *J. Physiol.* **163**, 13.

[119] NEEDHAM C.D., ROGAN M.C. & McDONALD J. (1954) Normal standards for lung volumes, intrapulmonary gas-mixing and maximum breathing capacity. *Thorax* **9**, 313.

[120] NEERGAARD K. (1929) Neue Auffassungen über einen Grundbegriff der Atemmechanik. Die Retraktionskraft der Lunge, abhängig von der Oberflächenspannung in der Alveolen. *Z. Ges. Exp. Med.* **66**, 373.

[121] NEGUS V. (1967) The function of mucus: a hypothesis. *Proc. roy. Soc. Med.* **60**, 75.

[122] NEWHOUSE M.T., BECKLAKE M.R., MACKLEM P.I. & McGREGOR M. (1964) Effect of alterations in end-tidal CO_2 tensions on flow resistance. *J. appl. Physiol.* **19**, 745.

[123] OLITZKI L. (1948) Mucin as a resistance lowering substance. *Bact. Rev.* **12**, 149.

[124] PAINTAL A.S. (1957) The location and excitation of pulmonary deflation receptors by chemical substances. *Quart. J. exp. Physiol.* **42**, 56.

[125] PALMER D.M. (1936) The lung of a human foetus of 170 mm C.R. length. *Am. J. Anat.* **58**, 59.

[126] PAPPENHEIMER J.R., FENCL V., HEISEY S.R. & HELD D. (1965) Role of cerebral fluids in control of respiration as studied in unanaesthetized goats. *Am. J. Physiol.* **208**, 436.

[127] PARCHET V.N. & BAUMGARTNER P. (1953) Bronchial temperature after laryngectomy. *Proc. 5th intern. Congr. Otol. Rhinol. Laryngol.*, Amsterdam, p. 495.

[128] PATTLE R.E. (1955) Properties, function and origin of the alveolar lining layer. *Nature (Lond.)* **175**, 1125.

[129] PERLMAN H.B. (1939) The Eustachian tube: abnormal patency and normal physiologic state. *Arch. Otolar.* **30**, 212.

[130] PERLMAN H.B. (1943) Quantitative tubal function. *Arch. Otolar.* **38**, 453.

[131] PICKRELL K.L. (1938) The effect of alcohol intoxication and ether anaesthesia on resistance to pneumococcal infection. *Bull. Johns Hopkins Hosp.* **63**, 238.

[132] PLUM F., BROWN H.W. & SNOEP E. (1962) Neurologic significance of posthyperventilation apnoea. *J. Am. med. Ass.* **181**, 1050.

[133] PRATT P.C. (1958) Pulmonary capillary proliferation induced by oxygen inhalation. *Amer. J. Path.* **34**, 1033.

[134] RADFORD E.P.Jr. (1957) Recent studies of mechanical properties of mammalian lungs, in *Tissue Elasticity*, ed. Remington J.W., p. 177. The American Physiological Society, Washington, D.C.

[135] RAHN H. & FENN W.O. (1955) *A graphical analysis of the Respiratory Gas Exchange: the O_2–CO_2 diagram*. The American Physiological Society, Washington.

[136] RALL J.E. GILBERT N.C. & TRUMP R. (1945) Certain aspects of the bronchial reflexes obtained by stimulation of the nasal pharynx. *J. Lab. clin. Med.* **30**, 953.

[137] RATTO O., BRISCOE W.A., MORTON J.W. & COMROE J.H.Jr. (1955) Anoxemia secondary to polycythemia and polycythemia secondary to anoxemia. *Am. J. Med.* **19**, 958.

[138] REID LYNNE (1967a) *The Pathology of Emphysema*. London, Lloyd-Luke.

[139] REID LYNNE (1967b) Mucus in respiratory disease. *Proc. roy. Soc. Med.* **60**, 78.

[140] REMINGTON J.S., VOSTI K.L., LIETZE A. & ZIMMERMAN, A.L. (1964) Serum proteins and antibody activity in human nasal secretions. *J. clin. Invest.* **43**, 1613.

[141] REUCK A.V.S. DE & O'CONNOR M. (Eds.) (1962) Ciba Foundation Symposium on *Pulmonary Structure and Function*. London, Churchill.

[142] RHODIN J.A.G. (1966) Ultrastructure and function of the human tracheal mucosa. *Am. Rev. resp. Dis.* **93**, Suppl. 1.

[143] ROBIN E.D., FORKNER C.E., BROMBERG P.A., CROTEAU J.R. & TRAVIS D.M. (1960) Alveolar gas exchange in clinical pulmonary embolism. *New Engl. J. Med.* **262**, 283.

[144] SAID S.I., THOMPSON W.T.Jr., PATTERSON, J.L.Jr. & BRUMMER D.L. (1960) Shunting effect of extreme impairment of pulmonary diffusion. *Bull. Johns Hopkins Hosp.* **105**, 255.

[145] SCHULZ H. (1962) Some remarks on the submicroscopic anatomy and pathology of the blood–air pathway in the lung, in Ciba Foundation Symposium on *Pulmonary Structure and Function*, ed. de Reuck and O'Connor, p. 205. Boston, Little, Brown.

[146] SEIFERT E. (1928) Über den feineren Bau des

Mediastinums. Ein Beitrag zur Frage des Künstlichen Pneumothorax. *Arch. klin. Chir.* **151**, 237.

[147] SEVERINGHAUS, J.W., SWENSON E.W., FINLEY T.N., LATEGOLA M.T. & WILLIAMS J. (1961) Unilateral hypoventilation produced in dogs by occluding one pulmonary artery. *J. appl. Physiol.* **16**, 53.

[148] SEVERINGHAUS J.W. & MITCHELL R.A. (1962) Ondine's curse—failure of respiratory automaticity while awake. *Clin. Res.* **10**, 122.

[149] SEVERINGHAUS J.W. (1962) Electrodes for blood and gas P_{CO_2}, Pa_{O_2} and blood pH. *Acta anaesth. scand., Suppl.* **11**, 207.

[150] SEVERINGHAUS J.W. (1965) The regulation of ventilation at rest, in *Breathlessness*, ed. Howell, J.B.L. & Campbell E.J.M., Oxford, Blackwell Scientific Publications.

[151] SIEKER H.O., ESTES E.H.Jr., KELSER G.A. & McINTOSH H.D. (1955) A cardiopulmonary syndrome associated with extreme obesity. *J. clin. Invest.* **34**, 916.

[152] SIMKINS C.A. (1943) Functional anatomy of the Eustachian tube. *Arch. Otolar.* **38**, 476.

[153] SLEIGH M.A. (1966) Some aspects of the comparative physiology of cilia. *Am. Rev. resp. Dis.* **93**, Suppl. 16.

[154] SPALDING J.M.K. & SMITH A.C. (1963) *Clinical Practice and Physiology of Artificial Respiration.* Oxford, Blackwell Scientific Publications.

[155] STEINER R.E., LAWS J.W., GILBERT J. & McDONNELL M.J. (1960) Radiological lung function studies. *Lancet* ii, 1051.

[156] STILLMAN E.G. (1924) Persistence of inspired bacteria in the lungs of alcoholized mice. *J. exp. Med.* **40**, 353.

[157] STOREY W.S. & STAUB N.C. (1962) Ventilation of terminal air units. *J. appl. Physiol.* **17**, 391.

[158] SWENSON E.W., FINLEY T.N. & GUZMAN S.V. (1961) Unilateral hypoventilation in man during occlusion of one pulmonary artery, *J. clin. Invest.* **40**, 828.

[159] SWENSSON S.A. & FEYCHTING H. (1960) Viewpoints on the technique in respirator treatment of the newborn and infants. *Acta anaesth. scand.* **17**, Suppl. 6.

[160] Symposium on *Emphysema and the 'Chronic Bronchitis' Syndrome* (1959) Aspen, Colorado, **80**, *Am. Rev. resp. Dis.* 1.

[161] THOMAS D.P., STEIN M., GUREWICH V. & ASHFORD T.P. (1966) Pathophysiologic role of platelets in pulmonary embolism. *Proc. Fed. Am. Soc. Exp. Biol.* **25**, 2, Part 1.

[162] THOMSEN K.A. (1955) Eustachian tube function tested by employment of impedance measuring. *Acta Otolar.* **45**, 252.

[163] TOBIN C.E. (1954) Lymphatics of the pulmonary alveoli. *Anat. Rec.* **120**, 625.

[164] TOBIN C.E. (1959) Pulmonary lymphatics with reference to emphysema. *Am. Rev. resp. Dis.* **80**, Suppl., July 50.

[165] TRENCHARD D., NOBLE M.I.M. & GUZ A. (1967) Serum carbonic acid pK^1 abnormalities in patients with acid-base disturbances. *Clin. Sci.* **32**, 189.

[166] TURNER-WARWICK M. (1963) The capillary systemic-pulmonary anastomoses. *Thorax* **18**, 225.

[167] USHER R. (1961) Respiratory distress syndrome of prematurity, in *Pediatric Clinics of North America*. Ed. Mackay R.J., p. 525. Philadelphia, Saunders.

[168] WEIBEL E.R. & GOMEZ D.M. (1962a) Architecture of the human lung. *Science* **187**, 577.

[169] WEIBEL E.R. & GOMEZ D.M. (1962b) A principle for counting tissue structure on random sections. *J. appl. Physiol.* **17**, 343.

[170] WEIBEL E.R. (1963) *Morphometry of the Human Lung*. New York, Academic Press.

[171] WEST J.B. (1963a) Blood-flow, ventilation and gas exchange in the lung. *Lancet* ii, 1055.

[172] WEST J.B. (1963b) Distribution of gas and blood in normal lungs. *Br. med. Bull.* **19**, 53.

[173] WEST J.B. (1963c) Regional differences in gas exchange in the lung of erect man. *J. appl. Physiol.* **17**, 893.

[174] WIDDICOMBE J.G. (1954) Receptors in the trachea and bronchi of the cat. *J. Physiol. (Lond.)* **123**, 71.

[175] WIDDICOMBE J.G. (1963) Regulation of tracheobronchial smooth muscle, *Physiol. Rev.* **43**, 1.

[176] WIDDICOMBE J.G. & NADEL J.A. (1963) Reflex effects of lung inflation on tracheal volume. *J. appl. Physiol.* **18**, 681.

[177] WIDDICOMBE J.G. (1964) Respiratory reflexes in *Handbook of Physiology*, Section 3, Vol. 1, Chapter 24. American Physiological Society, Washington.

[178] WIDDICOMBE J.G. (1966) The regulation of bronchial calibre, in *Advances in Respiratory Physiology*, ed. Caro C.G. London, Arnold.

[179] WRIGHT B.M. & McKERROW C.B. (1959) Maximum forced expiratory flow rate as a measure of ventilatory capacity. *Br. med. J.* ii, 1041.

CHAPTER 2

The Epidemiology of Respiratory Disease

In this chapter a brief account will be given of the general rôle of epidemiology in respiratory disease and of the importance of this group of diseases as a cause of disability and death. The epidemiology of individual diseases is outlined in the appropriate chapters.

In recent years the term 'epidemiology' has been used in a broader sense than formerly, being applied not only to the study of epidemics of infectious disease but to the general statistical approach to disease in the community. In this sense epidemiology has a valuable part to play in defining the prevalence and mortality of different diseases, which in turn assists the planning of medical services to deal with them. Moreover the trends in mortality and prevalence provide a measure of the success of those services in achieving prevention and cure. A dramatic example is tuberculosis (p. 164), in which the figures for mortality and notification, and their rise in the 1939–45 war in Britain and elsewhere, provided the challenge and stimulated the response, both in the provision of services and in the search for new methods. The gratifying subsequent decline witnessed the success of the new methods and of their application in practice. Moreover the contrast between the rate of decline in different countries has demonstrated the importance of having not only effective methods available but also of seeing that they are effectively applied (chap. 10).

If the individualist clinician concedes the rôle of recorder to epidemiology, perhaps with no great burgeoning of interest, he can hardly withhold enthusiasm from the remarkable contributions which epidemiological studies have made in recent years to knowledge of the causation of respiratory and other diseases. For instance, far the most important evidence for the dominating effect of cigarette smoking in the aetiology of lung cancer (p. 519) and chronic bronchitis (p. 305) has been epidemiological. Epidemiological techniques have also incriminated atmospheric pollution as an important contributory factor in chronic bronchitis (p. 307) and perhaps to a lesser extent in lung cancer (p. 522). A brief indication of the sort of techniques which have been used in these studies is given later in this chapter.

MORTALITY AND PREVALENCE OF RESPIRATORY DISEASES

In most countries upper respiratory tract infections are of great importance as a cause of minor disability. It seems possible that the rate of disability in Britain may be greater than in some other countries because of our troublesome winter climate, our high rate of atmospheric pollution and our large number of chronic bronchitics in whom an upper respiratory infection may have more troublesome consequences than in normal people. We

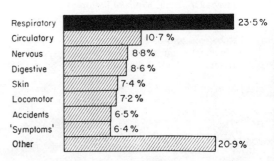

FIG. 2.1. Conditions for which general practitioners are consulted. Figures for Britain derived from a sample survey reported in *Studies on Medical and Population Subjects No. 14. Morbidity Statistics from General Practice*, Vol. 1. Her Majesty's Stationery Office, London 1958.

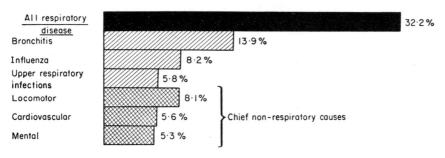

FIG. 2.2. Chief causes of absence from work in England, Wales and Scotland: year ending June 1962. Diagram based on *Report on an Enquiry into the Incidence of Incapacity for Work, Part II*. Her Majesty's Stationery Office, London 1965.

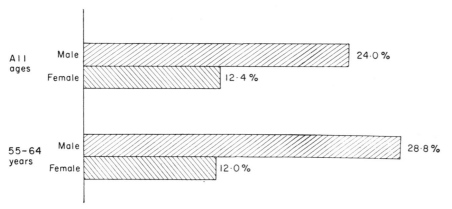

FIG. 2.3. Percentage deaths in England and Wales in 1963 due to respiratory causes. (Calculated from the Registrar General's figures.)

know of no comparative figures and it may be that our sufferings from minor respiratory illness, in comparison to others, are less than we imagine. Nevertheless it is certain that Britain's high rate of atmospheric pollution and formidable cigarette consumption result in a disastrous and preventable toll from chronic and fatal respiratory diseases, such as chronic bronchitis (p. 307) and lung cancer (p. 518), for both of which Britain has the highest figures in the world.

MEDICAL CONSULTATION AND LOSS OF WORK

It is not therefore surprising to find that nearly a quarter of all consultations in general practice in Britain are for respiratory diseases (fig. 2.1), a much higher rate than for any other group of disorders. Respiratory diseases account for nearly a third of absences from work in Britain (fig. 2.2), a figure nearly 4 times greater than that for the next largest disease group.

MORTALITY FROM RESPIRATORY DISEASES

As would be expected from what has been said, respiratory diseases are an important cause of death in Britain, especially in males and especially in the later years of working life. In England and Wales in 1963, 24% of deaths in males of all ages, and 28·8% of deaths in males aged 55–64, were due to respiratory causes, about twice the female figures (fig. 2.3). The diseases principally concerned are shown in figs. 2.4. & 2.5. Lung

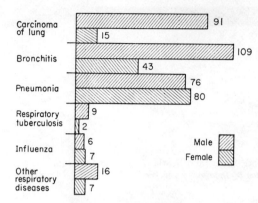

FIG. 2.4. Death rates (per 100,000 population) from respiratory diseases England and Wales 1963: all ages. (Figures from Registrar General's Report.)

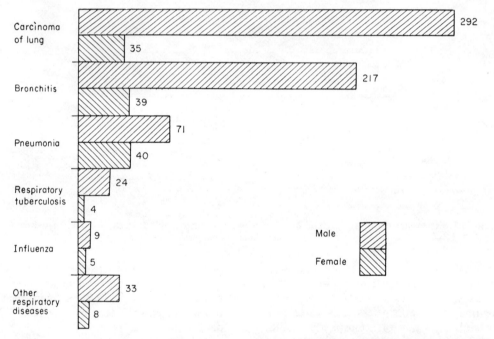

FIG. 2.5. Death rates (per 100,000 population) from respiratory diseases England and Wales 1963: ages 55–64. (Figures from Registrar General's Report.)

cancer and bronchitis bulk large in males, both in those of all ages and in those aged 55–64; pneumonia is an important cause of mortality only in old people (p. 140).

HOSPITAL BEDS

In a survey in Scotland respiratory diseases were responsible for more hospital admissions than any other group of disorders (fig. 2.6).

The same would probably be true elsewhere in Britain.

EPIDEMIOLOGICAL METHODS IN THE INVESTIGATION OF CAUSES OF RESPIRATORY DISEASE

In man it is not always possible to establish the cause of a disease directly and unequi-

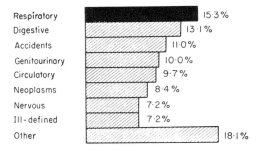

Respiratory	15·3%
Digestive	13·1%
Accidents	11·0%
Genitourinary	10·0%
Circulatory	9·7%
Neoplasms	8·4%
Nervous	7·2%
Ill-defined	7·2%
Other	18·1%

FIG. 2.6. Hospital in-patient discharges, or deaths, in Scotland 1963. (Figures derived from *Scottish Hospital In-patient Statistics 1963*: Scottish Home and Health Department.)

vocally. The most elegant example of direct proof is perhaps tuberculosis. Robert Koch, the discoverer of the tubercle bacillus, suggested that, to establish an infecting agent as causative, it must be consistently isolated from patients with the disease, must cause the disease if introduced into experimental animals and must be consistently recoverable from the experimental lesions ('Koch's postulates'). He himself fulfilled all these criteria for tuberculosis. For various reasons, including the lack of experimental animals susceptible to a number of human infections, such a convincing demonstration is not often possible even in diseases due to an infecting agent. Moreover, it has become clear that in some diseases a number of aetiological factors are at work. In chronic bronchitis, for instance, these include cigarette smoking, atmospheric pollution and infecting agents (p. 308). Sorting out the relative importance of the different factors may be very difficult.

In a number of respiratory (and of some other) diseases the evidence may have to be indirect. The initial step is to investigate a possible *association* between the suspected factor and the disease. Obviously one has to be very careful in assuming guilt from association. Any apparent association must be tested in all sorts of ways before assuming a causal relationship. Lung cancer has greatly increased in Britain since the introduction of cigarette smoking but it would be highly dangerous, on this evidence alone, to assume a causal relationship; the consumption of bananas and the manufacture of gramophone records may have increased impressively in the same period. But when it is found that cigarette consumption has been very much higher in patients with lung cancer than in those of the same age, sex and social background without the disease and that this pattern is found in many countries; when individuals record their smoking habits when healthy, are then followed up and there appears to be a close relationship between the number of cigarettes smoked per day and the chances of later developing lung cancer; when this is also repeated in more than one country; when the national cigarette consumption seems, in international comparisons of mortality, to be closely related to deaths from lung cancer; then this cumulative evidence leads to an overwhelming probability that there is not only an association but that it is causal (p. 519).

In seeking causal factors in disease the method of *sample survey* has been increasingly used in recent years, particularly in investigating chronic bronchitis. The population of the area to be investigated is first defined, preferably by a specific census held for the purpose or, less satisfactorily, from such data as electoral rolls. A relatively small sample is then selected. It may be confined to a particular age group in which the disease is known to be prevalent; in investigating chronic bronchitis the age group 40–64 is often chosen. Within this group a sample is selected designed to be representative of the population in terms of such social factors as housing and occupation. The sample is then investigated to determine whether these individuals have chronic bronchitis, employing a standard questionnaire (one designed by the British Medical Research Council has been used extensively in Britain and elsewhere). Simple respiratory function tests and sputum investigation may also be carried out and questions asked about smoking and other possible causative factors, such as occupation. A sample survey may be confined to a particular occupation. For instance the prevalence of bronchitis in transport drivers has been investigated by similar methods in London and Bergen, in order to compare two towns with very different degrees of atmospheric pollution. Of course other factors such as cigarette smoking have to be taken into account.

CONCLUSION

In this short section it has not been possible to do more than to draw the reader's attention to the very great contribution which epidemiology may make to the understanding of respiratory diseases and their causation. This understanding may in turn lead to better means for prevention, palliation and cure. Much, of course, still remains to be done and the causes of many respiratory diseases are still incompletely elucidated. This section has also sought to make clear the great amount of disability, suffering and death due to respiratory disease, at least in Britain. As will be shown in individual chapters, much of this could be prevented if society as a whole, and the individuals which make up society, could be persuaded fully to apply the measures which are obviously indicated by the advances in knowledge made in recent years.

CHAPTER 3

Common Clinical Manifestations in Respiratory Disease

This chapter consists of a brief revision of symptoms and physical signs in respiratory disease. It may be omitted by any experienced clinician.

Pulmonary diseases may give rise to both general and respiratory manifestations. Respiratory manifestations include cough, sputum, dyspnoea, wheeze and pleuritic pain.

COUGH

The physiology of cough has already been described (p. 23). Clinically cough is perhaps the commonest manifestation of respiratory disease. So common is it among cigarette smokers that many of them regard a morning cough as 'normal'. Nevertheless it is risky to assume that the cough is merely due to cigarette smoking; the chest should be x-rayed to exclude underlying disease and the x-ray should be repeated if at any time the cough worsens. Cough is a frequent symptom in upper respiratory infections, but if it does not clear within 3 weeks a chest x-ray should be taken in order to exclude tuberculosis, carcinoma of the bronchus or other serious pulmonary disease.

The commonest stimulus to cough is the formation of sputum in the respiratory tract and the cough process is an essential element in keeping the tract clear. Cough suppression can therefore be dangerous if much sputum is being formed. Indeed cough suppressants are seldom justified except when an 'unproductive cough' is due to irritation of the upper respiratory tract or in advanced malignant disease when the patient's comfort is more important than his safety. The cough reflex can be initiated by a wide variety of stimuli, varying from touch to irritant gases. Sensitivity is increased by inflammation of the mucous membrane. An exotic stimulus may be initiated by irritation of the external auditory meatus and outer aspect of the eardrum, which receive a nerve supply from the vagus. We have known a paroxysm of coughing, induced by toilet of otitis externa, cause a spontaneous pneumothorax.

SPUTUM

The normal adult produces about 100 ml of mucus from his respiratory tract in a day. When excess mucus is formed the normal process of removal may be ineffective and accumulation of mucus may occur, so that the mucous membrane is stimulated and the mucus coughed up as sputum. Sputum may be formed in response to any sort of insult to the mucous membrane of the bronchi, physical, chemical or infective. The offending element tends to be diluted, buffered and coughed away. When there is inflammation of the respiratory tract, pus cells and other inflammatory products reach the sputum either through the bronchial wall or from the alveoli, depending on the site of infection. Haemorrhage may cause streaking of the sputum with fresh blood. An acute haemorrhagic exudate in the alveoli, as in pneumonia, may result in brown particles of altered blood, the so-called 'rusty sputum' (p. 120).

The *macroscopic appearances* of sputum which are of clinical importance may be classified as follows: (1) mucoid, (2) black, (3) purulent, (4) blood stained, (5) rusty, (6) containing plugs or casts. These subdivisions are not mutually exclusive. Sputum, for instance, may obviously be both purulent and blood stained. The appearances are most easily appreciated if the sputum is coughed into a glass container. *Mucoid* sputum is clear or white. *Black* sputum may be mucoid sputum flecked with detritus of cigarette smoke or atmospheric smoke; these are the common types. Coalminers' sputum may contain coal dust and patients with coalminer's pneumoconiosis may occasionally cough up tarry material derived from areas of progressive massive fibrosis (p. 474). *Purulent* sputum may contain a variable amount of pus mixed with mucus. When there is not much pus it is often referred to as 'mucopurulent'. It is useful for the clinician to accustom himself to classifying the amount of pus by eye, either estimating the approximate percentage or dividing into 'less than a third pus', 'a third to two-thirds' or 'over two-thirds'. Purulent sputum is usually yellow but if it has been stagnant, as may happen when the patient has had a long sleep, it may be green owing to the action of verdoperoxidase derived from neutrophils.

Blood stained sputum varies from small streaks to gross haemoptysis. It is always an indication for investigation, with particular reference to carcinoma and tuberculosis, though in many cases no explanation is found for casual slight blood streaking. *Rusty sputum* occurs mainly in lobar pneumonia (p. 120). *Plugs* or *casts* may be found in asthmatic pulmonary eosinophilia (p. 429).

In chronic conditions such as chronic bronchitis or bronchiectasis *measurement of the amount of sputum* produced each 24 hours, or in the first hour after waking, is a useful means of comparing patients and estimating progress.

Microscopically the most important elements which may be identified in the sputum are bacteria (p. 88), pus cells, eosinophils and malignant cells (p. 534). Certain other elements which are occasionally of diagnostic value will be mentioned under the heading of individual diseases. The presence of *eosinophils* suggests an allergic process; they are commonly found in asthma (p. 409) and pulmonary eosinophilia (p. 425).

DYSPNOEA

Dyspnoea is a term used to indicate subjective awareness of disturbance of breathing. The relevant physiological disturbances have been discussed in chapter 1. Several possible classifications are given on pp. 53–54. Dyspnoea may be divided clinically into four main categories:

(1) The commonest is a sense of *discomfort* on breathing, as in patients with airways obstruction due to chronic bronchitis or asthma, with restrictive lung disease, with left ventricular failure, or with mechanical embarrassment such as pleural effusion or pneumothorax.

(2) In dry pleurisy dyspnoea is due to *pain* on breathing.

(3) In such conditions as metabolic acidosis or anaemia the patient may be aware of *more rapid* or *deeper respiration* without suffering actual discomfort.

(4) Occasionally patients suffering from neurosis may become *conscious* of the normally unconscious process of breathing, may feel difficulty 'in getting the air down into the lungs' and indulge in sighing respirations from time to time.

A patient is conscious of dyspnoea if the effort of breathing or the volume of air he has to move is disproportionate to the exercise he is taking—the 'inappropriateness' of his respiratory effort. Some patients who are found to have severe respiratory impairment may be unaware of it because they do not normally test their respiratory reserve. In fact it is the usual clinical experience in chronic diseases to find that the patient only begins to complain of dyspnoea when his respiratory reserve is already quite severely impaired.

WHEEZE

Patients with airways obstruction due to chronic bronchitis or asthma often complain of wheeze, a musical sound usually mainly heard on expiration. The noise is made by air blowing through narrowed bronchi; as the bronchi become shorter and narrower on expiration the noise is mainly expiratory. Generalized narrowing of bronchi may be due to mucus in the bronchial lumen, swelling or oedema of the bronchial mucous membrane or spasm of the bronchial muscle. The exact preponderance of each of these factors in the different diseases or in different patients is still uncertain. The patient may occasionally be aware of localized wheeze if a large bronchus is partially obstructed by a neoplasm, foreign body or localized inflammation.

STRIDOR

Stridor is a somewhat musical noise caused by obstruction in the trachea or larynx. It is usually inspiratory because of the more rapid air flow during inspiration. It may occur with a variety of neoplastic or inflammatory conditions.

CHEST PAIN

The most important form of chest pain is *pleuritic pain*, associated with dry pleurisy, which may be due to many conditions. It is characteristically worse on breathing and coughing and can usually be accurately localized by the patient. The pain of *intercostal fibrositis* occurs mainly on coughing, rather than breathing, and local tenderness is found. A *cough fracture* causes local pain and tenderness over the affected area, as does the relatively rare *costochondritis*. *Intrathoracic neoplasms* sometimes give rise to a deep ache. Pain in the chest may also be due to *coronary insufficiency* or be referred from *abdominal organs*, such as the gall bladder, or from *spinal lesions*. Differential diagnosis is discussed in the section on pleurisy (p. 264).

PHYSICAL SIGNS IN PULMONARY DISEASE

A full account of physical signs in pulmonary disease must be sought in the appropriate textbooks, though in practice physical signs are best learned at the bedside. In this section a brief account will be given of those which are of greatest practical value.

Radiology has now become an essential part of the examination of the chest. Disease, for instance tuberculosis, may cause quite gross radiological changes without being detectable on clinical examination. On the other hand in such conditions as bronchitis or asthma there may be grossly abnormal physical signs with little change in the x-ray. The two means of examination are therefore complementary. The detection of rhonchi, crepitations and pleural rub by auscultation provide the most important diagnostic information which cannot be obtained radiographically. Whether a patient's chest should be x-rayed is usually decided from the history but sometimes unexpectedly abnormal physical signs in a patient with very minor complaints may give a clue that important abnormalities are present in the lungs or pleura.

GENERAL OBSERVATION OF THE PATIENT

The patient may be observed to be *breathless*, either at rest or after the effort of undressing. There may be *wheeze* (p. 108) or stridor (p. 95). If he has chronic bronchitis or emphysema he may breathe with '*pursed lips*' (p. 313). If the history suggests an acute illness, and if there is a history of chest pain, the *alae nasi* may be moving with respiration, as may occur in pneumonia. In pneumonia or pleurisy the respirations may be rapid and shallow and there may be a sudden *catch* in *breathing* if the patient takes a deep breath, owing to pleuritic pain. He may be cyanosed.

Cyanosis (p. 44) means 'blueness'. In the majority of cases this is due to an increased proportion of reduced haemoglobin compared to oxyhaemoglobin in the arterial blood, though it can occasionally be associated with methaemoglobinaemia or sulphaemoglobinaemia. Cyanosis is not easy to judge unless it is severe, and the arterial oxygen saturation is under 85%. Observer error is high. Closest agreement between observers and closest agreement with objective measurement of arterial oxygen saturation are found when cyanosis is estimated by observation of the tongue [1].

Sweating, *coarse tremor* or *twitching*, *drowsiness* or *coma* may be observed in patients who have *hypercapnia* as well as the *hypoxaemia* associated with cyanosis. In severe hypoxaemia there may be mental confusion.

In pulmonary disease *finger clubbing* is most frequently found associated with *neoplasms* (usually bronchial carcinoma but sometimes a benign neoplasm such as pleural fibroma), or with *chronic septic conditions*, such as lung abscess, empyema or the more severe degrees of bronchiectasis. Slight clubbing may be present with relatively severe pulmonary tuberculosis but grosser clubbing only occurs with *long standing tuberculosis* in patients who are producing large quantities of purulent sputum. A rare cause of clubbing and cyanosis is *arteriovenous fistula* of the lung.

Palpation of the neck from in front may reveal enlarged *cervical lymph glands*, but a thorough examination of the cervical region is best made from behind, as a preliminary to the examination of the posterior aspect of the chest (see below). Before the anterior chest is examined both axillae and the epitrochlear regions should be palpated for enlarged lymph nodes.

THE ANTERIOR CHEST

INSPECTION

Inspection will reveal the rate and type of respiration and any chest deformities. *Decreased movement* of the chest on one side may indicate the possibility of underlying disease and the symmetry should also be observed. Undue flattening or indrawing beneath one of the clavicles may indicate long standing fibrosis at an apex. A sunken and immobile hemithorax, the so-called '*frozen chest*', may indicate the immobilization of a lung by grossly thickened pleura. In chronic bronchitis, emphysema and asthma the chest is often '*barrel shaped*' because of the distension of the lungs by airways obstruction. *Scars* of thoracotomy or empyema drainage should also be noted. The *apex beat* may be visible.

PALPATION

The position of the *trachea* should be identified. Deviation of the trachea is the main indication of lateral shift of the upper mediastinum. Deviation of the *apex beat* and the cardiac dullness are the main indications of shift of the lower mediastinum (fig. 3.1).

If the patient has complained of *pain in the chest* he should be asked to point to the site of the pain with one finger and the area should be carefully palpated to determine whether there is local tenderness. *Tenderness* precisely over a rib may suggest a fracture, due to coughing or trauma, or a secondary deposit. Tenderness over intercostal muscles may indicate intercostal fibrositis. Nevertheless tenderness is sometimes present over the site of pleurisy so that the results of palpation should be interpreted with caution and other physical signs taken into account.

PERCUSSION

It is particularly important to determine the upper level of the *liver dullness*, which is most easily done in the midclavicular line on the right side. With quiet breathing and the patient lying in bed liver dullness normally lies at the level of the 6th rib. Deviation of the dullness downwards is indicative of *lung inflation*, due to emphysema or airways obstruction. Many conditions in the lungs or pleura cause *impaired percussion note* (fig. 3.1). If there is gross deviation of the mediastinum the *cardiac dullness* may be shifted to the left or the right.

VOCAL FREMITUS

The only value of this crude sign is to help to distinguish dullness on percussion due either to underlying consolidation or to pleural effusion. Fremitus is decreased in pleural effusion, increased or normal in consolidation.

CAUSES OF DEVIATION OF MEDIASTINUM

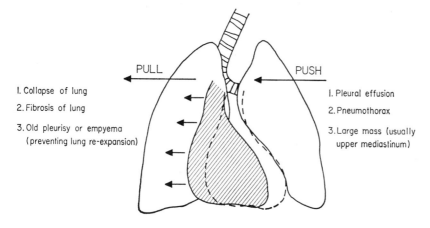

PULL

1. Collapse of lung
2. Fibrosis of lung
3. Old pleurisy or empyema
   (preventing lung re-expansion)

PUSH

1. Pleural effusion
2. Pneumothorax
3. Large mass (usually
   upper mediastinum)

CAUSES OF DULLNESS TO PERCUSSION

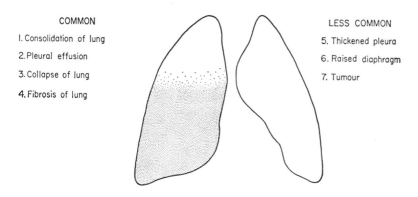

COMMON

1. Consolidation of lung
2. Pleural effusion
3. Collapse of lung
4. Fibrosis of lung

LESS COMMON

5. Thickened pleura
6. Raised diaphragm
7. Tumour

FIG. 3.1. Causes of deviation of mediastinum and causes of dullness to percussion.

AUSCULTATION

As already indicated, auscultation is the most important means of examining the chest, as it may give information which cannot be derived from an x-ray.

BREATH SOUNDS

In listening to the breath sounds, note should be taken of the *duration* of inspiration and expiration relative to one another, the *pitch* of inspiration and expiration relative to one another and the *general quality* of the sounds. In *bronchial breathing* the general quality of the sound is harsh or blowing, the duration of expiration is as long or longer than that of inspiration and the pitch of the expiratory sound is as high or higher than that of inspiration. Bronchial breathing is the noise that respiration makes in the bronchi, which on auscultation is normally damped down and lost by the buffering effect of the air filled alveoli. Bronchial breathing is heard over the chest wall when various abnormal conditions facilitate the conveyance of the bronchial sounds to the surface (fig. 3.2.).

When in doubt about the presence of bronchial breathing one should test for *whispering pectoriloquy* which is an inseparable physical sign.

CAUSES OF BRONCHIAL BREATHING

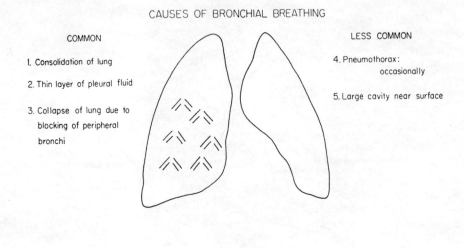

COMMON

1. Consolidation of lung

2. Thin layer of pleural fluid

3. Collapse of lung due to
   blocking of peripheral
   bronchi

LESS COMMON

4. Pneumothorax:
        occasionally

5. Large cavity near surface

CAUSES OF CREPITATIONS

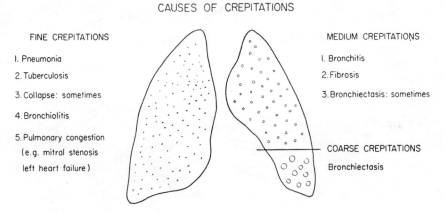

FINE CREPITATIONS

1. Pneumonia
2. Tuberculosis
3. Collapse: sometimes
4. Bronchiolitis
5. Pulmonary congestion
   (e.g. mitral stenosis
   left heart failure)

MEDIUM CREPITATIONS

1. Bronchitis
2. Fibrosis
3. Bronchiectasis: sometimes

COARSE CREPITATIONS

Bronchiectasis

CAUSES OF RHONCHI

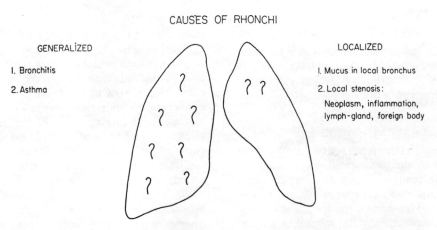

GENERALIZED

1. Bronchitis
2. Asthma

LOCALIZED

1. Mucus in local bronchus
2. Local stenosis:
   Neoplasm, inflammation,
   lymph-gland, foreign body

FIG. 3.2. Causes of bronchial breathing, causes of crepitations and causes of rhonchi.

ADDED SOUNDS IN THE CHEST

There are 3 main types of added sounds in the chest, crepitations, rhonchi and the sound of a pleural rub. Clicking sounds are also occasionally heard.

Crepitations (fig. 3.2.) are discontinuous sounds, made either by the opening up of alveoli filled with exudate or by air bubbling through mucus in bronchi of various sizes. Fine crepitations are probably derived from the alveoli; medium, which are more bubbling in quality, from the small bronchi; and coarse either from large bronchi or from bronchiectatic dilatations of peripheral bronchi.

Rhonchi (fig. 3.2) are somewhat musical noises made by air passing through the moist bronchial tubes, particularly if they are narrowed. As the bronchi are narrower on expiration rhonchi are most commonly expiratory. A *pleural rub* may be difficult to identify. When pleuritic pain is present the patient should be asked to indicate with one finger the maximum site of the pain and careful auscultation should be carried out over this area. A fine pleural rub is usually heard at the extreme end of inspiration and may be difficult to distinguish from crepitations, except that the latter are likely to be altered by coughing. Other types of rub may be like the creaking of leather or the rubbing of sandpaper. *Clicking sounds* associated with the heart beat may be heard in left spontaneous pneumothorax, usually to the left of the sternum, due to the heart, as it beats, alternately occluding and opening a small, overlying, airfilled pleural pocket (p. 445). Occasionally a somewhat similar sound, also in time with the heart beat, may be due to the beat causing a wave in a small effusion complicating a pneumothorax. Rarely a clicking sound on auscultation may be due to the slipping of a displaced costal cartilage, usually of the 8th or 9th rib (p. 623).

Vocal resonance is not a helpful physical sign. Information derived from it can usually be obtained at least as well by other means.

THE POSTERIOR CHEST

Before proceeding to examine the posterior aspect of the chest the *neck* should be palpated for enlarged cervical lymph glands. In chest disease the region behind the clavicle and immediately lateral to the sternomastoid muscle is the most important. It is best examined with the index finger from behind, the patient's head being deviated to the same side in order to relax the muscle. The remainder of the retroclavicular area, the tonsillar and submandibular areas and the anterior and posterior triangles should also be carefully palpated.

Examination of the rest of the posterior chest should proceed on similar lines to that of the anterior chest. Owing to the thickness of the muscle *percussion* has to be firmer than over the anterior chest wall. Because of the thick muscle layers dullness at the apices should only be asserted if the difference between the two sides is clear cut.

REFERENCE

[1] MEDD W.E., FRENCH E.B. & WYLLIE V.McA. (1959) Cyanosis as a guide to arterial oxygen desaturation. *Thorax* **14**, 247.

CHAPTER 4

Diagnostic Procedures in Respiratory Disease

RADIOGRAPHY

RADIOGRAPHIC PROJECTIONS

The value of the chest x-ray in the investigation of a patient with respiratory disease needs no emphasis. The *posteroanterior* (PA) is the standard view, taken with the x-ray tube between 5 and 6 ft from the subject and with the film against the front of the chest. In this projection the size of the heart shadow approximates to the actual size. The *anteroposterior* view, used if the patient is too sick to be out of bed, is taken with the source of rays usually nearer the subject and with the film against his back. There is more divergence of the rays with this technique and the heart size is, therefore, exaggerated. Scatter of rays in a patient with actual cardiomegaly may result in appearances indistinguishable from left pleural effusion. For precise anatomical localization a *lateral* film is necessary. A *lordotic view* (*apical projection*) raises the clavicles clear of the lung and may be valuable in revealing or defining apical lesions.

In the posteroanterior and anteroposterior views radiographic description utilizes the convention of 'lung zones'.

LUNG ZONES

The lung fields are subdivided into zones which are defined as follows:

Upper zone

That area of the lung in the chest radiograph which extends from the apex to a horizontal line through the lower border of the 2nd ribs at their junction with the costal cartilages.

Mid zone

That area of lung between the lower border of the upper zone and a horizontal line through the lower border of the 4th ribs at their junction with the costal cartilages.

Lower zone

That area of lung between the lower border of the mid zone and the hemidiaphragm.

It will be evident that the upper zone is reduced in size in the lordotic position; the lower zone is then proportionately increased. The patient with kyphosis has an increased upper lung zone and a reduced lower zone.

EXAMINATION OF THE PA CHEST FILM

It is useful to observe a regular system of examination of the PA chest film:

(1) *Positioning*. The distance is noted between the vertebral spine (or lateral edge of the vertebral body) and the medial end of the clavicle on each side. This will show if there is rotation to one side which may make a normal hilar opacity appear more prominent or explain an apparent deviation of the mediastinum or an apparent difference in transradiancy in the 2 lung fields.

(2) Examination of the *soft tissue shadows* for:

(a) Absence of breast shadow due to previous mastectomy. This might give a clue to the cause of later pulmonary or pleural abnormality.

(b) Foreign body, e.g. presence of shrapnel from a previous war wound might explain appearances suggesting pleural thickening due to an old haemothorax.

(c) Calcification in neck or axillary glands, suggesting previous tuberculous infection.

(d) Opacity extending beyond the confines of the lungs, e.g. lipoma of chest wall; clothes; long hair in women, which may simulate apical tuberculous disease.

(e) Subcutaneous emphysema.

(3) Examination of the *bony cage* for:

(a) Congenital or acquired deformity, e.g. scoliosis: pectus excavatum ('funnel chest', shown by a more vertical direction of the anterior ribs associated with displacement of the heart, usually to the left); unilateral contraction from previous pleural fibrosis. Cervical ribs, rib fractures and previous rib resection for thoracotomy or drainage of empyema are also noted.

(b) Osteolytic areas suggesting tumour metastases.

(c) Notching of ribs in coarctation of aorta (p. 624).

(d) Periostitis from adjacent infection, particularly actinomycosis (p. 290).

(4) The *position of the trachea* is noted; it is normally deviated slightly to the right.

(5) The *upper mediastinum* and aorta are scanned for abnormalities, e.g. intrathoracic thyroid, upper mediastinal adenopathy, enlarged paratracheal lymph nodes, aortic aneurysm.

(6) The *heart shadow* is observed for enlargement or abnormality of outline and a deliberate effort is made to observe whether there is any abnormal shadow, e.g. collapsed left lower lobe or hiatus hernia, concealed *behind the heart* where it is readily overlooked.

(7) *Hemidiaphragms, costophrenic and cardiophrenic angles.* The relative positions of the hemidiaphragms are noted and the smoothness of their outline. The left is normally 1 to 2 cm lower than the right. The *costophrenic angles* are examined for evidence of pleural thickening or effusion. Opacities in the *cardiophrenic angle* may be due to:

(a) Lesions, including collapse, of the middle lobe, or either lower lobe, or of the lingular segment of the left upper lobe.

(b) Hiatus hernia.

(c) Pleuropericardial cyst, more commonly on the right.

(d) Pericardial fat in the obese.

(e) Prominent inferior vena cava opacity on the right.

(8) The *hila* of the lung need to be carefully examined. Since bronchial carcinoma frequently arises at the hilum this part of the x-ray is particularly important. Interpretation may not be easy owing to the overlap of pulmonary vessels and the influence of rotation of the chest on the appearance of the hilar shadows. Bilateral enlargement is usually due either to dilatation of pulmonary arteries or to bilateral hilar adenopathy. In the former, the proximal vessels are also enlarged. Unilateral enlargement is most often due to neoplasm, though sometimes to adenopathy (e.g. a primary tuberculous complex in a child or metastatic neoplasm in an adult). Aneurysm of a pulmonary artery occasionally occurs. Rotation as an explanation of slight enlargement must always be excluded and it must be remembered that a lateral film may show that an apparent hilar mass in fact lies in the apex of the lower lobe. Elevation of one or both hila is most often due to apical fibrosis. Unilateral depression is most often caused by collapse of a lower lobe.

(9) The position of the *transverse fissure* is noted. This is normally present at the level of the 4th costal cartilage anteriorly. The lower end of the *oblique fissure* may rarely be seen in the PA film in the normal as a 1–2 cm crescentic line, concave medially, meeting the diaphragm about the junction of the lateral and middle thirds. Occasionally the upper part of a thickened fissure may be seen outlining the apex of the lower lobe to the right of the hilum. It is even rarer to see it on the left.

(10) The *lung fields* are then inspected, carefully comparing the zones on each side.

EXAMINATION OF THE LATERAL
CHEST FILM

(1) *Positioning.* In the lateral chest film significant rotation is indicated by the appearances of the sternum; abnormality such as pectus excavatum is noted.

(2) The *soft tissues*, particularly the arm folds, are defined in order to exclude possible fallacy in interpretation of pulmonary opacities in relation to these.

(3) *Bony cage*. The spine and ribs are examined for fractures, osteolytic lesions and osteoporosis.

(4) The *heart* and the *aorta* are examined for abnormalities such as pericardial calcification (perhaps not evident in the PA film) and aortic aneurysm. Sometimes the aorta is only visible where it crosses other shadows; the curved border of the arch could be mistaken for a tumour. The aortic shadow becomes more readily visible with age. The inferior vena cava, entering the heart, must not be mistaken for segmental collapse.

(5) *The hemidiaphragms*. In the lateral film the left hemidiaphragm is distinguished by the presence of the stomach gas bubble. Collapse of upper or middle lobes tends to cause a rise in the anterior part of the diaphragm, collapse of the lower lobe a rise in the posterior part. The latter may be visible only in the lateral film.

(6) The *oblique fissure* should cut the hemidiaphragm at a point anterior to the junction of the anterior and middle thirds. If an apparent oblique fissure lies parallel to rib shadows, it probably is in fact the margin of a rib and not the fissure. The *transverse fissure* is more or less horizontal at the level of the centre of the right hilum. Shrinkage of lung due to collapse or fibrosis causes appropriate deviation of one or both fissures.

(7) *The hilum*. Although often difficult to interpret, hilar adenopathy or the shadow of a hilar tumour may be confirmed.

(8) The lateral film gives the precise *anatomical situation of a pulmonary lesion*. An apparent 'hilar' opacity may be shown in the lateral film to be in the apex of the lower lobe.

The lateral film is essential for the demonstration of the location of mediastinal lesions and interlobar effusion. The transradiancy of the area in front and above the heart should equal that between the lower heart and the spine. If it does not, one or other is abnormal.

PREVIOUS CHEST FILMS

It is frequently of great value to obtain any previous chest x-ray for comparison. Several large cities in Britain have conducted a mass miniature radiography campaign which has provided a reference point for future radiographic comparison.

OTHER RADIOGRAPHIC TECHNIQUES

(1) *Penetrated views* may be useful, particularly for better definition of doubtful lesions in the mediastinum and the spine, or lesions obscured by the heart, breast shadow, effusions or diaphragm. Calcification and opaque foreign bodies may also be seen better by this technique. The value of the *lordotic view* has already been mentioned. *Oblique views* may be helpful for specific problems, the angle of rotation being determined by the problem in hand. For example, a lower lobe collapse or calcification of heart valves is seen best at 45° rotation whereas 60–70° will show the heart and aorta to better advantage [17]. The *lateral decubitus view* may demonstrate nonencysted pleural effusion and is particularly helpful in infrapulmonary effusions.

(2) *Macroradiography* gives magnification of the image and is valuable in cases with doubtful miliary type shadowing, e.g. sarcoidosis, pneumoconiosis. The technique involves increasing the distance between the patient and the x-ray film. The blurring this would normally produce is avoided by using an x-ray tube with a very small 'focal spot' of 0·3 mm [4].

(3) *Tomography* (anteroposterior or lateral) provides films of sections of the lungs at different depths. Tomography may confirm the presence of cavitation and may be particularly useful in the evaluation of solid lesions. A tuberculoma may be differentiated from a carcinoma if calcification or 'satellite lesions' (distinct from the main mass) are found. Tomography may also be helpful in suspected hilar enlargement, small pulmonary metastases, arteriovenous malformations and, sometimes, mediastinal masses.

(4) *Bronchography*. The introduction of opaque iodized oil into the bronchi after preliminary anaesthesia (local or general) outlines the bronchial tree and confirms the presence of bronchiectasis (p. 352), and anomalies of the bronchial tree. Bronchography is of little value in the diagnosis of carcinoma

because of the difficulty of interpretation of the findings. Bronchography distinguishes a middle lobe collapse/consolidation from interlobar effusion in the lower end of the right oblique fissure (p. 266).

Among indications for bronchography are *suspected bronchiectasis* (e.g. at site of recurrent pleurisy and/or pneumonia), known *bronchiectasis* in order to define the site and extent when surgical treatment is under consideration, *haemoptysis unexplained by other methods* including bronchoscopy, and *unilateral transradiancy* (McLeod's syndrome, p. 327). Although there are characteristic bronchographic appearances in chronic bronchitis (p. 319) it is rarely necessary to perform bronchography purely for diagnosis.

Since the contrast medium contains iodine a history of iodine hypersensitivity contraindicates bronchography; so also does severe reduction of lung function.

(5) *Barium swallow*. Left atrial enlargement may be confirmed in the right anterior oblique view of the barium filled oesophagus. Deviation of the barium outlined oesophagus by tumour or secondary glands may be seen in the PA or lateral views.

(6) *Fluoroscopy* or *screening* allows examination of the heart, lungs and diaphragm in the dynamic state. Absent or reduced cardiac pulsation may suggest pericardial effusion. Paradoxical movement of a hemidiaphragm on sniffing indicates phrenic paralysis, e.g. from tumour (p. 531), or as a consequence of pulmonary infarction (p. 462) or eventration (p. 635).

Apart from the conditions mentioned, fluoroscopy may be helpful in the investigation of the dynamics of bullae and obstructive emphysema (e.g. mediastinal swing away from the affected side on expiration), the movement of intrathoracic fluid (in effusion), the investigation of arteriovenous fistulae (p. 559), assessment of cardiac chamber size and, in combination with barium swallow, the detection of diaphragmatic hernias or of abnormalities in swallowing (e.g. megaoesophagus) in cases suspected of 'spillover' pneumonia.

(7) *Angiography*. In angiography contrast medium is injected into a peripheral vein, or centrally by a cardiac catheter, to outline the pulmonary arteries. The systemic circulation can be visualized by the technique of thoracic aortography performed by injection of contrast medium through an arterial catheter.

Indications for pulmonary angiography, which is not frequently employed, include pulmonary embolism (p. 460), and hilar enlargement when there is difficulty in distinguishing between pulmonary artery dilatation or aneurysm and hilar adenopathy. When there is doubt about aortic aneurysm angiography may be indicated although clot in an aneurysm may prevent entry of the contrast medium and so give the appearance of a solid lesion. Congenital anomalies of the heart and great vessels, and arteriovenous malformations, are other indications for thoracic angiography.

Injection of contrast medium intracostally outlines the azygos vein. This technique of *azygography* has been occasionally used in the demonstration of central mediastinal metastases in which case the azygos vein may fail to fill.

(8) *Diagnostic pneumothorax and pneumoperitoneum*. Pneumothorax may help in the differential diagnosis of pleural lesions. It is not without risk and is now rarely employed. Its most common use is in demonstrating pleural tumours if these have not resulted in pleurodesis.

Pneumoperitoneum is most helpful in relation to diaphragmatic lesions. For example, an infrapulmonary loculated effusion may be defined and a localized diaphragmatic herniation clearly shown to be subdiaphragmatic in origin.

(9) The chest radiograph after induction of *pneumomediastinum* may outline doubtful hilar and mediastinal lymphadenopathy with greater clarity than the standard PA film. It is rarely necessary for the evaluation of other mediastinal abnormalities and is seldom used.

(10) *Miniature radiography* is used on a large scale as a screening procedure, especially for tuberculosis (p. 189). The 100 mm film, which in Britain has largely replaced the

earlier 35 mm film, is highly satisfactory and gives definition which compares favourably with the standard large film. Being cut film rather than roll film it is easily filed with the patient's records. In many countries 70 mm roll film is the standard one for mass radiography. It gives a quality which, for reading, is intermediate between 35 mm and 100 mm film.

EXAMINATION OF BRONCHIAL SECRETIONS

This is one of the most important techniques in the differential diagnosis of pulmonary disease. The indications are mentioned in the various sections of this book but the techniques may be briefly summarized here.

SPUTUM

Sputum examination is of great value in diagnosis.

Direct smear examination

Previous antibiotic treatment may invalidate the results of culture but pathogenic bacteria may still be visible on smear examination. This may give invaluable information in patients with severe respiratory infection and determine the antibiotic policy (p. 88). Direct smear examination for tubercle bacilli is a standard method of diagnosis. The significance of eosinophils in the sputum is discussed elsewhere (p. 425). Asbestos bodies in the sputum may confirm a diagnosis of asbestosis. Rarely rupture of a hydatid cyst may allow recovery of hooklets from the sputum (p. 368). Amoebic lung abscess (p. 361) may establish connection with a bronchus and *Entamoeba histolytica* may be recognized in the characteristic sputum.

Sputum cytology

Smear examination for malignant cells is a valuable method of diagnosis in skilled hands. It is discussed on p. 534.

Sputum culture

Sputum culture is of great importance in respiratory infections, both for diagnosis, and by the use of drug resistance tests, as a guide to therapy. It is important to indicate to the bacteriologist the likely diagnosis since this may determine the type of culture to be employed, e.g. for tubercle bacilli, or anaerobic culture in lung abscess or for actinomycetes. Sputum culture for fungi requires special media (p. 286).

Laryngeal swabs

Laryngeal swabs are used for the culture of tubercle bacilli (p. 226), and sometimes for the culture of organisms in the diagnosis of pneumonia when the patient has no sputum.

Gastric aspiration

Gastric aspiration is, in most hands, more sensitive than laryngeal swab in the culture of tubercle bacilli though repeated swabs may be equally good. Direct smear examination may also be useful (p. 226).

Pharyngeal or tonsillar swabs

These swabs are useful in the diagnosis of bacterial or viral infection, especially in children.

The cough plate

The cough plate is mainly used in the diagnosis of whooping cough in children.

Guinea pig inoculation

Guinea pig inoculation may be required to recover tubercle bacilli from the sputum or other body fluids. It is a particularly sensitive technique, though repeated culture may be as good. It may also be used to measure virulence or pathogenicity of acid-fast bacilli.

TUBERCULIN TESTING

This is one of the most important ancillary diagnostic techniques. Methods of testing and the interpretation of results are discussed on p. 288. The tuberculin test, though often of considerable value, is all too often omitted in tackling a difficult diagnostic problem.

OTHER DIAGNOSTIC SKIN TESTS

These may be useful in the evaluation of disease due to atypical mycobacteria (p. 260), histoplasmosis (p. 292), coccidioidomycosis (p. 291), blastomycosis (p. 294), brucellosis (p. 126), sarcoidosis (p. 379), hydatid disease (p. 366) and berylliosis (p. 498).

LARYNGOSCOPY

Inspection of the vocal cords directly or indirectly may confirm suspicion of recurrent laryngeal nerve paralysis, most commonly due to bronchial carcinoma. The appearances are described on p. 3. Tumours or various forms of inflammation may cause hoarseness or, occasionally, stridor.

BRONCHOSCOPY [20]

VALUE

Direct visualization of the bronchial tree under local or general anaesthesia is needed mainly for the diagnosis of bronchial carcinoma. Vision is possible as far as the segmental bronchi and tumours can be seen if they affect the bronchial tree at or above this level. Peripheral tumours cannot be seen. Secondary lymph node metastasis may cause bulging or actual erosion of the larger bronchi, or widening and distortion of the main carina. By means of special forceps specimens of tissue can be taken for histological examination. Apart from bronchial biopsy, bronchoscopy permits the collection of bronchial secretions for microbiological examination, particularly for tubercle bacilli.

Other indications for bronchoscopy include haemoptysis of undetermined aetiology (even with a normal x-ray), stridor, suspected bronchial rupture, a positive sputum for *M. tuberculosis* with a negative x-ray (when endobronchial tuberculosis may be found, (p. 218)), and positive sputum cytology for mitotic cells in the absence of x-ray abnormality.

The appearances of many lesions, as viewed with the bronchoscope, are beautifully illustrated by Stradling [20].

Bronchoscopy may be used in the treatment of certain conditions, e.g. respiratory failure with inability to cough up secretions (p. 342), lung abscess (p. 159), removal of foreign body.

Caution should be observed at bronchoscopy when there is

(1) cardiac arrhythmia, which may be worsened by the procedure,

(2) severe respiratory failure when the investigation is usually academic in any case,

(3) a lesion with the characteristics of adenoma, biopsy of which may result in severe bleeding and

(4) when stenosis of a main bronchus is so severe that any bleeding from biopsy would result in total occlusion and pulmonary collapse.

PULMONARY FUNCTION STUDIES

The various tests employed and their indications are detailed in chapter 1.

BIOPSY PROCEDURES
(other than bronchoscopic)

PLEURAL BIOPSY

Biopsy of the parietal pleura by the punch technique [1, 6, 11 & 22] has greatly reduced the need for direct inspection and biopsy of pleural lesions by thoracoscopy. The introduction of the Abram's pleural biopsy punch, in which the biopsy is made by a lateral orifice, has made biopsy of the parietal pleura such an easy procedure that it is commonly coupled with pleural aspiration as a routine measure. Pleural biopsy is of greatest value in pleural malignancy when positive results may be obtained in 40–60% of cases. If the pleura is suspected of being involved in a malignant process and an initial pleural biopsy is negative, a second or even a third attempt should be made in different sites as tumour implants may be situated irregularly on the pleura. In tuberculous pleurisy positive results from a pleural biopsy may be obtained in an even higher percentage of cases (70–80%) but the relative value of the procedure is less in this condition as other features usually combine to indicate tuberculosis as the probable diagnosis. Pleural biopsy with the Abram's punch is only employed when there is an associated pleural effusion. Sufficient fluid is aspirated for diagnostic purposes and to relieve dyspnoea and, while there is still some residual fluid, the biopsy is made. The best results are obtained by moving the needle almost tangentially to the chest wall while still remaining within the pleural cavity. Pleural biopsy performed at right angle to the chest wall commonly yields intercostal muscle only. Parietal pleural tumour without effusion may be biopsied by the Vim–Silverman or Menghini needle.

THORACOSCOPY

Thoracoscopy to examine the pleural surfaces after the introduction of air into the pleural space is only necessary if examination of the pleural aspirate and pleural biopsy are unhelpful.

BIOPSY OF OTHER TISSUES

Biopsy of other tissues may assist in the diagnosis of respiratory disease, e.g. lymph nodes (usually cervical) in sarcoidosis (p. 386), reticulosis, or lung cancer (p. 530). 'Blind' biopsy of nonpalpable scalene nodes is rarely profitable except, perhaps, in sarcoidosis (p. 386). A significant node in other diseases is virtually always palpable [10].

MEDIASTINOSCOPY

Biopsy of diseased mediastinal glands through a small incision in the suprasternal notch (mediastinoscopy) is being increasingly employed [2, 3, 5, 7, 8, 9, 12, 13, 14, 15 & 21].

LUNG BIOPSY

The main value of lung biopsy is in diffuse lung disease not diagnosable by other methods. Formal biopsy is usually employed for the diagnosis of diffuse lung disease only when other methods of diagnosis have failed. Open lung biopsy by formal thoractomy was the only satisfactory method until recently. This is never undertaken lightly because of the morbidity and mortality, small though these are. The threshold for lung biopsy has been lowered by the introduction of a high speed air drill [19]. This employs a rotating trephine, 2·95 mm in external diameter, driven at 15,000 revolutions per minute by a compressed air drill. Steel and Winstanley [19] reported successful biopsies in 75% of 91 cases. Examples included cases of alveolar proteinosis, beryllium granuloma and allergic vasculitis. Complications (chiefly pneumothorax and slight haemoptysis) occurred in 18 patients (20%) but were never serious. We have used this technique in unusual cases of sarcoidosis and in one case of asbestosis when the discovery of asbestos bodies confirmed the diagnosis.

Percutaneous needle biopsy of the lung is sometimes employed in the diagnosis of a large pulmonary lesion adjacent to the pleura, using a Vim–Silverman [18] or Menghini needle. This technique is indicated if exploratory thoracotomy is contra-indicated and a diagnosis is necessary, particularly to prove the presence of an inoperable tumour for which x-ray treatment may be given. A theoretical hazard is the seeding of malignant cells along the course of the needle but this is not at all common. Pneumothorax occurred in 40% of 61 patients reported by Smith [18] but a positive histological diagnosis was made in 64% of the whole series and in 73% of the 41 patients with diffuse lung disease.

CYTOLOGY OF PLEURAL FLUID

Examination of pleural fluid for malignant cells requires particular skill and experience but may be very helpful when done by an expert. It is considered further on p. 280.

SEROLOGICAL TESTS

These are of particular value in rheumatoid lung (p. 578) and Caplan's syndrome (p. 474), systemic lupus erythematosus (p. 581), glandular fever (p. 130) and acute rheumatic fever (p. 577). Diagnostic titres may be found in bacterial (e.g. brucellosis, typhoid), viral, rickettsial and mycoplasmal infections.

BIOCHEMICAL TESTS

A number of biochemical tests are useful in the study of respiratory disease and are listed in the various sections. Hypercalcaemia and hypercalciuria may occur in some cases of sarcoidosis (p. 384) and berylliosis (p. 498). Biochemical and hormonal abnormalities may be found in bronchogenic carcinoma (p. 531). Gammaglobulins may be raised in chronic infectious disease, collagenosis, lymphomata, sarcoidosis and, particularly, in myeloma. A very high erythrocyte sedimentation rate (ESR) should raise the possibility of associated myeloma, especially if there are other features such as recurrent pneumonia. Hypogammaglobulinaemia (p. 119) predisposes to recurrent bacterial infections. Reference is made to the serum amylase level in the pleural complications of acute pancreatitis on p. 267. The serum glutamic oxalacetic transaminase (SGOT) may be helpful in the diagnosis of malignant pleural effusion. The serum lactic dehydrogenase (SLDH) was at one time thought to be characteristically raised in pulmonary embolism but this has been disproved [16]. The carcinoid syndrome may result in elevation of the blood serotonin and urinary 5-hydroxyindole acetic acid (5-HIAA) (p. 556). The raised sweat sodium or chloride may be helpful in the diagnosis of cystic fibrosis in children (p. 592).

ELECTROCARDIOGRAPHY

Evidence of right heart strain may be found in chronic *cor pulmonale* but is often absent (p. 315). Ischaemic changes or those of left ventricular hypertrophy may be present in patients presenting with acute pulmonary oedema. Severe pulmonary embolism may show abnormalities in the form of right heart strain (p. 459) or arrhythmias (p. 462).

REFERENCES

[1] ABRAMS L.D. (1958) A pleural biopsy punch. *Lancet* i, 30.

[2] BERGH N.P. (1964) Mediastinal exploration by technique of Carlens. *Dis. Chest* 46, 399.

[3] CARLENS E. (1959) Mediastinoscopy: a method for inspection and tissue biopsy in the superior mediastinum. *Dis. Chest* 36, 343.

[4] CARSTAIRS L.S. (1967) Macroradiography of the lungs in sarcoidosis. *Proc. roy. Soc. Med.*, 60, 991.

[5] ELLIOT R.C., BOYD A.D., SNYDER W. & MEESE E.H. (1967) Mediastinoscopy: a valuable diagnostic procedure of intrathoracic lesions. *Am. Rev. resp. Dis.* 96, 981.

[6] HAMPSON F. & KARLISH A.J. (1961) Needle biopsy of the pleura in the diagnosis of pleural effusion. *Quart. J. Med.*, N.S. 30, 249.

[7] KNOCHE E. & RINK H. (1963) *Mediastinoscopy: Bioptic Exploration of the Superior Mediastinum according to E. Carlens* (German text). Stuttgart, F.K. Schattauer.

[8] KOSKINEN O. & LINDEN L.W.F. (1964) Mediastinoscopy in mediastinal surgery. *Ann. Otol.* 73, 111.

[9] LACQUET L.K. (1964) Mediastinoscopy (Dutch text). *Leuvens. genesk. T.* 3, 116.

[10] LECKIE W.J.H., MCCORMACK R.J.M. & WALBAUM P.R. (1963) The case against routine scalene node biopsy in bronchial carcinoma. *Lancet* i, 853.

[11] MESTITZ P., PURVES M.J. & POLLARD A.C. (1958) Pleural biopsy in the diagnosis of pleural effusion. A report of 200 cases. *Lancet* ii, 1349.

[12] PALVA T. (1965) *Mediastinoscopy*. Chicago, Year Book Publishers.

[13] PALVA T. & VIKARI S. (1961) Mediastinoscopy. *J. thorac. cardiovasc. Surg.* 42, 206.

[14] PEARSON F.G. (1965) Mediastinoscopy: a method of biopsy in the superior mediastinum. *J. thorac. cardiovasc. Surg.* 49, 11.

[15] REYNDERS H. (1964) Mediastinoscopy in bronchogenic carcinoma. *Dis. Chest* 45, 606.

[16] SCHONELL M.E., CROMPTON G.K., FORSHALL J.M. & WHITBY L.G. (1966) Failure to differentiate pulmonary infarction from pneumonia by biochemical tests. *Br. med. J.* i, 1146.

[17] SIMON G. (1962) *Principles of Chest X-ray Diagnosis*, 2nd Edition. London, Butterworths.

[18] SMITH W.G. (1964) Needle biopsy of the lung. *Thorax* 19, 68.

[19] STEEL S.J. & WINSTANLEY D.P. (1967) Lung biopsy with a high-speed air drill. *Thorax* 22, 286.

[20] STRADLING P. (1968) *Diagnostic Bronchoscopy*. London, Livingstone.

[21] VAN DER SCHAAR P.J. & VAN ZANTEN M.E. (1965) Experience with mediastinoscopy. *Thorax* 20, 211.

[22] WEISS W. (1958) Needle biopsy of the parietal pleura in tuberculosis. *Am. Rev. Tuberc.* 78, 17.

CHAPTER 5

Some Principles of Chemotherapy

THEORETICAL CONSIDERATIONS

On the whole chemotherapy is an empirical subject, depending on trial and error in the discovery of new therapeutic agents. Nevertheless, scientific theory is gradually catching up with empirically discovered fact and is defining the mode of action of drugs and certain principles in their clinical use. With the great success of powerful antibiotics in most infections the clinician may be tempted to neglect the underlying theory. In the majority of cases his patients will pay no major penalty for this but in a proportion the problem can only be solved by deeper knowledge. It is impossible in this chapter to do more than outline some basic principles in chemotherapy which may be of use and interest to the physician concerned with respiratory diseases.

SITES OF ACTION OF CHEMOTHERAPEUTIC AGENTS

The sites of action of many drugs are still unknown but with the advances in molecular biology knowledge has greatly increased in the last few years. Indeed the specific actions of antibiotics, many of them too toxic for clinical use, are now employed by molecular biologists as research tools in the analysis of cell metabolism. Most drugs whose site of action has been determined affect bacteria either by interfering with protein synthesis or by damaging the bacterial cell wall [1].

INTERFERENCE WITH PROTEIN SYNTHESIS

The action of certain antibiotics on protein synthesis in bacteria is summarized diagrammatically in fig. 5.1. The genetic coding for the synthesis of proteins is carried on the DNA of the cell. Appropriate sections of this coding are conveyed to the ribosome, where protein synthesis occurs, by means of messenger RNA (mRNA). This process is interfered with by *chloramphenicol*. The relevant amino acids needed for protein synthesis are carried to the ribosome by transfer RNA (tRNA). Magnesium ions are required for this process. *Tetracycline* interferes with the action of tRNA, possibly partly by acting as a chelating agent for magnesium. *Streptomycin*, *kanamycin* and *neomycin* apparently have direct action on the ribosome; they cause it to misread the genetic code and so to manufacture wrong proteins, with resulting enzyme deficiencies in the bacterial cell. Streptomycin probably acts on a specific portion of the ribosome (30S portion), which is absent from streptomycin resistant strains. The synthesis of the 30S portion is probably conditioned by a single gene locus with multiple alleles, a fact which is relevant to acquired streptomycin resistance. *Erythromycin* and *lincomycin* are known to inhibit bacterial protein synthesis but their site of action is unknown.

ACTION ON BACTERIAL CELL WALL AND CELL MEMBRANE

The action of antibiotics on bacterial cell wall and cell membrane is summarized in fig. 5.2. *Penicillin* is thought to affect the synthesis of a mucopolysaccharide which is necessary to provide energy in the bacterial cell wall. As a result the osmotic barrier of the cell wall is damaged. The cell absorbs water and bursts. The action therefore is bactericidal. *Ampicillin* and *methicillin* also affect the cell wall but the site of action is unknown. *Polymyxin* and *colistin* probably act on the cell membrane. *Cycloserine* interferes with an enzyme which synthesizes a precursor to the mucopolypeptide of the cell wall. *Nystatin* and *amphotericin B* are bound to a specific sterol in the bacterial membrane.

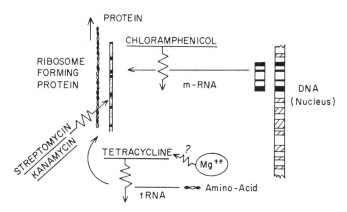

FIG. 5.1. *Antibiotics affecting protein synthesis* (see text): Chloramphenicol interferes with the conveyance of the DNA coding, transmitted *via* messenger RNA (mRNA) to the ribosomes where new protein is manufactured. Tetracycline interferes with the conveyance of aminoacids to the ribosome, a process carried out by transfer RNA (tRNA); the drug may act partly by functioning as a chelating agent for magnesium ions which are probably essential to the process. Streptomycin and kanamycin affect a particular section of the ribosome and cause the manufacture of incorrect proteins (data from Carter and McCarty 1966).

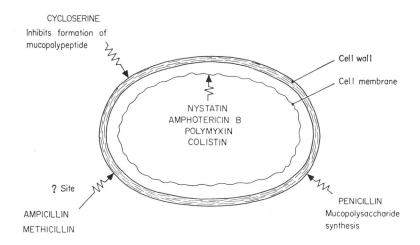

FIG. 5.2. *Action of antibiotics on bacterial cell wall and cell membrane:* Penicillin interferes with the cell wall. Ampicillin and methicillin affect the cell wall in a manner still undetermined. Polymyxin and colistin act on the membrane in the manner of a detergent and alter its properties. Cycloserine affects an enzyme concerned with the synthesis of a precursor to the cell wall mucopolypeptide. Nystatin and amphotericin are bound to a specific sterol in the bacterial membrane (data from Carter and McCarty 1966).

BACTERICIDAL AND BACTERIOSTATIC DRUGS

The contrast between bactericidal and bacteriostatic drug action is shown in fig. 5.3 & 5.4. Bactericidal drugs (fig. 5.3) kill relatively quickly, some, like streptomycin, by causing the cell to make incorrect proteins leading to metabolic poisoning; others, like penicillin, by damaging the cell wall and disrupting the cell. Bactericidal drugs may be able to eliminate bacteria relatively quickly but will of course be aided in this by the body's defences. Bacteriostatic drugs only inhibit growth and reproduction, possibly, as is suggested by the site of action of such drugs as chloramphenicol and tetracycline, by blocking the synthesis of fresh proteins. With bacteriostatic drugs the body's defences may

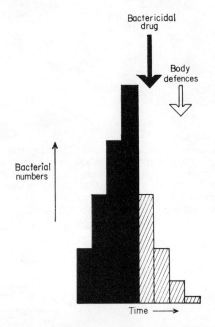

FIG. 5.3. *Action of a bactericidal drug:* The ascending columns on the left are a symbolic representation of an increasing bacterial population in the patient as his illness develops. When a bactericidal drug is given this directly kills the bacteria and, with the aid of the body's defences, eliminates them.

be necessary to eliminate the bacteria completely (fig. 5.4). If the drug is stopped prematurely the residual bacteria may multiply again and cause further symptoms.

The main chemotherapeutic agents which are used in respiratory diseases may be roughly classified into 2 groups of drugs as follows:

Bactericidal	*Bacteriostatic*
Ampicillin	Chloramphenicol
Carbenicillin	Erythromycin
Cephaloridine	Novobiocin
Cloxacillin	Sulphonamides
Colistin	Tetracyclines
Gentamicin	

Bactericidal
Kanamycin
Lincomycin
Methicillin
Penicillin
Polymyxin
Streptomycin

The difference between the 2 types of drugs is to some extent relative. If organisms are prevented from growing for long enough they are likely to die from inanition. In addition, by controlling the virulence of the antigen,

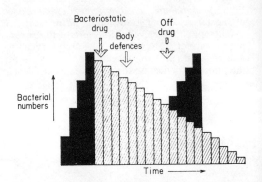

FIG. 5.4. *Action of a bacteriostatic drug:* A bacteriostatic drug prevents the bacteria growing but does not directly kill them. With the aid of the body's defences the numbers are gradually diminished and the bacteria may be finally eliminated. But if the drug is discontinued prematurely the organisms may proliferate once more, causing clinical relapse.

bacteriostatic drugs may enable the body's defences to be increased by active immunity; the weakened organisms may stimulate immunity without damaging the host. Some bacteriostatic drugs, such as erythromycin, may become bactericidal if given in big enough concentrations. In general the rate of killing by bactericidal drugs increases with increasing concentration.

PERSISTERS

In vitro even high concentrations of a bactericidal drug may fail to eliminate sensitive bacteria. For instance if a large inoculum of penicillin sensitive staphylococci is placed in a medium containing high concentrations of penicillin, it will be found after some days that some staphylococci can still be sub-cultured and that they remain fully penicillin sensitive. As might be expected, the more active the cell metabolism the more likely is an antibiotic to damage the cell. Persistence is therefore more likely to occur when the bacterial population has passed the stage of logarithmic increase, so that persisters are commoner in old bacterial populations and in pus. This phenomenon probably also explains the very long duration of chemo-therapy which is necessary in tuberculosis. Although tubercle bacilli can be killed in a few days by chemotherapy *in vitro* it may take 18 months to achieve the same effect in the body (p. 239). Presumably a small pro-portion of the bacterial population is not in an active metabolic stage and therefore persists in a relatively dormant form. If the organisms begin active metabolism they are killed by chemotherapy; if they remain dor-mant they ultimately die from inanition, per-haps with some assistance from the body's defences. It is often suggested that organisms may be protected from the action of anti-biotics if they are isolated in fibrous tissue where the antibiotics may not penetrate. One must remember that the body's metabolites must reach such cells and *a priori* there seems no good reason why antibiotics should not do so also. It may be that the more important factor is that bacteria in these situations are in a relatively dormant phase and therefore not readily killed. There is good *in vitro* evidence that the more rapid the antibacterial effect the less likely are persisters to emerge. It may be that the greater effectiveness of high doses of penicillin in such conditions as lung abscess or actinomycosis is due to the pre-vention of persistence rather than to increased penetration of the antibiotic. Besides tuber-culosis it is possible that relapse in chronic bronchitis and bronchiectasis, associated with infection by *H. influenzae*, may be due to the phenomenon of persistence. Although not, of course, a respiratory problem, bacterial endocarditis is a notorious example of the same process.

4—R.D.

SYNERGISM AND ANTAGONISM

In *in vitro* studies it has been found that, if marginal concentrations of bactericidal drugs are used together, the bactericidal effect may be dramatically better than the additive effect of the two drugs used independently. A similar phenomenon has been demonstrated with experimental infections [5]. The effect depends partly on the strain of organisms used. Clinically the utilization of 2 bacteri-cidal drugs in combination is mainly im-portant in the treatment of infections which are difficult to eliminate [3]. The most impressive example is probably the superiority of penicillin plus streptomycin in the treat-ment of enterococcal bacterial endocarditis. The use of the same combination to treat bronchial infection with *H. influenzae* in bronchitis and bronchiectasis is another possible instance. Streptomycin plus isoniazid in tuberculosis probably have a synergistic effect, as well as preventing the emergence of drug resistance to both drugs. In general there is virtually never a synergistic effect between bacteriostatic drugs; the effect is purely additive. In fact, clinically a more than ade-quate dose of both drugs is usually given, so that the effect is equivalent only to that of the more powerful component, the second drug making no additional contribution.

In carefully designed *in vitro* and *in vivo* experiments a bacteriostatic drug can be shown, with some organisms and some drugs, to diminish or antagonize the effect of a bactericidal drug given in a marginally effective dose [3 & 5]. However, such an-tagonism is very unlikely to be important in clinical practice, as the dose of drugs used is normally well above the marginal level at which such antagonism occurs [6].

DRUG RESISTANCE

It is important to differentiate between various types of drug resistance as the difference is very relevant to therapy and pre-vention. Drug resistance may be conveniently classified into 3 groups:

(1) *natural* drug resistance occurring in

organisms which have never been exposed to the drug,

(2) *acquired* drug resistance which results from exposure of the organisms to the drug, and

(3) *transferred* drug resistance by which organisms owing to their resistance to genetic elements may transfer resistance to a sensitive species; *transduction* of genetic material endowing resistance may also occur by means of bacteriophage.

NATURAL DRUG RESISTANCE

Organisms may be naturally drug resistant because they do not depend on a particular metabolic process which is attacked by the chemotherapeutic agent to which they are resistant. Alternatively, as in the case of penicillin, certain species, such as *E. coli*, may be resistant because they produce an enzyme, penicillinase, which destroys the antibiotic concerned. As far as is known at present this is mainly relevant to penicillin and related drugs.

Natural resistance may be confined to particular strains within the species. The most notorious example is that of staphylococci among which an increasing number of strains have been shown to be penicillin resistant, owing to the production of penicillinase. The prevalence of drug resistant strains or species in an environment, such as a hospital, depends on the previous use of the drugs in that environment. In the case of staphylococci, when penicillin was first discovered, naturally penicillin resistant strains were extremely rare. Repeated surveys after the drug came into use showed a steady increase in the proportion of penicillinase producing strains isolated in any individual hospital. These strains were of different phage type from the original sensitive strains, indicating that the penicillin resistant strains had been put at a biological advantage compared to the penicillin sensitive ones which gradually became eliminated from the hospital environment. When a patient initially had a penicillin sensitive staphylococcus and a penicillin resistant one was subsequently isolated, this was due to superinfection, as could be shown by the difference in

phage type. Exactly the same phenomenon has been found if any other antibiotic has come into regular use in a particular environment; the number of strains of resistant staphylococci steadily increases. For this reason it is very important to keep such drugs as cloxacillin in reserve and to use them only when a particular strain of staphylococcus has been shown to be resistant to the more usual antibiotics or, in a desperate case in which one is unable to wait for the results of the resistance tests, only until the results of those tests become available. It is our own custom, when possible, to treat such patients in isolation in order to minimize the risk of encouraging resistant strains in the environment. The hospital environment, and the skin, sputum, etc. of the individual patient, do not remain sterile. Elimination of pathogenic bacteria from the sputum or other excreta leaves an ecological vacuum which will be filled either by harmless or by harmful organisms which must be resistant to the antibiotic the patient is receiving. This explains the increasing problem of infection by species resistant to the usual antibiotics, such as *Proteus* and *Pseudomonas pyocyanea*.

ACQUIRED DRUG RESISTANCE

Acquired drug resistance is due to the exposure of a strain of bacteria to a drug. A strain of bacteria infecting the patient may become resistant during treatment. There has in the past been some controversy as to whether acquired resistance is due to encouragement of growth of naturally occurring *resistant mutants* or to *adaptation* of the strain to the drug. It is now generally thought that the former is the more likely process. (See review by Mitchison [10].)

Chemotherapeutic agents may be conveniently classified into 2 groups, to one of which resistance may be very rapidly acquired, to the other of which it is only relatively slowly acquired [10]. In the case of *slowly acquired resistance*, if organisms are repeatedly subcultured in increasing concentrations of a drug, subculturing on each occasion from the highest tube in which growth occurs, the degree of resistance may be slowly increased, as shown diagrammatically in fig. 5.5. This small-step increase is probably due to mutations occurring in a number of genes, each of which conditions a slight increase in resistance. In the case of penicillin, certain organisms such as pneumococci which have been made

resistant in this way may lose their pathogenicity, but this does not hold with all species. Acquired drug resistance of this type is relatively rare in the individual patient though it may gradually occur in a community if the drug is extensively used.

If the *in vitro* procedure is repeated with certain other drugs, such as streptomycin, quite high degrees of resistance may be obtained, even on the first subculture. Such *rapidly acquired resistance* is probably due to mutations in more powerful genes which confer a considerable degree of resistance [10], as shown symbolically in fig. 5.5. This type of resistance is of great clinical importance and always a potential danger in the individual patient when such drugs are used. In general strains rendered resistant in this way do not readily revert to sensitivity. Such reversion is commoner with erythromycin than with other drugs.

Antibiotics used in treating chest disease may be roughly classified as follows:

Drugs to which resistance rapidly acquired

Capreomycin
Erythromycin
Isoniazid
Kanamycin
Novobiocin
P.A.S.
Pyrazinamide
Streptomycin
Viomycin

Drugs to which resistance only slowly acquired

Chloramphenicol
Colistin
Cycloserine
Gentamicin
Lincomycin
Penicillin
Polymyxin
Tetracycline

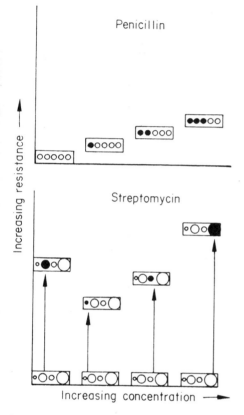

FIG. 5.5. *Multiple step and single step resistance development in bacteria:* Resistance to penicillin may be gradually induced *in vitro*, as shown above, by culturing in a series of media containing ascending concentrations of the drug, and successively subculturing from the highest concentration in which there is bacterial growth. Such multiple step resistance seldom occurs clinically and is of little importance (see text). On the other hand a similar *in vitro* experiment with streptomycin and certain other drugs often results in sudden rapid increases in resistance, probably due to selection of organisms undergoing a single mutation in a gene which confers a high degree of resistance. This is of great clinical importance. (Reproduced by courtesy of the Editors, Proc. Roy. Soc. Med.)

It will be noted that most of the drugs used in tuberculosis belong to the group to which resistance may be rapidly acquired, but the same phenomenon occurs if they are used to treat other infections.

Rapidly acquired resistance may be *prevented* by using 2 or more drugs in combination. An example of the mechanism of such prevention is shown diagrammatically in figs. 5.6 & 5.7. This applies, for instance, to the combined use of streptomycin and isoniazid in tuberculosis. In a large population of tubercle bacilli approximately one in a million bacilli are naturally occurring isoniazid resistant mutants. If isoniazid is used

a second patient, who may be found to have resistant bacilli in spite of never having received the drug ('*primary*' drug resistance).

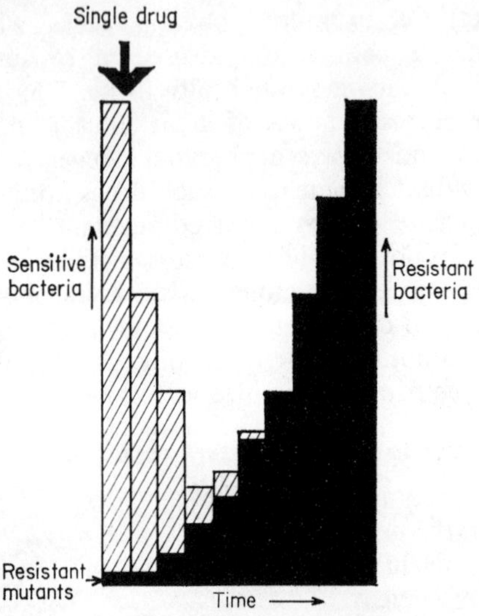

In the initial population of the original patient (fig. 5.7) approximately 1 in 10^7 bacilli will be mutants naturally resistant to

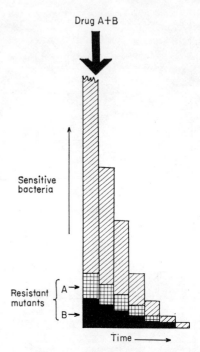

FIG. 5.6. *Acquired resistance in single drug therapy*: The drug will eliminate the sensitive part of the bacterial population but will not affect the resistant mutants which will thus be at a biological advantage. If the body's defences are inadequate, the small resistant minority may proliferate and replace the original sensitive majority.

FIG. 5.7. *Prevention of resistance with combined chemotherapy*: If 2 drugs are used, both will act on the major part of the population sensitive to both. In addition drug A will act on the mutants resistant to drug B, and *vice versa*. Both the sensitive population and the resistant mutants are thereby eliminated.

alone in a patient with a large population of bacilli approximately 1 in 10^6 of his organisms will be already resistant to the drug. The drug will eliminate the isoniazid sensitive bacilli which form the very great majority of the population. The resistant bacilli, which are unaffected by the drug, will be at a biological advantage and, if the size of the initial population is big enough and if the patient's defences are poor, may grow up and replace the original sensitive population. What is more, these bacilli may then be passed on to

streptomycin. If streptomycin is given alone exactly the same thing is liable to happen as in the case of isoniazid. But, if both the drugs are given together they will both affect the large majority of the bacilli which are sensitive to both drugs; in fact the two drugs probably act synergistically. More important still, the isoniazid resistant mutants will be eliminated by the streptomycin and the streptomycin resistant mutants by the isoniazid, so preventing the emergence of a resistant population. Although there is a theoretical risk that a small proportion of mutants may be simultaneously resistant to both drugs, this is a multiple of the chances of resistance to each individual drug; that is to say only 1 in 10^{13} mutants is likely to be doubly resistant. A patient must have a very large population of bacilli to have many of these organisms. Presumably in almost all, if not all, patients doubly resistant mutants are so rare that they are readily eliminated by the patient's own defences, as drug resistance virtually never emerges if these 2 drugs are used in proper combination on an initially sensitive population (p. 236). Of course if the 2 drugs are used *successively* instead of *concurrently* the population may become resistant first to one drug and then to the second.

If drugs are used in an inadequate combination, such as streptomycin twice a week with daily isoniazid, there may be time for isoniazid resistant mutants to multiply during the time when they are not exposed to adequate concentration of streptomycin. Although resistance is not likely to emerge in such a high proportion of patients as if isoniazid were given alone, such a combination does result in an appreciable proportion of failures of therapy, with the emergence of bacilli which are at first isoniazid resistant and later become streptomycin resistant. Because the resistant mutants are initially to some extent suppressed, resistance is likely to emerge later than when the drug is given alone.

Tubercle bacilli are relatively slow growing bacteria and, even when a drug is used alone, resistant organisms usually emerge clinically about 6–8 weeks after starting treatment, although they may do so as early as 2 weeks or, if inadequate combinations of drugs are used, only after a number of months. But with quickly growing organisms, such as initially streptomycin sensitive gram negative bacilli, drug resistance may emerge in 24 or 48 hours if streptomycin is given alone. Clinically it is most important that, if any of the drugs to which resistance is rapidly acquired are used, they should be given in combination with a 2nd drug to which the organism is sensitive or is likely to be sensitive in order to prevent the emergence of resistance.

TRANSFERRED RESISTANCE

This phenomenon, which has also been called '*infectious*' *drug resistance*, has been relatively recently reported, originally by Japanese workers [12]. It has been found, both in animals and man, that genetic elements conferring drug resistance, indeed often multiple drug resistance, may be transferred from the cells of resistant individuals in strains of nonpathogenic bacteria (such as *E. coli*) to other previously sensitive, pathogenic gram negative species such as Salmonella (see review by Datta [2]). The resistant nonpathogenic individuals may have originally acquired their resistance from another resistant and pathogenic strain. The mechanism is a fascinating one from the biological point of view [9] but cannot be elaborated here. So far this phenomenon has mainly been shown to be of clinical and epidemiological interest in gram negative intestinal infections but the subject is being very actively pursued and it may well prove to be of clinical importance in any part of the body where resistant and sensitive strains can exist side by side, as may occur in the respiratory tract.

TRANSDUCTION OF RESISTANCE

Resistance can be conveyed from a resistant to a sensitive strain by means of a bacteriophage which carries genetic material, usually extrachromosomal (plasmids), from one organism to the other. Penicillinase production and other forms of resistance can be conferred in this way. The phenomenon has been studied mainly in staphylococci and has been demonstrated both *in vitro* [8] and in experimental animals [11]. Its clinical significance is at present uncertain but it seems probable that it has contributed to the increased prevalence of penicillin resistant staphylococci in hospitals.

CROSS RESISTANCE BETWEEN DRUGS

By 'cross resistance' is meant that if a strain is resistant to one drug it is also resistant to another. Cross resistance between drugs commonly used in chest diseases may be summarized as follows:

(1) *Tetracyclines.* There is virtually complete

cross resistance between all types of tetra-cyclines.

(2) *Tetracyclines and chloramphenicol.* This may occur with gram negative bacilli but is unusual with gram positive.

(3) *Methicillin, cloxacillin and cephalori-dine.* There is virtually complete cross resistance between methicillin and cloxa-cillin. It is relatively common, although the extent has not yet been precisely defined, for organisms resistant to these drugs to be also resistant to cephaloridine and *vice versa.* These are the most vital reserve drugs for treating infections with staphylococci resis-tant to the commoner drugs, so that in our view they should all be kept in reserve and only used when there are very specific indica-tions. The chief of these is infection with staphylococci known or suspected to be resistant to the commoner antibiotics.

(4) *Erythromycin, oleandomycin, carbomy-cin, spiramycin* and *lincomycin.* Cross resis-tance between these various antibiotics is relatively common *in vitro,* but less often found clinically.

(5) *Erythromycin* and *chloramphenicol.* In staphylococci there is said sometimes to be cross resistance between these drugs.

(6) *Kanamycin, neomycin, framycetin, paro-momycin, gentamicin.* There is frequently cross resistance between these drugs. It is said that organisms which are resistant to them are also resistant to streptomycin but not *vice versa.* Cross resistance in this group has mainly been demonstrated by *in vitro* induction of resistance and does not necessarily occur clinically. In any individual clinical problem, therefore, cross resistance should not be assumed but should be tested.

(7) *Ethionamide* and *thioacetazone.* Cross resistance between these drugs may occur (p. 248).

SOME PRACTICAL CONSIDERATIONS

USE OF THE LABORATORY

The use of the bacteriological laboratory for identifying causative organisms and determin-ing their sensitivity to chemotherapeutic agents tends to be taken for granted but the limitations of laboratory investigation in practice are often forgotten. Frequent con-sultation between the clinician and his bacteriological colleague will enable the former to use the laboratory much more intelligently and the latter to adapt his tech-nique to yield information of real value to the clinician. In an acute illness, such as pneumonia, the clinician must make a deci-sion about treatment immediately on diag-nosis and cannot wait for the results of cultures. The physician and bacteriologist should become accustomed to examining a *smear of the sputum* immediately in such cases, particularly if severe. It is often possible to decide whether the pneumonia is likely to be due to pneumococci, staphylococci or *Klebsiella pneumoniae* (Friedländer's bacillus) as a result of examining the smear (p. 136).

The laboratory may fail to identify the actual causal organism either because of *previous chemotherapy* or because of *technical deficiencies.* Even a single dose of an anti-biotic may result in inability to culture pneumococci, though they may sometimes be seen on direct smear of the sputum. The fre-quency with which two common respiratory pathogens, pneumococci and *H. influenzae,* are identified is very dependent on technical methods. Culture in an atmosphere of 10% CO_2 substantially increases the isolation rate of both species, while mouse inoculation may increase the isolation rate of pneumococci in pneumonia by as much as 50% [4].

The sputum is virtually never sterile. If a pathogen has been eliminated by chemo-therapy it is likely to be replaced by either pathogenic or nonpathogenic organisms re-sistant to the drug in use. The presence of pathogenic organisms in these circumstances does not necessarily indicate that they are the cause of the patient's disease. All too often a patient's treatment is changed because a few resistant staphylococci or *K. pneumoniae* have been grown from a sputum specimen sent to the laboratory after the patient has already started treatment. If there is the slightest doubt the matter should be discussed with the bacteriologist. In general little notice need be taken of such a result if the patient is apparently responding to treatment. If he is not responding to treatment it is important to know whether the positive culture consists of just a few colonies or of confluent growth. Major growth makes it more likely that a resistant species is in fact responsible for the patient's condition. *Proteus* and yeasts are frequently found in the sputum in patients who have already received chemotherapy. They are seldom of clinical significance and *Proteus* grows so explosively *in vitro* that it is likely to obscure any pathogens that may be present.

The disc *resistance tests* which are used as a routine in most laboratories for nontuberculous bacteria appear to be reliable enough for most clinical purposes, providing the disc contains the correct concentration of the drug; in some countries, at least, not all those commercially available are reliable. In complex infections due to organisms resistant to most of the commoner antibiotics tube dilution or other special methods [3] may have to be used and the bacteriologist, in consultation with the clinician, may be able to determine whether a combination of drugs will be useful. There has been very much less investigation of the quantitative significance of drug resistance in nontuberculous respiratory infection but in general it seems that organisms showing any degree of resistance on disc testing are unlikely to respond to the drug in question. In tuberculosis the quantitative aspects of resistance testing are most important and methods of testing must be used which will reveal even the lowest degree of drug resistance (p. 239).

If the clinician uses the bacteriological laboratory with due regard to the practical considerations outlined, and to the theoretical background sketched in the earlier part of this chapter, he should be able to avoid inundating the laboratory with the vast number of unnecessary specimens with which most laboratories now have to cope. This will give the bacteriologist and his staff time to make really careful studies on relevant specimens. In any difficult case of chest infection, especially if it is not responding to the treatment given, the clinician is failing in his duty if he has not discussed the problem with the bacteriologist.

THE CHOICE OF CHEMOTHERAPEUTIC AGENT

As already mentioned, in many acute infections treatment has to be initiated before the precise bacteriology is known. If the clinician does not obtain assistance from a direct smear examination of the sputum he will usually choose the drugs which are likely to be effective against the commonest cause of the relevant condition. It can be initially assumed that most pneumonias are caused by the pneumococcus and are therefore susceptible to penicillin, but if the patient is desperately ill the clinician may have to increase his insurance by widening his therapeutic attack (p. 138). In acute exacerbations of bronchitis bacteriology carried out at any level below the optimum is of little value and often the clinician must assume that the pneumococcus or *H. influenzae* is likely to be responsible, as has been repeatedly shown under research conditions (p. 323). The value of direct smear examination has been already mentioned.

If the organism has been identified but the results of resistance tests are not yet available the drug must be chosen on the basis of likely sensitivity. In a particular locality it may be known that a certain pattern of resistance is probable because of previous antibiotic policy in that area and the results of resistance tests on local strains. The appropriate drugs for treating infections with various organisms which may attack the respiratory system are outlined in table 5.1 (p. 90).

COMBINATIONS OF DRUGS

From what has been said above (p. 83) it will be obvious that there are only relatively limited indications for using combinations of drugs in respiratory infections. Some indications are outlined below:

(1) To *increase the effect* in infections difficult to eliminate. In general this is a matter of using two bactericidal drugs for their synergistic effect. In the respiratory tract a good

TABLE 5.1

Indications for the Main Chemotherapeutic Agents

N.B. Where numbers are given in brackets they indicate the order of preference. Data derived from many authors and from personal experience.

Infecting organism	Penicillin	Streptomycin	Tetracyclines	Remarks
Actinomyces	DRUG OF CHOICE (4 mega units/day)	Sometimes effective	Effective	Give penicillin at least 6 weeks
Bacteroides fusiformis necrophorus melanogenicus	DRUG OF CHOICE	Not effective	Effective	
Brucella species	Not effective	? with tetracycline	DRUG OF CHOICE	Continue at least 3 weeks
Candida albicans	Not effective	Not effective	Not effective	Nystatin or fungistatin: effective mouth and intestine
Escherichia coli	Not effective	Effective (combine with sulphonamides)	Effective	1. Colistin: some strains 2. Cephaloridine: some strains 3. Kanamycin 4. Cycloserine
Fungi pathogenic	Not effective	Not effective	Not effective	Natamycin inhalations (Aspergillus) Amphotericin B (Histoplasmosis, etc.) Nystatin
Haemophilus influenzae	Sometimes effective: best with streptomycin or 3 mega b.d.	Effective with penicillin DRUG OF CHOICE	Effective	1. Ampicillin 2. Erythromycin + novobiocin 3. Cephaloridine 4. Chloramphenicol: toxicity
Haemophilus pertussis	Not effective	Not effective	Probably effective early	
Klebsiella pneumoniae (Friedländer's bacillus)	Not effective (but strains vary)	DRUG OF CHOICE (with chloramphenicol or tetracycline)	Some strains (with streptomycin)	1. Colistin 2. Cephaloridine: some strains 3. Ampicillin: some strains
Mycoplasma pneumoniae	Not effective	Not effective	DRUG OF CHOICE	
Pasteurella pestis	Not effective	DRUG OF CHOICE (early)	Probably effective early	Tetracycline intravenously and orally initially
Pneumococcus	DRUG OF CHOICE (1)	Weakly effective (4)	Effective (3) (occasional resistant strains)	Erythromycin (2) best alternative to penicillin

TABLE 5.1—*continued*

Infecting organism	Penicillin	Streptomycin	Tetracyclines	Remarks
Proteus	Sometimes effective (large doses)	DRUG OF CHOICE (with chloramphenicol)	Sometimes effective (strains vary)	1. Cephaloridine: *P. mirabilis* only 2. Ampicillin: some strains 3. Colistin: occasional strain 4. Gentamicin: some strains 5. Sulphonamides + polymyxin 6. Chloramphenicol + tetracycline may be effective 7. Kanamycin 8. Carbenicillin
Pseudomonas pyocyanea or *aeruginosa*	Not effective	May be effective with polymyxin	Sometimes effective (strains vary)	1. Colistin 2. Gentamicin: severe cases (ototoxicity) 3. Tetracycline or streptomycin + polymyxin (? or colistin) 4. Carbenicillin
Rickettsia (including Q Fever)	Probably not effective	Probably not effective	DRUG OF CHOICE	? Chloramphenicol
Staphylococcus Pyogenes	DRUG OF CHOICE (if sensitive)	Partially effective	Effective	1. Severe illness (sensitivity unknown) or penicillin resistant; penicillin + cloxacillin (or methicillin) 2. Cephaloridine 3. Erythromycin + novobiocin 4. Lincomycin
Streptococcus pyogenes (haemolytic)	DRUG OF CHOICE	Many strains now resistant	Many strains now resistant	Erythromycin best alternative to penicillin
Streptococcus viridans	DRUG OF CHOICE (4 mega units/ day) Sometimes with streptomycin	Partially effective. Sometimes with penicillin	Effective (but not for endocarditis)	Penicillin + streptomycin for more resistant strains
Vincent's organisms (*Borrelia* species) and see '*Bacteroides*'	DRUG OF CHOICE	Partially effective	Probably effective	
Viruses ornithosis psittacosis	Probably effective	Probably not effective	DRUG OF CHOICE	

example is the use of penicillin plus strepto-mycin in *H. influenzae* infections associated with bronchitis or bronchiectasis. Debilitated patients may be infected with drug resistant gram-negative organisms in hospital and these may sometimes produce septicaemia. In such cases the bacteriologist should be asked to carry out very careful *in vitro* tests to deter-mine the best combination of drugs to use [3].

(2) The use of combinations of drugs to *prevent the emergence of drug resistant organisms* is essential whenever the clinician uses one of the drugs to which resistance may rapidly develop. In tuberculosis drugs should always be given in combination as almost all antituberculosis drugs may give rise to acquired resistance (p. 236). The value of streptomycin plus chloramphenicol or tetra-cycline in pneumonia due to *K. pneumoniae* is another important example. If erythromycin is used to treat staphylococcal infection it should always be combined with a second drug, often novobiocin.

(3) In our view it is always worth while treating an infection due to *penicillin resistant staphylococci* with penicillin in addition to cloxacillin or methicillin. These organisms are only resistant to penicillin because of their production of penicillinase. If their meta-bolism can be diminished by the use of cloxacillin or methicillin less penicillinase may be produced and the organisms become sensi-tive to the surviving penicillin. If the penicillin is enabled to reach the staphylococci it is a more effective drug than cloxacillin or methi-cillin. Penicillin should, for obvious reasons, be given in as big a dose as possible.

(4) In certain very severe acute infections it may be necessary to give more than one drug because the cause of the infection has not yet been determined. For instance, in a desperately ill case of pneumonia it may be advisable to give both penicillin and cloxa-cillin (p. 137) as it may not be known whether the pneumonia is pneumococcal or staphylo-coccal and whether the staphylococci, if present, are penicillin sensitive.

CONCLUSION

It is hoped that this chapter has persuaded the reader of the value of some theoretical knowledge regarding chemotherapy and the importance of weighing up all the relevant factors before initiating or changing treat-ment.

GENERAL REFERENCES

GARROD L.P. & O'GRADY F. (1968) *Antibiotic and Chemotherapy*, 2nd Edition. London, Livingstone.
LORIAN V. (1966) *Antibiotics and Chemotherapeutic Agents in Clinical and Laboratory Practice*. Springfield, Illinois, Charles C. Thomas.

REFERENCES

[1] CARTER W. & McCARTY K.S. (1966) Molecular mechanisms of antibiotic action. *Ann. int. Med.* **64**, 1087.
[2] DATTA NAOMI (1965) Infectious drug resistance. *Br. med. Bull.* **21**, 254.
[3] GARROD L.P. & WATERWORTH P.M. (1962) Methods of testing combined antibiotic bacteri-cidal action and the significance of the results. *J. clin. Path.* **15**, 328.
[4] HUMPHREY J.H., JOULES H. & VAN DER WALT E.D. (1948) Pneumonia in North-West London 1942–44. *Thorax* **3**, 112.
[5] JAWETZ E. & GUNNISON J.B. (1953) Antibiotic synergism and antagonism: an assessment of the problem. *Pharm. Rev.* **5**, 175.
[6] JAWETZ E. (1964) Principles of antimicrobial therapy. *Modern Treatment* **1**, 819.
[7] McDERMOTT W. (1958) Microbial persistence. *Yale J. biol. Med.* **30**, 257.
[8] McDONALD SHEILA (1966) Transduction of antibiotic resistance in *Staphylococcus aureus*. *Lancet* ii, 1107.
[9] MEYNELL ELINOR & DATTA NAOMI (1967) Mutant drug resistant factors of high trans-missibility. *Nature* **214**, 885.
[10] MITCHISON D.A. (1962) Microbial genetics and chemotherapy. *Br. med. Bull.* **18**, 74.
[11] NOVICK R.P. & MORSE S.I. (1967) *In vivo* transmission of drug resistance factors between strains of *Staphylococcus aureus*. *J. exp. Med.* **125**, 45.
[12] WATANABE T. (1963) Infective heredity of multiple drug resistance in bacteria. *Bact. Rev.* **27**, 87.

CHAPTER 6

Upper Respiratory Tract Infections, Acute Tracheitis and Bronchitis

Upper respiratory tract infections are by far the commonest diseases in Britain, accounting for approximately 50% of the time lost from work through acute illness. In recent years it has become clear that the large majority are viral infections and an attempt at classification is now feasible.

Most of the major advances in knowledge of viral respiratory diseases have resulted from the development and availability of laboratory techniques. Modern virological studies may be said to have stemmed from the successful cultivation of polioviruses *in vitro* after the 1939–45 war [16]. The application of these and related techniques for diagnostic and epidemiological purposes led to the discovery of many viruses which were shown to be the cause of disease so that now over 100 different viruses are known to be capable of causing upper respiratory tract infections (table 6.1).

Respiratory viruses lack specificity in the sense that one virus does not produce one disease as, for example, measles virus produces measles. Upper respiratory tract infections can be grouped into a number of fairly well defined clinical syndromes which have aetiological associations involving both host and virus. For instance, respiratory syncytial virus causes bronchiolitis or pneumonia in children but usually only a common cold in adults. Presumably the adult's possession of antibodies confers a protection lacking in the child encountering the disease for the first time. This may be why viral infections are generally more serious in children than in adults.

Viruses of entirely different taxonomic groups may cause similar clinical syndromes (table 6.2); conversely, most respiratory viruses are capable of producing a spectrum of clinical pictures ranging from the common cold to pneumonia. To add to the complexity, a small fraction of acute infective respiratory disease results from simultaneous infection by multiple agents.

At the bedside the clinician can do no more than hint at the probable aetiological agent concerned in respiratory viral infection and laboratory studies are essential for precise aetiological diagnosis. Combined clinical and virological studies have, however, indicated that certain clinical syndromes are more likely to be caused by particular viruses.

SYNDROMES IN VIRAL INFECTIONS OF THE UPPER RESPIRATORY TRACT

There are 6 recognizable clinical pictures of viral infection of the upper respiratory tract (table 6.2). It will be seen that there are no hard and fast boundaries between the various syndromes.

(1) *The coryzal syndrome* (or common cold, p. 100). The coryzal syndrome is characterized by increased nasal discharge, sneezing, nasal obstruction, and sometimes watering of the eyes and slight conjunctivitis. The nasal discharge, at first watery or mucoid, later becomes purulent. Obstruction of the maxillary sinuses and Eustachian tubes by mucosal oedema often causes discomfort, and sometimes actual pain, in the face or ear. 'Sore throat' in the coryzal syndrome is usually a dry or rough sensation on the posterior part of the soft palate or the uvula and it is often the first symptom, heralding the onset of a cold. Systemic upset may occur with headache, malaise, muscular aching, lassitude and chilliness, but the symptoms are seldom severe. Fever is uncommon.

(2) *The pharyngeal syndrome*. The dominant symptom is sore throat which may be

TABLE 6.1

Viruses* causing Upper Respiratory Tract Infections

ADENOVIRUSES—31 serotypes recognized by neutralization tests.
Common antigen detected by CFT.

REOVIRUSES—3 serotypes.

PICORNAVIRUSES (pico = very small; RNA = ribonucleic acid)—No group antigen. Very many serotypes.

(a) *Rhinoviruses* (over 80 serotypes known)

Inactivated at pH5. Grow best at 33°C.
Found in nose and pharynx but not in faeces.
Subdivided into M type (grow in cells derived from monkeys as well as human cells) and H type (grow in human but not in monkey cells)

(b) *Enteroviruses*

Found in faeces and pharynx but rarely in nose.

1. Polioviruses (may sometimes cause systemic upset with nose and throat symptoms in contacts of patients with poliomyelitis)
2. Coxsackie A viruses (> 24 serotypes)
3. Coxsackie B viruses (6 serotypes)
4. Echoviruses—('*Enteric Cytopathic Human Orphan*'. When isolated from man were still 'in search of a disease', hence 'orphan') (> 30 serotypes). Types 11, 20 and 28 known to give URT infections.

MYXOVIRUSES (so named because of affinity for mucous surfaces)

(a) *Influenza viruses*

1. Influenza A. Common CF nucleoprotein antigen. Subgrouped by surface protein antigens into A0, A1 and A2 (or A Asian).
2. Influenza B. Common antigen distinct from that of A virus. Subgroups not clearly defined.
3. Influenza C. Only 1 serotype known.

(b) *Parainfluenza and respiratory syncytial viruses*

1. Five parainfluenza viruses, serologically distinct but related distantly to mumps virus.
2. Respiratory syncytial virus (named because of syncytia produced in infected cultures).

* All contain RNA as nucleic acid except adenoviruses which contain DNA.

TABLE 6.2

Principal Viruses Associated with Upper Respiratory Syndromes

Syndrome	Principal viruses
1. Common Cold	Rhinovirus Parainfluenza I & II ECHO 28 Coxsackie A21 Respiratory Syncytial Virus
2. Pharyngeal Syndrome and	Adenovirus Influenza
3. Pharyngo-Conjunctival Syndrome	Coxsackie ECHO Parainfluenza
4. Influenza	Influenza A, B & C
5. Herpangina	Coxsackie A
6. Croup	Parainfluenza I & II Respiratory Syncytial Virus Adenovirus Influenza

slight or severe. The pharynx is inflamed and the tonsils and adenoids enlarged, perhaps sufficiently to cause nasal obstruction which can sometimes occur quite rapidly. In severe cases patches of yellowish exudate may be seen on the tonsils and enlarged, tender, lymph nodes felt in the upper part of the neck. Cough is common but coryza slight or absent. General symptoms such as chills, malaise, general aching, headache and mild pyrexia are common. Hoarseness may occur. The infecting organisms are generally adenoviruses but the pharyngeal syndrome can also be caused by influenza, Coxsackie, ECHO and parainfluenza viruses.

Infectious mononucleosis sometimes bears a close resemblance to the pharyngeal syndrome although the lymphadenopathy is likely to spread to groups other than the cervical, and the white cell count and the Paul–Bunnell test may confirm the diagnosis.

Acute streptococcal sore throat causes more severe general and local effects as a rule. The purulent exudate on the tonsil is more extensive and the throat swab culture will generally yield Group A beta haemolytic streptococci. Sore throat of viral or streptococcal aetiology may however be indistinguishable clinically.

3. *The pharyngoconjunctival syndrome.* The pharyngoconjunctival syndrome is simply a variant of the pharyngeal syndrome caused by the same viruses. The onset is usually marked by pharyngeal symptoms to which conjunctivitis is subsequently added, generally but not invariably bilateral, accompanied by photophobia and sometimes pain in the eyeballs. Sometimes conjunctivitis appears first and it may outlast the other symptoms by one or two weeks. Systemic upset is mild and lasts a few days only. Epidemics of the pharyngoconjunctival syndrome are fairly common in the spring and summer among schoolchildren and in holiday camps.

(4) *The influenza syndrome* (see influenza, p. 104). The dominant feature of the influenza syndrome is severe constitutional disturbance. The symptoms—chills, fever, prostration, headache, generalized muscular pain, malaise and anorexia—tend to develop with startling suddenness and later on cough, sore throat and retrosternal ache generally make their appearance. While the influenza syndrome can be mild enough to pass for the coryzal syndrome or pharyngeal syndrome it can also be a severe and devastating illness. The worst cases, those encountered during pandemics, may owe something of their severity to superadded bacterial infection. In the last pandemic, influenza virus A in partnership with *Staphylococcus pyogenes* was responsible for a necrotizing tracheobronchitis which was often fatal. In Britain minor epidemics of influenza are experienced every year beginning in midwinter and reaching their peak sometime between January and March. Most of the cases are due to influenza virus A and B; C virus appears to be uncommon.

(5) *The herpangina syndrome.* This is a brief illness, caused by Coxsackie A viruses, which generally affects children and is characterized by pharyngeal and sometimes oral and gingival vesicles which become punched out ulcers with congested margins. Sore throat, fever and headache may also be present.

(6) *Acute obstructive laryngotracheobronchitis* (croup syndrome). The croup syndrome is a serious condition affecting small children and characterized by cough, dyspnoea and inspiratory stridor associated with cyanosis and a variable amount of systemic upset. The illness often begins with common cold symptoms and after becoming established tends to progress rapidly to severe airways obstruction with marked use of accessory muscles and indrawing of the lower intercostal spaces on inspiration. These alarming features will generally subside almost as quickly as they arise, although a residuum of mild respiratory infection may persist for a few days. Forbes recognizes 4 stages of severity of the illness [17]. Inspiratory stridor may be succeeded by continuous stridor and in the third stage anoxia, pallor and extreme restlessness herald a 4th stage of respiratory failure with cyanosis which may compel tracheostomy. The illness may be fatal in the young child under 2 years of age [15].

The condition is most commonly due to infection with parainfluenza viruses 1 and 2, respiratory syncytical virus, adenoviruses and influenza viruses. Influenza viruses are most often met with in older children. Bacterial superinfection with haemolytic streptococci and staphylococci sometimes occurs. Treatment consists of warm humid inhalations from a steam kettle and mild sedation with chloral hydrate. A lack of response to treatment within 24 hours calls for the use of one of the tetracycline drugs or erythromycin to combat a possible secondary bacterial infection. Severe obstruction may demand tracheostomy and the earlier this is carried out the better. Usually tracheostomy is required for less than a week and if all goes well after the first day or two complete recovery may be expected.

A form of croup associated with *Haemophilus influenzae* Type B infection [1] results from supraglottic oedema due to inflammation of the epiglottis and aryepiglottic folds.

Hoarseness and aphonia which may be features of viral croup do not occur since the larynx is not primarily involved.

LABORATORY DIAGNOSIS OF VIRAL UPPER RESPIRATORY TRACT INFECTIONS

COLLECTION AND CARE OF SPECIMENS

Since the duration of excretion of some viruses is short, specimens should be taken as early as possible in the illness and conveyed to the laboratory on wet ice without delay. It cannot be overemphasized that close cooperation between clinician and virologist will ensure that the proper specimens are obtained and forwarded to the laboratory in such a way that these have the best possible chance of giving positive information. In general, nasal or pharyngeal washings are more likely to give higher yields of virus than throat swabs but the latter are more easily obtained and if taken vigorously usually prove satisfactory. For infections caused by enterovirus specimens of faeces are likely to yield more virus than rectal swabs. All swabs should be taken on a wooden stick and broken off immediately into transport medium such as Hank's BSS. Skim milk is stated to be a satisfactory alternative to transport medium [3]. Throat swabs are only of value if taken early in the disease, i.e. up to 5 days after onset, while enterovirus is detectable in the faeces for considerably longer.

The thermal stability of the different viruses varies greatly. Enteroviruses may be kept at +4°C for weeks and at −20°C almost indefinitely. Viruses such as respiratory syncytial virus and parainfluenza viruses are, however, extremely labile and are best isolated by inoculation into tissue culture either at the bedside or within an hour or so of the specimen being taken.

When specimens are taken at night they may be kept at +4°C until morning when cultures can be set up. Should there be further delay the specimens should be 'snap frozen' with a mixture of dry ice and acetone and stored at −70°C. Pharyngeal and rectal swab fluid and nasopharyngeal washings are first treated with antibiotics and then inoculated directly into tissue culture. Postmortem material and faeces are made into 10–15% suspensions then centrifuged and treated with antibiotics before inoculation into tissue culture.

VIRAL ISOLATION (table 6.3)

TISSUE CULTURE

There is no universal tissue culture for viruses. Hence it is usual for laboratories to employ 2 or 3 different culture systems. Cultures may

TABLE 6.3.

Isolation of Commoner Respiratory Viruses
(Time taken and media commonly used)

	Time	Medium
Influenza	3–21 days	Eggs: monkey kidney
Parainfluenza	3–21 days	Monkey kidney
Adenovirus	3–30 days	HeLa cells
Rhinovirus	1–2 months	Embryo kidney WI.33
R.S. virus	5–21 days	HeLa cells

be primary, continuous or semicontinuous. Primary cultures are derived directly from animal or human organs or tissues, e.g. monkey kidney (MK), human embryonic lung or kidney, human amnion, or human embryo nasal or tracheal epithelium [28 & 64]. Embryonic tissues are specially susceptible to viruses, possibly because of the absence of interferon. Most continuous cultures are heteroploid, having been derived originally from malignant tissues, e.g. HeLa and Hep 2, or from amnion or foetal lung cells. Continuous cultures can be propagated indefinitely by subculture. These are affected by many viruses and are generally the most useful form of culture because they are so readily available. The cells of semicontinuous culture systems (e.g. human embryonic fibroblasts) [23] retain the normal diploid karyotype and may be subcultured 30 to 50 times before degenerating or losing their diploid character. These cultures are very susceptible to certain picornaviruses (table 6.1). Tissue culture cells are first trypsinized and then seeded into culture tubes with an appropriate growth medium. Cell growth results in a confluent monolayer which is inoculated with the specimen. The presence of virus may be detected by direct or indirect methods.

Direct. Many viruses exert a cytopathic effect (CPE) on the nutrient cells (e.g. adenoviruses, picornaviruses) or may stimulate growth in a particular way (e.g. respiratory syncytial virus).

Indirect. When no CPE is produced virus may be detected by haemadsorption or interference phenomena. For example, myxoviruses such as influenza and parainfluenza produce little CPE on primary isolation in MK but if a dilute suspension of red cells is added to the culture these adhere to the cell surface and combine with haemagglutinating virus-specific material. This is known as haemadsorption [66].

Some viruses which produce no CPE or haemadsorption may be detected by the phenomenon of virus interference. This is the phenomenon in which a cell which supports the growth of one virus cannot support the growth of a second virus which has been added to the culture. The method was used in the early studies of rhinoviruses [27].

PLAQUE TECHNIQUES

Inoculated cell cultures may be covered with a medium containing agar so that virus can spread only from cell to cell and not through the medium. Thus replication of one viable virus particle results in plaque formation of damaged, destroyed or altered cells which gives a quantitative measure of the virus content of the inoculum. The technique is particularly useful for detection of enteroviruses. Plaques are difficult to produce with viruses such as influenza which will only multiply if a high degree of oxygenation is present such as can only be produced by rolling or shaking in a fluid overlay. The shape of the plaque produced by some viruses is characteristic and mixed viral infections may be recognized in this way.

Both direct and indirect techniques may be confirmed by serological neutralization, haem-adsorption inhibition or complement fixation tests.

SEROLOGICAL STUDIES

Viral antibodies are detected by neutralization, complement fixation or, in some cases, by haemadsorption inhibition tests. Neutralizing antibody tends to persist for prolonged periods providing a variable degree of protection against further infection. The experience of different population groups with regard to exposure to different viruses may be assessed by the detection of neutralizing antibodies. Haemadsorption inhibition tests, which are widely used to identify cultures infected with influenza and parainfluenza viruses, probably detect antibodies very closely related to those demonstrated by neutralization tests. Complement fixation tests are not always as sensitive as neutralization tests but are especially valuable in the diagnosis of respiratory infections since the antigens are easily prepared and results are quickly obtained.

The commonest clinical test for respiratory viral infections is the demonstration of a 4-fold increase in antibody titres in serum specimens taken at the outset of the illness and again 10–14 days later. This is at present impracticable for the many varieties of rhinovirus. As has already been stated, certain of the viruses may be cultured from throat washings or nasal secretions or faeces early in the disease. Rises in titre of antibodies common to antigenically related viruses, e.g. parainfluenza and mumps viruses, sometimes make it difficult to be certain of the precise aetiological agent if virus has not actually been isolated, and if the clinical features fail to differentiate the diseases.

RAPID DIAGNOSIS OF VIRAL INFECTIONS
IMMUNOFLUORESCENT TECHNIQUES

Fluorescent antibody staining of secretions is a promising development, and diagnosis of influenza and respiratory syncytial virus as well as mycoplasma and rickettsial infections has been made within 2–5 hours of obtaining specimens [25 & 39]. Specimens must be obtained early in the infection and high titre specific sera must be available in order to reduce non-specific fluorescence. The technical expertise required by these techniques is considerable.

ELECTRONMICROSCOPY

This has great possibilities for the early diagnosis of viral infections particularly since the introduction of newer techniques [53]. Generally, however, specimens must contain a large amount of virus for this technique to be useful. Thus it is of great value in such problems as smallpox. Its place in viral respiratory infection has still to be defined.

At the present stage of development the techniques available for rapid diagnosis of viral infections have not been shown to be useful in upper respiratory tract infections since respiratory viruses tend to be relatively sparse making identification of extracellular forms in respiratory secretions difficult. The technique of ultra-thin sections is still under study but may find a place in the rapid diagnosis of viral pneumonia.

THE VIROLOGY LABORATORY AND THE CLINICIAN

Lack of contact between clinicians and virologists has meant that clinical virology as a subject is practised in few places [44]. The lack of antiviral therapeutic agents is, of course, one of the important reasons for this. Others include the rather esoteric nature of virological technology which is constantly evolving and, most importantly, the fact that diagnostic procedures usually take so long to complete that results seldom influence the management of patients who are acutely ill.

Until antiviral remedies become available the diagnostic laboratory can best be used to study specific problems. Epidemiological data of great value may be obtained by investigating the rôle of different agents from year to year and in various types of communities, so defining the extent of infections and the public health problems they create. The clinician must be prepared to become increasingly involved with respiratory virology by providing well documented clinical data and the virologist must concentrate on increasing the sensitivity and speed of his diagnostic procedures.

EPIDEMIOLOGY OF UPPER RESPIRATORY TRACT INFECTIONS

Clinical epidemiology provides information about the basic patterns of upper respiratory tract infections with which the results of laboratory studies have to be matched. Precise information regarding the occurrence of acute respiratory infections in the population as a whole is difficult to obtain since there is no regular scheme of notification of the commoner infections. The Social Security surveys based on claims for sickness benefit in adults have been of little epidemiological value except in relation to epidemics of influenza which result in a sudden increase in claims [57]. Equivalent information for school children obtained from the records of school attendances gives incomplete information for similar reasons. It is, however, possible by these methods to recognize a waxing and waning of acute respiratory illnesses as a whole although the aetiological agents are not usually known precisely unless specific laboratory studies are undertaken. A method of monitoring viral respiratory infection which is becoming increasingly useful is the regular reporting to an information centre of microorganisms identified in peripheral laboratories, as has been done in Britain in recent years. Correlation with the clinical data has frequently yielded valuable information. For example, this method implicated Coxsackie B5 infection as the cause of widespread outbreaks of a variety of illnesses including respiratory symptoms, meningitis, myalgia and gastrointestinal symptoms during the summer of 1965 [47].

In Britain the return of children to school in September after the summer holidays always results in an increase in upper respiratory infections. The close contact between children in school promotes the spread of viruses and other susceptible members of the family may be affected. This upsurge of viral infection may result in exacerbation of chronic respiratory disease as a result of viruses introduced to the home by schoolchildren, but in general exacerbations of chronic bronchitis tend to occur later when fogs are more common. The early part of December is frequently a time when respiratory viral illness is less in evidence with the possible exception of respiratory syncytial infection in children, but early in the New Year it is common to have a sudden increase in acute respiratory illnesses in adults. Influenza tends to build up from endemic foci at this time [58] although peak infection is more likely in February or early March. Other viral infections occur sporadically, though sometimes in epidemics, usually small. In March–April a further wave of viral infections occurs and after this there is a fall in incidence to its lowest in July and August. The epidemiology of upper respiratory viral infections is discussed in detail by Stuart-Harris [57] and Tyrrell [65].

Although much useful information has already been gleaned, knowledge of the importance of viruses in upper respiratory tract disease as a whole is still incomplete. This applies particularly to children. Most of the children who have been studied have been sufficiently ill to be admitted to hospital or to be seen at clinics or by the family doctor. Until recently there was an important gap in knowledge concerning the large group of children with upper respiratory infections who are not ill enough to be off school or to see their doctor. An important contribution towards filling this gap has been made by Pereira and her colleagues [45]. These workers studied a well housed primary school in North West London over a period of 2 years. Any child thought to have a cold had nose and throat swabs taken. The cooperation was very good and there was a steady rate of sampling throughout the observation period. Not surprisingly there was more success in collecting specimens from the older children aged 10–11 than from the younger aged 4–5. Despite this the proportion of positive isolations (8% overall) was approximately the same in all age groups. Influenza, parainfluenza or respiratory syncytial virus was obtained from 22 illnesses and rhinoviruses from 23. Herpes simplex virus was isolated in 8 and mycoplasma pneumoniae (not strictly a virus) in 2. Of those children from whom

virus isolation was positive 50 had nasal discharge, 11 had sore throat and 22 a cough. Six children showed infection with influenza A2 but only 4 of these had mild nasal symptoms; 5 of 7 children infected with respiratory syncytial virus did not require to be off school. In all there were 59 illnesses (8%) in which a virus was isolated but in only 12 did this lead to an absence from school, usually less than 3 days. As expected, the epidemics of common infections of childhood such as measles led to waves of absence from school but, these apart, 10% of all children lost some time from school at other times in the year due to upper respiratory infection. The aggregate effect of minor upper respiratory tract infection in the child was estimated as an average of about 1–2 weeks of lost schooling per child per year. There is, of course, the additional and unmeasured problem of reduced attention and energy of children still able to be at school but with mild viral infections.

An interesting comparison can be made between the frequency of detection of viral infection in these mild cases compared to that in those investigated by similar techniques in general practice and in hospital [49]. Pereira and her colleagues found virus or other pathogen in only 8%. This contrasts with 30% detected in more serious illnesses [49]. The general pattern of virus isolation in the 2 studies was very similar and it would be reasonable to conclude that there is a smaller chance of recovering viruses from mild illnesses than from severe ones. The possible explanation that some of the illnesses might be due to bacteria rather than viruses is not supported by other work. It has been suggested that the isolation rate could be improved by using organ cultures of human respiratory epithelium to recover fastidious viruses [14]. It is also possible that paired sera tested for antibodies would have indicated a higher incidence of viral infections but this technique would have destroyed the cooperation on which the study by Pereira and her colleagues depended.

Huebner has described the environment of children as one 'shimmering with viruses' [57]. This has been supported by numerous studies. Moffet and Cramblett [43] studied all children attending a 'well baby clinic' in a low income group in North Carolina. A third of the children had colds and a few diarrhoea. The viruses found were mostly enteroviruses —Coxsackie A9, B4, ECHO 19 and others. Adenoviruses Types 1, 2, 3 or 5 were found in a third of the children. Virus was found in 54 of 303 cultures from children without symptoms and from 99 of 524 children with symptoms. There seems little doubt that most of the infection was acquired from other children, for viruses were seldom recovered from the babies' mothers. Nasal discharges probably helped the spread of some of the nonpathogenic viruses. An increasing number of adenoviruses in children from 1 to 6 months of age was thought to be related to the decline in maternal antibodies. Viruses were recovered 10 times less frequently from older children than from infants. It seemed that, although some infants had clinical illnesses due to the viruses they excreted, more commonly the viruses were present without symptoms.

The largest study of an orphan population, aged 6 to 18 months, was that by Huebner and his colleagues at Bethesda, who isolated adenoviruses, enteroviruses, parainfluenza viruses and respiratory syncytial viruses from many children [57]. Certain serotypes of enteroviruses and adenoviruses were as often recovered from well as from ill children. Most respiratory viruses, however, were isolated at times when clinical illnesses were evident. Studies in boarding schools and the armed services also show that there is a higher correlation between illness and the laboratory detection of viruses during outbreaks of acute respiratory illnesses. The fever associated with other viral infection in older children and young adults frequently leads to confusion with true influenza [57].

THE COMMON COLD

AETIOLOGY

Kruse [34] in 1914 first showed coryza could be transmitted to volunteers by the intranasal inoculation of bacteria free filtrates of the nasal secretions from a patient suffering from the disease. Dochez and his colleagues (1926–1936) extended Kruse's work in a series of carefully controlled experimental transmissions to human volunteers and chimpanzees which led to the conclusion that colds were viral infections [8, 9 & 10]. Formal proof was delayed until after the second world war when the discovery that poliovirus could be grown in cultured human kidney cells made possible the isolation of common cold viruses by similar methods, though special conditions of temperature and pH were necessary. Tyrrell and Parsons [63] cultivated viruses with cytopathic effects in human embryo tissue cultures from the nasal secretions of adults with clinical colds. These are now known as rhinoviruses which, with the enteroviruses, constitute the group picornaviruses [41].

It is now agreed that many viruses can cause the common cold, but that it is most often due to infection by *rhinoviruses*, a group which flourish at a temperature of 33°C and a pH of 6·8, approximating to the conditions found in the anterior nares. Other viruses capable of causing the common cold include parainfluenza virus 1 and 2, respiratory syncytial virus, ECHO 28 and Coxsackie A21. Indeed almost all the respiratory viruses when instilled into the nose of volunteers can give a coryzal illness.

The part played by *bacterial infection* is still debated. It has been found that the bacterial flora of the nasopharynx remains unchanged for the first few days of the illness and thereafter shows a quantitative change, with increased numbers particularly of pneumococci and *H. influenzae*. Antibiotic treatment hastens resolution of the illness (p. 104). The available evidence thus suggests that bacteria are not concerned with the genesis of the infection but that as secondary invaders they exercise an important influence on the severity and duration of the illness and on the development of complications [65].

EPIDEMIOLOGY

The complexity of the epidemiological background has been revealed by the results of serological studies and of studies based on clinical observation and statistical analysis of cases occurring in different communities. Serological studies of the important rhinovirus group show that there are at least 80 antigenically distinct strains of virus which spread slowly among the children in a community, each strain predominating for a few weeks at a time, so that a wide range of protective antibodies is not acquired until adolescence. It seems probable that, after loss of maternal antibody in the first few months of life, newly formed antibodies against rhinoviruses develop one by one in response to an infection by a series of different antigenic types [65]. Neutralizing antibody against any type is usually found in about two-thirds of adults [65]. The greatest rise in antibody titre appears to occur during adolescence [31, 51, 59 & 62]. The distribution of M rhinoviruses is world-wide [61] and they have been found even in such isolated places as Tristan da Cunha [60]. It appears that antibody responses to H rhinoviruses are smaller and do not last so long as those against M strains.

Although rhinoviruses have been recovered from all age groups at all seasons of the year they are more commonly found in patients with clinical features of coryza and in adolescents and adults, which may imply that rhinovirus infections in the very young may be 'diluted' by infections with the many other viruses which affect infants and young children. Several different strains of rhinovirus may be recovered within a relatively short space of time even in relatively confined communities [22 & 33]. Certain strains may disappear from a community only to return several years later [21],

The multiplicity of strains of rhinovirus ensures that the state of protection of an open community is never sufficient to prevent recurring outbreaks of colds. The converse is seen in a closed community; it comes to terms with its own viruses and remains free from colds so long as its isolation is maintained. In Spitzbergen, after contact with the outer world is lost at the beginning of winter, colds gradually die out only to recur again when the first boat arrives in early spring with its unintended cargo of fresh viruses ('boat cold').

Arctic explorers have been known to develop colds after unpacking stored clothes which, presumably, harboured virus. The reservoir of rhinovirus infection would not seem to be that of latent infection of the herd but a constantly moving one in the form of a continuous change of infection throughout the population. There is some evidence that apparently healthy individuals may be the means of dissemination of colds.

Clinical and statistical studies on the incidence of colds in what might be called standard communities provide information on the spread of infection within the community. In a *rural community* it is found that schoolchildren have colds 3 times more often than adults living in households with no schoolchildren, and that the presence of schoolchildren in a household doubles the number of colds suffered by the adult and preschool child members [35]. In an *urban community* adults under 30 are relatively susceptible whereas those over 40 are relatively resistant. Wives and mothers have more colds if there are children in the house. Among office workers those with colds do not very commonly infect their contacts at work; cross infection is less frequent than might have been supposed [37].

Seasonal variation in the incidence of colds is a matter of common experience. The rise in the autumn, the peak in the winter months, and the fluctuations persisting to the end of spring are all confirmed statistically. Chilling *per se* will not lead to the development of a cold in the absence of infection and does not influence the incidence of positive 'takes' in volunteers. It has been shown, however, that intranasal inoculation of virus in women at the time of ovulation results in an increased susceptibility to colds if they are simultaneously chilled [13]. This interesting observation stands in isolation for the moment since it has not been shown to have any counterpart in the natural history of the disease.

FACTORS AFFECTING THE SPREAD OF COLDS

Accurate information about the transmission of upper respiratory tract viruses is as yet fragmentary but the following facts may be listed:

(1) Noisy classrooms and overcrowding in the home are more important than direct transmission of droplet spray [46].

(2) In rural areas colds are usually introduced to the home by schoolchildren, and in crowded urban areas by pre-school-children [35].

(3) Spread in the working environment may be as much by those with subclinical colds or by fomites as by people with obvious colds.

(4) The highest attack rate is at age 2–4 when there are several children in the family and at age 5–6 when an only child first goes to school. The incidence falls sharply after age 7 and again in later life over 40. To some extent this may be a matter of exposure since volunteers appear to be experimentally susceptible at all ages.

(5) Although the most important aetiological agents are the rhinoviruses, the myxoviruses are common causes of colds in adults and often cause lower respiratory tract disease in children. The myxoviruses spread very effectively among children [5, 32 & 56]. Respiratory syncytial and parainfluenza 3 viruses probably affect all children in the first year or two and parainfluenza 1 and 2 attack most of them a few years later. Parainfluenza 3 appears to be present in communities most of the year but parainfluenza 1 and respiratory syncytial virus cause sharp winter outbreaks. Respiratory syncytial virus is recognized clinically because it causes bronchiolitis in infants.

(6) It is not known if viruses survive between epidemics by affecting a few people all the time or by persisting in symptomless carriers. It is certain that some children continue to shed parainfluenza 3 virus for a long time but family outbreaks of illness with the parainfluenza viruses do not last much longer than those associated with rhinoviruses. Adenovirus and enterovirus infections cause prolonged family outbreaks of respiratory disease and the virus is discharged for many weeks, particularly in the faeces.

(7) Respiratory viruses associated with colds spread easily throughout the world. This explains the fact that antibodies to these viruses are detected as commonly in tropical as in temperate areas of the world [11 & 61]. It also explains why young students coming from tropical areas to Britain have no more colds than British students [48].

(8) Studies in the Common Cold Research Unit in Salisbury with Coxsackie A21 virus which causes colds show that an infected individual has a 1 in 5 chance of infecting his closest contacts. Virus is present in high concentration only at the outset, with a greater concentration in nasal secretions than in pharyngeal secretions and saliva. The amount of virus expelled during talking and coughing is small and although sneezing and blowing the nose disperse large amounts of infected material nearly all of it falls to the floor or is retained in the handkerchief and only an estimated 0.1% is in the form of airborne droplets capable of spreading infection by inhalation. Even this small amount of virus is unstable and is rapidly inactivated. Moreover, nasal secretions expelled during sneezing and blowing the nose are soon dispersed in the air and are, therefore, effective only at a very short range. Volunteers can be infected by this means if they inhale the suspended droplets through the nose but infection is much less easily achieved if the droplets are only allowed to reach the throat or the conjunctiva.

(9) The manner in which seasonal and climatic factors affect the incidence of colds is not clear but a correlation between a fall in temperature and the onset of colds 2 or 3 days later has been established and a relation to humidity is regarded as probable [38]. It is still uncertain whether or not the dissemination, survival or uptake of virus is influenced by temperature changes and whether or not a fall in temperature makes subclinical infection manifest.

PATHOLOGICAL EFFECTS OF COLDS

Since colds are rarely fatal, there is a dearth of postmortem studies of the nasopharyngeal epithelium in this condition. Nevertheless, the effects of viruses on ciliated epithelium had been studied long before precise information about the causative agents was available. In 1930 Hilding examined the nasal epithelium in colds by scrapings, biopsies and smears of nasal secretions [26]. An initial oedema was followed by shedding of columnar epithelial cells which was almost complete by the third day leaving only the cells in the deepest layer from which regeneration occurred over a fortnight. Similar changes were later reported in experimental infection of ferrets with influenza virus [18] and in natural and experimental colds using more modern staining techniques [4 & 30]. Organ cultures of nasal epithelium infected with rhinoviruses have shown focal rather than general destruction of ciliated epithelium [65].

Although there is no animal model for study of the pathical effects of rhinoviruses a close approximation is the ferret infected with respiratory syncytial virus which causes a virtually asymptomatic infection in this animal. Coates and Chanock observed increase in number and progressive distention of goblet cells in the nasal epithelium between the 2nd and 6th day after infection [6]. Desquamation of superficial cells occurred in a patchy fashion and by the 5th day multinucleate cells containing eosinophil inclusions were seen, resembling those found in tissue cultures. Coincidentally there was disorganization of the submucosa and infiltration with lymphocytes and polymorphs. Complete restoration of the epithelium took 1 month. Infection with respiratory syncytial virus and parainfluenza viruses in man probably follow a similar pathological pattern.

CLINICAL FEATURES

Experimental studies in volunteers have shown that the incubation period is 2–3 days for rhinoviruses and about 4 days for respiratory syncytial virus and parainfluenza viruses. There is little difference clinically between colds due to the different viruses. The duration of the common cold is extremely variable. The systemic upset, sneezing and sore throat seldom last for more than 1 or 2 days but nasal discharge and cough sometimes persist for 3 weeks or even longer. Extension of the infection beyond the nasopharynx is common, giving rise to sinusitis, otitis media, bronchitis or pneumonia. These complications are due to secondary bacterial infection of tissues already damaged by the viral infection and they usually resolve promptly under treatment with appropriate antibiotics. An attack of the common cold may exacerbate chronic infections of sinuses, middle ear and bronchi, and in patients with chronic heart disease may be enough to precipitate heart failure.

The Common Cold Research Unit, Salisbury have graded the severity of colds in volunteers into 4 groups:

(1) *Abortive colds*. In this group the respiratory symptoms are so slight and transient as to be scarcely recognizable except in experimental conditions.

(2) *Mild colds*. Here nasal secretion and upper respiratory symptoms do occur but subside within 2 to 4 days. Systemic upset is rare.

(3) *Moderate colds*. In addition to local symptoms systemic upset occurs—headache, malaise, perhaps fever, shivering and sweating—and symptoms last longer, up to 1 week.

(4) *Severe colds*. Marked respiratory symptoms, mainly nasal but frequently cough, are linked with systemic upset which may be sufficiently severe to warrant bed rest.

The presence or absence of fever may also be used to grade the severity of colds.

DIFFERENTIAL DIAGNOSIS

The diagnosis of colds rarely presents difficulty. Paroxysmal rhinorrhoea of the seasonal or perennial variety may be mistaken for the features of coryza but progression to purulent infection of the nasopharynx does not occur and precipitating factors (grass pollen in hay fever; dusts, fumes, atmospheric changes, etc. in perennial rhinorrhoea) may be recognized. The onset of measles may be confused with a cold but the true diagnosis will soon be apparent.

PREVENTION

A strictly maintained isolation of cases would doubtless prevent dissemination of the infection but it is seldom practicable. The face masks worn on occasion by hospital staff, nursing mothers and others may serve to remind those concerned of the source of infection but probably do little to reduce the dissemination of virus. The use of antiseptic aerosols [36] and ultraviolet radiation in offices and classrooms fails to reduce the incidence of colds. Antiviral vaccines to be useful must be specific for the infecting strain of virus and no vaccine effective against all the strains of all the upper respiratory tract viruses has yet been, or is likely to be, prepared.

TREATMENT

The prevalence of secondary bacterial infection has prompted studies of the prophylactic use of antibiotics given at the outset of the illness. Ritchie [50] reported a significant reduction in the duration of symptoms following the use of autogenous vaccine and, in another series, the administration of tetracycline (15 mg twice a day in a lozenge for 3 days at the beginning of prodromal symptoms). The latter has been confirmed in a further trial [40]. Present opinion favours restricting the prophylactic use of antibiotics to patients at special risk because of cardiac or respiratory disease. There is no dispute about the wisdom of giving antibiotics when complications develop.

It is known that mycoplasmal organisms are capable of causing an illness indistinguishable from the common cold and if this illness were known to be prevalent tetracycline, or one of its analogues, would be the drug of choice. At the present time, however, the place of mycoplasmal infection in this and other fields is still under investigation.

Ciliary activity is already impaired in the common cold and local vasoconstrictors are, if anything, likely to delay healing. The same objection applies to medicated inhalations. If, however, nasal blockage or the features of Eustachian or sinus catarrh are prominent vasoconstrictor nasal sprays or drops and inhalations of menthol or tinct.benz.co. may give temporary symptomatic relief.

In general it is advisable to keep children in a warm atmosphere, or in bed if ill, until the acute phase subsides. Whether an adult should remain off work will be decided by the amount of systemic upset and whether or not complications have developed. He should at least aim at getting to bed early while symptoms persist.

Although certain substances are now known which can specifically prevent the multiplication of many of the viruses which cause colds none is sufficiently developed for general use. The present status of specific treatment of respiratory viruses is reviewed by Tyrrell [65].

INFLUENZA

Influenza is a highly infectious disease of the respiratory tract caused by the influenza group of myxoviruses of which there are 3 varieties—A, B and C influenza viruses. It is endemic in all countries but epidemic outbreaks due to either A or B virus tend to occur irregularly, and pandemics due to virus A approximately every 30 years. The outbreaks are precipitated by the emergence of mutant forms of the viruses with altered antigenic components. Mutational change of this sort is common among the influenza viruses and accounts in part for the spread of the disease in a supposedly immune population. The pandemics are the ultimate expression of this property. The last three pandemics were in 1957–58, 1918–19 and 1889–92 but earlier visitations are recorded and influenza takes its name from its cyclical recurrence of pandemics which suggested to 17th century observers the 'influence' of the stars.

In epidemic influenza the attack rate is usually less than in the pandemic variety; the illness is commonly less severe and complications are less frequent and less serious except in those with chronic respiratory or cardiac disease. Characteristically influenza occurs explosively and the rapidity of spread is such that all the members of a household may become ill during a single week. This is a distinctive feature; few virus diseases can compete with influenza in rapidity of spread. Transference of the virus from person to person is presumed to occur in the same way as it does in colds.

THE EPIDEMIOLOGY OF INFLUENZA

Influenza A virus was discovered in 1933, influenza B in 1940 and influenza C in 1947. Influenza A virus was first identified in 1933 when nasopharyngeal washings from patients with clinical influenza in Britain were shown to produce a mild febrile disease when inoculated into ferrets intranasally [54]. The virus could be transmitted serially in ferrets and could be passed to mice in which it produced a more severe illness [2]. It was found that the virus of swine influenza produced similar effects in ferrets and mice. An antigenic similarity between the human and swine influenza virus seemed probable on the basis of immunity studies in the ferret. So far as human influenza was concerned it was shown that the virus alone could result in the classical clinical picture in volunteers and the long held belief that *H. influenzae* was aetiologically related was disproved [55].

Influenza B was detected during an epidemic in New York in 1940 [19] and was shown to have no serological relationship with any of the virus strains previously recognized. In 1946 a variant of A virus termed A1 appeared and spread rapidly over the world in 1947. Influenza C was first recovered in 1947 [58].

Thus the original influenza A was displaced in 1946–47 by an antigenically distinct strain (A1) which caused outbreaks of influenza of varying severity all over the world until 1957 when the first strains of another variant of the A family were recovered in the Kwei-Chow Province of South-East China. This new virus which was designated Asian or A2 virus was responsible for the pandemic which swept the world in 1957–58. Since then influenza A outbreaks have all been with the A2 virus and, from previous experience, it is expected that this virus will persist for several years yet.

Influenza B infection has usually resulted in moderate epidemics only and the mortality has always been much less than from influenza A. There is antigenic diversity in the B virus family but the various serotypes have not been accurately classified. C virus has only been recovered from sporadic cases or found incidentally during influenza A epidemics

[20]. Only one serotype is known and unlike viruses A and B is not thought to be a cause of epidemic respiratory illness [7].

There is some evidence that when a new antigenic strain of influenza virus displaces another, pockets of infection due to the earlier virus may persist for a few years [29].

It has never been possible to foretell the antigenic variation on which the effects of influenza virus infection depend. Serological studies with swine virus antibodies have given indirect evidence that the 1918 epidemic may have been due to a virus identical with that causing swine influenza in later years and first recovered by Shope in America [52]. This modern counterpart of the Gadarene swine is still, however, a theoretical concept and only time will tell the true relationship of pig influenza to the human form of the disease. The evidence is reviewed in detail by Stuart-Harris [57].

PATHOGENESIS AND PATHOLOGY

The inhaled influenza virus adheres to and invades respiratory epithelial cells whose metabolic processes it utilizes for the production of more virus. Whether the infected cells survive or succumb depends on the extent to which their metabolism is deranged in serving the ends of virus proliferation. Such, in fact, is the nature of 'virulence' in virus infection. The more virulent the virus the greater the amount of epithelial cell destruction and the more severe the pathological lesions and clinical manifestations. The pathological changes begin with sloughing of the damaged epithelium in the trachea and bronchi, accompanied by local congestion and fluid exudation. Bacterial infection of denuded surfaces and of the fluid and cellular débris blocking the bronchioles often occurs and is the main factor in determining the subsequent course of events.

While the epithelial lesions in the trachea and bronchi in influenza are similar to those found in the experimental animal [67], the lesions in the lungs are not so easy to interpret because of the effect of secondary bacterial invasion. That fatal influenzal pneumonia can occur without associated bacterial infection was demonstrated during the 1957–58 epidemic [24]. Alveolar cells were shown to undergo cytopathic changes and there was capillary thrombosis, necrosis of capillary walls and serous exudation into alveoli. In patients who survived longer, evidence of regeneration of the epithelium was demonstrated in alveoli and in respiratory bronchioles. The response to antibacterial chemotherapy, however, shows that bacteria most commonly determine the severity and the outcome of the disease.

H. influenzae, the commonest bacterial invader in the ordinary case of influenza, produces little more than a general worsening of the lesions. The Group A beta haemolytic streptococcus which was the cause of many deaths from pneumonia and empyema in the 1918 pandemic is seldom encountered today, and streptococcal lesions when they occur tend to be much less severe than those of the pandemic cases. *Staphylococcus pyogenes* was the principal bacterial invader in the 1957 pandemic and is still the commonest cause of bacterial complications in severe cases of influenza. Infection of the denuded epithelial surfaces by *Staphylococcus pyogenes* leads to a combination of inflammation and necrosis so that the affected areas are covered by a membranous slough. More or less uniform involvement of the mucosa may occur from larynx to bronchi (laryngotracheobronchitis) or one region may be more severely affected than another (tracheitis, p. 108, bronchitis or bronchiolitis, p. 108). Aspiration of infected material into the alveoli leads to staphylococcal pneumonia (p. 121). Some of the patients who survived staphylococcal pneumonia during the 1957–58 pandemic have been left with some degree of bronchiectasis and tend to suffer from respiratory symptoms during the winter months.

CLINICAL FEATURES

After a short incubation period of about 48 hours the classical case of influenza begins abruptly with malaise, chills, fever, headache and a slight cough. These symptoms are soon followed by generalized muscular aches, marked prostration, anorexia and sometimes vomiting. The clinical picture is dominated by the constitutional disturbance with nothing more than slight nasal obstruction and mild sore throat to point to respiratory involvement. The face is flushed, the conjunctivae reddened and the pharynx may show slight injection. In the average uncomplicated case the fever subsides in 2–4 days and the other symptoms rapidly follow suit, except perhaps the cough which may persist and become productive, with sputum which provides evidence of secondary bacterial infection. The younger the patient the less definite the clinical picture. Small children may appear only to have a bad cold, older children only a bad sore throat; in a single family common cold, sore throat, pharyngitis, tracheitis and croup may result from infection by the same influenza virus. Convalescence is not protracted except in the middle aged or elderly and in those with chronic respiratory or cardiac disease. Postinfluenzal depression is a recognized entity, but varies greatly in degree and is seldom serious. Loss of the sense of smell may rarely be a permanent residuum. Patients with residual lower respiratory tract infection, as indicated by the presence of rhonchi or crepitations on auscultation, may continue to have cough and expectoration throughout convalescence. Not infrequently an initial febrile incident subsides and the patient improves temporarily only to have a recurrence of symptoms. Relapse may be related to the development of secondary bacterial infection.

Variable symptoms include epistaxis, which is relatively more common in children, aching of the eyes on movement or photophobia, dizziness and insomnia. Meningism and diarrhoea are uncommon and should suggest other diagnoses.

The development of necrotizing laryngotracheobronchitis may result in a dramatic worsening of the illness with extreme respiratory distress and cyanosis. Patients with this complication may sometimes require emergency bronchoscopy to clear the airways and tracheostomy may be necessary to keep them clear.

The development of influenzal pneumonia is usually sudden. The details are dealt with elsewhere (p. 129) but mention should be made of the most serious complications affecting the circulatory system which include peripheral circulatory failure, pericarditis and myocarditis.

OTHER COMPLICATIONS OF INFLUENZA

Lesions outside the respiratory tract are uncommon but among the rare complications may be mentioned sinusitis, otitis media, encephalopathy, organic dementia, pericarditis and cardiac arrhythmia. Sinusitis and otitis media occurring during influenza are more likely to be due to recrudescence of chronic infection than to primary bacterial infection. Organic dementia occurs at the height of the illness and need not occasion undue alarm since complete recovery is the rule. Cardiac arrhythymia usually takes the form of auricular fibrillation in elderly patients with ischaemic heart disease.

DIFFERENTIAL DIAGNOSIS

In epidemics and pandemics the diagnosis is usually obvious. At other times it may be a matter of conjecture for it is seldom practicable to set in train the laboratory investigations necessary to prove that the short pyrexial illness was due to infection by influenza virus. More important than a precise virological diagnosis is a recognition of bacterial superinfection, for the antibiotic plan of campaign must be based on the knowledge of what organisms are present.

In order to exclude complications of influenza or alternative primary disease a chest radiograph should be taken if symptoms persist for more than a week. Serious pulmonary disease, particularly tuberculosis and carcinoma, may masquerade as 'recurrent influenza'—a diagnosis which should never be accepted without question.

PREVENTION

Antiviral vaccine must be specific for the particular organism causing the epidemic or pandemic if it is to be effective. If the antigenic constitution of the virus can be determined sufficiently early (e.g. as in 1957 when the pandemic began in the Far East and took some weeks to spread westwards) an antiviral vaccine is a valuable protective measure with an efficacy of around 60%. While it is generally agreed that those at special risk by virtue of chronic disease, or members of the Health Services, should be offered vaccine if there is sufficient forewarning of a pandemic, there seems little chance that epidemic influenza will be prevented in a community unless the whole of the susceptible population is immunized. An attempt at the latter may be justifiable in pandemics with high attack rates.

The duration of protection with inactivated vaccines is short and continued prophylaxis requires annual inoculation. The Ministry of Health Advisory Committee [42] recommend patients with chronic pulmonary, heart and renal disease, and certain other debilitating illnesses such as diabetes, as suitable for annual inoculation with saline vaccine. Experience with oil adjuvant vaccine is insufficient to define the duration of protection; it is possible that reinoculation may only be required every 3 or 4 years [57].

Attempts to develop effective live influenza vaccines have met difficulties due to the fact that passage of virus in the laboratory leads to overattenuation and loss of immunogenicity. This applies particularly to A virus [68]. Apart from vaccination there are no means at present available for control of the disease.

Infection of man from animal reservoirs has not been proved but remains a possibility (p. 105). It is also possible that new strains may emerge as a result of hybridization in nature between human and animal strains. There may be some significance in the fact that B viruses, which are much less common in the animal kingdom than A viruses, show considerably less antigenic variation [68]. The monitoring of influenza virus strain variation by virological laboratories throughout the world is likely to prove valuable in forecasting future pandemics.

TREATMENT

The uncomplicated case needs only supportive treatment. Some will be appropriately treated by simple remedies, such as aspirin and a hot drink. Cough may be treated with a suppressant drug such as pholcodine and insomnia by an appropriate hypnotic. Antibiotics are probably unnecessary unless there is a history of otitis media or lower respiratory tract infection but if pus appears in the sputum an oral antibiotic such as tetracycline or erythromycin (0·25 g 6-hourly) may be given. Early administration of antibiotics and admission to hospital may be necessary when there are severe respiratory complications. The treatment of influenzal staphylococcal pneumonia is described elsewhere (p. 138).

ACUTE TRACHEITIS AND BRONCHITIS

AETIOLOGY

Pyogenic infection of the trachea and bronchi is a common complication of the upper respiratory tract viral syndromes, in particular coryza and influenza, and regularly accompanies more severe attacks of measles and whooping cough. Apart from these infections the commonest cause of acute bronchitis is exacerbation of chronic bronchitis. The common infecting organisms are the *pneumococcus* and *Haemophilus influenzae*. *Staphylococcus pyogenes* may be the invader when the condition complicates influenza.

In children recurrent acute bronchitis may rarely be a manifestation of mucoviscidosis (p. 592) or hypogammaglobulinaemia (p. 140).

CLINICAL FEATURES

Superimposed on the features of the primary illness an irritating dry cough associated with retrosternal soreness or even pain indicates the development of tracheitis. Atmospheric changes such as moving from a warm atmosphere to a cold one exaggerate the symptoms. Tracheitis produces no abnormal physical signs in the lungs but with extension of infection to the bronchi the features of airways obstruction become evident in the form of bilateral rhonchi of low or medium pitch, with occasional coarse crepitations. With further extension to the finer bronchi or even alveoli the rhonchi become progressively

more high pitched and crepitations more predominant.

Involvement of the bronchi is associated with the development of tightness in the chest, wheezy respiration and variable dyspnoea. The sputum usually becomes mucopurulent and occasionally is flecked with blood. The further the progression down the respiratory tract the greater the systemic upset and the more severe the symptoms. The clinical range extends from a mild afebrile disturbance with cough and upper chest discomfort lasting a day or two to a severe illness characterized by fever, polymorph leucocytosis, dyspnoea and cyanosis, indicating bronchiolitis or lobular pneumonia. Severe illness occurs mainly among the very young, the very old, the debilitated and those with chronic bronchitis. An acute exacerbation of bronchitis or pneumonia is the commonest factor precipitating congestive cardiac failure in the chronic bronchitic.

DIFFERENTIAL DIAGNOSIS

The diagnosis is seldom in doubt particularly when the clinical picture is fully developed. Rarely bronchial carcinoma with glandular involvement encroaching on both main bronchi may present with features similar to those of acute bronchitis. Pulmonary tuberculosis may also occasionally masquerade as recurrent acute bronchitis. The chest radiograph distinguishes both of these conditions from acute bronchitis in which there are no abnormal radiographic features.

TREATMENT

When infection is confined to the trachea the avoidance of temperature change in the surroundings and the use of a simple cough sedative containing codeine, pholcodine or methadone may suffice. In cases of acute bronchitis with purulent sputum antibiotic treatment should be begun early, particularly if it is known that chronic heart or lung disease is also present. In these patients tetracycline 0·25 g to 0·5 g 4 times daily or a combination of penicillin 1 mega unit twice daily along with streptomycin sulphate 1 g twice daily may be given for a 7 day course or, alternatively, ampicillin 0·25 g 4 times daily. Inhalations from a steam kettle may have a very soothing effect particularly in the young child or in the adult with viscid secretions which are difficult to cough up. Broncho-spasm accompanying acute bronchitis may justify the use of bronchodilator drugs and, in the severe case, a short course of predniso-lone.

Severe acute bronchiolitis in children is usually caused by respiratory syncytial virus. Hypoxia rapidly develops and oxygen is the principal treatment, together with attention to fluid and acid–base balance.

The appearance of the sputum is the best guide to the efficacy of antibiotic treatment in acute bronchitis. If the sputum is still purulent after 7 days of treatment it means that the antibiotic in use is ineffective and should be changed [12]. Before doing so the sputum should be examined bacteriologically to make sure that the pus is not due to a new infection by organisms such as *Staphylococcus pyogenes* or *Klebsiella pneumoniae* for which specific antibiotic treatment will be required; nonpathogenic bacteria, even if resistant to the antibiotic in use, should be ignored.

REFERENCES

[1] ALEXANDER H.E., ELLIS C. & LEIDY D. (1942) Treatment of type-specific *Haemophilus influenzae* infections in infancy and childhood. *J. Paediat.* 20, 673.

[2] ANDREWES C.H., LAIDLAW P.P. & SMITH W. (1934) The susceptibility of mice to the viruses of human and swine influenza. *Lancet* ii, 859.

[3] BANATVALA J.E. (1967) Advances in virology. *Proc. roy. Soc. Med.* 60, 637.

[4] BRYAN W.T.K. & BRYAN M.P. (1953) Structural changes in the ciliated epithelial cells during the common cold. *Trans. Am. Acad. Ophthal. Otolaryng.* 57, 247.

[5] CHANOCK R.M., PARROTT R.H., JOHNSON K.M. KAPIANA Z. & BELL J.A. (1963). Myxoviruses: parainfluenza. *Am. Rev. resp. Dis.* 88, 152.

[6] COATES H.V. & CHANOCK R.M. (1962) Experimental infection with respiratory syncytial virus in several species of animals. *Am. J. Hyg.* 76, 302.

[7] DeMEIO J.L., WOOLRIDGE R.L., WHITESIDE J.E. & SEAL J.R. (1955) Epidemic influenza B and C in navy recruits 1953–54. II. Antigenic studies on influenza type C. *Proc. Soc. exp. Biol.* (*N.Y.*) 88, 436.

[8] DOCHEZ A.R., SHIBLEY G.S. & MILLS K.C. (1930) Studies in common cold; experimental transmission of common cold to anthropod apes and human beings by means of filtrable agent. *J. exp. Med.* 52, 701.

[9] DOCHEZ A.R., MILLS K.C. & KNEELAND Y.Jr. (1931) Study of virus of common cold and its cultivation in tissue medium. *Proc. Soc. exp. Biol.* (*N.Y.*) 28, 513.

[10] DOCHEZ A.R., MILLS K.C. & KNEELAND Y.Jr. (1936) Studies on common cold; cultivation of virus in tissue medium. *J. exp. Med.* 63, 559.

[11] DOGGETT J.E. (1965) Antibodies to respiratory syncytial virus in human sera from different regions of the world. *Bull. Wld. Hlth Org.* 32 849.

[12] DOUGLAS A.C., SOMNER A.R., MARKS B.L. & GRANT I.W.B. (1957) Effect of antibiotics on purulent sputum. *Lancet* ii, 214.

[13] DOWLING H.F., JACKSON G.G. & INOUYE T. (1957) Transmission of the experimental common cold in volunteers. II. The effect of certain host factors upon susceptibility. *J. Lab. clin. Med.* 50, 516.

[14] Editorial (1968) Sniffly schoolchildren. *Br. med. J.* i, 400.

[15] EMERY J.L. (1952) Acute laryngo-tracheo-bronchitis in children. *Br. med. J.* ii, 1067.

[16] ENDERS G.F., WELLER T.H. & ROBBINS F.C. (1949) Cultivation of the Lansing strain of poliomyelitis virus in cultures of various human embryonic tissues. *Science* 109, 225.

[17] FORBES G.A. (1961) Croup and its management. *Br. med. J.* i, 389.

[18] FRANCIS T.Jr. & STUART-HARRIS C.H. (1938) Studies on nasal histology of epidemic influenza virus infection in ferret; development and repair of nasal lesion. *J. exp. Med.* 68, 789.

[19] FRANCIS T.Jr. (1940) A new type of virus from epidemic influenza. *Science* 92, 405.

[20] FRANCIS T.Jr., QUILLIGAN J.J.Jr. & MINUSE E. (1950) Identification of another epidemic respiratory disease. *Science* 112, 495.

[21] HAMRE D. & PROCKNOW J.J. (1961) Virological studies on acute respiratory disease in young adults. I. Isolation of ECHO 28. *Proc. Soc. exp. Biol.* (*N.Y.*) 107, 770.

[22] HAMRE D. & PROCKNOW J.J. (1963) Virological studies on common colds among young adult medical students. *Am. Rev. resp. Dis.* 88, Part 2, 277.

[23] HAYFLOCK L. & MOORHEAD P.S. (1961). The serial cultivation of human diploid cell lines. *Exp. Cell. Res.* 25, 585.

[24] HERS J.F.Ph. MASUREL N. & MULDER J. (1958) Bacteriology and histopathology of the respiratory tract and lungs in fatal Asian influenza. *Lancet* ii, 1141.

[25] HERS J.F.Ph. (1963) Fluorescent antibody

technique in respiratory virus diseases. *Am. Rev. resp. Dis.* **88**, Part 2, 316.

[26] HILDING A. (1930) Common cold. *Arch. Otolaryng.* **12**, 133.

[27] HITCHCOCK T. & TYRRELL D.A.J. (1960) Some virus isolations from common colds. II. Virus interference in tissue cultures. *Lancet* i, 237.

[28] HOORN B. & TYRRELL D.A.J. (1966) A new virus cultivated only in organ cultures of human ciliated epithelium. *Arch. ges. Virusforsch.* **18**, 210.

[29] ISAACS A., HART R.J.C. & LAW V.G. (1962) Influenza viruses 1957–60. *Bull. Wld Hlth Org.* **26**, 253.

[30] JACKSON G.G., DOWLING H.F., ANDERSON I.O., RIFF L., SAPORTA J. & TURK M. (1960) Susceptibility and immunology to common upper respiratory viral infections—the common cold. *Ann. intern. Med.* **53**, 719.

[31] JOHNSON K.M. & ROSEN L. (1963) Characteristics of five newly recognized enteroviruses recovered from the human oropharynx. *Am. J. Hyg.* **77**, 15.

[32] KAPIKIAN A.Z. (1961) An outbreak of febrile illness and pneumonia associated with respiratory syncytial virus infection. *Am. J. Hyg.* **74**, 234.

[33] KENDALL E.J.C., BYNOE M.L. & TYRRELL D.A.J. (1962) Virus isolations from common colds occurring in a residential school. *Br. med. J.* ii, 82.

[34] KRUSE W. (1914) Die Erreger von Husten und Schnupfen. *Münch. med. Wschr.* **61**, 1547.

[35] LIDWELL O.M. & SOMMERVILLE T. (1951) Observations on the incidence and distribution of the common cold in a rural community during 1948 and 1949. *J. Hyg. (Lond.)* **49**. 365.

[36] LIDWELL O.M. & WILLIAMS R.E.O. (1954) Trial of hexylresorcinol as air disinfectant for prevention of colds in office workers. *Br. med. J.* ii, 959.

[37] LIDWELL O.M. & WILLIAMS R.E.O. (1961) The epidemiology of the common cold. I and II. *J. Hyg. (Lond.)* **59**, 309, 321.

[38] LIDWELL O.M., MORGAN R.W. & WILLIAMS R.E.O. (1965) The epidemiology of the common cold. IV. The effect of weather. *J. Hyg. (Lond.)* **63**, 427.

[39] LIU C.E. (1956) Rapid diagnosis of human influenza infection from nasal smears by means of fluorescein-labelled antibody. *Proc. Soc. exp. Biol. (N.Y.)* **92**, 883.

[40] McKERROW C.B., OLDHAM P.D. & THOMSON S. (1961) Antibiotics and the common cold. *Lancet* i, 185.

[41] MELNICK J.L., COCKBURN W.C., DALLDORF G., GARD S., GEAR J.H.S., HAMMON W.McD., KAPLAN M.M., NAGLER F.B., OKER-BLOM N., RHODES A.J., SABIN A.B., VERLINDE J.B. & VON MAGNUS H. (1963) Picornavirus group. *Virology* **19**, 114.

[42] Ministry of Health Advisory Committee (1963).

[43] MOFFET H.L. & CRAMBLETT H.G. (1962). Viral isolations and illnesses in young infants attending a well-baby clinic. *New Engl. J. Med.* **267**, 1213.

[44] OSWALD N.C. (1967) Clinician's approach to respiratory viruses. *Br. med. J.* **3**, 35.

[45] PEREIRA M.S., ANDREWS B.E. & GARDNER S.B. (1967) A study on the virus aetiology of mild respiratory infections in the primary school child. *J. Hyg. (Lond.)* **65**, 475.

[46] REID D.D. (1958). Environmental factors in respiratory disease. *Lancet* i, 1237.

[47] Report to the Director of the Public Health Laboratory Service from various laboratories in the United Kingdom (1967). Coxsackie B5 virus infections during 1965. *Br. med. J.* **4**, 575.

[48] Report to the Medical Research Council's Committee on the Aetiology of Chronic Bronchitis (1964). An investigation into the differences in respiratory illness in overseas and United Kingdom students. *Br. J. prev. soc. Med.* **18**, 174.

[49] Report of the Medical Research Council Working Party (1965) A collaborative study of the aetiology of acute respiratory infection in Britain 1961–64. *Br. med. J.* ii, 319.

[50] RITCHIE J.M. (1958) Antibiotics in small doses for the common cold. *Lancet* i, 615, 618.

[51] SCHILD J.C. & HOBSON D. (1962) Neutralizing antibody levels in human sera with the HGP and B632 strains of common cold virus. *Br. J. exp. Path.* **43**, 288.

[52] SHOPE R.E. (1931) Swine influenza III. Filtration experiments and aetiology. *J. exp. Med.* **54**, 373.

[53] SMITH K.O. & MELNICK J.L. (1962) Recognition and quantitation of herpesvirus particles in human vesicular lesions. *Science* **137**, 543.

[54] SMITH W., ANDREWES C.H. & LAIDLAW P.P. (1933) A virus obtained from influenza patients. *Lancet* ii, 68.

[55] SMITH W. & STUART-HARRIS C.H. (1936) Influenza infection of man from the ferret. *Lancet* ii, 121.

[56] STARK J.E., HEALTH R.B. & PETO S. (1964) A study of the antibodies against parainfluenza viruses in children's sera. *Arch. ges. Virusforsch.* **14**, 160.

[57] STUART-HARRIS C.H. (1965) *Influenza and Other Virus Infections of the Respiratory Tract*, 2nd Edition. London, Arnold.

[58] TAYLOR, R.M. (1949) Studies on survival of influenza virus between epidemics and antigenic virulence of the virus. *Am. J. pub. Hlth* **39**, 171.

[59] TAYLOR-ROBINSON D. & TYRRELL D.A.J. (1962) Serological studies on some viruses isolated from common colds. *Br. J. exp. Path.* **43**, 264.

[60] TAYLOR-ROBINSON, D. & TYRRELL D.A.J.

(1963) Virus diseases on Tristan da Cunha. *Trans. roy. Soc. trop. Med. Hyg.* **57**, 19.

[61] TAYLOR-ROBINSON D. (1965) Respiratory virus antibodies in human sera from different regions of the world. *Bull. Wld Hlth Org.* **32**, 833.

[62] TYRRELL D.A.J. & BYNOE M.L. (1958) Inoculation of volunteers with J.H. strain of new respiratory virus. *Lancet* **ii**, 931.

[63] TYRRELL D.A.J. & PARSONS R. (1960) Some Virus isolations from common colds. III. Cytopathic effects in tissue cultures. *Lancet* **i**, 239.

[64] TYRRELL D.A.J. & BYNOE M.L. (1965) Cultiva-tion of a novel type of common cold virus in organ cultures. *Br. med. J.* **i**, 1467.

[65] TYRRELL D.A.J. (1965) *Common Colds and Related Diseases.* London, Arnold.

[66] Vogel J. & SHELOKOV A. (1957) Adsorption-haemagglutination test for influenza virus in monkey tissue cultures. *Science* **126**, 358.

[67] WALCH D.J., DIETLIEN L.F., LOW F.N., BURCH G.E. & MOGABGAB W.J. (1961) Bronchotrach-eal response in human influenza. *Arch. intern. Med.* **108**, 376.

[68] World Health Organization Chronicle (1967) Vaccines against viral diseases **21**, 95.

CHAPTER 7

Pneumonia

DEFINITION

As commonly used, the term 'pneumonia' indicates an inflammation, in general acute, of the substance of the lungs. The term 'pneumonitis' is synonymous, though it has been most often applied to mild segmental pneumonia; it is best avoided. Clinically a diagnosis of pneumonia depends either on the detection of physical signs or of radiological evidence of consolidation.

CLASSIFICATION AND AETIOLOGY OF PNEUMONIA

Although lobar consolidation is most commonly pneumococcal any anatomical type of pneumonia can on occasion be produced by virtually any of the established aetiological agents. Diagnosis should therefore be both aetiological and anatomical. One should speak, for instance, of a pneumococcal or staphylococcal lobar pneumonia, a segmental pneumonia due to psittacosis virus, or of a staphylococcal lobular pneumonia complicating viral influenza.

ANATOMICAL CLASSIFICATION

It is convenient to classify pneumonias into
 (1) lobar
 (2) segmental
 (3) lobular which, when it is bilateral, is often termed 'bronchopneumonia'.

AETIOLOGICAL CLASSIFICATION

THE DETERMINATION OF AETIOLOGICAL AGENTS

Most pneumonias are due to infective agents, though chemical or allergic pneumonias can occur. Certain aetiological agents are well established as causes of pneumonia, others are uncertain or rare. The isolation of a viral or bacterial species from a patient's sputum does not necessarily mean that that species is the cause of the pneumonia. This is particularly true of *H. influenzae* or *E. coli* in adults or of enteroviruses in children. It is uncertain whether the ordinary commensals of the upper respiratory tract can on occasion cause a pneumonia. The purulent phase of the common cold is probably due to proliferation of the common commensals, especially *N. catarrhalis* and *Str. viridans* [83]. Some pneumonias, especially in the debilitated, the elderly or those with preceding disease such as chronic bronchitis, seem to behave both clinically and therapeutically as bacterial pneumonias, but no established pathogen can be isolated. It is possible that an impairment of the patient's defences has allowed upper respiratory commensals to reach the lower respiratory tract and there proliferate and become pathogenic. *Str. viridans* has certainly been shown, by culture from blood, pleural fluid or lung at autopsy, to be capable of producing pneumonia [89 & 99]. Nevertheless if the best techniques are used in patients who have not had previous chemotherapy it is only in a very small proportion that a causative organism cannot be identified. Bath et al. found that failure to identify a bacterial pathogen was most often associated with previous chemotherapy [10]. Viral infection or technical error could have explained most other failures, though in a few bronchitics none of these factors could be adduced. Only in 10% of failures was there no obvious explanation. Nevertheless in ordinary clinical practice it is undoubted that many pathogens are missed owing to deficiencies in technique (p. 88).

If the patient has already received chemotherapy it may be difficult to identify the causative organism. Pneumococci, in particular, disappear rapidly from the sputum and blood ; they are sometimes still detectable on direct smear even though they fail to grow on culture. One must remember that if a patient has already received an antibiotic it is probable that only organisms resistant to that antibiotic will survive in the sputum and these organisms may not necessarily be related to the original pneumonia. For instance, the isolation of *E. coli* resistant to penicillin from a patient who has already received 2 days' penicillin is no evidence that this organism is aetiologically important. Again if a few colonies of resistant staphylococci are isolated from a patient who has already received an antibiotic it is more likely to be a casual contaminant than the cause of the pneumonia.

Particular care is required in viral isolation. In the past, specimens have often been kept at low temperature pending examination but this has now been shown to inactivate respiratory syncytial virus and perhaps others. At present precise aetiological diagnosis in viral pneumonia is usually retrospective because of the time taken to isolate the virus and because the 4-fold rise in serological titre, which is usually regarded as significant, is often achieved only during convalescence. More rapid methods are being developed and it is possible that immunofluorescent techniques may soon allow the direct and immediate identification of specific viruses in the sputum or other specimen [8]. Doane *et al.* have described the immediate identification of parainfluenza virus in nasopharyngeal secretions both by electron microscopy and by haemagglutination [23].

Multiple pathogens are often identified in cases of pneumonia. The isolation from the same patient of both *Str. pneumoniae* and *H. influenzae* is relatively common [10]. In patients ill enough to be admitted to hospital it is frequent to find evidence of both viral and bacterial infection. More than one virus is not uncommonly identified [25] and a bacterial pathogen may also be found. In such cases it is difficult to be certain which is the primary infection but as most viruses mainly affect the upper respiratory tract it is probable that, in general, it is the viral infection which prepares the way for bacterial pneumonia, as has long been recognized in the case of influenza and measles.

Fungi may occasionally cause pneumonia. Changes which may be regarded as pneumonic may occur in certain *allergic* and *collagen* diseases. Rarely the aspiration or inhalation of certain *fluids, fumes* or *poisonous gases* may give rise to pneumonia, or perhaps more accurately to pulmonary oedema which may become secondarily infected. Pneumonia may also be caused by *x-radiation*.

CAUSAL AGENTS IN PNEUMONIA

The main bacteria causing pneumonia are *Streptococcus pneumoniae, Staphylococcus Pyogenes, Klebsiella pneumoniae, Bordetella pertussis* and *Mycobacterium tuberculosis. Respiratory syncytial* (RS) *virus* is probably the most important viral cause of pneumonia in infants. Secondary bacterial infection often causes pneumonia in patients with *measles* and *influenza* and sometimes in those with other viral infections in the upper respiratory tract, particularly parainfluenza. These viruses may occasionally themselves cause pneumonia and this is relatively common in the psittacosis/ornithosis group. *Mycoplasma pneumoniae* may cause epidemics, particularly in communities of young people as in military barracks, but also occurs endemically. Q fever (*R. burneti*) causes pneumonia in some parts of Britain and in many other areas in the world. *Actinomyces israeli* and other fungi cause pneumonia relatively rarely.

The following is an extended list of causal agents. *The less important are given in parenthesis.*

BACTERIAL PNEUMONIAS

Common
> *Streptococcus pneumoniae:* Pneumococcus (p. 119).
> *Staphylococcus pyogenes* (p. 121).
> *Mycobacterium tuberculosis* (p. 122).

Uncommon
> *Klebsiella pneumoniae:* Friedländer's bacillus (p. 122).

(*Haemophilus influenzae*) (p. 122).
(*Escherichia coli*) (p. 122).
(*Pseudomonas aeruginosa* or *pyocyanea*) (p. 122).
(*Bacteroides*) (p. 122).
(*Streptococcus pyogenes*) (p. 122).
(*Streptococcus viridans*) (p. 122).

AS A MANIFESTATION OF A SPECIFIC
BACTERIAL DISEASE
Common
    Pertussis: *Bordetella pertussis* (p. 126).
    (Typhoid-paratyphoid: *Salmonella typhi* and *paratyphi*) (p. 126).
    (Brucellosis: *Brucella abortus* and *melitensis*) (p. 126).

Uncommon
    (Plague: *Pasteurella pestis*) (p. 127).
    (Tularaemia: *Pasteurella tularensis*): (p. 127).
    (Anthrax: *Bacillus anthracis*); (p. 127).
    (Leptospirosis: *Leptospira icterohaemorrhagiae* or *canicola*) (p. 127).

VIRAL PNEUMONIAS

PNEUMONIA COMMONLY COMPLICATING
INFECTION
Psittacosis-ornithosis group (p. 128).
Respiratory syncytial virus (p. 129).
Influenza: Pneumonia usually bacterial (p. 129).
Measles: Pneumonia usually bacterial (p. 129).
Cytomegalovirus (p. 129).

PNEUMONIA OCCASIONALLY
COMPLICATING INFECTION
Most viral infections of upper respiratory tract, including
Common
    Adenoviruses (p. 130).
    Parainfluenza viruses (p. 130).
    Rhinoviruses (p. 130).

Uncommon
    (Varicella: chicken-pox) (p. 130).
    (Herpes zoster) (p. 130).
    (Smallpox) (p. 130).

(Lymphocytic choriomeningitis) (p. 130).
(Infectious mononucleosis) (p. 130).

RICKETTSIAL PNEUMONIAS
(Complicating louse-borne, murine or scrub typhus) (p. 131).
Q fever: *Rickettsia burneti* (p. 131).

MYCOPLASMAL PNEUMONIAS
Mycoplasma pneumoniae (p. 131).
Erythema multiforme exudativum: Stevens-Johnson syndrome (p. 588).

PNEUMONIAS DUE TO YEASTS,
FUNGI AND PROTOZOA
Common
    Actinomycosis: *Actinomyces israelii* (p. 289).
    (Nocardiasis: *Nocardia asteroides*) (p. 290).
    (Aspergillosis: *Aspergillus fumigatus* (p. 286).

Uncommon
    (Coccidioidomycosis: *Coccidioides immitis*) (p. 291).
    (Histoplasmosis: *Histoplasma capsulatum*) (p. 292).
    (*Pneumocystis carinii*) (p. 141).
    (*Toxoplasma gondii*) (p. 362).

ALLERGIC PNEUMONIAS AND
PNEUMONIAS COMPLICATING COLLAGEN
DISEASES
Pulmonary eosinophilia (including polyarteritis nodosa and Wegener's syndrome) (p. 425).
(Rheumatic fever) (p. 577).
(Rheumatoid disease) (p. 578).
(Disseminated lupus erythematosus) (p. 581).

CHEMICAL PNEUMONIAS
Common
    Aspiration of vomit (p. 146).
    (Dysphagic pneumonia) (p. 146).
    (Toxic gases and smokes) (p. 489).
    (Lipoid pneumonia) (p. 142).

Uncommon
    (Manganese) (p. 492).
    (Beryllium) (p. 498).
    (Aspiration of volatile hydrocarbons such as petrol) (p. 144).

(RADIATION PNEUMONIA) (p. 144)

PATHOGENESIS OF PNEUMONIA

PNEUMOCOCCAL PNEUMONIA

Pneumococci are classified into about 80 antigenic 'types'. These have been divided into 2 groups, 'infective' types (types 1, 2, 3, 6, 7, 14 and 19), commonly isolated from cases of pneumonia, and 'carrier' types which more rarely cause pneumonia. Pneumococci are present in the nasopharynx in 20–40% of the normal population and almost everyone carries a pneumococcus from time to time [94]. In most individuals the latter are the 'carrier' types but 'infective' types are found in some normal people. The carrier rate of 'infective' types may increase during epidemics of pneumonia and is found to be higher in those with colds. It seems that infective types of pneumococci in the nasopharynx of carriers may cause pneumonia in the carrier himself or may be passed on to others. The distinction between the infective and the commoner carrier types is only relative. Lobar pneumonia is more often caused by infective types of pneumococci but carrier types are sometimes responsible. Type 3 pneumococci tend to cause particularly severe illness and this type has the highest mortality [6]. In patients with bronchopneumonia the frequency of the different types of pneumococcus is similar to that in healthy carriers [110].

To cause pneumonia it is not enough for pneumococci to reach the nasopharynx. Experimental work in monkeys shows that it is necessary to introduce the organisms directly into the trachea [15]. Other experimental work supports the view that pneumococci are more likely to become established in the lung and cause pneumonia if they are aspirated in mucus from the upper respiratory tract. The mucus protects the bacteria from the body's defences and allows them to proliferate (p. 16). The body reacts by an intensive outpouring of oedema fluid and the pneumococci spread in this fluid from alveolus to alveolus, either through the interalveolar pores or by the bronchial tree [84 & 111]. The

initial spread from the upper to the lower respiratory tract is facilitated by exposure to cold [84], by alcoholic intoxication or by anaesthesia [74]. Experimental evidence makes it relatively certain that pneumococci reach the blood stream from the alveolar capillaries.

OTHER LOBAR PNEUMONIA

The pathogenesis of lobar pneumonia due to other bacteria is similar to that of pneumococcal, though both *Staphylococcus pyogenes* and *Klebsiella pneumoniae* (Friedländer's bacillus) are more liable to cause tissue necrosis and lung abscess. Subsequent fibrosis is also more common with *K. pneumoniae* infection [86].

SEGMENTAL PNEUMONIA

Anatomical limitation of pneumonia to a segment may be due to the infecting bacteria being less potent stimulators of oedema fluid. No doubt the relation between the virulence of the infecting organisms and the host defences also plays a part. Pneumococci are particularly powerful stimulators of oedema fluid and this may account for their tendency to cause spread throughout a lobe.

Routine x-ray after relatively minor upper respiratory tract infections often reveals segmental or subsegmental shadows even though lower respiratory symptoms have been mild. This type of pneumonia has been referred to as 'benign aspiration pneumonia' to indicate that the main factor is a mechanical one with aspirated mucus entering a segmental bronchus. The spread of the infecting organisms is limited either by their small numbers, by their lack of virulence or by the strength of the host defences. The term 'aspiration pneumonia' is unsatisfactory as most pneumonias, including severe lobar pneumonia, originate in aspiration. It is better to use the term 'mild segmental' or 'mild subsegmental' pneumonia.

LOBULAR PNEUMONIA AND BRONCHOPNEUMONIA

Localized lobular pneumonia is often a mild infection and may depend on the aspiration of mucus into a number of small peripheral bronchi where further spread is limited by the factors mentioned. Bilateral lobular pneumonia is often associated with severe bronchitis. In this case the infected mucus originates in the bronchi and spreads peripherally into alveolar tissue. Nevertheless extensive lobular pneumonia may occasionally occur without obvious bronchitis. It can be associated with *Mycoplasma pneumoniae*, streptococci or staphylococci.

EPIDEMIOLOGY

Much of what has been said in the section on pathogenesis is relevant to the epidemiology of pneumonia. *Epidemics* of *viral infections*, such as respiratory syncytial (R.S.) virus in children or influenza in adults, are likely to be associated with an increased attack rate of pneumonia. Sometimes the pneumonia is caused by the virus itself, which is probably the case in bronchopneumonia complicating infection with R.S. virus. Sometimes, as in influenza, the viral infection lowers the patient's resistance and facilitates bacterial invasion of the lung. Severe *atmospheric*

pollution, such as the great London fog of 1952, is often accompanied by a significant increase in attack rate from pneumonia. The mode of action is uncertain, but probably the pollutant lowers the patient's resistance to bacterial pathogens and perhaps interferes with ciliary action. The *winter prevalence* of pneumonia is probably related to greater overcrowding indoors, poorer ventilation, greater atmospheric pollution and possibly to the effect of cold in facilitating infection of the lower respiratory tract.

The trends of *pneumonia mortality* since 1944, by age and sex, are given in figs. 7.1 & 7.2. It will be seen that the main changes are the decrease of infant mortality, perhaps associated with improving social conditions as well as with the increasing use of antibiotics, and the rise in mortality in the very old. The latter need not be taken too seriously, being probably mainly a terminal event in the elderly and a convenient label on the death certificate. In the other age groups the introduction of the newer antibiotics after 1945 seems to have contributed little that had not already been achieved by penicillin and the

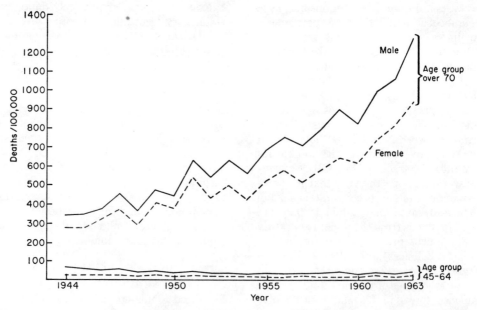

Fig. 7.1. Pneumonia mortality England and Wales 1944–63, for males and females of age groups 45 and over.

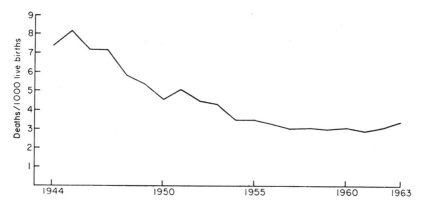

FIG. 7.2. Pneumonia mortality in infants, England and Wales 1944-63.

sulphonamides, although in individual patients the newer antibiotics may on occasion be life saving. At all ages males have a higher mortality than females.

PATHOLOGY [90]

PNEUMOCOCCAL PNEUMONIA

The pathology of pneumococcal pneumonia will be only briefly summarized as it is very familiar. The earliest stage consists of a spreading inflammatory oedema teeming with organisms, a stage naturally seldom seen in man. This proceeds to the stage of red hepatization in which the affected lobe is firm, airless and red in colour, often with petechiae beneath the pleura which frequently shows a thin coat of fibrin. The smaller bronchi in the affected lobe are also plugged with fibrin. Microscopically the alveoli are filled with red blood cells and fibrin, but there are relatively few neutrophils. The alveolar capillaries are intensely congested. The bronchial arteries are blocked proximal to the affected lobe though they appear to open up again during the third stage, that of grey hepatization. Section of the lung during this stage shows a greyish yellow appearance. Microscopically the alveoli are stuffed with large numbers of neutrophils and relatively few red blood cells. The alveolar capillaries are less obvious than during red hepatization and the pulmonary arterioles may become thrombosed. The neutrophils phagocytose the pneumococci but

apparently do not kill them. As resolution proceeds the alveoli are invaded by macrophages, probably derived from the capillary vascular endothelium, which engulf both the leucocytes and their contained pneumococci.

STAPHYLOCOCCAL PNEUMONIA

In fatal staphylococcal pneumonia complicating viral influenza the lungs are usually dark red in colour and intensely oedematous. The mucous membrane of the bronchi is highly inflamed and often sloughs. The cut surface of the lung exudes haemorrhagic fluid on gentle pressure and there may be considerable haemorrhage. Microscopically there is destruction of the bronchial mucous membrane with intensive infiltration with neutrophils. The alveoli are filled with exudate and may contain hyaline membranes and a variable number of neutrophils. In less acute cases there may be patchy bronchopneumonia showing as a grey-yellow consolidation around pus-containing bronchi, and, microscopically, as massive neutrophil infiltration of the alveoli. These patches may break down to form abscess cavities of variable size. Fatal *lobular* or *bronchopneumonia* due to *other bacteria* shows a similar picture.

KLEBSIELLA PNEUMONIAE PNEUMONIA

In pneumonia due to *Klebsiella pneumoniae* the oedema fluid is said to be particularly viscid and the initial exudate to be mononuclear. Later, alveolar destruction is accompanied by neutrophil infiltration and later still the reaction may become more chronic with granulation tissue and fibrosis. Both abscess formation and empyema may occur.

VIRAL, MYCOPLASMAL AND RICKETTSIAL PNEUMONIAS

Patients dying with viral pneumonias frequently have secondary bacterial infection, in which case the pathology is similar to that of the bacterial pneumonias already mentioned. In pure rickettsial or viral pneumonias there is often alveolar oedema with variable numbers of intra-alveolar macrophages and with proliferation of the alveolar lining cells. There is frequently interstitial infiltration with lymphocytes and sometimes with plasma cells and macrophages. In some of the viral pneumonias, such as influenza, necrosis of the alveolar wall may occur. Where the oedema is less marked there may be hyaline membrane formation. Sometimes there may be giant cells, as in measles pneumonia. Inclusion bodies may be found in the alveolar lining cells in psittacosis, measles and in infection with cytomegalovirus. In acute influenza, as mentioned above, there is severe damage to the bronchial epithelium with oedema and lymphocyte infiltration of the walls and sloughing of the mucous membrane. Lesser degrees of this phenomenon may be found in other viral pneumonias.

Certain pathological characteristics of some of the other specific pneumonias will be mentioned in the appropriate sections.

FUNCTIONAL ABNORMALITY

LOBAR PNEUMONIA

In the early stages of lobar pneumonia the affected lobe is perfused with blood but, owing to the alveolar exudate, little gas exchange takes place. There is therefore a shunt of unoxygenated blood from the right to left resulting in cyanosis, decreased Pa,o_2 and Sa,o_2 [54]. Later the blood flow through the lobe, and the consequent shunt, probably decreases. Delirium is said to be closely related to the degree of hypoxaemia [9].

If the ventilatory reserve is normal the unaffected parts of the lung will be hyperventilated and there will be no retention of carbon dioxide; Pa,co_2 may even be reduced. Increased Pa,co_2 may occur in patients with other conditions, such as chronic bronchitis or spinal deformity, which prevent effective compensation. If several lobes are involved the remaining lung, even if normal, may be insufficient for compensation. Marshall and Christie [60] showed increased rigidity of the lung in lobar pneumonia, in fact more than could be accounted for by the demonstrable consolidation, so that it seemed that there was more widespread abnormality than was clinically obvious. They calculated that reduced tidal volume and increased respiratory rate was the most economic pattern of breathing in terms of work, even if tidal volume was not limited by pleuritic pain.

LOBULAR AND BRONCHOPNEUMONIA

In bronchopneumonia the effect on the blood gases will depend on

(1) the extent of the consolidation, which will affect the arterial oxygen saturation, and

(2) the ventilation of the remaining lung, which may affect both oxygen uptake and carbon dioxide loss.

The diminished arterial oxygen saturation may be further worsened by the effect of pyrexia in shifting the oxygen dissociation curve to the right, that is to say less oxygen combines with haemoglobin at any given partial pressure of oxygen in the plasma [54]. Bronchopneumonia frequently occurs in those with chronic bronchitis who, because of airways obstruction, may have difficulty in hyperventilating their unconsolidated alveoli. Both oxygen unsaturation and carbon dioxide retention are therefore common in such patients.

CLINICAL FEATURES

PREDISPOSING FACTORS

It has already been mentioned that experimentally, exposure to *cold* facilitates the passage of mucus containing pneumococci from the upper respiratory tract to the lower [84]. Clinically, exposure to cold may predispose in the same way. When working in a military hospital during the war the writer was impressed by the wave of admissions with pneumonia after each fresh batch of recruits was exposed to its first experience of sleeping out in the wet and the cold. In *postoperative pneumonia* (p. 135), particularly common after abdominal operations, the effect of the anaesthetic in impairing the respiratory defences, decreased diaphragmatic movement and the limitation of cough by pain or sedation are important factors, but the attack rate is much higher in cigarette smokers who are likely to have some degree of preceding chronic bronchitis [22 & 91]. *Alcohol* may also predispose to pneumonia [74], partly by its direct suppression of the respiratory reflexes, partly by its depression of the body's reaction to infection (p. 24) and partly perhaps by the secondary effect of cold if the individual with alcoholic vasodilatation has 'slept it off' under conditions which would not be selected by most of us when sober.

A high proportion of patients with pneumonia give a history of a common cold or other *upper respiratory tract infection* preceding the onset of the acute symptoms of pneumonia. Sometimes the organism which caused the 'cold' may be the same as that which later caused the pneumonia, sometimes the effect may be that of lowering the patient's defences, both general and local, sometimes the cold may only act by producing the mucus in which organisms can be aspirated into the lower respiratory tract.

Chronic bronchitis and *bronchiectasis* are important predisposing factors in pneumonia. Infected material is particularly liable to be aspirated into the lower respiratory tract if there is chronic *infection of the sinuses*, and recurrent attacks of pneumonia, often of the segmental variety, have been described in *obstruction of the oesophagus*, particularly achalasia (p. 146).

Two conditions which interfere with normal antibody manufacture, *myelomatosis* and *hypogammaglobulinaemia*, predispose to recurrent pneumonia (p. 140). To these may be added *'heavy chain disease'* [32 & 69], with abnormal globulin production, clinical manifestations similar to a reticulosis and a particular susceptibility to recurrent pneumonia. Pneumonia may, of course, complicate the chronic bronchial infection of *mucoviscidosis* (p. 592).

Any interference with the defences of the respiratory tract or the normal drainage of the lung is liable to predispose to pneumonia. For instance, *carcinoma of the bronchus* or an aspirated *foreign body* may first present clinically as a complicating pneumonia. It has been already mentioned that postoperative pneumonia is commoner in cigarette smokers and it seems likely that *cigarette smoking* predisposes to pneumonia in general, certainly in those in whom cigarette smoking has caused chronic bronchitis, but possibly in others who have only minimal bronchitic symptoms. The body's general resistance may, of course, be lowered by any severe *debilitating illness* or by the use of *corticosteroid drugs*.

Age is an important predisposing factor. Pneumonia, especially severe pneumonia, is commoner in older people, even in the absence of such predisposing conditions as chronic bronchitis. Presumably the main factor is the general waning of the body's defensive capacity.

PNEUMOCOCCAL LOBAR PNEUMONIA

Pneumococcal lobar pneumonia is the classical type of pneumonia and will first be described, the different characteristics of other pneumonias being mentioned later.

ONSET

As mentioned above, there is often a preceding history of common cold or other upper respiratory infection. At any time, but usually within a week of the onset of the cold, the patient may rather rapidly become much more ill, perhaps with an initial *rigor*, but in any case with a sharp *rise* in *temperature*, usually in the region of 101–103°F (38·5–39·5°C) but sometimes higher or lower. At the same time he will usually develop *pleuritic pain* over the affected lobe. He may appreciate that he is breathing rapidly and he will certainly appreciate that he is feeling ill. There may be an initial dry, *painful cough* but he will soon begin to cough up sputum. Classically the *sputum* in pneumococcal lobar pneumonia is 'rusty' in colour, the rustiness being due to particles of altered blood from the areas of red hepatization in the lung. The sputum is often viscid and difficult to cough up, which adds to the patient's pain. It is by no means always rusty; quite commonly it is purulent or slightly blood stained. Often the patient develops labial *herpes simplex* within the first few days.

Not all cases of pneumococcal lobar pneumonia develop exactly as outlined above. In a number of cases there is no overt preceding upper respiratory tract infection and the *sudden onset* may come 'out of the blue'. Sometimes, particularly after a cold, the onset may be more insidious and it may be some days before the patient appreciates that he is really ill.

COURSE

Before specific chemotherapy was available the patient remained ill with a high fever for 5 to 10 days. Then, if he had survived, the temperature would subside rapidly by so-called 'crisis', or perhaps more slowly by 'lysis'. Nowadays this process is almost always cut short by treatment.

PHYSICAL SIGNS

On examination the patient is often *flushed* and *cyanosed*. He will be *breathing rapidly* and shallowly. Sometimes it can be seen that his *alae nasi* are moving with inspiration and expiration. There may be labial *herpes simplex*. His *temperature* and *pulse* will be raised. On *examination of the chest* it may be observed that the affected side is *moving less* and that, if he is asked to take a deep breath, there is a sudden catch as he feels the pleuritic pain. The affected lobe will be *dull* to percussion, sometimes very dull. One may be left in doubt as to whether the dullness represents fluid. In that case it is worth testing for *vocal fremitus* which is usually normal or exaggerated in a lobar consolidation but diminished when fluid is present. The patient should be asked to point with one finger to the site of the maximal pleuritic pain and the examiner should listen carefully for a *rub* in this area. In the early stages the patient frequently is unable to take a breath deep enough for the rub to be detected but the tell-tale catch in the breathing is sufficient to indicate pleural involvement. *Bronchial breathing* may be present over the whole or a part of the lobe. *Whispering pectoriloquy* will be detected in the same areas.

There are rarely important physical signs elsewhere, apart from the complications of pneumonia, but the *spleen* is occasionally *palpable*.

RADIOLOGY (figs. 7.3–7.5)

Any lobe may be involved in pneumococcal lobar pneumonia. Although the lower lobes are more frequently affected, upper lobe or

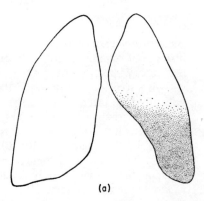
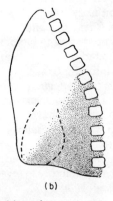

(a)   (b)

FIG. 7.3. Lobar pneumonia left lower lobe: PA and lateral.

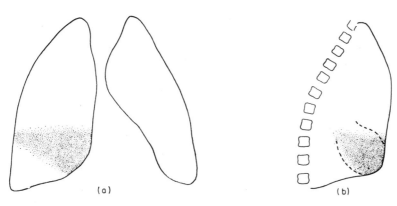

FIG. 7.4. Lobar pneumonia middle lobe.

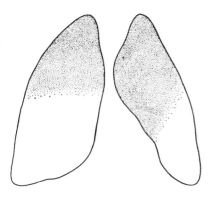

FIG. 7.5. Bilateral upper lobe pneumonia due to Type 3 pneumococcus.

total white blood cell count does not often exceed 30,000 and is more frequently 12,000–15,000/mm³. In general the count tends to be proportional to the extent of the consolidation but there are many exceptions. Leucocytosis may be absent in very ill patients; this is regarded as an adverse prognostic sign. There is sometimes an eosinophilia in convalescence. The erythrocyte sedimentation rate is usually raised and may be very high. A rate of 100 mm or more per hour is not uncommon, though of course it decreases in convalescence. A high rate persisting over many weeks should indicate a search for some other underlying condition such as mylomatosis or a collagen disease.

DIAGNOSIS

Diagnosis and differential diagnosis of pneumococcal pneumonia is considered with that of other pneumonias on p. 133.

OTHER BACTERIAL LOBAR PNEUMONIAS

STAPHYLOCOCCAL LOBAR PNEUMONIA

Staphylococcal lobar pneumonia is the next most common type of lobar pneumonia after pneumococcal, although it is comparatively infrequent except during epidemics of influenza. The pneumonia can be very severe, especially if it complicates viral influenza, when it may be fatal within a few hours. Many cases of staphylococcal pneumonia do not differ appreciably in their clinical course

middle lobe pneumonia is quite common. Radiologically a hazy, relatively uniform shadow is seen in the area corresponding to the anatomical situation of the affected lobe (p. 6). The density varies according to the intensity of the exudate. The exact anatomical distribution is more easily determined by a lateral film, if the patient is well enough to have one, but the posteroanterior film, combined with physical examination, usually suffices for localization. The shadowing does not always include the whole lobe. If most of the lobe is involved the pneumonia is usually classified as of lobar distribution.

HAEMATOLOGICAL EFFECTS

A neutrophil leucocytosis is usual in pneumococcal and other bacterial pneumonias. The from pneumococcal, but *abscess formation* is more common and may dominate the picture (p. 161). The abscesses are usually thin-walled and may be cyst-like on the x-ray. In children they not uncommonly rupture into the pleura to produce *pneumothorax* or *pyopneumothorax*. This is less common in adults, in whom it has been suggested that corticosteroid therapy may predispose to this complication [67].

TUBERCULOUS LOBAR PNEUMONIA

Although a patient with tuberculosis lobar pneumonia usually gives a history of a more gradual onset than in other types of bacterial pneumonia, this is not always the case and the disease may in the first place resemble one of the more common types, though the white blood count is not usually raised. All patients diagnosed clinically as pneumonia should have the sputum examined for tubercle bacilli.

PNEUMONIA DUE TO KLEBSIELLA PNEUMONIAE (Friedländer's bacillus)

These pneumonias are comparatively rare (0·5–4% of all pneumonias) but are usually very severe. In most reported series the mortality is 20–50% [53], some of this probably being due to failure to make an early aetiological diagnosis and to adjust treatment accordingly. Most cases are in middle aged or elderly males, not uncommonly with chronic alcoholism or some other chronic disease. The upper lobes, or more than one lobe, are more often affected than in pneumococcal pneumonia. Radiologically the lobe may appear to bulge owing to the intensive inflammatory exudate. The blood culture may be positive. There is a strong tendency to *abscess formation* (p. 161) and complication by empyema [80]. The *sputum* may be viscid, jelly-like and blood-stained, but may be purulent or rusty. The pneumonia may become gradually transformed into a chronic fibrocavernous condition, with low fever and purulent sputum. Clinically and radiologically it may resemble pulmonary tuberculosis, especially if it is bilateral. This condition may last for weeks or months, it may ultimately

clear up with or without residual fibrosis and bronchiectasis, or it may end fatally. It may be complicated by empyema, pericarditis or even meningitis.

PNEUMONIA DUE TO OTHER GRAM NEGATIVE BACILLI

H. influenzae is often associated with chronic bronchitis and bronchiectasis. Nevertheless it is seldom the only pathogen found in pneumonia, though its significance has occasionally been confirmed by positive blood culture [21 & 38]. It is not uncommonly found with *Str. pneumoniae*, especially in patients with preceding chronic bronchitis [10]. Other gram negative bacteria are relatively rare causes of pneumonia in Britain, though perhaps commoner in North America [102]. *E. coli*, *Pseudomonas aeruginosa* (or *pyocyanea*), *Bacteroides* and even *Proteus* have been incriminated. We have already cautioned about attributing pneumonia to such organisms in patients who have previously received chemotherapy (p. 84) but on occasion their aetiological rôle has been attested in previously untreated patients by positive culture from pleural fluid or blood, as well as from sputum [102]. Most such cases occur in individuals with other chronic diseases. Corticosteroid therapy or inhalation therapy are among the predisposing factors [75].

STREPTOCOCCUS PYOGENES PNEUMONIA

Pneumonia due to *Streptococcus pyogenes* complicated some of the earlier influenza epidemics in this country but is now rarely seen. When it occurs it is usually of the bronchopneumonic type.

STREPTOCOCCUS VIRIDANS PNEUMONIA

Although it has been shown that pneumonia caused by *Streptococcus viridans* can occur, as cultures from lung, pleural effusion and blood have been positive in individual patients [89 & 99], with most patients it would be difficult to prove as the organism is commonly found in sputum or laryngeal swabs from normal people. It may be that some of the pneumonias occurring in the elderly, in which no other accepted pathogen has been identified, may be due to *Streptococcus viridans* and this organism might well be involved in some of the milder segmental pneumonias to be discussed below. At present such a view is purely speculative.

throughout both lung fields. Much more common are multiple patchy shadows at both bases, sometimes throughout both lungs. The size of the individual shadows is variable, usually between 0·5 and 3 cm in diameter, and

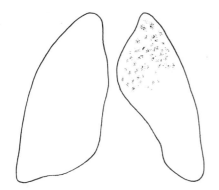

FIG. 7.6. Lobular pneumonia left upper lobe simulating tuberculosis. Cleared in 2 weeks with tetracycline.

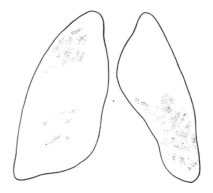

FIG. 7.8. Lobular pneumonia (bronchopneumonia): Influenza A. No pathogenic bacteria isolated.

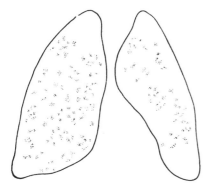

FIG. 7.7. Diffuse lobular pneumonia accompanying measles and simulating coarse miliary tuberculosis. Cleared in 10 days with penicillin.

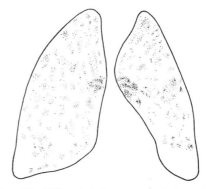

FIG. 7.9. Diffuse lobular pneumonia in patient with chronic bronchitis and emphysema.

LOBULAR PNEUMONIA, INCLUDING BRONCHO-PNEUMONIA (figs. 7.6 –7.9)

ANATOMICAL TYPES

Radiologically, patchy lobular shadows may be confined to one segment, in which case the aetiological and clinical features are similar to those of segmental pneumonia (p. 124). Occasionally small ill-defined shadows, a few millimetres in diameter, are scattered diffusely

the margins ill defined. The shadows are not necessarily symmetrical. It is this type of pneumonia with bilateral patchy shadows in the x-ray which is usually referred to as bronchopneumonia.

AETIOLOGICAL FACTORS

The diffuse type of fine lobular pneumonia is comparatively rare, but can be associated with bacterial, viral or mycoplasmal infections. Basal or diffuse coarse lobular shadowing (bronchopneumonia) usually complicates an exacerbation of chronic bronchitis but may follow any attack of severe bronchitis, especially if this is associated with viral influenza. *H. influenzae*, pneumococci or staphylococci may be the causal organisms and bronchopneumonia may also occur with viral and rickettsial infections.

The old or debilitated may develop a somewhat insidious type of patchy bilateral basal pneumonia, the so-called '*hypostatic*' pneumonia, probably due to the invasion of retained secretions and basal oedema by normal upper respiratory tract flora. Such an infection may by itself be sufficient to carry off a severely debilitated patient but often the diagnosis, *post mortem* or *ante mortem*, is only an incident in the terminal phase of some other disease.

CLINICAL FEATURES

The clinical features of *localized lobular pneumonia* are similar to those of segmental pneumonia (p. 124). Patients with *diffuse fine lobular pneumonia* are often severely ill. Their symptoms may be mainly febrile and toxic, but there is usually at least some cough with or without sputum. In bacterial infection the latter may be purulent. Diffuse fine crepitations may be audible in the chest but sometimes there are few physical signs.

Bronchopneumonia is very common. Clinically bronchopneumonia is differentiated from severe bronchitis either by the presence of *patchy bronchial breathing* or by the presence of patchy shadows on the chest x-ray. The initial symptoms are those of acute bronchitis. As bronchopneumonia supervenes the patient becomes more ill and more breathless. *Cyanosis* increases. The patient with advanced chronic bronchitis may, owing to decreased alveolar ventilation, retain carbon dioxide. *Temperature*, *pulse* and *respiratory rate* will be raised, there may be *confusion* due to hypoxia, or *coma* due to CO_2 retention. The latter may also cause a *coarse tremor*. The *sputum* is likely to be purulent, sometimes blood flecked. The patient may sound *bubbly* and have obvious difficulty in getting rid of his secretions. In the chest the *physical signs*

are largely those of bronchitis (p. 108) but, in the presence of bronchopneumonia, these usually include medium or fine *basal crepitations*. There may be local areas of *diminished breath sounds* or *bronchial breathing*, but the areas of consolidation are not usually large enough to produce impairment of percussion note. Occasionally there is pleural involvement, with *pleuritic pain* and a *pleural rub*.

In a patient with advanced chronic bronchitis an attack of bronchopneumonia may precipitate *cor pulmonale*, indicated by raised jugular venous pressure, oedema and sometimes by enlargement and tenderness of the liver (p. 318).

As already indicated, in old and debilitated people basal bronchopneumonia, associated with poor drainage of alveolar exudate and viscid secretions from the bases of the lungs, may be insidious with relatively little distress and little rise in temperature.

SEGMENTAL AND SUBSEGMENTAL PNEUMONIA
(figs. 7.10–7.13)

In recent years it has become a common and very proper practice to refer patients for x-ray who have had colds, influenza or other upper

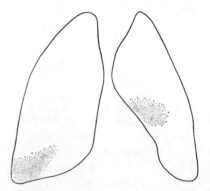

FIG. 7.10. Bilateral segmental pneumonia. 'Influenza' followed by purulent sputum. Cleared within 3 weeks.

respiratory tract infections which have been rather more severe than usual, have lasted longer than usual, or have been accompanied by cough. As a result it has been found that

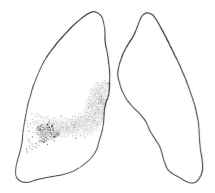

Fig. 7.11. Segmental pneumonia right lower lobe in young boy with history of tuberculosis contact and mimicking primary tuberculosis. Shadows cleared in 1 week without treatment.

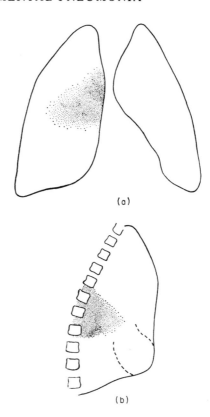

(a)

(b)

Fig. 7.12. Pneumonia apical segment right lower lobe. 'Influenza' 3 weeks previously. No significant increase in mild chronic bronchitic symptoms. Cleared rapidly with penicillin.

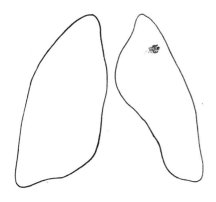

Fig. 7.13. Subsegmental pneumonia left upper lobe mimicking tuberculosis. Cleared rapidly.

segmental pneumonia very frequently complicates these upper respiratory infections. The x-ray appearance is very variable. The opacity may occupy a complete segment or a part of a segment, or it may be lobular in distribution within the segment. Usually only one segment is involved, sometimes more than one.

ANATOMICAL DISTRIBUTION

It is probable that the radiological appearances derive from mucus aspirated from the upper respiratory tract, often during sleep. The shadows are therefore commonly seen in segments to which mucus will gravitate in the sleeping position. The axillary subsegments of the anterior and posterior segments of the upper lobes are often affected, as are the apical segments of the lower lobes and the lateral segment of the middle lobe. However, basal segments may also be involved. It is unusual for the apical segments of the upper lobes to be affected, but this is occasionally seen.

AETIOLOGY

It seems probable that in many cases the changes are largely due to mechanical factors and that the rhinoviruses or commensal organisms which may be present in the aspirated mucus may play relatively little part in producing the radiological changes. But segmental pneumonia may be caused by any of the aetiological agents associated with pneumonia.

CLINICAL FEATURES

The great majority of cases of segmental pneumonia are mild and there is *little beyond the radiological changes*, and perhaps the presence of *cough* with or without sputum, to indicate that the patient has had anything more than an upper respiratory infection, sometimes quite a mild one. It is this mild type of segmental pneumonia which has been called 'benign aspiration pneumonia', to indicate the minor clinical manifestations and the largely mechanical origin of the lung changes. Usually by the time a patient has had his x-ray there is *little to be found clinically in the chest*, although there may sometimes be some local diminution of breath sounds and inspiratory crepitations. This type of mild segmental pneumonia may be seen at any age and is comparatively common in young people.

If the pathogen is a more virulent one, such as the pneumococcus or the staphylococcus, the symptoms may be more severe. A positive blood culture for pneumococcus may sometimes be found in the presence of only a relatively small lesion on the x-ray. Similarly

a patient with Q fever or psittacosis may sometimes be much iller than the extent of the radiological lesions might lead one to expect.

Clinically the *course* of a benign segmental pneumonia is much the same as that of the original upper respiratory infection. Radiologically the shadows will usually be found to have shown some clearance within a fortnight and they usually clear completely within 3 or 4 weeks.

PNEUMONIAS COMPLICATING SPECIFIC BACTERIAL DISEASES

PERTUSSIS

Pneumonia complicating pertussis is often due to secondary invasion by pathogenic bacteria although occasionally to *Bordetella pertussis* itself [81 & 110]. The pneumonia may be of any of the 3 main anatomical types.

TYPHOID-PARATYPHOID

Secondary bacterial pneumonia may complicate typhoid or paratyphoid or may occur as an extension of the bronchitis which may be part of the typhoid picture. Huckstep found some evidence of pneumonia in 15% of cases of typhoid but severe lobar pneumonia in only 3% [43]. During an epidemic we have seen a number of cases of pneumonia in which routine blood culture unexpectedly grew paratyphoid bacilli.

BRUCELLOSIS

Cough, sputum, haemoptysis, hoarseness, pleuritic pain, consolidation and pleural effusion have been reported in brucellosis [11]. X-rays have been described as showing 'hilar infiltration' or 'generalized peribronchial infiltration' [11], bronchopneumonia or 'vague irregular infiltrations' [35]. Single, or multiple localized, pulmonary granulomata have also been recorded [106]. Histologically the lesions may closely resemble sarcoidosis, with epithelioid cells, giant cells, plasma cells and lymphocytes [35]. Although leucopenia is usual in brucellosis, leucocytosis may occur with respiratory infection [35]. The recommended treatment is tetracycline 0·5 g 4 times daily for at least 3 weeks.

PLAGUE

Pneumonic plague, with spread of respiratory infection from person to person and, in some epidemics, an extremely high mortality, is one of the most dreaded manifestations of the disease. Initially the patient may be very much iller than the extent of clinical signs in the chest would suggest but consolidation may then rapidly develop. He may begin to cough bloody frothy sputum and death often occurs within 3 days. A devastating epidemic of this type swept Manchuria in 1910–11 but fortunately more recent outbreaks of pneumonic plague have had a much lower mortality and seem to have been less infectious. Pneumonia may also complicate bubonic plague and increases the gravity of the prognosis. Streptomycin, tetracycline and chloramphenicol have been highly effective if given within the first 15 hours [55]. Streptomycin 1 g and tetracycline 1 g, both 4-hourly, would be suitable initial therapy. The first tetracycline dose should be intravenous.

TULARAEMIA

Pneumonia is a relatively common complication of tularaemia and laboratory workers may develop the disease as a primary pneumonia due to inhalation of *Pasteurella tularensis*. Mediastinal gland enlargement and pleural effusions are common.

ANTHRAX

Pneumonia in anthrax usually occurs from the inhalation of spores of *Bacillus anthracis* from infected wool (Woolsorter's Disease) or from hides or furs.

LEPTOSPIROSIS

This may occasionally be complicated by a specific pneumonia [3].

With the exception of pneumonia associated with pertussis the above conditions are seldom seen in Britain. Enteric fever, brucellosis and leptospirosis occur from time to time; anthrax is extremely rare and plague and tularaemia virtually unknown.

VIRAL AND PRESUMED VIRAL PNEUMONIAS

In certain viral infections pneumonia is a common complication. This is true of the *psittacosis–ornithosis* group of viruses. In infants *respiratory syncytial virus* frequently causes bronchiolitis which may give rise to fine lobular shadows on the x-ray. Adenoviruses, influenza and parainfluenza viruses, and *Mycoplasma pneumoniae* are rarer causes of this syndrome [72]. Pneumonia due to the virus itself may occasionally occur in *influenza* (p. 129) and in *measles*, but most pneumonias complicating these two conditions are bacterial.

Pneumonia may complicate infection with *adenoviruses* [25 & 72], *parainfluenza viruses* [72] and perhaps *rhinoviruses*, but usually in these conditions the pneumonia is either a mild segmental one, in which simple aspiration of mucus may be more important than the virulence of the organisms, or the dominant factor is secondary bacterial infection. Naturally the former is commoner in domiciliary practice and the latter in hospital practice. Infection can occur with more than one virus at the same time.

CLINICAL CHARACTERISTICS

If the characteristics are examined of large numbers of pneumonias proved to be primarily due to viruses, *Mycoplasma pneumoniae* or *Rickettsia burneti*, and without secondary bacterial infection, a suggestive clinical picture emerges, but there are many exceptions in individual cases. The typical picture is more often seen in outbreaks, particularly in the armed forces and in general practice; in the absence of bacterial superinfection patients are not often ill enough to require admission to civilian hospitals. When the pneumonia is a bacterial one complicating an initial viral infection the clinical manifestations will be largely those of the bacterial pneumonia, unless, as sometimes happens, there is an interval of comparative wellbeing between the initial viral infection and the subsequent bacterial pneumonia.

In primary viral pneumonia the presenting symptoms may be predominantly *general* and *febrile*, with *headache, general aches, prostration* and *fever*. There may be little in the way of respiratory symptoms or physical signs and the pneumonic element in the disease may be discovered only when a routine x-ray of the chest is taken as part of the investigation of the pyrexia. Respiratory symptoms, if present, may be somewhat different from those of a bacterial pneumonia. The *cough* may be *paroxysmal*, the *sputum* mucoid or blood-stained. There is seldom pleuritic pain; pain, if present, is often retrosternal. *Physical signs* in the chest may be scanty, perhaps with some localized diminution in breath sounds or a few crepitations; sometimes there are no obvious physical signs at all. The *white blood count* is normal though it may be raised in convalescence.

Nevertheless, as already mentioned, there are many exceptions to this picture. Although a patient with predominantly febrile symptoms whose x-ray shows pneumonic shadows, may prove to have a pneumonia due to infection with a virus or mycoplasma, or to have Q fever, many patients with symptoms no different from those with bacterial pneumonia may also turn out to have a viral infection with or without an added bacterial element.

The physician must beware of a too facile tendency to diagnose 'viral pneumonia'. All too often an unusual appearance of a chest x-ray is passed off as a 'viral pneumonia' without other supporting evidence, whereas in fact the shadow may be due to carcinoma of the bronchus or to pulmonary infarct. 'Viral pneumonia' must not be used as a diagnostic wastepaper basket.

PSITTACOSIS–ORNITHOSIS
[12 & 64]

The term 'psittacosis' was originally used for a disease caught from parrots. Later the term 'ornithosis' was introduced when it was known that a very similar disease was caused by a closely related or identical virus derived from other birds, including pigeons, ducks, turkeys and fulmars. The disease occurs particularly in pigeon fanciers (but is different from 'pigeon fancier's lung', p. 504) and in those concerned with the care of parrots. After an initial illness, which may not be severe, the birds may be carriers of the virus for long periods and infection occurs from dust derived from the excreta or feathers.

CLINICAL FEATURES

The typical picture is that described for viral pneumonia (p. 127), but there are wide variations in severity. Although a high mortality occurred in earlier epidemics, and infection from parrots seems to result in more severe disease than infection from other birds, serological examination has shown that infections may be quite mild and even sub-clinical. The *incubation period* is usually 7–14 days, occasionally up to 28 days. If untreated the pyrexia usually lasts 1–2 weeks but the disease may pursue a low grade course over several months. The pulse is said to be relatively slow. *X-ray* may show broncho-pneumonia, single or multiple segmental opacities or even lobar pneumonia [92] but abnormal shadows may not be present until the end of the first week of the illness. The *spleen* and *liver* are occasionally enlarged. Scanty 'rose spots' may occur on the skin of the abdomen. The development of a typhoid state, coma, cyanosis or a rising pulse rate are ominous signs carrying a poor prognosis.

DIAGNOSIS

The diagnosis may be suspected in a clinically compatible case with a history of contact with birds. The virus may be isolated from the blood in the 1st week of illness by inoculation into mice or incubated eggs. It may also be obtained from sputum. Serologically the complement fixation test is the best. False positive W.R. and Kahn tests may occur [92].

TREATMENT

The virus is susceptible to *tetracycline*. Very large doses are said to suppress or delay the antibody response: 0·5 g 3 times daily has been recommended as the optimum dose [65]. Penicillin and chloramphenicol are less effective.

RESPIRATORY SYNCYTIAL VIRUS [16, 36 & 42]

Investigations over the last few years in several countries have shown that respiratory syncytial virus infection is one of the commonest causes of severe respiratory infection in infants and young children, although in adults infection may result in no more than upper respiratory tract symptoms. In young children there is frequently *bronchiolitis* or *bronchopneumonia*. The main manifestations are *coryza, cough, wheezing respiration* resembling asthma, and *fever*. Occasionally there may be an *erythematous rash*. The disease often occurs in winter epidemics. The virus is not susceptible to any chemotherapeutic agent at present known [31]. It is reasonable therefore to withhold chemotherapy in the milder cases of bronchiolitis in children but, as the diagnosis usually has to be made retrospectively, more severe cases may be treated with penicillin or tetracycline for the first 48 hours. The antibiotic may then be stopped unless pathogenic bacteria have been isolated [27]. If there is definite radiological pneumonia and one cannot exlude a bacterial cause at this stage the antibiotic should be continued.

INFLUENZA

Pneumonia complicating viral influenza is commonly bacterial, though in the 1957 pandemic some fatal cases were recorded apparently due to pure viral pneumonia [40 & 95]. Pneumococci are probably the commonest complicating organisms, but *Staphylococcus Pyogenes* has been much the most frequent pathogen isolated from fatal cases in recent years [38 & 77]. Such cases may be fulminating and cause death within a few hours, or the patient may remain critically ill over days or weeks. Sometimes the trachea or larynx may be obstructed by sloughed mucous membrane. We have observed almost complete necrosis of the entire visible bronchial mucous membrane at bronchoscopy. Such very severe cases are mainly seen during major epidemics. Their treatment is dealt with on p. 138.

MEASLES

Most pneumonia complicating measles is bacterial, but the pneumonia is sometimes viral. Pure measles pneumonia is associated with bronchopneumonic or miliary shadows in the x-ray and histologically with the presence of giant cells [66]. At one time '*giant cell pneumonia*' of children was thought to be a specific disease. It is an interstitial pneumonia characterized by multinucleate giant cells with cytoplasmic and nuclear inclusion bodies, aggregations of mononuclear cells and proliferation of alveolar lining cells. It usually affects children with other chronic disease, such as leukaemia or mucoviscidosis. There is now good evidence that this type of pneumonia is caused by measles virus [26].

CYTOMEGALOVIRUS

Recent serological studies suggest that infection with cytomegalovirus, presumably largely subclinical, is relatively common. About a third of adults have acquired antibodies [93]. Actual disease due to this virus is rare. Except in the newborn and in very young infants it seldom occurs except in patients already suffering from some other debilitating disease, especially reticulosis or leukaemia and especially when corticosteroid or cytotoxic drugs have been used [112]. Histologically the condition is characterized by large cells containing acidophil inclusion bodies in their nuclei. The *newborn infant* is usually infected *in utero* by virus derived from the symptom free mother. The disease is severe and often fatal, the presenting features being *jaundice, hepatosplenomegaly, purpura, thrombocytopenia* and *haemolytic anaemia*. The *brain* is often affected and survivors are usually mentally retarded. Pathologically the lungs are almost always affected both in infants and in the rare adult cases. In adults the virus may cause a disease resembling infectious mononucleosis but without pharyngitis or lymphadenopathy [52]. Both in infants and affected adults there may be a secondary pneumonia due to *Pneumocystis carinii* (p. 141). The disease may occur in localized form affecting the *salivary glands* only or, in older children and adults, the lungs. No effective treatment is known.

ADENOVIRUSES, PARAINFLUENZA VIRUSES AND RHINOVIRUSES

Pneumonia may sometimes complicate infection with adenoviruses, especially in children [16]. It may complicate infection with parainfluenzal viruses in either children or adults, although, at least in the latter, the pneumonia may be due to bacterial secondary infection. The position regarding the common cold viruses is not fully explored.

VARICELLA (Chicken-pox)

Pneumonia due to the varicella virus may complicate severe chicken-pox in adults [51]. The attack rate is said to be 4·2% in all varicella cases but as high as 38% in adults [73]. Pneumonic symptoms begin 2–5 days after the eruption. Severe respiratory distress, cough, chest pain, and often cyanosis and haemoptysis, are typical, but milder cases occur. The x-ray shows diffuse nodular infiltration which eventually may leave a residuum of miliary calcification [1 & 57]. Varicella may also be complicated by bacterial pneumonia.

HERPES ZOSTER

Herpes zoster is thought to be due to the same virus as chicken-pox, expressing itself in an individual with partial immunity. Herpes zoster is commoner in patients with leukaemia or reticuloses and in those receiving corticosteroids; in such cases generalized zoster occasionally occurs. Pleural friction, pleural effusion and radiological shadows in the lung have been described on the ipsilateral side in patients with intercostal zoster. Severe necrotizing pneumonia has been reported in generalized zoster. It is uncertain whether these pulmonary complications are all directly due to the virus, but typical intracellular inclusions have been demonstrated in at least 2 cases [73].

SMALLPOX

Pneumonia may complicate smallpox, especially in fatal cases. It is usually due to secondary bacterial infection.

LYMPHOCYTIC CHORIOMENINGITIS

This virus can produce pneumonia in guinea pigs and monkeys [2]. Pneumonia has been described in human cases and the virus has been isolated from consolidated lung at autopsy [88]. In a series of 79 patients Adair *et al.* [2] noted sore throat and cough in over a fifth and lung crepitations in 2, but in no case was there radiological evidence of pneumonia. It seems, therefore, to be a rare complication, but may occur in the course of a generalized disease due to the virus, not necessarily accompanied by meningitis [88].

INFECTIOUS MONONUCLEOSIS (Glandular fever)

Enlargement of the intrathoracic lymph glands is surprisingly rare in infectious mononucleosis [87]. Abnormal pulmonary shadows have been occasionally described but Hoagland [41] found no lower respiratory tract manifestations in 200 cases and is critical of the diagnostic criteria used in reports in the literature of various unusual manifestations of the disease. Pneumonia directly due to the unknown agent of infectious mononucleosis must be rare, if it occurs at all.

RICKETTSIAL PNEUMONIAS

Q FEVER

HISTORY [96]

The term 'Q fever' is derived from 'Query' fever, a name given at the stage when the causal organism had not been identified. It was first described in Queensland, Australia among meat and cattle workers and the causal organism, now called *Rickettsia* (or *Coxiella*) *burneti*, was identified in 1937. Shortly afterwards the same organism was isolated from ticks in Montana, U.S.A., where it was shown that a disease could be conveyed to man. During the 1939–45 war epidemics of Q fever appeared among troops in Italy and the Balkans. Shortly after the war outbreaks in cattle workers were reported in the U.S.A. Subsequently Q fever has been recognized in many parts of the world, including Britain.

AETIOLOGY AND EPIDEMIOLOGY

Infection in man is probably mainly derived from *cows* or *sheep*. Although infected animals excrete rickettsia in the milk, pasteurization probably prevents infection by this route and it seems likely that most human infection comes from *dust-laden air* with infection derived from hides, straw, etc. Explosive outbreaks have been reported mainly in abattoir workers, and sometimes under somewhat exotic conditions, such as when a number of students at an Art College were infected from dust derived from straw used for packing a statue! In clinical practice in Britain occasional cases will be found if all patients with pneumonia or unidentified pyrexia undergo routine investigation for the disease.

CLINICAL FEATURES

The *incubation period* is 2 to 3 weeks. The *symptoms* and *physical signs* correspond closely to those already outlined for viral pneumonias (p. 127). *Radiological change* is variable. Usually the lesions are segmental or subsegmental and are not uncommonly multiple. Sometimes almost a whole lobe may be involved. The *white blood count* is normal. The *duration* of the illness varies from a few days to 3 weeks or more with recovery in the great majority of cases; occasionally it may run a chronic course of several months [85]. Some of these chronic cases develop cerebral or peripheral complications possibly due to chronic vasculitis. Rarely there may be *rickettsial endocarditis* with the organisms present in vegetations on the heart valves [5, 28 & 50].

DIAGNOSIS

Largely febrile symptoms accompanied by radiological changes may suggest a viral, rickettsial or mycoplasmal pneumonia, but the nature of this usually has to be identified retrospectively by comparing the titres of agglutinating or complement-fixing antibodies in paired sera taken early in the illness and repeated after 3 weeks or so. An attempt may be made to isolate the rickettsia by inoculation of blood or sputum into guinea pigs, mice or eggs.

TREATMENT

Tetracycline is the drug of choice and should be given in doses of 0·5 to 1 g 4 times daily according to severity.

TYPHUS

Pneumonia may complicate louse borne or scrub typhus, and be seen occasionally in the less severe murine form.

MYCOPLASMAL PNEUMONIA

HISTORY, AETIOLOGY AND EPIDEMIOLOGY

Among members of the United States Forces, and to a lesser extent of the British Forces, during the 1939–45 war outbreaks of pneumonia occurred, with characteristics similar to those described above for viral pneumonia (p. 127) and differing from those then accepted for bacterial pneumonia. The term 'primary atypical pneumonia' was coined for the syndrome, but this curious phrase is illogical and has been used in a number of different senses, so that it is best abandoned. It was soon found that in certain outbreaks serum from patients agglutinated human group O red cells in the cold ('*cold agglutinins*'). A number of the patients also developed agglutinins to a non-haemolytic streptococcus ('*Streptococcus MG*') although evidence accumulated that this streptococcus had no causal relationship to the disease. Respiratory disease, often mild, could be transmitted to volunteers by means of filtered nasal washings. Eaton transferred the agent (later known as 'Eaton's agent') to hamsters and cotton rats, which developed pneumonia, but for a number of years these results were doubted, owing to the spontaneous occurrence of viral pneumonias in these animals. More recently, by the use of fluorescent antibody techniques, the agent was demonstrated to be present in the lesions of inoculated chick embryos and cotton rats and antibodies were demonstrated in convalescent serum from patients. More recently still, it has been shown that the organism concerned is not in fact a virus, although it is filter passing, but belongs to a group of organisms now known as the *Mycoplasmata* which can be cultured on cell-free media and are the smallest known free living organisms [17]. A number of different species of mycoplasmata are found as saprophytes in man but only *Mycoplasma pneumoniae* has so far been shown to cause disease, although other pathogenic species affect animals. The disease occurred on a large scale in wartime armies. It has since been reported in outbreaks among recruits and in institutions, and occasionally in general practice [30]. An outbreak is not usually a sharp epidemic but an increased incidence occurring throughout the year, with a peak in autumn and early winter. There is often a cyclic incidence with a peak every 4 or 5 years [17 & 29]. In hospital practice we ourselves have seen a fairly steady trickle of sporadic cases, many with associated bacterial pneumonia. A figure of 10–16% of all pneumonic illnesses has been quoted from Britain and Finland [17]. The majority of cases occur

between late childhood and the age of 30. Pneumonia is said to result from infection in only 3–10% of infected persons [17].

CLINICAL FEATURES

The *incubation period* is 1–3 weeks, usually about 12 days. The *symptoms* and *physical signs* often resemble those described for viral pneumonia (p. 127) but may be similar to those of bacterial pneumonia which may indeed sometimes coincide, particularly in the more severe cases which are admitted to hospital. In the absence of bacterial complication the *white blood count* is usually normal. *Radiological changes* are very variable. Segmental or subsegmental shadows are the most common, but lobar pneumonia may occur and occasionally miliary lobular shadows may be seen. A few severe cases may develop *haemolytic anaemia* or *meningism*.

DIAGNOSIS

Although a 'viral' pneumonia may be suspected clinically, the diagnosis is usually made retrospectively on serological grounds. The exact nature of the cold agglutinins, so often present in the disease, is uncertain, but the test is a useful simple diagnostic one. Cold agglutinins are more likely to occur if the illness is severe and have been present in 33–76% of reported series: 72–92% of all those with cold agglutinins are found to have evidence of infection with *M. pneumoniae* [17]. Agglutinins to *Streptococcus MG* are less often found than cold agglutinins, but may be common in certain outbreaks [4]. Their relationship to the disease is obscure; there is no evidence of an antigen common to the 2 organisms [59]. Antibodies to *Mycoplasma pneumoniae* have now been detected by the indirect fluorescent antibody technique and by tests for growth inhibition, indirect haemagglutination or complement fixation [17]. In special laboratories attempts may be made to isolate the organism by the inoculation of embryonated eggs or tissue cultures; it often persists into convalescence and has been isolated as late as 45 days after the onset of symptoms [17].

PREVENTION

A vaccine is now available and has been effective in volunteers. It might be justifiable to use it in groups or institutions showing a high attack rate of the disease [17].

TREATMENT

Mycoplasma pneumoniae is susceptible to tetracycline which has been shown to be effective in a controlled trial [49]. A dose of 0·5 to 1·0 g 4 times daily should be given according to severity.

THE DIAGNOSIS OF PNEUMONIA

There are two phases in the diagnosis of pneumonia—the decision as to whether a pneumonia is present and the decision as to what sort of pneumonia it is.

In defining the *type of pneumonia*, both an anatomical and an aetiological diagnosis is required. In the case of lobar pneumonia the former is usually readily made by physical signs in the chest, but in general the precise anatomical diagnosis is best made by a lateral chest radiograph. A complete investigation involves taking *sputum* for direct examination and culture for bacteria (including tubercle bacilli), viruses, mycoplasmata and rickettsia, together with *pharyngeal swabs* for the same purpose and *laryngeal swabs* for bacterial culture. *Blood* is taken for bacterial culture and for serology and a *white blood count* is carried out. In many centres such elaborate investigation is not possible, but the sputum should certainly be sent at the earliest possible moment for direct smear examination and culture. Laryngeal swabs should be taken if sputum is unobtainable; as a result of the stimulation of the cough reflex a good specimen of sputum is often produced. Blood culture is positive in 20–30% of severe cases of pneumococcal pneumonia, and occasionally in other infections; it is well worth carrying out.

Although staphylococci and *Klebsiella pneumoniae* are relatively easy to isolate, pneumococci and *Haemophilus influenzae* re-quire special care. If a patient has had any previous chemotherapy pneumococci may not be grown, although they may be seen in smears of the sputum. Culture in an atmosphere of 10% carbon dioxide increases the isolation rate of both pneumococci and *H. influenzae*. Isolation of the latter is increased by culture on chocolate agar and the former by intraperitoneal mouse inoculation of sputum [44]. Blood culture is often positive in severe cases [6 & 10], sometimes when sputum culture is negative.

DIFFERENTIAL DIAGNOSIS

In many cases the history of an upper respiratory tract infection followed by a fairly sudden increase of malaise, fever and perhaps pleuritic pain will be good *a priori* evidence for pneumonia, which may then be confirmed by the physical signs and x-ray of the chest. Nevertheless, the physician must bear in mind the possibility that the more recent symptoms may be due to a *pulmonary infarct*, resulting from the relative immobilization of the patient during an upper respiratory tract infection. Sudden onset, haemoptysis and the absence of pus from the sputum will favour infarct as will, of course, evidence of peripheral thrombophlebitis, although the latter may only appear a number of days after the initial incident. More than one incident of pleuritic pain, or the appearance of a new pulmonary shadow while under treatment for pneumonia, strongly suggests the possibility of infarct. When there has only been a single incident it is sometimes impossible to say whether the patient has suffered from pneumonia or infarct.

In pneumonia due to viruses, to *Rickettsia burneti* or *Mycoplasma pneumoniae*, and with no bacterial component, the initial symptoms may be largely febrile and general. The existence of a pneumonia may only be demonstrated by the chest radiograph taken as part of the routine investigation of a pyrexia. Here again the question of pulmonary infarct may arise but the persistence of pyrexia favours pneumonia.

The differentiation of *lobar pneumonia* from *tuberculous pleural effusion* may be difficult in the initial stages, especially as lobar pneumonia may be complicated by pleural effusion. A preliminary upper respiratory tract infection is less likely in the tuberculous effusion and cough and sputum are less obvious features. The sputum is unlikely to be purulent. In the early stages, when there is only a thin layer of fluid, examination of the chest may, in a pleural effusion, reveal bronchial breathing and other physical signs corresponding to those of a lobar pneumonia. In the chest radiograph, rise of the opacity in the axilla is suggestive of fluid, but this may of course be present as a complication of the pneumonia. In a tuberculous effusion the white count is likely to be normal and the aspirated fluid may be considerable in volume and largely lymphocytic, whereas a smaller volume of fluid is usually present in an effusion complicating pneumonia and the cells are neutrophils or degenerate. Pleural biopsy may also help.

Patients with *carcinoma* of the *bronchus* may present with pneumonia affecting the ill-drained lung beyond the carcinoma. Because of the inflammatory exudate the lung may not show collapse and the infection usually, but not always, responds to simple antibiotic therapy. An obvious superimposed hilar shadow on the x-ray may give a clue to the underlying diagnosis, but in many cases this is only established by precautionary bronchoscopy in a patient in whom the abnormal radiographic shadows have been slow to clear. Much less commonly the same sequence of events may be seen in a patient who has aspirated a *foreign body* into the bronchus.

Bronchopneumonia is only differentiated from *severe bronchitis* by the greater illness of the patient and by clinical or radiological evidence of pneumonic patches in the lungs. Serious diagnostic problems do not often arise but in the rare diffuse lobular pneumonia with miliary shadows the differentiation from *miliary tuberculosis* may be a problem. As in miliary tuberculosis, the symptoms may be largely febrile rather than respiratory. The *tuberculin test* may be unhelpful as it can be negative in the presence of miliary tuberculosis and in any case if the patient is severely

ill there is no time to wait for the results. If diffuse lobular shadowing is due to a viral infection the *white blood count* may be normal as in miliary tuberculosis. *Radiologically*, in pneumonia the individual shadows are usually less well defined and less dense than in miliary tuberculosis, but the differentiation may not be absolute. The patient should always be examined for *choroidal tubercles* which are virtually pathognomonic of miliary tuberculosis, but if this is negative and the patient is very ill it may be necessary to treat for both conditions and to make a final decision later. The later decision will be made on the basis of the x-ray. This should be repeated weekly. Pneumonic shadowing will begin to clear in 1–2 weeks and should be clear by 3–4 weeks. Miliary shadowing is unlikely even to begin to clear in less than 4 weeks. Clearance may take 3–4 months or longer.

In the more severe *segmental pneumonias* the diagnostic problems are similar to those of lobar pneumonia, with *bronchial carcinoma* and *pulmonary infarct* important in the differential diagnosis and *tuberculosis* always to be borne in mind. In the less severe segmental pneumonias in young people the main differential diagnosis is tuberculosis. By the time the x-ray is taken in convalescence the white blood count is usually of little value. A tuberculin test may be worth doing, as a strongly positive test is in favour of tuberculosis. If the condition is a pneumonic one, the relevant organisms are unlikely to be still present in the sputum and examination is usually a waste of time, but the sputum should be examined for tubercle bacilli. By far the most important measure is to *repeat* the *chest x-ray* after an interval of 2–3 weeks. By that time shadows due to pneumonia will always have improved or cleared, whereas shadows due to tuberculosis will be unchanged.

In an older person, especially if he is a smoker, the question of *bronchial carcinoma* will arise. If the history is suggestive, bronchoscopy should be carried out straight away. Otherwise it is justifiable to wait for 2–3 weeks to see whether the shadows clear; if they do not, bronchoscopy should be done.

If the symptoms are largely febrile rather

than respiratory, and pneumonic shadows are found on the routine x-ray film, the question of a viral, mycoplasmal or rickettsial pneumonia arises. The specific diagnosis of these conditions has usually to be retrospective, but the possibility of such a pneumonia has certain therapeutic implications (p. 138).

PREVENTION OF PNEUMONIA

In general the prevalence of pneumonia would probably be reduced by attacking some of the predisposing factors mentioned in the section on epidemiology (p. 118), such as poor ventilation, overcrowding, atmospheric pollution, cigarette smoking and overindulgence in alcohol. Soldiers, and others exposed to bad weather and cold, should have adequate clothing and be gradually adapted to the rigours they have to face. Severe upper respiratory infections, especially in predisposed persons such as bronchitics, should receive prompt chemotherapy.

There is evidence from a controlled trial that in thoracic operations *preoperative treatment with penicillin* does reduce the attack rate and mortality of postoperative pneumonia [18]. Thulbourne and Young [101] found no benefit in a controlled trial of prophylactic penicillin in abdominal operations, even in those with preexisting chronic bronchitis but there were few in the latter category. In a more recent controlled trial Collins *et al.* found a reduction of 50% in serious chest complications if penicillin and streptomycin were given for 5 days, starting the day before the operation [19]. The incidence of postoperative lung complications is much higher in those with even mild chronic bronchitis. The importance of identifying such patients before operation, by screening for airways resistance with routine measurement of FEV and FVC, has been emphasized [22 & 91]. *Pre- and postoperative postural coughing* in such patients substantially reduces the risk of lung complications [71 & 100]. The results are less satisfactory if physiotherapy is only given postoperatively [100]. Whether prophylactic penicillin would also help is uncertain. It showed no benefit in Thulborne

and Young's series [101] already quoted or in a controlled trial in patients operated on for inguinal hernia [70].

The argument against giving prophylactic antibiotics before operations is that, if continued as a long term policy, infective complications are likely to be due to organisms resistant to the antibiotic used and therefore difficult to treat. It seems reasonable therefore to adopt the policy of carrying out a preoperative FEV and FVC in all patients undergoing nonemergency abdominal and thoracic operations. All those with an FEV/FVC ratio below 70% should have intensive breathing exercises and postural coughing before and after operation and should stop smoking. Infective complications should be treated as they arise.

Patients on high dosage of corticosteroids have a reduced resistance to infection. Staphylococcal pneumonia is a recognized risk. Such patients are best treated in isolation using barrier nursing methods to prevent the intrusion of pathogenic staphylococci into their environment.

There is evidence that *immunization with pneumococcal capsular polysaccharides* does give some protection against pneumococcal pneumonia. A single injection of mixed polysaccharides substantially reduced the attack rate among army recruits [56] and both attack rate and mortality in an old people's home [46], In most communities the attack rate is too small to justify such a form of prophylaxis but it might be justifiable in a community in which, for some reason, pneumococcal pneumonia was particularly frequent.

TREATMENT OF PNEUMONIA

Whether a patient with pneumonia should be treated in hospital depends on the severity of the disease and the care available in the home. An alert family doctor will probably abort many pneumonias by initiating chemotherapy as soon as a simple upper respiratory infection appears to be becoming more severe than usual. A previously fit person with mild or moderate pneumonia, with little cyanosis and good home conditions, may be managed at home, but a severe case or any patient thought to need oxygen should certainly be sent to hospital.

LOBAR PNEUMONIA

The treatment of lobar pneumonia comprises general management, the control of pleuritic pain, chemotherapy, the use of oxygen, and breathing exercises to ensure the restoration of lung function.

GENERAL MANAGEMENT

Patients should be nursed in the most comfortable position, which is often propped up at an angle of about 45°. The patient is liable to lose fluid, partly from his overbreathing and partly from sweating, so that he must receive copious fluids. In the acute stage he will probably only be able to take the lightest food but can gradually return to a full diet as he improves. It has been shown that the use of a bedpan requires more physical effort than a commode so that the latter is better. Active movement of the legs should be carried out several times a day to reduce the risk of deep venous thrombosis.

PLEURITIC PAIN

Although a hotwater bottle at the site of the pain may be some comfort analgesics are almost always necessary. Severe pleuritic pain is most distressing to the patient and morphia in a dose of 15 mg subcutaneously is entirely justifiable in the early stage of lobar pneumonia, provided there is no contraindication. The most important contraindication is a history of chronic bronchitis, especially if there is evidence that the patient has been previously breathless. If the patient sounds bubbly and his cough reflex seems depressed, this is also a reason for caution, but in general there is little contraindication in the early stage of lobar pneumonia in a previously fit individual, although the dose should be lowered to 10 mg in old people.

In patients with a bronchitic history and profuse secretions which are difficult to clear the pain may have to be controlled by less powerful analgesics such as aspirin 0·6 to 0·9 g or paracetamol 0·5 to 1 g by the mouth so as to avoid depression of the respiratory and cough centres. Dihydrocodeine bitartrate 30 mg by the mouth or 50 mg intramuscularly is a valuable analgesic but is liable to cause some depression of the respiratory centre in higher dosage. It may be valuable in intermediate cases in which morphia is thought to carry some risk.

Patients who have to have these less effective analgesics will need a sedative in addition, at least at night. The safest is probably chloral in the form of dichloralphenazone, two 650 mg tablets.

OXYGEN

Any patient with lobar pneumonia and signs of cyanosis should be treated with oxygen. In the absence of chronic bronchitis this should be given in high concentration. If there is a history of chronic bronchitis, especially if this has been severe, the concentration should be carefully controlled (p. 345). Although the oxygen will have no effect on the parts of the lung which are perfused but unventilated it will increase the concentration of oxygen in any partially ventilated alveoli and so ensure the maximum uptake.

CHEMOTHERAPY

The majority of cases of *lobar pneumonia* are due to pneumococci, which are virtually always susceptible to penicillin and usually to tetracycline and ampicillin. In the straightforward case, not desperately ill, and when the causative organism is unknown, treatment may be begun with benzylpenicillin 1 mega unit twice daily intramuscularly, or tetracycline 0·5 g 4 times daily, or ampicillin 0·25 g 4 times daily. A controlled therapeutic trial has shown that ampicillin in this dose is as good as penicillin plus streptomycin [20]; it is probable, but not proved, that tetracycline would be equally good. One of the oral drugs is obviously more convenient for treatment at home.

In hospital it may be possible to obtain some information about the causative organism by examination of a direct smear of the sputum. If *pneumococci* are identified or no obvious pathogens are found, treatment should be initiated with one of the above drugs; any previous antibiotic treatment may have caused the disappearance of pneumococci from the sputum. If the direct smear of the sputum shows obvious *staphylococci*, treatment may have to be modified, as a number of strains of staphylococci are resistant to penicillin, especially if the pneumonia has arisen in hospital. Until the results of resistance tests are available cloxacillin should be given in a dose of 500 mg 6-hourly on an empty stomach by the mouth, or 250 mg 6 hourly by intramuscular injection if the patient is very ill. As cloxacillin is much less potent than penicillin in penicillin sensitive staphylocci, benzylpenicillin should be given as well in a dose of 1 mega unit 6 hourly. If the staphylococci prove to be penicillin resistant it is worth while continuing both drugs for reasons already outlined (p. 92). It is a good rule, if it can be implemented, that any patient with potentially resistant staphylococci should be nursed in isolation.

If a direct smear of sputum shows capsulated gram negative bacilli, the possibility of pneumonia due to *Klebsiella pneumoniae* must be considered. If the organisms are numerous in the sputum and the patient has had no previous chemotherapy, this possibility must be regarded as a serious one, particularly if he is very ill. *Klebsiella pneumoniae* is almost always initially sensitive to streptomycin, usually to chloramphenicol and sometimes to tetracycline. Streptomycin should be given, as it is bactericidal, but should be combined with a second drug to prevent the emergence of resistance (p. 86). Because of the potential seriousness of this type of pneumonia it is permissible to take the small risk of blood dyscrasia and give chloramphenicol as the second drug. Streptomycin should be given in a dose of 0·5 or 1 g intramuscularly 6 hourly, depending on the severity of the illness, and combined with chloramphenicol 0·5–1 g 6 hourly by the mouth. Resistance tests should also be carried out to tetracycline, cephaloridine and ampicillin and the drug combination modified if

necessary. If only a few capsulated gram negative organisms are seen, and particularly if there has been previous chemotherapy which might have eliminated pneumococci or staphylococci and allowed survival of or superinfection by *K. pneumoniae* which might not, in fact, be causal, it is wise to cover the possibility of *Klebsiella* pneumonia by giving the drugs as indicated, but to add benzylpenicillin in case a causal pneumococcus has been missed.

In most cases of pneumonia the patient will begin to respond within the first 24 hours and will then gradually improve with fall of temperature and diminution of symptoms. Chemotherapy should be continued for 3 or 4 days after the temperature has become normal. 7–10 days' treatment is usually adequate. Initial intramuscular penicillin may be replaced by oral phenoxymethylpenicillin as the patient improves.

If the patient is a chronic bronchitic, *H. influenzae* will often be present in the respiratory tract and may contribute to the pneumonia so that many physicians combine intramuscular penicillin with streptomycin 0·5 g twice daily, the 2 drugs acting synergistically on this organism.

FAILURE TO RESPOND TO TREATMENT WITHIN 36–48 HOURS

Failure to respond to treatment within 36–48 hours may be due to a mistaken diagnosis of pneumonia, to an organism resistant to the drug or drugs in use or to a slow response of a susceptible organism. The most important *diagnostic errors* are to regard as pneumonia what is really a tuberculous pleural effusion or a pulmonary infarct. Differential diagnosis has already been discussed (p. 133). Pneumonia may also occur beyond a bronchial obstruction, such as a carcinoma of the bronchus or a foreign body (p. 119). The pyrexia of such a pneumonia usually responds to treatment, suspicion being later aroused by failure of radiographic clearing. Occasionally pyrexia persists in such cases; a suspicious hilar shadow or failure to detect another cause for the persistent fever should lead to bronchoscopy.

If initial treatment was with penicillin, the most likely *resistant bacteria* which might cause failure to respond are *Staphylococci, M. tuberculosis* or *K. pneumoniae* in that order. *Staphylococci* and *Klebsiella* are readily cultured; the result should be available within 24 hours and lead to the appropriate adjustments in chemotherapy (p. 90). Any patient with pneumonia should always have his sputum examined for tubercle bacilli. If his pneumonia fails to respond to initial treatment further sputa should be examined.

Failure to respond to penicillin may be due to *viral, mycoplasmal* or *rickettsial* infection. Some indication of this possibility may sometimes be obtained from the history, but not always so. If no other cause for the failure to respond has been found it is reasonable to treat the patient with tetracycline as *Mycoplasma pneumoniae, Rickettsia burneti* and viruses of the ornithosis group are all susceptible to this drug.

DESPERATELY ILL PATIENT

Sometimes the patient may be first seen at a very advanced stage, when he appears as if he may die within 24 hours. This may be due to his being first seen late in the disease or to an overwhelming infection, as in a staphylococcal pneumonia complicating viral influenza. The correct chemotherapy is vital and it is most important for a smear of the sputum to be examined immediately. This may identify the causal organism and the appropriate chemotherapy should be given. If the examination is unhelpful, or sputum is difficult to obtain, *benzylpenicillin* and *cloxacillin* should be given intramuscularly, as this will cover both the possibility of staphylococcal and pneumococcal pneumonia. In addition, benzylpenicillin 1 mega unit can be given intravenously 4 hourly if there is *peripheral circulatory failure*. If the systolic blood pressure is below 100 mm Hg it is justifiable to give hydrocortisone hemisuccinate in a dosage of 10 mg/hour as 30 mg added to 500 ml of dextran infusion fluid. In pneumonia complicating severe influenza the larynx and upper trachea may be blocked by sloughed mucous membrane, so that bronchoscopy followed by tracheostomy may be required.

CONVALESCENCE

As soon as the patient's fever has subsided he should begin to sit up in a chair and thereafter gradually increase his activities. When the temperature has been normal for a couple of days breathing exercises should be begun with the aim of clearing the lung of inflammatory products as soon as possible and ensuring return to full function. The chest should be x-rayed weekly. In younger patients the film usually returns to normal within 2–6 weeks. In the elderly it may take longer; the average was 6 weeks in a group of our patients over the age of 60. Any undue delay should raise the suspicion of an underlying carcinoma of the bronchus and bronchoscopy should be carried out. The duration of convalescence before returning to work will depend on the patient's age, the severity of the illness and the nature of his work.

BRONCHOPNEUMONIA

The most important ways in which the treatment of bronchopneumonia differs from that of lobar pneumonia are in the particular care which must be taken over the use of sedatives and oxygen. It is important to clear the bronchi of increased secretions and it is therefore most important not to suppress the cough reflex. Morphia should be avoided and a mild sedative such as chloral given if necessary (p. 136). Fortunately pleuritic pain is not often a problem; if present it can be dealt with by simple analgesics (p. 136). The principles of oxygen therapy are similar to those in exacerbations of chronic bronchitis, of which the bronchopneumonia is often only an extension (p. 345).

The chemotherapy used need not differ greatly from that of lobar pneumonia, but because of the more frequent rôle of *H. influenzae* benzyl penicillin 1 mega unit may be combined with streptomycin 0·5 g twice daily; in very ill patients the penicillin may be given 4 times daily. In moderate or mild cases tetracycline or ampicillin may be substituted (p. 136).

SEGMENTAL AND LOCALIZED LOBULAR PNEUMONIA

If a patient with segmental or localized lobular pneumonia is moderately or severely ill he should be treated in the same way as for lobar pneumonia (p. 136). Usually he is not severely ill and the pneumonia may not be diagnosed until an x-ray is taken in convalescence. By this time the main consideration is to exclude other conditions (p. 134) but tetracycline or ampicillin (p. 136) may be given if the patient still has important symptoms.

NONBACTERIAL PNEUMONIA

The general management of these pneumonias is similar to that of the bacterial pneumonias. The chemotherapy of pneumonias due to the larger viruses (p. 128), the rickettsiae (p. 131) and to *Mycoplasma pneumoniae* (p. 133) is dealt with under the individual headings. A definitive diagnosis is not usually made during the acute stage; the handling of a patient in whom a nonbacterial aetiology is probable has already been outlined on p. 138.

COMPLICATIONS OF PNEUMONIA

Herpes labialis often develops in the first few days of pneumococcal pneumonia.

Pleural effusion and empyema. Empyema (p. 151) was formerly a common complication of pneumococcal pneumonia. With modern chemotherapy it is now rare. In one series it occurred in only 3·4% of over 500 cases with positive blood culture [6]. Pleural effusion is common. The effusion is usually not large. It may be detected by physical examination; stony dullness and decreased vocal fremitus are suggestive. In the x-ray an opacity running upwards in the axilla indicates that fluid is present. The fluid is yellow and often slightly turbid. It may contain neutrophils or degenerate cells and is usually sterile. A moderate effusion is better aspirated in order to avoid pleural thickening; a small one may be left to clear spontaneously. A large effusion accompanying a pneumonia suggests the possibility of an underlying neoplasm. If there is any doubt of the diagnosis a pleural biopsy should be done.

Lung abscess (p. 161) is a common complication of pneumonia due to staphylococci or *Klebsiella pneumoniae*, but is relatively rare in pneumococcal pneumonia. *Spontaneous pneumothorax* tends to complicate staphylococcal pneumonia, especially if there is abscess formation (p. 161) and especially in children. It is occasionally seen in other pneumonias. *Pericarditis, endocarditis, septic arthritis, peritonitis* and *meningitis* are rare complications of pneumonia, especially pneumococcal [6] or staphylococcal. They are more likely in those with positive blood culture.

Peripheral thrombophlebitis (p. 464) is relatively common. Its prevention has already been discussed. The patient's legs should be examined daily so that anticoagulant therapy can be initiated if indicated.

Jaundice occasionally complicates pneumonia; there were 13 cases among 2807 patients with pneumonia in one series [37]. In pneumococcal pneumonia it may be due to breakdown of red cells in the stage of red hepatization, but probably also to toxic or anoxic liver damage. It is an indication of severe disease. Haemolytic anaemia may complicate cases of mycoplasmal pneumonia in which there is a high titre of cold agglutinins.

Meningism is occasionally seen, especially with apical pneumonias. It is commoner in children.

Mental confusion and occasionally *schizophrenic symptoms* may sometimes complicate the acute toxic stage of pneumonia. Hypoxaemia may be the main factor [9].

Uraemia and acute glomerulonephritis. A raised blood urea is not uncommon in the acute stages of pneumonia but subsides in convalescence. We have seen severe glomerulonephritis complicate pneumococcal pneumonia.

Circulatory failure may occur in severe pneumonia, due to toxic injury to the peripheral vessels and perhaps to the cardiac muscle. The peripheral vessels lose their tone, the blood pressure falls and the limbs become cold and clammy. Such patients are desperately ill. Their treatment has been dealt with on p. 138.

PROGNOSIS OF PNEUMONIA

Obviously the more severe the disease the worse the prognosis. The nature of the organism is important. *Staphylococcal pneumonia* complicating epidemic influenza has a deservedly grim reputation. The high mortality of pneumonia due to *Klebsiella pneumoniae* has already been mentioned. *Type 3* is the most lethal of the pneumococcal strains. Pneumonia is more dangerous in patients with other diseases, especially *chronic bronchitis*, in

young infants and in *old age*. In the individual patient with bacterial pneumonia a *low* or *a very high white blood cell count*, a *positive blood culture* or *jaundice* are indications of severity.

Nevertheless with modern chemotherapy the prognosis for recovery is excellent. The mortality obviously depends on the type of case treated. Hospitals mostly admit the more seriously ill patients, with a high proportion of bronchitics and old people. Even in such series and in influenza epidemics the mortality is not usually more than 10%.

On the other hand less is known about residual disability after pneumonia. Fry [33] in general practice found that twice as many patients had persistent or recurrent respiratory symptoms after an attack of lobar pneumonia as before; this was particularly true of smokers in the lower economic groups. Although residual disability was much less common after segmental pneumonia, it was relatively common in those who had had a previous chest illness.

UNRESOLVED AND CHRONIC SUPPURATIVE PNEUMONIA

Although the great majority of pneumococcal pneumonias resolve completely residual fibrosis sometimes occurs, particularly after pneumonia due to staphylococci or *Klebsiella pneumoniae* and especially if there has been abscess formation. In the absence of abscess formation, neoplasm or tuberculosis, Israel and his colleagues [46] found radiographic shadows persisting beyond 8 weeks in only 1 out of 139 patients; relatively slow resolution was commoner in older patients and in

diabetics. In the pre-chemotherapy era patients were sometimes seen with persistent purulent sputum, continuous or recurrent fever and shadowing in the x-ray which might spread to new areas of the same lung, the whole illness extending over months and sometimes having a fatal outcome (*chronic suppurative pneumonia*). Such cases are now very rare, presumably because intensive chemotherapy cuts the disease short.

RECURRENT PNEUMONIA

Recurrence of two or more attacks of 'pneumonia' within weeks should make the physician doubt the diagnosis. Recurrent *pulmonary infarct* is the commonest alternative (p. 460). If there are asthmatic symptoms, or eosinophilia, *pulmonary eosinophilia* (p. 425) may be considered. Recurrence over a longer period suggests either a general factor reducing resistance or a local pre-

disposing cause. Chronic bronchitis, a very common predisposing condition, is obvious enough. Less usual and less obvious are *hypogammaglobulinaemia*, *myelomatosis*, 'heavy chain disease' and *disseminated lupus erythematosis* (p. 581). Among local predisposing causes are recurrent *aspiration* from infected sinuses, from a pharyngeal pouch or from an obstructed oesophagus. A patient with achalasia of the cardia may sometimes present in this way without any complaint of dysphagia (p. 146). Recurrent pneumonia at the same site, or series of sites, suggests the possibility of underlying *bronchial tumour* or *bronchiectasis*. We have on a number of occasions seen recurrent localized pneumonia or pleurisy as the only manifestation of a small area of bronchiectasis.

PNEUMONIAS DUE TO YEASTS, FUNGI AND PROTOZOA

Pneumonia due to *Pneumocystis carinii* is described below. For other pneumonias in these categories see p. 284.

PNEUMOCYSTIS CARINII PNEUMONIA

AETIOLOGY AND EPIDEMIOLOGY

This organism is probably a protozoon but possibly a fungus [34]. It occurs in a wide variety of animals, mainly as a saprophyte. Proof of the association with pneumonia in man depends mainly on its frequent histological demonstration in a somewhat specific form of pneumonia and on the finding of positive complement fixation tests in some cases. The disease affects in particular the newborn, especially premature infants. It is more common in institutions. It has been extensively described in central and eastern Europe, but cases have now been reported from most parts of the world [34]. In infants the disease occurs especially between the 4th and 16th week of life with a probable incubation period of about 40 days. Adults may also be affected, usually those with a background of chronic disease, such as leukaemia or lymphadenoma, or who have been treated with high doses of corticosteroids, cytotoxic drugs or radiotherapy [82]. Congenital hypogammaglobulinaemia is a predisposing factor both in adults and children. Associated infection with cytomegalovirus is relatively frequent, probably because of the widespread presence of both agents in the environment and of common predisposing factors [34 & 82]. Multiple cases have been described in a single family [61 & 105].

PATHOLOGY

Macroscopically the lungs show varying degrees of consolidation. The diagnostic feature is the presence of intra-alveolar clumps of foamy eosinophil material containing the characteristic cysts which are round or oval and about 5 µ in diameter. These are often demonstrable with haematoxylin and eosin staining but sometimes are best seen with silver staining or on smears of lungs rather than in histological sections. Interstitial emphysema may be present in infants. The inflammatory reaction is variable. There is often alveolar cell hyperplasia and usually interstitial invasion with lymphocytes and plasma cells. In fact, before the causal organism was identified this was often known as 'plasma cell' pneumonia of infants.

FUNCTIONAL ABNORMALITY

As with other forms of pneumonia in which the remaining lung is relatively normal the Pa,O_2 is usually decreased but the Pa,CO_2 may be normal or even decreased [82].

CLINICAL FEATURES

In infants the onset is often insidious and characterized by restlessness and poor feeding. There is often no initial fever and even later only low pyrexia. Gradually the infant develops greater respiratory distress and obvious cyanosis. Cough, which is usually slight initially, becomes a more marked feature. Physical signs in the chest may be absent or minimal, consisting of a few scattered crepitations or sometimes small areas of consolidation. In outbreaks in institutions some infants may have mild disease with slight symptoms and transient radiological shadows. In adults the characteristics are low grade fever, dyspnoea, dry cough and cyanosis. Physical signs are minimal. These features may continue for many weeks.

The characteristic radiological feature is bilateral midzone perihilar shadowing which may later spread to include the bases and the whole lung fields. There is usually no pleural reaction but interstitial emphysema, either subcutaneous or mediastinal, may be seen in infants.

DIAGNOSIS
The typical radiological shadows with the relative absence of physical signs in an infant or in an adult with one of the predisposing conditions, should suggest the possibility of the diagnosis. The diagnosis in life has only comparatively seldom been made by sputum or tracheal smears but the organism has been demonstrated by lung puncture or lung biopsy. It has even occasionally been found in a thick smear of the peripheral blood. It cannot be cultured at present. A complement fixation test, using the dried lungs of fatal cases, has been described but its value is doubtful [34 & 82].

TREATMENT
The best results seem to have been reported with pentamidine isethionate, an antiprotozoal agent. The dose is 4 mg/kg in a single daily intramuscular dose for 10–14 days. It is claimed that this treatment has reduced the mortality in infants in Hungary from 50 to 5% [47 & 61].

PROGNOSIS
It is difficult to be sure of the overall prognosis as many of the patients have only been diagnosed at postmortem and other patients may well have recovered without a specific diagnosis having been made. In institutional outbreaks the mortality has been quoted as 20–50% [61] but treatment with pentamidine is said to have reduced this to a much lower figure.

ALLERGIC PNEUMONIAS AND PNEUMONIAS COMPLICATING COLLAGEN DISEASES

For these see sections elsewhere: Pulmonary eosinophilia and related pneumonias (p. 425), rheumatic fever (p. 577), rheumatoid disease (p. 578), disseminated lupus erythematosis (p. 581).

CHEMICAL PNEUMONIA

PNEUMONIA DUE TO IRRITANT GASES, SMOKE OR METAL FUMES

Pneumonias due to these causes are mainly occupational and are dealt with on p. 489.

LIPOID PNEUMONIA

Two types of lipoid pneumonia have to be distinguished, *exogenous* in which the fatty or oily material is inhaled and *endogenous*, in which it is deposited from the tissues. In the latter are included fat embolism (p. 457), and lipoid histiocytic diseases (Histiocytosis X, p. 572).

EXOGENOUS LIPOID PNEUMONIA

PATHOGENESIS AND PATHOLOGY [90]
The inhaled oil may be mineral, vegetable or animal. The most common is liquid paraffin taken as an aperient or used in nasal drops. Diesel oil was inhaled by shipwrecked sailors during the war [108]. Codliver oil or milk feeds may be inhaled by children. Most cases occur in infants or the elderly, especially if the latter are suffering from chronic neurological or other disability. The effect of various types of oils on the lung was investigated by Pinkerton [76]. Mineral oils are chemically inert and are rapidly emulsified and engulfed

by macrophages. Some are eventually taken up by the lymphatics but any residuum may ultimately give rise to fibrosis. Most vegetable oils, such as olive oil, become emulsified, are not hydrolysed by the lung lipases and cause little damage to the lung. They are removed mainly by expectoration. Animal fats are hydrolysed by the lung lipases and the liberated fatty acids, in addition to any present in the original material, produce severe inflammatory reaction [76 & 90].

In infants and the elderly aspiration tends to occur when the individual is lying down. The oil is often distributed throughout the lung causing diffuse interstitial pneumonia and intraalveolar exudate. In the intermediate ages the inhaled material is more likely to be localized to one part of the lung resulting in a dense fibrotic mass looking like a carcinoma on the x-ray. Liquid paraffin is the most frequent cause of this type of lesion. Spencer [90] differentiates a series of stages ranging from an acute polymorphonuclear and haemorrhagic stage after inhaling a milk feed, through a stage of macrophage and giant cell proliferation, to destruction of the lung architecture and fibrosis. Saprophytic mycobacteria may be inhaled with the milk and are perhaps responsible for some of the extensive damage caused by lipoid pneumonia complicating achalasia of the cardia.

FUNCTIONAL ABNORMALITY

Diffuse lipoid pneumonia is said to give rise to a restrictive type of lesion with decreased Pa,O_2 on exercise and decreased transfer factor for carbon monoxide, without airways obstruction [107].

CLINICAL FEATURES

Patients with radiological lesions due to lipoid pneumonia may have very little in the way of symptoms or physical signs but cough, sputum and dyspnoea may occur and there may be basal crepitations, particularly in the elderly [103].

RADIOLOGY

In the early stages the chest film is said to show rosette-like clumps of small nodules [107]. If the lesion is diffuse there is usually basal interstitial fibrosis with 'white lines like cotton threads separated by tiny bullae' [87]. Sometimes there are multiple granulomata giving a miliary appearance in addition to the reticular shadows. The appearance may be very like the interstitial fibrosis of collagen diseases. Occasionally there is a large localized mass suggesting a carcinoma.

DIAGNOSIS

The patient seldom volunteers information which might lead the clinician to diagnose exogenous lipoid pneumonia. In any suggestive case the physician should therefore make enquiries about nasal drops, liquid paraffin for constipation, etc. Appropriate staining or fluorescent microscopy may demonstrate oil- or fat-laden macrophages [107], but these are not necessarily specific and may occur in other chronic inflammations. Lung biopsy or lung aspiration has been occasionally undertaken and the localized form of granuloma has often been removed surgically as a possible carcinoma.

PREVENTION AND TREATMENT

It is now realized that the routine use of mineral oil in nasal drops or laxatives is undesirable. It is particularly important to avoid this in old and disabled people in whom aspiration is more likely. When there are no important symptoms diagnosis by x-ray should lead to stopping the use of mineral oil. Secondary infection will require treatment if it occurs.

ENDOGENOUS LIPOID PNEUMONIA
('Cholesterol pneumonitis')

PATHOGENESIS AND PATHOLOGY

This condition is primarily a localized lesion giving a greyish or yellowish appearance on macroscopic section and dominated microscopically by the presence of large numbers of cholesterol-containing macrophages in the alveoli and alveolar walls. The nuclei of the macrophages are central and the cytoplasm

stains brilliantly with Sudan dyes [97]. Proliferation of the alveolar endothelium and
various degrees of intralobular fibrosis may
also be present. Such a lesion may complicate
a carcinoma or other obstructive lesion of the
bronchus, or chronic lung abscess, bronchiectasis or x-radiation [98] but may occur in the
absence of any of these [56 & 97]. Experimentally a similar lesion was produced in
rabbits by introducing infection with gram
negative organisms in animals fed on diets
resulting in a high serum cholesterol. Slight
lesions could be obtained even in the absence
of high blood cholesterol [104]. It was suggested that as the pH fell in inflamed areas
there was flocculation and precipitation of the
lipid systems.

CLINICAL FEATURES
These include cough, sputum, haemoptysis
and chest pain. *Radiologically* the localized
shadow, unaltered over a period, suggests
the possibility of a bronchial carcinoma and
in most patients the correct diagnosis has
only been made on a resected specimen.

DIAGNOSIS
It seems possible that the diagnosis might
sometimes be suspected by finding suggestive
cells in the sputum, but this would not necessarily exclude the presence of a chronic
inflammatory lesion of this kind beyond a
carcinoma.

TREATMENT
In most cases the possibility of a carcinoma
cannot be excluded. A frozen section at
thoracotomy may permit the diagnosis to
be made in the theatre and allow a more
limited resection than might be necessary in
the case of a carcinoma. Because of the
necessity of excluding the latter, and the uncertain prognosis, the lesion is best resected.

PNEUMONIA DUE TO
PETROLEUM, PARAFFIN
(KEROSENE), ETC.

This type of pneumonia is usually due to
inhalation during accidental ingestion [79]

or aspiration of vomit after ingestion. It is
naturally commoner in children. The inhaled
material causes acute oedema, inflammation
and bronchospasm. Inhalation of petrol
vapour has mainly mental and neurological
effects but may also cause pneumonia [45].
Absorption of petrol or paraffin from the lung
may cause damage in the liver, kidney, heart
and central nervous system, with shock,
convulsions, coma and death. If the patient
survives the acute period there are usually
signs of pneumonia, accompanied by fever,
which in most cases clears in 7–10 days but
occasionally runs a prolonged course [63],
sometimes with recurrent shadows in the
chest x-ray. The radiological changes are
usually bilateral and in the midzones or
bases. There has been some controversy over
the desirability of gastric lavage which was
thought to increase the liability to aspirate
the material which has a low surface tension.
Olstad and Lord [68] concluded that the
incidence of pneumonia was lower in patients
who had had gastric lavage or vomited, or
both, but Baldachin and Melmed [67], who
avoided lavage, had only 1 death in 200 cases.
The general view at present is that lavage
should be avoided [62]. Oxygen should be
given. There is evidence that corticosteroids
may help to tide the patient over the acute
stage though relapse may occur if they are
stopped prematurely [63].

RADIATION PNEUMONIA

DEFINITION
An inflammation of the lung induced by
radiation, usually that used for radiotherapy.

PATHOGENESIS
Radiation pneumonia, sufficient to produce
symptoms, occurs particularly after wide field
radiation for reticuloses or lung metastases
[109]. On the other hand the most common
type is that arising after radiation for carcinoma of the breast. As this is purely localized
it may give rise to few symptoms. The reaction is limited to the area which has actually
been irradiated and therefore the condition
is usually only severe when irradiation has

affected both sides. The effect varies with the size of the radiation dose, the amount of lung which has been irradiated and the rate of administration. It is more likely to occur in thin individuals. It has also been reported after radioactive iodine therapy of carcinoma of the thyroid with pulmonary metastases [78].

PATHOLOGY

The alveolar walls are thickened by lymphocyte infiltration and fibrosis. The alveolar lining cells are swollen; there may be hyaline membrane formation and the alveoli may contain desquamated alveolar cells, macrophages and organizing exudate. Lipoid pneumonia may occur [109]. There may be thrombosis of small vessels.

FUNCTIONAL ABNORMALITY

Radiation pneumonia results in a restrictive abnormality (p. 51). The spirogram may show 'door step breathing', the end inspiratory trace having a flat squared off top owing to loss of elasticity of the lung and the sudden cessation of inspiration as the lung reaches the limit of its compliance on inspiration.

CLINICAL FEATURES

There is an interval varying between 1 and 16 weeks, with a mean of 4 weeks, between the finish of the radiotherapy and the onset of radiological and clinical features of radiation pneumonia. With slighter lesions in the lungs, as demonstrated radiologically, there may be no clinical symptoms. Dyspnoea is the dominant symptom and increases rapidly. After recovery there is gradual decrease in dyspnoea over a period of weeks but most patients are left with some permanent functional impairment. About 50% of patients have dry cough, worse on exercise or deep breathing. Patients who develop radiation pneumonia often have dysphagia due to radiation oesophagitis but this has usually disappeared before the onset of the lung symptoms. Pain from rib fractures, due to radiation damage, may also occur. There is usually no fever and relatively few physical signs in the chest although diminished percussion note

and breath sounds, or inspiratory crepitations, may occur. The erythrocyte sedimentation rate is usually increased [109].

RADIOLOGY

In acute stages the most common appearance resembles bilateral pulmonary oedema, with maximum opacities in the midzones, particularly round the hila [109]. The opacity is usually not completely opaque and linear interstitial thickening may be visible through it. The pleura usually becomes thickened, particularly on the mediastinal side [87]. Later there may be coarse fibrosis. The ribs may show signs of radiation necrosis or fractures.

PROGNOSIS

Radiation pneumonia sufficient to give rise to symptoms of dyspnoea can be life-threatening. Seven out of 49 of Whitfield et al.'s patients died [109].

PREVENTION AND TREATMENT

It has been suggested that it would be worth while giving corticosteroids prophylactically to patients who are having wide field radiotherapy which includes both lungs, but there are considerable differences of opinion in the literature as to whether this measure is in fact of value and no controlled trials have come to our notice (see discussion by Douglas [24]). It has been suggested, as a result of experimental work on animals, that anticoagulant therapy might be useful as the lung lesion is supposed at least partly to be due to thrombosis of small vessels. Once again clinical experience has produced no unequivocal evidence of the value of this measure [109].

Corticosteroid drugs should always be given in the acute stage. They may result in dramatic relief of symptoms but may also fail to be effective. Much probably depends on the actual amount of lung damage. At least 10 mg of prednisolone 4 times daily should be given, gradually reducing the dose once success is achieved. Corticosteroids should be continued for at least 3 months at the minimal dose which controls symptoms. The patient should be nursed in isolation to avoid secondary infection [24]. Any secondary infection which occurs should be enthusiastically treated. The patient should be put at rest and given oxygen in high concentration.

PNEUMONIA FROM INHALATION FROM THE UPPER GASTROINTESTINAL TRACT
[13 & 14]

PATHOGENESIS

Inhalation from the upper gastrointestinal tract is liable to occur particularly in infants and old people, in those with neurological lesions of the bulbar apparatus, in those under sedation and during or after anaesthesia or alcohol intoxication. Inhalation may occur from the following sources:

(1) Inhalation of vomit after anaesthesia or intoxication.

(2) Inhalation of milk feeds, codliver oil or mineral oils (see 'Lipoid Pneumonia', p. 142).

(3) Pharyngeal diverticulum.

(4) Achalasia of the cardia, the commonest condition causing this syndrome.

(5) Hiatus hernia.

(6) Oesophageal strictures, benign or malignant, especially carcinoma of the upper third when it causes vocal cord paralysis [13].

In patients without neurological lesions aspiration may occur because of relaxation of the oesophagopharyngeal sphincter during sleep.

PATHOLOGY

In Belcher's series [13], which included a survey of the previous literature, lung abscess was the commonest manifestation. Belsey [14] writing 11 years later found that recurrent pneumonia was much more common. He attributed the difference to advances in dental hygiene and chemotherapy. The pneumonia may be acute, recurrent or chronic. Aspiration of vomit is particularly liable to give rise to an acute haemorrhagic pneumonia, which may be rapidly fatal. Recurrent aspiration may give rise to lipoid pneumonia (p. 142) and there may be gross local fibrosis and bronchiectasis. Some localized lesions may

strongly suggest carcinoma of the bronchus on clinical and radiological grounds. Atelectasis is relatively rare. It has been suggested that it may occur after aspiration of a bolus or perhaps due to pressure on the main bronchus by the dilated oesophagus in cases with achalasia of the cardia or oesophageal stricture [13].

FUNCTIONAL ABNORMALITY

Multiple diffuse lesions with fibrosis are likely to give rise to a restrictive lesion. Aspiration of vomit may result in acute 'bronchospasm' and airways obstruction. Localized lesions may result in appropriate diminution of overall lung function.

CLINICAL FEATURES

Inhaled vomit may give rise to a very severe haemorrhagic pneumonia with gross pulmonary oedema and haemoptysis. The clinical features of lipoid pneumonia secondary to aspiration of milk feed, codliver oil, liquid paraffin, etc. are dealt with on p. 142. Recurrent inhalation from the oesophagus may be more cryptic. Often the patient does not volunteer any history of dysphagia, though he may acknowledge this if asked direct questions. Nevertheless the achalasia may be asymptomatic and may only be detected by recognizing the dilated oesophagus on the straight x-ray of the chest. In any patient where the incidents could be due to oesophageal lesions direct questions should be asked and a barium swallow should form part of the investigation. Patients may present with recurrent cough and sputum. There may be radiological or clinical evidence of pneumonia ('dysphagic pneumonitis') but sometimes there is only recurrent tracheobronchitis due to repeated aspiration of oesophageal contents. Small recurrent haemoptyses may be the only manifestation. Sometimes the blood stained sputum contains acid-fast bacilli which do not prove to be tubercle bacilli [14]. Inhalation of this type is one of the recognized causes of recurrent pneumonia (p. 140). Chronic fibrosis may give rise to dyspnoea and even clubbing. Sometimes radiological abnormality may be accompanied by no clinical disability.

RADIOLOGY

Although there may be a wide variety of intrapulmonary opacities the typical appearance is of bilateral midzone opacities, often more on the right. The opacities may be ill-defined and nonhomogeneous, later with evidence of fibrosis. Evidence of a dilated oesophagus may be seen with a convex shadow to the right of the mediastinum, often most visible in the upper mediastinum but differentiated from an unfolded aorta by the continuation of the convex shadow below the origin of the aorta. The accumulated food within the esophagus gives a granular appearance on the x-ray similar to that of faeces seen in an abdominal film. Sometimes a fluid level is seen in the oesophagus, usually just above the *left* sternoclavicular joint [13 & 87].

PREVENTION AND TREATMENT

Once the basic condition is recognized its treatment should prevent further pulmonary episodes.

REFERENCES

[1] ABRAHAMS E.W., EVANS C., KNYVETT A.F. & STRINGER R.E. (1964) Varicella pneumonia: a possible cause of subsequent pulmonary calcification. *Med. J. Aust.* 2, 781.

[2] ADAIR C.V., GAULD R.T. & SMADEL J.E. (1953) Aseptic meningitis, a disease of diverse etiology: clinical and etiologic studies on 854 cases. *Ann. intern. Med.* 39, 675.

[3] ALSTON J.M. & BROOM J.C. (1958) *Leptospirosis in Man and Animals*. London, Livingstone.

[4] ANDERSON T.B. (1960) Pneumonia with antibodies to *Streptococcus MG. Lancet* i, 1375.

[5] ANDREWS P.S. & MARMION B.P. (1959) Chronic Q Fever. 2. Morbid anatomical and bacteriological findings in a patient with endocarditis. *Br. med. J.* ii, 893.

[6] AUSTRIAN R. & GOLD J. (1964) Pneumococcal bacteremia with especial reference to bacteremic pneumococcal pneumonia. *Ann. intern. Med.* 60, 759.

[7] BALDACHIN B.J. & MELMED R.N. (1964) Clinical and therapeutic aspects of kerosene poisoning: a series of 200 cases. *Br. med J.* ii, 28.

[8] BANATVALA J.E. (1967) Clinical virology today. *Proc. roy. Soc. Med.* 60, 637.

[9] BATES D.V. & CHRISTIE R.V. (1964) *Respiratory Function in Disease. An Introduction to the Integrated Study of the Lung*. Philadelphia, Saunders.

[10] BATH J.C.J.L., BOISSARD G.P.B., CALDER MARGARET A. & MOFFAT MARGARET A. (1964) Pneumonia in hospital practice in Edinburgh. *Br. J. Dis. Chest* 58, 1.

[11] BEATTY O.E. (1937) Manifestations of undulant fever in the respiratory tract. *Am. Rev. Tuberc.* 36, 283.

[12] BEDSON S.P. (1961) Psittacosis-lymphogranuloma venereum group (the Castaneda-positive viruses). Ed. Bedson S., Downie A.W., MacCallum F.O. & Stuart-Harris C.H. In *Virus and Rickettsial Diseases of Man*, (1961). 3rd Edition. London, Arnold.

[13] BELCHER J.R. (1949) The pulmonary complications of dysphagia. *Thorax* 4, 44.

[14] BELSEY R. (1960) The pulmonary complications of oesophageal disease. *Br. J. Dis. Chest* 54, 342.

[15] BLAKE F.G. & CECIL R.L. (1920) Pathology and pathogenesis of pneumococcal lobar pneumonia in monkeys. *J. exp. Med.* 31, 445.

[16] CHANOCK R.M. & PARROTT R.H. (1965) Acute respiratory disease in infancy and childhood: Present understanding and prospects for prevention. *Pediatrics* 36, 21.

[17] CHANOCK R.M. (1965) Mycoplasma infections of man. *New Engl. J. Med.* 273, 1199 and 1257.

[18] CITRON K.M. (1965) Controlled trial of prophylactic penicillin in thoracic surgery. *Thorax* 20, 18.

[19] COLLINS C.D., DARKE C.S. & KNOWELDEN J. (1958) Chest complications after upper abdominal surgery: their anticipation and prevention. *Br. med. J.* i, 401.

[20] CROFTON EILEEN (1966) Ampicillin in the treatment of pneumonia. A cooperative controlled trial. *Br. med. J.* i, 1329.

[21] CROWELL J. & LOUBE S.D. (1954) Primary *Hemophilus influenzae* pneumonia. Report of four cases. *Arch. intern. Med.* 93, 921.

[22] DIAMENT M.L. & PALMER K.N.V. (1967) Spirometry for preoperative assessment of airways resistance. *Lancet* i, 1251.

[23] DOANE F.W., CHATIYANONDA K., MCLEAN D.M., ANDERSON N., BANNATYNE R.M. & RHODES A.J. (1967) Rapid laboratory diagnosis of paramyxovirus infections by electron microscopy *Lancet* ii, 751.

[24] DOUGLAS A.C. (1959) Treatment of radiation pneumonitis with prednisolone. *Br. J. Dis. Chest* 53, 346.

[25] DOWLING H.F. & LEFKOWITZ L.B.Jr. (1963) Clinical syndromes in adults caused by respiratory viruses. *Am. Rev. resp. Dis.* 88, Suppl. 61.

[26] EDITORIAL LANCET (1960) Giant-cell pneumonia. *Lancet* i, 214.

[27] ELDERKIN F.M., GARDNER P.S., TURK D.C. & WHITE ANITA C. (1965) Aetiology and management of bronchiolitis and pneumonia in childhood. *Br. med. J.* ii, 722.

[28] EVANS A.D., POWELL D.E.B. & BURRELL C.D. (1959) Fatal endocarditis associated with Q Fever. *Lancet* i, 864.

[29] EVANS A.S., ALLEN VIRGINIA & SUELTMANN SUZANNE (1967) *Mycoplasma pneumoniae* infections in University of Wisconsin students. *Am. Rev. resp. Dis.* 96, 237.

[30] FEIZI T., MACLEAN H., SOMMERVILLE R.G. & SELWYN J.G. (1966) An epidemic of respiratory disease caused by *Mycoplasma pneumoniae*. *Proc. roy. Soc. Med.* 59, 1109.

[31] FIELD C.M.B., CONNOLLY J.H., MURTAGH G., SLATTERY CLAIRE M. & TURKINGTON E.E. (1966) Antibiotic treatment of epidemic bronchiolitis—a double-blind trial. *Br. med. J.* i, 83.

[32] FRANKLIN E.C., LOWENSTEIN J., BIGELOW B. & MELTZER M. (1964) Heavy chain disease. A new disorder of serum γ-globulins. *Am. J. Med.* 37, 332.

[33] FRY J. (1960) Fate of 424 patients with pneumonia and bronchitis. *Br. med. J.* ii, 1483.

[34] GAJDUSEK D.C. (1957) *Pneumocystis carinii*—etiologic agent of interstitial plasma cell pneumonia of premature and young infants. *Pediatrics* 19, 543.

[35] GANADO W. (1965) Human brucellosis—some clinical observations. *Scot. med. J.* 10, 451.

[36] GARDNER P.S., ELDERKIN F.M. & WALL A.H. (1964) Serological study of respiratory syncytial virus infections in infancy and childhood. *Br. med. J.* ii, 1570.

[37] GERSHONOWITZ G. (1963) Jaundice associated with pneumonia (In Hebrew). *Dapim Reffuim* 22, 316 (summarized *Excerpta Med.* (1964) 18, 1246).

[38] GOLDSTEIN E., DALY A. KATHLEEN & SEAMANS CAROL (1967) *Haemophilus influenzae* as a cause of adult pneumonia. *Ann. intern. Med.* 66, 35.

[39] HERS J.F.P., GOSLINGS W.R.O., MASUREL N. & MULDER J. (1957) Death from Asiatic influenza in the Netherlands. *Lancet* ii, 1164.

[40] HERS J.F.P., MASUREL N. & MULDER J. (1958) Bacteriology and histopathology of the respiratory tract and lungs in fatal Asian influenza. *Lancet* ii, 1141.

[41] HOAGLAND R.J. (1960) The clinical manifestations of infectious mononucleosis. A report of two hundred cases. *Am. J. med. Sci.* 240, 21.

[42] HOLZEL A., PARKER L., PATTERSON W.H., CARTMEL D., WHITE L.L.R., PURDY ROSEMARY, THOMPSON K.M. & TOBIN J.O'H. (1965) Virus isolations from throats of children admitted to hospital with respiratory and other diseases. Manchester 1962–64. *Br. med. J.* i, 614.

[43] HUCKSTEP R.L. (1962) *Typhoid Fever and Other Salmonella Infections*. London, Livingstone.

[44] HUMPHREY J.H. JOULES H. & VAN DER WALT E.D. (1948) Pneumonia in North-West London, 1942–44: 1. Bacterial pneumonias. *Thorax* 3, 112.

[45] HUSBAND A.W. & GELFAND M. (1952) Petrol pneumonia. *Lancet* ii, 320.

[46] ISRAEL H.L., WEISS W., EISENBERG G.M., STRANDNESS D.E. & FLIPPIN H.F. (1956) Delayed resolution of pneumonias. *Med. Clin. N. Am.* 40, 1291.

[47] IVÁDY G., PÁLDY L. & UNGER G. (1963) Weitere Erfahrungen bei der Behandlung der interstitiellen plasmacellurären Pneumonie mit Pentomidin. *Mschr. Kinderheilk.* 111, 297, Quoted Rifkind et al. (1966).

[48] KAUFMAN P. (1947) Pneumonia in old age. Active immunization against pneumonia with pneumococcus polysaccharide: Results of a six year study. *Arch. intern. Med.* 79, 518.

[49] KINGSTON J.R., CHANOCK R.M., MUFSON M.A., HELLMAN L.P., JAMES W.D., FOX H.H., MANKO M.A. & BOYERS J. (1961) Eaton agent pneumonia. *J. Am. med. Ass.* 176, 118.

[50] KRISTINSSON A. & BENTALL H.H. (1967) Medical and surgical treatment of Q fever endocarditis. *Lancet* ii, 693.

[51] KRUGMAN S., GOODRICH C.H. & WARD R. (1957) Primary varicella pneumonia. *New Engl. J. Med.* 257, 843.

[52] LAMB S.G. & STERN H. (1966) Cytomegalovirus mononucleosis with jaundice as presenting sign. *Lancet* ii, 1003.

[53] LAMPE W.T. (1964) *Klebsiella* pneumonia. A review of forty-five cases and re-evaluation of the incidence and antibiotic sensitivities. *Dis. Chest* 46, 499.

[54] LUCHSINGER P.C. & MOSER K.M. (1960) *Respiration: Physiologic Principles and the Clinical Applications*. St. Louis, Mosby.

[55] McCRUMB F.R.Jr., MERCIER S., ROBIC J., BOUILLAT M., SMADEL J.E., WOODWARD T.E., & GOODNER K. (1953) Chloramphenicol and terramycin in the treatment of pneumonic plague. *Am. J. Med.* 14, 284.

[56] McDONALD J.R. & HODGSON C.H. (1954) The problem of lipoid pneumonia or granuloma of the lung. *Med. Clin. N. Am.* 38, 989.

[57] MACKAY J.B. & CAIRNEY P. (1960) Pulmonary calcification following varicella. *N.Z. med. J.* 59, 453.

[58] MACLEOD C.M., HODGES R.G., HEIDELBERGER M. & BERNHARD W.G. (1945) Prevention of pneumococcal pneumonia by immunization with specific capsular polysaccharides. *J. exp. Med.* 82, 445.

[59] MARMION B.P. & HERS J.F.P. (1963) Observations on Eaton primary atypical pneumonia agent and analogous problems in animals. *Am. Rev. resp. Dis.* **88**, Suppl., 198.

[60] MARSHALL R. & CHRISTIE R.V. (1954) The viscoelastic properties of the lungs in acute pneumonia. *Clin. Sci.* **13**, 403.

[61] MARSHALL W.C., WESTON H.J. & BODIAN M. (1964) *Pneumocystis carinii* pneumonia and congenital hypogammaglobulinaemia. *Arch. Dis. Child* **39**, 18.

[62] MATTHEW H. & LAWSON A.A.H. (1967) *Treatment of Common Acute Poisonings.* London, Livingstone.

[63] MAYCOCK R.L., BOZORGNIA N. & ZINSSER H.F. (1961) Kerosene pneumonitis treated with adrenal steroids. *Ann. intern. Med.* **54**, 559.

[64] MEYER K.F. (1959a) Psittacosis-ornithosis. In *Viral and Rickettsial Infections of Man,* ed. Rivers T.M. & Horsfall, F.L., 3rd Edition. Philadelphia, Lippincott.

[65] MEYER K.F. (1959b) Some general remarks and new observations on ornithosis and psittacosis. *Bull. Wld. Hlth. Org.* **20**, 101.

[66] MILLES G. (1945) Measles pneumonia (with a note on the giant cells of measles). *Am. J. clin. Path.* **15**, 334.

[67] OLESEN K.H. & QUAADE F. (1961) Pneumothorax accompanying staphylococcal pneumonia in patients treated with steroids. *Lancet* i, 535.

[68] OLSTAD, R.B. & LORD R.M. (1952) Kerosene intoxication. *Am. J. Dis. Child* **83**, 446.

[69] OSSERMAN E.F. & TAKATSUKI K. (1964) Clinical and immunochemical studies of four cases of heavy (Hγ^2) chain disease. *Am. J. Med.* **37**, 351.

[70] PALMER K.N.V. & SELLICK B.A. (1952) Effect of procaine penicillin and breathing exercises in postoperative pulmonary complications. *Lancet* i, 345.

[71] PALMER K.N.V. & SELLICK B.A. (1953) Prevention of postoperative pulmonary atelectasis. *Lancet* i, 164.

[72] PARROTT R.H., VARGOSKO A.J., KIM H.W. & CHANOCK R.M. (1963) Clinical syndromes among children. *Am. Rev. resp. Dis.* **88**, Suppl. 73.

[73] PEK S. & GIKAS P.W. (1965) Pneumonia due to herpes zoster. Report of a case and review of the literature. *Ann. intern. Med.* **62**, 350.

[74] PICKRELL K.L. (1938) The effect of alcoholic intoxication and ether anaesthesia on resistance to pneumococcal infection. *Bull. Johns Hopkins Hosp.* **63**, 238.

[75] PIERCE A.K., EDMONSON E.B., McGEE G., KETCHERSID J., LOUDON R.G. & SANFORD J.P. (1966) An analysis of factors predisposing to gram negative bacillary necrotizing pneumonia *Am. Rev. resp. Dis.* **94**, 309.

[76] PINKERTON H. (1928) The reaction to oils and fats in the lung. *Arch. Path.* **5**, 380.

[77] PUBLIC HEALTH LABORATORY SERVICE (1958) Deaths from Asian influenza, 1957. *Br. med. J.* i, 915.

[78] RALL J.E., ALPERS J.B., LEWALLEN C.G., SONENBERG M., BERMAN M. & RAWSON R.W. (1957) Radiation pneumonitis and fibrosis: A complication of radioiodine treatment of pulmonary metastases from cancer of the thyroid. *J. clin. Endocr.* **17**, 1263.

[79] REED E.S., LEIKIN S. & KERMAN H.D. (1950) Kerosene intoxication. *Am. J. Dis. Child.* **79**, 623.

[80] REID J.M., BARCLAY R.S., STEVENSON J.G., WELSH T.M. & McSWAN N. (1967) Empyema due to *Klebsiella pneumoniae. Thorax* **22**, 170.

[81] RICH A. (1932) On the etiology and pathogenesis of whooping cough. *Bull. Johns Hopkins Hosp.* **51**, 346.

[82] RIFKIND D., FARIS T.D. & HILL R.B.Jr. (1966) *Pneumocystis carinii* pneumonia. Studies on the diagnosis and treatment. *Ann. intern. Med.* **65**, 942.

[83] RITCHIE J.M. (1958) Autogenous vaccine in prophylaxis of the common cold. *Lancet* i, 615.

[84] ROBERTSON O.H. (1938) Recent studies on experimental lobar pneumonia: Pathogenesis, recovery and immunity. *J. Am. med. Ass.* **111**, 1432.

[85] ROBSON A.O. & SHIMMIN C.D.G.L. (1959) Chronic Q Fever. 1. Clinical aspects of a patient with endocarditis. *Br. med. J.* ii, 980.

[86] SALE L.P. & WOOD W.B. (1947) The pathogenesis of experimental Friedländer's bacillus pneumonia. *J. exp. Med.* **86**, 239.

[87] SHANKS S.C. & KERLEY P. (1962) *A Textbook of X-ray Diagnosis by British Authors.* 3rd Edition, Vol. II. London, Lewis.

[88] SMADEL J.E., GREEN R.H., PALTAUF R.M. & GONZALES T.A. (1942) Lymphocytic choriomeningitis: Two human fatalities following an unusual febrile illness. *Proc. Soc. exp. Biol. and Med.* **49**, 683.

[89] SOLOMON S. & KALKSTEIN M. (1943) Pneumonia due to the *Streptococcus viridans. Am. J. med. Sci.* **205**, 765.

[90] SPENCER H. (1962) *Pathology of the Lung.* Oxford, Pergamon Press.

[91] STEIN M., KOOTA G.M., SIMON M. & FRANK H.A. (1962) Pulmonary evaluation of surgical patients. *J. Am. med. Ass.* **181**, 765.

[92] STENSTRÖM R., JANSSON E. & WAGER O. (1962) Ornithosis pneumonia with special reference to roentgenological lung findings. *Acta med. scand.* **171**, 349.

[93] STERN H. & ELEK S.D. (1965) The incidence of infection with cytomegalovirus in a normal population. A serological study in Greater London. *J. Hyg., Camb.* **63**, 79.

[94] STRAKER EDITH, HILL A.B. & LOVELL R.

(1939) *A study of the Nasopharyngeal Bacterial Flora of Different Groups of Persons observed in London and South-East England during the years 1930 to 1937. Rep. publ. Hlth. med. Subj. Lond. Minist. Hlth.*, No. 90.

[95] STUART-HARRIS C.H. (1961a) Clinical characteristics: Twenty years of influenza epidemics. *Am. Rev. resp. Dis.* **83**, *Suppl.* 54.

[96] STUART-HARRIS C.H. (1961b) The rickettsial diseases. In *Virus and Rickettsial Diseases of Man.* Ed. Bedson S., Downie A.W., MacCallum F.O. and Stuart-Harris C.H., 3rd Edition. London, Arnold.

[97] SULLIVAN J.J.Jr., FERRARO L.R., MANGIARDI J.L. & JOHNSON E.K. (1961) Cholesterol pneumonitis. *Dis. Chest* **39**, 71.

[98] SUNDBERG R.H., KIRSCHNER K.E. & BROWN M.J. (1959) Evaluation of lipoid pneumonia. *Dis. Chest* **36**, 594.

[99] THOMAS H.M. (1943) The rôle of alpha hemolytic streptococcus in pneumonia. *Bull. Johns Hopkins Hosp.* **72**, 218.

[100] THORÉN L. (1954) Postoperative pulmonary complications. Observations on their prevention by means of physiotherapy. *Acta chir. scand.* **107**, 193.

[101] THULBORNE T. & YOUNG M.H. (1962) Prophylactic penicillin and postoperative chest infections. *Lancet* **ii**, 907.

[102] TILLOTSON J.R. & LERNER A.M. (1966) Pneumonias caused by gram negative bacilli. *Medicine* **45**, 65.

[103] VOLK B.W., NATHANSON L., LOSNER S.,

[104] WADDELL W.R., SNIFFEN R.C. & WHYTEHEAD L.L. (1954) The etiology of chronic interstitial pneumonitis associated with lipid deposition. An experimental study. *J. thorac. Surg.* **28**, 134.

[105] WATANABE J.M., CHINCHINIAN H., WEITZ C. & MCILVANIE S.K. (1965) *Pneumocystis carinii* pneumonia in a family. *J. Am. med. Assoc.* **193**, 685.

[106] WEED L.A., SLOSS P.T. & CLAGETT O.T. (1956) Chronic localized pulmonary brucellosis. *J. Am. med. Assoc.* **161**, 1044.

[107] WEILL H., FERRANS V.J., GAY R.M. & ZISKIND M.M. (1964) Early lipoid pneumonia. Roentgenologic, anatomic and physiologic characteristics. *Am. J. Med.* **36**, 370.

[108] WEISSMAN H. (1951) Lipoid pneumonia: a report of two cases. *Am. Rev. Tuberc.* **64**, 572.

[109] WHITFIELD A.G.W., BOND W.H. & KUNKLER P.B. (1963) Radiation damage to thoracic tissues. *Thorax* **18**, 371.

[110] WILSON G.S. & MILES A.A. (1964) *Topley & Wilson's Principles of Bacteriology and Immunity*, 5th Edition, Vol. II. London, Arnold.

[111] WOOD W.B. (1941) Studies on the mechanism of recovery in pneumococcal pneumonia. *J. exp. Med.* **73**, 201.

[112] WONG T.W. & WARNER NANCY E. (1962) Cytomegalic inclusion disease in adults. Report of 14 cases with review of literature. *Arch. Path.* **74**, 403.

[113] KNYVETT, A.F. (1966): The Pulmonary lesions of Chickenpox Q.J.M. July 1966: No 139, P. 313.

CHAPTER 8

Empyema

DEFINITION AND VARIETIES

Empyema is a purulent pleural effusion. As with effusions of the nonpurulent variety, empyema may be in the general pleural space or encysted (p. 266). The condition can be acute or chronic. Modern chemotherapy has made empyema relatively rare.

AETIOLOGY

The commonest cause of empyema is *extension of infection from the lung* but infection can also reach the pleura by *penetrating chest wounds* (less commonly than expected unless a foreign body is retained), as a *complication of thoracic surgery*, from *contiguous infection* (e.g. subphrenic abscess), or as a rare complication of *pyaemia* or *septicaemia* when small subpleural abscesses rupture into the pleura [2].

Pneumonia (p. 139), *lung abscess* (p. 158) and *bronchiectasis* (p. 353) are the commonest conditions associated with empyema. Pneumonia or lung abscess may, of course, be secondary to *bronchial neoplasm* (p. 156). *Perforation of the oesophagus* due to foreign body, oesophagitis, or following oesophagoscopy or leakage at the site of a suture line may result in mediastinitis (p. 616) and empyema, more commonly on the left side. Postoperative empyema may also result from fistula formation and *leakage from lung* or *bronchus*. *Tuberculous empyema* is now rare in Britain. *Actinomycosis, amoebiasis* and *fungal infections* are rare causes of empyema. Empyema has been described as a complication of paragonimiasis [7].

The commonest infecting organisms are *Staphylococcus pyogenes*, the *pneumococcus*, the group A *betahaemolytic streptococcus* and *anaerobic streptococci*. Enterococci and coliform organisms may be found in empyema following subphrenic abscess. In infants the staphylococcus, usually penicillin resistant, is the commonest cause of empyema [3, 4 & 6]. In the adult the causal organism may not be identified in at least a quarter of cases, mainly due to the fact that antibiotic treatment has been begun by the time the diagnosis is made. When the condition complicates specific pneumonias the organism responsible is often isolated in pure culture. When associated with lung abscess or bronchiectasis mixed infections may be found. In a series of 18 cases of empyema associated with ruptured lung abscess in adults treated over the period 1957–62 Nicks found causal organisms in 11 and no growth on culture in 7 [5]. In 3 of the 11 in which organisms were isolated mixed infections were found; in the others the infecting organisms were *pneumococci, Staphylococcus pyogenes* and *haemolytic streptococci*. Mixed organisms may include *anaerobic streptococci*, and Vincent's-type organisms are commonly present when the empyema fluid is foul smelling. Penetrating injuries of the chest which retain foreign bodies may be associated with *Cl. welchii* infection.

PATHOLOGY

Infection of the pleura results in exudation of highly proteinous fluid containing increasing numbers of polymorphs. If the exudate becomes frankly purulent the condition is now an empyema. Depending on whether or not adhesions are present, empyema may involve the whole pleural space or be localized. Adhesions which limit an empyema may preexist or may develop as a local defence mechanism. Partial suppression of pleural infection by antibiotic treatment appears to be a factor in promoting the formation of adhesions. Fibrinous adhesions occur relatively early in pneumococcal infection. The fibrinolysin produced by streptococci results in pus remaining free in the space for much longer. The effect of staphylococcal infection is somewhere in between. Fluid may continue to collect in a localized empyema, compressing adjacent lung and displacing the mediastinum.

The inflammatory process subsides following adequate aspiration or drainage and appropriate antibiotic treatment. The pleural surfaces come together and fuse to form adhesions which permanently obliterate the pleural space. In a successfully treated acute empyema the pleural deposits are gradually absorbed over a period of a few months to leave a pleura of almost normal consistency. Empyema may be complicated by pneumothorax when an abscess or staphylococcal cyst has ruptured into the pleural space (*pyopneumothorax*) or by eruption of pus into the lung and communication with a bronchus giving rise to a *bronchopleural fistula* or into the chest wall resulting in the so-called *empyema necessitatis*.

The pathological process in acute and chronic empyema is a continuum and there is no clear demarcation between them. Successive deposition of fibrin and enmeshed cellular debris on the pleural surfaces results in the formation of a pleural peel which is most marked on the parietal pleura. Organization of the fibrinous peel is evident in the deeper layers after about a week and progresses so long as pus is present. Fibrinous scarring extends through the pleura to involve the interstitium of the lung to a variable degree. The term 'pleural thickening' is misleading in this context since the pleura itself is not thickened. The pleural rind finally becomes almost avascular and can be stripped off from the pleura at operation (decortication).

CLINICAL AND RADIOGRAPHIC FEATURES

ACUTE EMPYEMA

Failure of a pneumonia to show expected improvement with appropriate chemotherapy should raise the possibility of the development of effusion which may have become purulent (p. 139). This is the clinical setting in which the diagnosis of empyema is generally made nowadays. To the clinical features of the primary condition those of acute empyema become added, namely fever, perhaps with rigors, pleuritic chest pain and, in time, loss of weight. There is usually a leucocytosis in the range of 15,000 to 20,000 per mm^3. Physical examination shows the signs of pleural effusion (p. 266) and this is confirmed by the chest x-ray. Most empyemata lie in the posterolateral aspect of the pleural space and aspiration in this area yields pus of varying degrees of thickness. Culture of the fluid may reveal the causal organism but coincidental chemotherapy often suppresses growth. Lack of bacterial growth on ordinary culture media may also mean that the empyema is due to tuberculosis, or very rarely to actinomycosis.

Empyema complicating staphylococcal pneumonia in infants may become a pyopneumothorax, recognized by a sudden deterioration associated with increased dyspnoea.

If the acute phase of empyema is unrecognized the pain tends to subside but toxaemia persists along with a swinging temperature, insomnia, poor appetite and anaemia. Finger clubbing may develop within 2–3 weeks of the onset. Failure to aspirate pus may result in its presenting as an abscess of the chest wall, commonly in relation to the costochondral junction of the 5th rib. This is the empyema necessitatis which may erupt through the skin to form a chronic sinus.

Bronchopleural fistula is heralded by increase in cough and sputum which may be blood-stained. Communication with a bronchus results in the sudden coughing up of large amounts of pus. If the ability to cough is impaired for any reason the sudden flooding of the bronchial tree may prove fatal. Following the formation of a bronchopleural fistula the severity of cough and the amount of purulent sputum varies with the patient's position, being less when lying on the affected side.

The x-ray shows a uniform opacity, free in the pleural space or localized by adhesions. A large empyema causes a dense opacity over the whole of one hemithorax. Smaller empyemata usually extend upwards from the diaphragm in the paravertebral gutter. Encysted fluid may occur in any site, sometimes in the upper part of the pleural space. Interlobar empyema is rare and is nearly always associated with pus elsewhere in the pleural space. It appears as an elliptical density in the line of one of the fissures in the lateral chest x-ray. Mediastinal empyema is extremely rare. This causes a dense rounded opacity in the PA film continuous with the normal mediastinal opacity. PA and lateral views should always be taken to determine accurately the site of an empyema.

When a bronchopleural fistula develops a fluid level appears. Other causes of a fluid level associated with empyema are the introduction of air, at aspiration or through a wound of the chest wall, and infection by gas-producing organisms such as *Cl. welchii*. Gas-producing infections frequently result in multiple fluid levels because of fibrinous adhesions.

CHRONIC EMPYEMA

When pus persists in the pleural cavity and the process of obliteration of the space ceases an empyema has become chronic. It has already been mentioned that the transition from acute to chronic empyema has no clear demarcation and in the sense that a slowly resolving acute empyema should not be termed chronic the distinction between the two is only loosely related to duration. Nevertheless it is usually a fact that an empyema persisting longer than 3 months is chronic. The causes of chronic empyema are:

(1) *Failure to recognize an acute empyema* or *ineffective drainage* when a diagnosis has been made. Between them these are much the most common causes of chronic empyema.

(2) *Chronic forms of infection*, particularly tuberculosis and actinomycosis, which may have no clearly defined acute stage. Biopsy of the empyema wall gives the diagnosis in these two conditions and is more reliable for im-

mediate diagnosis than examination of the discharge for tubercle bacilli or the sulphur granules of actinomycosis, although these should always be looked for.

(3) *Chronic bacterial lung infection* in the form of lung abscess or bronchiectasis which results in shrunken fibrotic lung which cannot expand to fill the cavity.

(4) *Lung cancer* with abscess formation and pleural involvement. Bronchoscopy and pleural biopsy are the important investigations.

(5) *Bronchopleural fistula* resulting from lung abscess, trauma of the lung or rupture of an infected lung cyst. This permits repeated reinfection of the pleural space.

(6) *Foreign body* in the pleural cavity, e.g. drainage tube, clothing, swabs or missile. A rib sequestrum may be included in this group. Removal is necessary before healing can proceed.

(7) *Inadequate drainage of a subphrenic abscess* complicated by empyema. A sinogram may be helpful.

Persistent respiratory symptoms such as cough, chest discomfort or actual pain and purulent sputum, together with recurrent pyrexia, poor appetite, loss of weight and marked normocytic, normochromic anaemia make up the clinical picture. Finger clubbing is usually present and pleural fibrosis finally results in chest wall deformity. The chest movement on the affected side is restricted, the ribs are flattened and crowded and there may be scoliosis to the affected side, especially in the younger patient. The pull of the fibrosing pleura on the periosteum of the ribs results in these becoming triangular in shape and they may overlap [1]. If the cause of chronicity is inefficient drainage of an acute empyema, a sinus will be present which drains continuously or intermittently. In the latter case the patient feels unwell with chest pain and fever when the sinus is closed. These features subside when the sinus opens and discharges dammed-up fluid. Sometimes bleeding occurs from the empyema cavity when the aetiology is tuberculosis or lung cancer or when a drainage tube erodes an intercostal vessel. When a bronchopleural fistula exists air can be heard or felt blowing through a patent sinus during coughing. If the sinus is closed, posturing the patient on the opposite side results in coughing up of pus from the pleural space.

The chest x-ray shows a dense pleural opacity, crowding of the ribs and elevation of the diaphragm on the affected side. Periostitis may be seen on the inner aspect of the ribs. This is especially marked in actinomycosis but can result from any chronic pleural infection. Incomplete drainage or the presence of a bronchopleural fistula will result in a fluid level. Sometimes the thick wall of the pleural cavity can be seen above the fluid. Because of the density of the empyema opacity a retained foreign body may not be visible. Progressive fibrosis results in contraction of the affected hemithorax with crowding of the ribs, scoliosis, elevation of the diaphragm and shift of the mediastinum to the affected side. As a very late development calcification may occur in the hemithorax.

Secondary amyloidosis is prone to develop in cases of longstanding empyema.

Spontaneous cure over the course of years is a theoretical consideration since it implies failure of diagnosis and lack of treatment. Slow fibrosis and obliteration of the cavity will occur in time, assisted in rare cases by rupture of the empyema into a bronchus and evacuation of the pus by coughing.

DIAGNOSIS

It is important to be alive to the possibility of empyema. Persistence or recrudescence of respiratory symptoms and toxaemia in the course of a pneumonia should always bring empyema to mind. The chest x-ray may show unequivocal evidence of fluid but the precise diagnosis rests on the demonstration of pus in the pleural space by aspiration through a wide bore needle. The thinner the pus the easier it is to aspirate. It may be very difficult to aspirate the thick pus in a chronic empyema. Diagnostic aspiration should always be attempted if the clinical picture is suggestive. The pleural aspirate should be sent for cyto-logical and bacteriological examination including sensitivity tests of any organism isolated.

Differential diagnosis must be made from *delayed resolution of pneumonia* (p. 140) and *lung abscess* (p. 158), principally by the finding of stony dullness, the x-ray appearances and, most importantly, pleural aspiration. *Lung collapse* is not associated with stony dullness and mediastinal displacement is to the side of the lesion. When fever and toxaemia predominate and physical and radiographic signs are not clear cut, other causes of systemic upset, particularly *septicaemia* and *bacterial endocarditis*, should be excluded. It is important to remember that empyema may only be one manifestation of serious generalized disease. For example, it may complicate septicaemia in a child who may also have otitis media or meningitis or pericarditis.

When a patient presents with a chronic empyema bacteriological investigations may be required for tuberculosis, actinomycosis, fungal infections or even amoebiasis. Bronchoscopy should also be carried out to exclude bronchial carcinoma or an inhaled foreign body. Intrapleural foreign body is rare but this possibility should be remembered. Bronchopleural fistula is demonstrated by injecting 2 ml of 1% methylene blue into the empyema and examining the sputum for the dye. Bronchography may confirm and accurately localize the presence of a bronchopleural fistula. It also demonstrates underlying bronchiectasis although interpretation is often difficult in the presence of an empyema.

TREATMENT [1]

The aims of treatment are control of infection, removal of pus and obliteration of the empyema space. For an empyema containing *thin pus* the initial treatment consists of repeated aspiration to dryness combined with oral or parenteral administration of an appropriate antibiotic which may also be injected into the pleural cavity. These measures will usually result in cure but if the empyema persists and the pus remains thin, treatment by intercostal catheter drainage through an underwater seal must be carried out.

Chronic empyemata containing *thick pus* require surgical treatment on a larger scale. Excision of the empyema is indicated for patients in good condition with no serious lung disease such as bronchiectasis, neoplasm or suppuration due to a foreign body. Thickened pleura is removed by decortication and any bronchopleural fistula closed by suture. Drainage by rib resection must be performed in patients too ill to withstand excision; a causal lung lesion may need to be resected later. Rarely a persistent empyema space requires thoracoplasty as a last resort.

Chemotherapy appropriate to the causal organism must be continued for several weeks in cases of pyogenic infection and for at least 18 months in tuberculous cases. Amoebic and actinomycotic empyemata usually respond to repeated aspiration and systemic emetine (65 mg/day) and penicillin (10 mega units/day) respectively. Sometimes open drainage proves necessary.

Empyema complicating bronchial carcinoma usually means that the tumour is inoperable. The patient's comfort is the most important consideration and this is best served by occasional aspiration with instillation of antibiotic. Because of the associated discomfort drainage procedures should be avoided at all costs in this context.

Fibrinolytic enzymes have proved unhelpful in the management of chronic empyema.

REFERENCES

[1] EDWARDS F.R. (1966) *Foundations of Thoracic Surgery*. London, Livingstone.
[2] HAY D.R. (1960) Pulmonary manifestations of staphylococcal pyaemia. *Thorax* **15**, 82.
[3] HOFFMAN E. (1961) Empyema in childhood. *Thorax* **16**, 128.
[4] MACAULAY D. (1952) Pneumonia and empyema in children. *Arch. Dis. Childh.* **27**, 107.
[5] NICKS R. (1964) Empyema and ruptured lung abscess in adults. *Thorax* **19**, 492.
[6] RAVITCH M.M. & FEIN R. (1961) The changing picture of pneumonia and empyema in children. *J. Am. med. Ass.* **175**, 1039.
[7] SHU-NGOEH KOO & DJE-DI WOO (1949) Pleural paragonimiasis complicated by empyema thoracis. *Chin. med. J.* **67**, 211.

CHAPTER 9

Lung Abscess

DEFINITION

In the strict sense all lesions due to suppuration and necrosis in the substance of the lung should rank as abscesses. Some, however, cannot conveniently be separated for descriptive purposes from the diseases of which they are a part. In this group are abscesses due to tuberculosis, fungal infections, necrosis in malignant tumours and infected cysts. With these and other specific conditions excluded the term lung abscess is customarily restricted to necrotic, suppurative, cavitated lesions due to infection by pyogenic organisms.

AETIOLOGY

The different modes of infection subdivide lung abscesses into those due to:

(1) infection arising in or spread by the respiratory passages,
(2) pyaemia and infected pulmonary infarcts,
(3) complications of certain types of pneumonia,
(4) traumatic injury to the lung,
(5) rarely, extension from a subdiaphragmatic source of infection.

The incidence of lung abscess as thus defined is steadily falling owing to the wider use of chemotherapy and to improved anaesthetic techniques with consequent reduction in postoperative pulmonary complications—a fruitful cause of lung abscess in the past.

LUNG ABSCESS DUE TO INFECTION FROM THE RESPIRATORY PASSAGES ('ASPIRATION ABSCESS')

This is the commonest form of abscess and occurs when organisms from the upper respiratory tract become established in the lung through the operation of a variety of predisposing factors. The organisms are a mixed population from the flora of the mouth, nose and throat and may include aerobic and anaerobic streptococci, staphylococci, pneumococci, fusiform bacilli, spirochaetes and occasionally proteus and clostridia. The predisposing factors are:

A. *Pre-existing sources of infection in the respiratory tract*
   (1) Sinusitis.
   (2) Oral infection, e.g. pyorrhoea, tartar masses (about 80% of patients with an aspiration abscess also have gross dental sepsis) [6].
   (3) Infected laryngeal tumour.
   (4) Chronic bronchitis and bronchiectasis.
   (5) Bronchogenic carcinoma with associated infection.

B. *Breakdown of normal defence mechanism* (see 'The defences of the respiratory tract' (p. 24)).

   (1) *Larynx*
      (a) laryngeal palsy.
      (b) unconscious states—coma, anaesthesia, sleep, alcohol, epilepsy, following electroconvulsion therapy [7].
   (2) *Cricopharyngeal sphincter*
      (a) achalasia.
      (b) carcinoma of oesophagus.
   (3) *Inefficient expectoration*
      (a) postoperative and post-traumatic chest and abdominal pain,
      (b) debility and immobility, particularly in older patients.
   (4) *Defective ciliary action*, e.g. chronic bronchitis, the effects of general anaesthesia.

C. Mechanical obstruction

(1) *Aspiration* of blood clot, pus, fragments of tooth, tissue or tumour may occur as a complication of tonsillectomy and oral and dental operations, particularly when general anaesthesia has been employed. Food and foreign bodies (e.g. peanuts, pins, coins, etc.) may be aspirated from the mouth into the trachea with a sudden uncontrolled inspiration. In patients with achalasia or carcinoma of the oesophagus 'spill over' aspiration carries food or infected material into the trachea.

Because the right main bronchus is more in line with the trachea than the left, aspirated material tends to pass from the trachea to the right lung. 'Aspiration abscesses' are, therefore, commoner in the right lung and are characteristically situated in the axillary subsegments of the upper lobe and the apical segment of the lower lobe, these being the dependent parts of the lung when the patient is lying, respectively, on his side and on his back [4]. The corresponding segments of the left lung are next in frequency but any segment in either lung may be the site of an aspiration abscess on occasion.

(2) *Tumour of bronchus* (p. 517). A tumour obstructing a bronchus may be the cause of a lung abscess if the stagnant secretions in the obstructed segment become infected.

It will be seen that several factors predisposing to the development of lung abscess may coexist in the same patient.

Abscess is particularly liable to develop when the organisms enter the respiratory passages along with particulate material which can plug a small bronchus causing an area of collapse which becomes infected and so the site of abscess formation. Inhaled bacteria alone give rise to pneumonia; inhaled infected fluid such as vomit results finally in diffuse bronchopneumonia.

PATHOLOGY

Aspiration abscesses begin as local infections in bronchi or bronchioles of a size corresponding to that of the aspirated material. Suppuration and necrosis, aided by the effects of bronchial obstruction and often by the presence of foreign material, carry the lesion into the lung parenchyma and granulation tissue forms along the advancing edge. Extension to the pleura is common because of the peripheral situation of most of these abscesses but the granulation tissue barrier which develops in advance of the expanding abscess usually prevents infection of the pleural cavity. Pleurisy, pleural effusion and adhesions may result from the presence of reactive granulation tissue on the pleural surface but empyema is rare in 'aspiration abscess' [2]. If rupture into the pleural sac is rare, rupture into the bronchi is common. The partial evacuation of the abscess which follows does lead to some local healing and fibrosis but an abscess of some standing is characteristically multiloculated with fistulous openings into several bronchi.

As the organisms die out and the necrotic contents are evacuated or absorbed the granulation tissue in the wall of the abscess becomes fibrosed and epithelial cells from neighbouring bronchi grow in to provide the cavity with a lining of more or less normal bronchial epithelium although sometimes metaplastic squamous epithelium develops instead. Small abscesses may shrink and disappear in fibrous scar tissue but the larger ones persist. Inadequate drainage, persistence of infection and perhaps lack of treatment may prolong the chronic stage to a point where the greater part of a lobe or lung is replaced by a honeycomb of cystic spaces and fistulous tracks with thick, fibrous walls lined by shaggy, necrotic membranes in which the infection smoulders on. The lesion at this stage is less a chronic abscess than a variety of chronic suppurative pneumonia. Abscesses may flare up here and there in the larger lesion and it will be noted that chronic suppurative pneumonia due to other causes may itself be a source of lung abscess. In most cases these processes are cut short by treatment.

CLINICAL FEATURES

The features of associated disease (e.g. bronchial carcinoma) may be evident.

SYMPTOMS

In the typical case symptoms appear one to three days after the inhalation of infected material. *Malaise* and *fever* with chills or even rigors are common early features which are followed by *cough* accompanied perhaps by *pleuritic pain* or a deep-seated chest ache. At this stage some cases are likely to be mistaken for pneumonia and started on antibiotic treatment. In the absence of treatment the further progress of the disease results in *systemic effects* with fever, frank pleurisy and perhaps dyspnoea and cyanosis, continuing and worsening over a period of about ten days after which the patient characteristically coughs up a *large amount of pus* which may be foul smelling due to anaerobic bacteria and in which a small amount of blood is frequently present. The diagnosis will now be clear.

Other cases are less typical in their mode of onset and clinical course. Thus on the one hand the disease may begin abruptly, presenting as a devastating pneumonia with copious, purulent sputum and recurrent haemoptysis, while on the other the onset may be insidious with symptoms suggesting a mild attack of influenza. The clinical course is sometimes influenced by inadequate antibiotic treatment, for example in cases diagnosed as early pneumonia. After a period of improvement under antibiotic treatment these cases may then relapse with recurrent fever and haemoptysis, the cause of which—a thick-walled, chronic abscess—will now be seen in the chest radiograph.

Cases in which the clinical features simulate those of pneumonia with post-pneumonic effusion or empyema are also not uncommon. Errors in diagnosis will be minimized if it is remembered that respiratory infections failing to resolve after a week's treatment with the appropriate antibiotic and associated with persisting fever, abundant purulent sputum and recurrent haemoptysis may be due to lung abscess.

Rupture of an abscess into the pleura is associated with severe pleuritic pain and dyspnoea and signs and symptoms of empyema or pyopneumothorax.

PHYSICAL SIGNS

It is unusual for the classical signs of cavitation to be elicited over a lung abscess. The commonest physical signs are dullness on percussion and impaired breath sounds, perhaps with added crepitations and transient pleural friction. At a later stage the signs of pleural effusion, or less commonly pneumothorax with associated effusion, may appear.

Finger clubbing may develop within a few weeks, particularly when effective bronchial drainage has not been established.

LABORATORY FINDINGS

The white cell count is almost invariably increased in lung abscess and may be as high as 20–30,000/mm^3. The sputum contains pus macroscopically and fusiform bacilli and spirochaetes may be found on microscopic examination if penicillin has not been given beforehand. Aerobic culture commonly yields mixed respiratory organisms only; anaerobic culture may demonstrate anaerobic streptococci. It is always prudent to request anaerobic culture, especially if the sputum is foul smelling.

RADIOGRAPHIC APPEARANCES

The chest radiograph at first shows a pneumonic opacity only but later the opacity develops a cavity in which a fluid level may appear, indicating that the abscess has established connection with a bronchus. It may be difficult to distinguish radiographically between a large lung abscess and a localized empyema with bronchopleural fistula.

COMPLICATIONS OF LUNG ABSCESS

Complications which may occur in the acute stage are haemoptysis which may be severe, extension of infection to other parts of the lung, cerebral abscess following septic thrombosis in pulmonary veins, and rupture into the pleural cavity. All are uncommon, particularly since the advent of antibiotics. Early diagnosis of acute lung abscess and effective treatment at all stages of the disease combine to make chronic lung abscess and its complications of cachexia, anaemia and amyloidosis as rare today as they were common in the past.

DIFFERENTIAL DIAGNOSIS OF LUNG ABSCESS

The commoner conditions to be distinguished from lung abscess are:

(1) *Cavitated bronchial carcinoma* (nearly always squamous cell carcinoma). The cavity wall, which consists of tumour and not granulation tissue, is generally thickened and irregular (p. 527). Some cavitated carcinomas, nevertheless, have very thin walls. These are the carcinomas which have been all but eaten away by necrosis. Bronchoscopy and sputum cytology may help in the differential diagnosis. It should always be remembered that squamous carcinoma of the bronchus is the commonest cause of a cavitated opacity in the chest radiograph in men over the age of fifty in Britain.

(2) *Tuberculosis* (p. 216) *and fungal infections* (p. 284). The organisms will be detected on bacteriological examination. In Britain actinomycosis is the commonest fungal infection associated with lung necrosis. Elsewhere blastomycosis, coccidioidomycosis and histoplasmosis may cause cavitated lung lesions.

(3) *Infected pulmonary bulla with a fluid level* (p. 330). There is less consolidation in the surrounding lung. Comparison with a previous chest radiograph will be helpful.

(4) *Infected lung cyst, particularly bronchogenic* (p. 615) *and hydatid* (p. 366). As for 3. The presence of the cyst may be known from a previous chest radiograph.

(5) *Pulmonary haematoma.* A history of trauma to the chest will suggest the diagnosis. Cough is slight or absent and sputum, if present, is not purulent. Spontaneous cure can usually be expected in a few weeks.

(6) *Cavitated pneumoconiosis* (p. 476). The patient's occupation suggests the diagnosis and the radiograph shows background simple pneumoconiosis as well as the cavitated opacity.

(7) *Hiatus hernia.* Retrosternal pain and heartburn, made worse on bending, the situation of the lesion and the absence of respiratory symptoms or systemic upset suggest the diagnosis which is confirmed by barium examination.

PREVENTION

Foci of infection in the respiratory tract should be eradicated. Circumstances favouring aspiration of blood, pus or stomach contents should be avoided, e.g. appropriate precautions during tonsillectomy or teeth extraction; ensuring that the stomach is empty before general anaesthesia. If it is thought that aspiration of septic material has occurred prophylactic penicillin should be given. If there is any suspicion of a foreign body having been aspirated bronchoscopy *must* be carried out.

TREATMENT

Chemotherapy, bronchoscopy, postural drainage and surgery may be required according to circumstances in the individual case.

A. *Chemotherapy.* Penicillin is the most useful antibiotic in the common forms of lung abscess, although its use should be governed by the result of bacteriological examination. A dosage of 1–2 mega units twice or three times daily should be given by intramuscular injection until the clinical state and the radiographic appearances are satisfactory (usually four to six weeks). Towards the end of the period a change to oral phenoxymethyl-penicillin (250 mg 4 times daily) may be desirable.

Chemotherapy will cure most cases, often with little residual scarring.

B. *Bronchoscopy.* Apart from its diagnostic value in excluding carcinoma and foreign body aspiration, bronchoscopy is also a useful therapeutic measure. It enables tenacious secretions to be aspirated and the draining bronchus to be accurately localized. This may be helpful in planning postural drainage although the lateral x-ray is usually sufficient for precise anatomical localization of lung abscesses. It should be stressed that the diagnostic rôle of bronchoscopy in the management of lung abscess is by far the most important.

C. *Postural drainage* should be planned so as to secure gravitational drainage of the abscess as effectively as possible. Heavy percussion by the physiotherapist may assist the process.

D. *Surgical treatment*. This will rarely be required if adequate chemotherapy has been given.

(1) Lobectomy may be necessary:

(a) if medical treatment has failed to do more than convert an acute lung abscess into a chronic one.

(b) at a later date, if, after bacteriological cure has been achieved, the functionless, bronchiectatic residuum of scarred lung gives rise to significant symptoms.

(2) Thoracotomy must be carried out to establish the diagnosis if cavitated carcinoma cannot be excluded by other means.

(3) Lung abscess due to suppuration distal to bronchial carcinoma must be treated surgically if there are no contra-indications to thoracotomy (p. 51).

(4) Empyema developing as a complication of lung abscess may require surgical drainage (p. 155).

Results of treatment

To some extent the management of lung abscess parallels that of pulmonary tuberculosis since confidence in the efficacy of chemotherapy grew with experience, finally becoming the treatment of choice and displacing almost completely the surgical treatment which had previously been the mainstay. In 1936, when external surgical drainage was standard treatment and complications such as empyema and brain abscess were frequent a representative mortality was 34% [1]. Sulphonamides did little to influence the mortality but improved surgical drainage resulted in a marked fall in mortality to 4% for acute abscesses although the mortality for the more chronic forms remained high at around 23% [8]. The advent of penicillin so altered the picture that by 1955 Shoemaker and his colleagues [9] could affirm that simple lung abscess was essentially a 'medical' disease. Purposeful management, however, is no less necessary now that a broad range of antibiotics is available [3]. A study by Fifer and his co-workers [5] found that unfavourable factors included delay in starting treatment, a large abscess (over 37 cm^2), fever persisting beyond 3 weeks, permanent bronchial disease such as bronchostenosis, coexisting diabetes mellitus and imperfect antibiotic treatment because of penicillin resistant organisms. The commonest predisposing factor in the series was alcoholism but the prognosis in alcoholics appeared to be as good as in others. Average duration of treatment was 5 weeks in medically treated cases and 7 weeks for those in whom surgery was necessary.

LUNG ABSCESSES DUE TO PYAEMIA AND INFECTED PULMONARY INFARCTS

Pyaemia and septic venous embolism are variants of the same pathological process. In pyaemia the venous blood is infected from septic thrombi in capillaries and small venules. The same lesions occurring in larger veins are the cause of septic embolism. Infected material carried to the lungs from either source can give rise to multiple abscesses, most of which are peripherally situated. Some of the abscesses are likely to lie very close to the pleura and are thus liable to erupt into the pleural cavity. In adults the risk is minimized by the thickness of the pleura but in infants the pleura is too thin to withstand infection, and rupture into the pleural cavity with ensuing pyopneumothorax is a common complication. In pyaemic lung abscess the systemic effects usually overshadow the pulmonary condition unless pyopneumothorax develops.

Pulmonary infarcts due to noninfected emboli may occasionally develop into abscesses if they subsequently become infected but this very seldom happens. The route of infection is probably by bronchioles which have survived infarction because of their independent blood supply.

The organisms in abscesses derived from infected pulmonary infarcts are the usual mixed bacterial flora of the respiratory tract. Those in lung abscesses due to pyaemia or septic emboli are generally staphylococci.

When bacterial endarteritis complicates patent ductus arteriosus infected fragments may enter the pulmonary circulation and cause embolic lung abscesses.

LUNG ABSCESS AS A COMPLICATION OF PNEUMONIA

Necrosis in the consolidated areas is an occasional complication of pneumococcal pneumonia (p. 139) and is probably due to thrombosis of pulmonary vessels—capillaries in 'red hepatization' and arterioles in 'grey hepatization'.

Lung abscesses are much more frequent complications in *staphylococcal pneumonia* (p. 122) and the lesions are usually multiple and bilateral. Infants with staphylococcal pneumonia develop very characteristic lesions. Cavities formed by necrosis in consolidated areas tend to become inflated during crying to form cystic spaces which, by distorting the bronchi, give rise to a valvular mechanism allowing air to enter the cysts during inspira-

tion but hindering its escape during expiration. The cysts rapidly enlarge and frequently rupture into the pleural cavity; pyopneumothorax then ensues.

In *Klebsiella pneumonia* (p. 122), like staphylococcal pneumonia, there is a marked tendency for abscess formation in the consolidated area which in Klebsiella pneumonia is generally confined to one lobe.

The lung abscesses developing as complications of pneumonia will, if untreated, pass into a chronic stage and ultimately into the condition of chronic suppurative pneumonia. The process is the same as that described already in the later stages of aspiration abscesses.

LUNG ABSCESS DUE TO TRAUMATIC INJURY

Injury of the lung through open chest wounds, with or without the implantation of foreign material, may be followed by an abscess. The same result can occur after a closed chest

injury resulting in lung haemorrhage, the haematoma so formed subsequently becoming infected via the respiratory passages.

LUNG ABSCESS DUE TO SUBDIAPHRAGMATIC INFECTION

Amoebae (*Entamoeba histolytica*) infecting the colon commonly enter the portal vein and are carried to the liver where they give rise to an amoebic abscess, almost invariably situated in the right lobe. As the abscess enlarges reactive granulation tissue develops binding the liver to the diaphragm and the diaphragm to the lung. Depending on the rate of progress of the condition the amoebic infection may sometimes rupture into the lung with the development of abscess formation.

Subdiaphragmatic abscesses resulting from

infection of the peritoneal cavity, usually after perforation of a viscus, rarely penetrate the diaphragm and still more rarely enter the lung. Lung abscesses arising in this way are likely to be infected by coliform organisms and perhaps by clostridia.

REFERENCES

[1] ALLEN C.I. & BLACKMAN J.F. (1936) Treatment of lung abscess. *J. thorac. Surg.* 6, 156.
[2] BARRETT N.R. (1944) Lung abscess; pathology and diagnosis of certain types. *Lancet* ii, 647.

[3] BROCK R.C. (1952) *Lung Abscess*. Oxford.
[4] BROCK R.C., HODGKISS F. & JONES H.O. (1942) Bronchial embolism and posture in relation to lung abscess. *Guy's Hospital Rep.* **91**, 131.
[5] FIFER W.R., HASEBYE K., CHEDISTER C. & MILLER M. (1961) Primary lung abscess—analysis of therapy and results in 55 cases. *Arch. intern. Med.* **107**, 668.
[6] FLAVELL G. (1966) Lung abscess. *Br. med. J.* **1**, 1032.

[7] KWALWASSER S., MONROE R.R. & NEANDER J.F. (1950) Lung abscess as complication of electro-shock therapy. *Am. J. Psychiat.* **106**, 750.
[8] NEUHOF H., TOUROFF A.S.W. & AUFSES A.H. (1941) Surgical treatment by drainage of sub-acute and chronic putrid abscesses of lung. *Ann. Surg.* **113**, 209.
[9] SHOEMAKER E.H., YOW E.M. & BYRD W.C. (1955) Antibiotic therapy for primary pulmonary abscesses. *Arch. intern. Med.* **96**, 683.

CHAPTER 10

Epidemiology and Prevention of Pulmonary Tuberculosis

INTRODUCTION

With the increased control of malaria tuberculosis has become the world's most important communicable disease. This is easily forgotten in economically developed countries where the mortality has fallen dramatically and there has been an appreciable fall in morbidity, although in fact there are very great differences between different developed countries and within these countries the problem is often larger than is generally recognized [129]. In economically developing countries the disease is one of the principal causes of suffering and death. What evidence is available suggests that there may have been some improvement in the last decade, though the problem remains formidable [129]. Pulmonary tuberculosis is much the most important manifestation of the disease, both because it is far the most common and because patients with pulmonary tuberculosis are the principal sources of infection. The World Health Organisation estimates that there are at least 10–20 million cases of active tuberculosis in the world today and that some 1–2 million people die of the disease every year. More than three-quarters of the cases are in the developing countries [129].

With the development of modern transport and the frequency with which people now move about the world, no country can afford to regard tuberculosis as a purely parochial problem. The relatively high degree of control of tuberculosis in economically developed countries is mainly due to the use of effective chemotherapy, and drug resistance at present is not a major difficulty. But in the economically developing countries drug resistance is becoming a very formidable challenge and, with movement of populations, this problem could well spread to the economically developed countries and result in a type of

tuberculosis which will be very difficult to control with present methods of treatment. The complete control of tuberculosis on a world-wide basis is therefore in everyone's interest.

HISTORY

Tuberculosis is a disease of great antiquity. What were almost certainly tuberculous lesions have been found in the vertebrae of neolithic man in Europe, and of Egyptian mummies perhaps as early as 3700 B.C. [89]. In the early writings pulmonary tuberculosis may well have been confused with other pulmonary diseases but it seems certain that the disease was common in the Hellenic and Roman periods, and in ancient India and China. Tuberculous lymphadenitis ('scrofula') appears to have been widespread throughout mediaeval Europe. In Europe and North America tuberculosis, already a prevalent disease, seems to have increased disastrously during the industrial revolution, reaching its peak in England in the late 18th century and then gradually diminishing, probably as a result of the increasing standards of living and the elimination of the more susceptible members of the population [35] (fig. 10.1). In the last 15 years chemotherapy, BCG and improved medical services have impressively accelerated the decline of the disease in economically developed countries although in developing countries the situation remains grim.

Some of the more remote areas—parts of rural Ireland, the Highlands of Scotland, central Africa and the Himalayas—have probably only been reached by tuberculosis in the recent past. Adolescents and young adults from these comparatively virgin populations are particularly liable to develop acute, rapidly progressive tuberculosis when they come to work in the infected environment of great cities.

Tuberculosis is, of course, an infectious disease caused by the tubercle bacillus. Up to very recently most people in Western Europe and America, indeed most people in the world, were infected at some time in their lives [53]. Fortunately, owing to the good defences of the host and perhaps to the small number of infecting bacilli, the vast majority

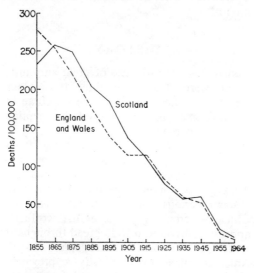

FIG. 10.1. Decennial death rates for respiratory tuberculosis in Scotland and in England and Wales 1855–1964.

of people overcame the invaders without any important evidence of illness. In a small proportion the infecting dose was so large, or the host resistance so poor, that clinical tuberculosis resulted.

MEASUREMENT OF THE EXTENT OF TUBERCULOSIS IN THE COMMUNITY

The measurement of the size of the tuberculosis problem in a community is of importance not only in the planning of antituberculosis services but also in assessing their success. For this purpose the following measurements may be used: (1) mortality rate, (2) notifica-

tion rate, (3) prevalence, (4) attack rate, (5) tuberculin positivity rate.

In economically developed communities *mortality rate* has long been available. In the pre-chemotherapy period, in spite of some drawbacks, it was a reasonable reflection of the prevalence of the disease; now it is a poor index of the prevalence but mortality trends provide some indication of the efficacy of the services. In developing countries mortality figures are likely to be unreliable, if available at all. In an individual community or country the *notification rate* may be useful but standards of notification are very variable, though, if confined to the bacteriologically positive, may provide an index of comparison. Well designed *prevalence* studies on a sample basis are useful in developing and perhaps in developed countries as an assessment of the initial problem but are more difficult to use for continuous assessment. *Attack rates* are even more difficult to measure reliably. The rate of *tuberculin positivity* at a standard age, say 13–14, is a useful index of the amount of infection in the community and can be utilized in most types of society, but is subject to a number of technical reservations. These various kinds of measurement, and their application to certain communities, will now be examined in more detail.

MORTALITY

The *decennial mortality* in England and Wales and in Scotland since causes of death were first reported in the mid-nineteenth century is shown in fig. 10.1. It will be seen that there has been a marked overall decrease. The major factors in this decrease have probably been the improvement of the host resistance by the gradually rising standard of living and by the survival and procreation of individuals with a higher natural resistance to the disease. The improvement of housing and working conditions, and the provision of facilities for isolating at least some of the most infectious patients, has presumably also decreased the risk of receiving a high infecting dose. More detailed *annual figures* are shown in fig. 10.2. Increase of mortality during the two World Wars is obvious and the rapid

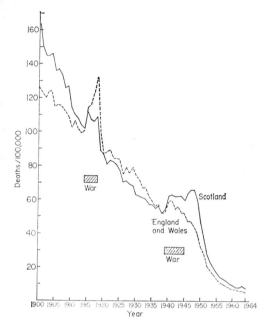

FIG. 10.2. Death rates for respiratory tuberculosis in Scotland and in England and Wales 1900–64.

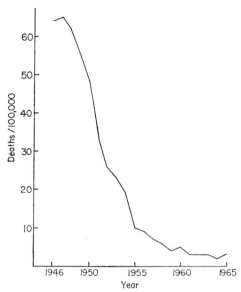

FIG. 10.3. Death rates for respiratory tuberculosis in Edinburgh 1946–65.

decrease following the introduction of chemotherapy in 1947. The effect in a single community, that of Edinburgh, is shown in fig. 10.3. The initial impact of chemotherapy on the mortality is well illustrated in fig. 10.4 where the ratio between *notification rate and death rate* is shown for Edinburgh and certain other British cities in the early years after development of chemotherapy and before there had been an impressive fall in notifications. It will be noted that before the introduction of chemotherapy there was approximately 1 death for every 2 notifications, converted within a few years to 1 death for every 14 notifications, although the ratio becomes less dramatic as chemotherapy and other preventive measures result in a decrease of new cases of tuberculosis. It will be seen from figs. 10.5 & 10.6 that the *fall in mortality* has been particularly marked in the *younger age groups*. The fall is less in older people, particularly males, where problems of other diseases, diminished respiratory reserve, alcoholism and misdiagnosis complicate the picture.

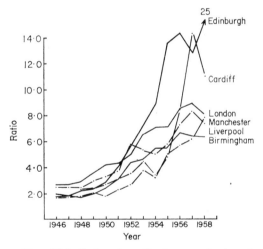

FIG. 10.4. *Ratio of notifications to deaths of pulmonary tuberculosis in certain British cities:* Note that previous to 1947 there was approximately one death for every two notifications in each of these cities. (Between 1929 and 1938 the ratio of deaths to notifications in Edinburgh varied from 1.6 to 1.8.) The Edinburgh figure for 1958 is influenced by a major mass radiography campaign which resulted in a very large number of notifications. (Courtesy of Editor, British Medical Journal).

An analysis of all the deaths from pulmonary tuberculosis in Edinburgh, a town of approximately half a million inhabitants in 1965, showed that there were 8 males and 6 females. All except one were over the age of

relatively moribund condition at diagnosis. No less than 5 of these patients, undiagnosed or only diagnosed very late, had miliary tuberculosis. Several had inactive tuberculosis at the time of death, death being a late result

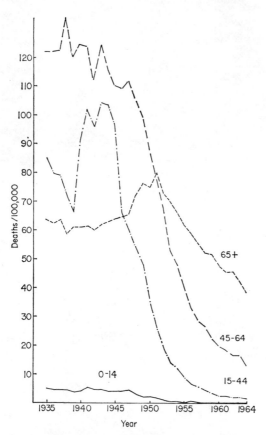

FIG. 10.5. Respiratory tuberculosis mortality by age groups. England and Wales 1935–64. Males. Note the figures for males aged 15–44 between 1940–45 are not a true reflection of the actual mortality, because of the large number of males away from home in the armed forces at that period. It will be seen that there has been a very much greater decrease in mortality in the younger than in the older age groups.

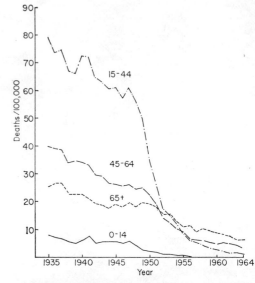

FIG. 10.6 Respiratory tuberculosis mortality by age groups. England and Wales 1935–64. Females. Note the very great fall in mortality in young women and the slower fall in the older age groups.

of *cor pulmonale* or chronic bronchitis in a patient whose lungs had been severely damaged by previous tuberculosis which had been arrested by chemotherapy. Only one died with resistant organisms as a result of previous unsatisfactory treatment.

Finally, some *international comparisons* of mortality are made in fig. 10.7. It will be seen that there are quite considerable differences in mortality between different economically developed countries. Between these countries mortality data are probably reasonably comparable, although in economically underdeveloped countries (fig. 10.8) the data are probably less reliable. The differences between economically developed countries probably reflect historical and social factors as well as the quality of the medical services.

45. Six were only diagnosed at postmortem, indicating the difficulties of diagnosis which may be encountered in patients admitted moribund but also indicating some failure in the diagnostic services. Two were notified only within a month of death, indicating a

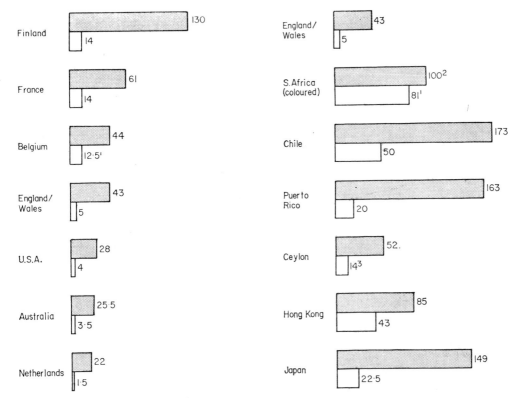

FIG. 10.7. Mortality per 100,000 population for respiratory tuberculosis in 'economically developed' countries. Dark columns represent mortality for 1947–49, light columns for 1964. Adapted from W.H.O. (1966) *Epidemiol. vital Statist. Rep.*, **19**, 182.
Note: [1]1963.

FIG. 10.8. Mortality per 100,000 population for respiratory tuberculosis in 'economically developing' countries. Dark columns represent mortality for 1947–49, light columns for 1963. Adapted from W.H.O. (1966) *Epidemiol. vital Statist. Rep.* **19**, 182.
Notes: [1]1961. [2]1957–59. [3]1962.

NOTIFICATION

Notification of pulmonary tuberculosis has been compulsory in Britain only during this century. The patient is supposed to be notified either when he is, because of infectiousness, a danger to other people or when his tuberculosis requires an alteration in his way of life. The latter is nowadays interpreted to include the necessity for chemotherapy. A notification on the basis of positive bacteriological findings is fairly straightforward although of course it depends partly on the intensity with which tubercle bacilli are sought. Nevertheless such a definition would include only a proportion of patients with active disease requiring treatment. In Edinburgh in recent years only about 50–60% of notified patients have a positive sputum. Experience has shown that the grounds for decision as to whether a case has active disease requiring treatment varies very much from area to area and even from doctor to doctor. It is therefore much more difficult to make comparative studies of notification rates between different areas and different countries, unless figures are confined to those in whom tubercle bacilli have been identified. Even this depends on the methods used and the number of specimens examined.

Notification rates for pulmonary tuberculosis in Britain are shown in fig. 10.9. As with mortality the rises in the two world wars are

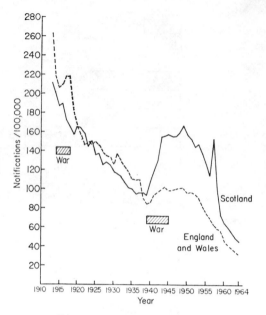

FIG. 10.9. Notification rates for respiratory tuberculosis in Scotland and in England and Wales 1913–64.

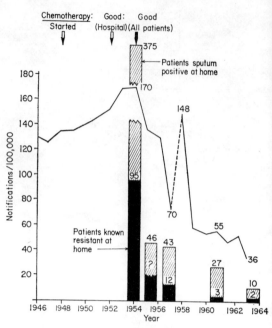

FIG. 10.10. Notification rates for respiratory tuberculosis in Edinburgh 1946–64. Interrupted line indicates major mass radiography campaign in 1958. Arrows show evolution from initial chemotherapy with streptomycin (first arrow) to 'good' chemotherapy (by present standards), applied first to hospital patients only (second arrow) and finally to all patients (third arrow). Columns show totals for known sputum positive patients out of hospital and the numbers of patients out of hospital with known resistant organisms. Population of Edinburgh approximately 500,000. Note dramatic fall in notification rate after institution of 'good' chemotherapy for all known patients.

obvious, particularly in the Second World War in Scotland, and the marked reduction in recent years. The potential effect of chemotherapy in preventing the spread of disease is illustrated in fig. 10.10 in the case of Edinburgh. The introduction of chemotherapy had little effect on notification to begin with. At this time there was considerable shortage of hospital beds. Although good chemotherapy was given to hospital patients from 1952 it was not until 1954 that the organization of the service resulted in the best available chemotherapy being given to patients both in and out of hospital. The better use of hospital beds resulted in the virtual abolition of waiting lists within a year and a very great reduction in the number of patients with a positive sputum out of hospital. It will be noted that in 1954 there were quite a large number of patients with resistant organisms out of hospital but that in subsequent years these were very greatly reduced. The original patients were either salvaged with surgery and such reserve drugs as were available at that time, or died. With universal good chemo-

therapy no new cases with resistant organisms were created and the resistance problem became negligible.

The decrease in notifications has been very much greater in the younger than the older age groups (figs. 10.11a & 10.11b). It will be seen that there has been relatively little fall in the notification rates in men over the age of 55. There has also been little fall in women over the age of 55, although the number in this age group in females has always been very small. One must presume that the better treatment of infectious cases has reduced the new infections in younger people—with some

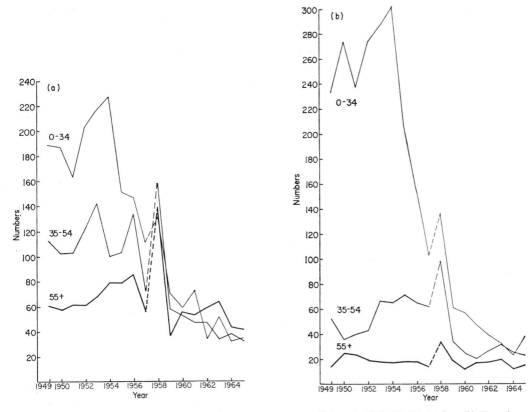

FIG. 10.11. Notification of respiratory tuberculosis by age. Edinburgh 1949–65. (a) Males, (b) Females.
Note: Interrupted line indicates major mass radiography campaign in 1958.

small contribution from BCG—and that most cases in older people result from the breakdown of infections acquired many years previously.

PREVALENCE

The number of active cases of pulmonary tuberculosis present in a community at any one time is very difficult to estimate accurately. The *ideal method* would be to institute miniature radiography, tuberculin testing and, where relevant, bacteriological investigation of the entire population. This has seldom or never been done. In the major centres of population in Scotland an intensive mass radiography campaign was carried out in the years 1957 and 1958. In these areas 68% of the population over the age of 15 (75% in the urban areas) were x-rayed in a comparatively

short period and the great majority of patients with abnormal shadows were clinically investigated. The prevalent rate of active cases for the population surveyed was 2·35 per 1000, 3·69 in Glasgow and 1·69 per 1000 in Edinburgh [81]. These surveys have not been repeated but, if one can judge by changes in the notification rate, it is probable that the prevalence has substantially decreased since that time.

A less exacting technique is to carry out *sample surveys* on a random sample of the population, although this requires careful preparation to ensure that the sample is truly representative. The World Health Organisation has sponsored a number of such surveys in different parts of the world, mainly in economically underdeveloped countries [100]. Figures for such countries have varied from approximately 5 to 50 per 1000 population, the higher figure being particularly characteristic of the Far East. A national survey carried out in India in 1955–58 [63] showed figures for active and probably active cases varying from 13 to 25; for bacteriologically positive cases from 2 to 8 per 1000. One of the surprises of this survey was that the prevalence of tuberculosis in the rural areas, at least those that could be reached by survey teams, was of the same order as in the cities. In underdeveloped countries such prevalence studies are the only effective way of measuring the extent of the tuberculosis problem.

ATTACK RATE

As a measure of tuberculosis control the attack rate of the disease is theoretically better than the mortality rate, which is affected so much by treatment and case fatality; and than the prevalence, which is affected both by the attack rate and the case fatality rate. But the attack rate in a community can only be estimated by x-raying a high proportion of the population on at least two occasions at an interval of one or more years, with subsequent clinical investigation to establish the diagnosis. This has not often been done in Britain. Cochrane and his colleagues [23] in the early 1950s carried out surveys in a Welsh mining valley and found that the attack rate was much higher in both sexes under the age of 35, with a maximum in the 15–24 age group and a much higher rate in contacts of a known case. The overall annual attack rate was 0·9 per 1000 population in females and 2·0 in non-mining males, though the latter was probably too high an estimate owing to the absence of fit young men on military service. Their figures were somewhat similar to those estimated by Springett [113] on the basis of mass radiographic information for London in the period 1946–49 (about 1·9 per 1000 for males and 0·6 for females). Springett also found the highest rate was in the 15–24 age group in both sexes. It is probable that, with the increasing control of tuberculosis, the attack rate is now lower in young people. In the period 1957–58 Geddes [49] in Glasgow found the rate in men over 45

(0·9 per 1000) almost as high as in young male adults (1·2 per 1000).

In a small town and surrounding villages in India Frimodt-Møller [46] found the annual attack rate as low as 0·44 per 1000 though the inclusion of 'inactive' lesions would have raised it to 2·8 for males and 2·4 for females. The susceptibility of young people was much less obvious than in Europe, the highest rate being in the 30–49 age group in females and the 'over 50' group in males. There was evidence of a long delay between first infection and the emergence of disease.

MEASUREMENT OF INFECTION (TUBERCULIN TESTING)

The basis of the tuberculin test is the fact that, coincident with the development of the primary tuberculous lesion, the patient becomes hypersensitive to a protein fraction of the tubercle bacillus. This hypersensitivity can be detected by introducing tuberculin into the skin with a resultant reaction of the delayed type [99]. A positive reaction was formerly considered to indicate a previous infection with the tubercle bacillus, although not necessarily the presence of tuberculous disease. This view now has to be modified. In the course of the investigations by the World Health Organisation it was shown that there was a variation in different parts of the world in the proportion of the population showing weak reactions to tuberculin, although patients with actual tuberculous disease nearly always showed strong reactions. If the size of the reactions among the general population was plotted against the frequency it was found that in many countries there was a bimodal distribution, a large number of people having small reactions, a relatively small number having intermediate reactions, and then a second peak of frequency of larger reactions [38, 92 & 127]. In consequence it was suggested that there were 2 sorts of reaction to the tuberculin tests: a *specific* reaction, indicating previous infection with the tubercle bacillus and manifested by a larger skin response, and a *nonspecific* reaction, manifested by a smaller response to tuberculin and due to infection by some unknown organism.

As mentioned, there is considerable geographical variation. The W.H.O. studies suggested that nonspecific sensitivity ranged from less than 10% in Denmark and North U.S.A. to over 90% in the Phillipines, the Sudan and Vietnam. It was relatively high, with a figure of 70–80%, in some parts of India, and relatively low, between 20 and 30%, in England and Mexico. Though in temperate and subtropical regions it was relatively easy to differentiate between weak (nonspecific) and strong (specific) reactions, there was considerable overlap in tropical areas [92]. These studies were done in children. It was found that as the children grew older an increasing proportion of them transferred into the group with specific hypersensitivity, in which the greater reaction would obscure any co-existing nonspecific hypersensitivity. Very detailed studies have been carried out in the U.S.A. [39] where a relatively high prevalence of nonspecific reactions has been found in the southeast diminishing towards the north and west.

In seeking for the cause of the nonspecific reactions it was natural first to examine the possibility that they derived from infection with other mycobacteria. It has been shown that infection of guinea pigs with *M. avium* and a number of different strains of 'anonymous' mycobacteria (p. 259) results in low degrees of reaction to mammalian tuberculin [39]. 'Tuberculins' have been prepared from a number of these organisms. Comparative testing in man has shown that there is considerable cross reaction between the different tuberculins. In consequence it is difficult to say whether one or more of the organisms concerned, or indeed some other unrelated organism, is responsible for nonspecific hypersensitivity, although in U.S. navy recruits tuberculin made from a scotochromogen isolated from the cervical lymph gland of a child (PPD-G) gave reactions in almost half [39]. In the exploration of the problem of nonspecific reactions most of the testing has been done either with avian tuberculin (PPD-A) or with PPD-B prepared from the Battey strain of Group III anonymous mycobacteria (p. 259). Comparative testing in

Britain confirms that in an important proportion of schoolchildren and young adults weak reactions are more likely to be of nontuberculous origin [16, 50, 55, 119 & 120]. Sutherland and his colleagues [120] conclude that 'it would appear that in a group of subjects who have all had an infection with mammalian tubercle bacilli (such as old people in Great Britain, or those who have had BCG vaccination anywhere) low grade tuberculin sensitivity to human tuberculin may be interpreted as due to mammalian infection, whatever sources of non-mammalian infection there may be. However, in a group of which only a proportion has been infected with mammalian tubercle bacilli (such as young people in Great Britain), the greater part of any low grade sensitivity to human tuberculin may well represent cross reactions to infections other than those due to mammalian tubercle bacilli'. They are referring to sensitivity elicited only by intradermal injection of 0·1 ml of 1:100 dilution of Old Tuberculin (100 tuberculin units).

TUBERCULINS

The confusion caused to what had been thought to be a relatively simple epidemiological test by the discovery of nonspecific reactions has been added to by the realization of the complexities of mammalian tuberculin. Tuberculins are difficult to standardize and even standardized and purified tuberculins, such as those prepared independently in the United States (PPD-S) and for the World Health Organization in Denmark (PPD-RT23)) may give different results in practice [24].

The original tuberculin most widely used was Koch's Old Tuberculin (OT). This was derived by evaporation from filtrate of cultures of *M. tuberculosis* at first in glycerol broth, later in synthetic medium. It was a relatively crude material. The active principle in the tuberculin reaction was found to reside in protein, and a purified protein derivative (PPD) was first prepared by Siebert and her colleagues in 1934 [105]. The purity is only relative as small quantities of lipids, polysaccharides and nucleic acids are also present. It has subsequently been found that there are problems in keeping PPD because of its adsorption onto glass. Although this can be mitigated by the use of small quantities of detergent this may itself have an influence on the reaction [123]. In consequence of this problem the international unit (TU) has been defined by the World Health Organisation in terms of Old Tuberculin and is contained in 0·00001 ml of the international Standard Old Tuberculin. A large batch of standardized PPD (PPD-RT23) has been produced in Denmark for international use and has been extensively employed by W.H.O. in international projects. The United States has its own standard PPD (PPD-S) and so has Britain (PPD-Weybridge). It has certainly been shown that PPD-S and PPD-RT23 are not equivalent [24] and the same may well hold for PPD-RT23 and PPD-Weybridge.

In the present stage of knowledge one must accept that in individuals with relatively weak reactions the different tuberculins may give different percentages of positivity and this may vary in different parts of the world. Nevertheless, tests with any of these tuberculins are likely to detect the more strongly positive reactions associated with recent or active tuberculous infection, although one or the other may fail to detect, to a varying extent, nonspecific reactions or weak reactions from old and waning tuberculous infection, such as are relatively common in the old.

The international standard avian tuberculin (PPD-A) is prepared for W.H.O. by the Central Veterinary Laboratory, Weybridge and is contained in 0·00002 mg of this PPD [94]. The other tuberculin which has been widely used in comparative testing, both in the study of nonspecific reactions and in the diagnosis of patients with infection with 'anonymous' mycobacteria (p. 259) has been that derived from a strain of Group III mycobacteria isolated from a patient at Battey Hospital in Georgia, U.S.A. (PPD-B). Tuberculins derived from other mycobacteria are under study in an attempt to find methods of defining the organism responsible for nonspecific sensitivity in different parts of the world [40 & 69].

TECHNIQUE OF TUBERCULIN TESTING

A number of methods of tuberculin testing have been used in the past. The original scarification test of von Pirquet has now been superseded and the Moro tuberculin ointment, at one time popular for tests in children, has been shown to be unreliable. The great majority of tuberculin testing for epidemiological purposes which has been carried out, especially by the World Health Organisation, has employed the Mantoux test. In Britain the multipuncture test devised by Heaf has been very widely used in recent years. In the United States another multipuncture test, the Tine test, has also been used. In view of the problem of nonspecific tuberculin sensitivity (p. 170), for research purposes it may now be necessary to use multiple tuberculins and the Mantoux technique.

The *Mantoux test* is performed on the volar surface of the forearm by injecting intradermally with a fine needle the appropriate dose of tuberculin contained in 0·1 ml of diluent. The latter is normally a buffer solution. The World Health Organisation uses an isotonic phosphate buffered saline at pH 7·38 to which 0·05 part per 1000 of a detergent (Tween 80) has been added [94]. For epidemiological work the standard dose used in most international work has been 5 TU, though W.H.O. is now recommending 1 TU [93]. A separate syringe should be employed for each concentration of tuberculin. The test is read at 48 to 72 hours. The reaction usually consists of both induration and erythema. Erythema is disregarded and the diameter of the induration is measured. The thickness of the induration should be at least 1 mm. At one time a diameter above 6 mm was regarded as due to previous tuberculous infection but it is now realized that some of these reactions may be nonspecific and only reactions above 10 mm are regarded as almost always of tuberculous origin. Smaller diameters should nevertheless be recorded because of possible significance with regard to infection with nontuberculous mycobacteria.

The *multipuncture test* of Heaf is carried out with an instrument which carries a small plate to which are fixed short steel needles. On release of a spring the 6 needles puncture the skin to a depth of 2 mm; adjustment allowing penetration of only 1 mm may be used in children. A small drop of testing fluid is first placed on the skin of the forearm with a rod or dropper. The skin is tensed with the left hand and the instrument applied with the right. The tuberculin used is either PPD in a strength of 2 mg per ml or pure OT to which 1 drop of 1:1000 adrenaline has been added to each ml. This test is best read between 72 hours and 6 days. The latter is often a convenient time. The reactions are graded as follows: *Grade I* shows at least 4 separated papules; in *Grade II* the papules are confluent to form a ring; in *Grade III* the ring is filled in in the centre and induration may spread outwards from the ring (see Pagel et al. [94] p. 271 for further details.) The advantage of the multipuncture test is that it is readily tolerated by small children, it requires relatively little skill and the concentrated tuberculin keeps well. It has been shown that this test detects approximately the same proportions of tuberculin reactions in the population as the Mantoux test with 5 TU followed by 100 TU [15]. At the time the latter study was carried out it was not realized that nonspecific reactions to tuberculin might be occurring in Britain. It is now known that reactions which are positive with the Mantoux test to 100 TU, but negative to 5 TU, often indicate a nonspecific origin. A re-analysis of the data from the British Tuberculosis Association's study [15] has suggested that there may be some difficulty, with present knowledge, in deciding whether reactions to the multipuncture test of Grade I or Grade II strength are specific or nonspecific [36]. Further studies have suggested that Grades I and II reactions are not usually associated with infection by virulent tubercle bacilli and may be due to other mycobacteria [50]. In Edinburgh since 1956 there has been a very considerable decrease in Grade III reactions but very much less reduction in the Grades I and II, which is consistent with the same view.

TUBERCULIN TINE TEST

This test is a multiple puncture test introduced by Rosenthal [101]. The test is carried out with disposable units. Each unit carries four prongs or 'tines' 2 mm in length mounted on a disc. The tines have been dipped in Old Tuberculin and subsequently sterilized. The sterile tines are mounted on a plastic base from which they are removed immediately before use. The tines are pressed on the skin of the volar surface of the forearm to form 4 puncture sites. The test is read in 48 to 72 hours and a 2 mm or greater palpable induration around one or more of the puncture sites is approximately equivalent to a 5 mm reaction to the 5 TU Mantoux test [6, 21 & 83]. Most investigations have been in children; in adults the tine test has given a higher percentage of positives than the Mantoux [1]. The test is rapid, convenient and acceptable but expensive if used on a large scale. A certain amount of experience with it has been accumulated in the United States [1 & 80] and it is said to be satisfactory. In Britain comparison has been made with the Heaf Multipuncture test [4, 42 & 51]. Disagreement between the two tests has been found, mainly consisting in a negative tine with a positive Heaf. This is not necessarily a disadvantage as the weaker reactions to the Heaf test may well be nonspecific.

The *value of tuberculin testing* for *diagnostic purposes* in clinical work will be considered on p. 181. For *epidemiological purposes* it is used as a measure of the prevalence of tuberculous infection in the community and of the success of methods of control, as well as for determining those who require BCG. Although tuberculin testing of a whole population, or a random sample of a population, may be used to indicate the amount of tuberculous infection in the community and the age of infection, the testing of schoolchildren of a standard age was formerly regarded as one of the simplest methods of following the progress of tuberculosis control. Thirteen to 14 year old schoolchildren are tested annually as a preliminary to administering BCG (p. 184) and this gives very valuable comparative data. The prevalence of positive tests provides a comparison between different communities and a decrease is a measure of the success of control. Unfortunately, because of nonspecific reactions (p. 171), interpretation is subject to considerable reservations, at least so far as the weaker reactions are concerned. In making comparisons it is probably wise to include only the proportion of children who show a positive reaction of at least 10 mm to 5TU in the Mantoux test [92] or Grade III reaction in a Heaf multipuncture test. A dose as low as 1 TU, with 10 mm as the crucial diameter, has recently been advocated [93] but less information of its value is so far available.

Formerly BCG vaccination was given only to those who were negative to the Mantoux test, sometimes with 10 or 100 TU. Present knowledge would suggest that a number of these children, perhaps a high percentage, had not in fact been infected with the tubercle bacillus (see above). Although there is slight evidence that such non-tuberculous infection might provide some degree of protection against later tuberculous infection, it is probably desirable that such individuals should be vaccinated. Now that it is known that vaccinating individuals who are already tuberculin positive carries no particular disadvantages [128] a case may be made for vaccinating all children who give a reaction of less than 10 mm to 5 TU by the Mantoux test or less than Grade III reaction by the Heaf multipuncture test.

CONCLUSIONS

One may conclude that mortality and notification rates, in spite of their drawbacks and inaccuracies, are useful measures in developed countries. Sample *prevalence studies* have an important place, especially in planning services in developing countries. Studies of attack rate are not usually practicable. When an agreed standard of *specific tuberculin positivity* has been generally accepted and a uniform method is used this will surely be an excellent monitor of community infection but is at present still subject to many qualifications.

Our methods of measurement in this field are still far from perfect and we must meantime use what is available in a constructive but critical way in order to obtain the best possible picture of the tuberculosis problem and of our success in combating it.

FACTORS RELEVANT TO THE DEVELOPMENT OF TUBERCULOUS DISEASE

As tuberculosis is an infectious disease the following factors have to be considered:

(1) *Sources of infection*
 (a) man (p. 177): (i) sputum; (ii) other excreta.
 (b) animals (p. 176): (i) milk; (ii) respiratory or other excreta of cats, dogs, cows, etc.
(2) *Size of infecting dose* (p. 177).
(3) *Virulence of infecting tubercle bacilli* (p. 175).
(4) *Defences of the host*. This is sometimes referred to as 'the resistance complex', because of the many variables which may affect it, including the following:

 (a) *genetic* (p. 181),
 (b) *physiological* (p. 182), including the effects of age, sex and pregnancy,
 (c) *environmental* (p. 183), including nutrition, occupation and living conditions,
 (d) *toxic* (p. 183), including the effects of alcohol and tobacco,
 (e) *immunological* (p. 184), including the protective effect of a previous primary tuberculous infection and artificial immunity with BCG vaccine (p. 184),
 (f) the debilitating effect of other *conditions* such as diabetes, gastrectomy, etc.,
 (g) *psychological* factors (p. 187).

Prevention of tuberculosis
Prevention of tuberculosis consists of action to deal with the factors which are responsible for tuberculous disease. The factors relevant to prevention may be summarized as follows:

(1) *Prevention of infection*
 (a) prevention of infection from sputum by
 (i) *case finding* by means of miniature radiography (p. 179), sputum exam-

ination (p. 181) and tuberculin testing (p. 181);

(ii) *isolation* and effective *treatment* of patients (p. 178);

(iii) reducing the chances of infection from an unknown case by *better ventilation* and *avoidance* of *overcrowding* at home, at work, in public transport and in places of entertainment.

(b) prevention of infection from milk by building up *tuberculosis free herds* of *cattle* and by *pasteurization* of milk (p. 177).

(c) prevention of infection from other animals—relatively unimportant but some measures of control desirable.

(2) *Increasing host defences*

(a) *general social measures* to increase the standard of living; good nutrition, good housing, adequate sleep, exercise and fresh air.

(b) specific raising of host resistance by *BCG vaccination* (p. 184).

(3) prevention of disease in infected subjects by *chemoprophylaxis*.

Some of these factors will now be considered in more detail.

SOURCES OF INFECTION

Four types of *Mycobacterium tuberculosis* are recognized, *human, bovine, murine* and *avian*. Only the human and bovine are of major clinical importance. The rare infections with avian mycobacteria will be considered in the section on 'anonymous' mycobacterial disease (p. 259). Artificial intradermal infection with murine mycobacteria has been used as a substitute for BCG prophylactic vaccination (p. 184), but does not cause human disease.

VIRULENCE OF TUBERCLE BACILLI

There is little difference in virulence between European strains of human and bovine tubercle bacilli. Up to recently it was considered that there was in fact very little variation in virulence between any strains of either group but investigations by Mitchison and his colleagues [87] have shown that as

many as two-thirds of strains of human tubercle bacilli isolated in South India have a diminished virulence for guinea pigs and probably for man, compared both with strains isolated in Britain and with other strains prevalent in India. Cultures from Thailand were intermediate in virulence between British and Indian strains. All East African cultures tested and almost all of those from Hong Kong were similar to British strains. Later studies [88] suggest that the maximal number of strains with diminished virulence occurs in South India, the frequency decreasing with samples taken in Pakistan, Afghanistan and Iran and also eastwards to Hong Kong. Some less virulent strains were also found in East Africa. The bacilli with diminished virulence showed greater susceptibility to hydrogen peroxide than virulent strains but, in contrast to isoniazid resistant strains, there was no correlation with catalase activity (see below).

Strains of tubercle bacilli rendered highly *isoniazid resistant* are often found to have lost the capacity to produce the enzyme catalase, in contrast to sensitive strains. Inoculation of guinea pigs with these highly resistant strains often results only in a regressive local lesion, although it is of interest that Zaidi and his colleagues [131] were able to produce progressive pulmonary tuberculosis in guinea pigs by the intratracheal injection of isoniazid resistant tubercle bacilli and coalmine dust, each of which were comparatively innocuous alone. A similar contrast between the virulence of an isoniazid sensitive strain of tubercle bacilli and the same strain rendered artificially resistant has been shown in the case of monkeys [9, & 103]. However, even in completely catalase negative resistant strains the degree of pathogenicity varies from strain to strain.

Three types of evidence suggest that this phenomenon is not of great clinical importance.

(1) In man isoniazid resistant strains isolated from the sputum often have a mixed degree of resistance, highly isoniazid resistant and relatively avirulent organisms being mixed with fully virulent bacilli which have a lower degree of resistance or are even

sensitive. Such mixed strains injected into a guinea pig cause death sooner or later.

(2) Primary infection with highly isoniazid resistant bacilli has been demonstrated in man, even though it is possible that such organisms spread less readily than fully sensitive strains.

(3) Patients whose bacilli have been rendered highly resistant by mistreatment often deteriorated and died before the introduction of the newer chemotherapeutic agents. From the clinical and epidemiological point of view, therefore, it is as important to prevent the development of isoniazid resistance as of any other form of drug resistance. For an excellent review of this subject see Kreis [70].

VIABILITY OF TUBERCLE BACILLI

Tubercle bacilli can survive in the dark for months or years. On the other hand they are highly susceptible to sunlight. As a convenient approximation it can be said that direct sunlight kills tubercle bacilli in 5 minutes, but that in a north light they may survive for more than 5 hours. In the dark bacilli may survive for 5 months or more [111]. The use of direct sunlight is a convenient method of killing tubercle bacilli in the tropics where it is probable that most disease is spread at night or in dark houses. In sputum bacilli may resist even 5% phenol for several hours [29]. 1% sodium hypochlorate liquefies sputum and kills tubercle bacilli rapidly, but has to be used in a glass jar as it corrodes metal and is also liable to bleach dyed material if it is dropped on it. Tubercle bacilli are also, of course, rapidly destroyed by heat, in 20 minutes at 60°C and in 5 minutes at 70°C. Patients should use paper handkerchiefs which are burnt. Steam sterilization is said to be best for clothes. Woollens and blankets are best sterilized by dry heat, 250°F for 30 minutes; cottons or kapok toys by dry heat at 300–400°F for 30 minutes. Exposure to air and sunlight is a very reasonable substitute.

BOVINE TUBERCULOSIS

Human infection by bovine bacilli was at one time widespread in Britain and Europe owing to the extensive infection of cattle and spread to man through infected milk. Cowmen were also sometimes infected by the respiratory route [22]. Cats and dogs were liable to the disease, either from infected cow's milk or occasionally from human sources. It is difficult to know whether these animals in turn infected man [45, 57, 72 & 112].

Bovine tubercle bacilli are as virulent for man as are human tubercle bacilli. Bacteriologically there are three useful differences between human and bovine bacilli:

(1) Bovine bacilli grow better in the absence, human in the presence, of glycerine. As the latter is used in routine cultures bovine bacilli may be suspected by their dysgonic growth.

(2) Bovine bacilli are highly virulent for rabbits; human bacilli produce local lesions only.

(3) All human strains are niacin-positive, usually strongly so, whereas bovine give only weak reactions and 'anonymous' mycobacteria, with minor exceptions, are negative [121 & 125].

TYPE OF DISEASE

In the past tuberculosis due to bovine bacilli was often nonpulmonary because milk infection was naturally more frequent in childhood. Because of the age of infection haematogenous tuberculosis was common. With milk infection the primary lesion was often in the tonsils, giving rise to a glandular component in the cervical lymph glands; or in the intestines, with a glandular component in the mesenteric lymph glands and sometimes secondary abdominal tuberculosis. Because of the route of infection pulmonary disease was uncommon unless it arose by the haematogenous route or from direct contact with cows.

PRESENT IMPORTANCE

By the end of 1960 all herds of cows in Britain were said to be virtually free from tuberculosis, although occasionally there may be a local breakdown of control and a small epidemic. Bovine tubercle bacilli are still occasionally isolated from older patients who were previously infected, usually from lesions in lymph glands or kidneys. In a national survey in Britain in 1963 bovine bacilli were cultured from 0·2% of newly diagnosed cases of respiratory tuberculosis [75] and from just over 1% of cases from the more rural areas of West Scotland in 1963–65 [7]. Bovine tuberculosis has been virtually abolished in all Scandinavian countries, except for relapse of old disease, but it is still an important, although diminishing, problem in many other European countries. It has been virtually abolished in North America. Bovine tuberculosis is thought to be unimportant in most tropical and economically developing countries, either because milk is not drunk or, if it is, it is boiled first.

METHODS OF ESTIMATING THE RISK OF BOVINE TUBERCULOSIS IN A COMMUNITY

The most effective method is to type tubercle bacilli isolated from patients, especially from nonpulmonary disease and from children. Isolation surveys may also be carried out on milk samples and on autopsies of cattle at slaughter houses. Tuberculin surveys of cattle are the method of control now widely used but it must be remembered that cattle can develop small abortive lesions if infected from human sources by human tubercle bacilli. This is liable to confuse the issue in tuberculin testing and it is wise if all cattle handlers have their chests x-rayed regularly. Rough guides to the effectiveness of the control of milk may be obtained by following the notification of abdominal tuberculosis, which is mainly due to intestinal infection, or the incidence of tuberculosis in children under 5. During the period when bovine tuberculosis was coming under control in Britain there were marked contrasts in both these respects between controlled and uncontrolled areas [27].

METHODS OF COMBATING BOVINE TUBERCULOSIS

Bovine tuberculosis has been brought under control in many countries by two methods, the pasteurization of milk and the building up of 'attested' herds of tuberculin negative cattle. In Britain the latter was achieved by financial inducements to farmers, free tuberculin testing and the slaughter of tuberculin positive cattle during the later stages of the campaign [82]. Bovine tuberculosis remains a problem in some eastern European countries where collectivization of farms has resulted in large numbers of cattle being kept together indoors.

MAN AS A SOURCE OF TUBERCULOUS INFECTION

With the control of bovine tuberculosis in many countries man has become virtually the only origin of infection. The sputum is far the most important source of tubercle bacilli. Infected urine and discharges from sinuses, etc. are theoretical dangers but are undoubtedly far less important. The greatest danger is the patient whose *sputum* is positive on *direct smear*. He may cough up 1000 million or more bacilli per day. Those whose sputum is positive only on *culture*, or who have no sputum but from whom positive cultures may be obtained in gastric lavage or laryngeal swab, are very much less of a danger. In a study of contacts, Shaw and Wynn Williams [109] showed that among child contacts of patients whose sputum was positive on direct smear 65% were tuberculin positive compared to 28% of contacts of patients only positive on culture from sputum, gastric lavage or laryngeal swab; the figure for contacts of culture negative patients was 18% compared to 22% of non contacts of the same age. The percentage of child contacts showing active tuberculosis was 17% for contacts of patients with sputum positive on direct smear, 2·6% for contacts of those positive only on culture and 0·9% for contacts of culture negative patients. It may be concluded that patients who are only positive on culture are a relatively unimportant infectious risk although a study by Loudon and his colleagues [76] suggested that these patients may also be dangerous if a cavity is present on the x-ray.

There is a good deal of evidence that children with *primary pulmonary tuberculosis* without sputum are not an infectious risk of any importance. For instance, Hyge [62] in a school epidemic in Denmark observed 32 tuberculin negative siblings who had been in contact with patients with primary tuberculosis, gastric lavage positive, for 6 months; all remained tuberculin negative. The infectiousness of an undiagnosed patient with sputum positive on direct smear is well illustrated in the studies by Gedde–Dahl [48]. Similar instances of high infectiousness of an individual have been reported elsewhere [74]. One of Gedde–Dahl's particularly striking cases was that of a young sailor home on leave for a month, clinically well but with a cough and later found to have sputum positive on direct smear and a cavity on the x-ray, who infected 22 people previously tuberculin negative, most of whom developed clinical tuberculosis. The careful studies in the Tuberculosis Chemotherapy Unit in Madras have shown the very rapid *decrease* of *infectiousness* in *treated patients*. Even under grim slum conditions the attack rate of tuberculosis in contacts after the start of treatment of the index case was no greater in the families of those treated at home than in the families of those treated for a year in hospital [66].

Considering human sources of infection from the preventive point of view it is convenient to divide these into those belonging to the *known* pool of infection and to the *unknown* pool of infection. The known pool of infection consists of diagnosed patients with a positive sputum, to which might perhaps be added *potential infectors*, those known to have pulmonary changes due to tuberculosis on x-ray but from whom tubercle bacilli have not been isolated. In economically developed countries efficient therapeutic service should render all these patients negative and cut off the source of infection. The problem is a more difficult one in economically underdeveloped countries and every effort should be made to provide the best chemotherapy at least for the highly dangerous patients whose sputum is positive on direct smear. Although the Madras studies have not shown that it is strictly necessary, it is a wise precaution in countries where tuberculosis beds are readily available to treat in hospital at least all those whose sputum is positive on direct smear

until they become negative. The dramatic effect of good chemotherapy on the notification rate has been illustrated for Edinburgh in fig. 10.10. In developing countries it should be remembered that from the purely public health point of view partial treatment may be worse than useless. It is likely to keep the patient alive and infectious, perhaps with resistant organisms. For economic reasons it will often be necessary to give less than perfect treatment, with an increased risk of failure. Chemotherapeutic policy must be designed to minimize this risk (p. 234). Carefully controlled trials from the Madras Centre [31] have shown that, provided reasonable chemotherapy is given, treatment at home can be just as effective as treatment in hospital, so that only a very limited number of beds need be provided for emergencies, the money saved being utilized for the most important preventive measures, *chemotherapy* and *BCG*.

The *unknown pool of infection* is dealt with in 2 ways:

(1) environmental hygiene to reduce the chance of infection by unknown infectious cases;

(2) case finding to reduce the size of the unknown pool to a minimum.

ENVIRONMENTAL HYGIENE

This consists of three major measures:

(1) The *avoidance of overcrowding* in the home, at work, in public transport and in places of public entertainment. Glasgow studies by Stein [116] showed that domestic overcrowding correlated better with the notification and mortality rates of tuberculosis than any other measurable social factor. Studies by Stewart and Hughes [118] in the boot and shoe industry in Northampton suggested that multiple small rooms provided safer working conditions than a few large rooms, because of the reduction of the number of individuals with whom a potential infector came in contact. In public transport and in places of entertainment the effect of overcrowding can to some extent be mitigated by effective ventilation.

(2) *Ventilation.* In temperate or cold

climates adequate ventilation must be combined with adequate heating. In tropical climates the good ventilation of houses, especially at night, should be quite feasible and the population, and especially patients, should be encouraged to sleep in the open air.

(3) *Spitting*. Social pressures are fortunately diminishing the spitting habit in economically developed countries, although in some areas a good deal of propaganda is still necessary, especially in older males. In a number of countries spitting is encouraged by the chewing of betelnut. Besides the danger of spreading tuberculosis and other diseases this habit is also liable to give rise to cancer of the cheek and intensive efforts should be made to discourage it.

CASE FINDING

Three techniques are available for case finding:

(1) radiology;
(2) sputum examination;
(3) tuberculin testing followed by (1) and (2) in positives or strong positives.

The present value of case finding in the antituberculosis campaign is very different in economically developed and economically developing countries. In developed countries where there are adequate therapeutic services case finding should be maximal, the ultimate aim being to eliminate tuberculosis. In developing countries therapeutic services are at present overstretched and the value of case finding is therefore debatable. There is little advantage in identifying patients with tuberculosis unless one can treat them. Case finding will therefore be considered separately for each type of country.

MINIATURE RADIOGRAPHY

Miniature radiography (photofluorography) is the most widely used method of case finding in economically developed countries. The *ideal technique* would be to survey the whole adult community every year. An attempt is being made to do this in East Germany but most governments are not prepared to meet the expense involved. A substitute for universal annual surveys is the community survey repeated at intervals which will vary according to the tuberculosis problem. Examples of '*super surveys*' were the series carried out in the more populous areas of Scotland in 1957–58 in which the whole of the Scottish Mass Radiography service and a considerable proportion of the English were mobilized for short intensive surveys accompanied by great propaganda efforts and much voluntary assistance. For instance, in Edinburgh 276,526 people were x-rayed by 27 machines in a 5 week period and, adding patients who had been x-rayed in hospitals during the previous 3 months, 84% of the adult population was surveyed on a voluntary basis [106]. It is doubtful whether, with the far more satisfactory position in tuberculosis, such a survey could now be successfully repeated. In *routine community surveys* with smaller populations successful response is usually obtained from only 25–50% of the population, although the percentage can be increased by intensive home visiting. The actual amount of tuberculosis is probably higher among those who do not volunteer. For this reason compulsory surveys have been carried out for a number of years in Norway and in certain States of Australia. In these countries compulsion has the backing of public opinion but in many countries it is still not accepted.

With the limited facilities available it is important that, *between surveys*, miniature radiography facilities should be used to the best advantage. The service should be concentrated on x-raying two major groups in the population:

(1) *High yield groups*, those groups in the population known to have a prevalence of tuberculosis above the average;
(2) '*Danger*' *groups*, consisting of persons who, by reason of their work, are particularly likely to infect others.

High yield groups
These may be classified as follows:

(1) *Symptom group*. This consists of patients who have symptoms, however mild, which could be due to pulmonary tuberculosis (p.

219). It has been found very valuable to have in each community a static miniature x-ray apparatus to which general practitioners can very readily refer patients for x-ray. The yield of active tuberculosis among such individuals is 8–10 times the average yield in mass radiography.

(2) *Home contacts of known cases.* Here again the prevalence of tuberculosis is well above the average (p. 189).

(3) *Hospital in-patients*, and *perhaps hospital outpatients*. Several surveys have suggested that the routine x-raying of hospital patients, whatever the cause of their attendance or admission, gives an incidence of tuberculosis appreciably higher than the average. Every big hospital should have a miniature apparatus and an attempt should be made to carry out these surveys. Miniature films are so much cheaper than large films that the survey would probably be an economy. In practice it is difficult to ensure that every patient is x-rayed.

(4) *Home contacts of tuberculin positive school entrants.* Several surveys have suggested that the prevalence of tuberculosis in this group is higher than in the general population but we were unable to confirm this in Edinburgh and the method has tended to fall into disuse in recent years.

(5) *Inhabitants of lodging houses, prisons and mental institutions.* The inhabitants of lodging houses and prisons tend to come from the lower social groups and to have a relatively high prevalence of tuberculosis [58, 84 & 104]. Every effort should be made to x-ray them regularly. An x-ray of the chest should be a routine part of the medical examination of every man admitted to prison, although unfortunately in Britain it is not. Mental institutions formerly had a high prevalence of tuberculosis; the routine x-raying of patients and staff has now, at least in some areas, reduced this to negligible proportions.

(6) *Immigrants.* In Britain immigrants from the Indian subcontinent have particularly high tuberculosis notification rates [5, 115, 18 86 & 117]. Immigrants should preferably be x-rayed in their country of origin, but, if not, as soon as possible after arrival. [73].

(7) *Middle aged and elderly men* form one of the important residual reservoirs of tuberculosis, besides having a high attack-rate of bronchial carcinoma. Every effort should be made to x-ray men of this age-group on the slightest medical excuse.

'*Danger*' groups

Among those whose work is particularly liable to bring them into contact with susceptible individuals may be listed the following:

(1) schoolteachers and other school employees,
  (2) all those working with children,
  (3) all hospital employees,
  (4) doctors and dentists,
  (5) ticket collectors and bus conductors,
  (6) shop assistants and cashiers,
  (7) waiters and other food servers,
  (8) barmen,
  (9) hairdressers.

In all these groups it is desirable that regular x-ray should be a condition of employment. In Edinburgh, after considerable efforts, this has been achieved in the case of schoolteachers and transport workers. There is no national policy in Britain as a whole although in certain countries routine radiography is compulsory for at least some of these groups. This is an aspect of prevention which greatly needs to be developed.

Miniature radiography policy should be kept under constant review, usually by consultation between the doctor in charge of the service, the chest physician and the medical officer of health. If there is a particular spate of new cases in one geographical area or in one place of work the radiography service should move in and intensive efforts should be made to x-ray all possible sources of infection.

In *economically developing countries*, for reasons which have already been outlined, miniature radiography cannot be used to the same extent, partly because of its expense, partly because of the inaccessibility of many of the areas, and partly because the therapeutic services would at present be unable to cope with the added load of cases discovered.

In such areas miniature radiography might be used in the first place to carry out *sample surveys* in order to determine the prevalence of the tuberculosis in the community and form a base-line for the success of future control measures. The limited number of machines might then be used as an economic way of x-raying patients with symptoms. As the therapeutic services develop, miniature radiography could be extended, perhaps at first to special groups who may have treatment privileges, such as government employees, and later more widely. Case finding should never be allowed to outrun the capacity of the therapeutic services to deal with the patients found. Otherwise the whole service will get into disrepute with the public and make future preventive measures more difficult of acceptance.

SPUTUM EXAMINATION AS A CASE FINDING METHOD

Direct smear examination of sputum is a very useful method of case finding in developing countries because it is relatively cheap, saving the cost of x-ray equipment and film; because technicians are easily trained for the work; because it can be readily done in areas not accessible to an x-ray van; and finally because the method picks up the most infectious cases. It has been found by surveys in India that if the sputum is examined of all individuals in a community complaining of chest symptoms a high proportion of the infectious cases of pulmonary tuberculosis will be identified [129]. In these countries sputum examination is therefore the best method both for case finding and for the control of treatment. The technique is less applicable to developed countries but even here it has been found that middle aged or elderly men, who would not be bothered to come for a miniature x-ray, are prepared to produce a specimen of sputum in a container left at their home. In this way cases of tuberculosis may be discovered among the less cooperative members of the community [108].

TUBERCULIN TESTING

Tuberculin testing as a method of case finding is mainly applicable in an area in which there is a low infection rate and in which BCG has not been used extensively, for of course BCG will result in a positive tuberculin test. The method has been found useful for tracing local epidemics in isolated communities on the West coast of Norway [48] and has been advocated in the Middle West of the United States where the tuberculin rate of communities is low and where BCG is not used [91]. Because of the justifiably wide use of BCG this technique is at present only applicable to a very few communities. The many problems associated with tuberculin testing have already been mentioned (p. 170).

HOST DEFENCES: THE RESISTANCE COMPLEX

A brief summary of certain of the factors which contribute to the resistance complex has been given on p. 174. Some of these factors will now be considered individually.

GENETIC FACTORS

(1) *Racial.* At one time it was thought that races without a long history of tuberculosis were particularly liable to develop very rapidly fatal disease. The liability of individuals from rural Ireland, the Highlands of Scotland, Central Africa and the remoter areas of the Himalayas has already been mentioned (p. 163). The high attack rate of French Senegalese troops brought to France in the 1914–18 war and of Africans in urban slums is notorious. There is evidence to suggest that shipwrecked sailors in the early nineteenth century who were used as rations by the cannibals of the South Seas Islands achieved a posthumous revenge by infecting their consumers with tubercle bacilli and producing a devastating epidemic of the disease. Nevertheless, it is difficult to differentiate between racial susceptibility and environmental conditions. In most of the instances quoted the racial groups were also subjected to marked environmental stresses which could have affected their resistance to the disease. In New York, American negroes, who have long been exposed to tuberculosis and often live in poor environmental conditions, had a

tuberculosis morbidity 4 times higher than whites. Yet under the same environmental conditions in New York mental hospitals there was little racial difference in morbidity among long stay patients [67]. Nevertheless, in spite of the difficulty in assessment and the complicating environmental factors, it seems highly probable that virgin populations, previously unexposed to tuberculosis, have indeed a lower resistance to the disease. Europeans and Chinese, long exposed to the disease, have probably acquired increased resistance by natural selection.

(2) *Other genetic factors.* Twin studies have suggested genetic differences between individuals in their resistance to the disease. Diehl and Verschuer [32] found similar reactions to the disease in 65% of 52 monozygotic pairs of twins compared to 25% of 125 dizygotic pairs. Kallmann and Reisner [65] found that when one twin developed tuberculosis the disease occurred in the other 3 times more often in the case of monozygotic than of dizygotic twins. Simonds [110] carried out a very careful twin survey in Britain and critically reviewed the previous literature. Although she confirmed a higher tuberculosis rate in monozygotic than dizygotic twins, she concluded that this could be explained by the closer contact between monozygotic twins. She believed that biases in selection probably vitiated some of the previous surveys. The occurrence of disease in families was attributed, before the discovery of the tubercle bacillus, to a hereditary factor but it is now considered that the increasing chance of infection is by far the more important influence. In general, therefore, genetic factors are not of great importance.

PHYSIOLOGICAL FACTORS

Age and *sex* are inter-related after puberty although there is little difference between the sexes up to puberty. Primary infection with the tubercle bacillus *up to the age of 1 year* is particularly likely to be complicated by the acute haematogenous forms of the disease, miliary tuberculosis and tuberculous meningitis. Such complications have been recorded in as many as 16% of first infections at this age [96].

This risk diminishes sharply after the age of 1, although primary pulmonary disease and the more chronic haematogenous forms, such as bone and joint disease, are still an appreciable risk. The risk of serious disease is probably at its lowest between the *ages of 5 and puberty* [99]. Progressive pulmonary tuberculosis is unusual under the age of puberty in children of European stock although it may occur in African or Indian children. *After puberty* the risk of acute or chronic haematogenous disease, as the result of primary infection, is very much less but the risks of progressive pulmonary disease become much higher (p. 197). Among young adults susceptibility, as judged by the attack rate of pulmonary tuberculosis, is probably equal in the 2 sexes [23 & 113] but in the pre-chemotherapy era *female mortality* and *morbidity* waned rapidly after the age of 40. In *males* the mortality and morbidity from pulmonary tuberculosis remained high throughout life [114]. Since the introduction of chemotherapy and the development of better protective measures there have been very great falls in mortality and morbidity in the younger age groups in both sexes but both have been considerably less affected in middle aged and elderly males (figs. 10.5, 10.6, 10.11 & 10.12). There are probably several reasons for the residual pool of disease in *older men:*

(1) These men are survivors of a generation which had a higher susceptibility to tuberculosis throughout all age groups, probably because of the social conditions in which they were reared [114].

(2) Older children and young adults are now protected in Britain by BCG.

(3) Chemotherapy of infectious cases has reduced the chances of young people being infected; older people were previously infected at a time when the prevalence of tuberculosis in the community was high.

(4) The deleterious effect of tobacco smoking and alcohol on resistance to tuberculosis applies mainly to older males (p. 184).

Pregnancy

It is controversial how far pregnancy and

parturition have an adverse effect on resistance to tuberculosis. Previously it was relatively common for young mothers to develop severe tuberculosis after parturition and for this reason routine x-rays are usually taken in pregnancy. In order to minimize radiation risk these, in Britain, are normally taken on a large film. It has been shown that under ideal conditions pregnancy and parturition are not an undue strain, but in any case, provided the diagnosis is made, any possible lowering of resistance is mainly of academic interest as chemotherapy can deal effectively with the disease.

ENVIRONMENTAL FACTORS

It is difficult to isolate the various environmental influences which may affect resistance to tuberculosis because a number of adverse factors tend to be found together. The following may be considered.

(1) *Nutrition.* Protein and fats are usually considered important protective foods. During the blockade of Germany in 1914–18 there was a much bigger rise in tuberculous mortality in Saxon and Prussian industrial towns, where food shortage was severe, than in rural Bavaria. In the last year of the 1939–45 war there was an enormous rise in mortality in the occupied area of Holland where the population was starving. One of the most impressive pieces of evidence regarding the effect of nutrition was the sudden increase in mortality from the disease in French prisoners of war in Germany after the cessation of Red Cross food parcels in 1944 following the invasion of France by the allies. At the time there was no other obvious change in the environment of the prisoners.

(2) *Housing conditions.* It has already been pointed out that overcrowding increases the chances of infection but poor housing conditions probably also lower resistance to the disease although this is difficult to prove.

(3) *Occupation.* At one time certain occupations in Britain, such as the *boot and shoe industry*, *tailoring* and *printing*, had a high morbidity and mortality from tuberculosis. It was thought that such occupations, which were less exacting physically, might have attracted less fit people which would include those with active tuberculosis and that infectious individuals might be able to stay at work for a longer period, and in consequence infect more people, than in more exacting trades [118]. Since the concentration of miniature radiography on these occupations the incidence is no higher than in the general population. It is known that occupations giving rise to a risk of pulmonary *silicosis*, such as masons, quarry workers and knife grinders, carried in the past a high mortality from tuberculosis. Silicosis appeared to have a specific effect in lowering resistance to the disease. Although the notification rate of pulmonary tuberculosis in *coal miners* was below the average and there was some evidence of a decreased attack rate [23], the disease, when it occurred, appeared to be particularly difficult to control in those who developed progressive massive fibrosis as a result of coal workers' pneumoconiosis and were, by present standards, inadequately treated. Nevertheless, it has now been shown that, provided proper chemotherapy is used, the disease responds as well as in patients without pneumoconiosis [98]. At one time it was thought that progressive massive fibrosis was a form of tuberculosis but this is now regarded as improbable (p. 474). *Barmen* have a high morbidity and mortality from tuberculosis, probably partly because of their alcoholic intake but perhaps partly because of the greater chance of infection from their clients and the attraction of a physically unexacting job for a patient rendered less fit by cryptic tuberculosis.

(4) *Toxic factors.* The relatively high incidence of tuberculosis in *alcoholics* is well known. Brown and Campbell [19] found a much higher alcohol consumption among 100 male Australian patients with tuberculosis than in matched controls and concluded that correlation with excess alcohol was greater than with excess cigarette smoking. They have also reviewed the previous evidence. The effect may be due to resultant malnutrition, to direct lowering of resistance or to correlation with poverty and other adverse social factors. Lowe [77] and Edwards [37] have shown that

in patients with pulmonary tuberculosis over the age of 30 of both sexes there is a highly significant deficiency of nonsmokers and light smokers, and an excess of *moderate* and *heavy smokers* compared to controls of the same age suffering from other diseases. Doll and Hill [33] have shown that mortality from pulmonary tuberculosis among doctors increased with the number of cigarettes smoked, though the association did not attain statistical significance. Studies of the ratio in mortality between males and females in cohorts born at different periods over the last 100 years show a steady increase of the male:female mortality ratio, beginning with the cohorts, the males of which would have been exposed to increased cigarette smoking in the 1914–18 war. These findings are also consistent with an adverse effect of tobacco [28]. *Corticosteroid drugs* may lower resistance to the disease. Tuberculosis is a well known complication in patients on long term corticosteroid drugs, especially if these are given in large doses. This is due to the nonspecific depression of the patient's resistance against infection. Such patients should have their chests x-rayed at intervals. If there is evidence of potentially active tuberculosis in the x-ray of the chest anti-tuberculosis chemotherapy should be given at the same time as the corticosteroids.

(5) *Immunological factors.* Animal experiments have long suggested a greatly increased resistance to re-infection if an animal has had a previous primary complex. In the Prophit Survey carried out in England before and during the 1939–45 war [30], in which nurses and young adults were subjected to annual tuberculin tests, those tuberculin-negative, that is to say uninfected at the start of the study, had a much higher rate of later active pulmonary tuberculosis than those initially positive and with a clear x-ray. Most of the latter had presumably already overcome a primary tuberculous infection, often at the less dangerous period before puberty. The annual rate of cases of active tuberculosis per 1000 persons in the survey was 7·3 for all who were tuberculin positive at entry compared to 23·1 for those who were tuberculin negative on entry. Similarly in the 7½–10 year follow-up by the Medical Research Council of 14 year old schoolchildren admitted to a BCG trial the annual rate of notification of tuberculosis per 1000 participants was 1·91 in those tuberculin negative on entry to the the the trial and unvaccinated, compared to 1·25 in those with tuberculin tests positive to 3 tuberculin units and 0·81 in those positive only to 100 tuberculin units [14]. It will be seen that there was less difference between the tuberculin negative and the tuberculin positive than in the Prophit Survey but the exposure of the participants in the BCG trial to tuberculous infection was probably less than among the nurses included in the Prophit Survey and followed during a war. The lower attack rate in those who were only weakly positive to tuberculin might be because these individuals had more effectively overcome a primary infection or because the weak tuberculin positivity was due to infection with some nontuberculous organism which nevertheless conveyed a certain protection against tuberculosis (nonspecific tuberculin positivity). At the present time it is uncertain which, if either, of these explanations is correct [14].

Experimental studies on host resistance have been extensively pursued [79 & 126] but cannot be summarized here.

ARTIFICIAL IMMUNITY: BCG AND VOLE BACILLUS VACCINATION

The theory of BCG and vole bacillus vaccination is similar to that of smallpox vaccination; the artificial induction of a lesion due to a nonvirulent organism which gives protection against later infection with a virulent organism. Although vole bacillus vaccination has been shown to give protection of a similar order to BCG, it has the disadvantage that when a relatively high dose of bacilli is used there is an appreciable incidence of local lupoid reaction. When a lower dose is used the proportion of individuals whose tuberculin test converts from negative to positive is relatively small, in spite of giving a high degree of protection against the disease. Tuberculin conversion is a useful check on the efficacy of a vaccine so that the low rate of conversion has a disadvantage in practice [12 & 14]. Vole bacillus vaccination will not therefore be considered further.

HISTORY

'BCG' stands for 'Bacille-Calmette-Guérin'. This was originally a bovine strain of *M. tuberculosis* which was grown in the laboratory by these French workers for many years, mainly on sauton-potato and bile/potato medium. It was found gradually to lose its virulence for laboratory animals and was first used orally in infants in France in 1922. The popularity of the vaccine received a major setback in the Lübeck disaster of 1930 when contamination of a vaccine with virulent tubercle bacilli led to the death of a large number of infants in Germany. The vaccine is now always prepared in special laboratories where major precautions are taken against the introduction of any virulent strains. Vaccination was initially by the oral route but in the 1930s inoculation was introduced in Scandinavia. Although a good deal of evidence accumulated regarding the efficacy of the vaccine, the only really well controlled trial carried out in the prewar years was that by Aronson and his wife in North American Indian children [3]. Highly suggestive results were obtained by Sergent and Ducros-Rougebief [107] who vaccinated the newly born in families which had already lost at least one child from tuberculosis. Later postwar controlled trials are reviewed briefly below.

As a result of their previous experience an international BCG campaign was initiated by the Scandinavian countries in devastated Europe in the immediate postwar period. It was later taken over by the World Health Organisation and extended to North African and Asiatic countries. BCG was first introduced into Britain for groups at special risk, such as nurses, medical students and contacts of tuberculous patients, in 1949. The major controlled trial by the British Medical Research Council in school-leavers was launched in 1950 and from 1954 most local authorities in Britain began the voluntary vaccination of school leavers. Children are now vaccinated

in many European countries, but at varying ages and with varying completeness of cover. In the United States, where a controlled trial on persons of European and negro stock has been less successful [95] and where there has been a vocal opposition, the vaccine is used comparatively little. In Britain, infants are vaccinated in maternity hospitals in a few high prevalence areas and vaccine is offered as a routine to contacts of notified cases of tuberculosis and to nurses and medical students. In most communities local authorities arrange for vaccination, on a voluntary basis, of prospective school leavers at the age of 13, although central sanction has been given to lower this age to 10 if tuberculin positivity rates are unduly high in the 13 year old children. In tropical and developing countries the extent to which the campaign, initiated either by the World Health Organisation or locally, has been carried on later varies from place to place. In Brazil oral vaccination of children is widespread but there is little evidence of its efficacy. Oral vaccination at one time was also widespread in the U.S.S.R. but it appears that there is now some return to the intradermal method.

TYPES OF VACCINE

It is known that there may be very great differences between different strains of BCG and different products. These must be carefully standardized; if the vaccine is too 'virulent' there is a higher incidence of complications; if it is too 'weak' the tuberculin conversion rate may be decreased and probably the efficacy of the vaccine impaired. The vaccine must also be given under carefully controlled conditions as the organisms are very susceptible to daylight or sunlight. For many years the standard vaccine was a 'wet' vaccine, freshly prepared, which had to be given within a week or less of preparation. In recent years 'freeze dried' vaccine has been developed. It has the great advantage that it can be kept for much longer periods. It must be kept at a temperature of less than 6°C, when it maintains its efficacy for up to one year, although deterioration is unlikely at a temperature up to 20°C for short periods of up to a week during transit. Deterioration may occur within a day or two at temperatures up to 37°C, which may be found in very hot climates [13 & 130].

TECHNIQUES OF ADMINISTRATION

Both types of vaccine have in the past usually been given by the intradermal injection of 0·1 ml in the lower deltoid area. In infants the dose may be divided into two 0·05 ml injections, given on either arm. Recently a technique of vaccination with a multiple puncture instrument, which requires less skill, has been developed. Using freeze dried vaccine, vaccination by an instrument giving 20 punctures on 2 adjacent areas of the skin has resulted in tuberculin positivity rates at 10–13 weeks and at 9–11 months after vaccination similar to those obtained by the intradermal method [17]. Intradermal injection by a compressed air jet has now been described and is found to be acceptable to schoolchildren. An initial trial gave results comparable to those with the standard method of intradermal injection with a needle [52].

With intradermal injection a papule appears in 3–4 weeks which usually remains for a number of weeks and may ulcerate slightly and discharge. There is sometimes slight enlargement of the draining lymph glands. The tuberculin test should become positive within 3 months, with 'wet' vaccine usually within 6 weeks, with 'freeze-dried' rather later.

COMPLICATIONS

The complications of BCG are very few. Local secondary infection may occur and occasionally gives rise to an abscess or to swollen and tender draining lymph glands, sometimes with a resultant abscess. Cold abscess of the draining glands may occur. Local lupoid reactions are very rare, most often under an occlusive dressing. Erythema nodosum has occasionally been recorded. In the world literature there are 4 deaths which appear to have been due to BCG. These have occurred among more than 100 million people who have received the vaccine and must have been due to some very unusual peculiarity in the individual. Complications of any kind should occur in well under 2% of vaccinated individuals.

EVIDENCE OF EFFICACY

There have been 4 well controlled trials of BCG. The first was carried out by Aronson and his wife on North American Indians in 1936–38 and showed a high degree of protection which has persisted for 20 years. The mortality rate for tuberculosis in the unvaccinated control group was reduced by 82% [3]. The second by Rosenthal and his colleagues [101] in Chicago infants in 1937–48 gave a 74% protection over 12–23 years. In 1950–52 the British Medical Research Council launched a controlled trial in 56,000 urban school leavers who have now been followed up for 7½–10 years [14]. A 79% reduction in tuberculosis in the vaccinated group was achieved, the annual attack rate of tuberculosis in this group being 0·40 per 1000 participants compared with 1·91 among those in the initially tuberculin negative unvaccinated group. In South India Frimodt-Møller [47] obtained a 62% reduction in attack rate. A controlled trial carried out by the United States Public Health Service in Puerto Rico and in the southern United States has shown much less satisfactory results [25 & 95]. It is uncertain whether the difference is due to a difference in vaccine, to the prevalence of low degrees of tuberculin sensitivity in the area which might itself have given some protection, to the low attack rate in tuberculin negative controls or to circumstances connected with the design of the trial [56]. However, the British and Indian trials have certainly indicated that, with an effective vaccine, a high degree of protection can be achieved. A study of age-specific attack rates in three Scandinavian countries, where mass BCG is given at different ages, has shown the attack rates to be markedly more favourable following vaccination [10].

BCG vaccination, therefore, is one of the most important and one of the cheapest methods of tuberculosis prevention. In economically developed countries the British system of vaccinating school leavers and those at special risk (p. 180) is a reasonable one.

Countries with a low tuberculosis rate may be able to forego vaccination but, in these days of world travel, the risk to those going abroad tuberculin negative must be remembered. In economically developing countries BCG is probably one of the cheapest and most effective methods of tuberculosis control (p. 190).

INFLUENCE OF OTHER DISEASES

Any debilitating disease may predispose to tuberculosis. The association with *diabetes* is particularly notorious and the outlook for patients with both diseases before chemotherapy became available was grim [58 & 124]. Patients with diabetes should be tuberculin tested and, if negative, given BCG. An annual chest x-ray is a wise precaution and this should be repeated if there is any unexpected difficulty in diabetes control. With modern chemotherapy the results of treatment are as good as in non-diabetics [78]. The association with *pneumoconiosis* has already been mentioned (p. 183). Tuberculosis may complicate or simulate leukaemia (p. 212). The risk of developing pulmonary tuberculosis after partial *gastrectomy* is well known [2 & 122]; malnutrition may contribute and smoking may be a linking factor. A routine preoperative x-ray is desirable.

PSYCHOLOGICAL FACTORS

It has been suggested that emotional factors may contribute to the development of clinical tuberculosis. Kissen [68] in a blind comparison with a control series found a much higher incidence of a 'broken love link' (loss of near relative, broken marriage, etc.) in those diagnosed as tuberculous. The formerly high incidence in mental hospitals was probably due to hygienic conditions rather than poor host resistance. For a brief but balanced discussion see Pagel et al. [94].

CHEMOPROPHYLAXIS

Chemoprophylaxis is the giving of chemotherapy to prevent the development of tuberculous disease. It has been divided into 2 groups, *primary chemoprophylaxis*, the giving of chemotherapy to individuals who have not so far been infected; and *secondary*

prophylaxis, the use of chemotherapy in individuals whose only evidence of tuberculosis is a positive tuberculin test, in order to prevent the later development of disease. The term has also sometimes been used for the administration of chemotherapy to patients with radiological evidence of doubtfully active pulmonary lesions or primary pulmonary tuberculosis, but this is best regarded as therapy (p. 235). In certain communities with a high prevalence of tuberculosis there have been trials of mass chemoprophylaxis with isoniazid applied to the whole population, in which case all three groups have been included [26, 54 & 60]. Such mass prophylaxis has resulted in diminution of the amount of tuberculosis in the treated group when special care was taken to ensure that a high proportion of the population took their drugs. In the Alaskan trial [26] a year's prophylaxis resulted in a 60% reduction in disease, persisting for at least 5 years. Nevertheless it is probably not a justifiable procedure in most developing countries where it is difficult to provide drugs for patients with known active disease and where it would be very difficult to ensure efficient drug taking. In the Alaskan trial 10 cases were prevented for every year of personnel time, a forbidding expense in less affluent countries. Present evidence suggests that the emergence of isoniazid resistant strains in those developing the disease is not an important drawback to this method of prevention. The question of a possible carcinogenetic effect of isoniazid is not yet completely resolved, but it is doubtful whether this very theoretical risk (p. 241) would alone justify discarding the method.

PRIMARY CHEMOPROPHYLAXIS

The use of isoniazid to prevent disease in individuals who have not previously been infected is based on the value of isoniazid in preventing infection in experimental animals [8, 11, 43, 71 & 97]. The very rapid decrease of infectiousness in the treated index case [66] makes the method in general unnecessary although in some parts of the world where it may be impossible to separate a suckling child from a tuberculous mother, as separation would lead to death from malnutrition, it may be justified to give the infant isoniazid and isoniazid resistant BCG [11], the isoniazid being continued until the mother is sputum negative [34, 61 & 64].

SECONDARY CHEMOPROPHYLAXIS

The use of chemotherapy in individuals whose only evidence of disease is their positive tuberculin test is more controversial. The breakdown rate in infected infants is high [85] and studies by the U.S. Public Health Service in contacts have shown that prophylactic chemotherapy with isoniazid alone for a year can substantially reduce the rate of later development of tuberculosis [44 & 90]. A more intermittent régime has been somewhat less successful in Greenland Eskimos [60]. Between the ages of 5 and puberty the risk of breakdown is so comparatively small that very large numbers of cases would have to be treated to prevent a small number. It is doubtful whether prophylactic chemotherapy is justified as a routine, although it might be in a known recent conversion in a child who has been exposed to a very infectious index case. Japanese experience in contact households has also been less successful [20].

Extensive tuberculin testing is carried out in schoolchildren aged 13–14 in a number of countries. A proportion of these will give strongly positive reactions and the question arises whether these individuals should have prophylactic chemotherapy. In the British Medical Research Council studies of BCG the annual incidence of tuberculosis in children with a 15 mm induration or more to 3 TU was 3·67 per 1000 per annum in the first 2½ years. The implication is that a thousand children would have to be treated to prevent between 10 and 12 cases, even if the prophylaxis was 100% successful. It is unlikely to be so; a trial in household contacts in Kenya showed no benefit to the tuberculin reactors [41]. When one remembers that the actual cases are most likely to occur in families which will be least conscientious in giving the chemotherapy it seems highly doubtful whether the expense and organization necessary to apply chemo-

prophylaxis to this group on a national scale is worth while. It is more practicable to keep the individuals under regular x-ray survey and to treat at once if there is any evidence of a lesion. Nevertheless it may be argued that it would be appropriate to treat an individual with a strongly positive tuberculin test who was known to have recently converted to positive, especially if he was also known to have been exposed to a very infectious case.

Most chemoprophylaxis has been carried out with isoniazid alone. Certainly combined chemotherapy would be impracticable on a mass scale. Some animal experiments suggest a risk of isoniazid resistant strains emerging [71 & 97] though the Greenland experience is slightly reassuring [60]. In the Alaskan trial [26] resistant strains were few and were thought not to have been clinically important. The latter has not been our own clinical experience (p. 236) and therefore it is our practice, in treating an individual case, always to give PAS and isoniazid. In *developing countries*, where it is difficult to provide sufficient drugs to treat known cases, chemoprophylaxis seems quite unjustifiable except perhaps in infants.

Theoretically mass chemoprophylaxis to middle aged and elderly men might prevent the most important component of the tuberculosis problem in *developed countries*. This certainly requires further exploration but we are very far from achieving acceptable methods of administering the drugs to such people on a large scale.

THE ANTI-TUBERCULOSIS CAMPAIGN

We are now in a position to summarize the basic requirements of the anti-tuberculosis campaign, but it will be clear from much in the above discussion that the methods have to be quite different in economically developed and economically developing countries.

ECONOMICALLY DEVELOPED COUNTRIES

In economically developed countries the aim should be the *eradication* of tuberculosis. It has been suggested that tuberculosis could be regarded as virtually eradicated at a stage when not more than 1% of 13–14 year old schoolchildren are tuberculin positive. Now that so much is known about nonspecific tuberculin positivity (p. 171) this objective is rather less well defined and one would have to modify it to suggest that not more than 1% of such schoolchildren should have a positive test likely to be due to infection with mammalian tubercle bacilli.

We now undoubtedly have the tools to eliminate tuberculosis, but the rate at which it will be eliminated will depend on the money and effort which society as a whole is prepared to put into the job as well as on the quality of the people concerned with carrying it out. The main measures are as follows:

(1) The control of infection from cow's *milk* by pasteurization and the building up of tuberculin tested herds (p. 177).

(2) *Effective treatment* to render infectious or potentially infectious individuals noninfectious (p. 234).

(3) Identification of all infectious or potentially infectious individuals, mainly by *miniature radiography* (p. 179).

(4) *BCG* (p. 184).

SUCCESS DEPENDS ON

(1) The provision of trained clinicians, public health workers and bacteriologists with proper facilities.

(2) The intelligent use of available mass miniature radiography facilities.

(3) Efficient organization, with close cooperation between preventive and therapeutic services.

(4) Efficient public relations designed to obtain the full cooperation from the entire community. Teamwork is essential to this task; individualism can never achieve more than partial success. *Diagnostic and therapeutic services* should be based on the chest clinic or the chest department of a general hospital. Efficient notification of new cases is essential. It is highly desirable that the same team of clinicians deals with the patient both as an outpatient and inpatient. As the chest

services in most developed countries are concerned with other diseases besides tuberculosis there is much less risk of error if all cases likely to be highly infectious, that is all with obvious cavities on the x-ray or a positive sputum on direct smear, are admitted to hospital at least until negative on direct smear and preferably until negative on culture. New cases which are not likely to be infectious may be treated at work without interfering with their lives in any other way but require very close supervision to ensure that treatment is fully taken. The patient's cooperation must be ensured by personal interest and by proper medical social care. There must be adequate financial provision for the sick person and his family, and adequate care of children if the mother is the patient.

PREVENTION STEMMING FROM THE PATIENT

Domestic contacts of all ages should be examined. In the conditions obtaining in many developed countries tuberculin testing is probably desirable at all ages and BCG should be given to the negatives. Often in Britain those who are initially tuberculin negative have been re-examined in six weeks' time, in case they are in the incubation period when first examined, and the tuberculin test repeated. If it is still negative BCG is given. This latent period was mainly designed to protect the reputation of BCG. It is probable that it could now be dispensed with and BCG given at the first attendance if the individual is tuberculin negative. Tuberculin testing should be repeated 3 months after BCG is given. If the test is strongly positive it may be suspected that the individual was in the incubation period when first tested and he should then be x-rayed. Otherwise child contacts who are initially tuberculin negative need not have a chest x-ray. The positives should be x-rayed. If adequate facilities exist x-ray should be repeated after 3–6 months. Thereafter, if the index case has received adequate treatment, there is little point in further examination [76]. If the individual is in contact with a noncooperative patient who is not receiving adequate treatment then he should be re-examined at 3–6 monthly intervals. The decision as to whether to examine *work contacts* of the index case is best made on an individual basis, depending on the likely infectiousness of the index case or the known occurrence of more than one case at the same place of work. It is a useful measure to keep a list of all notified cases by place of work. If multiple cases are occurring a major effort should be made to x-ray all employees. Similarly notifications should be classified by place of residence and intensive local efforts made if any particular area shows a high notification rate.

Aftercare

With proper treatment most patients can return to their former work unless extensive lung damage has resulted in insufficient respiratory reserve for hard physical work. 'Rehabilitation' services, important when treatment was inefficient, are now hardly required for tuberculosis.

Prevention in the community

The defences of the members of the community against disease will be raised by general economic improvement and social advance, and by health education to encourage consumption of proper foods, adequate exercise and sleep, fresh air, etc. The defences can be specifically enhanced by the use of BCG in school leavers, contacts and groups at special risk (p. 184). *Infection* can be prevented by *milk control* (p. 177) and an *adequate casefinding programme* (p. 179). The latter presents the preventive services with their major challenge at the present time. Whether *chemoprophylaxis* (p. 187) will later find a place is still uncertain.

ECONOMICALLY DEVELOPING COUNTRIES [128]

In economically developing countries the outlook is very different. In all such countries the problem is a vast one and finance and staff are inadequate. It follows that the finance and staff available must be used to the best advantage and nothing must be wasted. The *main measures* are:

(1) *BCG* to increase the resistance of the community and individuals, which should be first applied on a mass scale and then on a continuing basis through the normal health services, with statistical control to ensure cover of a high proportion of the community (p. 184). It should be given at the earliest possible age.

(2) *Case finding*, which should never outrun the capacity of the therapeutic services to treat effectively the cases found, and should in the first place be mainly concentrated on symptom groups with *direct smear sputum examination* as the main tool (p. 181). *Miniature radiography* should initially be used for helping to define the problem and later perhaps for limited use in special groups where the cases found can be adequately treated (p. 180).

(3) *Chemotherapy*. The provision of mass chemotherapy for infectious cases is a preventive tool second only to BCG as well as being the best way of obtaining the cooperation of the public. *Special methods* of chemotherapy have to be employed, for economic reasons, in developing countries (p. 250). Chemotherapy is at present grossly abused in most developing countries and by keeping patients alive and infectious by a series of short courses—and often alive, infectious and with drug resistant organisms—is frequently doing more harm than good. In consequence primary drug resistance is a major problem. *Bad chemotherapy* arises from ignorance by doctors about correct drug combinations, prescription by nondoctors and, in the past, the mistaken idea that isoniazid resistant tubercle bacilli were nonvirulent for man. *Poor supply* arrangements often result in doctors being unable to give the treatment which they know is required. The adequate and regular supply of the basic agents, isoniazid, streptomycin and thiacetazone is a first priority and, where doctors have been trained to use chemotherapy properly, it should not be available to untrained doctors or direct to the public. Treatment may be controlled by *sputum smear* only. Culture is not strictly essential but a few *reference laboratories* in each country should be equipped to

carry out both culture and resistance tests on a sample basis in order to review the resistance problem. These laboratories might be associated with a few *training centres* which could specialize in the treatment of resistant cases. It may be that only these centres should have access to second line drugs. The great majority of patients should be *treated at home* or *at work* and only a few beds made available for emergencies.

ORGANIZATION

The first essential is enthusiastic *medical leaders*. Enthusiasm, organizing ability and personality are more important than academic attainment. Finance should primarily be spent on such leaders and their training, on the provision of drugs and on BCG. It should not be wasted on hospitals or sanatoria, on expensive chest clinics or elaborate x-ray equipment. *Supporting staff* are usually relatively cheap and can be trained *ad hoc*. Nothing should be done by a doctor which can be done by technicians trained for the particular job. The conscientiousness of the latter can often be maintained by their working in pairs, by unexpected sample checks and by feeding in, for instance, known positive smears into any series which a technician is asked to examine. Much can be done by simple *social work* by social workers trained *ad hoc*. Patients are often far more cooperative than is alleged if their personal problems can be sympathetically dealt with. Doctors cannot have the time to do this but much can be done by a humane social worker with a good personality.

A World Health Organization scheme in South India has shown that with a population of 1·5 million in an area of some 4000 square miles (10,360 km²) a single team of six workers (doctor, public health nurse, laboratory technician, x-ray technician, BCG team-leader and statistical clerk) has been able to mobilize the already existing health services and to discover 5000 cases in the first year and 2500 in each of the next two. More than 60% completed more than one year of treatment, in spite of a previously very large defaulter rate. Vaccination coverage increased to over 70% of those eligible; 1 team of 6 technicians vaccinated over 100,000 people in a year [129]. Such an achievement shows what is possible with good leadership.

CONCLUSION

In many developing countries there is an acute emergency in tuberculosis control. If the use of chemotherapy is not regulated and put into trained hands much of the tuberculosis occurring in these countries may prove untreatable by present methods. Prevention will then become increasingly difficult.

REFERENCES

[1] AFFRONTI L.F., PARLETT R.C., PIERSON F. & ANELLO C. (1967) An epidemiologic comparative study in Delaware of the tine and Mantoux tests. *Am. Rev. resp. Dis.* **95**, 81.

[2] ALLISON S.T. (1955) Pulmonary tuberculosis after subtotal gastrectomy. *New Eng. J. Med.* **252**, 862.

[3] ARONSON, J.D., ARONSON CHARLOTTE F. & TAYLOR HELEN C. (1958) A twenty-year appraisal of BCG vaccination in tuberculosis. *A.M.A. Arch. intern. Med.* **101**, 881.

[4] ARTHUR A.B. & WHITE J.E.W. (1965) An evaluation of a disposable tuberculin test in children. *Tubercle, Lond.* **46**, 126.

[5] ASPIN J. (1962) Tuberculosis among Indian immigrants to a Midland industrial area. *Br. med. J.* i, 1386.

[6] BADGER T.L., BREITWIESER E. Ruth & MUENCH H. (1963) Tuberculin tine test. Multiple puncture intradermal technique compared with PPD-S, intermediate strength (5 TU). *Am. Rev. resp. Dis.* **87**, 338.

[7] BARRIE J.D. & BRUCE L.G. (1966) Human infections with bovine tuberculosis in the West of Scotland, 1963–65. *Scot med. J.* **11**, 436.

[8] BARTMANN K. (1964) Newer experimental data on chemoprophylaxis with special regard to the influence of treatment on acquired immunity. *Bull. internat. Un. Tuberc.* **35**, 87.

[9] BERNARD E., KREIS B., THIERY J. & LE JOUBIOUX E. (1955) Perte chez le singe au pouvoir pathogène des bacilles tuberculeux résistantes à l'isoniazide. *Bull. Acad. nat. Méd.* **139**, 462.

[10] BJARVEIT K. & WAALER H. (1965) Some evidence of the efficacy of mass BCG vaccination. *Bull. Wld Hlth Org.* **33**, 289.

[11] BJERKEDAL T. & PALMER C.E. (1966) Isoniazid prophylaxis in experimental tuberculosis.

Comparison of a single versus multiple daily doses. *Scand. J. resp. Dis*. **47**, 131.

[12] BRITISH MEDICAL RESEARCH COUNCIL (1959) BCG and vole bacillus vaccines in the prevention of tuberculosis in adolescents. *Br. med. J*. **ii**, 379.

[13] BRITISH MEDICAL RESEARCH COUNCIL (1960) Freeze dried BCG vaccine. Stability of vaccine under different conditions of storage and persistence of tuberculin sensitivity in school children after vaccination. *Br. med. J*. **ii**, 979.

[14] BRITISH MEDICAL RESEARCH COUNCIL (1963) BCG and vole bacillus vaccines in the prevention of tuberculosis in adolescence and early adult life. *Br. med. J*. **i**, 973.

[15] BRITISH TUBERCULOSIS ASSOCIATION (1959) A single tuberculin test for epidemiological use: a comparison of the Mantoux and Heaf tests. *Tubercle, Lond*. **40**, 317.

[16] BRITISH TUBERCULOSIS ASSOCIATION (1963) Sensitivity to human and avian tuberculin among schoolchildren in England and Wales. *Tubercle, Lond*. **44**, 119.

[17] BRITISH TUBERCULOSIS ASSOCIATION (1965) BCG vaccination by multiple-puncture: Third Report. *Tubercle, Lond*. **46**, 111.

[18] BRITISH TUBERCULOSIS ASSOCIATION (1966) Tuberculosis among immigrants to England and Wales: A national survey in 1965. *Tubercle, Lond*. **47**, 145.

[19] BROWN K.E. & CAMPBELL A.H. (1961) Tobacco, alcohol and tuberculosis. *Br. J. Dis. Chest* **55** 150.

[20] BUSH O.B.Jr., SUGIMOTO M., FUJIL Y. & BROWN F.A. (1965) Isoniazid prophylaxis in contacts of persons with known tuberculosis. Second report. *Am. Rev. resp. Dis*. **92**, 732.

[21] CAPOBRES D.B., TOSH F.E., YATES J.L. & LANGELUTTIG H.V. (1962) Experience with the tuberculin tine test in a sanatorium. *J. Am. med. Ass*. **180**, 1130.

[22] CLARKE B.R. (1952) *Causes and Prevention of Tuberculosis*. Edinburgh, Livingstone.

[23] COCHRANE A.L., JARMAN T.F. & MIALL W.E. (1956) Factors influencing the attack rate of pulmonary tuberculosis. *Thorax*, **11**, 141.

[24] COMSTOCK G.W., EDWARDS LYDIA B., PHILIP R.N. & WINN W.A. (1964) A comparison in the United States of America of two tuberculins, PPD−S and RT23. *Bull. Wld Hlth Org*. **31**, 161.

[25] COMSTOCK G.W. & PALMER C.E. (1966) Long term results of BCG vaccination in the Southern United States. *Am. Rev. resp. Dis*. **93**, 171.

[26] COMSTOCK G.W., FEREBEE SHIRLEY H. & HAMMES L.M. (1967) A controlled trial of community-wide isoniazid prophylaxis in Alaska. *Am. Rev. resp. Dis*. **95**, 935.

[27] CROFTON J.W. (1961) Human tuberculosis. In *Tuberculosis in Animals*, ed. Ritchie J.N. &

Macrae W.D. *Symposia of Zoological Society of London*, No. 4, p. 57. London, Zoological Society of London.

[28] CROFTON EILEEN & CROFTON J. (1963) Influence of smoking on mortality from various diseases in Scotland and in England and Wales. An analysis by cohorts. *Br. med. J*. **ii**, 1161.

[29] CRUICKSHANK R., ed. (1965) *Medical Microbiology*, 11th Edition, p. 195. Edinburgh, Livingstone.

[30] DANIELS M., RIDEHALGH F., SPRINGETT V.H. & HALL I.M. (1948) *Tuberculosis in Young Adults: Report on the Prophit Tuberculosis Survey 1935–44*. London, Lewis.

[31] DAWSON J.J.Y., DEVADATTA S., FOX W., RADHAKRISHNA S., RAMAKRISHNAN C.V., SOMASUNDARAM P.R., STOTT H., TRIPATHY S.P. & VELU S. (1966) A 5 year study of patients with pulmonary tuberculosis in a current comparison of home and sanatorium treatment for 1 year with isoniazid plus PAS. *Bull. Wld Hlth Org*. **34**, 533.

[32] DIEHL K. & VERSCHUER O. VON (1930) Erbuntersuchungen an Tuberkulosen Zwillingen. *Beitr. Klin. Tuberk*. **75**, 206 and 214. Quoted Clarke (1952).

[33] DOLL R. & HILL A.B. (1964) Mortality in relation to smoking: Ten years' observations in British doctors. *Br. med. J*, **i**, 1399.

[34] DORMER B.A., HARRISON I., SWART J.A. & VIDOR S.R. (1959) Prophylactic isoniazid. Protection of infants in a tuberculosis hospital. *Lancet*, **ii**, 902.

[35] DUBOS R. & DUBOS J. (1953) *The White Plague: Tuberculosis, Man and Society*. London, Gollancz.

[36] EDITORIAL (1966) Tuberculin tests. *Tubercle, Lond*. **47**, 231.

[37] EDWARDS J.H. (1957) Contribution of cigarette smoking to respiratory disease. *Br. J. prev. soc. Med*. **11**, 10.

[38] EDWARDS PHYLLIS Q. & EDWARDS LYDIA B. (1960) Story of the tuberculin test. From an epidemiologic viewpoint. *Am. Rev. resp. Dis*. **81**, *Suppl*.

[39] EDWARDS LYDIA B. (1963) Current status of the tuberculin test. *Ann. N.Y. Acad. Sci*. **106**, 32.

[40] EDWARDS LYDIA B., HOPWOOD LOUISE & PALMER C.E. (1965) Identification of mycobacterial infections. *Bull. Wld Hlth Org*. **33**, 405.

[41] EGMOSE T., ANG'AWA J.O.W. & POTI S.J. (1965) The use of isoniazid among household contacts of open cases of pulmonary tuberculosis. *Bull. Wld Hlth Org*. **33**, 419.

[42] EMERSON P.A. & SHAW EILEEN M. (1964) A comparison of the Heaf and the 'tine' disposable multiple puncture tuberculin tests. *Tubercle, Lond*. **45**, 36.

[43] FEREBEE Shirley H. & PALMER C.E. (1956)

Prevention of experimental tuberculosis with isoniazid. *Am. Rev. Tuberc.* **73**, 1.

[44] FEREBEE SHIRLEY H. & MOUNT F.W. (1962) Tuberculosis morbidity in a controlled trial of the prophylactic use of isoniazid among household contacts. *Am. Rev. resp. Dis.* **85**, 490.

[45] FRANCIS J. (1958) *Tuberculosis in Animals and Man.* London, Cassell.

[46] FRIMODT-MØLLER J. (1960) A community-wide tuberculosis study in a South Indian rural population 1950–55. *Bull. Wld Hlth Org.* **22**, 61.

[47] FRIMODT-MØLLER J., THOMAS J. & PARTHA-SARATHY R. (1964) Observations on the protective effect of BCG vaccination in a South Indian rural population. *Bull. Wld Hlth Org.* **30**, 545.

[48] GEDDE-DAHL T. (1952) Tuberculous infection in the light of tuberculin matriculation. *Am. J. Hyg.* **56**, 139.

[49] GEDDES J.E. (1962) The eradication of tuberculosis. *Scot. med. J.* **7**, 300.

[50] GRIFFITH A.H., MARKS J. & RICHARDS M. (1963) Low grade sensitivity to tuberculin in schoolchildren. *Tubercle, Lond.* **44**, 135.

[51] GRIFFITH A.H. & KINSLEY BARBARA J. (1965) A comparison of the Heaf and tine tuberculin tests. *Tubercle, Lond.* **46**, 121.

[52] GRIFFITHS MARGARET I., DAVITT M.C., BRINDLE T.W. & HOLME T. (1965) Intradermal BCG vaccination by jet injection. *Br. med. J.* **ii**, 399.

[53] GROTH PETERSEN E., KNUDSEN J. & WILBEK E. (1959) Epidemiological basis of tuberculosis eradication in an advanced country. *Bull. Wld Hlth Org.* **21**, 5.

[54] GROTH-PETERSEN E., GAD U. & WILBEK E. (1964) The results of the chemoprophylactic trial in Greenland during the first 4 years. *Bull. internat. Un. Tuberc.* **35**, 116.

[55] HART P.D'A, MILLER C.L., SUTHERLAND I. & LESSLIE I.W. (1962) Sensitivity to avian and human old tuberculin in man in Great Britain. *Tubercle, Lond.* **43**, 268.

[56] HART P.D. (1967) Efficacy and applicability of mass BCG vaccination in tuberculosis control. *Br. med. J.* **i**, 587.

[57] HAWTHORNE V.M., JARRETT W.F.H., LAUDER I., MARTIN W.B. & ROBERTS G.B.S. (1957) Tuberculosis in man, dog and cat. *Br. med. J.* **ii**, 675.

[58] HAWTHORNE V.M. (1962) The eradication of tuberculosis. *Scot. med. J.* **7**, 303.

[59] HIMSWORTH H.P. (1938) Pulmonary tuberculosis complicating diabetes mellitus. *Quart. J. Med.* **31** (N.S.7), 373.

[60] HORWITZ O., PAYNE P.G. & WILBEK E. (1966) Epidemiological basis of tuberculosis eradication. 4. The isoniazid trial in Greenland. *Bull. Wld Hlth Org.* **35**, 555.

[61] HUTTON P.W. (1962) Tuberculosis in an African setting. The therapeutic problem. *Postgrad. med. J.*, **38**, 80.

[62] HYGE T.V. (1947) Epidemic of tuberculosis in a state school. *Acta tuberc. scand.* **21**, 1.

[63] INDIAN COUNCIL OF MEDICAL RESEARCH (1959) *Tuberculosis in India: A Sample Survey 1955–1958.* New Delhi, Special Report series No. 34.

[64] JENTGENS H. (1963) Zur Frage der konnatalen Tuberkulose. *Tuberkulosearzt*, **17**, 479.

[65] KALLMANN F.J. & REISNER D. (1943) Twin studies on the significance of genetic factors in tuberculosis. *Am. Rev. Tuberc.* **47**, 549.

[66] KAMAT S.R., DAWSON J.J.Y., DEVADATTA S., FOX W., JANARDHANAM B., RADHAKRISHNA S., RAMAKRISHNAN C.V., SOMASUNDARAM P.R., STOTT H. & VELU S. (1966) A controlled study of the influence of segregation of tuberculous patients for one year on the attack rate of tuberculosis in a 5-year period in close family contacts in South India. *Bull. Wld Hlth Org.* **34**, 517.

[67] KATZ J. & KUNOFSKY S. (1960) Environmental versus constitutional factors in the development of tuberculosis among negroes. *Am. Rev. resp. Dis.* **81**, 17.

[68] KISSEN D.A. (1958) *Emotional Factors in Pulmonary Tuberculosis.* London, Tavistock Publications.

[69] KLARE K.C. ABELES H., ARONSOHN M.H., CHAVES A.D., GLASS R. & ROBINS A.B. (1967) The prevalence of atypical mycobacterial tuberculin sensitivity in a selected population in New York City. *Am. Rev. resp. Dis.* **95**, 103.

[70] KREIS B. (1966) *Résistance et survivance du bacille tuberculeux aux médications anti-bacillaires.* Chapter X: Résistance et pouvoir pathogène. Paris, Masson.

[71] LAMBERT H.P. (1959) The chemoprophylaxis of tuberculosis. A review. *Am. Rev. resp. Dis.* **80**, 648.

[72] LAUDER I.M. (1961) Tuberculosis in dogs and cats. In *Tuberculosis in Animals*, ed. Ritchie J.N. and Macrae W.D. *Symposia of Zoological Society of London*, No. 4, p. 37. London, Zoological Society of London.

[73] LEADER (1965) Medical examination of immigrants. *Br. med. J.*, **ii**, 1381.

[74] LEADER (1966) Local outbreaks of tuberculosis. *Lancet* **i**, 805.

[75] LEFFORD M.J., MITCHISON D.A. & TALL R. (1966) Bacteriological aspects of the second national survey of primary drug resistance in pulmonary tuberculosis. *Tubercle, Lond.* **47**, 109.

[76] LOUDON R.G., WILLIAMSON J. & JOHNSON JOAN M. (1958) An analysis of 3,485 tuberculosis contacts in the city of Edinburgh during 1954–55. *Am. Rev. Tuberc.* **77**, 623.

[77] LOWE C.R. (1956) An association between smoking and respiratory tuberculosis. *Br. med. J.* **ii**, 1081.

[78] LUNTZ G.W.R.N. (1961) The prognosis of tuberculosis in diabetic patients. *Tubercle, Lond.* **42**, 379.

[79] LURIE M.B. (1964) *Resistance to Tuberculosis: Experimental Studies in Native and Acquired Defensive Mechanisms.* Cambridge, Mass., Harvard University Press.

[80] LYNCH H.J., TOSH F.E., DOTO I.L., PLACE V.A. & FURCOLOW M.L. (1961) A comparison of the intradermal intermediate PPD reaction with the tuberculin tine test in 5066 adults and children. *Am. Rev. resp. Dis.* **84**, 128.

[81] MACGREGOR I.M. (1961) *The Two-year Mass Radiography Campaign in Scotland 1957–58.* Edinburgh, H.M. Stationery Office.

[82] MACRAE W.D. (1961) The eradication of bovine tuberculosis in Great Britain. In *Tuberculosis in Animals*, ed. Ritchie J.N. and Macrae W.D. *Symposia of Zoological Society of London*, No. 4, p. 81. London, Zoological Society of London.

[83] MAHA G.E. (1962) Comparative study of tuberculin tine and Mantoux tests in 676 college stdents. *J. Am. med. Ass.* **182**, 304.

[84] MARSH K. (1957) Tuberculosis among the residents of hostels and lodging houses in London. *Lancet* i, 1136.

[85] MILLER F.J.W., SEAL R.M.E. & TAYLOR MARY D. (1963) *Tuberculosis in Children*, p. 76. London, Churchill.

[86] MILLER A.B., TALL R., FOX W., LEFFORD M.J. & MITCHISON D.A. (1966) Primary drug resistance in pulmonary tuberculosis in Great Britain: Second National Survey 1963. *Tubercle, Lond.* **47**, 92.

[87] MITCHISON D.A. (1964) The virulence of tubercle bacilli from patients with pulmonary tuberculosis in India and other countries. *Bull. int. Un. Tuberc.* **35**, 287.

[88] MITCHISON D.A. Personal communication.

[89] MORSE D., BROTHWELL D.R. & UCKO P.J. (1964) Tuberculosis in ancient Egypt. *Am. Rev. resp. Dis.* **90**, 524.

[90] MOUNT F.W. & FEREBEE SHIRLEY H. (1962) The effect of isoniazid prophylaxis on tuberculous morbidity among household contacts of previously known cases of tuberculosis. *Am. Rev. resp. Dis.* **85**, 821.

[91] MYERS J.A. (1959) *Tuberculosis and Other Communicable Diseases*, p. 19. Springfield, Illinois, Thomas.

[92] NYBOE J. (1960) The efficacy of the tuberculin test. An analysis based on results from 33 countries. *Bull. Wld Hlth Org.* **22**, 5.

[93] NYBOE J. (1964) Evidence in favour of a low dose for the tuberculin test. *Bull. Wld Hlth Org.* **30**, 529.

[94] PAGEL W., SIMMONDS F.A.H., MACDONALD N. & NASSAU E. (1964) *Pulmonary tuberculosis*, 4th Edition, p. 238. London, Oxford University Press.

[95] PALMER C.E., SHAW L.W. & COMSTOCK G.W. (1958) Community trials of BCG vaccination. *Am. Rev. Tuberc.* **77**, 877.

[96] PAYNE MILLICENT (1959) *Study of the natural history of primary tuberculosis in childhood with particular reference to the prevention of mortality and morbidity.* M.D. Thesis. University of Durham. Quoted Miller et al. (1963).

[97] PEIZER L.R., CHAVES A.D. & WIDELOCK D. (1957) The effects of early isoniazid treatment in experimental guinea pig tuberculosis. *Am. Rev. Tuberc.* **76**, 732.

[98] RAMSAY J.H.R. & PINES A. (1963) The late results of chemotherapy in pneumoconiosis complicated by tuberculosis. *Tubercle, Lond.* **44**, 476.

[99] RICH A.R. (1951) *The Pathogenesis of Tuberculosis*, 2nd Edition, p. 182. Oxford, Blackwell Scientific Publications.

[100] ROELSGAARD E., IVERSEN E. & BLØCHER C. (1964) Tuberculosis in tropical Africa. An epidemiological study. *Bull. Wld Hlth Org.* **30**, 459.

[101] ROSENTHAL S.R., LOEWINSOHN E., GRAHAM MARY L., LIVERIGHT DOROTHY, THORNE MARGARET C., JOHNSON VIOLET & BATSON H.C. (1961) BCG vaccination against tuberculosis in Chicago. A 20-year study statistically analyzed. *Pediatrics* **28**, 622.

[102] ROSENTHAL S.R. (1961) The disk-tine tuberculin test (dried tuberculin-disposable unit). *J. Am. med. Ass.* **177**, 452.

[103] SCHMIDT L.H., MIDDLEBROOK G., LINCOLN A.F. & MORSE W.C. (1955) Pathogenicity for monkeys of various isoniazid resistant strains of *M. tuberculosis. Trans. 14th Conf. Chemotherapy of Tuberculosis, Washington*, p. 214. Veterans Administration.

[104] SCOTT R., GASKELL P.G. & MORRELL D.C. (1966) Patients who reside in common lodging-houses. *Br. med. J.* ii, 1561.

[105] SEIBERT FLORENCE B., ARONSON J.D., KERCHEL J., CLARK L.T. & LONG E.R. (1934) The isolation and properties of the purified protein derivative of tuberculin. *Am. Rev. Tuberc.* **30**, 707.

[106] SEILER H.E., WELSTEAD A.G. & WILLIAMSON J. (1958) Report on Edinburgh x-ray campaign. *Tubercle, Lond.* **39**, 339.

[107] SERGENT E. & DUCROS-ROUGEBIEF H. (1944) Observations sur la prémunition antituberculeuse par le BCG en Algérie. (Familles d'enfants vaccinés après décès d'aînés non vaccinés). *Arch. Inst. Pasteur Alger.* **22**, 273.

[108] SHARP J.C.M. (1964) A tuberculosis sputum survey. *Med. Offr.* **112**, 316.

[109] SHAW J.B. & WYNN-WILLIAMS N. (1954) Infectivity of pulmonary tuberculosis in relation to sputum status. *Am. Rev. Tuberc.* **69**, 724.

[110] SIMONDS BARBARA (1963) *Tuberculosis in Twins*. London, Pitman.

[111] SOLTYS M.A. (1952) *Tubercle Bacillus and Laboratory Methods in Tuberculosis*. Edinburgh, Livingstone.

[112] SOLTYS M.A. (1958) Public health aspect of tuberculosis in domestic animals. *Br. med. J.* ii, 1133.

[113] SPRINGETT V.H. (1951) Results of re-examination by mass radiography. *Br. med. J.* ii, 144.

[114] SPRINGETT V.H. (1952) An interpretation of statistical trends in tuberculosis. *Lancet* i, 521.

[115] SPRINGETT V.H. (1964) Tuberculosis in immigrants. An analysis of notification rates in Birmingham 1960–62. *Lancet* i, 1091.

[116] STEIN LILLI (1952) Tuberculosis and the 'social complex' in Glasgow. *Br. J. soc. Med.* 6, 1.

[117] STEVENSON D.K. (1962) Tuberculosis in Pakistanis in Bradford. *Br. med. J.* i, 1382.

[118] STEWART ALICE & HUGHES J.P.W. (1951) Mass radiography findings in the Northamptonshire boot and shoe industry 1945–46. *Br. med. J.* i, 899.

[119] STEWART C.J. (1962) Sensitivity to human, bovine and avian PPDs and their relationship to human tuberculosis in East Anglia. *Tubercle, Lond.* 44, 456.

[120] SUTHERLAND I, MILLER C.L., HART P.D'A. & LESSLIE I.W. (1964) Further studies of sensitivity to avian and human old tuberculin in man. *Tubercle, Lond.* 45, 110.

[121] TARSHIS M.S. (1961) Further investigation of the usefulness of the niacin test for distinguishing human tubercle bacilli from other mycobacteria. *Am. J. clin. Path.* 35, 461.

[122] THORN P.A., BROOKES V.S. & WATERHOUSE J.A.H. (1956) Peptic ulcer, partial gastrectomy, and pulmonary tuberculosis *Br. med. J.* i, 603

[123] TOMAN K., POLANSKY F., HEJDOVA E. & STERBOVA E. (1965) Gelatin and tween 80 as stabilizing agents for tuberculin dilutions. *Bull. Wld Hlth Org.* 33, 365.

[124] TURNER-WARWICK MARGARET T. (1957) Pulmonary tuberculosis and diabetes mellitus. *Quart. J. Med.* 50, (N.S. 26), 31.

[125] WILSON G.S. & MILES A.A. (1964) *Topley & Wilson's Principles of Bacteriology and Immunity*, Vol. 1, p. 536. London, Arnold.

[126] WOLSTENHOLME G.E.W. & CAMERON MARGARET P. (eds.) (1955) *Ciba Foundation Symposium on Experimental Tuberculosis. Bacillus and Host. With an Addendum on Leprosy*. London, Churchill.

[127] W.H.O. TUBERCULOSIS RESEARCH OFFICE (1955) Further studies of geographical variation in naturally acquired tuberculin sensitivity. *Bull. Wld Hlth Org.* 22, 63.

[128] WORLD HEALTH ORGANIZATION (1964) *WHO Expert Committee on Tuberculosis: Eighth Report*.

[129] WORLD HEALTH ORGANIZATION (1965) *International Work in Tuberculosis 1949–64*.

[130] WORLD HEALTH ORGANIZATION (1966) Requirements for dried BCG vaccine. *Technical Report*, Series No. 329, p. 25.

[131] ZAIDI S.H., HARRISON C.V., KING E.J. & MITCHISON D.A. (1955) Experimental infective pneumoconiosis. III. Coal mine dust and isoniazid resistant tubercle bacilli of moderate virulence. *Br. J. exp. Path.* 36, 545.

CHAPTER 11

Primary Pulmonary Tuberculosis

CONGENITAL TUBERCULOSIS [4, 12, 14, 8, 1]

Congenital tuberculosis is very rare. Some 250 cases have been collected from the literature by a recent reviewer [12]. A primary complex (see below) in the foetal liver is proof that the tubercle bacillus reached the blood by the umbilical vein but a primary pulmonary lesion can occur by aspiration of amniotic fluid. In that case proof of a congenital lesion depends on finding tuberculous lesions in the foetus *in utero*, at birth or a few days afterwards. To label a case congenital there must be evidence that the mother also has active tuberculosis or at least a positive tuberculin test. Tuberculous lesions are usually found in the placenta if this has been fully examined. Congenital tuberculosis has occurred when the mother has been known to have had only a recent primary infection; in some cases there has been no obvious clinical disease.

Lesions in the infant are usually widespread. In several cases death has occurred after a sudden cyanotic attack in an infant a few days old. In others there has been deterioration setting in within a few days of birth with an enlarged liver and spleen. Obstructive jaundice may occur due to enlargement of lymph glands in the *porta hepatis*. Other cases present as an acute extensive bronchopneumonia, but the liver and spleen are usually enlarged. Direct smear examination of the gastric lavage may be positive. The tuberculin test may remain negative throughout.

If the mother is known or discovered to have tuberculosis the diagnosis in the infant may be suspected. Otherwise it may be difficult, although several cases of late diagnosis and successful treatment have been recorded [12]. Unless the mother is known to have drug resistant organisms the infant should be treated with streptomycin, PAS and isoniazid (p. 236). The latter can be given in doses as high as 45 mg/kg/day initially. If the infant is very ill corticosteroid drugs would also be justified (p. 242).

ACQUIRED PRIMARY PULMONARY TUBERCULOSIS

The first infection with the tubercle bacillus is known as 'primary' tuberculosis. In this first infection the draining lymph glands are involved in addition to the initial lesion. This combination of the two lesions is known as the 'primary complex'. All other tuberculous lesions are regarded as postprimary and are not, at least in Europeans, accompanied by major tuberculosis of the draining lymph glands.

Although primary tuberculosis was formerly relatively common in the intestine or tonsil, due to infection from milk, and may occur in various exotic sites [8], in the very great majority of cases the route of infection is by inhalation and consequently the primary lesion is pulmonary.

PATHOLOGY

The primary lesion is subpleural. In children it may occur in any part of the lung, though in adolescents and young adults there is some bias towards the upper zones [6]. Multiple primary lesions can occur.

When tubercle bacilli are first deposited in an *alveolus* there follows a serous or serofibrinous exudate containing neutrophils. After a short time the neutrophils disappear and are replaced by macrophages (epithelioid cells) which take up the tubercle bacilli. The intracellular tubercle bacilli may gradually disappear and the lesion clear. Alternatively the bacilli may multiply within the macrophages. After 3–8 weeks the individual develops hypersensitivity to tuberculoprotein as shown by the tuberculin test becoming positive. At this stage the macrophages rupture and release the tubercle bacilli. Thereafter in man, tubercle bacilli are less often found within cells.

At this time the classical pathological manifestations of tuberculosis may be found in varying proportions. These consist of a granulomatous lesion containing *epithelioid cells* derived from macrophages, *Langhans' giant cells* with multiple nuclei, *lymphocytes* and varying degrees of *fibrosis*. As a result of hypersensitivity necrosis may occur to a varying extent in the inflammatory tissue and also in the tissue of the lung. The peculiarly cheesy form of necrosis found in tuberculosis is known as *caseation* and the caseous tissue may later become *calcified*. Although calcium may start to be laid down within a few months it is not usually radiologically visible until more than a year has elapsed. If the lesion progresses the caseous tissue, owing to factors which are not well understood, may become liquefied to form purulent material. This material may be discharged into the air passages resulting in *cavitation* of the lesion. Cavitation, however, is usually regarded as one of the postprimary manifestations.

Experimental work with radioactive BCG has suggested [20] that within less than an hour of the tubercle bacilli reaching the lung bacilli are carried by the lymphatics to the draining *lymph glands* and often some into the *blood stream*. The bacilli which are held up in the draining lymph glands give rise to pathological changes similar to those taking place in the lung, the two lesions together forming the 'primary complex'.

Swollen lymph glands may compress neighbouring bronchi and later tuberculous granulation tissue may spread to involve the adjoining bronchial wall giving rise to *tuberculous bronchitis*. Quite frequently the gland may erode the bronchial wall and caseous material may be discharged directly from the gland into the bronchial lumen. The effect of tuberculous lymph glands on the adjacent bronchus may give rise to collapse, exudation or caseous pneumonia in the part of the lung supplied by the bronchus. These are some-times known collectively as 'epituberculosis' (p. 201).

FATE OF THE PRIMARY COMPLEX

In the great majority of individuals the primary focus *heals completely*, with or without calcification. Nevertheless studies of calcified primary lesions at postmortem have shown that tubercle bacilli could be isolated from as high a proportion as 20% [2]. In some cases the lesion is walled off, the tubercle bacilli cease to divide rapidly and the disease becomes *dormant*. However, subsequent decrease in the body's defences, as a result of puberty, starvation, psychological stress or other factors (p. 215), may result in the dormant lesion reawakening and giving rise to active postprimary pulmonary tuberculosis.

In a few individuals the primary lesion in the lung may be *actively progressive* from the beginning and merge directly into postprimary pulmonary tuberculosis. This is particularly liable to occur in adolescents or young adults. In countries such as India or Africa cavitary tuberculosis is not uncommon in young children; this is rare in those of European stock.

A more formidable result of a primary tuberculous lesion is the development of the *haematogenous forms*. These may either be of the acute type, miliary tuberculosis or tuberculous meningitis, which are more likely to occur in infants or young children (p. 207), or the more chronic type with local manifestations in the kidneys, bones, joints, etc.

Tuberculous pleural effusion (p. 272) in young people usually follows within a year of the primary lesion, *bronchial complications* (p. 200) within 6 to 9 months, *miliary tuberculosis* (p. 207) or *tuberculous meningitis* within a year, *bone* or *joint lesions* mostly within 3 years and *renal* and *skin lesions* mostly after more than 5 years [14].

CLINICAL MANIFESTATIONS OF PRIMARY TUBERCULOSIS OF THE LUNG

Radiological changes have been found at the time of tuberculin conversion, that is soon after first infection, in between 7 and 30% of young adults in different series, being higher in those exposed to a known source of infection [6 & 7]. In children radiological changes are probably less frequent. Radiographically *in adults* the lung component is usually more obvious and the glandular component of the primary complex may not be visualized. Although in children the lung component of the primary complex may be in any part of the lung, in adults it is more often in the upper zones. With the difficulty of detecting the glandular component radiologically, and the similarity of appearance to postprimary pulmonary tuberculosis, it is not easy to distinguish primary tuberculosis in adolescents or adults from postprimary tuberculosis, unless it is known that the tuberculin test has recently become positive. Primary pulmonary tuberculosis in adults will therefore be considered with postprimary and the remainder of this

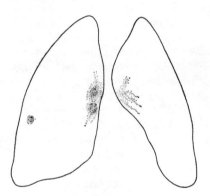

FIG. 11.1. Primary tuberculous complex in a child. Note small peripheral lesion in right midzone and enlarged hilar lymph node.

section will be concerned with primary tuberculosis in children. In children (fig. 11.1) the glandular component of the complex is often much more obvious radiologically and the lung component may in fact not be distinguishable.

SYMPTOMS

The great majority of primary tuberculous infections are probably *symptomless*, at least in adolescents and young adults [13 & 6]. The infection is usually overcome without the

individual being aware of any trouble. A proportion may experience a brief febrile incident at the time of tuberculin conversion which is passed off as 'influenza' or one of the brief fevers which are relatively common in childhood.

If the infection is a severe one, or host resistance is low, the child may appear to be vaguely unwell with *reduced appetite*, *fretfulness* and *failure* to *gain weight* normally. *Cough* is relatively unusual, but sometimes is paroxysmal and may be mistaken for whooping cough. This is usually due to pressure of lymph glands on bronchi, with or without invasion of the bronchial wall by granulation tissue. *Wheeze*, sometimes unilateral, occurs occasionally as a result of the same process. Children seldom bring up any sputum.

PHYSICAL SIGNS

In most cases there are *no detectable abnormal physical signs*. When the lesion is severe or extensive there may be the appearance of *general debility*. The child may be thin, pale and fretful. The *hair* may be less glossy than usual and the skin less elastic. In the *chest* there are usually no detectable physical signs but sometimes there may be a few local *crepitations* over a large lung component of the primary complex. More extensive physical signs may be present if there is 'epituberculosis' (see below). Occasionally pressure of glands on the bronchus may give rise to localized rhonchi.

DIAGNOSIS

The clinical manifestations of primary tuberculosis in children are vague and might well be due to numerous other causes. Primary tuberculosis should always be borne in mind when there is vague ill health. Such a suspicion is enhanced by a *history of contact* with an infectious case of tuberculosis either in the family or elsewhere. By the time there is clinical or radiological evidence of primary tuberculosis the *tuberculin test* is almost always positive to 5 or 10 TU (p. 172) and is usually strongly so. A negative test makes the diagnosis very unlikely.

Children's x-rays are often difficult to interpret. Where there is an obvious peripheral shadow in the lung together with enlarged hilar glands on one side, suspicion of a primary tuberculous complex will obviously arise. Every sort of variation may occur. The *lung component* may vary from a lesion which is so small as to be undetectable to a caseous pneumonia. The *lymph glandular component* is often invisible in adolescents or adults but may be very large, particularly in young children. Shadows in the apex of a lower lobe may simulate hilar lymph gland enlargement unless a lateral film is taken. The paratracheal glands may be enlarged. There may be radiological manifestations of '*epituberculosis*' (see below). In many cases there is a vague localized pneumonic shadow in the lung and it is uncertain whether this is due to a mild pneumonic process, perhaps following an upper respiratory tract infection, or to primary pulmonary tuberculosis. In this case the child may be re-x-rayed after 1–2 weeks, the tuberculin test being done in the meantime. If he is sufficiently unwell, oral penicillin may be given. After the interval a pneumonic shadow will almost always have changed for the better, but a tuberculous shadow will usually remain unaltered.

When there is a serious suspicion of primary pulmonary tuberculosis and the tuberculin test is positive, gastric lavage may be done with a view to obtaining bacteriological confirmation. A culture, of course, often takes 6 weeks but direct smear examination may be helpful. It is important to carry out gastric lavages where there is a suspicion that the child may have been infected with drug resistant tubercle bacilli or where there is serious doubt about the diagnosis. If the diagnosis is clear and the source of infection is known to harbour sensitive bacilli, a gastric lavage may cause the child unnecessary distress.

TREATMENT

There is some controversy as to the circumstances in which it is justifiable to give chemotherapy to a child whose *only manifestation* of tuberculosis is a *positive tuberculin test*. This problem has been discussed on p. 188. In any patient with a *radiographically visible lesion* the rate of complication by disseminated tuberculosis in the younger age group or by progressive pulmonary tuberculosis in those who have passed puberty, is so relatively high [15] that chemotherapy is mandatory in all cases.

CHEMOTHERAPY

In the first place it is important if possible to know the drug sensitivity of the organisms from the infector of the child. If the child is a known family contact this may be relatively easy but in a number of cases, of course, the source of infection is unknown. Acquired drug resistance is less likely to occur as a result of treating primary tuberculosis but the possibility cannot be excluded. In children it is desirable to avoid regular injections if this is possible. When the clinical and radiological manifestations are mild, and there is nothing to suggest that the child has been infected with a drug resistant organism, it is justifiable to treat with PAS and isoniazid from the beginning. Sodium PAS may be given in a dose of 300 mg/kg/day and isoniazid in a dose of 3 mg/kg/day, both drugs being administered in not more than two divided doses. It is often convenient to use the cachets containing both drugs (Sodium Aminosalicylate-Isoniazid Cachets BPC) and to empty these into milk, lemonade or jam. Palatable commercial preparations are also available. In hospital children are usually readily trained to take the drugs in solution. Children are seldom good at swallowing cachets whole.

If there is any probability of the infecting organisms being resistant to one of the drugs, or if the lesions are severe, it is wise to begin treatment with all 3 standard drugs, streptomycin being given in addition to PAS and isoniazid in a dose of 30 mg/kg/day in a single intramuscular injection. When the main clinical manifestations have subsided, and particularly if cultures from gastric lavages have shown that the organisms are fully sensitive to all three drugs, chemotherapy may be continued with PAS and isoniazid only. In some countries primary tuberculosis is treated with isoniazid alone, but the size of the risk of resistant organisms emerging is uncertain and it is wiser to use combined chemotherapy. Certainly our own experience with combined therapy is more satisfactory than that reported with isoniazid alone in the U.S. Public Health Service trial [15] but there may have been other differences between the groups which could account for their less satisfactory results. Although combined chemotherapy is therefore recommended in an economically developed country the risk of resistance emerging is small enough for single drug therapy perhaps to be justified in milder primary lesions in developing countries, though the extent of the local hazard of primary isoniazid resistance should be taken into account.

Chemotherapy should be continued for a minimum of one year. In many cases this is sufficient. If the response is slow or the lesions extensive it is wise to continue treatment up to 18 months or sometimes even longer.

LOCATION OF TREATMENT

It is desirable, if at all possible, not to separate the child from his mother. It is therefore much better to treat him at home. Sometimes the mother has difficulty in persuading the child to accept regular chemotherapy. In that case it may be useful to admit him to hospital for 1–2 weeks in order to get him used to taking the drugs. These can usually then be continued at home. If the mother is the source of infection and is ill, both she and her child may be admitted to hospital together.

BED REST

If the child is ill or febrile he should be kept in bed until the fever subsides and he is clinically improved. As soon as he is obviously improving he can be allowed up. A child who is not ill need never be put to bed. As long as chemotherapy is effectively administered bed rest is unnecessary for the healing of the disease.

THE EFFECT OF CHEMOTHERAPY

By the time the child is seen with primary tuberculosis there is probably considerable caseation in the lymph glands and chemotherapy usually has little obvious effect, the glands slowly subsiding over a number of months. When the lung component is a soft hazy shadow, and if it has spread locally, this may respond rather more rapidly. Certainly there is unlikely to be any progression of disease within the lung, although 'epituberculosis', which is largely mechanical in origin, may not be affected and fresh areas of the lung may actually be involved while the child is receiving chemotherapy (p. 201). The chief purpose of chemotherapy is to protect the child against the tuberculous complications of the primary lesion.

RELAPSE

When proper chemotherapy is prescribed and taken for 12–18 months as suggested, later relapse or tuberculous complications are virtually unknown.

USE OF CORTICOSTEROIDS

In general we have been unimpressed by the value of corticosteroids in the treatment of the primary complex. The glandular component usually seems to be unaffected, probably because caseation has already occurred. Others have had the same experience [11]. Nemir et al. [16] recorded significant advantage to corticosteroid treated cases in a controlled trial but did not clearly indicate whether there was a difference between those with and without segmental lesions. By analogy with postprimary pulmonary tuberculosis (p. 243) a large lung component no doubt would clear more quickly but there is little to be gained by this unless the child is clinically ill. Corticosteroid treatment probably has a place in treating bronchial complications (p. 243).

TRACHEAL AND BRONCHIAL COMPLICATIONS OF PRIMARY PULMONARY TUBERCULOSIS

As already mentioned, pressure by the enlarged parabronchial or paratracheal glands, or their erosion of the bronchial or tracheal wall, may give rise to wheeze or paroxysmal

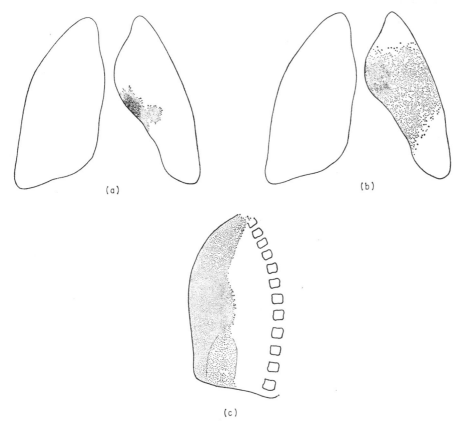

FIG. 11.2. (a) Primary tuberculous complex in girl aged 8. Note large hilar lymph node and possible peripheral component in left midzone. (b) 3 weeks later: collapse left upper lobe. (c) Left lateral film.

cough, sometimes with localized rhonchi. Occasionally the rupture of a caseous gland into the trachea, or the simultanous rupture of subcarinal glands into both main bronchi, may constitute an acute emergency requiring urgent bronchoscopy.

SEGMENTAL AND LOBAR LESIONS

Comparatively early in the study of tuberculosis in children it was recognized that children might have dense homogeneous shadows involving as much as a complete lobe of the lung yet the general condition might be comparatively good and the prognosis excellent. For this phenomenon the term 'epituberculosis' was coined by Eliasberg and Newland [9 & 10]. It is now realized that this radiological appearance (figs. 11.2 & 11.3) is usually either segmental or lobar and is associated with enlarged tuberculous lymph glands at the hilum. Because of the course of its bronchus, and the surrounding lymph glands, the middle lobe is often affected. It seems probable that the radiographic appearances may be caused by any of 3 pathological changes: collapse, inflammatory exudation with minimal caseation, or caseous pneumonia. Each may occur either alone or in combination with one or more of the others. *Collapse* is produced either by pressure of the gland on the bronchus, or by the spread of tuberculous granulation tissue into the bronchus with resultant stenosis, or by discharge of actual caseous material from the lymph gland through the damaged bronchial wall. Later the bronchial lesion may heal with a localized

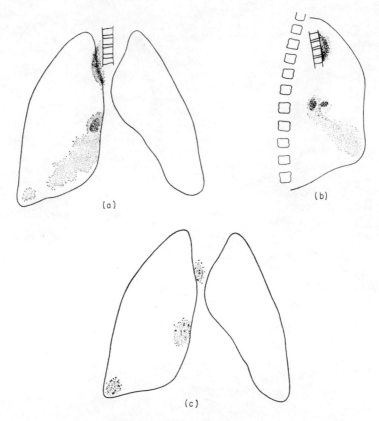

FIG. 11.3. (a) and (b) Collapse consolidation middle lobe in boy aged 4. Note enlargement of hilar and paratracheal lymph nodes and probable peripheral component (in right costophrenic angle) of primary tuberculous complex. (c) 4 years later: middle lobe re-expanded; calcification of components of primary complex.

scar or residual fibrous stenosis. The pathological evidence available suggests that the more common cause for the appearance is *inflammatory exudate*, either monocytic or actually polymorphonuclear. This is probably due to the discharge of caseous material into the bronchial lumen with aspiration into the relevant segment or lobe, followed by a brisk hypersensitivity reaction to the contained tuberculoprotein. It is not possible, on purely radiological grounds, to distinguish this appearance from *caseous pneumonia*, although the latter may later be implied from the development of calcification. In fact, caseous pneumonia appears to be very unusual, although small areas of caseation may occur. [5].

Clinically the *symptoms* do not differ importantly from those already outlined for primary tuberculosis, although naturally wheeze or a paroxysmal cough is rather more common. There may be remarkably few *physical signs* in the chest, in spite of formidable x-ray appearances, but dullness, diminished air entry, bronchial breathing or crepitations may occur. The latter is the commonest abnormal sign.

Treatment does not differ importantly from that for primary tuberculosis already outlined (p. 199) except for the use of corticosteroids. *Postural tipping* and coughing is desirable in an attempt to cough up as much as possible of the caseous material. If the child is not ill he should be encouraged to be up and running about. *Chemotherapy* will effectively prevent any important infectious complication and active exercise will make it more likely that the caseous material will be coughed up. *Bronchoscopy* is not usually a helpful procedure. Although the caseous material may be sucked out, more is usually soon discharged from the gland and bronchoscopy has to be frequently repeated. It may sometimes be necessary if secondary infection occurs beyond the bronchial block and drainage must be established as a matter of urgency. Segmental and lobar lesions, especially if recent, may respond to corticosteroid drugs given in addition to chemotherapy [11 & 16]. The daily dose should be equivalent to prednisolone 1–2 mg/kg. It should be continued for 4–6 weeks and then the dose gradually reduced over 2 weeks, resuming if there is any radiological or febrile relapse. It is also claimed that there is a reduction in the rate of residual bronchiectasis [11].

BRONCHIECTASIS AFTER PRIMARY PULMONARY TUBERCULOSIS

'Anatomical' bronchiectasis may occur following primary tuberculosis, especially when there have been lobar or segmental lesions. Roberts and Blair [19] conclude that distension by mucus, caseous tissue or secondary infection beyond the bronchial block is an important factor. Arteritis in bronchial vessels may also contribute. The incidence varies very much in different series, depending on the type of patient included [5]. Because the bronchiectasis is most often in the upper lobes, where it is well drained, secondary infection and clinical symptoms are comparatively rare, although commoner if the middle or lower lobes are involved. Gerbeaux and his colleagues [11] have shown that the earlier chemotherapy is started after appearance of a segmental shadow the less is the chance of subsequent bronchiectasis. The incidence is further reduced by giving corticosteroid drugs (p. 243). Brock [3] has described the late manifestations of bronchiectasis in the middle lobe in patients showing calcified areas in the lobe suggesting that the

bronchial lesions had their origin in a previous primary tuberculous infection.

OBSTRUCTIVE EMPHYSEMA

Occasionally the bronchus is so compressed as to result in a valve action, with air being admitted to a portion of the lung on inspiration but unable to escape on expiration. The segment or lobe may then become distended, sometimes with depression of the horizontal fissure or the diaphragm and deviation of the mediastinum on expiration. The phenomenon is best shown in an x-ray taken on expiration. In most series obstructive emphysema is rare and it is commoner in children under two years of age [14]. The symptoms are often similar to those already described above under the heading of 'Bronchial complications' (p. 200) although extreme distension of a lobe or even a lung may result in breathlessness. Unless there are severe symptoms bronchoscopy or surgical intervention is unnecessary and the condition resolves with chemotherapy without important residual damage. Corticosteroid drugs are worth a trial in an effort to relieve the valve action.

ERYTHEMA NODOSUM

Erythema nodosum is a hypersensitivity phenomenon which may accompany primary tuberculosis but is by no means specific to tuberculosis. In our own practice sarcoidosis is nowadays a much more frequent cause, owing to the low infection rate of tuberculosis in young people. Infection with haemolytic streptococci and treatment with drugs, particularly sulphathiazole, are other well known causes, although the latter drug is now relatively seldom used. The association of erythema nodosum with rheumatic fever may well be legendary as the joint complications of erythema nodosum may simulate rheumatic fever. Erythema nodosum has been described in a wide variety of other conditions, including coccidioidomycosis, histoplasmosis, cat-scratch disease, leprosy, etc., and with a wide variety of other drugs.

PATHOLOGY

Histologically the main lesions are subcutaneous, affecting the fat and the connective tissue septa. In the first few days there is dilatation of the blood vessels, oedema and infiltration with neutrophils. Histiocytes and lymphocytes are also seen and increase as the neutrophils diminish. Later there may be fibrinoid degeneration of the collagen and giant cells of the foreign body type appear, which may persist even for several months. The inflammatory changes are more marked round the veins than the arteries. Lesions have been described which are said to consist of groups of proliferated histiocytes with their oval nuclei radially disposed round a central cleft [14].

FREQUENCY

The frequency of erythema nodosum accompanying primary tuberculous infection seems to vary from country to country. Thompson [21] found an incidence of just over 1% in tuberculin positive children under 14 in Britain and it was 1·8% in 782 tuberculin conversions of young adults in the Prophit tuberculosis survey [6]. These figures are much lower than most of those from Scandinavia which have varied between 4·9 and 15% [5]. Erythema nodosum is said to be rare in dark skinned races but this may be due to the greater difficulty in identifying the characteristic eruption.

There is some variation with *age*. It is rare below the age of 7 and the frequency then increases up to puberty. It is more common in girls than boys at all ages but this discrepancy is even greater after puberty. In general the older the individual the greater the systemic upset.

RELATION TO THE TIME OF INFECTION

Tuberculin conversion is said to precede the eruption by a time varying from a few days to a fortnight, occasionally as long as a month. Fever may accompany the conversion and therefore precede the eruption [14]. Erythema nodosum is occasionally seen later in the primary infection or even in the postprimary phase.

CLINICAL FEATURES

The characteristic feature of erythema nodosum is the presence of tender, dusky-red, slightly *nodular lesions* on the anterior surface of the legs below the knee. On palpation the lesions feel as if they were deep to the skin rather than in it. They are usually 5–20 mm in diameter. The margins are ill-defined and the nodules may sometimes become confluent, usually in the region just above the ankles, to give an extensive, indurated, dusky-red area. A few lesions may sometimes be found on the anterior surfaces of the thighs, the extensor surfaces of the forearms and even, though rarely, on the forehead, nose, cheeks or ears. Over a week or so the red colour fades into purple and then brown. Some brownish pigment and induration may persist for several weeks. Recurrent crops of lesions may develop over a matter of weeks, sometimes much longer, but in most cases the condition subsides within a fortnight.

The amount of systemic reaction varies greatly. *Fever*, if present, often precedes the eruption by days, sometimes by a week or more. It may subside as the leg lesions clear but on occasion a high fever persists for several weeks accompanied by recurrent crops of nodules. High and prolonged fever seems commoner in older patients, the worst reactions being seen in women in their twenties or thirties. The latter are also more likely to develop *joint* changes. These may consist merely of pain in the larger joints, wrists, elbows, knees or ankles, but the joints are sometimes swollen, hot and tender and may be successively involved, mimicking rheumatic fever.

The main haematological change is in the erythrocyte sedimentation rate which is always raised and is often very high. A *leucocytosis* is sometimes seen.

DIAGNOSIS

The diagnosis of the *eruption* is not usually difficult unless the lesions are mainly confluent. Insect bites or Henoch-Schönlein purpura occasionally give rise to difficulty in younger children. The diagnosis of the *cause* may be more difficult. We are here concerned only with tuberculosis. The important initial procedure is the tuberculin test which is virtually always strongly positive in the tuberculous case. It is wise to give 1 TU as the first dose, as a severe reaction may follow a larger dose. If the Mantoux test is positive chest x-ray should follow. Radiological changes are commoner in children developing erythema nodosum at tuberculin conversion [14]. If the Mantoux is negative, or only weakly positive, other causes, such as sarcoidosis (p. 371) should be sought. If none is found it is well to keep the patient under observation for at least a year.

TREATMENT

If the chest x-ray suggests a diagnosis of primary tuberculosis the patient should be treated as already outlined (p. 199). Temperature and rash usually respond rapidly to chemotherapy and the child can be up and about as soon as he is well, though of course chemotherapy should be continued for at least a year. If the Mantoux test is strongly positive but the chest x-ray is normal a year's chemotherapy is still justifiable, as postprimary tuberculosis is more likely to develop when erythema nodosum complicates first infection. If fever and eruption fail to respond to chemotherapy the tuberculous diagnosis should be reviewed. We have never ourselves had to use corticosteroids in a tuberculous case, though we have had to do so in sarcoidosis (p. 388).

PHLYCTENULAR CONJUNCTIVITIS [14]

This condition is usually a hypersensitivity to the tubercle bacillus, though it may accompany sarcoidosis or infection with haemolytic streptococci. It is most often seen in children (of any age) with primary tuberculosis but, unlike erythema nodosum, is not necessarily confined to the early weeks after infection. It usually occurs within the first year [18] but may be seen even later. It has been reported after BCG vaccination [14]. It is commoner in children from a poor social environment and is said also to be more frequent in non-European communities in Africa and America [14].

CLINICAL FEATURES

Phlyctenular conjunctivitis is usually seen in one eye, but may occur in both, either simultaneously or successively. The attack begins with irritation, lachrymation and photophobia. The characteristic lesion is a small bleb 1–3 mm in diameter, which may be multiple, at the limbus. The bleb is shiny, yellowish or grey, with a characteristic sheaf of dilated vessels running out towards it from the edge of the conjunctival sac. The reaction subsides in a week or so but multiple crops may occur, either successively or at intervals.

DIAGNOSIS

Diagnosis has to be made from other types of conjunctivitis or from foreign bodies, but the lesion is characteristic and does not usually give rise to difficulty. Investigation of possible tuberculosis should be along the lines already indicated for erythema nodosum (p. 205).

TREATMENT

Any underlying tuberculosis should be treated with chemotherapy (p. 199). Locally the pupil is dilated with 0·25% atropine ointment; 1% hydrocortisone drops rapidly relieve the symptoms. Occasionally attacks continue to occur in spite of chemotherapy. In that case we have found desensitization to tuberculin a valuable measure [17].

PLEURAL EFFUSION

Pleural effusion may sometimes complicate primary pulmonary tuberculosis in children under the age of puberty. Such effusions are usually small and transient. Large pleural effusions are much commoner after puberty and are dealt with in detail elsewhere (p. 272).

GENERAL REFERENCES

BENTLEY F.J., GRZYBOWSKI S. & BENJAMIN B. (1954) *Tuberculosis in Childhood and Adolescence.* London, National Association for the Prevention of Tuberculosis.

MILLER F.J.W., SEAL R.M.E., TAYLOR MARY D., PROBERT W.R. & THOMAS D.M.E. (1963) *Tuberculosis in Children*. London, Churchill.

REFERENCES

[1] ARTHUR L. (1967) Congenital tuberculosis. *Proc. roy. Soc. Med.* **60**, 19.

[2] BLACKLOCK J.W.S. (1932) *Tuberculous Disease in Children: its Pathology and Bacteriology*. Med. Res. Counc. Spec. Rept Series No. 172. London, H.M.S.O.

[3] BROCK R.C. (1950) Post-tuberculous broncho-stenosis and bronchiectasis of the middle lobe. *Thorax* **5**, 5.

[4] CORNER BERYL D. & BROWN N.J. (1955) Congenital tuberculosis. Report of a case with necropsy findings in mother and child. *Thorax* **10**, 99.

[5] CROFTON J. (1954) Some problems in primary tuberculosis. *Br. med. Bull.* **10**, 125.

[6] DANIELS M., RIDEHALGH F., SPRINGETT V.H. & HALL I.M. (1948) *Tuberculosis in Young Adults*. Report on the Prophit Tuberculosis Survey 1935–44. London, Lewis.

[7] DAVIES P.D.B. (1961) The natural history of tuberculosis in children. *Tubercle, Lond.* **42**, Suppl.

[8] EDITORIAL (1965) Unusual primary tuberculosis. *Tubercle, Lond.* **46**, 420.

[9] ELIASBERG HELENE & NEULAND W. (1920) Die epituberkulöse Infiltration der Lunge bei tuberkulösen Sauglingen und Kindern. *Jber. Kinderheilk* **93**, 88.

[10] ELIASBERG HELENE & NEULAND W. (1921) Zur Klinik der epituberkulösen und gelatinösen Infiltration der kindlichen Lunge. *Ibid.* **94**, 102.

[11] GERBEAUX J., BACKLARD ARMELLE & COUVREUR J. (1965) Primary tuberculosis in childhood. Indications and contra-indications for corticosteroid therapy: Observations on 577 treated cases. *Am. J. Dis. Child* **110**, 507.

[12] JENTGENS H. (1963) Zur Frage der konnatalen Tuberkulose. *Tuberkulosearzt* **17**, 479.

[13] MALMROS H. & HEDVALL E. (1938) Studien über die Entstehung und Entwicklung der Lungentuberkulose. Leipzig, Barth.

[14] MILLER F.J.W., SEAL R.M.E., TAYLOR MARY D., PROBERT W.R. & THOMAS D.M.E. (1963) *Tuberculosis in Children*. London, Churchill.

[15] MOUNT F.W. & FEREBEE SHIRLEY H. (1961) Preventive effects of isoniazid in the treatment of primary tuberculosis in children. *New Engl. J. Med.* **265**, 713.

[16] NEMIR ROSA L., CARDONA J., VAZIR F. & TOLEDO R. (1967) Prednisolone as an adjunct in the chemotherapy of lymphnode-bronchial tuberculosis in childhood. A double blind study. II. Further term observation. *Am. Rev. resp. Dis.* **95**, 402.

[17] PINES A. (1959) Recurrent phlyctenular kerato-conjunctivitis treated by desensitization to tuberculin. *Br. med. J.* **i**, 689.

[18] PRICE DOROTHY & MCMANUS ADELINE (1943) Report on an investigation into phlyctenular ophthalmia. *Irish J. Med. Sci.* **215**, 602, quoted Miller et al. (1963).

[19] ROBERTS J.C. & BLAIR L.G. (1950) Bronchiectasis in primary tuberculous lesions associated with segmental collapse. *Lancet* **i**, 386.

[20] STRÖM L. (1955) A study of the cutaneous absorption of BCG vaccine labelled with radioactive phosphate in subjects with or without immunity. *Acta tuberc. scand.* **31**, 141.

[21] THOMPSON B.C. (1952) Discussion on the fate of the tuberculous primary complex. *Proc. roy. Soc. Med.* **45**, 741.

CHAPTER 12

Miliary Tuberculosis

Miliary tuberculosis is an illness produced by acute diffuse dissemination of tubercle bacilli via the blood stream. Although the overt case is relatively easily diagnosed, cryptic forms are not at all uncommon. In communities where tuberculosis is now greatly decreased these cryptic forms in older people contribute an important proportion of cases of miliary tuberculosis and are sometimes diagnosed only at postmortem. Even in a relatively sophisticated medical centre, 5 out of 17 deaths from pulmonary tuberculosis in one year were due to miliary tuberculosis; all were in old people; three were diagnosed only at postmortem and the other two very shortly before death (p. 166). As the disease is almost always fatal without adequate treatment and recovery is the rule if proper chemotherapy is given, the importance of making the diagnosis needs no emphasis.

PATHOGENESIS

When tuberculosis was widespread in the community young children were likely to be infected. The majority of cases of miliary tuberculosis closely followed the primary tuberculous infection, for young children are particularly susceptible to haematogenous spread (p. 197). If the infection is an overwhelming one and the patient's defences poor the haematogenous phase, occurring *via* the *lymphatics*, and the superior vena cava, which usually follows the primary tuberculous infection (p. 197), may be so overwhelming as to give rise to acute miliary tuberculosis. Sometimes this haematogenous dissemination results in the implantation of bacilli in a vessel wall to give a *caseous vasculitis* in the intima. This may in turn discharge bacilli into the blood stream. Such lesions are said to be commoner in the large veins, in the thoracic duct and less frequently in the arterial system, the aorta or endocardium [23]. Miliary dissemination may also follow *recrudescence* of an *old primary lesion* which may discharge itself into a vessel wall. Vascular invasion can probably also occur from *other active* post-primary lesions at any stage in the patient's career. The miliary tuberculosis which is now not uncommonly seen in middle aged and elderly people is presumably of this origin. Finally, miliary dissemination was once a dreaded complication of *surgical procedures* on tuberculous organs. Such procedures, when the diagnosis is known, should always be covered by effective chemotherapy. If the surgical procedure is a diagnostic one, when it is important not to kill the tubercle bacilli, chemotherapy should be started immediately after the operation, pending the result of the biopsy.

PREDISPOSING FACTORS

When tuberculosis was a common disease and children were frequently infected, a high proportion of cases occurred in *very young children* whose resistance to haematogenous dissemination is known to be poor (p. 197). In Debré's series [11] 22 out of 170 were aged less than one year and more than a third were aged less than 3 years. With the decrease in infection in children miliary tuberculosis in the child is now in some parts of the world a rarity, although cases continue to occur in adults. Debré found a higher rate in girls than in boys, but this was mainly in older children. *Measles* and *whooping cough* are well known predisposing factors; the diagnosis should be considered if either of these diseases is followed by unexplained fever. Miller and his colleagues [20] even found a number of cases following acute tonsillitis. *Chronic diseases,* such as leukaemia, may also predispose. Miliary tuberculosis may occur in patients receiving high doses of *corticosteroid* drugs, presumably because of lowering of resistance to the disease.

PATHOLOGY

In the commonest type of miliary tuberculosis the classical lesion is the focus of millet seed size, a few millimetres in diameter, which gives it its name. These lesions consist of clumps of epithelioid cells, lymphocytes and Langhans giant cells, often with central caseation. In the patient who has had a higher resistance, and in whom the lesions have persisted for a longer period, they may be larger and with greater central caseation. The distribution of the lesions in the body is variable. The lungs are virtually always affected, sometimes only microscopically. Involvement of spleen, liver and kidneys varies from case to case. Lesions may also occur in the serous sacs with resultant effusion. Bilateral pleural effusion is not uncommon; pericarditis, ascites or polyserositis may occur.

There is a rare acute malignant form of tuberculous septicaemia, sometimes known as the 'nonreactive' type, which occurs in adults and has a different pathology. Here the lesions are mainly necrotic, with no obvious tuberculous histology, and are teeming with tubercle bacilli. The spleen and liver may be enlarged and studded with irregular necrotic foci, usually less than 1 cm in diameter, or the foci may only be visible microscopically. Wedge-shaped infarct-like areas may be seen. Necrotic lesions may also occur in the bone marrow giving rise to various blood changes (p. 210) [23].

FUNCTIONAL ABNORMALITY

Few studies of abnormal function in miliary tuberculosis have been made. The main changes are probably reduced compliance, vital capacity and total lung capacity, together with diminished gas diffusion. Decrease of arterial oxygen tension and of carbon monoxide diffusing capacity have been demonstrated in individual cases [2].

CLINICAL FEATURES

There is nothing specific about the clinical presentation of miliary tuberculosis. An appreciable proportion of patients are first seen with *tuberculous meningitis*, this proportion varying with different series probably according to admission policy for the particular unit concerned. Tuberculous meningitis is not considered in this book. In the great majority of the remaining patients the presenting symptoms are *purely febrile* [11, 17 & 20]. *Cough* may occur from preceding primary infection (p. 198) but cough, breathlessness and cyanosis due to miliary disease are very late manifestations. In Miller's series [20] a number of patients were picked up merely on routine contact examination and Debré [11] emphasizes that miliary tuberculosis is commoner in children exposed to heavy infection in the home. A tuberculous lesion elsewhere may first bring the child to the doctor.

There is often a story of *gradual onset* of *vague ill-health*, perhaps with *loss* of *weight*. Sometimes this may have been due to a preceding primary infection and there may be temporary improvement with later relapse at the onset of the miliary tuberculosis. Sometimes the *onset* is relatively *sudden*. Patients are virtually always febrile, but there is nothing characteristic in the *fever* which may be irregular, regular or swinging. The pulse is usually raised. Except in the late stages the respiration rate is usually only raised in proportion to the pyrexia. Apart from these features there may often be no other abnormal physical signs. In particular it is unusual to find any physical signs in the *chest* until the late stages, when there may be diffuse fine crepitations. The *spleen* was enlarged in about half of the cases reported by Debré [11] and by Lincoln and Hould [17], although our own figures are lower. It is much less often palpable in adults with miliary tuberculosis. The *liver* may also be enlarged. The presence of *choroidal tubercles* is far the most important physical sign, because these are virtually pathognomonic. Illingworth and Lorber [16] reported their presence in 70 of 99 children with radiological evidence of miliary tuberculosis, with or without tuberculous meningitis. Debré [11] found them in 55 out of 58 cases of acute miliary tuberculosis but Miller and his colleagues [20] only in 11 out of 52. They are said to be commoner if tuberculous meningitis is also present. A search of the eye grounds is difficult in an irritable, ill child. If it is important from a diagnostic viewpoint the pupils should be dilated and the child given an anaesthetic as recommended by Illingworth and Lorber. The lesions are usually less than one-quarter of the diameter of the optic disc. Initially they are usually yellowish, a little shiny and give the impression of being slightly raised. Later they become flatter and may be very white in the centre, later still pigmented. There may be only 1 or 2 lesions or they may be very numerous. In a difficult case the eye grounds should be systematically searched 'round the clock'. In our experience choroidal tubercles are much less common in adults than in children. Miliary lesions of the *skin* may be seen very occasionally; macules, papules, vesicles and purpuric lesions have been described [24].

RADIOLOGY

It is important to recognize that the x-ray of the chest may be quite normal in the presence of miliary tuberculosis; the lesions may be too small to be seen. When the possibility of miliary tuberculosis is being considered the areas of the intercostal spaces should be examined very closely (plate 12.1), preferably with a very bright light behind the film, which should be well penetrated ('black'). This is the area where small miliary shadows can first be picked up. A lateral film may also be useful. In our experience it is much commoner in the adult than in the child to find a normal x-ray in the presence of miliary tuberculosis. When abnormal shadows are present they are usually fairly evenly distributed through both lung fields and may vary from faint shadows 1 or 2 mm in diameter to large dense shadows

up to 5 or 10 mm (plates 12.2 & 12.3). Most often all the shadows are of similar size. Evidence of a primary tuberculous complex, 'epituberculosis' or a postprimary lesion may be found. Bilateral pleural effusions may occur.

The clearance of the x-ray lesions under treatment may take a variable time. There is usually comparatively little change in less than a month. In most cases the x-ray clears in 3–4 months but, particularly if there are large lesions, clearance may take a year or more and there may be residual miliary calcification.

DIAGNOSIS

Diagnosis in the classical case with a febrile onset, *miliary shadows* in the x-ray and perhaps with *choroidal tubercles* and an enlarged *spleen*, is not difficult. In a child the history of *contact* with tuberculosis will obviously be valuable. The presence of an enlarged spleen may be suggestive, although of course this can occur in a number of other conditions. The *Mantoux test* should certainly be initiated. It is positive in the majority of cases of miliary tuberculosis, usually to 10 TU but sometimes only to 100 TU. However, it may be negative not only in patients with overwhelming disease but also in patients who are not particularly ill. In a very severe case the decision as to treatment may have to be made before the test can be read. *Gastric lavage* is often justifiable in a difficult case, although the result is only of immediate value if it is positive on direct smear, which is not very frequent.

If there is *fever* together with miliary shadows in the x-ray of the chest the only important differential diagnosis is from *lobular pneumonia* (p. 123). We have seen pneumonia due to haemolytic streptococci, staphylococci and mycoplasma mimicking miliary tuberculosis. The *white blood cell count* may be of some value; it is usually normal, with a leucopenia or with a relative lymphocytosis in miliary tuberculosis, although we have occasionally seen a leucocytosis. If the patient is very ill and serious doubt remains, antituberculosis chemotherapy may be started after sputum or gastric lavage has been sent both for tubercle bacilli and for other organisms and blood has been taken for virological examination. In addition to PAS and isoniazid, streptomycin may be given in two doses a day together with penicillin, in case the condition is pneumonic, perhaps with the addition of tetracycline in case the pneumonia is due to mycoplasma. The tuberculin test should also be initiated and the child's chest x-rayed weekly. A pneumonic lesion will usually start clearing within 1–2 weeks whereas a miliary lesion will take very much longer to subside. Corticosteroids are best avoided unless the patient is desperately ill, as they may confuse the issue by causing precocious clearing of miliary lesions.

Although sarcoidosis may produce miliary-like lesions on the x-ray, patients with pulmonary sarcoidosis are seldom febrile.

There is very much greater difficulty in diagnosing patients, usually adults and often middle aged or elderly, who present *only with fever*, with or without anaemia or other blood dyscrasia. These patients are usually less acutely ill; we have seen patients who have run a fever for many months before miliary shadows were detectable on the x-ray. Such patients will require full investigation for pyrexia of unknown origin but cryptic miliary tuberculosis must always be remembered as a common cause which is often missed [4]. Anaemia or other blood dyscrasia may or may not be present (p. 212). *Liver biopsy* should always be considered and the pathologist persuaded to examine a large number of

sections with great care. *Bone marrow* culture may prove positive but is of little value in the acute stage. *Bone marrow biopsy* [12 & 25] may be a very useful test, especially in individuals with a normal chest x-ray. The aspirated marrow should be sectioned and searched for tubercles and for tubercle bacilli. It should also be cultured.

In a number of cases the diagnosis may be very difficult. X-ray of chest may be normal, the tuberculin test only weakly positive or negative, there may be no abnormal physical signs. Pyrexia, with or without anaemia or leucopenia, may be the only manifestation. Liver and bone marrow biopsy may be unhelpful. Such difficult cases are much more common in adults than in children. If all other investigations for possible cause of the pyrexia are negative, it is important to treat the patient with PAS and isoniazid. Streptomycin should not be given initially as it may affect other causes of pyrexia; PAS and isoniazid are specific for tuberculosis. In most cases, where the underlying condition is miliary tuberculosis, the pyrexia will begin to respond within a few days, either dramatically or gradually (fig. 12.1). In our experience failure of the pyrexia to respond within 2 weeks usually suggests that the condition is not tuberculous. No patient with obscure pyrexia should be allowed to die without testing the effect of anti-tuberculosis chemotherapy.

PROGNOSIS

Before the introduction of chemotherapy virtually all cases of miliary tuberculosis died,

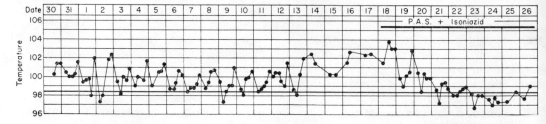

Fɪɢ. 12.1. Temperature chart of man aged 70 presenting with pyrexia and normocytic anaemia but a negative tuberculin test and no overt evidence of miliary tuberculosis. Response of pyrexia and anaemia to treatment with PAS and isoniazid.

although there were very occasional re-coveries. Most died within a few weeks, a small number after a number of months. In some of the more chronic cases there were periods of temporary remission [17]. There remains a risk of death in patients, either children or adults, admitted moribund. In a number of cases the diagnosis is still only made at autopsy. This is more likely in adults in whom a normal x-ray of the chest, in the presence of miliary tuberculosis, appears to be commoner than in children. If effective chemotherapy is given, supported if neces-sary by corticosteroid drugs, recovery should be the rule and later tuberculous complica-tions highly unlikely, apart from tuberculous lymphadenitis in a few cases (see below). Even when some of the cases received chemotherapy inadequate by present standards a high sur-vival rate and low complication rate has been recorded [18].

COMPLICATIONS OF MILIARY TUBERCULOSIS

TUBERCULOUS MENINGITIS

The proportion of children presenting with tuberculous meningitis in addition to miliary tuberculosis varies somewhat with the admis-sion policy for the particular unit but may be as high as 50%. In untreated cases terminal meningitis was formerly common. If menin-gitis is not present initially it virtually never complicates miliary tuberculosis treated with isoniazid.

PLEURAL EFFUSION AND POLYSEROSITIS

Miliary tuberculosis must be seriously con-sidered as a possibility in any patient who pre-sents with fever and bilateral pleural effusion. Disseminated lupus erythematosus is an im-portant alternative diagnosis. In addition to the above diagnostic measures, a pleural biopsy will be relevant as well as the examina-tion of the blood for antinuclear factor and LE cells. Miliary tuberculosis may also present with polyserositis, the pericardium and peri-toneal sacs being affected in addition to the pleural.

8—R.D.

CERVICAL LYMPHADENITIS

Tuberculous involvement of the cervical lymph nodes is sometimes seen at the time of diagnosis of miliary tuberculosis, but these nodes may become enlarged and fluctuant even during the course of treatment. It seems possible that this is a hypersensitive phenom-enon, due to the drainage of large amounts of tuberculoprotein into the lymph nodes. The tuberculoprotein is derived from the bacilli which are being killed in large numbers in the lung and thoracic nodes. Usually it is adequate merely to aspirate the nodes if they become fluctuant and to continue chemo-therapy as before. Corticosteroid drugs may be temporarily justifiable in an attempt to damp down the hypersensitive reaction. In the really difficult case desensitization to tuberculin may be worth while.

HYPOKALAEMIA [8]

Hypokalaemia may complicate miliary tuber-culosis, particularly in the middle aged and the elderly and particularly in women. All ill patients with miliary tuberculosis should have their electrolytes checked. The electrolytes may be normal when treatment starts but hypokalaemia may develop later, usually within the first couple of weeks but occasion-ally after several months. Any deterioration or unexplained weakness should lead to a check on the serum potassium. There is sometimes also a slight or moderate reduction in serum sodium. From the investigation of a number of patients we have concluded that the hypo-kalaemia is not due to any particular drug. The patients have often had a poor diet, owing to illness, for some time before admis-sion. Vomiting and diarrhoea, in most of our patients relatively mild, may have con-tributed to potassium loss. There may also have been some interference with the kidneys' capacity for preserving potassium as we have found appreciable quantities in the urine, in spite of a low serum level. It is particularly difficult to account for hypokalaemia occur-ring in convalescence. The most likely ex-planation may be that the building up of tissues after a severe illness results in a replacement of intracellular potassium at the expense of the extracellular, but this is purely speculative.

If the patient is very ill the potassium is best replaced by intravenous infusion. In our experience the response is better if sodium is given as well as potassium, even if the serum sodium appears normal. Potassium chloride injection (BP: 1·5 g in 10 ml, equal to 20 mEq/l) is diluted with 50 times its volume of 0·9% sodium chloride and given by slow intravenous drip at a rate not exceeding 20 mEq/hour. Up to 80 mEq may be given intravenously and then supplemented orally. In less severe cases potassium and sodium may be administered orally throughout. Potassium is best given as potassium chloride 8–12 g daily in divided doses, preferably as potassium chloride tablets. Sodium may be given as added salt in food or in capsules, 1–2 g 3 times daily.

BLOOD DYSCRASIAS

Patients with miliary tuberculosis who present with various forms of blood dyscrasia are often difficult diagnostic problems. They are usually adults, often middle aged or elderly. They are almost always febrile and the spleen is often, though not always, enlarged. The chest x-ray is usually normal. The diagnosis should always be considered in a febrile patient with an unexplained anaemia, with leukaemia (even if typical), or with other blood dyscrasia. Many, if not most, have been diagnosed only at postmortem. Perhaps half of the reported patients had the nonreactive form of miliary tuberculosis.

The commonest presentation is with *anaemia*, sometimes of *aplastic* type and sometimes with *pancytopenia* or with the emphasis on *leucopenia* or *agranulocytosis* [1, 6, 10, 19, 21 & 22]. Sometimes the reaction is *leukaemoid*, most often myelocytic but sometimes lymphatic or monocytic [15, 21, 22 & 26]. Differential diagnosis from true leukaemia may be difficult, especially as miliary tuberculosis may complicate leukaemia. The alkaline phosphatase of mature neutrophils is said to be normal in leukaemoid reactions in contradistinction to the reduction in true leukaemia, but the test has sometimes been misleading [15]. If there is any doubt it is important to treat the case as possibly tuberculous. A *leucoerythroblastic anaemia* with myelosclerosis has also been described [5, 7, 13 & 21]. *Purpura*, with decreased platelet count or of Henoch-Schönlein type, has fairly frequently been recorded and may be seen either as an isolated phenomenon or as part of a pancytopenia or leukaemoid reaction [3, 9 & 21]. In children purpura is seen more often than the other blood abnormalities. Finally *polycythaemia vera* has been described surprisingly often, usually with tuberculous splenomegaly, [14, 21 & 22] though it is uncertain which condition is primary.

In a number of cases the blood dyscrasia is obviously associated with bone-marrow involvement. In others pancytopenia may be due to hypersplenism, with a normal or hyperplastic marrow. In yet others the reaction may be due to a toxic (hypersensitivity) effect on the marrow.

In our experience, if the patient is successfully diagnosed, the condition usually responds well to *chemotherapy*. Cooper [6] describes a patient with pancytopenia whose blood changes failed to improve with three weeks' chemotherapy, but responded dramatically to subsequent splenectomy. If the diagnosis is certain the temporary addition of corticosteroid drugs to chemotherapy may be justified.

PREVENTION AND TREATMENT

Miliary tuberculosis is virtually unknown in children who have received BCG so that BCG given as early as possible in life is highly desirable in any community where the risk of infection in childhood is high (p. 184). For example in Hong Kong, with a very high prevalence of tuberculosis, miliary tuberculosis and tuberculous meningitis have dramatically decreased since the widespread introduction of BCG in infancy. Chemoprophylaxis for children in whom a positive tuberculin test has demonstrated that infection has occurred is likely to prevent the development of miliary tuberculosis as well as other tuberculous complications (p. 200). The same is true of all cases of primary tuberculosis with radiological evidence of disease. In adults the chemotherapy of known tuberculous lesions will prevent the development of miliary disease, but most cases of miliary tuberculosis in this age group now seen in developed countries have their origin in previously undiagnosed tuberculous lesions.

CHEMOTHERAPY

Chemotherapy should be along the lines already outlined for primary tuberculosis, though streptomycin, as well as PAS and isoniazid, should always be given initially and continued at least until the patient has been apyrexial for a month or so. In any case where there is reason to suspect that the patient may have been infected with resistant organisms appropriate modifications of chemotherapy should be made (p. 245). Our experience has not led us to think that a high dose of isoniazid is necessary, but in a very ill case it may be justifiable to start chemotherapy with a dose of 10 mg/kg/day, although this dose can be reduced to 3 mg/kg/day as soon as the temperature has been normal for a week or two. If the high dose is continued for more than a couple of weeks pyridoxine 10 mg/day should be added.

DURATION OF CHEMOTHERAPY

It is wise to continue chemotherapy for 18 months, at least in severe cases and those with large individual lesions on the x-ray, although at one time we treated a number of children with straightforward miliary tuberculosis for one year only without having had any relapse. Nevertheless in such a life-threatening disease it is better to give too much than too little. If the home conditions are good and one is confident that treatment will be effectively continued the child can be discharged as soon as he is clinically well and off corticosteroid drugs. In developing countries greater risks must often be taken but every effort should be made to supervise the chemotherapy as closely as possible.

CORTICOSTEROID DRUGS

Corticosteroid drugs are mandatory in any patient who is desperately ill, provided the diagnosis is reasonably certain, owing to the risk of death within the first few days. Corticosteroid drugs should 'detoxicate' the patient temporarily and give the chemotherapeutic agents time to take effect. In an adult prednisolone 10 mg 4 times daily may be given for the first few days in such a case, subsequently being lowered to 20 mg/day. We usually continue this dose for 4–6 weeks and then gradually reduce it by 5 mg every 5–7 days. If there is any return of symptoms or pyrexia corticosteroids are continued at the dose which gave control. In milder cases it is usually possible to take the patient off within 2 months but in some more severe cases the corticosteroid drugs have to be continued longer. In patients who are not desperately ill but are still ill enough to be miserable, corticosteroid drugs may be added to chemotherapy for purely humanitarian purposes, as the patient begins to feel better so much more quickly. In this case a dose of prednisolone 5 mg 4 times daily is adequate and the gradual reduction of dose can start in 3 or 4 weeks. In children, a dose of 2 mg/kg/day may be given to those under 2, 1·5 mg to children of 2–10 and 1 mg from 10–15. Corticosteroid therapy should not, of course, be given in a case where chemotherapy is being used as a diagnostic measure and it is best avoided when there is any uncertainty about the diagnosis.

HYPOKALAEMIA

The treatment of this complication has been outlined on p. 211.

BED REST

Bed rest is only necessary as long as the patient is feeling ill. He can be got up and about as soon as he feels sufficiently well. As soon as he is known to be no longer infectious and is feeling well he can return to work or school, but it is of course essential to ensure that chemotherapy is continued in the most conscientious manner.

REFERENCES

[1] BALL K., JOULES H. & PAGEL W. (1951) Acute tuberculous septicaemia with leucopenia. *Br. med. J.* ii, 869.

[2] BATES D.V. & CHRISTIE R.V. (1964) *Respiratory Function in Disease. An Introduction to the Integrated Study of the Lung.* p. 416. Philadelphia, Saunders.

[3] BENSAUDE R. & RIVET L. (1906) Purpura hémorrhagique et tuberculose. *Pr. méd.* 14, 469.

[4] BÖTTIGER L.E., NORDENSTAM H.H. & WESTER P.O. (1962) Disseminated tuberculosis as a cause of fever of obscure origin. *Lancet* i, 19.

[5] CHAPMAN C.B. & WHORTON C.M. (1946) Acute generalized miliary tuberculosis in adults. A clinico-pathological study based on 63 cases diagnosed at autopsy. *New Engl. J. Med.* 235, 239.

[6] COOPER W. (1959) Pancytopenia associated with disseminated tuberculosis. *Ann. int. Med.* 50, 1497.

[7] CRAIL W.H., ALT H.L. & NADLER W.H. (1948) Myelofibrosis associated with tuberculosis. A report of 4 cases. *Blood,* 3, 1426.

[8] CROFTON J., FRENCH E.B. & SANDLER A. (1956) Hypokalaemia in tuberculosis. *Tubercle, Lond.* 37, 81.

[9] DALGLEISH P.G. & ANSELL B.M. (1950) Anaphylactoid purpura in pulmonary tuberculosis. *Br. med. J.* i, 225.

[10] DAWBORN J.K. & COWLING D.C. (1961) Disseminated tuberculosis and bone marrow dyscrasias. *Australas. Ann. Med.* 10, 230

[11] DEBRÉ R. (1952) Miliary tuberculosis in children. *Lancet* ii, 545.

[12] EMERY J.L. & GIBBS N. (1954) Miliary tuberculosis of the bone marrow, with particular reference to the possibility of diagnostic aspiration biopsy. *Br. med. J.* ii, 842.

[13] FOUNTAIN J.R. (1954) Blood changes associated with disseminated tuberculosis. Report of 4 fatal cases with a review. *Br. med. J.* ii, 76.

[14] GUILD A.A. & ROBSON H.N. (1950) Polycythaemia vera with tuberculous splenomegaly. *Edin. med. J.* 57, 145.

[15] HUGHES J.T., JOHNSTONE R.M., SCOTT A.C. & STEWART, P.D. (1959) Leukaemoid reactions in disseminated tuberculosis. *J. clin. Path.* 12, 307.

[16] ILLINGWORTH R.S. & LORBER J. (1956) Tubercles of the choroid. *Arch. Dis. Childh.* 31, 467.

[17] LINCOLN EDITH M. & HOULD F. (1959) Results of specific treatment of miliary tuberculosis in children. A follow-up study of 63 patients treated with antimicrobial agents. *New Engl. J. Med.* 261, 113.

[18] LORBER J. (1966) The long term prognosis of generalized miliary tuberculosis in children. *Lancet* ii, 1447.

[19] MEDD W.E. & HAYHOE F.G.J. (1955) Tuberculous miliary necrosis with pancytopenia. *Quart. J. Med.* 48, (N.S. 24) 351.

[20] MILLER F.J.W., SEAL R.M.E. & TAYLOR MARY D. (1963) *Tuberculosis in Children.* London, Churchill.

[21] O'BRIEN J.R. (1954) Nonreactive tuberculosis. *J. clin. Path.* 7, 216.

[22] OSWALD N.C. (1963) Acute tuberculosis and granulocytic disorders. *Br. med. J.* ii, 1489.

[23] PAGEL W., SIMMONDS F.A.H., MACDONALD N. & NASSAU E. (1964) *Pulmonary Tuberculosis.* London, Oxford University Press.

[24] SAMMAN P.D. (1957) Skin lesions in diseases of the chest. *Br. J. Tuberc.* 51, 32.

[25] SCHLEICHER E.M. (1946) Miliary tuberculosis of the bone marrow. *Am. Rev. Tuberc.* 53, 115.

[26] TWOMEY J.J. & LEAVELL B.S. (1965) Leukaemoid reactions to tuberculosis. *Arch. int. Med.* 116, 21.

CHAPTER 13

Postprimary Pulmonary Tuberculosis

Postprimary pulmonary tuberculosis is by far the most important type of tuberculosis, partly because it is much the most frequent and partly because the resulting positive sputum is the main source of infection and responsible for the persistence of the disease in the community (p. 177).

PATHOGENESIS

Postprimary pulmonary tuberculosis may arise in any one of four ways:

(1) direct progression of a primary lesion,
(2) reactivation of a quiescent primary lesion,
(3) haematogenous spread to the lungs, and
(4) exogenous superinfection.

Progression of the primary lesion is most likely if the primary infection has occurred after puberty (p. 197). This is true particularly of those of European stock, although progressive primary lesions can certainly occur before puberty in Africans and Indians.

Reactivation of the primary lesion can occur at any time in the individual's life (p. 197). The original lesion may not have been visible radiographically and the only evidence that it has occurred may have been a positive tuberculin test. In children of school leaving age it has been found that those with strongly positive tests are at particular risk of later breakdown with pulmonary disease (p. 184). Waning of the individual's defences at any time in his life may result in development of postprimary pulmonary tuberculosis. The factors affecting these defences have been discussed in chapter 10. It is probable that the great majority of middle aged and elderly men who develop postprimary pulmonary tuberculosis do so as a result of a breakdown

of lesions contracted many years previously (p. 197).

Haematogenous spread of disease. When tubercle bacilli reach the lungs by the haematogenous route they do so mainly *via* lymphatic spread from the primary focus (p. 197), the bacilli thus reaching the right heart and being redistributed to the lungs by the pulmonary arteries. Scattered bilateral lesions evenly distributed in the upper zones are often attributed to haematogenous spread (p. 222), although this is difficult to prove. It is possible that bacilli may also be spread to the lungs *via* the bronchial arteries, the primary lesion having eroded a pulmonary vein and the bacilli being distributed by the left heart; naturally other organs besides the lungs are liable to be involved [32].

Exogenous superinfection. It is thought that in the majority of patients the primary lesion results in such considerable enhancement of the patient's defences (p. 184) as to prevent the development of disease if the patient is later infected with further tubercle bacilli. If such infection commonly resulted in disease one would have expected that patients with drug sensitive tubercle bacilli who were nursed in the same wards as those with drug resistant bacilli might sometimes be superinfected with resistant bacilli and that drug resistant lesions might develop in spite of the patient having received immaculate chemotherapy. Occasional cases suggestive of superinfection with resistant bacilli have been reported [40] but, considering the large number of patients at risk when individuals with drug resistant bacilli were common in tuberculosis wards, such an event appears to be extremely rare.

Of course it is not only primary tuberculous lesions which may lie dormant for months or years and then reactivate. A patient's defences may prove capable of dealing with a small, sometimes even with an extensive, post-primary lesion which may then remain dormant until some factor lowers the patient's defences and results in reactivation. Most cases of pulmonary tuberculosis arise either from a progressive primary lesion, in young people, or from reactivation of a dormant primary or postprimary lesion, in the middle-aged or elderly.

PATHOLOGY

The morbid anatomy of pulmonary tuberculosis depends on the complex interrelationship between tubercle bacilli on the one hand and the immunity and hypersensitivity of the host on the other. The manifestations may also be influenced by local conditions in the lung, such as the local concentration of oxygen and carbon dioxide, or the local blood flow. The relevant variables may not only be different topographically within the lung but also may change with time.

To the clinician the morbid anatomy is of particular interest in so far as it is reflected in the chest radiograph and thus influences problems of diagnosis, prognosis and treatment. The clinician must not forget that the basic enemy is the tubercle bacillus and that his objective is to identify that enemy and to destroy him. Interpretations of morbid anatomy are a means to that end and are not ends in themselves. In the same way the complexities of immunity in tuberculosis provide a fascinating intellectual challenge and were of compelling interest at a time when the patient's defences were the main hope for the defeat of the tubercle bacillus, but are of very much less practical interest now that we have means of destroying the bacillus directly. In consequence we propose only to give a brief outline of the morbid anatomy and pathology of tuberculosis. For fuller details the reader is referred to Rich [30], Canetti [5] and Pagel et al. [27]. Some problems of immunity have already been discussed (p. 184). The relevant data are summarized by Raffel [29] and dealt with at length by Rich [30].

HISTOLOGICAL TYPES OF LESIONS

There is considerable variety in the histological types of lesions which may be present in tuberculosis. The predominant histological type may vary from patient to patient and within the same lung. In the development of an individual lesion Canetti [5] recognizes a *pre-exudative phase* in which there is vasodilatation with swelling of the cells lining the alveoli. With appropriate staining methods numerous bacilli may be demonstrated and these are often intracellular. This is frequently succeeded by an *exudative phase* in which vasodilatation, oedema, fibrinous exudate, histiocytes, polymorphonuclear cells and lymphocytes occur in varying proportions. Bacilli in varying quantities are present in the exudative lesion and are particularly numerous if there is an important neutrophil component; in fact polymorphonuclear exudate is more likely, at least in experimental tuberculosis, if there is a large bacillary inoculum or poor host defences. In most cases the exudative lesion proceeds to *caseation*. The inflammatory cellular elements, and often those of the lung tissue also, become more homogeneous, lose their identity and gradually merge into the cheesy substance which gives its name to the process. Fibrinous exudate may be influenced in the same way. The chemistry of this particular form of necrosis is uncertain but caseation is nearly always preceded by an increase in the number of bacilli and it is probably largely a hypersensitivity phenomenon.

Around the edge of the caseation develop the so-called *productive* lesions, consisting initially of monocytes derived from the blood and local histiocytes both of which later evolve into the characteristic cell with a large pale nucleus known as the epithelioid cell. A number of these cells may fuse to form the characteristic Langhan's giant cell with multiple nuclei distributed around its periphery. There is often infiltration with lymphocytes, and sclerosis gradually develops. The epithelioid cells and giant cells may be aggregated into clumps to form the classical tubercles but may be merely distributed around the periphery of the caseous tissue.

Few bacilli are seen in the productive lesions and usually none in the sclerotic tissue.

If the lesion *regresses* the productive and sclerotic elements gradually replace the exudative. *Fibrosis* may increase around the periphery of the lesion and gradually invade it; central fibrosis may also occur. Caseous material may be reabsorbed but often becomes walled-off by fibrous tissue and *calcified*. There may later be actual bone formation. The benign developments in the caseous material are paralleled by a diminution in the number of bacilli. Investigations in the pre-chemotherapy era have shown that, although bacilli may quite often be seen microscopically in such old walled-off caseous material, cultures are often negative.

If on the other hand the lesion proves *progressive* the caseous material *liquefies* and discharges into a bronchus so that a *cavity* forms in the previously necrotic area. The actual mechanism responsible for the softening is uncertain. It is usually preceded by an increase in the number of bacilli. Canetti [5] recognizes two types of softening. In one, cracks appear in the caseous material and it appears to soften merely by the absorption of water without any invasion of cellular elements. In the other, the caseous material is invaded by polymorphonuclear cells. Whatever the mechanism of the softening, its occurrence is of great importance for the future of the disease. Not only does the liquid material from the softened caseum enter the bronchus and spread bacilli *via* the bronchial tree to other parts of the lung or, if coughed up, to other individuals but the cavity it leaves behind is a highly favourable breeding ground for bacilli which, through the connection of the bronchus to the bronchial tree, may continue to colonize other parts of the lung or the lungs of others.

The *wall of the cavity* is usually lined by softened caseous material containing very numerous bacilli, the greatest concentration of the latter being near the surface of the caseum, presumably owing to a better oxygen supply. The thickness of the caseous wall is very variable. Under treatment with chemotherapy the caseous element tends gradually to disappear, leaving, if the cavity remains open, only a thin fibrous rim. Although productive lesions may be found at the periphery of the caseous material they are sometimes scanty. Surrounding these is often a rim of fibrous tissue which may not be complete. Usually around the cavity lie atelectatic areas with alveoli diminished in size and with hypertrophy of the alveolar lining cells.

The cavity may be a mere necrotic hole in a mass of caseous tissue but it is very often influenced by *lesions in the draining bronchus*. Tuberculous inflammation in the bronchial mucous membrane may result in a check-valve mechanism whereby in deep breathing air may get into the cavity but be unable readily to get out. In this way the cavity may become distended and thin-walled. Such a blown up cavity is more likely to be surrounded by atelectatic lung. On the other hand the necrotic process in the bronchial wall may block the lumen completely, resulting in reabsorption of air within the cavity and its closure. Chemotherapy may result in suppression of the inflammatory process in the bronchus, reopening of its lumen and abolition of the check-valve, with consequent relaxation of tension within the cavity and its collapse and closure.

Canetti [5] recognizes three types of *peri-focal lesions* occurring around the exudative or caseous areas:

(1) oedema;
(2) haemorrhage, which may consist of 'haemorrhagic lakes' and be responsible for some cases of haemoptysis; and
(3) 'desquamating pneumonia' in which the alveolar lining cells swell up and are desquamated into the alveoli.

These three types of peri-focal reaction occur independently but all may be present in different parts of the same lung. Bacilli are few and the appearances are attributed to a hypersensitivity reaction to products of the neighbouring lesion.

Besides the peri-focal reactions there may be *secondary lesions* resulting from invasion of bronchi, bronchial arteries, pulmonary arteries or veins by the tuberculous process.

Tuberculous inflammation often spreads along the submucosal lymphatics in the bronchi producing a series of tubercles and there may be ulceration of the mucous membrane. Bacilli may perhaps also invade the bronchial mucous membrane from the surface. Erosion of the bronchial arteries may interfere with the nutrition of the muscle and elastic elements of the bronchial wall and result in *bronchiectasis*, which is common. The whole wall may sometimes be destroyed and only scraps of cartilage or muscle indicate that there was formerly a bronchus in the site. Sometimes the damaged bronchus encloses a mass of caseous material to form the so-called '*bronchial cold abscess*', one of the forms of solid rounded or elongated lesion which can be visible on the radiograph. Invasion of the *pulmonary arteries* may lead to diminution of function. Invasion of the pulmonary veins may have no significant local deleterious effect but may, as previously indicated (p. 215), lead to haematogenous spread.

MACROSCOPIC APPEARANCES

As might be expected from the multiplicity of the histological appearances, the macroscopic appearances of the lung are very variable. When tuberculous lesions are limited the *common sites* are the posterior segment of the upper lobe or the apical segment of the lower lobe. The most likely reason for this predilection is the decreased blood flow but relatively good ventilation of the upper lobes in the upright position. This results in a higher mean alveolar oxygen tension than in the lower lobes [1 & 7], thus favouring the growth of tubercle bacilli.

In severe disease there are usually parts of the lungs where the lesions are confluent, with large caseous areas and cavities. A whole lobe may be affected by *tuberculous pneumonia* with exudation and local caseation. There are often small round tubercles, a few millimetres in diameter, from which the disease derives its name. These may intervene between more massive lesions. In chronic disease there may be gross *fibrosis* with the distortion of septa or pulmonary arteries and deviation of

trachea or mediastinum. Wide areas of *calcification* may be recognized in the centre of the cheesy caseous material. Sometimes a pulmonary vessel may be seen running isolated across a cavity and forming a potential source of dangerous haemorrhage. Areas of *bronchiectasis* may be macroscopically obvious.

Cavities may be mere slits in caseous material, they may be large, sometimes multilocular, and with thick caseous walls, or they may be ballooned out and thin-walled. In a lung resected from a patient who has had prolonged chemotherapy a residual cavity may be lined by shiny fibrous tissue and there may be no histological evidence of tuberculosis even microscopically.

Fibrosis seems to be a process associated with the host's reaction to the infection and appears to be an unimportant part of the healing process under chemotherapy. In a controlled trial of corticosteroids and chemotherapy in pulmonary tuberculosis we reviewed a large series of x-rays taken before the start of treatment and at the end of one year of treatment. We were particularly concerned to detect whether there was less fibrosis in the patients who had received corticosteroid drugs. In fact, to our surprise, we were unable to convince ourselves that there was any fibrosis in either group which had not been present at the start of treatment except where a previous cavity had closed [14].

FUNCTIONAL ABNORMALITY

The functional abnormalities in pulmonary tuberculosis are well summarized by Birath [2] and reviewed by Bromberg and Robin [4]. The main abnormalities are

(1) *restrictive;*
(2) *obstructive*, due to
   (a) emphysema complicating fibrocaseous disease,
   (b) complicating bronchitis or, more rarely,
   (c) stenosis of a larger bronchus;
(3) *loss of lung parenchyma;*

(4) *rise in pulmonary artery pressure*, at first perhaps only on exercise, which is relatively common in patients with severe disease and extensive lung destruction [35 & 41].

Restrictive abnormalities (p. 51) were found particularly after old artificial pneumothoraces complicated by pleural thickening, but also after pleural effusion and fixation of the diaphragm by adhesions. They presumably occur with extensive fibrosis but here emphysema often dominates the picture.

Obstructive abnormalities, with decreased FEV and FEV/FVC ratios, decreased Pa,O_2 and increased Pa,CO_2, may occur with emphysema complicating extensive fibrocaseous disease. Studies in the U.S.A. and in Sweden have suggested that the extent and chronicity of the disease are the most important, though probably not the only, factors [3 & 17]. As might be expected, uneven gas distribution is likely to coexist [21]. In Britain chronic bronchitis, either independent from the tuberculosis or complicating it, may add to the disability. Stenosis of a large bronchus due to tuberculous granulation tissue, fibrosis, or a perforating lymph gland, may occasionally give rise to obstructive abnormality affecting a lobe or a whole lung. [2].

Loss of parenchyma obviously diminishes the respiratory reserve and, with hypoxaemia, leads to *raised pulmonary artery pressure*, at first on exercise and later at rest, and so eventually to *cor pulmonale*. This is a not uncommon mode of death, after an interval of months or years, in patients with extensive disease which has been arrested by chemotherapy. Investigation has shown that any detectable rise in pulmonary artery pressure during the convalescent phase carries a poor prognosis [41]. A rise during the acute phase in a patient with extensive exudative disease, which may respond excellently to chemotherapy, is less ominous if the patient can be successfully carried through the immediate crisis.

Diffusing capacity (transfer factor) may be impaired in acute pulmonary tuberculosis. Williams and his colleagues [42] found a good inverse correlation with the extent of radiological disease, using a single breath carbon monoxide method, though the amount of impairment was usually rather greater than might be expected radiologically. With treatment diffusing capacity improved *pari passu* with the x-ray.

Pulmonary blood flow: Radioisotope scanning of the lungs has shown that blood flow is often decreased to a greater extent than might be estimated from the x-ray, but the decrease tends to be reversed with treatment [20].

$\dot{V}/\dot{Q}$ abnormalities are mainly found in miliary tuberculosis (p. 208) and major shunts of unoxygenated blood only for 24 hours or so after collapse of a lobe; the pulmonary blood flow to the area decreases rapidly [2].

When pulmonary resection was an important component of the treatment of tuberculosis, pulmonary function tests were an essential part of preoperative assessment. Resection is now seldom indicated; nevertheless it could be argued that serial function tests are at least as important as serial radiology in assessing progress, provided the more vital infectious element is monitored by sputum examination. It would certainly be of great interest to determine, by a controlled trial, the value of corticosteroid drugs in minimizing residual functional disability (p. 243). For this purpose pulmonary diffusing capacity would be the best test. More work needs to be done in this field but the risk of infection in the laboratory must be borne in mind.

CLINICAL MANIFESTATIONS

SYMPTOMS

It is important to remember that miniature radiography has now demonstrated that active disease may be present in the lungs when the patient complains of *no symptoms* at all. Nevertheless mild debility may be of such gradual onset that the patient does not notice it and may deny symptoms, although he may later feel so much better after chemotherapy has been initiated that he realizes that previously he was unwell.

There is very little that is specific about the

symptoms of pulmonary tuberculosis. Most could be due to a number of other conditions. One of the points in the history which may make tuberculosis a possibility is the gradual onset of the symptoms over weeks or months. Even if the onset appears to be relatively sudden, questioning will often reveal that the patient has in fact been unwell for weeks or months previously. Of course, tuberculosis is not the only condition in which gradual onset occurs: the middle aged or elderly patient with carcinoma of the bronchus may give a very similar history.

Many patients with tuberculosis present with *general symptoms*, such as *tiredness*, feelings of *malaise*, or *loss of weight*. In more advanced cases the patient may have *febrile symptoms*. *Night sweats* are a classical symptom of tuberculosis, although nowadays in Britain rather uncommon. They also may be due to other conditions causing fever or merely to hot weather and too many blankets! Sometimes a patient will complain mainly of *mental symptoms*, such as irritability and difficulty in concentrating on his work. The doctor may initially consider that the symptoms are neurotic, but if such a neurosis is apparently of recent onset, with no previous history of neurotic symptoms, it is wise to have the chest x-rayed before dismissing an organic origin. Nor, indeed, are neurotics immune from tuberculosis.

Of course the majority of patients with tuberculosis who have any symptoms at all complain, at least on questioning, of symptoms related to the *respiratory system*. *Cough* is the outstanding manifestation. Cough is such a common accompaniment of cigarette smoking that many patients may ignore it, but anyone who has had a cough for more than three weeks, even if he attributes this entirely to cigarette smoking, should have his chest x-rayed. There is nothing specific about the *sputum* in tuberculosis. It may be virtually of any type: mucoid, purulent or blood stained. Frank *haemoptysis* is a classical symptom of pulmonary tuberculosis. It may vary from mere bloodstaining of the sputum, perhaps associated with the lakes of blood described histologically by Canetti [5] (p.

217), to the sudden eruption of half a litre or more of blood, occasionally immediately fatal. The latter of course is usually due to the erosion of an artery, either in a cavity wall or running across its lumen. *Pain in the chest* is a common symptom. Sometimes it is only a dull ache which is first experienced after the patient knows that he has an abnormal x-ray. Sometimes it is pleuritic. In other individuals the pain is primarily due to coughing which may cause 'fibrositis' of the intercostal muscle or even a cough fracture. If there is extensive pulmonary disease the patient may complain of *breathlessness*, but this is usually accompanied by cough, sputum and general symptoms. If there is severe tuberculous bronchitis, particularly local ulceration and narrowing of a major bronchus, the patient may complain of localized *wheeze*. It must be remembered that tuberculosis frequently occurs in heavy-smoking, middle aged or elderly males, who may also have chronic bronchitis. Such patients may have generalized wheeze.

It is not uncommon for a patient who is found to have pulmonary tuberculosis to complain of *recurrent colds* for a number of months before diagnosis. On close questioning these 'recurrent colds' may turn out to consist of exacerbations of cough, but sometimes they appear to consist of genuine coryza. Possibly the tuberculosis has lowered the patient's resistance to the rhinoviruses.

The patient may first come under medical care with an apparent *pneumonia*. Close questioning may or may not reveal that he has been previously unwell. The diagnosis of tuberculosis may only be made because the sputum is sent as a routine for examination for tubercle bacilli or because the fever fails to respond to routine treatment for pneumonia (p. 138). The development of acute tuberculosis following abdominal operations is notorious (p. 221). This will usually originate in a previously cryptic lesion and it is a wise precaution to have a miniature x-ray of all patients who are to undergo 'cold' abdominal surgery.

Loss of appetite is a common symptom which is often associated with *loss of weight*

It is not rare for a patient to be found to have pulmonary tuberculosis during the course of a barium meal examination on account of *dyspepsia*. Sometimes a peptic ulcer may also be found but more often not. It is possible that the dyspepsia is related to the tuberculosis, the general debility having in some way affected the gastro-intestinal tract. Certainly the coincidence is sufficiently frequent to make it advisable to take an x-ray of the chest in any patient who has sufficient dyspepsia to justify a barium meal. Any patient who has had a gastrectomy (p. 220) should have his chest x-rayed at least annually.

Amenorrhoea is relatively common in women with severe tuberculosis but occasionally it is the presenting complaint in a patient with few other symptoms.

In summary, the following are *common modes of presentation*:

(1) symptom-free; tuberculosis discovered at routine miniature radiography,

(2) 'smoker's cough' or other persistent cough which eventually leads to x-ray of the chest,

(3) recurrent colds and feeling run down,

(4) undue tiredness,

(5) unexplained loss of weight,

(6) pneumonia which turns out to be tuberculous,

(7) failure to recover adequately from an attack of 'influenza',

(8) haemoptysis,

(9) dyspepsia,

(10) in patients who have had previous gastrectomy for peptic ulcer.

PHYSICAL SIGNS

The *general condition* in pulmonary tuberculosis may be excellent, even with relatively advanced disease on the x-ray, but there may be pallor, a hectic flush or cachexia in advanced cases.

In Britain most cases are now discovered at an apyrexial stage but in more advanced cases there may be a varying degree of *fever*. Sometimes this consists of a slight evening pyrexia but higher irregular fever or even a swinging temperature, occasionally with peaks in the morning instead of the evening, may occur.

Pulse is usually raised in proportion to the pyrexia and *respiration* may be rapid in advanced cases.

Finger clubbing to an important degree is unusual except in chronic disease with purulent sputum. The presence of marked clubbing with a short history suggests another diagnosis, in particular carcinoma of the bronchus. Mild early clubbing is not uncommon with severe disease of short duration.

In the *chest* there are often no physical signs whatever, sometimes even in the presence of quite extensive radiological changes. The most common early abnormality consists of post-tussive crepitations in the upper zones or apices. When the disease is very advanced or pneumonic there may be physical signs of consolidation. In chronic disease deviation of the trachea or mediastinum may occur due to fibrosis. The classical physical signs of cavity (p. 70) are seldom found, even when a large cavity is detected on the x-ray, presumably because there is usually intervening aerated lung between the cavity and the stethoscope. Occasionally severe tuberculous bronchitis leads to stenosis of a large bronchus with resultant localized rhonchi. As tuberculosis is commoner in the upper zones of the lungs abnormal physical signs are also more likely in the upper zones.

In general, examination of the chest contributes relatively little to the diagnosis or assessment of pulmonary tuberculosis. Sputum examination and chest radiography are much more important. However, it is essential to conduct a general examination of the patient as there may be additional tuberculous lesions outside the chest.

RADIOLOGY

In an economically developed country in which radiological facilities are readily available any of the symptoms or physical signs already mentioned should be an indication to x-ray the chest. In economically developing countries this will often not be possible; sputum testing will have to be substituted, although this may fail to detect early cases. As already indicated, examination of the chest is relatively uninformative in pulmonary tuberculosis. Together with examination of the sputum, radiology is the major diagnostic weapon and a useful way of checking progress.

A *normal chest x-ray* almost, although not completely, excludes pulmonary tuberculosis. There are two provisos. In the first place it has been shown in a number of investigations that small radiological lesions are readily missed [6, 11, 39 & 43]. *Observer error* may be reduced by double reading by two independent observers or even by the same observer on two separate occasions. Secondly, it is possible very occasionally for a patient to have *localized tuberculous bronchitis* with a positive sputum and a normal x-ray. We have seen several such cases, one of whom had a repeatedly positive sputum, a localized wheeze and apparently normal bronchi within the limits of bronchoscopic visibility.

APPEARANCES SUGGESTIVE OF TUBERCULOSIS

It is seldom possible to make a completely confident diagnosis of pulmonary tuberculosis on radiological grounds alone, as almost all the manifestations of tuberculosis can be mimicked by other diseases. The following characteristics of a chest radiograph favour the diagnosis of tuberculosis:

(1) shadows mainly in the *upper zone*,

(2) *patchy* or *nodular* shadows,

(3) the presence of a *cavity* or cavities, although these of course can also occur in lung abscess, carcinoma, etc.,

(4) the presence of *calcification*, although a carcinoma or pneumonia may occur in an area of the lung where there is calcification due to tuberculosis,

(5) *bilateral shadows*, especially if these are in the upper zones,

(6) the *persistence* of the abnormal shadows without alteration in an x-ray repeated after several weeks; this helps to exclude a diagnosis of pneumonia or other acute infection.

CHARACTERISTIC RADIOLOGICAL APPEARANCES

Sketches of various characteristic x-ray appearances in tuberculosis are shown in figs. 13.1–13.11. These are by no means complete; there is a virtually endless spectrum of possible combinations. For instance, it is

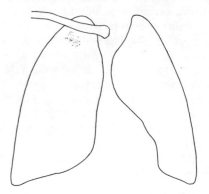

FIG. 13.1. Slight soft shadowing below clavicle. This could be pneumonic.

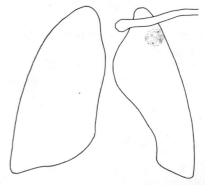

FIG. 13.2. Localized soft patchy shadows below clavicle. This could also be pneumonic.

common for chronic fibrotic tuberculosis to be complicated by acute spread of the disease. *Pathological interpretation* of the x-ray appearances has some value, although it is not always easy. At one time, when resection formed a common part of treatment of pulmonary tuberculosis, the authors and their colleagues made a practice of writing down in histological detail the probable morbid anatomy of a segment, lobe or lung about to be resected. Assessment was made by

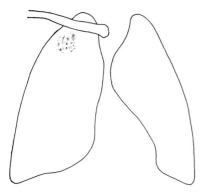

Fig. 13.3. Localized denser more nodular shadows. If dense white shadows indicate calcification, this is very suggestive of tuberculosis.

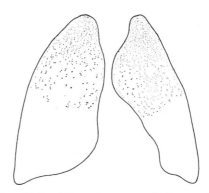

Fig. 13.6. Bilateral symmetrical mottled shadows, decreasing in size towards the mid zone. In successive x-rays over months may gradually extend towards the base. Probably of haematogenous origin.

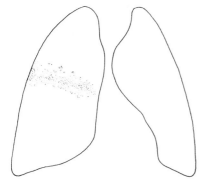

Fig. 13.4. Indefinite segmental shadow, perhaps with one or two satellite shadows. This could be pneumonic.

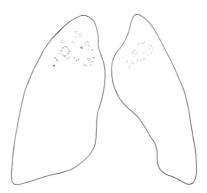

Fig. 13.7. Cavitated soft scattered shadows right upper zone with a little soft shadowing on left.

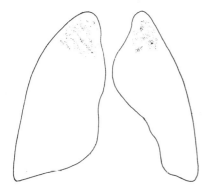

Fig. 13.5. Soft asymmetrical shadows both upper zones, with some linear shadows suggesting fibrosis.

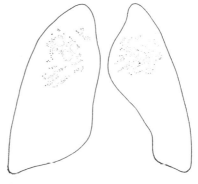

Fig. 13.8. Extensive bilateral acute exudative disease, largely confluent, with thin walled cavities.

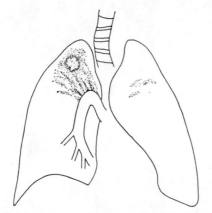

FIG. 13.9. Cavitated chronic fibrotic disease, mainly of right lung. Note elevation of right pulmonary artery and diaphragm, and deviation of trachea, by fibrosis.

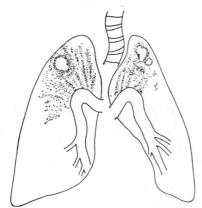

FIG. 13.10. Bilateral chronic cavitated fibrotic disease.

clinicians who had not been in charge of the patient. The first assessment was made on the film immediately before operation and then a second assessment when all the patient's films were available and also the details of his chemotherapy. It was found that there were frequent errors when only the preoperative film was available but that, with the complete chemotherapeutic history and complete series of x-rays, assessment of the possible pathology underlying the radiological shadows proved surprisingly accurate. *Soft confluent shadows* suggest an exudative process. If this is the only type of lesion ·present it is difficult to

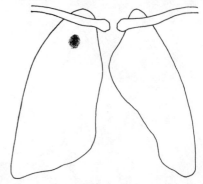

FIG. 13.11. 'Tuberculoma.' Rounded homogeneous shadow which could be a malignant or benign neoplasm. Calcification or satellite lesions may suggest tuberculosis.

distinguish it radiologically from a simple pneumonia unless serial x-rays are taken. *Linear shadows*, especially if they produce distortion of fissures, trachea, mediastinum or diaphragm, suggest fibrosis. *Caseation* cannot be directly diagnosed on the x-ray but caseation and productive lesions are almost always present in larger solid-looking areas. *Calcification* can be identified, if it is big enough, by the very dense white shadows; calcification is laid down in caseum for which it provides indirect evidence. Distended thin-walled *cavities* have their origin in a valvular process in the draining bronchus (p. 217). Excavations in a mass of caseous material may initially have irregular walls. These later become smoother, and, during chemotherapy, gradually thinner as caseous material is coughed up or absorbed. Such cavities may eventually come to resemble thin-walled bullae. A cavity may become 'blocked'. The draining bronchus may be obstructed and instead of the cavity collapsing it may become filled with purulent or caseous material, the so-called '*blocked cavity*'. This may sometimes be accompanied by increase in temperature and general symptoms. In the pre-chemotherapy era it was a perpetual threat to the patient in so far is it might reopen at any time and lead to spread of disease. With effective chemotherapy the lesion usually stabilizes in the same way as any other collection of caseous material [31].

Elongated translucent areas in the upper zones, seen particularly on tomography, may suggest *bronchiectasis*. This can be confirmed with bronchograms but there is usually little point in this; it does not affect treatment. Sometimes the bronchus becomes blocked and filled with caseous material and will form a '*bronchial cold abscess*' which may show as a solid looking elongated dense shadow, sometimes scalloped.

One of the purposes of *tomography* in pulmonary tuberculosis is to demonstrate the presence of cavities. At one time the presence of a cavity was very crucial to the prognosis. If the cavity remained unclosed the patient's prognosis was poor, the sputum usually continued to be positive and he was perpetually threatened with fresh spread of disease. It is still useful to know whether a cavity is present, even though the disease can be arrested in the presence of unclosed cavities. The persistence of an open cavity indicates a potentially large population of tubercle bacilli and chemotherapy should be correspondingly prolonged in order to ensure against relapse (p. 239).

If the diagnosis is doubtful tomography may reveal calcification which is not detected on the straight x-ray and so help to establish the diagnosis. In a 'tuberculoma' tomograms may reveal satellite lesions which make it more probable that the solid rounded shadow is in fact tuberculous.

CLASSIFICATION OF EXTENT OF THE DISEASE

For clinical and research purposes the classification of the National Tuberculosis Association of the U.S.A. [25] has proved useful. It is as follows:

'*Minimal*. Minimal lesions include those which are of slight to moderate density but which do not contain demonstrable cavitation. They may involve a small part of one or both lungs, but the total extent, regardless of distribution, should not exceed the volume of lung on one side which is present above the second chondrosternal junction and the spine of the fourth or the body of the fifth thoracic vertebra.'

'*Moderately advanced*. Moderately advanced lesions may be present in one or both lungs, but the total extent should not exceed the following limits: disseminated lesions of slight to moderate density which may extend throughout the total volume of one lung, or the equivalent in both lungs: dense and confluent lesions which are limited in extent to one third the volume of one lung; total diameter of cavitation, if present, must be less than 4 cm.'

'*Far advanced*. Lesions more extensive than moderately advanced.'

LABORATORY INVESTIGATIONS

SPUTUM EXAMINATION

Sputum examination is of great value in making the diagnosis of pulmonary tuberculosis and in following the patient's progress under treatment. Sputum should first be examined by direct smear. The fluorescence method allows large numbers of specimens to be examined rapidly [13]. Quantitative grading is of value in following progress, especially in research [8 & 23]. The results of these examinations are available more or less at once and are therefore very useful in diagnosis. Smear examination is often positive in more advanced disease but may be negative in less advanced. Sputum culture results usually only become available in 4–8 weeks. Guinea pig inoculation of the sputum is probably more sensitive than a single culture but multiple cultures in an individual case will be as effective as a single guinea pig inoculation. In any patient in whom the diagnosis is in doubt repeated smear and culture examinations should be carried out.

Sputum is sometimes negative, even when there are well-marked radiological shadows and perhaps symptoms. Direct smear examination is occasionally negative even in a patient with far advanced disease. Rarely even repeated cultures in such a patient may prove negative. Conversely it must be remembered that an unexpected positive culture or smear examination, in a patient whose clinical characteristics do not otherwise suggest tuberculosis, may be due to a laboratory error (such as contamination or a mistake about a name); alternatively an acute infectious process, or even neoplasm, in the lung may have eroded an old tuberculous focus. A single unexpected positive in an inappropriate clinical situation should not be given great weight unless repeated. Sputum examination, like all other examinations, must be considered in the total clinical context.

GASTRIC ASPIRATION [9]

The aspiration of the resting early morning juice is a useful way of finding tubercle bacilli in a patient who does not have sputum. The secretions from the lung, if not abundant, are often swallowed. Although at one time it was suggested that direct smear examinations of gastric juice were liable to be misleading, as nontuberculous acidfast bacilli often occurred in the food, investigation has shown that such an error is rare and that acidfast bacilli found in the resting juice are usually tubercle bacilli. The juice should also be cultured.

LARYNGEAL SWABS [9]

Laryngeal swabs are an alternative to aspirating gastric juice and are on the whole simpler to perform and less uncomfortable for the patient. The operator should be gowned and masked and the swabs taken in pairs. The first swab usually makes the patient cough and the second often collects the better specimen.

BRONCHIAL LAVAGE

Bronchial lavage probably gives more positive results than laryngeal swabs or gastric aspiration [19 & 28] but is not recommended owing to its danger to the operator. Aspiration at bronchoscopy, carried out for diagnosis, is sometimes indicated.

WHITE BLOOD CELL COUNT

The total count is usually normal or below normal. Increase of monocytes, decrease of lymphocytes or an increased proportion of immature neutrophils were at one time thought to be of value in assessing activity of the lesion or the prognosis but the findings are irregular and mainly unhelpful [24].

Rarely there may be a leucocytosis. In general a normal total white blood count in the presence of extensive pulmonary shadowing on the x-ray favours a diagnosis of tuberculosis rather than acute pneumonia or lung abscess. Nevertheless exceptions are not infrequent.

ERYTHROCYTE SEDIMENTATION RATE (ESR)

The ESR is a timehonoured investigation as an index of activity in tuberculosis. It has no diagnostic value, since it may be elevated in many infectious or neoplastic processes, and in practice is not a very useful index of activity. Active lesions may often be associated with a normal ESR. In one long term follow-up study of doubtfully active lesions extension of the x-ray shadowing or the presence of a positive sputum indicated definite activity in a number of patients. The ESR was measured as a routine but in not a single case did an elevation give warning that anything was going wrong [34]. We have consequently ceased to use it as a routine.

ANAEMIA

Moderate anaemia is not uncommon in severe pulmonary tuberculosis. Severe anaemia is rare unless there is amyloidosis, miliary spread, accompanying gastrointestinal tuberculosis or recurrent haemorrhage. Anaemia is often normocytic and improves as the disease improves. In women the anaemia may be of the iron-deficient type. This may also sometimes occur in men: accompanying peptic ulcer may be detected but sometimes there is no obvious source of blood loss. Macrocytic anaemia is said to occur very occasionally in association with very severe disease or severe blood loss [24]. The more bizarre blood dyscrasias are more often seen in miliary tuberculosis (p. 212) but may occasionally accompany severe pulmonary disease; in such a case it is difficult to be sure that there has not been a cryptic miliary spread.

LIVER FUNCTION TESTS

It is not uncommon to find liver function tests impaired in moderate or advanced pulmonary tuberculosis, usually improving as the patient progresses under chemotherapy. The cause is presumably toxicity, though of course hepatic lesions may be present. Certain chemotherapeutic agents may damage the liver so that it is important to ensure, before blaming a drug for liver damage, that liver function was not abnormal before the drug was started.

ASSESSMENT OF ACTIVITY IN PULMONARY TUBERCULOSIS

Abnormal shadows due to pulmonary tuberculosis are very common, especially in older people in economically developed countries and at all ages in developing countries. Individual clinicians often differ in deciding whether a particular lesion should be regarded as unimportant, requiring no further follow-up; of potential importance requiring follow-up to assess activity and the necessity for treatment; or requiring treatment forthwith. The facilities available will, of course, influence the physician's priorities. The following may give some guidance:

(1) A positive sputum, especially if repeated, certainly indicates activity and the necessity for treatment.

(2) The presence of symptoms, such as cough, tiredness or loss of weight, is suggestive that a radiological lesion is active.

(3) The detection of crepitations on auscultation, if persistent, is in favour of activity.

(4) There are certain radiological appearances which are suggestive: The existence of a cavity always indicates activity unless there has been effective previous treatment. Soft shadows, even if very small, are also suggestive. If shadows are extensive activity is very probable. Finally, any extension of shadows in serial x-rays suggests activity, unless it is due to intercurrent infection in which case it will rapidly clear.

(5) A raised erythrocyte sedimentation rate (ESR) may indicate activity but seldom proves a reliable guide.

Unless the lesion is purely calcified, experience has shown that there is a risk of breakdown in most lesions which are radiologically visible, although the risk varies with age and the type of lesions. The more extensive the lesion, the younger the patient, and the softer the shadow, the more likely is relapse with overtly active tuberculosis.

In a $3\frac{1}{2}$–4 year follow-up of the Danish Mass Campaign it was found that the annual breakdown rate with overt active tuberculosis was 2033 per 100,000 in those with definite and probably tuberculous lesions, compared to 110 in those with purely calcified lesions, 510 in those with fibrosis with or without calcification, 530 for those with 'questionable' shadows, 412 where the lesion was thought probably nontuberculous, 100 in those with 'pleural scars' and 50 in those with a positive tuberculin test but a normal chest film [12]. In each category the risk of breakdown diminished with age, much the highest risk being in the 15–24 age group, and the lowest over 45. Springett [37] showed that the risk increased with the size of the lesion. He confirmed the greater risk of breakdown in young people, especially women. A study by the Scottish Thoracic Society [34] also confirmed a higher breakdown rate in the young, those with larger lesions and in those with lesions showing no evidence of fibrosis.

The *tuberculin test* may be helpful. A strongly positive test is quite compatible with an inactive lesion but a negative or weakly positive one is not very likely in the presence of activity. Positivity may be depressed in very extensive disease and in the old. The complexities of the tuberculin reaction in tuberculosis are reviewed by O'Grady [26].

DIAGNOSIS

Tuberculosis is the great imitator and enters into the differential diagnosis of almost all chest diseases and of many diseases producing general symptoms of debility or fever. In countries in which tuberculosis is greatly diminished the possibility of the disease is sometimes too readily forgotten. Conversely, in countries where the disease is very common, respiratory abnormalities, particularly radiological, may be too readily assumed to be tuberculous. Investigations to exclude tuberculosis form part of the routine of diagnosis in most chest conditions, the intensity of the *diagnostic procedures* depending on the degree of suspicion. The following need to be considered:

(1) *Sputum examination* (p. 76)

Subject to the provisos already outlined (p. 225), the detection of tubercle bacilli on smear or culture usually indicates that the condition is tuberculous. Occasionally the acidfast bacilli prove to be 'anonymous' mycobacteria, the probability of this varying with the geographical area (p. 259). Direct smear examination is only positive when large numbers of bacilli are being excreted, so that a negative smear by no means excludes tuberculosis. A negative smear in the presence of extensive disease and cavitation makes the diagnosis less likely, particularly if the negatives are frequently repeated. Culture is usually positive in advanced disease although occasionally only after many attempts; it is frequently negative in early disease with limited radiological shadows. If there is no sputum but a reasonable suspicion of tuberculosis *gastric aspirations* or *laryngeal swabs* should be examined.

(2) *Tuberculin testing*

For clinical purposes the Mantoux test with 10 TU (0·1 ml of 1/1000 OT) is the most convenient for patients in hospital as it is read in 48–72 hours. For outpatients attending once weekly the Heaf multipuncture test is often convenient. Most patients of European origin with active tuberculosis react with an induration of 10 mm or more to 10 TU on the Mantoux test, though very ill patients or the elderly are sometimes only positive to 100 TU. If other factors support the diagnosis of tuberculosis a negative result with 10 TU would not be major contrary evidence. A test negative to 100 TU makes tuberculosis very unlikely, though there are very occasional individuals who appear to be anergic and fail to react to tuberculin in spite of proved active disease [15, 22 & 33]. It must be remembered that patients with miliary tuberculosis (p. 209)

and those desperately ill with tuberculosis or other diseases may have a negative test. Technical errors must not be forgotten. If tuberculosis seems a likely diagnosis and the tuberculin test is reported as negative, the test should be repeated.

The Heaf multipuncture test has rather less precision, but is convenient for outpatient use. Most patients with active disease have a Grade III test. Grade I or II positivity makes active tuberculosis less likely, with reservations similar to those regarding the Mantoux test.

(3) *White blood count*

This is only of value, for diagnostic purposes, if the patient is febrile and has cavitation or extensive shadowing on the chest x-ray. Leucocytosis makes bacterial pneumonia or lung abscess more likely than tuberculosis. In practice the white blood count is only useful in a minority of cases. When the patient is less ill and the radiological shadowing less extensive the count is often normal or high normal, even when due to nontuberculous bacterial infection.

Besides these routine investigations the *history* is sometimes of value. In tuberculosis the symptoms of malaise or cough are usually of *gradual onset* over weeks or months, whereas in acute infections the onset is over a matter of days. In the relevant age group a patient with carcinoma of the bronchus may, of course, have a very similar history to a patient with tuberculosis. A history of *contact* with tuberculosis may be of value, particularly in children or young people.

DIFFERENTIAL DIAGNOSIS

The most important conditions from which tuberculosis has to be distinguished are pneumonia, carcinoma of the bronchus, lung abscess and pulmonary infarct. In the differential diagnosis from *pneumonia* the problem is different in those with mild pneumonia, usually seen in an outpatient clinic in convalescence, and in those with more severe pneumonia admitted to hospital. As already pointed out, soft upper zone shadows on the radiograph may be due either to pneumonia or to tuberculosis. The patient with *mild segmental pneumonia* often gives a recent history of an upper respiratory tract infection or some relatively brief febrile episode. The patient with tuberculosis may have had no symptoms at all and have been picked up on routine radiography, or he may have had symptoms for a matter of months. A history of contact may be of value in young people. Routine investigation should include a tuberculin test and sputum examination for tubercle bacilli; examination of sputum for nontuberculous bacteria is usually of little value at this stage of the disease. The patient should be re-x-rayed in two to three weeks. If he has important symptoms he may be treated with tetracycline or oral penicillin in the meantime. After two to three weeks pneumonic shadows will have improved or cleared; shadows due to tuberculosis will be unchanged.

An apparent *acute bacterial pneumonia* admitted to hospital may sometimes prove to be tuberculous in origin. Every patient with pneumonia should have sputum examined for tubercle bacilli. If the pneumonia fails to respond to routine treatment (p. 138) and the aetiological diagnosis remains uncertain after several days, and especially if the white blood count is normal, further sputa should be sent for examination.

Differential diagnosis from *carcinoma of the bronchus* arises in the appropriate age group particularly if there is evidence of collapse. An isolated solid-looking shadow or an isolated cavitated shadow may also be carcinomatous. With a *lobar*, or *segmental*, lesion the hilar shadow should be carefully examined. Any enlargement should suggest the possibility of a carcinoma; if the sputum is negative on direct smear bronchoscopy should be carried out. If the appearances are particularly suspicious of carcinoma bronchoscopy should be done even if the sputum is positive; it is not uncommon for tuberculosis and carcinoma of the bronchus to coincide.

When there is an *isolated solid-looking* shadow, the presence of satellite lesions or of calcification, perhaps only detectable on tomography, is suggestive of tuberculosis. The sputum should be examined for tubercle

bacilli and malignant cells but may often be negative for both. The tuberculin test may be helpful. Bronchoscopy is usually unhelpful. It is often impossible to make a certain diagnosis and thoracotomy may have to be undertaken if the patient's respiratory function tests are good enough. Such a thoracotomy should be carried out under cover of antituberculosis chemotherapy. Frozen sections may be helpful at operation in order to decide the extent of the resection.

An *isolated cavity* may give rise to similar difficulties. Irregularity of the internal wall, and especially a polypoid protuberance into the interior, perhaps detectable only on tomography, is suggestive of carcinoma. Sputum examination for tubercle bacilli or for carcinoma cells may be helpful. Satellite lesions or calcification favour tuberculosis. If certain diagnosis cannot be achieved thoracotomy may be necessary. Cavitation may also of course occur as a lung abscess distal to a carcinoma of the bronchus which interferes with drainage. Here there will be some evidence of collapse or solidification of the lung and bronchoscopy is likely to be helpful. Although theoretically a cavitated carcinoma might produce shadows in the other lung, due to aspiration of infected material, in practice this seems to occur very seldom and bilateral shadows, unless they are solid-looking rounded lesions suggestive of metastases, are more often due to tuberculosis.

A patient with *lung abscess* is usually, but not always, iller than a patient with tuberculosis with lesions of similar radiological extent. If the cavity is due to tuberculosis it is likely that the sputum will be positive on direct smear, though this is by no means always the case. The history in lung abscess is often shorter and there is likely to be leucocytosis if the patient has a high fever. Multiple bilateral cavities may occur with blood-borne infection, for instance by staphylococci, but if there are such multiple cavities and severe illness the sputum is usually positive on direct smear should the condition be tuberculous. Inadequately treated pulmonary infection with *Klebsiella pneumoniae* may closely resemble chronic pulmonary tuberculosis

(p. 122). *Klebsiella* is usually readily cultured from the sputum. If a patient is significantly febrile he is likely to have a leucocytosis. Chronic pulmonary *actinomycosis* may also closely resemble chronic tuberculosis. Anaerobic culture is necessary to identify the organisms. There may be leucocytosis. The sputum of course will be negative for tubercle bacilli. The presence of periostitis of the ribs is strongly suggestive of actinomycosis (p. 290).

Upper zone *pulmonary infarcts*, especially if bilateral, may occasionally cause diagnostic difficulty. Routine investigations, the possible presence of a demonstrable origin of a pulmonary embolus and serial x-rays, which show relatively rapid change in the case of pulmonary infarcts, usually readily distinguish the two conditions.

A word should be added about the problem of *pneumoconiosis* complicated by tuberculosis. In general it is not possible to detect the complication of pneumoconiosis by tuberculosis on radiological grounds alone. When, because of symptoms or of deterioration in general condition, the possibility of tuberculosis has to be considered, intensive examination of the sputum is the most important step, although the tuberculin test may also be helpful.

Tuberculosis enters into the differential diagnosis of *many other pulmonary diseases*. The examination of the sputum for tubercle bacilli and tuberculin testing should in consequence be part of the routine investigation of every abnormal radiographic shadow.

In economically developing countries the relatively sophisticated diagnostic measures outlined will not usually be practicable. Sputum examination on direct smear is by far the most important investigation and this can often be supplemented by tuberculin testing. Radiology is often economically impossible. If an x-ray has been carried out and has shown a shadow the clinician must be cautious of assuming that this is tuberculous, as a diagnosis of tuberculosis implies prolonged treatment which should not be administered unnecessarily. If it has been possible to carry out one x-ray then it is usually possible to carry out a second one after 2–3 weeks. In most cases this will suffice to exclude a pneumonic process, which is the condition most likely to be confused with tuberculosis.

COMPLICATIONS

DRY PLEURISY

This is a relatively frequent complication of pulmonary tuberculosis. Pleuritic pain, as already mentioned, may be the presenting symptom and a rub may be heard.

PLEURAL EFFUSION

Pleural effusion is a not uncommon accompaniment, particularly of acute pulmonary tuberculosis. There is often fever, with or without dyspnoea, but a small or moderate pleural effusion may be present without any major general upset. The characteristics of the fluid are described elsewhere (p. 280).

TUBERCULOUS EMPYEMA

Formerly tuberculous empyema was most commonly found as a complication of artificial pneumothorax. With the abandonment of pneumothorax treatment empyema is comparatively rare. A pleural effusion complicating severe extensive exudative lesions sometimes becomes purulent to form an empyema. The conditioning factor is probably the number of tubercle bacilli in the effusion, polymorphonuclear exudate in tuberculosis usually signifying a reaction to a high concentration of organisms. A life-threatening emergency is the rupture of a tuberculous cavity into the pleura, resulting in tuberculous *pyopneumothorax*. This is usually a complication of acute cavitated exudative disease. The patient is very ill, febrile and dyspnoeic. The main differential diagnosis is from a ruptured staphylococcal abscess, but the latter is much commoner in children while the former is seen mainly in adults. Tubercle bacilli are usually found on direct smear in sputum or pleural pus. Occasionally the patient first presents when tuberculous empyema has become *localized* and *encysted*. Tubercle bacilli may be seen in sputum or pus, or the diagnosis may be established by pleural biopsy or by characteristic x-ray appearances of tuberculous lung infiltration.

TUBERCULOUS LARYNGITIS

This is occasionally seen in patients with a positive sputum and relatively severe disease. The initial symptom is hoarseness. Later there may be pain on swallowing which, when treatment was ineffective, often made the patient's last days an agonizing experience. Fortunately the disease responds rapidly to chemotherapy. Failure to do so, in the presence of sensitive organisms or improving lung disease, should lead to revision of the diagnosis; we have seen coexisting carcinoma of the larynx.

TUBERCULOSIS OF OTHER ORGANS

It must always be remembered that tuberculosis may not be confined to the lung. In the male the testes should be examined as a routine. Routine examination of the urine for tubercle bacilli is also advisable.

CHRONIC BRONCHITIS

Chronic bronchitis is a very common disease, especially in Britain, in males of the age which also shows the highest attack rate of pulmonary tuberculosis. It is not surprising therefore that the two diseases frequently coexist, especially as both may be related to smoking. The possibility that chronic bronchitis or asthma may predispose to tuberculosis has been considered [3 & 16] but we know of no convincing evidence for this. It has already been mentioned (p. 219) that diffuse airways obstruction is most frequently found in older patients with chronic diffuse pulmonary tuberculosis. In such patients there is often recurrent secondary infection and the clinical manifestations, apart from the radiological residua of the tuberculosis, are virtually identical with those of chronic bronchitis. In Sweden, where chronic bronchitis in pure form is relatively uncommon, Birath et al. [3] found that, unlike chronic bronchitis, airways obstruction in tuberculosis was as common in women as in men and that there was no relation to smoking habits, at least at the time of diagnosis.

COR PULMONALE

Cor pulmonale may complicate very severe acute or extensive chronic fibrocaseous tuberculosis, usually in the middle aged or elderly. In both types of disease heart failure is presumably due to loss of pulmonary vasculature and to the vasoconstrictive effect of hypoxia. In our experience *cor pulmonale* complicating acute disease can usually be reversed by intensive treatment if the patient can be carried through the immediate crisis. When heart failure complicates extensive fibrocaseous tuberculosis, especially late in treatment or after cessation of chemotherapy, the pathological changes are usually irreversible and the outlook proportionately graver. It has been found that any detectable rise in pulmonary artery pressure in the convalescent phase carries a poor prognosis [41]. With the success of chemotherapy an important proportion of the residual deaths from tuberculosis are due to *cor pulmonale* in patients with arrested disease. Early diagnosis of tuberculosis avoids this risk.

AMYLOIDOSIS

Formerly amyloidosis was a not uncommon complication of chronic pulmonary tuberculosis, usually in patients who had prolonged production of purulent sputum or chronic tuberculous empyema. With the introduction of chemotherapy it has become rare. The disease may manifest itself by enlargement of liver and spleen but there is usually profuse proteinuria, often with the full nephrotic syndrome leading ultimately to renal failure. Diagnosis may be made by the Congo red test but biopsy is more satisfactory. Rectal mucosal biopsy is quite frequently positive and is relatively simple to carry out. Liver or gum biopsies may also be positive but renal biopsy is almost always positive. Unless the kidney has been severely damaged the amyloidosis is often reversible if the tuberculous lesion is effectively treated. If there is tuberculous empyema it has usually been a chronic one and will require to be excised if the amyloid process is to be reversed. We have seen two cases of amyloidosis associated with an empyema concealed beneath an old thoraco-plasty.

ASPERGILLOSIS

Infection of healed open tuberculous cavities by *Aspergillus fumigatus* is now well recognized. The condition is discussed on p. 287.

CARCINOMA OF THE BRONCHUS

Carcinoma of the bronchus and pulmonary tuberculosis are both comparatively common in middle aged and elderly males. It is therefore not surprising that both diseases may occur in the same individual, either coincidentally or because carcinoma has opened up an old tuberculous focus and perhaps at the same time lowered the host resistance. The fact that both diseases are related to cigarette smoking is an additional linking factor. It has also been suggested that many cases of carcinoma of the bronchus originate in scars, which may be due to old tuberculosis [36]. Many more tuberculous patients are now, of course, living into the cancer age. Isoniazid has been shown to act as a carcinogen in certain particularly susceptible strains of mice [18] but there is no evidence at present that this is a significant factor in man. The other linking factors mentioned may well be sufficient to account for the known association which has been witnessed by several series [10 & 38].

HYPOKALAEMIA

Though commoner in miliary tuberculosis (p. 211), hypokalaemia may also complicate widespread acute pulmonary tuberculosis in the middle aged or elderly.

ANAEMIA

Anaemia in tuberculosis has been dealt with on p. 226.

REFERENCES

[1] BATES D.V. & CHRISTIE R.V. (1964) *Respiratory Function in Disease*, p. 98. Philadelphia, Saunders.

[2] BIRATH G. (1959) Forms of chronic cardio-pulmonary insufficiency in pulmonary tuber-culosis and their diagnosis. *Acta tuberc. scand. Suppl.* **47**, 32.

[3] BIRATH G., CARO J., MALMBERG R. & SIMONS-SON B.G. (1966) Airways obstruction in pulmonary tuberculosis. *Scand. J. resp. Dis.* **47**, 27.

[4] BROMBERG P.A. & ROBIN E.D. (1963) Abnormalities of lung function in tuberculosis. *Advances Tuberc. Res.* **12**, 1.

[5] CANETTI G. (1955) *The Tubercle Bacillus in the Pulmonary Lesion of Man.* New York, Springer Publishing Co.

[6] COCHRANE A.L. & GARLAND L.H. (1952) Observer error in the interpretation of chest films. An international investigation. *Lancet* **ii**, 505.

[7] CORPER H.J., LURIE M.B. & UYEI N. (1927) The variability of localization of tuberculosis in organs of different animals: III. The importance of the growth of tubercle bacilli as determined by gaseous tension. *Am. Rev. Tuberc.* **15**, 65.

[8] CROFTON J. (1964) The clinical evaluation of antituberculosis drugs. In *Chemotherapy of Tuberculosis*, ed. Barry V.C., p. 228. London, Butterworths.

[9] CRUICKSHANK R., Ed. (1965) *Medical Microbiology. A Guide to Laboratory Diagnosis and Control of Infection*, 11th Edition. Edinburgh, Livingstone.

[10] GLOYNE S. (1951). Pneumoconiosis. A histological survey of necropsy material in 1205 cases. *Lancet* **i**, 810.

[11] GROTH-PETERSEN E., LØVGREEN A. & THILLE-MANN J. (1952) On the reliability of the reading of photofluorograms and the value of dual reading. *Acta tuberc. scand.* **26**, 13.

[12] GROTH-PETERSEN E., KNUDSEN J. & WILBEK E. (1959) Epidemiological basis of tuberculosis eradication in an advanced country. *Bull. Wld Hlth Org.* **21**, 5.

[13] HOLST E., MITCHISON D.A. & RADHAKRISHNA S. (1959) Examination of smears for tubercle bacilli by fluorescence microscopy. *Ind. J. med. Res.* **47**, 495.

[14] HORNE N.W. (1960) Prednisolone in treatment of pulmonary tuberculosis: a controlled trial. Final report to the Research Committee of the Tuberculosis Society of Scotland. *Br. med. J.* **ii**, 1751.

[15] KENT D.C. & SCHWARTZ R. (1967) Active pulmonary tuberculosis with negative skin reactions. *Am. Rev. resp. Dis.* **95**, 411.

[16] KREUKNIET J. & ORIE N.G.M. (1961) Chronic bronchitis, bronchial asthma, a host factor in patients with pulmonary tuberculosis. *Allerg. Asthma* **7**, 220.

[17] LANCASTER J.F. & TOMASHEFSKI J.F. (1962) Tuberculosis—a cause of emphysema. *Am. Rev. resp. Dis.* **87**, 435.

[18] LEADER (1966) Isoniazid: How much a carcinogen? *Lancet* **ii**, 1452.

[19] LEES A.W., MILLER T.J.R. & ROBERTS G.B.S. (1955) Bronchial lavage for the recovery of the tubercle bacillus. Comparison with gastric lavage and laryngeal swabbing. *Lancet* **ii**, 800.

[20] LOPEZ-MAJANO V., WAGNER H.N., TOW D.E. & CHERNICK V. (1965) Radioisotope scanning of the lungs in pulmonary tuberculosis. *J. Am. med. Ass.* **194**, 1053.

[21] MALMBERG R., SIMONSSON B. & BERGLUND E. (1963) Airways obstruction and uneven gas distribution in the lung. *Thorax.* **18**, 168.

[22] MASCHER W. (1951) Tuberculin negative tuberculosis. *Am. Rev. Tuberc.* **63**, 501.

[23] MITCHISON D.A. (1966) Standard smears for grading the content of acid-fast bacilli in the sputum. *Tubercle, Lond.* **47**, 289.

[24] MULLER GULLI L. (1943) *Clinical Significance of the Blood in Tuberculosis.* New York, The Commonwealth Fund.

[25] NATIONAL TUBERCULOSIS ASSOCIATION OF THE U.S.A. (1961) *Diagnostic Standards and Classification of Tuberculosis.* New York, National Tuberculosis Association.

[26] O'GRADY F. (1967) Tuberculin reaction in tuberculosis. *Br. med. Bull.* **23**, 76.

[27] PAGEL W., SIMMONDS F.A.H., MACDONALD N. & NASSAU E. (1964) *Pulmonary Tuberculosis* London, Oxford University Press.

[28] PECORA D.V. (1959) A method of securing uncontaminated tracheal secretions for bacterial examination. *J. thorac. Surg.* **37**, 653.

[29] RAFFEL S. (1961) *Immunity*, 2nd Edition. New York, Appleton-Century-Crofts.

[30] RICH A.R. (1951) *The Pathogenesis of Tuberculosis*, 2nd Edition. Oxford, Blackwell Scientific Publications.

[31] ROSS J.D. & KAY D.T. (1956) A review of 138 cases of closure of tuberculous lung cavities under chemotherapy. *Thorax* **11**, 1.

[32] RUBIN E.H. (1939) Haematogenous tuberculosis in the adult. II. Haematogenous pulmonary tuberculosis. *Am. Rev. Tuberc.* **40**, 667.

[33] SCADDING J.G. (1956) Insensitivity to tuberculin in pulmonary tuberculosis. *Tubercle, Lond.* **37**, 371.

[34] SCOTTISH THORACIC SOCIETY (1963) A controlled trial of chemotherapy in pulmonary tuberculosis of doubtful activity: 5 year follow up. *Tubercle, Lond.* **44**, 39.

[35] SÖDERHOLM B. (1957) The hemodynamics of the lesser circulation in pulmonary tuberculosis. Effect of exercise, temporary pulmonary artery occlusion and operation. *Scand. J. clin. Lab. Invest.* **9**, Suppl. 26.

[36] SPENCER H. (1962) *Pathology of the Lung*, p. 645. London, Pergamon Press.

[37] SPRINGETT V.H. (1956) *Minimal Pulmonary Tuberculosis found by Mass Radiography (Fluorography).* London, Lewis.

[38] STEINITZ RUTH (1965) Pulmonary tuberculosis and carcinoma of the lung. A survey from two population-based disease registers. *Am. Rev. resp. Dis.* **92**, 758.

[39] STRADLING P. & JOHNSTON R.N. (1955) Reducing observer error in a 70 mm. chest radiography service for general practitioners. *Lancet* **i**, 1247.

[40] THOMAS O.F., BORTHWICK W.M., HORNE N.W. & CROFTON J.W. (1954) Infection with drug resistant tubercle bacilli. *Lancet* **i**, 1308.

[41] UGGLA L.G. (1957) Pulmonary hypertension in tuberculosis of the lungs. *Acta tuberc. scand.*, Supp. **41**, 1.

[42] WILLIAMS M.H., Jr., SERIFF N.S., AKYOL T. & YOO O.H. (1961) The diffusing capacity of the lung in acute pulmonary tuberculosis. *Am. Rev. resp. Dis.* **84**, 814.

[43] YERUSHALMY J. (1953) The reliability of chest roentgenography and its clinical implications. *Dis. Chest* **24**, 133.

CHAPTER 14

Treatment of Pulmonary Tuberculosis

INTRODUCTION

One of the most dramatic medical changes in the last 20 years has been the revolution in the outlook for the patient with tuberculosis. A tragic situation in which approximately 1 in every 2 newly diagnosed patients died, often after a grim downhill course of alternating stability and relapse, has been converted to one in which permanent recovery can theoretically be ensured for virtually every newly diagnosed case. Unfortunately this happy outcome is not simply attained. It depends on the physician prescribing precisely the correct chemotherapeutic regimen and the patient continuing to take it for many months after he has lost his symptoms. If wrong chemotherapy is given, owing to error by doctor or patient, drug resistant organisms are likely to emerge. This makes it very much more difficult to salvage the patient. Salvage may ultimately be achieved with newer drug combinations, though only at the expense of much skilled time, distress and discomfort for the patient and great economic cost. Moreover, the patient may pass on his resistant organisms to others (primary drug resistance). No physician is therefore justified in undertaking the care of tuberculous patients unless he is fully conversant with the problems of chemotherapy and is prepared to take the trouble to ensure that the patient takes his treatment meticulously and without interruption.

At one time the patient's recovery depended mainly on his own defences against his tubercle bacilli, so that the enhancement of these defences was attempted by bed rest, sanatorium treatment and other measures. Pneumothorax or thoracoplasty was used to rest the lung and substantial proportions of the patient's bacilli were removed, together with diseased lung, by resection. It is possible

that these methods did good, though the evidence in their favour was far from unequivocal. But they have been completely outdated by chemotherapy which is able to attack tubercle bacilli directly and to eliminate them, though surgery may still occasionally be required in some patients with resistant organisms and to deal with certain complications (p. 245).

In managing a patient with pulmonary tuberculosis the physician has to decide whether the clinical and radiological findings justify treatment and whether to treat him in hospital and, if so, for how long. He then has to decide what form of chemotherapy to use. For most recently diagnosed patients, whose tubercle bacilli are likely to be sensitive to the standard drugs, the decision regarding chemotherapy is not a very complex one, but for patients who have relapsed after previous treatment, who have had previous unsatisfactory chemotherapy or who are known to have drug resistant organisms, a great deal of thought may be required. In some patients the question of using corticosteroids may arise and in an occasional patient surgery may have to be considered. In every case a decision has to be made about the duration of chemotherapy. These various aspects will be taken up in the following pages. We shall also discuss the treatment of complications and the different approach required in economically developing countries where there is a shortage of money, staff and facilities for dealing with the disease.

TYPES OF PATIENT REQUIRING TREATMENT

In economically developed countries any patient who is considered to have active disease should receive chemotherapy. Although in many patients the symptoms, the radiological extent of disease and the finding

234

of tubercle bacilli in the sputum make it obvious that the disease is active and requires treatment, in many others the only evidence of the presence of disease is radiological and it may be impossible to say with certainty whether the disease is active. The term 'active' in this context is used to indicate that the disease is not permanently healed. Clearly in the individual case this judgment is a matter of probability and the various relevant factors have already been outlined (p. 227). In making the decision individual clinicians differ widely in their judgment. At one extreme the physician may treat almost every patient with a radiological lesion likely to be of tuberculous origin. If he does so, and ensures that the patient takes his drugs as directed, he should prevent later disease in most of his patients but at the expense of treating a large number of patients unnecessarily. The alternative is to keep the patient under observation with regular x-ray and to treat at once if there is any radiological deterioration or a positive sputum. The frequency of observation will depend on the clinician's assessment of the chances of later breakdown (p. 227).

It is impossible here to give absolute indications in this matter. A trial by the Scottish Thoracic Society [86] in patients with doubtfully active disease showed a substantial advantage, on a 5 year follow-up, to the treated group compared to the untreated controls. Nevertheless there were significant differences between subgroups and we would normally treat younger patients, those in whom there was no radiological evidence of chronicity, as judged by calcification or fibrosis, and any patient in whom the radiological changes, even if chronic, occupied an area of more than 10 cm² on the large x-ray film.

SANATORIUM, HOSPITAL AND BED REST

Sanatorium treatment was designed to increase the patient's defences against the disease. It depended on putting the patient in pleasant rural or mountainous surroundings, exposing him to a great deal of fresh air, feeding him well and later subjecting him to graded exercise as he recovered. No unequivocal evidence of its benefit is available and the success of chemotherapy now makes it an anachronism. Prolonged *bed rest* was another linchpin of treatment in the pre-chemotherapy era. In recent years a number of controlled trials and other suggestive evidence [22, 39, 92, 106, 108 & 112] have shown that the results of chemotherapy are just as good without bed rest as with it. In patients without gross cavitation and with sputum negative on direct smear a controlled trial by the Tuberculosis Society of Scotland [106] showed that patients who were treated without stopping work did as well as those who had a minimum of 3 months' bed rest and the same chemotherapy. A 5 year follow-up by the Tuberculosis Chemotherapy Centre, Madras [22] which compared the results of the same chemotherapy in patients either given a year's sanatorium treatment under good conditions or treated at home in the Madras slums, revealed no important differences between the two groups. Those treated at home had relatively little rest.

Very ill patients will of course require to be in bed but can be allowed up progressively as they improve. In economically developing countries a small number of beds may have to be made available for such patients but the great majority can be treated at home. In economically developed countries adequate hospital beds are available and a decision has to be made as to what type of patient should be admitted. Our own practice is to admit all patients who are ill, all those with extensive disease, all those with sputum positive on direct smear and most of those who, because of the radiological extent of their disease, are likely to prove an infectious risk. We also tend to admit patients whom we judge would be likely to be unreliable in taking their chemotherapy, so that they may have an initial period of assured treatment. It is true that the studies in Madras [22] have shown that such admission is not essential to the patient's recovery and that, once treatment is started, he very soon ceases to be an important infectious risk (p. 251). Nevertheless to obtain equal success with this more severe type of case, if treated at home, would involve a large, skilled and conscientious team giving frequent and detailed attention to the home treatment. Supervision on this scale is not usually available, even though reorientation of resources might make it so. The scheme we have outlined is not unduly expensive, not unduly hard on the individual patient and is more likely to ensure effective treatment for the patients who, both from their own individual point of view and from that of public health, are at greatest risk.

Patients who do not fall into the above categories we normally treat without any other interference with their lives than taking their chemotherapy and attending regularly at the outpatient clinic. For a patient admitted to hospital it is our own practice to examine the sputum weekly or fortnightly and to discharge him when 3 successive specimens have been found negative on culture, laryngeal swabs being taken if no sputum is available. Sputa are only reported as negative after they have been kept for 2 months. Most patients therefore remain in hospital for a minimum of 3 months and severe cases for a longer period. In individual cases it is justifiable to reduce this period if the patient is making satisfactory progress and there are good social reasons for an earlier discharge. On the other hand, it is wiser to prolong the hospital stay of less co-operative patients, even if the sputum has become negative, in order to ensure the longest possible period of supervised treatment.

STANDARD CHEMOTHERAPY

In countries in which there is no economic barrier to treatment isoniazid, streptomycin and the salts of para-aminosalicylic acid (PAS), in that order of efficacy, are the standard drugs for treating the disease. The order of efficacy has been established by various controlled clinical trials, in particular those by the British Medical Research Council [21, 60, 61, 62 & 63], and by general clinical experience. The value of thioacctazone*

* This name now recommended by the World Health Organisation.

(thiacetazone), as a substitute for PAS, has been established by controlled trials in Africa and India [27, 28, 29 & 104] but this substitution cannot yet be recommended for countries in which the use of PAS is economically possible [116].

Soon after the introduction of chemotherapy it was realized that tubercle bacilli readily acquired resistance to antituberculosis drugs. The mechanism is discussed elsewhere (p. 83). It was found possible greatly to reduce, or even to eliminate, the emergence of resistant organisms by using the drugs in the right doses and combinations [19, 21, 42, 60, 61, 62 & 63]. Unfortunately before the best drug combinations were established and generally used the tubercle bacilli of many patients had been made drug resistant and these patients had infected others with their resistant organisms. The latter, therefore, even when they had never received treatment, had organisms 'primarily' resistant to one or more of the standard drugs. Because drug resistance tests take 6–8 weeks to perform, the initial treatment for the individual patient has to be decided before it is known whether his organisms are primarily resistant or not. Treatment of a newly diagnosed patient has therefore to be designed to minimize the risk of his organisms acquiring resistance to a further drug should they prove to have been primarily resistant to one of the three standard medicaments. This is why, although certain double drug combinations are highly effective in preventing the emergence of acquired resistance, it is now standard practice to initiate treatment with all three drugs. Should the patient's organisms prove to have been primarily resistant to 1 of the 3, the other 2 drugs still form an effective combination to prevent the emergence of resistance to a second or third drug.

STANDARD DRUG COMBINATIONS FOR NEWLY DIAGNOSED PATIENTS

PATIENTS UNDER THE AGE OF 40 ADMITTED TO HOSPITAL
Streptomycin 1 g in a single injection daily plus isoniazid 100 mg orally twice daily plus

sodium PAS 5 g 3 times a day. This associates the most powerful drug combination, daily streptomycin and isoniazid, with a moderately high dose of PAS. If the patient's organisms are primarily resistant either to streptomycin or to isoniazid this dose of PAS should be sufficient to prevent resistance emerging to the remaining drug. The individual dose of sodium PAS should not be reduced below 5 g. In one of the earlier controlled trials it was shown that, if the total daily dose of PAS was given 4 times daily, a daily dose of 5 or 10 g was markedly inferior to 20 g in preventing the emergence of streptomycin resistant organisms [21]. On the other hand 5 g sodium PAS twice daily appeared to be as good as the same dose 4 times daily in preventing the emergence of isoniazid resistant organisms [63]. It seems likely therefore that it is the size of the individual dose of PAS which is important and it may well be, although it has not been proved, that the results might be just as good if PAS in the above combination were given in a dose of 5 g twice instead of 3 times daily. Indeed, in a trial in Madras the bacteriological results after 6 months were as good in a group receiving 6 g PAS with 200 mg isoniazid in a single morning dose as in a group receiving 5 g PAS and 100 mg isoniazid both twice daily [104]. There is much evidence, some of it indirect [115], to suggest that all 3 drugs could well be given in a single dose daily, a single dose of 10 g sodium PAS being combined with 200 mg isoniazid and 1 g streptomycin.

HOSPITAL PATIENTS OVER THE AGE OF 40

In this age group streptomycin is more likely to cause vestibular upset. A controlled trial has suggested that reduction of the dose to 0·75 g daily results in less frequent vestibular upset without loss of efficacy [48]. Alternatively, for a number of years we gave streptomycin 1 g 3 times weekly together with daily PAS and isoniazid. Theoretically if a patient had organisms primarily resistant to PAS this dose of intermittent streptomycin might not be sufficient to prevent isoniazid resistance but in practice we experienced no failures in many hundred cases. The risk therefore, if it is more than theoretical, must be very small. It has the advantage of decreasing the frequency of injections and this combination is therefore justifiable later in treatment and, for greater convenience, in outpatients.

HOSPITAL PATIENTS WHOSE ORGANISMS ARE KNOWN TO BE FULLY SENSITIVE TO THE STANDARD DRUGS

When the results of initial sensitivity tests have become available and the organisms are known to be fully sensitive to all drugs it is wise, in patients with severe disease, to continue with daily streptomycin and isoniazid, dropping the less powerful PAS. But if the patient is an older person who has been treated initially with streptomycin 3 times weekly both PAS and isoniazid must be continued, as intermittent streptomycin may be insufficient to prevent the emergence of isoniazid resistant organisms in all cases.

PATIENTS AFTER DISCHARGE FROM HOSPITAL

By the time a patient has been discharged from hospital it is normally known that his organisms were sensitive to the standard drugs. If it has not been possible to obtain a positive culture for testing, and his sputum has remained negative, it may be assumed that there is no great risk, even if his organisms are primarily resistant to one of the drugs. It is convenient therefore to continue with a combination of only 2 drugs. If the patient is judged to be a person who will fully cooperate in taking drugs regularly it is convenient to prescribe oral chemotherapy, a dose of 10 g sodium PAS and 200 mg isoniazid being given daily in 1 or 2 doses. It is advisable to give the drugs together in a single preparation, cachets or granules [32 & 37] often being used. If a patient is judged to be less reliable a useful alternative is to give streptomycin 1 g and isoniazid 14 mg/kg (or 900–1000 mg in a normal adult), together with pyridoxine 10 mg to combat possible isoniazid toxicity, all 3 drugs being given at the same time under supervision twice weekly. This has been shown [73 & 103] to be at least as effective a regimen as isoniazid and PAS in conventional doses.

OUTPATIENT TREATMENT OF NEWLY DIAGNOSED CASES

It will usually be less severely ill patients who are initially treated at home rather than in hospital. If for some reason a patient with advanced disease is to be treated at home, treatment should follow the lines already outlined. If a patient has less severe disease and the sputum is negative on direct smear there is little risk in initiating his treatment with streptomycin 1 g 3 times weekly, which is more convenient than daily injections, together with PAS and isoniazid as above. If negative cultures have been obtained at the end of 3 months, treatment can be continued with PAS and isoniazid daily, or streptomycin, isoniazid and pyridoxine twice weekly.

MODIFICATIONS OF STANDARD CHEMOTHERAPY

Many clinicians exceed the dose of 200 mg isoniazid daily suggested above. Extensive literature has shown that there is considerable variation among individuals in the rate at which isoniazid is metabolized, and a consequent variation in the period for which isoniazid is detectable, at what are theoretically inhibitory levels, in the blood (see review by Scottish Thoracic Society [85]). There is evidence that individuals may be divided roughly into slow and rapid metabolizers of isoniazid. It was at one time suggested that the dose of isoniazid should therefore be modified for the individual according to the speed with which the drug disappeared from the blood stream. In fact there have now been a number of controlled trials [85] which have failed to show more than a marginal, and statistically insignificant, advantage for high dosage isoniazid when used in combination with a second drug, even though a high dose gives better results if isoniazid is used alone [26 & 34]. Nevertheless, even alone, a dose above 9·6 mg/kg appears to convey no added benefit [102]. It may perhaps be justifiable to give high doses in the early stages of treatment of a patient with very severe disease, because of possible marginal advantage, but there is no reason to give a daily dose higher than 200 mg as a routine. Nevertheless, if streptomycin and isoniazid are given twice weekly, rather than daily, it is probable that the high dose of isoniazid recommended above is important in order to ensure a successful outcome in a high proportion of patients. A minimum dose of 300 mg is also required with thioacetazone (p. 247).

At one time a combination of streptomycin twice weekly together with daily isoniazid was widely used. This combination resulted in the emergence of isoniazid resistant organisms in some 13% of cases [63]. It should therefore never be used.

The importance of prescribing chemotherapy in strict accordance with the above recommendations for standard chemotherapy cannot be too strongly emphasized. Moreover it is equally important to ensure that there are no interruptions of treatment, except when there is really good evidence of definite toxicity. If there is evidence of toxicity to a specific drug the clinician must make certain that the patient receives an adequate alternative combination which will ensure that resistant organisms do not emerge. The trial of standard chemotherapy by the International Union against Tuberculosis [46] demonstrated the marked inferiority of results if treatment were interrupted or altered.

EVIDENCE FOR THE EFFICACY OF STANDARD CHEMOTHERAPY

The best evidence for the relative efficacy of different combinations of 2 standard drugs is to be found in the earlier trials of the British Medical Research Council [19, 62 & 63]. These trials indicated that the most powerful combination was daily streptomycin and isoniazid, which appeared to be superior to daily streptomycin and PAS and to daily PAS and isoniazid, although this superiority did not in all cases attain statistical significance. A regimen of intermittent streptomycin with daily isoniazid was shown to be inferior to the remainder. The results over 3–6 months with daily PAS and isoniazid in these earlier

Medical Research Council trials in Britain were appreciably better than the results of later trials in Africa and India in which treatment and observation continued for 1 year and the disease on average was more severe.

When the existence of primary drug resistance became obvious our own group, which had started in 1952 to utilize the results of the Medical Research Council trials but continuing treatment over much longer periods, began to initiate treatment with all 3 drugs as indicated above. As a result of this, and the development of methods of resistance testing capable of detecting even low degrees of clinically significant drug resistance [94], we were able to report sputum conversion to negative in almost all newly diagnosed patients with pulmonary tuberculosis whose organisms proved initially sensitive to at least 2 of the 3 standard drugs [17, 19, 42 & 81]. Similar results have been reported by Thomas et al. [97], Ibiapina et al. [45], Thibier et al. [96] and Russell et al. [82] and the claims have found substantial support in the large scale international trial, confined to far advanced pulmonary tuberculosis, conducted by the International Union against Tuberculosis [46].

RATE OF SPUTUM CONVERSION TO NEGATIVE

In a personal series of 452 hospital patients treated during a 10 year period approximately 50% had persistently negative cultures by 1 month, 80% by 3 months and 98% by 6 months, conversion having occurred in all patients by 10 months [19]. In other series positive cultures have been occasionally obtained up to a year. In a number of trials with frequent bacteriological examination [22, 64 & 73] isolated positive cultures, sometimes with resistant organisms, have been reported in the second year or later (on or off chemotherapy) but were said usually not to herald relapse. This has not been our experience, perhaps because of our more intensive early chemotherapy, our less intensive late bacteriology, or both. The rate of sputum conversion is of course related to the severity of the initial disease, conversion usually taking longer in patients with extensive cavitation and a large population of tubercle bacilli.

DURATION OF CHEMOTHERAPY AND RELATION TO RELAPSE

Some years ago [18] we compared the isolation of tubercle bacilli from lesions in lungs resected after different durations of chemotherapy and the relapse rate after different periods of chemotherapy, the data being derived from different investigations in Edinburgh. We found that the isolation of bacilli and the relapse rate ran parallel, the rate for isolation being slightly above that for relapse. Both rates dropped rapidly after one year's chemotherapy. The relapse and isolation rates were 2% and 1% respectively in patients who had received between 12 and 18 months' chemotherapy; both were reduced to nil in those who had received more than 18 months'. It is true that the number of lungs resected after more than 18 months' chemotherapy was small but some 260 cases, many with far advanced disease, had had more than 18 months' chemotherapy without relapse. Horne [42] reported 771 sputum positive patients treated in Edinburgh hospitals in the six years 1955–60 who had tubercle bacilli initially sensitive to at least 2 of the standard drugs. All became sputum negative and in only 2 did resistant organisms emerge, in both cases to isoniazid during a desensitization procedure. The relapse rate for this group was 2·1%. Using regimens of chemotherapy in which streptomycin either was not given or was given for a shorter period than that in most of the Edinburgh cases, the British Medical Research Council [64], in a trial in which the duration of chemotherapy was randomized in patients with chronic extensive pulmonary tuberculosis, showed a high relapse rate (62%) in patients receiving only 6 months' chemotherapy, an important rate (19%) in those receiving 1 year's treatment but a much lower rate (4%) in those who received 2 years'. The addition of a third year gave no added benefit.

From this and other evidence it is clear that no case of pulmonary tuberculosis should receive less than 1 year of chemotherapy. It is wise not to give less than 15 months even with minimal disease. Patients with moderately advanced disease should receive 18 months. Although it is possible that 18 months may be sufficient for the great majority of cases it is advisable, if one is seeking to have no relapses, to give those with far advanced disease, and those in whom there is a residual open cavity, a full 2 years. There is no evidence that continuation of treatment beyond 2 years confers added benefit [22 & 64].

TOXIC REACTIONS TO CHEMOTHERAPY
[4, 49, 66 & 90]

HYPERSENSITIVE REACTIONS

Allergic reactions to streptomycin and PAS are frequent, the latter being slightly commoner. Reactions to isoniazid are rare and virtually only occur if the patient has also become hypersensitive to the other 2 drugs. Hypersensitivity to streptomycin and PAS may develop simultaneously or successively. The incidence increases with the number of drugs used [90]. It is often reported that reactions are less common in races with darker skin, but this may be because rashes are less readily detected. The commonest manifestations are *fever* or *rash*, often both together. The rash is usually erythematous and often itchy. Less common are *enlargement of the lymph nodes* and *splenomegaly*. If a warning fever has been neglected *jaundice* may occur, particularly as a reaction to PAS. Raised serum transaminase is common in allergic reactions to the latter even without jaundice [89]. The reaction may be accompanied by *eosinophilia*, and *transient opacities* may be seen on the chest x-ray. If other warning signs are passed unrecognized the reaction may continue to *encephalopathy* or severe *depression* of the *bone marrow*; *exfoliative dermatitis* may also occur. *Albuminuria* is sometimes seen. In our experience the most severe reactions are commoner with PAS than with streptomycin.

Most reactions occur in the first 4 weeks after starting treatment, the commonest time being 2–3 weeks, but occasionally reactions are seen after several months, particularly rashes [49].

HYPOSENSITIZATION

It is a sensible rule that any new fever, or increase in fever, occurring in the first 4 weeks after starting chemotherapy should be regarded as due to an allergic reaction unless there is some other obvious reason. The first step is to stop the drugs. The fever will usually decrease within 24 hours. When the temperature has become normal and any skin reaction has cleared, *test doses* should be given in order to determine the drug or drugs to which the patient has become hypersensitive. If the reaction has not been a severe one the test dose can be half the standard dose, streptomycin 0·5 g, isoniazid 50 mg or PAS 2·5 g. If a patient is hypersensitive to the drug a rise in temperature, itchiness or rash will develop within 2 or 3 hours. It is best to start with the test dose of isoniazid as a reaction to this drug is less likely. If there is no reaction a full dose can be given in order to make certain. Isoniazid is then stopped and a streptomycin test dose is given, first a half dose and then, if there is no reaction, the full dose. If there is any reaction this is allowed to subside but must be followed by a test dose of PAS, as hypersensitivity may occur to both drugs. If the initial reaction has been very severe a smaller dose must be given. Streptomycin 0·1 g is usually low enough to prevent a severe reaction. With PAS a similar dose is usually low enough but if there is reason to feel particularly apprehensive a dose as low as 0·01 g can be given initially.

If the patient is only hypersensitive to 1 of the drugs the other 2 should be administered in the usual combination while hyposensitization proceeds. It is practicable and time saving to give the doses 12 hourly. Streptomycin may be given in an initial dose of 0·1 g and increased successively by 0·1 g until the full dose is reached. Should the patient have a reaction this must be allowed to subside and then the same dose, or a lower one if the reaction was severe, should be repeated. The initial dose of PAS can usually be 0·5 g but with severe reactions this may have to be lower, 0·1 g or even less. The dose can be increased successively by 0·5 g, or more slowly with severe reactions.

In our experience it is not very satisfactory to cover hyposensitization with corticosteroid drugs. They may suppress milder reactions but ultimately a severe reaction may develop in spite of the corticosteroids or may occur when the steroid therapy is withdrawn. It is better for the clinician to know exactly how the hyposensitization is proceeding so that he may make the necessary adjustments in dosage. Corticosteroid drugs may be used for a short time to control an unduly severe reaction in a patient in whom hyposensitization proves difficult.

If the patient is hypersensitive to both streptomycin and to PAS it is dangerous to combine a small dose of either of these drugs with isoniazid, owing to the risk of the emergence of isoniazid resistance, as has been reported [44]. In that case isoniazid should be combined with 1 or 2 second-line drugs (p. 247) while hyposensitization is proceeding.

Patients hypersensitive to isoniazid are always hypersensitive also to streptomycin and PAS, and usually highly so. In such a patient hyposensitization is likely to be a tedious and prolonged procedure. It is often best to start the patient on 3 second line drugs. After several weeks without any reaction to the new therapy, hyposensitization should be begun, first to isoniazid, then to streptomycin and finally to PAS. The reason for this order is that severe reactions are least likely with isoniazid and most likely with PAS. The initial dose of isoniazid should depend on the severity of the reaction to the test dose; it should be well below the smallest dose which produced a reaction.

OTHER TOXIC EFFECTS OF ISONIAZID

Isoniazid gives rise to very little toxicity. In high doses *peripheral neuritis* may occur, usually manifested by a burning sensation, pain or paraesthesia but sometimes by motor symptoms. It is very rare in patients receiving the normal dose of 200–300 mg daily, even when they are under-nourished but has occurred in as high a proportion as 13% in patients receiving approximately 8 to 10 mg/kg [23]. It is commoner in patients who inactivate isoniazid slowly [6 & 23]. The Madras workers [102] have shown that a relatively small dose of 6 mg of pyridoxine was sufficient to eliminate neuritis in patients receiving high doses of the drug daily. 10 mg is the more usual dose available for dispensing in Britain. It is only required when high doses are given as suggested above. *Pellagra* has complicated the administration of high doses of the drug in a malnourished population in South Africa and may occur very rarely even in an economically advanced country. It has been suggested that in *epileptics* there is increased risk of fits but we have experienced little trouble, using 200 mg daily. Impairment of concentration among intellectuals, sleepiness, wakefulness, encephalopathy and psychoses [1] have all been attributed to the drug. It is probable that some of the major manifestations may be due to the drug but minor symptoms are often subjective and unrelated. Isoniazid has been shown to be carcinogenic in mice [5]. It has been reported that patients with pulmonary tuberculosis have an excess incidence of carcinoma of the bronchus [93] but both excess of cigarette smoking and scarring are possible reasons for this and there is certainly no present evidence to incriminate isoniazid as a carcinogen in man [31].

OTHER TOXIC EFFECTS OF STREPTOMYCIN

Apart from hypersensitive reactions the main toxic effect of streptomycin is *vestibular damage*. The risk increases with the dose of the drug [7] and also with age [90]. The patient usually complains of giddiness. Damage to the vestibular apparatus is best shown by caloric tests [7] but a useful crude test for vestibular damage is to ask the patient to walk down a line, first with his eyes open and then with his eyes closed. He is much more unsteady with his eyes closed. Nystagmus may occasionally be demonstrated. Symptoms usually occur within the first 3 months but sometimes later [90]. If the drug is stopped at once the giddiness disappears in most cases over a matter of weeks but if streptomycin has been continued for some time after the start of symptoms damage may be permanent. In daylight the patient usually compensates for the loss by visual reflexes but he may have difficulty in the dark. The risk of vestibular upset is decreased in older people by reducing the dose to 0·75 g daily. In the very old, or those with renal impairment, we normally carry out serum estimations 24 hours after a dose. If the serum level is above 1 mcg per ml we decrease the dose accordingly, sometimes to as little as 0·25 g thrice weekly. It has been claimed that pantothenic acid given together with streptomycin reduces the damage to the vestibular apparatus but a controlled trial has not confirmed this claim [77]. In our experience deafness is almost unknown with streptomycin unless a patient has had previous impairment of hearing. Dihydrostreptomycin has been recommended as less damaging to the vestibular apparatus but undoubtedly is more likely to produce nerve deafness, which is usually permanent. In our opinion this drug should not be given.

There is thought to be a very slight risk that streptomycin, given to a mother during pregnancy, may cause vestibular damage in the foetus. Although the risk is a slight one, it is reasonable to avoid streptomycin during pregnancy if this can safely be done.

OTHER TOXIC EFFECTS OF PAS

The main side effects of PAS, apart from allergic reactions, are *gastrointestinal*. With confident handling by the doctor, PAS in the doses advocated does not normally result in nausea and vomiting. Naturally any suggestion that it may do so is liable to produce the symptoms. Nevertheless there are a few individuals who do not seem to be able to tolerate the drug. In these individuals severe diarrhoea is usually more of a problem than nausea and vomiting. In many cases initial diarrhoea diminishes if small doses of kaolin and opiates are given, the latter being later gradually withdrawn. Nevertheless in some individuals the diarrhoea is intolerable and another drug may have to be used; in our experience this is rare. *Malabsorption of Vitamin B12* as a

result of PAS therapy has been described [38] and we have ourselves seen instances, including fat malabsorption, reversing when the drug was stopped. In several series PAS has only had to be stopped because of side effects in very few, often well under 1%, of patients [26, 27, 28, 49, 90 & 100].

PAS has been shown to have an *antithyroid effect*, inhibiting the synthesis of thyroxin [57]. The thyroid may hypertrophy to overcome the effect and goitres may occasionally occur in patients who have had 6 months or more of PAS, although this is rarer with the lower doses now used. When larger doses of PAS were used actual myxoedema occasionally resulted. The manifestations disappear when PAS is stopped and can also be reversed by giving a small dose of thyroid or thyroxin if it is necessary to continue PAS.

Various *blood dyscrasias* have been rarely described with all three standard drugs, though some may have been related to the tuberculosis [65].

CORTICOSTEROID DRUGS
(see review by Horne [43])

EVIDENCE OF EFFICACY

After the early reports of florid tuberculosis developing in patients receiving corticosteroids for other diseases there was a natural reluctance to use these drugs in tuberculosis. Later, certain physicians employed corticosteroids to control allergic reactions to drugs and were impressed by the apparent favourable effect on the disease. As a result corticosteroids were used by a number of clinicians but widely differing results were reported. Some reported improvement, others deterioration. Although inadequate details were often given it seemed possible, reviewing the literature, that good results were obtained in patients who were receiving chemotherapy to which their organisms were sensitive and bad results when the corticosteroids were accompanied by ineffective chemotherapy. As a result a series of controlled trials were carried out in different countries. Newly diagnosed patients were treated with effective chemotherapy together with either prednisolone or, in some cases, ACTH [11, 12, 13, 41, 47, 58, 105 & 110]. Corticosteroid treatment was continued for periods varying between 5 weeks and 3 months. The use of less satisfactory chemotherapy or a low dose of steroids may explain certain discrepancies between some of the trials but in general the results may be summarized as follows:

Compared with control patients receiving the same chemotherapy those having corticosteroid drugs showed a much more *rapid subjective improvement, fall in temperature and erythrocyte sedimentation rate* and more rapid *gain in weight*. Radiologically, *exudative lesions* cleared more rapidly although there was no difference in the rate of cavity closure. Taken as a whole there was no evidence that the sputum became negative more quickly; in fact with the satisfactory chemotherapy used almost all patients had a negative sputum by 6 months and virtually all by a year; this applied to both groups.

In most of these trials the corticosteroid drugs have not been given for more than 3 months. Although, in the respects mentioned, the corticosteroid-treated group have been at an advantage in the earlier months the differences between the two groups tended to diminish as time went on. In the trial by the Tuberculosis Society of Scotland [41] the corticosteroid group was still at an advantage one year after the start of therapy but the difference was not statistically significant. In the British Tuberculosis Association trial [12] the corticosteroid group was still said to show an advantage after 2 years but the method of analysis was unsatisfactory. It seems doubtful, on present evidence, that corticosteroids reduce the *ultimate residua* from the disease.

No satisfactory long term controlled trial has been reported in which the ultimate effect of corticosteroid drugs on *respiratory function* could be assessed. The available evidence is reviewed by Horne [43]. Although it is by no means satisfactory it suggests that in patients with advanced exudative disease treatment with corticosteroids improves function during the earlier months, but no conclusion can be come to about the long term effect.

9—R.D.

INDICATIONS

From this evidence and from our own experience we consider that corticosteroids have a valuable part to play in patients who are admitted to hospital *desperately ill* with pulmonary tuberculosis and who are at risk of dying in the first few days or weeks, before chemotherapy can have its full effect. Corticosteroids enable the toxicity of the disease to be reduced in such cases and tide the patient over the period of high risk. In *other very ill patients*, even if not at immediate risk of dying, corticosteroids may be given in the early stages for purely humanitarian reasons. The patient feels better much more quickly.

DOSAGE

In most cases it is sufficient to give prednisolone 5 mg 4 times daily, although in very severe cases 30 or 40 mg may be given daily for the first few days. Our usual practice is to continue the full dose of 20 mg for 6 weeks or so and then gradually to reduce the dose, perhaps by 5 mg weekly. If there is any return of fever or major malaise the rate of reduction is slowed down.

It should be remembered that sometimes corticosteroids, used in these circumstances, may *suppress an allergic reaction* to chemotherapy which is revealed as the dose of corticosteroids is reduced. Hyposensitization may then be necessary at a late stage.

Corticosteroid drugs are also sometimes used to *control* a very severe *hypersensitive reaction* or to cover a *hyposensitization* procedure in a patient who is unusually susceptible to very small doses of drugs (p. 240). The danger of giving corticosteroids to such patients if they are not having effective chemotherapy must be appreciated. If necessary second line drugs may need to be given.

METHODS FOR DETECTING ANTITUBERCULOSIS DRUGS IN THE URINE

In earlier pages there has been frequent reference to urinary tests for antituberculosis drugs, as a control on the patient's conscientiousness in taking his therapy. Tests have mainly been carried out for PAS and isoniazid. The methods have been reviewed by Hobby [40], and, for isoniazid only, by Venkataraman et al. [111].

ISONIAZID

Venkataraman et al. recommended the Acetylisoniazid Test as the best. 'In a white porcelain plate with hemispherical depressions, 4 drops of urine, 4 drops of a 10% solution of potassium cyanide, followed by 10 drops of 10% chloramine T were added without shaking of the plate. The development of a pink or red colour indicated the presence of acetylisoniazid. The reagents used for this test were prepared at approximately weekly intervals and stored in the refrigerator at 4°C.' This test is positive in virtually all urines collected up to 12 hours after a dose of 100 mg isoniazid. A simpler but less sensitive test, using alkaline sodium nitroprusside and acetic acid as reagents, has been recently described [72].

PAS

In economically developed countries, where the minor expense can be borne, the most convenient test is to use the 'Phenistix' strips which are prepared for testing for phenylpyruvic acid in congenital phenylketonuria. The test end of the strip is dipped in a sample of urine. If PAS is present a colour change occurs varying from faint mauve to deep reddish-purple, according to the concentration of PAS. The strip changes colour immediately. There is cross reaction with salicylates, sulphonamides and possibly aminophylline [88]. This test is positive up to 12 hours after taking a dose of 5 g of PAS, and it is very quick and simple to use. This reaction is based on the ferric chloride reaction with PAS. When the strip cannot be afforded the test may be carried out directly as follows: A few drops of 1 N hydrochloric acid are added to 1 ml of urine. A 10% solution of ferric chloride is then added drop by drop. If PAS is present a purple colour is produced, the intensity varying with the concentration. There is a cross reaction with salicylates. This is a highly sensitive test which will be positive for at least 12 hours after the patient has taken 5 g of PAS. A simpler modification of this test has been suggested by Turner [107]. The patient merely wets a piece of blotting paper with his urine or it can be dipped into a urine container. One drop of 3% ferric chloride is then added to the wet blotting paper. If PAS is present a violet to violet-black spot is produced.

A very cheap test, using a small tablet containing anhydrous cobalt sulphate and no liquid reagents, has been described by Case [14].

ELECTROLYTE DISTURBANCES

Hypokalaemia [20] and other electrolyte disturbances are less common in pulmonary tuberculosis than in miliary tuberculosis (p. 211) but may occur in patients with very severe disease, especially in the elderly. In such patients the serum electrolytes should be checked on admission and if there is any suggestion of deterioration within the first few weeks after starting chemotherapy. If hypokalaemia is detected it should be dealt with along the same lines as in miliary tuberculosis (p. 212).

SPECIAL PROBLEMS AND COMPLICATIONS

There are certain problems about which the patient with pulmonary tuberculosis may require special advice. When the prognosis of the disease was poor the physician was often consulted about the question of *marriage*. It is of course rational to postpone marriage until the sputum is negative but otherwise there will be no particular barrier. If the patient is young it is reasonable to postpone *pregnancy* until chemotherapy is completed because of the possible very slight risks to the foetus. On the other hand if the patient has active disease and is pregnant the lesser risk is certainly to complete chemotherapy although streptomycin should be stopped as soon as the sputum is negative.

Patients who have had satisfactory treatment for pulmonary tuberculosis can return to any form of hard work, physical or mental, as long as their residual respiratory function is adequate for it. Patients are also quite capable of working in tropical climates. If the patient is likely to be exposed to particular strain this may be a reason for giving chemotherapy for 2 or 3 months longer than would normally be the case but we doubt if any patient needs more than 2 years' treatment [64].

Pleural effusion if it complicates overt pulmonary tuberculosis does not call for major modifications in treatment. If the effusion is large it may be aspirated and corticosteroid drugs may be given for a few weeks on the same lines as for simple tuberculous pleural effusion (p. 273). If a *tuberculous empyema* is seen in the acute stage, usually complicating a severe pulmonary lesion, it may be treated by simple aspiration, corticosteroids and chemotherapy on the same lines as a pleural effusion. A tuberculous pyopneumothorax (p. 272) resulting from a burst cavity is an acute emergency. Chemotherapy should be given at once and it is important to obtain lung expansion as soon as possible. In some cases this may be attained by simple aspiration of air and fluid but it may be necessary to insert a low intercostal tube, with underwater drainage, to aspirate both air and fluid. It is desirable to apply suction in order to close the pleural space as soon as possible.

Large residual cavities sometimes pose a problem. 70–80% of tuberculous cavities close under chemotherapy. Most of those that do not, cause little trouble, especially when situated in the upper lobe, but *haemorrhage, secondary bacterial infection* or infection with *Aspergillus fumigatus* resulting in an aspergilloma may cause difficulties with large cavities [25]. We certainly do not recommend routine surgery for such cavities but if, later on, complications prove troublesome and if the patient's respiratory function permits, resection may be indicated. Recurrent haemoptysis is sometimes troublesome even when the cavity appears to be completely healed and the sputum has been negative for many months. Any severe haemoptysis would justify emergency or preventive surgery if

respiratory function permits. An isolated incident of secondary bacterial infection may only require simple chemotherapy and we have known a long standing cavity close thereafter, presumably as a result of stenosis of the draining bronchus. Repeated troublesome infection may justify surgery. The treatment of complicating aspergilloma is dealt with on p. 288).

Haemoptysis is sometimes a problem in the early stages of treatment of pulmonary tuberculosis. Simple sedation and reassurance are usually all that is required. If the haemoptysis is a large one it is wise for the patient to lie on the affected side so as to minimize the risk of flooding the other lung. If much blood is lost a transfusion is occasionally necessary. Fatal haemoptyses are usually lethal within a matter of minutes. If the patient survives, conservative treatment is usually all that is necessary.

PATIENTS WHO HAVE HAD UNSATISFACTORY CHEMOTHERAPY

PATIENTS WITH RELAPSE, WITH PERSISTENTLY POSITIVE SPUTUM OR WITH KNOWN RESISTANT ORGANISMS

ASSESSMENT OF PROBABLE DRUG RESISTANCE ON CLINICAL GROUNDS

Patients with relapse or persistently positive sputum require very special consideration. It is most important to obtain as detailed information as possible about the previous chemotherapy. If possible one should know exactly what drugs have been given previously, and in what doses and combinations. The exact dates should be recorded so that the results of previous treatment may be compared with all available evidence regarding x-ray improvement or deterioration and the trends in sputum positivity. Every effort must be made to discover whether previous chemotherapy has not only been prescribed but has been taken as ordered.

Many relapses occur because the patient has simply not been given a sufficient period of chemotherapy. If, in his previous illness, he received one of the *standard drug combinations* (which should not have resulted in the emergence of resistant organisms) and if his sputum became negative under chemotherapy and his x-ray improved, then it is likely that, if he has later relapsed, his organisms will still be sensitive to the drugs previously given. On the other hand, if he has received previous chemotherapy with a *drug alone* it is possible that his organisms may now be resistant to that drug. If he has received an *unsatisfactory drug combination*, such as streptomycin twice weekly with daily isoniazid, his organisms may have become resistant first to isoniazid and later to streptomycin. If he has received a drug combination at a time when his organisms may have been *resistant to one of two drugs employed*, then they may later have become resistant to the second. If the patient's *sputum* has remained *positive* for *more than 6 months*, while he is alleged to have been receiving chemotherapy, it is likely that he has either not been taking his drugs as prescribed or his bacilli have become resistant to them. Radiological deterioration while under treatment has the same implications, provided that the deterioration is not due to some non-tuberculous cause.

If it is possible to tabulate the patient's previous chemotherapy, his sputum state and the x-ray changes the clinician can often guess fairly accurately to what drugs his organisms may now be resistant or whether they are likely to be resistant at all.

DRUG RESISTANCE TESTS

If possible these conclusions should be confirmed by drug resistance tests. Unfortunately there is no uniformity of opinion regarding the best available tests. As performed by our own bacteriological colleagues, methods similar to those used by the British Medical Research Council have proved satisfactory [94]. These methods involve a preliminary culture of the sputum and a resistance test carried out on a subculture (indirect method), using solid Löwenstein–Jensen medium and 2-fold drug dilutions. By these methods the results only become available 2–3 months after obtaining the sputum specimen. Direct

testing by inoculating the patient's sputum directly onto drug-containing medium may give a result in 3–4 weeks. If the patient's sputum is strongly positive on direct smear an early indication of drug resistance may be obtained [59 & 95]. We would accept the result of a direct test if it indicated that the patient's organisms were drug resistant but, in our present state of knowledge, we could not feel complete confidence in a report that the organisms were sensitive if there were any reason to suspect that they might not be. We would prefer to await the results of the indirect tests. Any degree of resistance above the normal biological variation should be regarded as potentially of clinical significance [94].

In any case in which there is reason from the chemotherapeutic history to suspect drug resistance, tests should be carried out on at least 3 separate cultures. Drug resistance to PAS in particular may be missed on a single test. Conversely, an unexpected report of drug resistance on a single culture should not be accepted uncritically. Errors can occur in the laboratory. All the relevant information should be assembled and the case discussed with the bacteriologist before any radical change in therapeutic policy is made as a result of such a report.

DESIGN OF A SUITABLE CHEMOTHERAPEUTIC REGIMEN

In spite of the inevitable delay in obtaining the results of resistance tests the clinician who has carried out a careful analysis along the lines indicated should be able to make an immediate decision on an appropriate initial chemotherapeutic regimen for his patient. If the history suggests that any of the standard drugs may be still effective they should be included in the therapeutic prescription but they should not be relied on to prevent resistance to other drugs, as the patient's organisms may prove to be in fact resistant. This means that it may be necessary, pending the results of resistance tests, to prescribe 4 or 5 drugs for the patient.

At this stage we will give a brief account of some of the reserve drugs now available and then proceed to discuss how they should be used. Sputum conversion should be permanently achieved and drug resistance avoided if treatment of newly diagnosed patients with standard drugs is given along the lines indicated above. Apart from the occasional patient who is unfortunate enough to have primary resistance to more than one drug, reserve drugs are only required for those who, by their own or the doctor's fault, have had poor previous chemotherapy. Unfortunately most of the reserve drugs have more side effects and are much more expensive than standard chemotherapy. Very careful handling of the patient and his problems is usually required to persuade him to persist with treatment for many months of discomfort, especially when his relapse, or the long-standing failure to control his disease, may have undermined his confidence in doctors.

RESERVE DRUGS AVAILABLE

In the following paragraphs a brief account will be given of the individual drugs available for treating patients with drug resistant tuberculosis. Subsequently appropriate drug combinations will be discussed.

THIOACETAZONE (thiacetazone)

This drug is one of the thiosemicarbazones. It is somewhat inappropriate to class it with the reserve drugs as it can now be accepted that, owing to its cheapness and relative effectiveness, it is a satisfactory substitute for PAS at least in certain developing countries (p. 250). It is given orally in a single dose of 150 mg daily. *Side effects* include nausea and vomiting, giddiness, rashes, jaundice and bone marrow suppression. A major international double-blind controlled trial of thioacetazone toxicity has been carried out on some 2000 patients, a regimen which included streptomycin, isoniazid and thioacetazone being compared with one in which only streptomycin and isoniazid were used [67]. Although the incidence of side effects was substantially higher in the group including thioacetazone it was comparable to the incidence of side-effects in other patients in whom streptomycin, PAS and isoniazid had been given simul-taneously. It was concluded that the toxicity of thioacetazone did not differ substantially from that of PAS. Of the serious side effects, jaundice and hepatitis had a very small and approximately equal incidence in both groups; 2 cases of agranulocytosis occurred in the thioacetazone group but these recovered rapidly. Gastrointestinal upsets, dizziness and giddiness were commoner in the thioacetazone group and there was some evidence that thioacetazone might have potentiated 8th nerve damage by streptomycin. Rashes occurred in 3·9% of the thioacetazone group compared to 1% of the controls but there was no case of exfoliative dermatitis. There was considerable difference from country to country in the incidence of side effects. It is concluded that in general the incidence is sufficiently low to make the drug quite acceptable as a substitute for PAS in developing countries but that, before the drug is introduced for mass treatment in any country, there should be a careful preliminary trial. There is evidence to suggest that toxicity may be high in British patients [74 & 75], but these reports were on a selected group. Strains from different countries seem to vary in their *sensitivity* to thioacetazone [68], though the clinical significance of this is still uncertain (p. 252). There is modified cross resistance with ethionamide (see below).

ETHIONAMIDE (alpha-ethylisothionicotinamide) and its modification

PROTHIONAMIDE

Ethionamide and prothionamide are powerful antituberculosis drugs which can be given orally [11, 52, 79 & 83]. It is desirable to give the drug in a dose of 0·5 g twice daily but some patients are unable to tolerate this. In that case a dose of 0·25 g may be given in the morning and 0·5 g last thing at night so that any gastrointestinal upset may not be noticed during sleep. A dose of 0·5 g is almost certainly inferior. There is some evidence of absorption if 0·5 g is given as a suppository. Nausea and nauseous eructations are often troublesome with ethionamide. Prothionamide causes less subjective side effects. Both drugs carry a slight and probably equal risk of liver toxicity. Other side effects which have been rarely reported are gynaecomastia, peripheral neuritis, impotence and acne. There is also a suggestion of a teratogenic effect and if possible it should be withheld from pregnant women. There appears to be some racial difference in gastrointestinal tolerance. The drug seems to be tolerated better in Africa and Asia than in Europe or America. Drug resistance develops rapidly and occasional strains appear to be primarily resistant [53]. It is effective against bovine tubercle bacilli. There is cross resistance with thioacetazone [3] although this is not complete. Some strains which have become resistant to thioacetazone are not resistant to ethionamide but the reverse does not hold.

PYRAZINAMIDE (pyrazinoic acid amide)

This is a powerful drug which can be given orally but has 2 major defects. Resistance to it develops very rapidly unless it is used in proper combinations and there is an important risk of liver toxicity which has occasionally proved fatal. We have normally given a total daily dose of 40 mg/kg/day divided into 2 doses with a maximum of 1·5 g twice daily. However, Toušek et al. [99] have reported highly satisfactory results when the drug was given in a triple combination using a dose of 0·5 g 3 times daily. It seems possible that this dose is sufficient. Patients should have liver function tests, preferably serum transaminase (SGOT) carried out fortnightly, at least for the first 6 months. A level of 40–80 units/ml should lead to a repeat test. If the rise persists or increases above 80 units the drug should be stopped. Pyrazinamide may cause diminished excretion of uric acid and the resultant elevation in serum uric acid may rarely result in joint pains resembling gout. A rash or fever due to hypersensitivity may occasionally be seen. Patients should be cautious in exposing themselves to sunshine as photosensitivity may result in erythema resembling sunburn. *Resistance tests* to pyrazinamide are very difficult as the drug only acts *in vitro* at a low pH. Primary (natural) resistance may occur and bovine

and nonhuman mycobacteria are normally resistant.

CYCLOSERINE

This is an antibiotic. It has a relatively weak effect against the tubercle bacillus when given alone but appears to be quite a valuable drug, preferably in a triple combination, in preventing resistance, for instance to ethionamide. It is given orally, if possible in a dose of 0·5 g twice a day but sometimes patients cannot tolerate more than 0·75 or 0·5 g. The main *toxic effects* [109] are on the nervous system. It may cause confusion, changes in behaviour or severe depression. A few cases of unexpected suicide have been reported. Patients and their relatives should be warned of this risk and advised to report any undue depression at once. Convulsions may also occur. It is better to avoid the drug if there is a history of epilepsy or major mental instability. *Resistance* appears to develop slowly but resistance tests are particularly difficult as clinically significant small rises in resistance tend to overlap the error of the method of testing.

VIOMYCIN, KANAMYCIN AND CAPREOMYCIN

These three drugs are all antibiotics which are poorly absorbed orally and have to be given by intramuscular injection. They were discovered in the order given. They are all relatively weak and all have potential toxicity on the 8th nerve and the kidney. Although there is not yet extensive experience with capreomycin it appears to be at least as effective as the other two and less toxic [10, 51, 55, 84 & 113]. It seems likely therefore to replace the others. The dose is 1 g in a single intramuscular injection daily. The toxicity with this dose appears to be low but the urine should be tested regularly for albumin and treatment should be stopped if there is any indication of deafness or giddiness. Although cross resistance between them is not constant it is frequent so that if a patient has had any of them previously the physician must remember that his organisms may be resistant to the others [80]. Drug resistance develops readily to all three drugs.

ETHAMBUTOL (dextro-2, 2'-ethylenediimino-di-1-butanol)

Ethambutol is an effective drug *in vitro* and in animals [50 & 98]. In man it has usually been given in combination so that judgment is more difficult but treatment of a limited number of patients with the drug alone [8 & 24] and experience with the drug in combination in chronic resistant cases [8, 16, 24, 51, 55 & 114] suggest that it is valuable and comparatively nontoxic. It is given orally. At first it was recommended that a single daily dose of 25 mg/kg be given for the first 60 days, followed by 15 mg/kg, but recently virtually no toxicity has been found with a dose of 20 mg/kg. The main *toxicity* is retrobulbar neuritis [51 & 54] which appears to be rare with the dose at present recommended. Nevertheless, pending more experience, patients should have a complete eye examination before starting the drug and visual acuity tests monthly. Any complaint of blurring of vision or difficulty in distinguishing colours should be investigated at once. So far recovery has been rapid when the drug is stopped. *Drug resistance* seems to develop relatively rapidly if ethambutol is given alone. Ethambutol has every promise of being a highly effective drug relatively free from toxicity and might even ultimately replace PAS in standard chemotherapy.

RIFAMYCIN AND 'RIFAMPICIN'

Rifamycin is an antibiotic first introduced in Italy [87]. It has a powerful action *in vitro* and in animals but in man it is rapidly metabolized by the liver [15 & 69]. It was found necessary to give the drug by intravenous infusion in order to obtain adequate blood levels, a considerable disadvantage. Little toxicity was observed. A modification 'rifampicin' has now been developed which is well absorbed by the mouth [15 & 70] and which may well find a place among the reserve drugs or even ultimately in standard therapy. A single daily dose of 450 mg may be given.

'ISOXYL' (4-4'-diisoamyloxythiocarbanilide)

This drug has been shown experimentally to have antituberculosis activity [36] and was claimed, in combination with streptomycin, to result in as rapid sputum conversion as isoniazid and to prevent streptomycin resistance, though less powerful in other respects [33]. A trial in Hong Kong, in combination with isoniazid, suggested that it was markedly inferior to PAS [71]. It has to be given in large doses, such as 6 g orally per day. Resistant organisms may emerge [51 & 71]. A review of the literature [30] certainly suggests that at present isoxyl has not established a firm place among the reserve drugs.

THE USE OF RESERVE REGIMENS IN PATIENTS WITH ORGANISMS RESISTANT TO STANDARD DRUGS

PATIENTS WITH BACILLI RESISTANT TO ALL THREE STANDARD DRUGS

There is a good deal of evidence to suggest that in such patients a triple drug regimen of reserve drugs has important advantages over one employing 2 drugs [9 & 99]. Excellent results have now been reported using ethionamide, pyrazinamide and cycloserine together, though very great efforts have to be made by the physician to persuade the patient to continue therapy in the face of side effects which are often troublesome, particularly nausea, a 'drugged feeling' and perhaps minor depression. Prothionamide should now be substituted for ethionamide. In those who can be persuaded to persist meticulously there has been a high degree of success [9, 76, 91 & 99]. As already mentioned, primary ethionamide and pyrazinamide resistance may occasionally occur, so there is a case for adding a fourth drug initially; capreomycin (perhaps, with further experience, rifampicin) is the most suitable. In spite of tests showing isoniazid resistance a proportion of the bacterial population may still be sensitive and there may even be some suppressive effect on resistant bacilli, so that isoniazid may be added, at least in the early months. It is best to give the maximum number of drugs initially, when the patient's bacillary population is high and to reduce them later, if one of the drugs is causing troublesome side effects, and when it is safer to do so.

If any of the above drugs are proving intolerable to the patient capreomycin or ethambutol may be substituted, as also if the organisms are known to be resistant to prothionamide or pyrazinamide. Indeed it may be that ethambutol, with further experience, will become a first choice, perhaps instead of cycloserine, the weakest of the trio suggested. It seems possible that oral rifamycin ('rifampicin') may also find a place.

As mentioned above (p. 249), one of the standard drugs may be used initially if there is a possibility that the patient's bacilli may still be sensitive to it; it can be stopped later if tests show this to be incorrect.

PATIENTS WHOSE BACILLI ARE ACTUALLY OR POSSIBLY RESISTANT TO TWO OF THE STANDARD DRUGS

In this case the remaining drug should be combined with pyrazinamide (or ethambutol) and prothionamide. If the remaining drug is PAS it may be advisable to avoid combining this with prothionamide as both may cause gastrointestinal symptoms. Prothionamide is probably more powerful and may be given with cycloserine (or ethambutol) and pyrazinamide.

PATIENTS WHOSE BACILLI ARE RESISTANT TO ONLY ONE OF THE STANDARD DRUGS

If this is PAS, daily streptomycin and isoniazid are indicated; if it is streptomycin, isoniazid may be given with PAS in mild cases, but in severe cases pyrazinamide or ethambutol should be added until the sputum is negative.

PATIENTS WHOSE BACILLI ARE ALSO RESISTANT TO RESERVE DRUGS

Some patients have received successive poor chemotherapy with standard and then with reserve drugs, so that their organisms are resistant to all three standard and most of the reserve medicaments. Fortunately most have not yet received ethambutol, and rifampicin is likely to be on the market before this book is published. We have had a number of successes in such patients (and so far no failures) by combining ethambutol and rifampicin with a 3rd reserve drug still available to the patient. There has been little toxicity.

MAINTENANCE OF CHEMOTHERAPY

For drugs with potentially dangerous side effects, such as pyrazinamide and prothionamide, liver function tests must be carried out meticulously and another drug substituted if there is evidence of important toxicity. Any abnormal reading should be checked by a second test before stopping the drug. On the other hand drugs are too often stopped because of tedious, but usually minor, side effects. It must be remembered that in most of these cases chemotherapy, with all its discomforts, stands between the patient and death. If the doctor is convinced of this he can usually carry the patient with him. Urine tests are available for pyrazinamide, cycloserine, ethionamide and certain other reserve drugs and provide a useful check that outpatients are taking their chemotherapy [40 & 78].

SURGERY

Resection should be considered if the patient's organisms are resistant to 2 or more of the standard drugs, the disease is localized and the respiratory function good, especially when the patient is young. It is wise to postpone operation until the sputum is negative, at least on smear, usually until 2–3 months after beginning treatment. Just in case resistant bacilli may have emerged but have not yet been detected, a further drug should be added over the operation. The resected lung should be cultured and the bacilli tested for resistance to all relevant drugs. In practice most patients with resistant bacilli have disease too extensive for resection.

TREATMENT OF TUBERCULOSIS IN ECONOMICALLY DEVELOPING COUNTRIES

ORGANIZATION

The problem of treating tuberculosis in economically developing countries is dominated by the shortage of money and trained personnel and by the formidable extent of the tuberculosis problem in most of these countries. The money available must therefore be spent to the best advantage. As already explained (p. 184), *BCG* is the most valuable preventive measure. It is important to have a few well informed and enthusiastic *leaders* who can apply the momentum to a treatment organization which is bound to be staffed by people with limited training. High priority must be given to the *provision of drugs* which is the most important single factor for the cure of the individual and the elimination of infectiousness. The available drugs must not be abused by inadequately trained doctors or untrained laymen. It is clearly foolish to spend valuable foreign exchange on importing drugs which are subsequently used only to produce temporary amelioration of symptoms and yet often result in drug resistant tubercle bacilli emerging. Where there are people trained to use the drugs properly only they should be allowed to prescribe them. Drug resistance is reaching such frightening proportions in some of these countries that close control of chemotherapy is essential to prevent a tuberculosis situation which may become unmanageable.

It has been shown that hospital treatment and bed rest are unnecessary (p. 235) so that only a few beds need to be provided for treating emergencies. Almost all patients should be *treated at home*, although in rural areas with widely scattered population it may prove practicable to bring the patients into a centre for a few weeks while chemotherapy is initiated and intensive propaganda is carried out to encourage the patient to persevere with his chemotherapy for the time necessary to prevent relapse. It is important to have efficient *supervisory teams* who will carry out propaganda among the patients and their relatives to ensure continued treatment, test urine for drugs (preferably at random and unexpectedly) to check that the patient is taking them, count pills or cachets for the same purpose and generally look after the patient's morale. In many areas these will have to be members of the ordinary health services who have had some special training in how to deal with tuberculosis. Mostly they will not be doctors but individuals trained *ad hoc* for the purpose. Conscientiousness can often be encouraged by arranging for them to work in pairs.

Diagnosis will mostly be made by means of *sputum smear* and sputum smears should continue to be made once a month while the patient is under chemotherapy. Continuation of positivity should necessitate special care to ensure that the patient is actually taking his drugs, although of course very ill patients may retain a positive smear for a number of months. Persistence of smear positivity beyond 6 months usually means either drug resistance or failure to take the treatment. Smear examination should be carried out by technicians, again preferably working in pairs. Their conscientiousness should be checked either by random sampling or by adding a number of known positives or negatives to the series they are examining. In the first place *culture* and *resistance tests* must be confined to one or more laboratories whose main responsibility is to carry out sample surveys of the prevalence of resistance.

Much can also be achieved by *medical social workers*, recruited and trained locally to deal with the particular local problems. It is surprising how much good can be done by a humane, intelligent person, with experience of other patients' problems and able to give simple advice to new patients. It is useful to have some person with a good personality to whom patients found to be irregular with their chemotherapy may be referred for intensive persuasion and encouragement. The general principle is that nothing should be done by a doctor which can be done by a technician trained for the purpose.

PATIENTS TO BE TREATED

Any patient whose sputum is found to be positive on smear is a candidate for treatment. Nevertheless, mistakes may be made and it is wise to have 2 positive smears before treatment is actually initiated. If an x-ray has been taken it may be difficult to be certain that the disease is tuberculosis unless the sputum is smear positive. If the sputum is negative and the film suggests the diagnosis of tuberculosis it is usually possible, if a film has been taken, to repeat it in 2–3 weeks in order to exclude pneumonia. If there is no change it may have to be assumed, under field conditions, that the disease is tuberculosis and treatment initiated, even though in some cases this may be an error. Tuberculin testing may help. Priority in treatment must always be given to sputum positive patients.

CHEMOTHERAPY

Extensive studies have been made in developing countries in the last 10 years, particularly by units associated with the British Medical Research Council, to find techniques of chemotherapy which are cheap and which can be employed on a mass scale. A considerable measure of success has been achieved but in most series success, even in those who continue treatment, does not reach a higher level than 85 to 90%. This is possibly because most regimens tested have consisted of 2 drugs, usually including isoniazid but excluding streptomycin. The 2 drug combination most extensively tested has been PAS and isoniazid but in recent years it has been shown in East Africa that the right doses of thioacetazone (thiacetazone) and isoniazid, given together in a single daily dose, produce as good results without a forbidding incidence of toxicity [27, 28 & 29] (p. 247). These results have now been confirmed in Madras, India [104], although in that series there were cases of exfoliative dermatitis. Although in India a number of strains of bacilli appear less sensitive than European strains [68] these tend to be of lower virulence and do not appear to influence the results of treatment. Less sensitive strains from Hong Kong have normal virulence and the clinical significance is less certain. Before accepting thioacetazone as standard treatment in a country, a carefully conducted pilot trial should be carried out.

A recent study in East Africa has shown the value of adding an initial period of streptomycin and the value of periodic home visits in the early stages of treatment, in diminishing the default rate in those who did not have an initial period of hospital treatment [29]; the results approach the 100% reached in some centres in developed countries.

Our own view is that the extra cost of giving a highly effective regimen in the early stages of treatment of patients with strongly positive sputum is probably justified by the reduction in the number of failures and in the number of patients who will be left with resistant organisms which they may pass on to others.

INITIAL CHEMOTHERAPY

In most developing countries there is a high rate of primary drug resistance. Often resistance is not truly primary, patients having frequently had chemotherapy previously though they deny it. In addition many patients, especially if selected because the sputum is positive on smear, have extensive disease and large bacterial populations. If further drug resistance is to be avoided it is highly desirable to initiate chemotherapy with 3 drugs. One of the 3 following regimens is suggested. They are given in order of preference.

(1) Streptomycin, PAS and isoniazid daily (p. 236), which has been established as the most successful drug combination. The disadvantage is expense and perhaps the difficulty of arranging for daily streptomycin injections.

(2) Streptomycin 0·75 g daily or, with slight added risk of failure, 3 times weekly, together with isoniazid 300 mg and thioacetazone 150 mg, both in a single dose daily. This has been shown to be highly successful in East Africa but is subject to the problems of toxicity of thioacetazone, and possibly to the diminished sensitivity of organisms, in certain countries (p. 247). It is importantly cheaper than (1).

(3) Streptomycin 1 g together with isoniazid 14 mg/kg, PAS 10 g and pyridoxine 6 mg, all given together, preferably under supervision, twice weekly. The value of twice weekly streptomycin, isoniazid and pyridoxine has been established (p. 237), but this does not allow for the possibility of primary drug resistance, the risks from which might be reduced by including PAS, although no actual

trial has been carried out. It is possible that substituting thioacetazone 150 mg for the PAS might be a cheaper alternative, but whether or not it would be inferior is not known.

One of these regimens should be given until the sputum is negative on smear. If it is economically impossible to do so one of the combinations in the succeeding section may be given but the failure rate will be appreciably higher, especially in those whose organisms are primarily resistant to one of the drugs.

MAINTENANCE CHEMOTHERAPY IN SEVERE CASES, OR INITIAL THERAPY IN THOSE WITH SMEAR NEGATIVE SPUTUM IF THE ABOVE ARE NOT FINANCIALLY POSSIBLE

When the sputum has become negative on smear, one of the following regimens should be substituted. They are given in order of preference.

(1) Streptomycin 1 g with isoniazid 14 mg/kg and pyridoxine 6 mg, all given together, preferably under supervision, twice weekly.

(2) PAS 5 g with isoniazid 0·1 g, both given twice daily.

(3) Isoniazid 0·3 g with thioacetazone 0·15 g, both given once daily in a single dose. This is almost as successful as PAS with isoniazid and very much cheaper. If the sputum is already negative on smear the risks of failure should be small.

Isoniazid alone in a single dose of 0·2 g daily may be substituted for one of the above combinations in the 2nd year of treatment, provided the patient is not left with an open cavity at the end of the first year. It has been shown [34] that the relapse rate is reduced in noncavitated but not in cavitated cases. The latter should continue the first year regimen. If x-rays are not available it might arbitrarily be suggested that isoniazid alone could be given in the 2nd year to patients whose sputum became negative on smear within the first 2 months. Isoniazid alone might also be justifiable in primary tuberculosis in children, if the economic situation were particularly difficult.

DURATION OF CHEMOTHERAPY

In patients whose sputum is negative on smear at the beginning of treatment a total of 12 months' chemotherapy will probably result in only a very small relapse rate. Those whose sputum is positive on smear should continue treatment for 18 months. This period should be sufficient to ensure against relapse in the great majority of cases so that any routine continuation beyond that period would seem economically unjustifiable. A continuation to 2 years may be defended in the occasional very severe case whose sputum has only become very slowly negative, though a greater risk of relapse in such cases has not been directly proved There is no added benefit from continuing treatment into a 3rd year [34].

THE CONTROL OF CHEMOTHERAPY

Except for a few emergencies the great majority of patients will need to be treated at home. The physician will have to discover the best method of ensuring conscientious drug taking in the particular community with which he deals. Right at the beginning it must be explained to the patient and his relatives that he will have to continue the drugs for very many months after he feels perfectly well. If at all possible the doctor should undertake this explanation personally but it should be reinforced by an assistant or assistants with good personality who should be trained to tackle the patient and his relatives in the early impressionable stage of the illness. The same point will have to be continually reiterated perhaps by broadcast talks in waiting rooms, by pamphlets if the patients are literate, etc. Supervised chemotherapy at the clinic is ideal. A careful record of attendances should be kept. If the patient begins to show irregularity then he should be referred for intense personal propaganda. A check on drug taking should be made by repeated urine testing for PAS or isoniazid (p. 243), pill counting and interviews with relatives. The physician should discover what local sanctions may be effective. For instance, in one area of East Africa, where the local Chiefs carried very considerable prestige, these were invited to a special meeting to discuss the problem of tuberculosis and were fully informed about the programme. Subsequently orderlies tested the urine of patients on PAS and isoniazid. Any patient whose urine showed default was reported to the Chief. This proved a very successful sanction and the cure rate was high. In other areas the Chiefs, for various social reasons, may be quite ineffective allies [56]. It has also been shown that home visits within a month of starting chemotherapy appreciably decreased the default rate in East Africa [29].

PATIENTS WHO HAVE HAD PREVIOUS CHEMOTHERAPY

In many areas only a limited range of drugs, indeed only those mentioned above, will be available. It therefore may not be possible to do more than give such a patient all 3 available drugs along the lines already mentioned. Should his organisms be already resistant to more than 1 of them the failure rate will be high but, if no other drugs are possible, it is the best that can be done. If a total of 4 or 5 drugs are available then the chemotherapeutic history, or the known local habits of treatment by unqualified practitioners, may enable a guess to be made as to the probable drug resistance and an appropriate drug combination may be designed, using whatever drugs are to hand. It is impossible to generalize but it may be practicable to make out a general plan to meet the known circumstances in a specific area. Even if isoniazid has been previously used, unless it is known that the patient's organisms are definitely resistant to it, it is worth adding this to any combination in view of the fact that some of the organisms may be sensitive and that this is the most powerful and one of the cheapest drugs.

RETURN TO WORK

Economically it is often essential that a patient who is in any way fit for work shall continue it. Otherwise his family may starve. Provided chemotherapy is prescribed and taken his infectiousness is very rapidly decreased and the risk to others is small.

GENERAL REFERENCES

BARRY V.C., Ed. (1964) *Chemotherapy of Tuberculosis*. London, Butterworths.

FOX W. (1963) Ambulatory chemotherapy in a developing country: clinical and epidemiological studies. *Adv. Tuberc. Res.* **12**, 28.

ROSS J.D. & HORNE N.W. (1969) *Modern Drug Treatment of Tuberculosis*. 4th Edition. London, Chest and Heart Association.

REFERENCES

[1] ADAMS P. & WHITE C. (1965) Isoniazid-induced encephalopathy. *Lancet* **i**, 680.

[2] ANGEL J.H., CHU L.S. & LYONS H.A. (1961) Corticotrophin in the treatment of tuberculosis. A controlled trial. *Arch. intern. Med.* **108**, 353.

[3] BARTMANN K. (1960) Kreuzresistenz zwischen α-Äthylthioisonicotinamid (1314Th) und Thiosemicarbazon (Conteben). *Tuberculosearzt* **14**, 525.

[4] BERTÉ S.J., DIMASE J.D. & CHRISTIANSON C.S. (1964) Isoniazid, para-amino-salicylic acid and streptomycin intolerance in 1774 patients. *Am. Rev. resp. Dis.* **90**, 598.

[5] BIANCIFIORI C. & SEVERI L. (1966) The relation of isoniazid (INH) and allied compounds to carcinogenesis in some species of small laboratory animals: a review. *Br. J. Cancer* **20**, 528.

[6] BIEHL J.P. & SKAVLEM J.H. (1953) Toxicity of isoniazid. *Am. Rev. Tuberc.* **68**, 296.

[7] BIGNALL J.R., CROFTON J. & THOMAS J.A.B. (1951) Effect of streptomycin on vestibular function *Br. med. J.* **i**, 554.

[8] BOBROWITZ I.D. & GOKULANATHAN K.S. (1965) Ethambutol in the retreatment of pulmonary tuberculosis. *Dis. Chest* **48**, 239.

[9] BÖZÖRMÉNYI M., FAUSZT I., BARÁT I. & SCHWEIGER O. (1965) A controlled clinical trial of ethionamide, cycloserine and pyrazinamide in previously treated patients with pulmonary tuberculosis. *Tubercle, Lond.* **46**, 143.

[10] BRAUN P.H. (1965) Results of clinical trial with capreomycin in 31 cases of fresh open lung tuberculosis. In *Proceedings of a Symposium on Capreomycin*, p. 43. London, Lilly.

[11] BRITISH TUBERCULOSIS ASSOCIATION (1961) An investigation of the value of ethionamide with pyrazinamide or cycloserine in the treatment of pulmonary tuberculosis. *Tubercle, Lond.* **42**, 269.

[12] BRITISH TUBERCULOSIS ASSOCIATION (1963) Trial of corticotrophin and prednisone with chemotherapy in pulmonary tuberculosis: a 2 year radiographic follow-up. *Tubercle, Lond.* **44**, 484.

[13] BROWNING R.H. (1961) Further observations

on prednisolone in the treatment of pulmonary tuberculosis. United States Public Health Service Tuberculosis Therapy Trial. *20th Research Conference in Pulmonary Disease, Veterans Adm. med. Bull.*, p. 267.

[14] CASE E.M. (1961) A new method for the detection of para-aminosalicylic acid in urine. *Tubercle, Lond.* **42**, 531.

[15] CLARK J. & WALLACE A. (1967) The susceptibility of mycobacteria to rifamide and rifampicin. *Tubercle, Lond.* **48**, 144.

[16] CORPE R.F. & BLALOCK F.A. (1965) Retreatment of drug resistant tuberculosis at Battey State Hospital. *Dis. Chest* **48**, 305.

[17] CROFTON J. (1958) 'Sputum conversion' and the metabolism of isoniazid. *Am. Rev. Tuberc.* **77**, 869.

[18] CROFTON J. (1960) Tuberculosis undefeated. *Br. med. J.* **ii**, 679.

[19] CROFTON J. (1964) Drug combinations in pulmonary tuberculosis with a brief review of commercial drug combinations. In *Proceedings of IIIrd International Congress on Chemotherapy*. Stuttgart, Georg Thieme Verlag.

[20] CROFTON J.W., FRENCH E.B. & SANDLER A. (1956) Hypokalaemia in tuberculosis. *Tubercle, Lond.* **37**, 81.

[21] DANIELS M. & HILL A.B. (1952) Chemotherapy of pulmonary tuberculosis in young adults. An analysis of the combined results of 3 Medical Research Council trials. *Br. med. J.* **i**, 1162.

[22] DAWSON J.J.Y., DEVADATTA S., FOX W. RADHAKRISHNA S., RAMAKRISHNAN C.V., SOMASUNDARAM P.R., STOTT H., TRIPATHY S.P. & VELU S. (1966) A 5 year study of patients with pulmonary tuberculosis in a concurrent comparison of home and sanatorium treatment for 1 year with isoniazid plus PAS. *Bull. Wld Hlth Org.* **34**, 533.

[23] DEVADATTA S., GANGADHARAM P.R.J., ANDREWS R.H., FOX W., RAMAKRISHNAN C.V., SELKON J.B. & VELU S. (1960) Peripheral neuritis due to isoniazid. *Bull. Wld Hlth Org.* **23**, 587.

[24] DONOMAE I. & YAMAMOTO K. (1966) Clinical evaluation of ethambutol in tuberculosis. *Ann. N.Y. Acad. Sci.* **135**, 849.

[25] DOUGLAS A.C. & HORNE N.W. (1956) Advanced pulmonary tuberculosis with persistent cavitation. Preliminary report on prolonged chemotherapy. *Br. med. J.* **i**, 375.

[26] EAST AFRICAN/BRITISH MEDICAL RESEARCH COUNCIL (1960) Comparative trial of isoniazid alone in low and high dosage and isoniazid plus PAS in the treatment of acute pulmonary tuberculosis in East Africans. *Tubercle, Lond.* **41**, 83.

[27] EAST AFRICAN/BRITISH MEDICAL RESEARCH COUNCIL (1960) Comparative trial of isoniazid in combination with thiacetazone or a substituted diphenylurea (Su 1906) or PAS in the treatment of acute pulmonary tuberculosis in East Africans. *Tubercle, Lond.* **41**, 399.

[28] EAST AFRICAN/BRITISH MEDICAL RESEARCH COUNCIL (1963) Isoniazid with thiacetazone in the treatment of pulmonary tuberculosis in East Africa—Second investigation. *Tubercle, Lond.* **44**, 301.

[29] EAST AFRICAN/BRITISH MEDICAL RESEARCH COUNCIL (1966) Isoniazid with thiacetazone (thioacetazone) in the treatment of pulmonary tuberculosis in East Africa—Third investigation. Effect of an initial streptomycin supplement. *Tubercle, Lond.* **47**, 1.

[30] EDITORIAL (1965) 'Isoxyl.' *Tubercle, Lond.* **46**, 298.

[31] EDITORIAL (1966) Isoniazid: how much a carcinogen? *Lancet* **ii**, 1452.

[32] EMERSON P.A. & KUPER S.W.A. (1964) PAS serum concentrations obtained with an adegrate granule preparation of PAS and isoniazid. *Tubercle, Lond.* **45**, 276.

[33] FAVEZ G. (1961) Essai thérapeutique du 4-4-diisoamyloxythiocarbanilide en tuberculose pulmonaire. *Schweiz Z. Tuberk.* **18**, 379.

[34] FOX W. (1963) Ambulatory chemotherapy in a developing country: clinical and epidemiological studies. *Adv. Tuberc. Res.* **12**, 28.

[35] FOX W. (1964) Realistic chemotherapeutic policies for tuberculosis in the developing countries. *Br. med. J.* **i**, 135.

[36] FREERKSEN E. & ROSENFELD MAGDALENA (1963) Zur experimentellen Wertermittlung des Tuberkulostaticums Isoxyl. *Beitr. Klin. Tuberk.* **127**, 386.

[37] GOW J.G. (1964) The blood levels of isoniazid and PAS when given together as adegrate granules. *Tubercle, Lond.* **45**, 274.

[38] HEINIVAARA O. & PALVA I.P. (1964) Malabsorption of Vitamin B12 during treatment with para-aminosalicylic acid. *Acta med. scand.* **175**, 469.

[39] HIRSCH J.G., SCHAEDLER R.W., PIERCE CYNTHIA H. & SMITH I.M. (1957) A study comparing the effects of bed rest and physical activity on recovery from pulmonary tuberculosis. *Am. Rev. Tuberc.* **75**, 359.

[40] HOBBY GLADYS L. (1964) Practical methods of detecting major antituberculosis drugs in the urine. *Adv. Tuberc. Res.* **13**, 98.

[41] HORNE N.W. (1960) Prednisolone in treatment of pulmonary tuberculosis. A controlled trial. Final report to the Research Committee of the Tuberculosis Society of Scotland. *Br. med. J.* **ii**, 1751.

[42] HORNE N.W. (1965) Chronic pulmonary tuberculosis: present problems. *Proceedings of the XVIIIth International Conference on Tuberculosis*. Excerpta Medica International Congress Series, No. 119, p. 172.

[43] HORNE N.W. (1966) A critical evaluation of

corticosteroids in tuberculosis. *Adv. Tuberc. Res.* **15**, 1.

[44] HORNE N.W. & GRANT I.W.B. (1963) Development of drug resistance to isoniazid during desensitization: A report of 2 cases. *Tubercle, Lond.* **44**, 180.

[45] IBIAPINA A., BETHLEM N., MAGARAO M.F., NEVES A., GOMES O., RIBEIRO DA SILVA NETTO A.F. & SANTIAGO A.C. (1962) O problema da resistencia bacteriana em tuberculose, em particular dos pacientes com B.K. resistentes a 2 ou 4 drogas 'standard'. *Rev. Serv. Nac. Tuberc.* **6**, 45.

[46] INTERNATIONAL UNION AGAINST TUBERCULOSIS (1964) An international investigation of the efficacy of chemotherapy in previously untreated patients with pulmonary tuberculosis. *Bull. internat. Un. Tuberc.* **34**, 80.

[47] JOHNSON J.R., TAYLOR B.C., MORRISSEY J.F., JENNE J.W. & MACDONALD F.M. (1965) Corticosteroids in pulmonary tuberculosis: I. Overall results in Madison-Minneapolis Veterans Administration hospitals steroid study. *Am. Rev. resp. Dis.* **92**, 376.

[48] JOHNSTON R.N., SMITH D.H., RITCHIE R.T. & LOCKHART W. (1964) Prolonged streptomycin and isoniazid for pulmonary tuberculosis. *Br. med. J.* i, 1679.

[49] KALINOWSKI S.Z., LLOYD T.W. & MOYES E.N. (1961) Complications in the chemotherapy of tuberculosis. A review with analysis of the experience of 3148 patients. *Am. Rev. resp. Dis.* **83**, 359.

[50] KARLSON A.G. (1961) Therapeutic effect of ethambutol(Dextro-2,2'-[ethylenediimino]di-l-butanol) on experimental tuberculosis in guinea pigs. *Amer. Rev. resp. Dis.* **84**, 902.

[51] KASS I. (1965) Chemotherapy regimens used in the retreatment of pulmonary tuberculosis. Part II. Observations on the efficacy of combinations of ethambutol, capreomycin and companion drugs, including 4-4-diisoamyl-oxythiosemicarbanilide. *Tubercle, Lond.* **46**, 160.

[52] LEES A.W. (1967) Ethionamide, 500 mg daily, plus isoniazid, 500 mg or 300 mg daily in previously untreated patients with pulmonary tuberculosis. *Am. Rev. resp. Dis.* **95**, 109.

[53] LEFFORD M.J. (1966) The ethionamide sensitivity of British pretreatment strains of *Mycobacterium tuberculosis*. *Tubercle, Lond.* **47**, 198.

[54] LEIBOLD J.E. (1966) The ocular toxicity of ethambutol and its relation to dose. *Ann. N.Y. Acad. Sci.* **135**, 904.

[55] LESTER W., FISCHER D.A. & DYE W.E. (1960) Evaluation of capreomycin and ethambutol in retreatment of pulmonary tuberculosis. *Ann. N.Y. Acad. Sci.* **135**, 890.

[56] MACFADYEN D.M., KLOPPER J.M.L. & SHONGWE S.P.N. (1963) Tuberculosis treatment in the Hlatikulu district of Swaziland. *Tubercle, Lond.* **44**, 82.

[57] MACGREGOR A.G. & SOMNER A.R. (1954) The antithyroid action of para-aminosalicylic acid. *Lancet* ii, 931.

[58] MCLEAN R.L., BURTON Z.C.Jr. & WARD ANNE (1962) Pulmonary function after acute pneumonic tuberculosis. Effects of methyl prednisolone. *Trans. 21st Research Conference in Pulmonary Diseases, Veterans Adm. Med. Bull.*, p. 30.

[59] MARKS J. & TAYLOR J. (1968) A rapid drug-sensitivity test for tubercle bacilli. *Tubercle, Lond.* **49**, 110.

[60] MEDICAL RESEARCH COUNCIL (1948) Streptomycin treatment of pulmonary tuberculosis. *Br. med. J.* ii, 769.

[61] MEDICAL RESEARCH COUNCIL (1952) The treatment of pulmonary tuberculosis with isoniazid. An interim report. *Br. med. J.* ii, 735.

[62] MEDICAL RESEARCH COUNCIL (1953) Isoniazid in combination with streptomycin or with PAS in the treatment of pulmonary tuberculosis. *Br. med. J.* ii, 1005.

[63] MEDICAL RESEARCH COUNCIL (1955) Various combinations of isoniazid with streptomycin or with PAS in the treatment of pulmonary tuberculosis. *Br. med. J.* i, 435.

[64] MEDICAL RESEARCH COUNCIL (1962) Longterm chemotherapy in the treatment of chronic pulmonary tuberculosis with cavitation. *Tubercle, Lond.* **43**, 201.

[65] MEYLER L. (1963) Antibacterial agents. A. Tuberculostatics. In *Side Effects of Drugs as Reported in the Medical Literature of the World*, p. 131. Amsterdam, Excerpta Medica Foundation.

[66] MEYLER L., Ed. (1966) Chemotherapeutic Drugs. A. Tuberculostatics. In *Side Effects of Drugs. Adverse Reactions as Reported in the Medical Literature of the World 1963–1965*, p. 256. Amsterdam, Excerpta Medica Foundation.

[67] MILLER A.B., FOX W. & TALL RUTH (1966) An international cooperative investigation into thiacetazone (thioacetazone) side-effects. *Tubercle, Lond.* **47**, 33.

[68] MITCHISON D.A. & LLOYD JANET (1964) Comparison of sensitivity to thiacetazone of tubercle bacilli from patients in Britain, East Africa, South India and Hong Kong. *Tubercle, Lond.* **45**, 360.

[69] MONALDI V., GURCI G. & NITTI V. (1961) La rifomicina SV: nuovo antibiotico contro il micobatterio della tuberculosi. Nota preliminare. *Arch. tisiol.* **16**, 361.

[70] MONCALVO F., FURESZ S. & MOREO G. Preliminary clinical observations on rifaldazine in pulmonary tuberculosis. To be published.

[71] MOODIE A.S., AQUINAS SISTER M. & FOORD R.D. (1964) Controlled clinical trial of 4-4-

diisoamyloxythiocarbanilide in the treatment of pulmonary tuberculosis. *Tubercle, Lond.* **45**, 192.

[72] NAGESWARA RAO K.V., EIDUS L., JACOB C.V. RADHAKRISHNA S. & TRIPATHY S.P. (1967) Sodium nitroprusside test for the detection of isoniazid and acetylisoniazid in urine. *Tubercle, Lond.* **48**, 45.

[73] NAZARETH O., DEVADATTA S., EVANS C., FOX W., JANARDHANAM B., MENON N.K., RADHAKRISHNA S., RAMAKRISHNAN C.V., STOTT H., TRIPATHY S.P. & VELU S. (1966) A 2-year follow-up of patients with quiescent pulmonary tuberculosis following a year of chemotherapy with an intermittent (twice weekly) regimen of isoniazid plus streptomycin or a daily regimen of isoniazid plus PAS. *Tubercle, Lond.* **47**, 178.

[74] PINES A. (1964) Thiacetazone toxicity in British patients. *Tubercle, Lond.* **45**, 188.

[75] PINES A. (1964) Thiacetazone in British patients. *Tubercle, Lond.* **45**, 392.

[76] PINES A. (1965) Treatment of pulmonary tuberculosis with cultures resistant to 2 or more drugs: a series of 44 patients. *Tubercle, Lond.* **46**, 131.

[77] RALEIGH J.W. (1959) Highlights of the 18th Veterans Administration—Armed Forces Conference on the Chemotherapy of Tuberculosis. *Antibiot. Chemother.* **9**, 238.

[78] RAO K.V.N., EIDUS L., JACOB C.V. & TRIPATHY S.P. (1965) A simple test for detection of pyrazinamide and cycloserine in urine. *Tubercle, Lond.* **46**, 199.

[79] RIST N., GRUMBACH FRANÇOISE & LIBERMANN D. (1959) Experiments on the antituberculous activity of alpha-ethyl-thioisonicotinamide. *Am. Rev. resp. Dis.* **79**, 1.

[80] RIST N. & GRUMBACH FRANÇOISE (1965) Antituberculous activity of capreomycin *in vitro* and in mice and cross-resistance against capreomycin, viomycin and kanamycin in *in vitro* and clinical studies. In *Proceedings of a Symposium on Capreomycin*, p. 19. London, Lilly.

[81] ROSS J.D., HORNE N.W., GRANT I.W.B. & CROFTON J.W. (1958) Hospital treatment of pulmonary tuberculosis. *Br. med. J.* **i**, 237.

[82] RUSSELL W.F.Jr., KASS I., HEATON ANGELINE D., DRESSLER S.H. & MIDDLEBROOK G. (1959) Combined drug treatment in tuberculosis. III. Clinical application of the principles of appropriate and adequate chemotherapy to the treatment of pulmonary tuberculosis. *J. clin. Invest.* **38**, 1366.

[83] SCHWARTZ W.S. (1966) Comparison of ethionamide with isoniazid in original treatment cases of pulmonary tuberculosis. XIV. A report of the Veterans Administrations—Armed Forces comparative study. *Am. Rev. resp. Dis.* **93**, 685.

[84] SCHWARTZ W.S. (1966) Capreomycin compared with streptomycin in original treatment of pulmonary tuberculosis. *Am. Rev. resp. Dis.* **94**, 858.

[85] SCOTTISH THORACIC SOCIETY (1962) High and low isoniazid dosage in the combined drug treatment of pulmonary tuberculosis. *Tubercle, Lond.* **43**, 130.

[86] SCOTTISH THORACIC SOCIETY (1963) A controlled trial of chemotherapy in pulmonary tuberculosis of doubtful activity. 5-year follow-up. *Tubercle, Lond.* **44**, 39.

[87] SENSI P. (1964) A family of new antibiotics, the rifamycins. In *Research Progress in Organic, Biological and Medicinal Chemistry*, Vol. I. Milan, Società Editoriale Farmaceutica.

[88] SIMPSON J.McD. (1961) The detection of urinary para-aminosalicylic acid with 'Phenistix' reagent strips. *Tubercle, Lond.* **42**, 107.

[89] SMITH J.M. & SPRINGETT V.H. (1966) Serum transaminase levels during treatment with isoniazid, streptomycin and PAS. *Tubercle, Lond.* **47**, 245.

[90] SMITH J.M. & ZIRK M.M. (1961) Toxic and allergic drug reactions during the treatment of tuberculosis. *Tubercle, Lond.* **42**, 287.

[91] SOMNER A.R. & BRACE A.A. (1966) Late results of treatment of chronic drug resistant pulmonary tuberculosis. *Br. med. J.* **i**, 775.

[92] SPRIGGS E.A., BRACE, A.A. & JONES MURIEL (1961) Rest and exercise in pulmonary tuberculosis: a controlled study. *Tubercle, Lond.* **42**, 267.

[93] STEINITZ RUTH (1965) Pulmonary tuberculosis and carcinoma of the lung. A survey from two population-based disease registers. *Am. Rev. resp. Dis.* **92**, 758.

[94] STEWART SHEILA M. & CROFTON J.W. (1964) The clinical significance of low degrees of drug resistance in pulmonary tuberculosis. *Am. Rev. resp. Dis.* **89**, 811.

[95] STEWART SHEILA M. & BURNET M. EILEEN (1968) The detection of streptomycin, PAS and isoniazid resistant tubercle bacilli by the direct method. *Tubercle, Lond.* **49**, 217.

[96] THIBIER R., LEPEUPLE A., VIVIEN J.N. & GROSSET J. (1963) Résultats de la chimiothérapie chez 221 malades atteints de tuberculose pulmonaire à bacilles initialement sensibles aux antibiotiques majeurs. *Rev. Tuberc.* **27**, 541.

[97] THOMAS H.E., FORBES D.E.P., LUNTZ G.R.W.N., ROSS H.J.T., MORRISON SMITH J. & SPRINGETT V.H. (1960) 100% sputum conversion in newly diagnosed pulmonary tuberculosis. *Lancet* **ii**, 1185.

[98] THOMAS J.P., BAUGHN C.O., WILKINSON R.G. & SHEPHERD R.G. (1961) A new synthetic compound with antituberculous activity in mice: Ethambutol (Dextro-2,2'-(ethylenediimino)-di-1-butanol). *Am. Rev. resp. Dis.* **83**, 891.

[99] TOUŠEK J., JANČIK E., ZELENKA M. & JANČI-KOVA-MÁKOVÁ (1967) The results of treatment in patients with cultures resistant to strepto-mycin, isoniazid and PAS: a 5 year follow up. Tubercle, Lond. 48, 27.

[100] TUBERCULOSIS CHEMOTHERAPY CENTRE, MAD-RAS (1959) A concurrent comparison of home and sanatorium treatment of pulmonary tuberculosis in South India. Bull. Wld Hlth Org. 21, 51.

[101] TUBERCULOSIS CHEMOTHERAPY CENTRE, MADRAS (1960) A concurrent comparison of isoniazid plus PAS with 3 regimens of isoniazid alone in the domiciliary treatment of pulmonary tuberculosis in South India. Bull. Wld Hlth Org. 23, 535.

[102] TUBERCULOSIS CHEMOTHERAPY CENTRE, MADRAS (1963) The prevention and treatment of isoniazid toxicity in the therapy of pul-monary tuberculosis: 2. An assessment of the prophylactic effect of pyridoxine in low dosage. Bull. Wld Hlth Org. 29, 457.

[103] TUBERCULOSIS CHEMOTHERAPY CENTRE, MADRAS (1964) A concurrent comparison of intermittent (twice weekly) isoniazid plus streptomycin and daily isoniazid plus PAS in the domiciliary treatment of pulmonary tuberculosis. Bull. Wld Hlth Org. 31, 247.

[104] TUBERCULOSIS CHEMOTHERAPY CENTRE, MADRAS (1966) Isoniazid plus thioacetazone compared with 2 regimens of isoniazid plus PAS in the domiciliary treatment of pulmon-ary tuberculosis in South Indian patients. Bull. Wld Hlth Org. 34, 483.

[105] TUBERCULOSIS SOCIETY OF SCOTLAND (1957) Prednisolone in the treatment of pulmonary tuberculosis. A controlled trial. A preliminary report. Br. med. J. ii, 1131.

[106] TUBERCULOSIS SOCIETY OF SCOTLAND (1960) The treatment of pulmonary tuberculosis at work: a controlled trial. Tubercle, Lond. 41, 161.

[107] TURNER P.P. (1959) Simplification of the ferric chloride test for PAS in urine. Br. med. J. i, 1514.

[108] TYRRELL W.F. (1956) Bed rest in treatment of pulmonary tuberculosis. Lancet ii, 821.

[109] UNITED STATES PUBLIC HEALTH SERVICE (1956) A pilot study of cycloserine toxicity. Am. Rev. Tuberc. 74, 196.

[110] UNITED STATES PUBLIC HEALTH SERVICE (1965) Prednisolone in the treatment of pulmonary tuberculosis. Am. Rev. resp. Dis. 91, 329.

[111] VENKATARAMAN P., EIDUS L., RAMACHAND-RAN K. & TRIPATHY S.P. (1965) A comparison of various methods for the detection of isoniazid and its metabolites in urine. Tubercle, Lond. 46, 262.

[112] WIER J.A., TAYLOR R.L. & FRASER R.S. (1957) The ambulatory treatment of patients hos-pitalized with pulmonary tuberculosis. Ann. intern. Med. 47, 762.

[113] WILSON T.M. (1965) Capreomycin in the treatment of tuberculosis. In Proceedings of a Symposium on Capreomycin, p. 6. London, Lilly.

[114] WILSON T.M., LODGE KATHLEEN, HESLING CONSTANCE M. & HUNT L.B. (1966) Etham-butol in the treatment of pulmonary tuber-culosis. Clin. Trials J. 3, 361.

[115] WILSON J.L. & LAMPE W.T. (1964) Single daily dose regimen of isoniazid and PAS in the treatment of pulmonary tuberculosis. Am. Rev. resp. Dis. 89, 756.

[116] WORLD HEALTH ORGANISATION (1967) Tuber-culosis control in Europe. W.H.O. Chronicle 21, 155.

CHAPTER 15

Pulmonary Disease due to "Atypical" Mycobacteria*

It is probable that pulmonary disease due to mycobacteria other than *M. tuberculosis* and *M. bovis* has been occurring for many years though usually mistaken for tuberculosis. More recently the closer study of patients whose bacilli were found resistant to the standard drugs has made physicians realise that some of the resistant strains are not in fact classical tubercle bacilli. Although certain of these strains have now been classified as separate species, others await definition and it is convenient to consider the group as a whole. For the group the terms 'anonymous' and 'unclassified' have also been used, but it has recently been agreed [13] that for the present 'atypical' should be the standard term.

CLASSIFICATION

The classification suggested by Runyon [19] is convenient and generally accepted.

Group I: Photochromogens

Colonies are cream or buff in the dark but produce a yellow or orange pigment on exposure to light. May give rise to a relatively benign type of human pulmonary disease. Usually sensitive to high concentrations of streptomycin, PAS and isoniazid and said always to be sensitive to thiosemicarbazones [14]. It is probable that all strains isolated from man belong to a single species which has now been designated *Mycobacterium kansasii haudoroy* [13]. Capable of producing disease in mice.

Group II: Scotochromogens

Probably a series of different species which

* For a good review of the problem see Lester [13]; for bacteriological reviews see Wilson and Miles [26] and Kovacs [10].

have in common the production of yellow, orange or reddish pigment in the dark. Rarely cause human disease; isolations from man are usually transient. Resistant to all the usual chemotherapeutic agents, including thiosemicarbazones. Nonpathogenic for laboratory animals.

Group III: Nonchromogens

Probably a heterogeneous group. Some strains closely resemble *M. avium*, differing mainly in pathogenicity for birds. Colonies mainly smooth but rough, and even pigmented, variants occur [10]. Most frequent type reported in human disease is so-called 'Battey-bacillus', because first identified in Battey State Hospital, Georgia. In some parts of the world relatively important cause of human pulmonary disease; disseminated disease has been reported. Resistant to most standard and reserve chemotherapeutic drugs. May produce lesions in mice.

Group IV: Rapid growers

A heterogeneous group, including defined species such as *M. smegmatis*, *M. fortuitum*, *M. phlei*, *M. ulcerans* and *M. balnei*. Human disease rare; usually superficial lesions such as skin ulcerations with *M. ulcerans* and *M. balnei*.

All groups, except an occasional strain in Group IV [1], are niacin negative. This is therefore a very useful test in distinguishing these strains from *M. tuberculosis*.

ESTABLISHING SIGNIFICANCE IN HUMAN DISEASE

Little significance attaches to casual isolation. Only if there is repeated isolation in the presence of clinically compatible disease

259

should the organism be regarded as probably of aetiological importance. Differential skin testing with 'tuberculins' derived from the various strains may prove a diagnostic aid [9 & 16].

GEOGRAPHICAL DISTRIBUTION AND SOURCES OF INFECTION

No evidence of man-to-man infection has been found with any of these organisms. It is probable that, at least in the affected areas, atypical mycobacteria are widespread in nature. Organisms of Group III have been isolated from apparently healthy pigs in Australia [21] and in the U.S.A. [20]. They have also been isolated from soil, milk, water and dust [18 & 21]. Chapman et al. [4] have suggested that milk may play a part in dissemination, having isolated strains of Group II, III and IV from many samples of raw milk.

The varying frequency of nonspecific tuberculin reactions in different parts of the world might suggest a varying risk of human disease due to atypical mycobacteria, but the extent of the problem has yet to be defined. In the U.S.A. disease due to the Battey bacillus (Group III) is relatively common in the Southeastern States, diminishing to the North and West. Cases due to Group I have mainly been reported from the Middle West and the South. Groups II and IV seldom give rise to disease. In Britain a number of cases have been reported [8, 14, 15 & 23]. A British Public Health Laboratory Service Report [17], surveying newly diagnosed cases, recorded 1·9% of atypical mycobacteria, mainly Groups I and III. In the British Medical Research Council's national survey of primary drug resistance [12], 1·6% of isolations were atypical mycobacteria, mostly Group I but a few Group III. Disease due to Group III organisms is relatively common in Western Australia and in Queensland [10]. It is probable that it also occurs in other parts of the world with varying frequency. Kovacs suggests that there is a reciprocal distribution of the Battey strain and *M. avium* in nature.

PREDISPOSING FACTORS

The evidence suggests that atypical mycobacteria are of relatively low virulence. Most cases of pulmonary disease have occurred in individuals over the age of 50, usually males and often with evidence of preceding chronic bronchitis, silicosis, coalminers' pneumoconiosis or tuberculosis [2, 8 & 22].

PATHOLOGY

This is very similar to that of chronic indolent pulmonary tuberculosis. In Group I infections acute pneumonic lesions are said to be less common than in tuberculosis and submucosal endobronchitis more so [13].

CLINICAL FEATURES

Pulmonary disease is usually due to Group I or Group III bacilli; it is rare with Group II and virtually unknown with Group IV. The clinical features do not differ importantly from pulmonary tuberculosis except that acute forms are unusual. Chronic fibrocaseous disease with cavitation is common. In Group I suppurative cervical adenitis has been seen in children [3, 7 & 9] and renal lesions have been recorded [13]. In addition to pulmonary lesions involvement of lymph glands may also be found in Group III infections and very occasional cases of dissemination have been recorded, chiefly in children [24 & 25]. In a personal case in a 13 year old girl [20A] there were lesions in mesenteric lymph glands, peritoneum, spleen, liver, lungs and numerous bones. This particular case was probably due to *M. avium*, which is best considered a member of Group III [10].

Group II bacilli may cause suppurative lymphadenitis in children and possibly pulmonary disease very occasionally. Group IV organisms are mainly saprophytes but may cause skin lesions.

TREATMENT

Careful drug resistance tests should be carried out with as many drugs as possible.

Group I cases are said to respond to full doses of streptomycin, PAS and isoniazid, using all 3 drugs. Isoniazid should be used in a dose of at least 8 mg/kg/day and streptomycin in a dose of 0·5–1 g given daily. A success rate as high as 83% has been recorded [13]. Viomycin and ethionamide have been recommended for failures on the standard therapy but careful testing followed by treatment with at least 3 drugs to which the bacilli are sensitive *in vitro* would seem wiser than an empirical attack. Resection may be justified with localized lesions and a high success rate has been reported [11]. Group II infections, if requiring treatment, may respond to erythromycin.

The treatment of Group III infections is unsatisfactory since the organisms are usually resistant to all agents at present available. Corpe [5] reports only 25% showing a favourable response, although Smyth [22] achieved sputum conversion in 41% on medical treatment. When feasible, resection seems to give the best hope of cure [5 & 11]. The outlook in general is much worse than in pulmonary tuberculosis, at least with Group III infections; 28% of Smyth's patients died.

Guy and Chapman [6] and Tinne [23] have reported susceptibility of Group I and III to erythromycin *in vitro*. Tinne states that all 4 groups are susceptible but Guy and Chapman that Group II species are less so. Tinne also reports susceptibility of all groups to chloramphenicol. Keay and Edmond [9] were impressed with the clinical response of 3 cases of cervical lymphadenitis, at least one of them due to *M. avium*, to erythromycin.

REFERENCES

[1] BÖNICKE R. (1965) The occurrence of atypical mycobacteria in the environment of man and animals. *Bull. Int. Un. Tuberc.* 37, 361.

[2] CAMPAGNA M. & GREENBERG H.B. (1964) Epidemiology and clinical course of 41 patients treated for pulmonary disease due to unclassified mycobacteria. *Dis. Chest* 46, 282.

[3] CHAPMAN J.S., Ed. (1960) *The Anonymous Mycobacteria in Human disease.* Springfield, Illinois, Thomas.

[4] CHAPMAN J.S., BERNARD JOANNA S. & SPEIGHT M. (1965) Isolation of mycobacteria from raw milk. *Am. Rev. resp. Dis.* 91, 351.

[5] CORPE R.F. (1964) Clinical aspects, medical and surgical, in the management of Battey-type pulmonary disease. *Dis. Chest* 45, 380.

[6] GUY L. RUTH & CHAPMAN J.S. (1961) Susceptibility *in vitro* of unclassified mycobacteria to commonly used antimicrobials. *Am. Rev. resp. Dis.* 84, 746.

[7] HSU KATHARINE H.K. (1962) Nontuberculous mycobacterial infections in children. A preliminary clinical and epidemiologic study. *J. Pediat.* 60, 705.

[8] KAMAT S.R., ROSSITER C.E. & GILSON J.C. (1961) A retrospective clinical study of pulmonary disease due to 'anonymous mycobacteria' in Wales. *Thorax* 16, 297.

[9] KEAY A.J. & EDMOND ELISABETH (1966) Differential Mantoux testing in the diagnosis of atypical mycobacterial infection in children. *Lancet* ii, 1425.

[10] KOVACS N. (1965) New bacteriological, epidemiological and clinical aspects of 'anonymous' ('atypical') mycobacteria. *Bull. Int. Un. Tuberc.* 37, 351.

[11] LAW S.W. (1965) Surgical treatment of atypical mycobacterial disease. A survey of experience in Veterans Administration hospitals. *Dis. Chest* 47, 296.

[12] LEFFORD M.J., MITCHISON D.A. & TALL RUTH (1966) Bacteriological aspects of the second national survey of primary drug resistance in pulmonary tuberculosis. *Tubercle, Lond.* 47, 109.

[13] LESTER W. (1966) Unclassified mycobacterial diseases. *Ann. Rev. Med.* 17, 351.

[14] MARKS J. & TROLLOPE D.R. (1960) A study of 'anonymous' mycobacteria. I. Introduction; colonial characteristics and morphology; growth rates: biochemical tests. *Tubercle, Lond.* 41, 51.

[15] NASSAU E. & HAMILTON G.M. (1957) Atypical mycobacteria in human pulmonary disease. *Tubercle, Lond.* 38, 387.

[16] PALMER C.E. & LONG MARY W. (1966) Effects of vaccination with atypical mycobacteria on BCG vaccination and tuberculosis. *Am. Rev. resp. Dis.* 94, 553.

[17] PUBLIC HEALTH LABORATORY SERVICE REPORT (1961) Drug resistance in untreated pulmonary tuberculosis in England and Wales during 1960. *Tubercle, Lond.* 42, 308.

[18] RODDA GWENDA M.J. & SINGER E. (1963) Nonspecific sensitization to Old Tuberculin: cultural studies. *Tubercle, Lond.* 44, 251.

[19] RUNYON E.H. (1959) Anonymous mycobacteria in pulmonary disease. *Med. Clin. N. Am.* 43, 272.

[20] SCAMMON LOIS A., PICKETT M.J., FROMAN S. & WILL D.W. (1963) Nonchromogenic acidfast bacilli isolated from tuberculous swine. *Am. Rev. resp. Dis.* 87, 97.

[20A] SCHONELL M.E., CROFTON J.W., STUART A.E. & WALLACE A. (1968) Disseminated infection

with *Mycobacterium avium*. *Tubercle, Lond.*
49, 12.

[21] SMYTH J.T., KOVACS N. & HARRIS W.P. (1964)
Pulmonary disease due to unclassified mycobacteria (Battey type): Report of 14 cases with
histological confirmation. *Tubercle, Lond.*, **45**,
223.

[22] SMYTH J.T. (1965) *Infection of Adults by Anony-
mous Mycobacteria Group III (Battey type) in
Western Australia*. M.D. Thesis: University of
Western Australia.

[23] TINNE J.E. (1965) Human infections with
atypical mycobacteria. *Scot. med. J.* **10**, 413.

[24] VAN DER HOEVEN L.H., RUTTEN F.J. & VAN
DER SAR A. (1958) An unusual acidfast bacillus
causing systemic disease and death in a child.
With special reference to disseminated osteo-
myelitis and intracellular parasitism. *Am. J. clin.
Path.* **29**, 433.

[25] VOLINI F., COLTON ROSEMARY & LESTER W.
(1965) Disseminated infection caused by Battey
type mycobacteria. *Am. J. clin. Path.* **43**,
39.

[26] WILSON G.S. & MILES A.A. (1964) *Topley &
Wilson's Principles of Bacteriology and Immunity*. 5th Edition, p 569. London, Arnold.

CHAPTER 16

Pleurisy and Pleural Effusion

The anatomy of the pleura is outlined in Chapter 1.

PLEURAL PAIN

While the visceral pleura is insensitive to pain the parietal pleura is exquisitely sensitive. Pain of pleural origin is referred to the chest wall and is accurately localized to the site overlying the lesion except when the diaphragmatic pleura is involved. Diaphragmatic pleurisy causes pain in the shoulder or abdomen, the former being referred from the central part of the diaphragm through the phrenic nerve, the latter from the peripheral part through spinal segments whose surface representation overlaps the abdomen. Lesions involving visceral pleura alone (i.e. strictly interlobar lesions) are painless.

PLEURAL FLUID

The visceral and parietal layers of pleura are separated by a thin lubricating film of fluid which is kept in being by a balanced rate of capillary filtration and lymphatic drainage. It is comparable to ordinary interstitial fluid and subject to the same pathological disturbances. The factors which predispose to accumulation of pleural fluid (pleural effusion) are as follows:

GENERAL

Sodium or protein imbalance (e.g. *congestive cardiac failure, nephrotic syndrome*).

LOCAL

(1) Increased pressure in pulmonary capillaries, e.g. *acute left ventricular failure, pulmonary venous thrombosis*.

(2) Increased permeability of pleural capillaries, e.g. *inflammatory* lesions.

(3) Decreased pleural lymphatic drainage,

e.g. *inflammation* or *thickening* of *parietal pleura*; *tumour infiltration* of *lymphatics*.

The *protein content of the fluid* is low in (1), higher in (3) because delayed drainage allows protein entering with the capillary filtrate to accumulate, and highest in (2) because a greatly increased amount of protein escapes from the capillaries in inflamed areas.

Fluid in the pleural space may also be *pus* (empyema, p. 151), *blood* (haemothorax) or *chyle*. Chylothorax (p. 276) is due to involvement of the thoracic or right lymphatic duct by trauma, surgical accident or malignancy. Along with malignant involvement of the pleura, and pulmonary infarction complicated by mitral stenosis or congestive cardiac failure, it is one of the causes of prolonged pleural effusion.

DRY OR FIBRINOUS PLEURISY

Simple bruising of the parietal pleura in traumatic injury to the chest can cause dry or fibrinous pleurisy but with this exception it is almost invariably due to disease in the underlying lung. Rare causes are rheumatoid arthritis and systemic lupus erythematosus; more commonly these are associated with pleural effusion.

The first mild inflammatory changes in the visceral pleura covering the lung lesion are painless, but when the adjacent parietal pleura becomes congested and swollen every movement of that part of the chest wall results in the classical symptom of stabbing pain. Ordinary respiration is often restricted because of the pain; deep breathing and coughing always make it worse, and it is sometimes brought on by twisting and bending movements. In pneumonia the combination of increased rate of respiration and pleuritic pain reduces respiratory effort to a succession of short, grunting inspirations. The commoner causes of fibrinous pleurisy are *pneumonia* (p. 119) (in the pneumococcal variety pleurisy is almost a constant feature), *pulmonary infarction* (p. 460), *bronchial carcinoma* (p. 525), *lung abscess* (p. 158) and, with diminishing frequency, *pulmonary tuberculosis* (p. 270). A history of *recurrent dry pleurisy* on the same side suggests a diagnosis of bronchiectasis (p. 353).

Epidemic myalgia ('Bornholm' disease) due to infection by Coxsackie B virus is sometimes associated with dry pleurisy, rarely with small pleural effusions. This illness, which is of all degrees of severity, occurs mostly in late summer and autumn, sometimes in epidemics. Any age group may be affected but the condition is commoner in young adults and children. In very young children Coxsackie B virus infection may result in neurological as well as respiratory symptoms and some may present with convulsions [46]. Neurological symptoms are rare in the adult. Findlay and Howard [36] showed that the incubation period was 2 days in experimental transmission but clinical studies have shown longer incubation periods of 3–5 days. The illness commonly begins with fever and upper respiratory symptoms such as sore throat or coryza, which may virtually subside only to return with increased severity. The classical stabbing pain then develops in the chest or upper abdomen and movement of the thorax, including respiration, evokes extreme pain. The chest muscles are tender to palpation on the affected side and true pleurisy further limits respiration; pain in the shoulder from diaphragmatic pleurisy is common. Cough is not a feature. Sometimes the pain of the myositis and pleurisy is so severe as to preclude even attempts at eating during the acute phase. The chest radiograph is usually normal but sometimes blunting of the costophrenic angle may occur. Fever is not invariable and when present is usually low grade; the ESR is normal or only very slightly raised. Examination of the peripheral blood is not helpful.

The illness usually lasts about a week in the acute phase with chest pain rapidly diminishing thereafter. Some cases may be complicated by pericarditis [43].

The diagnosis may be made by virus isolation from throat washings or stools during the acute phase or by the demonstration in paired sera of a rising titre of complement-fixing and neutralizing antibodies to one of the Coxsackie B viruses.

There is no specific treatment. The severity of the chest pain frequently demands analgesics.

In a case with clinical evidence of one or other of the above diseases the diagnosis of fibrinous pleurisy is formally established by the finding of *pleural friction* on physical examination. The distinction from fine crepitations is not easy but it is probably permissible to interpret dubious sounds as due to pleural friction if the patient also has characteristic pleural pain. In *diaphragmatic fibrinous pleurisy* no friction sounds are heard and the pain may be felt in the shoulder or abdomen. The pleuritic quality of the pain and the relative immobility of the chest on the affected side owing to the reduced diaphragmatic movement help to establish the diagnosis.

Fibrinous pleurisy usually resolves or progresses to pleural effusion but occasionally it persists for a long period or indefinitely as a friction sound, like creaking of leather, heard on auscultation or sometimes palpable, but unaccompanied by pleural pain. The common finding of pleural adhesions at autopsy or thoracotomy in cases without a history of pleurisy suggests that fibrinous pleurisy is much commoner than clinical experience would suggest.

DIAGNOSIS

Dry pleurisy may have to be distinguished from a variety of other causes of chest pain, including *intercostal myalgia, herpes zoster* before the rash has become evident, *rib fracture* and *costochondritis* (p. 624). In none of these is pleural friction present. Sometimes the pain of *acute upper abdominal disease* may simulate dry pleurisy.

TREATMENT

This is essentially treatment of the primary lesion although pleurisy *per se* may require special consideration with regard to relief of pain. Local heat from a hot water bottle, kaolin poultice or electric pad, and morphine, lesser analgesics or splinting of the chest with firm strapping are measures which can be adopted to relieve the pain but due regard must be paid to the underlying lung condition. In chronic lung disease, for example, the danger of depression of respiration by morphine and the retention of secretions by immobilizing the chest would have to be taken into account. The correct position of the patient in bed is the one which is most comfortable for breathing and most patients will find it out for themselves. It will be found that many choose to lie on the affected side.

PLEURAL EFFUSION

DEFINITION

A pleural effusion is an accumulation of fluid in the pleural space as a result of excessive transudation or exudation from the pleural surfaces. Pleural effusion is a sign of disease and not a diagnosis in itself.

DYNAMICS OF THE PLEURAL FLUID

The pressure variation within the pleural space in health and in disease is discussed in Chapter 1. The pleural fluid is also in a highly dynamic state, being constantly absorbed and replenished. In the normal resting subject the sum total of the processes of formation and removal of pleural fluid is only a few millilitres, sufficient to wet the pleural surfaces. Studies in animals [24 & 27] and in man [101] have shown that the movement of fluid into and out of the pleural space is accelerated by increased lung movements. Furthermore, there is a differential turnover of the constituents of the pleural fluid. Thus between 30 and 75% of the water content is exchanged each hour [22]. Protein is absorbed from the pleural space by the lymphatics only (principally those of the lower mediastinal pleura) [14] and the rate of turnover is much less than that of water and electrolytes. Curtice and Simmonds [26] showed that protein injected into the pleural cavity of cats can be almost entirely recovered from the lymphatics,

75% of which drain into the right lymphatic duct and 25% into the thoracic duct. The costal, diaphragmatic and visceral pleura appear to absorb protein poorly [27].

Burke [14] showed that particulate matter introduced into the pleural space of guinea pigs drains to the parasternal and para-aortic lymph nodes. This transport is increased by exercise. Using graphite Lemon and Higgins [56] showed that when the lymph nodes became choked the flow of particulate matter ceased. Fluid absorption was also decreased and fluid tended to accumulate in the pleural space.

Leckie and Tothill [55] have studied the rate of albumin turnover in various types of pleural effusion. The colloid osmotic pressure of plasma is mainly related to the albumin concentration and the transcapillary exchange rates of albumin and globulin have a constant relationship, similar to that of their diffusion coefficients. Thus investigation of the movement of albumin reflects the total pattern of protein kinetics in effusions. Using radio-iodinated human serum albumin injected into the effusions these workers showed that the rate of protein loss from the pleural space was reduced in all conditions other than those which primarily involved the visceral pleura. Inflammatory pleural effusion, from whatever cause, resulted as much from decreased pleural absorption of protein as from increased vascular leak. Tumour involving the parietal pleura obstructed drainage of protein. Corticosteroids were shown to reduce the albumin turnover and it was suggested that this resulted from reduction in permeability of the blood capillaries and probably also of the lymphatic capillaries. They estimated that the albumin turnover through a pleural cavity normally exceeds 1 g per 24 hours.

DETECTION OF PLEURAL EFFUSION

Amounts less than 100 ml are probably undetectable by any means. 100–300 ml will probably, but not certainly, be detected in chest radiographs, while for an effusion to be apparent on clinical examination it must have a volume of at least 500 ml.

PHYSICAL FINDINGS

Pleural effusion may be (a) in the general pleural space, (b) loculated, in the general pleural space or interlobar, or (c) infrapulmonary, simulating a raised hemidiaphragm. If the effusion is in the general pleural space and is sufficiently large the physical signs are characteristic. These are: (a) restriction of respiratory movement on the affected side, (b) marked (stony) dullness on percussion, (c) diminution or absence of breath sounds and of vocal resonance and fremitus. At the upper level of dullness, which sweeps upwards towards the axilla, bronchial breathing (conducted through the relaxed lung) may be heard.

With small effusions the signs are best elicited at the base posteriorly. Large effusions will displace the trachea and apex beat to the opposite side.

Effusions loculated within the fissures may not be detectable on physical examination if there is no associated effusion in the general pleural space. Infrapulmonary effusions may be clinically indistinguishable from a fixed elevation of the hemidiaphragm.

RADIOGRAPHIC APPEARANCES

Pleural effusions usually present as dense, homogeneous opacities. A very small effusion may only be represented by obliteration of a costophrenic angle. A moderate-sized effusion appears as a triangular lateral opacity with the base obscuring the hemidiaphragm and with a curved upper border, concave medially, extending upwards in the axilla. The upper border may be obscured by an underlying parenchymal lesion or an interlobar collection of fluid. The latter may sometimes be confused with a pulmonary mass ('vanishing pulmonary tumour'). A large effusion may obscure the whole hemithorax and displace the heart and trachea to the opposite side.

Davis and his colleagues have produced physical, experimental and clinical evidence to suggest that the upper limit of a free pleural effusion is not S-shaped but is, in fact, horizontal. The level of this limit is indicated approximately by the highest point of dullness to percussion and by the apex of the axillary opacity in the PA film. The curve upwards in the x-ray occurs because the greatest depth of fluid is in the axilla. These workers suggested that the x-ray signs of fluid are misleading and that clinical signs are more accurate in determining the extent of an effusion since successful aspiration may be achieved at a level above the x-ray shadow of fluid [28].

A moderate-sized or small pleural effusion if not loculated and not too viscid can be observed to alter in shape and position when x-rays are taken with the patient in different positions. The effusion may be distinguished from pleural thickening by the simple expedient of comparing the chest x-ray taken with the patient upright with that taken in the lateral recumbent position. Fluid is not usually truly encysted in infrapulmonary effusion and if the patient lies on the affected side for some minutes before the film is taken it will usually be found that a certain amount of the fluid will gravitate so as to lie along the lateral chest wall. With a truly encysted right infrapulmonary effusion it may be necessary to induce a pneumoperitoneum to distinguish it from a raised hemidiaphragm. On the left side the distinction may be made by observing the position of the stomach gas bubble, created artificially if necessary by giving sodium bicarbonate.

Occasionally a thin ('lamellar') effusion at the periphery of the hemithorax may extend from the costophrenic angle to the apex.

A very thin layer of fluid in the general pleural space may not be recognizable in the lateral chest radiograph. The lateral film is, of course, essential for accurate localization of interlobar effusion. The rounded outlines of an interlobar effusion usually indicate the diagnosis. Commonly there is also evidence of pleural reaction in the general pleural space. On rare occasions bronchography may be required to distinguish a loculated effusion in the lower part of the right oblique fissure from a consolidated right middle lobe.

TRANSUDATES AND EXUDATES

It is convenient and clinically useful to classify pleural effusions as transudates or exudates.

The distinction between them is made chiefly on the protein content, transudates containing less than and exudates more than 3g% [103]. The specific gravity of the fluid is another but less reliable distinguishing feature, transudates having a specific gravity of less than 1.015 while exudates usually exceed this figure. In general the 2 types of fluid possess different physical properties but overlapping tends to blur the contrast between them. In practice, therefore, neither protein content nor specific gravity is relied upon to make differentiation, which is usually not difficult on clinical grounds.

Pleural transudates are clear or faintly yellow watery fluids; exudates are dark yellow or amber, slightly cloudy fluids which often clot on standing in a specimen jar. Transudates are often bilateral; exudates are usually unilateral. A collection of transudate fluid in the pleural cavity is called a *hydrothorax*.

PRINCIPAL CAUSES OF HYDROTHORAX

(1) *Congestive cardiac failure* is by far the commonest cause. The effusion is unilateral to begin with, more often on the right side than the left, and it becomes bilateral if the heart failure worsens. The diagnosis will be suggested by the usual evidence of cardiac disease but in a doubtful case the cardiac origin of an effusion can be accepted if the effusion is controlled by diuretic treatment.

(2) *Hypoproteinaemia* leading to pathological increase in tissue fluid may result in peripheral oedema, ascites and pleural transudates. In Britain the nephrotic syndrome is the commonest cause of pleural effusions in this category. Hepatic cirrhosis and severe anaemia are other causes.

(3) *Constrictive pericarditis.* Hydrothorax results from the combined effect of congestive cardiac failure and hypoproteinaemia due to liver damage from congestive cardiac failure. Gross congestive failure with a radiographically small heart should suggest the diagnosis. Calcification of the pericardium may not be seen in the PA film and a lateral view is essential.

(4) *Meigs' syndrome* [65]. Some ovarian tumours, usually benign fibromata but occasionally malignant tumours of various types, give rise to ascites and hydrothorax which disappear if the tumour is removed. The hydrothorax is usually on the right side but may be bilateral. No satisfactory explanation of the phenomenon is yet available. Some cases of hydrothorax complicating ascites have been shown to be due to a defect in the diaphragm [32, 38 & 42]. This may explain the hydrothorax in some cases of Meigs' syndrome but proof is lacking.

(5) *Myxoedema* may occasionally give rise to pleural effusion as well as pericardial effusion and ascites, all evidently due to endocrine disturbance since they are resistant to digitalis and diuretics but disappear after treatment with thyroxin.

PLEURAL EXUDATES

In Britain the commonest causes of pleural exudates are *bacterial pneumonias*, *pulmonary infarction* and *secondary pleural malignancy*. *Tuberculosis* is less frequent but is still common in some countries. *Subphrenic infections*, *collagen disorders* and *fungal infections* are relatively uncommon. Among the unusual causes may be mentioned:

(1) The *postmyocardial infarction syndrome* occurs in a small proportion of cases days or weeks after the acute incident and consists of fever, pericarditis and sometimes pneumonia and pleural effusion with the characteristics of an exudate [30]. It is said to occur in 3–4% of myocardial infarctions and to respond to corticosteroid therapy. It may be difficult to distinguish from pulmonary infarction complicating myocardial infarction.

(2) *Acute pancreatitis.* Absorption of peritoneal fluid from the upper abdomen may result in a pleural effusion, generally on the left side, often bloodstained and distinguished from all other pleural effusions by its high content of amylase. The amylase concentration in the pleural fluid is higher than the level in the serum [76].

In a study of the pleuropulmonary complications of pancreatitis Kaye [52] found radiographic abnormality in 55% of 58 cases. He discusses the possible mechanisms of the pleural effusion complicating pancreatitis and lists the following, any of which may occur in individual cases:

(a) Direct contact of pancreatic enzymes with the diaphragm.

(b) Haematogenous carriage of pancreatic enzymes to the pleura.

(c) Direct movement of fluid from abdomen to thorax by (1) natural hiatus; (2) diaphragmatic perforation by a pancreatic pseudocyst; (3) transfer of fluid into pleural cavity by transdiaphragmatic lymphatics.

(3) *Primary pleural tumour* is an uncommon but important cause of pleural exudation. All primary pleural tumours are rare but malignant primary tumours of the pleura are apparently increasing with the increasing opportunities for exposure to asbestos dust (p. 484). Pleural effusion accompanying a primary pleural tumour is generally a sign that the tumour is malignant.

Diffuse malignant mesothelioma characteristically gives rise to a massive bloodstained effusion. Clinical features include cough, chest pain, dyspnoea and a bulging hemithorax which moves poorly or not at all. There may be muscle wasting and sensory loss over the chest wall. The diagnosis may be made by cytological examination of the pleural aspirate or needle biopsy of the pleura. Sometimes it is only made at thoracotomy or even at autopsy. The tumour may spread to mediastinal and axillary lymph glands. Only rarely does it metastasize more widely [62]. In some cases a tumour of the same type is present in the peritoneal cavity as well.

Pleural effusion occasionally complicates *localized benign mesothelioma* of the pleura [21 & 48].

POSTPNEUMONIC PLEURAL EFFUSION

The pleural reaction which so frequently accompanies bacterial pneumonias may progress to pleural effusion and this complication should always be suspected if fever persists despite appropriate chemotherapy. Usually there will be recognizable preceding features of pneumonia. The white cell count is usually raised somewhat but because it usually sits on the fence it is seldom helpful in differential diagnosis unless the effusion has become an empyema.

In postpneumonic effusions the fluid is amber or straw-coloured, possibly turbid and on microscopic examination the predominant cell is the neutrophil polymorph. The patient is nearly always having antibiotic treatment when the effusion develops and it is not common for the causal organism to be cultured from the fluid. Nevertheless these effusions must always be regarded as potential empyemata and should be aspirated to dryness at once. The temperature rapidly returns to normal after removal of the fluid, which is almost always achieved with a single aspiration. If the organism is resistant to the antibiotic used (e.g. *Staph. pyogenes*) the effusion soon becomes purulent (empyema), bacteriological examination is positive and the white cell count rises to a higher level.

Bronchial neoplasm may be complicated by postpneumonic pleural effusion in conjunction with a pneumonic lesion distal to the site of obstruction. Failure of the effusion to recur after aspiration suggests that it is of the simple, postpneumonic serous variety and not due to malignant invasion of the pleura.

Pleural effusion only rarely complicates *viral pneumonia*. Usually it is small and often undetectable clinically [96]. Effusions have been described in association with influenza A infection [95], ornithosis [95] and Coxsackie B5 infection [43]. Although pleural effusion may, therefore, complicate viral pneumonia in a small percentage of cases the diagnosis can only be made comfortably if the usual virological studies corroborate recent infection.

PLEURAL EFFUSION COMPLICATING PULMONARY INFARCTION

Pleural involvement in pulmonary infarction is almost invariable and pleuritic pain is the most constant clinical feature. Pleural effusion commonly develops and in some cases may be the only radiographic abnormality. The clinical and radiographic features and the frequent difficulty in diagnosis are discussed elsewhere (p. 461). The effusion is usually small to moderate in size, and self-limiting.

Fluid may be bloodstained but more commonly it is clear and yellow in colour. Aspiration is seldom required and it is rare for more than a single withdrawal to be necessary, unless the pulmonary infarction complicates mitral stenosis or congestive cardiac failure in which case the effusion may be persistent or recurrent.

The cytology is usually pleomorphic with eosinophils (p. 280) constituting from 5 to 50% of the cells. Spriggs [86] showed that mesothelial cells are frequently present, sometimes constituting 20–30% of the total cell count. The diagnosis of effusion complicating pulmonary infarction depends, however, on the features suggesting the primary disease and not on the characteristics of the effusion or the pleural biopsy.

MALIGNANT PLEURAL EFFUSION

(A) *Primary pleural neoplasm* is rare (p. 268).

(B) *Secondary pleural malignancy* is common.

(1) *Bronchial carcinoma* (p. 517) is the commonest cause of malignant pleural effusion. In most cases the presence of a bronchial carcinoma will have been established already on clinical or other grounds but sometimes the effusion is the first manifestation. If, as often happens, it develops rapidly over several days, increasing dyspnoea will be a prominent feature, but in cases in which the effusion develops gradually it may have scarcely any effect on the symptoms already present.

(2) *Metastatic pleural tumours* derived from *extrathoracic primary growth* (of *breast, pancreas, uterus, stomach,* etc.) often cause pleural effusions which may be bilateral. The primary tumour may be obvious when the effusion develops, or it may be so small as to escape detection, or in other cases (particularly in breast carcinoma) it may have been removed years ago and the onset of pleural effusion brings to an end a long period of well-being and apparent cure. Chest radiographs taken after aspiration of the fluid may reveal tumour metastases in the lung which had previously been obscured by the opacity due to the fluid.

(3) *Lymphatic carcinomatosis.* Bilateral effusions in cases of lymphatic carcinomatosis increase still more the unremitting, progressive dyspnoea due to the 'stiff lung' effect of widespread lymphatic permeation by tumour.

(4) *Lymphomata.* Hodgkin's disease, lymphosarcoma and certain other lymphomata cause pleural effusion, often bilateral, as a result of metastatic involvement of pleura, lung or lymph nodes. The diagnosis will often be assisted by radiographic evidence of enlarged mediastinal lymph nodes and by the other features of the disease such as generalized lymphadenopathy, hepatomegaly, splenomegaly, fever and anaemia.

Malignant pleural effusions have 2 special characteristics: the fluid is often *bloodstained* and it *recurs promptly after aspiration*. The second feature is seldom lacking, but the fluid may be clear or yellowish rather than bloodstained. Cytological examination of the fluid may show malignant cells, in clumps or singly. The absence of malignant cells does not exclude malignancy since tumours do not always shed their cells. It is important to recognize that the value of the method is directly related to the training and experience of the pathologist who examines the fluid.

The cause of the effusion is exudation from tumour cells, or obstruction of venous or lymphatic drainage, or both. Large effusions cause severe dyspnoea and may prove fatal from respiratory failure. Repeated pleural aspirations may sometimes result in the manifestations of protein depletion if the patient survives long enough. Always there are the discomforts of troublesome cough and chest pain.

TREATMENT OF MALIGNANT PLEURAL EFFUSION

While it is true that malignant effusions due to metastases from hormone-sensitive breast carcinoma may be controlled, sometimes for long periods, by appropriate treatment (oestrogens, corticosteroids, etc.) and that the occasional mesothelioma may be resected *in toto* there is no gainsaying the fact that the treatment of malignant pleural effusions is purely palliative. The best that can be hoped for in the vast majority of cases is a reduction in the rate of reaccumulation of fluid and this is sometimes achieved for a few months by the instillation of nitrogen mustard (20 mg) into the pleural space. The other alternatives, including thiotepa and radioisotopes such as gold-198 or yttrium-90, give no better results. In some cases of advanced ovarian carcinoma oral chlorambucil is worth a trial [102] and we have had one recent case in which this treatment was brilliantly successful. In the common context of malignant pleural effusion complicating a bronchial carcinoma our usual practice is to instil nitrogen mustard after initial aspiration and to give prednisolone, which has been shown experimentally to reduce the reaccumulation of the effusion [55]. The eutonic effect of prednisolone is also beneficial.

Attempts to secure pleurodesis and so prevent fluid reaccumulation have been advocated and even pleurectomy has been used [49] although most clinicians would feel that this is unnecessarily radical and unwarranted. A simple, quick and apparently effective method of pleurodesis using talc in an aerosol has been described by Adler and Tappole [1]. All the fluid is aspirated from the pleural space through a cannula and the small catheter of the aerosol unit is then inserted until it just projects into the space. By moving the tip of the catheter in several directions as the aerosol is sprayed the talc is diffused over the pleural surfaces. The procedure is stated to take less than $\frac{1}{2}$ minute. A large drainage tube is left *in situ* for 2–3 days to ensure that the pleural space is kept free from fluid during the process of pleurodesis. This simple technique merits further trial [31].

TUBERCULOUS PLEURAL EFFUSION

The cause of the effusion is an exudative inflammation in the pleura occurring when tuberculous material enters the pleural space of an individual who has become hypersensitive to tuberculoprotein from previous infection. The demonstration that effusion could occur by the introduction of dead tubercle bacilli into the pleural space of guinea pigs already hypersensitive to tuberculin supported the concept of a mainly allergic response, but the recent techniques of pleural biopsy have

shown that actual infection with miliary tubercles of the pleura is usually present. Thus the allergic component in tuberculous pleural effusion is probably no more important than in tuberculous lesions elsewhere.

In the past, tuberculous pleural effusion most often followed rupture of a caseous primary focus or a caseous lymph node into the pleural space with subsequent seeding of tubercles on the pleura. The condition was uncommon below the age of 5 after which the frequency increased to reach a peak in adolescence. Pleural effusion complicating primary tuberculosis before adolescence is usually transient. The classical tuberculous pleural effusion was seen in adolescents and young adults.

With the decline of natural primary infection in Britain pleural effusion has become much less common. Pleural effusion now occurs most often in older patients who may or may not have scarred lung lesions. At one time the effusion was a common complication of pneumothorax therapy. Bilateral effusions may be due to miliary tuberculosis which is now seen more commonly in the elderly.

Primary tuberculosis with pleural effusion is still seen on rare occasions and it should be remembered that a history of successful BCG vaccination, although it makes the diagnosis unlikely, does not exclude it.

Effusions nearly always occur on the same side as the primary focus and enlarged tracheobronchial lymph nodes [92 & 59]. In these cases effusion is fairly certainly due to direct extension to the pleura from a subpleural primary focus or from caseous lymph nodes [33].

Two forms of tuberculous pleurisy have been described by Auerbach [6]:

(a) Caseous tuberculosis of pleura. Fibrin is first deposited over the epithelial lining and tuberculous granulation tissue with caseation extends from the subepithelial area to involve the pleura and the fibrinous exudate. Almost complete healing may occur but sometimes organization results in fibrothorax and perhaps calcification.

(b) Miliary tuberculosis of pleura. The

pleural surfaces are studded with small tuberculous granulomata which develop beneath the pleural membrane and which provoke localized fibrinous exudate. Complete healing usually occurs with chemotherapy.

TUBERCULOUS PLEURAL EFFUSION COMPLICATING PRIMARY TUBERCULOSIS

In the High Wood survey [11] 5% of 317 children of all ages admitted with simple primary pulmonary tuberculosis developed an effusion. Pleural effusion was uncommon below the age of 5. In the over 5 group there were 13 cases of effusion out of 183 (7%). 10% of these were males and 4% females. The writers indicated that these figures did not necessarily represent the true risk of pleural effusion occurring in children undergoing primary infection. The incidence of pleural effusion may be higher among children showing radiographic abnormality due to primary infection than among those who do not and the High Wood study was concerned with those who had radiographic abnormality. Also there was an average waiting period of over 3 months before children with simple primary tuberculosis were admitted and a number of cases of pleural effusion must have developed during the waiting period and would then be classified as pleural effusion on admission and not as simple primary tuberculosis. Nevertheless, these 2 factors might have counterbalanced each other to some extent and the report suggested that a figure of 7% was a reasonable estimate of the risk of pleural effusion occuring in children over 5 with simple primary tuberculosis. It was shown that in the few cases under 5 the sex incidence was almost equal but that boys predominated in the over 5 age group.

Pleural effusion has a fairly constant time relationship to primary infection, most cases occurring 3–6 months after infection [98 & 99] or at most within 1 year [93]. Occasionally the initial primary infection goes unrecognized and by the time effusion is diagnosed the lung fields are clear. This type of effusion was previously referred to as 'idiopathic'. Like primary infection the effusion is rather more common on the right side. In the High Wood survey 119 were right-sided, 98 left-sided and 9 bilateral. The right-sided predominance was also noted by Landau [54] and Thompson [92].

In most children the onset of effusion was acute and in the majority accompanied by characteristic pleural pain. When pain was absent the clinical picture was that of a febrile illness with malaise, anorexia and general debility. Rarely, a large effusion developed silently while the child continued normal activities. Untreated, the fever usually lasted about 3 weeks; the ESR usually remained high much longer and sometimes remained elevated for a few months.

The amount of fluid was variable but most often only one third to one half of the lung field was covered by fluid [11]. The rate of absorption was also variable but in general took 3 or 4 months in the days before effective antituberculosis chemotherapy. Commonly only obliteration of the costophrenic angle was the sole evidence of recent effusion and sometimes even this disappeared completely. Frequently there was radiographic evidence of primary pulmonary tuberculosis in the form of enlarged hilar glands, a primary complex or a segmental lesion or all three. The primary lesions may be obscured by the fluid initially and only become visible after spontaneous absorption or aspiration. In the majority of cases the only residuum several years later was obliteration of the costophrenic angle but in a few there was pleural thickening with contraction of the affected hemithorax. Occasionally pleural calcification was evident. The underlying primary lesions behaved in the ordinary way, the primary complex resolving or becoming calcified, and segmental lesions usually showing contraction and subsequent re-aeration.

The diagnosis of primary tuberculous pleural effusion in the child is usually easy. Pleural effusion occurring in a tuberculin positive child should be regarded as tuberculous until proved otherwise. As with other forms of tuberculous pleural effusion the lymphocyte is the predominant cell. Pleural biopsy is commonly positive and culture of sufficiently large amounts of pleural aspirate yields tubercle bacilli in a high proportion of cases.

CLASSICAL ADOLESCENT PLEURAL EFFUSION

This is now quite uncommon in Britain since the introduction of widespread BCG vaccination and because of the reduced pool of tuberculous infection. In the classical case in an adolescent or young adult the illness usually begins with pleuritic pain and fever, sometimes after a few weeks of general ill health, but occasionally slowly progressive dyspnoea is the only manifestation of the disease. Pleural friction may be heard while the effusion is still small, and in some cases recurrent episodes of dry pleurisy precede the onset of pleurisy with effusion. Patients with recurrent pleuritic pain should always be watched for at least 6 months to make sure that the pleurisy is not tuberculous. Patients who are left untreated because of an error in diagnosis may lose their symptoms in a few weeks and all clinical and radiographic disease in a few months, but 20–30% of them will develop pulmonary tuberculosis within 5 years. It is clearly important to establish the diagnosis and to start antituberculosis chemotherapy at an early stage.

Aside from the significance of untreated tuberculous pleural effusion in relation to the subsequent development of chronic pulmonary tuberculosis, the condition is a potentially serious one because of the tendency to the development of pleural fibrosis and pleural adhesion resulting in a restrictive pattern of ventilatory dysfunction (p. 51) (fig. 16.1). This is more likely to occur in the adolescent or the adult than in the child. The early treatment of the condition will prevent these sequelae.

Laboratory aids to diagnosis include the white blood count, the tuberculin test, examination of the pleural fluid and pleural biopsy. In a typical case the white cell count is normal, the tuberculin reaction strongly positive and the pleural fluid contains lymphocytes. Films from the centrifuged deposit may demonstrate the tubercle bacillus but only on rare occasions. Tubercle bacilli may sometimes be isolated by culture of the fluid and the more that is sent for examination the higher the success rate. Needle biopsy of the parietal pleura provides histological evidence of tuberculous granulation tissue in 70–80% and should always be done if the diagnosis is in doubt. The tuberculin test has a quantitative

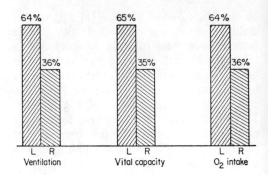

FIG. 16.1. Unilateral pleural thickening. Results of bronchospirometry.

value in that failure to react to 1:1000 Old Tuberculin virtually excludes tuberculosis. In this type of pleural effusion the lung fields are commonly clear.

TUBERCULOUS PLEURAL EFFUSION COMPLICATING ESTABLISHED PULMONARY OR EXTRAPULMONARY TUBERCULOSIS

Rupture of a cavity results in pneumothorax and effusion which may proceed to empyema. Underlying pulmonary disease may be clearly demonstrated, with cavities and positive sputum. Sometimes, however, the lung lesions may appear radiographically inactive. When *pneumothorax* was commonly employed in treatment, pleural effusion which sometimes progressed to empyema was a frequent complication, often resulting in gross fibrothorax.

With the development of antituberculosis chemotherapy the incidence of effusion complicating active postprimary pulmonary tuberculosis has become extremely small.

Occasionally a *paravertebral abscess* associated with tuberculosis of the thoracic vertebrae abuts on the parietal pleura and results in pleural effusion, which sometimes is bilateral and may progress to empyema [13, 69 & 89]. Early *tuberculosis osteitis of a rib* may be complicated by pleural effusion. The character of the fluid is initially as described in adolescent pleural effusion except that the tendency to develop frank empyema is much greater.

TREATMENT

When tuberculous pleural effusion is a relatively early complication of primary infection the aims of treatment are to *relieve symptoms*, to *prevent the subsequent development of other tuberculous lesions*, e.g. chronic pulmonary tuberculosis, bone and joint and renal disease, and to *prevent fibrothorax.* Cases complicating rupture of a tuberculous cavity will also require treatment as for pneumothorax (p. 446).

Aspiration of the pleural fluid to dryness and the giving of *antituberculosis chemotherapy* should suffice to cure the tuberculous infection and also to prevent the development of pleural fibrosis. Aspiration of the pleural exudate seldom needs to be repeated more than 2 or 3 times. *Corticosteroid drugs* are useful in preventing adhesions and aiding absorption of fluid and can be given as a routine (prednisolone 5 mg 4 times daily for 2 or 3 weeks followed by decreasing dosage over a further 2–4 weeks according to severity) if the diagnosis is clear. Corticosteroids should certainly be given if the effusion is extensive, if the systemic upset is marked or if loculation of the effusion has occurred. A study by Menon [66] has clearly shown the value of corticosteroid therapy in aiding absorption of fluid and in reducing residual pleural thickening. Other studies have shown similar results [5 & 71]. There is no need to inject corticosteroids intrapleurally. Antituberculosis chemotherapy is also given in the usual way and it is no longer considered necessary to insert streptomycin into the pleural space. Most patients can leave hospital within 3–6 weeks to continue chemotherapy on an ambulant basis for a total period of 18 months. The patient should be encouraged to practise deep breathing exercises during the early stages.

PLEURAL EFFUSION AS A COMPLICATION OF SUBPHRENIC INFECTION

Subphrenic abscess. The effusion accompanies or follows the development of subphrenic abscess in cases of perforated *peptic ulcer, appendicitis, cholecystitis* or *malignant neoplasms* of *stomach or colon.* Fluid from the effusion contains polymorphs but usually no organisms initially as the effusion is due to the spread of inflammation rather than infection through the diaphragm. If diagnosis and treatment are delayed, however, the infecting organism may reach the pleura and the effusion becomes an empyema. This may occur in about a quarter of the cases [47]. The condition may occur at any age but because of the type of primary lesion it is most common in the 4th or 5th decades. The usual organisms include coliforms, streptococci and gas-forming bacteria. Sometimes when subphrenic abscess occurs as part of a pyaemic process the causal organism is *Staph. pyogenes.* Gas-forming organisms may outline the diaphragm by a rim of gas but more commonly this occurs from air escaping from a ruptured viscus. In the rare cases in which signs of pleural effusion are not attended by clinical evidence of abdominal disease the radiographic appearance of a fluid level under a raised hemidiaphragm allows a confident diagnosis to be made of pleural effusion secondary to subphrenic abscess. Treatment is urgently required to prevent the development of empyema and consists of aspiration of the pleural effusion, evacuation of the abdominal abscess, and appropriate antibiotic therapy.

HEPATIC AMOEBIASIS

Hepatic amoebiasis may be complicated by a right-sided effusion. Not uncommonly, however, the diaphragmatic pleura and the adjacent visceral pleura become adherent. Rupture of the hepatic abscess into the lower or middle lobe may then occur, sometimes establishing bronchial communication and being coughed up. Amoebae may be found in the sputum. Treatment with emetine should be begun immediately on suspicion of the development of amoebic hepatitis.

PLEURAL EFFUSION IN COLLAGEN DISORDERS

(1) *Acute rheumatic fever*: Acute rheumatic fever is accompanied by fibrinous pleurisy and pleural effusion in about 10% of cases. The effusion is usually transient and may be slight or moderate, unilateral or bilateral. The fluid contains polymorphs and lymphocytes but is sterile. These cases are often complicated by pericarditis and pneumonic lesions (p. 577), all of which, together with the pleural effusion, make their appearance when the disease is clinically well established. The effusion is usually small and subsides along with the other features of the primary disease. The effusion usually requires no treatment but rarely a large effusion compels aspiration and the use of systemic corticosteroids as well as salicylate therapy.

Effusions of transudate type, free from inflammatory cells, are also encountered in severe cases of acute rheumatic fever with congestive cardiac failure.

(2) Pleural effusion as a complication of *rheumatoid arthritis* is commoner in males than in females. It may be the first manifestation of the disease or may develop after the disease has become clinically obvious. The effusion is usually unilateral and tends to run a protracted course over many months, recurring after aspiration but to a gradually diminishing extent. The fluid is pale or dark yellow, grey or opalescent, has the characteristics of exudate and has a low glucose content. The effusion is presumably due to rheumatoid disease of the pleura and in some cases proof is obtained by the finding of pleural nodules, visible at thoracoscopy, which have the same histological appearance as the familiar rheumatoid nodule of subcutaneous tissues. In a case without other features of rheumatoid arthritis the diagnosis is supported by the finding of rheumatoid factor in the serum.

A series reported by Walker and Wright [97] included 12 right sided effusions, 6 left

sided and 4 bilateral. The effusions were of all degrees of size from little more than blunting of the costophrenic angle to an opacity obscuring half the hemithorax. In most cases the fluid occupied between one third and one half the hemithorax. Differential cell counts showed predominance of lymphocytes in 6, polymorphs in 3 and in the remaining 4 the cells were mixed. Punch biopsy of the parietal pleura was helpful in only 4 of 11 cases.

In most instances of rheumatoid pleural effusion there is no evidence of underlying rheumatoid lung disease.

Several authors have reported a high incidence of pleural adhesions at autopsy [4, 7, 37, 84 & 91]. The histological changes have been nonspecific, however, and the relationship to the rheumatoid process is uncertain. Although it is widely held that attacks of dry pleurisy are more frequent in rheumatoid subjects this is not supported in the one comprehensive controlled investigation by Short et al. [82].

(3) *Systemic lupus erythematosus*, preeminently a disease of young females, can give rise to pleural effusion which is usually bilateral and sometimes presents in recurring form as a first manifestation of the disease. LE bodies are sometimes seen in cells from the pleural fluid but otherwise there is nothing distinctive about the effusion or the pleural biopsy and the diagnosis rests on the exclusion of other causes of pleural effusion, the demonstration of LE cells in the blood and the presence of specific features of systemic lupus (p. 583). The chest x-ray may show the features of pericardial effusion, interstitial pulmonary oedema, areas of segmental collapse, diffuse nodular opacities or patchy pneumonic shadowing.

(4) In *polyarteritis nodosa* (p. 434) involvement of the pleural blood vessels in the widespread disease process may give rise to pleural effusion. Pulmonary lesions (diffuse reticular fibrosis, multiple nodules, infarction or pneumonic infiltration) may be seen in the chest x-ray and asthma may be included in the clinical features, but in general the diagnosis depends on finding evidence of multisystem involvement.

(5) Pleural effusion has been reported in a few cases of *scleroderma* (p. 585) and *dermatomyositis* (p. 587).

PLEURAL EFFUSION IN FUNGAL INFECTIONS (p. 284)

Any fungal infection causing lung abscess or pneumonic consolidation may cause pleurisy or pleural effusion at the same time. *Actinomycosis* (p. 289), the only primary fungal infection of the lungs likely to be encountered in Britain, involves the pleura in a less fortuitous manner since the lesions characteristically develop beneath the pleura in the lower lobes. Pleurisy and pleural effusion appear at an early stage in the disease but empyema and chest wall infection soon follow and the diagnosis may not be made until the organism, *Actinomyces israelii*, is identified in the discharge from chest wall sinuses. *Actinomycosis israelii* is microaerophilic but will grow in the ordinary anaerobic culture media. Earlier diagnosis is sometimes possible if the x-ray shows periosteal thickening in the ribs near the pleural opacity since actinomycotic periostitis commonly accompanies the pleural lesions.

Pleural effusion may occur in primary *coccidioidomycosis* (p. 291). Usually there is associated pneumonia and hilar adenopathy although the parenchymal lesion may be obscured by the fluid. The diagnosis is suggested by the clinical features and a positive skin test and is proved by positive cultures or serological evidence of recent infection. Coccidioidal empyema may result when a chronic cavity ruptures into the pleural space.

Blastomycosis (p. 294) may result in pleural reaction with thickening but effusion is uncommon. Pleural effusion is rare in *histoplasmosis* (p. 292) and *cryptococcosis* (p. 290).

EOSINOPHILIC PLEURAL EFFUSION [12]

Pleural fluid in eosinophilia has been the subject of relatively few reports [15]. The condition is not a disease entity, but rather an interesting laboratory finding. It has been variously defined according to the numbers of eosinophils in the differential count of the pleural aspirate. As little as 5% have been

10—R.D.

accepted by some writers as significant [60]; others have required as many as 20% of the total count [75 & 86]. Most workers now consider the higher level to be more realistic since small amounts of eosinophils may be present without significance and only transiently in a large variety of conditions.

INCIDENCE AND AETIOLOGY

The incidence is not known with certainty but estimates have been made from 1 to 8% of all pleural effusions [9, 20, 45, 50, 70, 75 & 86]. Most reported cases have been in males [20 & 45]. Symptoms depend on the nature of the primary disease and the local effects of the effusion.

It is convenient to distinguish those eosinophil pleural effusions with blood eosinophilia and those without blood eosinophilia although exceptions occur in both groups. Accompanying blood eosinophilia is said to suggest that the effusion is secondary to Löffler's syndrome, polyarteritis nodosa, tropical eosinophilia, hydatid disease (although only inconstantly associated with blood eosinophilia) or Hodgkin's disease. When blood eosinophilia is absent pulmonary infarction, pneumonia, carcinoma or trauma are the more likely primary causes. Amoebiasis rarely causes significant blood eosinophilia although eosinophilic effusion can occur as a complication of amoebic abscess in the liver [23 & 29]. Sterile eosinophilic pleural effusion complicating lobar pneumonia was described in 1916 by Bayne-Jones [9]. Subsequent reports show that an eosinophil count of about 12% can occur in this condition, the count being higher when the patient has been treated with antibiotics [80]. More recently viral infections have been implicated but only in influenza and ornithosis have the reports been convincing [20]. Most writers agree that tuberculosis is not a likely cause of eosinophilic pleurisy [45, 50 & 75] and certainly other aetiologies should be sought before making a diagnosis of tuberculous pleural effusion in this circumstance. Histoplasmosis and coccidioidomycosis have been described as causing eosinophilic effusion on rare occasions [25].

CAUSES OF PLEURAL EOSINOPHILIA

Schwartz in 1914 [79] suggested that foreign protein or degradation products might stimulate the production of eosinophils. Inert substances such as oil can also be eosinophilotactic. A large number of substances have been shown experimentally to result in eosinophilic pleural effusion when introduced into the pleural space. These include iodine, chalk, nucleic acid, pilocarpine, egg albumin, gold salts, hydatid fluids, extracts of parasites and even saline [86]. A particularly powerful stimulus to eosinophil production is a protein or protein carbohydrate compound in the stroma of the red blood cell, and blood in the pleural space is probably the commonest cause of significant eosinophilia in a pleural effusion [17, 18 & 19]. Any condition producing blood in the pleural space, e.g. pulmonary infarction or trauma, may result in an eosinophilic effusion. But despite the fact that malignant effusions are frequently bloodstained, pleural eosinophilia is remarkably uncommon [86].

When collagen disorders are associated with eosinophilic effusions there is usually a coincident blood eosinophilia. Pleural effusion complicating acute rheumatism and typical rheumatoid arthritis have on occasion been found to contain significant numbers of eosinophils [44 & 74].

The rôle of eosinophilia in inflammation has been suggested by Archer [3] who has pointed out that eosinophils are attracted into tissue by raised concentrations of histamine and that eosinophils have an antagonistic action towards both histamine and 5-hydroxytryptamine. It has also been suggested that pleural eosinophilia may occur as a rebound phenomenon after adrenal cortical stress [90].

The rôle of the eosinophil in antibody production remains obscure. Speirs [85] has postulated that the eosinophil is an intermediary in the formation of antibody. On the other hand Litt [57] and Sabesin [77] considered that eosinophil accumulation is a phenomenon secondary to the presence of immune complexes. More recently fibrinolysin has been demonstrated in eosinophil granules [8]. The precise significance of these findings is not yet known. The actual rôle of eosinophils in pleural fluid remains a matter for speculation. The significance of eosinophilia is also discussed on p. 280.

DIAGNOSIS

The eosinophilic nature of the fluid is revealed at aspiration. Pleural biopsy in most cases will only show nonspecific changes. The chest x-ray may show evidence of one or other of the causal diseases and examination of the peripheral blood may show an eosinophilia. Routine investigations should include examination for ANF and the LE cell phenomenon, examination of the sputum for aspergilli, and stool examination to exclude ascariasis or other helminth or amoebic infections. When amoebiasis is seriously suspected sigmoidoscopy should be carried out but may not be helpful. When hydatid disease is a possibility the Casoni test, complement fixation and precipitin tests should be performed. Eosinophils in a pleural effusion are most commonly due to blood and when this occurs in the absence of blood eosinophilia the clinical problem is to determine the cause of the bloodstained effusion. Sometimes bronchoscopy may be necessary to exclude bronchial carcinoma.

TREATMENT

This depends on the primary disease and is discussed in the various sections dealing with these.

CHYLOTHORAX

Anatomical and physiological considerations: In general the thoracic duct receives the lymph from both sides of the body below the diaphragm and the left side above the diaphragm. It begins in the abdomen as a dilatation called the *cisterna chyli*, which lies on the front of the upper 2 lumbar vertebrae between the aorta and the right crus of the diaphragm. The duct passes upwards through the aortic opening of the diaphragm, ascends in the posterior mediastinum, first behind the diaphragm and then behind the oesophagus, inclining to the left at the 5th thoracic vertebra to ascend in the superior mediastinum closely applied to the left side of the oesophagus. Entering the root of the neck it turns laterally between the carotid sheath and the vertebral artery, turns downwards in front of the subclavian artery and enters the venous system at the junction of the left internal jugular and subclavian veins. This is the course found in more than 50% of cases. In the remainder, 2 or more ducts are present at some stage in its course [51]. The right lymphatic duct which is very small, perhaps only 1 cm long, is formed from the union of the right jugular lymph trunk which receives the lymph from the right half of the head and neck and the right subclavian trunk. The union occurs at the medial margin of the *scalenus anterior* above the subclavian artery, and the right lymphatic duct descends across the front of the first part of the subclavian artery to end at the junction of the right jugular and subclavian veins. The right bronchomediastinal lymph trunk gathers lymph from the right half of the thorax. It ascends along the right margin of the oesophagus into the neck and usually joins the right lymphatic duct but may enter the innominate vein independently.

Cross communications of the bronchomediastinal trunk with the thoracic duct occur and many anastomoses exist between the thoracic duct and the azygos, intercostal and lumbar veins. Thus the main thoracic duct can safely be ligated at any point in its thoracic or cervical course [53]. The amount of chyle produced daily varies greatly. It is much increased by meals with a high fat content. It is reduced in starvation and increased by drinking water. It has been estimated that the volume may reach 2·5 1 per 24 hours [100]. When chylothorax develops, chest aspiration may remove as much as 2 1 of chyle per day with consequent depletion of protein, fat and fat-soluble vitamins, water and electrolytes.

AETIOLOGY AND INCIDENCE OF CHYLOTHORAX

Although it is a comparatively rare condition the incidence of chylothorax is increasing. In a comprehensive review of the literature to 1936 Shakelford and Fisher [81] found 41 cases. Lampson [53] recorded 18 cases from 1936 to 1948 and Goorwitch [41] described a further 31 cases from 1948 to 1954. Reviewing the literature between 1953 and 1957 Schmidt [78] published details of 92 cases, the most recent and largest series recorded. Schmidt considered the increase in incidence to be mainly the result of *surgical trauma* during intrathoracic operations because of the great increase in this form of surgery. Maloney and Spencer [61] reviewing 2660 thoracic operations in the Johns Hopkins Hospital reported 13 cases of chylothorax after surgery. A comparable incidence was reported by Steiger *et al.* [88] and they concluded that operations close to the left subclavian artery were most likely to be complicated by chylothorax.

Other types of trauma are occasionally responsible. Chylothorax has been known to result from sudden hyperextension of the spine which may rupture the duct just above the diaphragm [68]. Rupture has also followed falls, compression injuries of the trunk, severe blows on the chest or abdomen, blast, rib fractures and rarely severe bouts of vomiting or coughing. All of these causes are, however, extremely uncommon. Other causes include gunshot and stab wounds and operative procedures in the neck, particularly block dissection of lymph glands and scalene node biopsy [41]. If the injury is recognized at the time of operation ligation of the duct results in no untoward effects [72].

Chylothorax occurs rarely in infancy. This may result from *birth injury* or from *congenital abnormality* of the thoracic duct system resulting in multiple fistulae [35 & 73].

The commonest nontraumatic cause of chylothorax is *malignant involvement of the thoracic duct* or *left subclavian vein*. This may occur from a variety of tumours, with metastatic deposits from carcinoma of the stomach high on the list. Follicular lymphoma is particularly associated with chylothorax [39]. Other *rarer causes* include tuberculous mediastinal lymph glands, filariasis, thrombosis of the left subclavian vein, aneurysms of the thoracic aorta and benign lymphangioma of the thoracic duct. Very rarely chylothorax has complicated chylous ascites although the thoracic duct has been intact [34]. The mechanism of this is unknown although chyle may pass through the oeso-phageal opening into the mediastinum and thereafter rupture into the pleural space.

CLINICAL FEATURES

A latent interval between rupture of the thoracic duct and the development of chylous effusion of between 2 and 10 days is common. This has been explained by accumulation of chyle in the posterior mediastinal pleura, usually on the right side at the base of the pulmonary ligament [81]. Rarely the latent period is considerably longer and a case has been reported with a latent period of 11 months [94]. When the latent period has been longer, such as the $6\frac{1}{2}$ years described by Beatty [10], it seems probable that scar tissue has developed as a result of the original injury making the duct unyielding and there-fore liable to rupture from further trivial trauma.

Chylothorax usually presents with sudden onset of breathlessness and the physical signs of an extensive pleural effusion. There may be a mild fever but toxaemia is not a feature. There is nothing to distinguish chylothorax radiographically and the diagnosis is made by the demonstration of the characteristic fluid on pleural aspiration. The effusion rapidly reforms after aspiration and requires repeated aspiration. As a consequence hypo-proteinaemia and lymphopenia develop [58]. Because of the depletion of essential food ele-ments the patient rapidly becomes emaciated, thirsty, and in consequence polyuric. Death occurs unless the fistula heals or is closed.

COMPLICATIONS

In common with other causes of chronic pleural effusion a fibrinous peel may develop over the pleural surface, that over the visceral pleura restricting the lung movement [64]. Complicating pneumothorax is rare, and em-pyema has never been reported.

DIAGNOSIS

Aspiration reveals the characteristic fluid. Immediately after injury the chyle may be mildly bloodstained; later it is white and oily. There may be a superficial resemblance to pus but differentiation is usually easy. Sometimes diagnosis has to be made from the opalescent effusion due to *cholesterol* crystals which cause a shimmering exudate and which occur in longstanding effusions of whatever aetio-logy; tuberculosis, carcinoma and the nephro-tic syndrome are the commoner causes. *Chyliform effusions* look milky due to fat globules derived from degenerating cells in longstanding encysted effusions with a high cell content. Tuberculosis and carcinoma are the usual causes. On microscopy large num-bers of degenerating cells, principally lym-phocytes, are seen in addition to free fat globules. The features of the primary con-dition commonly suffice to differentiate from true chylothorax. Absolute differentiation is confirmed by asking the patient to eat a fat stained with a lipophilic dye. Aspiration of the pleural fluid next morning will show discoloration of the fluid if the condition is truly a chylothorax.

TREATMENT

Opinions are divided as to the best manage-ment. Since Lampson [53] performed the first successful ligation of the thoracic duct for chylothorax this method has proved safe and effective and numerous series testify to this. Because there is about a 50% chance of spontaneous closure of the fistula, conserva-tive treatment by repeated aspiration should first be tried [63]. A time limit has to be placed on conservative treatment because of the fairly rapid deterioration of the patient's general condition through inanition. Gingell [40] has advocated a more active approach with a view to reducing hospitalization and preventing the development of inanition and fibrothorax. He advocates insufflation of iodized talc to promote a pleurodesis, com-bined with suction drainage of the pleural cavity. He has found this method highly suc-cessful in that the lung remains fully expanded and fusion of the pleural surfaces prevents further accumulation of chyle. He suggests that insufflation should be done as soon as the diagnosis is made.

INVESTIGATION OF PLEURAL EFFUSION

While many of the causes of pleural effusion can be accurately deduced from the clinical features of the case (e.g. congestive cardiac failure) in other patients diagnosis may be difficult without examination of the fluid and pleural biopsy. Pleural aspiration and biopsy can now be carried out together without difficulty by the use of Abrams' pleural biopsy punch (p. 77). Pleural biopsy is particularly effective in the diagnosis of malignant disease of the pleura, histological confirmation being obtained in 40–60% of cases, if not at the first attempt then at the second or third, sampling other areas of pleura. Cases of tuberculous pleurisy yield even a higher success rate, up to 80%, although the value of pleural biopsy in this condition is lessened by the fact that other effective methods of diagnosis are available. Pleural biopsy by the punch technique has greatly reduced the need for thoracoscopy in the evaluation of diseases of the pleura.

When performing pleural aspiration, besides sending specimens for bacteriological examination (p. 268) and cytology (p. 269), it is wise to take an extra specimen of fluid and to keep this in the ward as a record of the macroscopic appearances.

COMPLICATIONS OF PLEURAL ASPIRATION

(1) *Removal of too much fluid too quickly* has been known to lead to pulmonary oedema and even death. Usually this is heralded by the patient complaining of chest discomfort and cough which may progress to the coughing up of typical oedema fluid. At the earliest sign of discomfort the aspiration should be discontinued. Usually up to 600 ml at a time can be safely withdrawn.

(2) *When the lung is bound down by pleural fibrosis* and cannot re-expand freely, aspiration may result in a high negative intrapleural pressure which can interfere with venous filling and result in circulatory collapse [2 & 67]. Usually the feel of the pull on the syringe plunger indicates the development of this complication and the patient begins to cough and complain of tightness in the chest. Again this complication reflects too rapid aspiration of the pleural fluid.

(3) *Air embolism and pleural shock.* Tearing of the visceral pleura or puncture of a superficial vessel may allow air to enter the pulmonary venous system through the needle or more commonly from neighbouring alveoli. This emergency is treated by laying the patient with the head lower than the feet and the right side uppermost, positions which reduce the risk of air entering the cerebral and coronary arteries.

Probably most cases of reported pleural shock are really episodes of air embolism. Nevertheless, vagal inhibition through pleural puncture appears to have been the cause of death in some cases [83].

(4) *Rupture of intercostal vessel.* This is rare and can be avoided by always keeping the aspirating needle as near as possible to the upper edge of the lower rib. It is particularly important to remember this while making pleural biopsy with the Abrams' punch.

CHARACTERISTICS OF THE PLEURAL ASPIRATE

(1) *Macroscopic appearance.* The fluid of an exudate is usually yellowish in colour, varying from straw to amber, and clear, although if the cell count is high it may be cloudy. Transudates are paler and more watery than exudates and much less liable to clot on standing. Blood in the fluid changes the colour in a range from bright red to brown, depending on the time the blood has been present. The so called 'bloody tap' which occurs when the needle transfixes an intercostal vessel is recognized by the blood in the first fluid drawn and the progressive loss of colour as aspiration proceeds. *Haemorrhagic effusions* are uniformly coloured in all specimens and occur characteristically in *malignant disease of the pleura, pulmonary infarction* and in *injury to the chest* although they may also

be encountered in *leukaemia, hepatic cirrhosis* and rarely in tuberculosis. The paramount position of malignant disease as a cause of haemorrhagic effusion needs to be stressed; no other diagnosis should be entertained until malignant disease has been excluded.

A milky appearance probably means that the fluid contains *chyle* (p. 276) which will be more evident if the patient has had a meal shortly before the aspiration. *Purulent fluid* in cases of frank empyema is easily recognized but lesser degrees of infection give the fluid a cloudiness which may be indistinguishable from that due to mere cellularity. A shimmering, satin sheen is the sign of *cholesterol* in the fluid and an indication of chronicity but of nothing else; it has nothing to do with the cause of the effusion.

(2) The significance of the *protein content* and to a lesser extent the *specific gravity* in distinguishing exudates from transudates has been mentioned already.

(3) *Cytological examination* of the effusion is of primary importance. A citrated specimen should be sent for a differential white cell count. *Polymorphs* as the predominant cells favour a bacterial infection, usually a post-pneumonic effusion. The *lymphocyte* is the characteristic cell of tuberculous pleural effusion. Cytological examination of the pleural fluid for *malignant cells* is often done as a routine but even experts may have difficulty in distinguishing between malignant cells and serosal cells.

Eosinophilia in the pleural fluid may be encountered in a number of conditions (p. 275) including collagen disorders, but is usually only significant when there is coincident blood eosinophilia. The commonest cause of eosinophils in the pleural fluid is *extravasated* blood (p. 276). *Serosal* cells are stated to be rarely found in appreciable numbers in tuberculous effusion [87] and this fact may be of contributory value in the differential diagnosis between a malignant and a tuberculous effusion. The finding is not, however, wholly reliable.

(4) *Chemical studies* of pleural effusion are rarely of diagnostic significance. Nevertheless certain chemical investigations may yield data

of contributory value in assessing the probability in any particular case of pleural effusion. *Fat droplets* may be demonstrated in chylothorax. The value of estimating the *protein content* has already been mentioned. Effusions due to rheumatoid arthritis may have a *low glucose content*, often less than 20 mg %. The reason for this has not been satisfactorily explained [16].

The *amylase* concentration in a left pleural effusion complicating acute pancreatitis may be much in excess of the concentration in the serum, perhaps 50 times as much. The finding is diagnostic [76] (p. 267).

(5) *Bacteriological culture* is essential for a precise aetiological diagnosis of those pleural effusions complicating infections. The appropriate method of culture will be employed according to the degree of suspicion attaching to the clinical features of the case. With regard to tuberculosis it is important to submit as much fluid as possible for examination, the positivity rate for culture being proportional to the volume of the specimen examined. Anaerobic culture is essential for the demonstration of actinomyces.

REFERENCES

[1] ADLER R.H. & TAPPOLE B.W. (1967) Recurrent malignant pleural effusions and talc powder aerosol treatment. *Surgery* **62**, 1000.
[2] ALPCHULE M.D. & ZAMCHECK N. (1944) The effects of pleural effusion on respiration and circulation in man. *J. clin. Invest.* **23**, 85.
[3] ARCHER R.K. (1963) *The Eosinophil Leukocytes*. Philadelphia, Davies.
[4] ARONOFF A., BYWATERS E.G.L. & FEARNLEY G.R. (1955) Lung lesions in rheumatoid arthritis. *Br. med. J.* **ii**, 228.
[5] ASPIN J. & O'HARA H. (1958) Steroid treated tuberculous pleural effusions. *Br. J. Tuberc.* **52**, 81.
[6] AUERBACH O. (1950) Pleural, peritoneal and pericardial tuberculosis. *Am. Rev. Tuberc.* **61**, 845.
[7] BAGGENSTOSS A.H. & ROSENBERG E.F. (1943) Visceral lesions associated with chronic infectious (rheumatoid) arthritis. *Arch. Path.* **35**, 503.
[8] BARNHART M.I. & RIDDLE J.M. (1963) Cellular localization of profibrinolysin (plasminogen). *Blood* **21**, 306.
[9] BAYNE-JONES S. (1916) Pleural eosinophilia:

with report of a case. *Bull. Johns Hopkins Hosp.* **27**, 12.

[10] BEATTY O.A. (1936) Chylothorax: case report. *J. thorac Surg.* **6**, 221.

[11] BENTLEY F.J. & GRZYBOWSKI S. (1954) *Tuberculosis in Childhood and Adolescence.* London, The National Association for the Prevention of Tuberculosis.

[12] BOWER G. (1967) Eosinophilic pleural effusion. *Am. Rev. resp. Dis.* **95**, 746.

[13] BROOKS W.D.W. (1942) Paravertebral abscess with rupture into the pleura or lung. *Br. J. Tuberc.* **36**, 49.

[14] BURKE H.E. (1959) The lymphatics which drain the potential space between the visceral and parietal pleura. *Am. Rev. Tuberc.* **79**, 52.

[15] CAMPBELL G.D. & WEBB W.R. (1964) Eosinophilic pleural effusion. *Am. Rev. resp. Dis.* **90**, 194.

[16] CARR D.T. & McGUCKIN W.F. (1968) Pleural fluid glucose. *Am. Rev. resp. Dis.* **97**, 302.

[17] CHAPMAN J.S. (1955) The reaction of serous cavities to blood. *J. lab. clin. Med.* **46**, 48.

[18] CHAPMAN J.S. & REYNOLDS R.C. (1958) Eosinophilic response to intraperitoneal blood. *J. lab. clin. Med.* **51**, 516.

[19] CHAPMAN J.S. (1961) Effects of solvents on eosinophilic stimulating substance of erythrocyte stroma. *Proc. Soc. exp. biol. Med.* **108**, 566.

[20] CHRETIEN J. & OLIO G. (1963) Les pleurésies à éosinophiles. *Poumon Coeur*, **19**, 19.

[21] CLAGETT O.T., McDONALD J.R. & SCHMIDT H.W. (1952) Localized benign mesothelioma of the pleura. *J. thorac. Surg.* **24**, 213.

[22] CLAUS R.H., YACOUBIA N.H. & BARKER H.G. (1957) Dynamics of pleural effusions. *Surg. Forum* **7**, 201.

[23] CORDIER V. & MORENES L. (1930) Eosinophilie pleurale symptomatique d'abscès hepatique amoebian évacué par vomique. Constatation d'*Entamoeba dysenteriae* dans l'expectoration. *C. R. Soc. Biol. Paris.* **104**, 198.

[24] CUNNINGHAM R.S. (1926) The physiology of the serous membranes. *Physiol. Rev.* **6**, 242.

[25] CURRAN W.S. & WILLIAMS A.W. (1963) Eosinophilic pleural effusion. *Arch. intern. Med.* (*Chicago*) **111**, 809.

[26] CURTICE F.C. & SIMMONDS W.J. (1949) Absorption of fluid from the pleural cavity of rabbits and cats. *J. Physiol.* (*Lond.*) **109**, 117.

[27] CURTICE F.C. & SIMMONDS W.J. (1954) Physiological significance of lymph drainage of serous cavities in lungs. *Physiol. Rev.* **34**, 419.

[28] DAVIS S., GARDNER F. & QVIST G. (1963) The shape of a pleural effusion. *Br. med. J.* **i**, 436.

[29] DE LAVERGE V., ABEL E. & DEPENEDETTI R. (1930) Eosinophilie pleurale au cours d'abcès amibien du poumon. *Bull. et Mém. Soc. méd. Hôp. Paris*, p. 593.

[30] DRESSLER W. (1959) Postmyocardial infarction syndrome. *Arch. intern. Med.* **103**, 28.

[31] EDITORIAL (1968) Malignant pleural effusion. *Br. med. J.* **3**, 202.

[32] EMERSON P.A. & DAVIES J.H. (1955) Hydrothorax complicating ascites. *Lancet* **i**, 487.

[33] ERWIN G.S. (1944) Pleural effusions arising from tuberculous tracheal bronchial adenitis (primary effusions). *Tubercle* (*Lond.*) **25**, 44.

[34] EVANS H.W. (1960) Painless chronic pancreatitis, chylo-ascites and chylothorax. *Am. J. med. Sci.* **240**, 494.

[35] FEINERMAN B.E., BURKE E.C. & OLSEN A.M. (1957) Chylothorax in infancy. *Proc. Mayo Clin.* **32**, 314.

[36] FINDLAY G.M. & HOWARD E.M. (1950) Coxsackie viruses and Bornholm disease. *Br. med. J.* **i**, 1233.

[37] FINGERMAN D.L. & ANDRUS F.C. (1943) Visceral lesions associated with rheumatoid arthritis. *Ann. rheum. Dis.* **3**, 168.

[38] FROTHINGHAM J.R. (1942) Cirrhosis of the liver complicated by persistent right hydrothorax and ascites. Report of an unusual case. *New Engl. J. Med.* **226**, 679.

[39] GALL E.A. & MALLORY T.B. (1942) Malignant lymphoma. *Am. J. Path.* **18**, 381.

[40] GINGELL J.C. (1965) Treatment of chylothorax by producing pleurodesis using iodised talc. *Thorax* **20**, 261.

[41] GOORWITCH J. (1955) Traumatic chylothorax and thoracic duct ligation. *J. thorac. Surg.* **29**, 467.

[42] GOODMAN S. (1937) Pleural ascites: the result of traumatic rupture of the diaphragm in a case of latent hepatic cirrhosis. *J. Am. med. Ass.* **109**, 1980.

[43] GORDON R.B., LENNETT E.H. & SANDROCK R.S. (1959) The varied clinical manifestations of Coxsackie virus infection. *Arch. intern. Med.* **103**, 63.

[44] GRIFFITH G.C., PHILLIPS A.W. & ASHER C. (1946) Pneumonitis occurring in rheumatic fever. *Am. J. med. Sci.* **212**, 22.

[45] GUHL R. (1957) Über pleurale Eosinophilie; die sogenannte Eosinophilic Pleuritis. *Schweiz. med. Wschr.* **26**, 838.

[46] HANSON L.A., LUNDGREN S., LYCKE E., STRANNEGARD O. & WINBERG J. (1966) Clinical and serological observations in cases of Coxsackie B3 infections in early infancy. *Acta paediat.* (*Stockholm*) **55**, 577.

[47] HARLEY H.R.S. (1949) Subphrenic abscess. *Thorax* **4**, 1.

[48] HAWTHORNE H.R. & FORBESE A.S. (1950) Benign fibroma of the pleura: report of a case. *Dis. Chest* **17**, 588.

[49] JENSIK R., CAGLE J.R.Jr., MILLOY F., PERLIA C., TAYLOR S., KOFMAN S. & BEATTIE E.J. Jr. (1963) Pleurectomy in the treatment of pleural

effusion due to metastatic malignancy. *J. thorac. cardiovasc. Surg.* **46**, 322.

[50] JARVINEN K.A.J. & KAHANPAA A. (1959) Prognosis in cases with eosinophilic pleural effusion. *Acta med. scand.* **164**, 245.

[51] KAUSEL H.W., REEVE P.S., STEIN A.A., ALLEY R.A. & STRANAHAN A. (1957) Anatomic and pathologic studies of the thoracic duct. *J. thorac. Surg.* **34**, 631.

[52] KAYE M.D. (1968) Pleuropulmonary complications of pancreatitis. *Thorax* **23**, 297.

[53] LAMPSON R.S. (1948) Traumatic chylothorax: a review of the literature and report of a case treated by mediastinal ligation of the thoracic duct. *J. thorac. Surg.* **17**, 778.

[54] LANDAU N. (1949) A study of tuberculous pleural effusion in Indian children and adults. *Tubercle* **30**, 26.

[55] LECKIE W.J.H. & TOTHILL P. (1965) Albumin turnover in pleural effusions. *Clin. Sci.* **29**, 339.

[56] LEMON W.S. & HIGGINS G.M. (1929) Lymphatic absorption of particulate matter through the normal and the paralysed diaphragm. An experimental study. *Am. J. med. Sci.* **178**, 538.

[57] LITT M. (1961) Studies in experimental eosinophilia. III. The induction of peritoneal eosinophilia by the passive transfer of serum antibody. *J. Immun.* **87**, 522.

[58] LOWMAN R.M., HOOGERHYDE J., WATERS L.L. & GRANT C. (1951) Traumatic chylothorax. The roentgen aspects of this problem. *Am. J. Roentgenol.* **65**, 529.

[59] MACKAY-DICK J. & ROTHNIE N.G. (1954) Serous primary pleural effusion in young adults. *Tubercle, Lond.* **25**, 182.

[60] MACMURRAY F.G., KATZ S. & ZIMMERMAN H.J. (1950) Pleural fluid eosinophils. *New Engl. J. Med.* **243**, 330.

[61] MALONEY J.V.Jr. & SPENCER F.C. (1956) The nonoperative treatment of traumatic chylothorax. *Surgery* **40**, 121.

[62] MANFREDI F., ROSENBAUM D. & CHILDRESS R.H. (1965) Diffuse malignant mesothelioma of the pleura. *Am. Rev. resp. Dis.* **92**, 269.

[63] MAURER E.R. (1956) Complete extirpation of the thoracic duct *J. Am. med. Ass.* **61**, 135.

[64] MEAD R.H., HEAD J.R. & MOEN C.W. (1950) Management of chylothorax. *J. thorac. Surg.* **19**, 709.

[65] MEIGS J.V. (1954) Fibroma of the ovary with ascites and hydrothorax—Meigs' syndrome. *Am. J. Obstet. Gynec.* **67**, 962.

[66] MENON N.K. (1964) Steroid therapy in tuberculous pleural effusion. *Tubercle, Lond.* **45**, 17.

[67] MORLAND A. (1949) Pleural shock. *Lancet* ii, 1021.

[68] NOWAK S.J.G. & BARTON P.N. (1941) Chylothorax: report of a case arrested by phrenicectomy. *J. thorac. Surg.* **10**, 628.

[69] ORNSTEIN G.C. & ULMER D. (1935) Tuberculous caries of vertebral bodies. *Quart. Bull. Sea View Hosp.* **1**, 3.

[70] PADDOCK F.K. (1940) The diagnostic significance of serous fluids in disease. *New Engl. J. Med.* **223**, 1010.

[71] PALEY S.S., MIHALAY J.P., MAIS E.L., GITTENS S.A. & LUPINI B. (1959) Prednisone in the treatment of pleural effusions. *Am. Rev. Tuberc.* **79**, 307.

[72] PRICE THOMAS C. & CLELAND W.P. (1942) Extrafascial apicolysis with thoracoplasty: indications, technique and complications. *Br. J. Tuberc.* **36**, 109.

[73] RANDOLPH J.G. & GROSS R.E. (1957) Congenital chylothorax. *Arch. Surg. Chicago* **74**, 405.

[74] ROBERTSON R.F. (1952). Primary tuberculous pleural effusion in older age groups. *Br. med. J.* i, 133.

[75] ROBERTSON R.F. (1954) Pleural eosinophilia. *Br. J. Tuberc.* **48**, 111.

[76] ROSEMAN D.M., KOWLESSAR O.D. & SLEISENGER M.H.A. (1960) Pulmonary manifestations of pancreatitis. *New Engl. J. Med.* **263**, 294.

[77] SABESIN S.M. (1963) A function of the eosinophil; phagocytosis of antigen–antibody complexes. *Proc. Soc. exp. Biol. Med.* **112**, 667.

[78] SCHMIDT A. (1959) Chylothorax: review of 5 years' cases in the literature and report of a case. *Acta chir. scand.* **118**, 5.

[79] SCHWARTZ E. (1914) Lehre von allgemeiner und ortlicher Eosinophilie. *Ergebn. allg. Path.* **17**, 137.

[80] SCOTT T.F.McN. & FINLAND M. (1934) The cytology of pleural effusions in pneumonia studied with a supravital technique. *Am. J. med. Sci.* **188**, 322.

[81] SHAKELFORD R.T. & FISHER A.M. (1938) Traumatic chylothorax. *Sth. med. J., Nashville.*

[82] SHORT C.L., BAUER W. & REYNOLDS W.E. (1957) *Rheumatoid Arthritis.* Cambridge, Mass. Harvard University Press.

[83] SIMPSON K. (1949) Death from vagal inhibition. *Lancet* i, 558.

[84] SINCLAIR R.J.T. & CRUICKSHANK B. (1956) A clinical and pathological study of 16 cases of rheumatoid arthritis with extensive visceral involvement. *Quart. J. Med.* **25**, 313.

[85] SPEIRS R.A.S. (1958) A theory of antibody formation involving eosinophils and reticuloendothelial cells. *Nature (Lond.)* **191**, 681.

[86] SPRIGGS A.I. (1957) *The Cytology of Effusions.* p. 9. London, Heinemann.

[87] SPRIGGS A.I. & BODDINGTON M.M. (1960) Absence of mesothelial cells from tuberculous pleural effusions. *Thorax* **15**, 169.

[88] STEIGER Z., WEINBERG M. & FELL E.H. (1960) Postoperative chylothorax. *Am. J. Surg.* **100**, 8.

[89] STEVENSON F.H. (1960) Pulmonary and pleural complications of Pott's disease. *Proc. roy. Soc. Med.* **53**, 938.

[90] SULAVIK S. & KATZ S. (1963) *Pleural Effusion.* Springfield, Ill., Thomas.

[91] TALBOTT J.A. & CALKINS E. (1964) Pulmonary involvement of rheumatoid arthritis. *J. Am. med. Ass.* **189**, 911.

[92] THOMPSON B.C. (1946) Pathogenesis of pleurisy with effusion. Clinical, epidemiological and follow up study of 190 cases. *Am. Rev. Tuberc.* **54**, 349.

[93] THOMSPON B.C. (1949) Studies in primary pleurisy with effusion. *Br. med. J.* **ii**, 841.

[94] THORNE P.S. (1958) Traumatic chylothorax. *Tubercle, Lond.* **39**, 229.

[95] TURIAF J., MARLAND P., BASSET G. & LORTHOLARY P. (1959) Les pleurésies et les pericardites virales. *Poumon,* **15**, 449.

[96] TURNER R.W.D. (1945) Atypical pneumonia. *Lancet* **i**, 493.

[97] WALKER W.C. & WRIGHT V. (1967) Rheumatoid pleuritis and other rheumatoid diseases. *Ann. rheum. Dis.* **26**, 467.

[98] WALLGREN A. (1929) Pathogenesis of acute serofibrinous pleurisy. *Am. J. Dis. Childh.* **38**, 829.

[99] WALLGREN A. (1948) The timetable of tuberculosis. *Tubercle* **29**, 245.

[100] WATNE A.L., HATIBOGLU I. & MOORE G.E. (1960) A clinical and autopsy study of tumour cells in the thoracic duct lymph. *Surg. Gynec. Obstet.* **110**, 339.

[101] YAMADA S. (1933) Über die seröse Flüssigkeit in der Pleurahöhle der gesunden Menschen. *Z. ges. exp. Med.* **90**, 342.

[102] ZELENIK J.S., HALPERN A.J. & WILLIAMS D.W. (1964) Treatment of neoplastic effusions with chlorambucil. *Obstet. Gynec.* **23**, 703.

[103] ZINNEMAN H.H., JOHNSON G.J. & LYON R.H. (1957) Proteins and mucoproteins in pleural effusions. *Am. Rev. Tuberc.* **76**, 247.

CHAPTER 17

Fungal Infections of the Lung [86 & 94]

The reported incidence of infections due to fungi has increased in recent years. This is probably due to increased awareness and the consequent search for fungal infection by appropriate techniques, and also to the promotion of fungal growth by certain modern treatments, in particular the use of wide spectrum antibiotics, corticosteroids and radiomimetic drugs. Well known factors predisposing to some fungal infections are severe chronic diseases, including malignant disease. The increasing longevity in most populations must add to the incidence. Though relatively uncommon compared with bacterial and viral infections, fungal infections are important since treatment is available for at least some of them and failure to treat may be fatal. Moreover the risks of some fungal infections may be reduced by attention to certain therapeutic principles. For example candidiasis is frequently iatrogenic when ablating or prolonged chemotherapy creates an ecological vacuum into which the fungus may enter and exert its own pathogenic effects.

Although several fungi tend to be geographically isolated, the ease and speed of modern travel make it possible for the physician to encounter fungal infection usually met with only in distant lands. Consequently it is possible that the hazard to laboratory workers will increase.

CLASSIFICATION OF FUNGI ASSOCIATED WITH PULMONARY DISEASE

Riddell [86] has classified the pulmonary mycoses as follows:

(1) Infections due to actinomycetes (filamentous organisms of bacterial dimensions)
    (a) actinomycosis
    (b) nocardiosis
These are not true fungal infections but are conveniently discussed here).

(2) Infections due to yeasts and yeast-like fungi:
    (a) candidiasis (moniliasis)
    (b) cryptococcosis (torulosis)

(3) Infections due to filamentous fungi:
    (a) aspergillosis
    (b) mucormycosis.

(4) Infections due to dimorphic fungi:
    (a) coccidioidomycosis
    (b) histoplasmosis
    (c) North and South American blastomycosis
    (d) sporotrichosis.

The mycoses encountered in Britain are principally aspergillosis, candidiasis, actinomycosis and cryptococcosis. Histoplasmosis, coccidioidomycosis and blastomycosis have a relatively restricted geographical distribution but may be met with in travellers from endemic areas or in laboratory workers handling specimens from these areas.

EPIDEMIOLOGY

With the exceptions of actinomycosis and candidiasis the pulmonary mycoses are acquired by inhalation of spores. Nearly all fungi are soil organisms and some require specific natural conditions which limit their distribution as pathogens (e.g. coccidioides, blastomyces). Others are ubiquitous and world-wide in distribution (e.g. aspergillus, cryptococcus). Curiously, despite the ease with which spores can be disseminated, there is no evidence of direct transmission from person to person as a rule. The only record of this is an epidemic of coccidioidomycosis occurring in 6 persons in whom case to case transmission seemed probable [30]. Group infections may, of course, occur in endemic areas. Undoubtedly the fact that many pulmonary fungal infections are subclinical has explained the failure to recognize them in the past.

Both *Actinomyces israelii* and *Candida albicans*, respectively the causative agents of actinomycosis and candidiasis, are obligatory parasites, existing in symbiotic relationship with the human host until certain predispositions, mainly devitalizing processes, allow them to become invasive and cause pathological changes. *A. israelii* exists commonly in human mouths and contact by kissing, such as occurs between mother and child, ensures perpetuation of this relationship between the organism and man in succeeding generations [2]. Usually mechanical trauma is necessary to allow *A. israelii* to become pathogenic.

C. albicans is variably present in the normal flora of the skin, mouth, vagina and intestine. Candidiasis is an example of 'opportunistic' infection and is predisposed to by chronic debilitating diseases, the use of wide spectrum antibiotics and corticosteroid therapy. The defence mechanisms which normally keep the organism in check become less effective and the normal saprophyte becomes a pathogen. It has been shown that an antibody to *C. albicans* exists in human blood after the age of 6–8 months and that this factor is deficient in acute leukaemia, the late stages of chronic leukaemias, the malignant reticuloses, multiple myeloma and erythremic myelosis [91 & 92].

The fungi responsible for histoplasmosis, coccidioidomycosis, cryptococcosis and aspergillosis are soil organisms. Spores are produced in the soil and carried by the wind, infections being then acquired by inhalation [2]. Only 2 species of fungi recognized as causing airborne pulmonary mycoses have not, so far, been detected in the soil. These are *Blastomyces dermatitidis* and *Paracoccidioides brasiliensis* [94].

The geographical distribution of *Coccidioides immitis* is limited by climatic conditions [65]. Infection with this organism occurs in the southwestern parts of the U.S.A., Mexico and Venezuela which are the only areas in which the condition is met with endemically. For example a high incidence has been found in some southwestern American Indian tribes living in reservations situated in dusty, desert areas [96]. The movement of individuals or of contaminated materials to other parts of the world may, however, result in isolated reports of infection elsewhere and the infection may be acquired in the laboratory since it is highly infectious [73, 100 & 103].

Following the isolation of the organism from the soil by Emmons in 1942 [35] it has been shown that growth is promoted by high summer temperatures, mild winters, high humidity, a certain altitude and a characteristic flora of which the cresote bush is an important component [94]. Fungal growth appears to be more prolific near the burrows of rodents and it is thought that the excrement is the important promoting factor [33].

Histoplasma capsulatum and *Cryptococcus neoformans* also depend on certain characteristics of soil. *H. capsulatum* was originally isolated from the soil by Emmons [36]. Soil contaminated by chicken and bat excreta is particularly suitable for growth. Thus acute histoplasmosis has been traced to soil fertilized by chicken manure [57], to the dust of a silo tower [63], to derelict houses where starlings have congregated, and to caves inhabited by bats [3, 39 & 59]. So-called 'cave disease' is an influenza-like illness due to *H. capsulatum* [14 & 70] encountered in cave explorers in Venezuela and South Africa.

In endemic areas (the north and central United States, Argentine, Brazil, Venezuela and parts of Africa) as many as 80% of the population may show a positive reaction to histoplasmin skin tests [32]. In Britain and Eire such skin testing as has been performed has given negative results [71 & 72]. The 20 or so cases reported in Britain have all been infected in endemic zones. One such case was reported by one of us [24]. It is interesting that several years may elapse after primary infection before clinical histoplasmosis develops [52, 61 & 82].

Once known as torulosis [23 & 60], infection with *Cryptococcus neoformans*, or cryptococcosis, occurs sporadically all over the world. While the organism has been isolated from fruit and milk [15] the commonest association is with pigeon excreta [37, 38 & 77]. Bovine mastitis may sometimes be due to cryptococcal infection [53 & 97].

Blastomycosis is endemic in central and southeastern parts of the U.S.A. and in South America. North American blastomycosis is due to *Blastomyces dermatitidis* and South American to *Paracoccidioides brasiliensis*.

Sporotrichosis due to *Sporotrichum schenckii* occurs sporadically in various parts of the world but mainly in areas with hot climates. Most commonly it produces indolent skin lesions: primary pulmonary sporotrichosis is uncommon [25, 83 & 88].

The distribution of aspergillosis and mucormycosis is world-wide; the first is a relatively common condition, the second is rare.

INCIDENCE OF PULMONARY MYCOSES

Precise figures for the incidence of any of the pulmonary mycoses are not available. It is thought that the increasing use of wide spectrum antibiotics and corticosteroid therapy has increased the number of infections with *C. albicans*. Local infections involving the mouth, oesophagus, intestine and vagina are frequent but systemic candidiasis, endocarditis and pulmonary candidiasis are rare. In a review of the literature up to 1962 Winner and Hurley [120] refer to 20 cases of systemic candidiasis in children and 33 in adults.

Actinomycosis occurs in all countries but is relatively uncommon, particularly since the introduction of penicillin which has made the chronic form of the disease with sinus formation a rarity.

In endemic areas infection with coccidioidomycosis is almost 100% although perhaps only 20% will have a clinical illness leading to a diagnosis [40].

The high incidence of histoplasmin skin sensitivity in endemic areas has already been mentioned. Again, only a proportion of skin reactors to histoplasmin (about 25%) have clinical disease and of these the vast majority present with a nonspecific influenza-like ill-

ness; only about 0·2% develop systemic histoplasmosis [94].

A. fumigatus has been reported in about 10% of patients with bronchitis and in greater numbers of asthmatic patients (p. 405) [78 & 87]. *A. fumigatus* is a frequent laboratory contaminant, however, and its isolation does not necessarily imply pathogenicity. Nevertheless, repeated positive cultures are suggestive. There is good evidence that bronchopulmonary aspergillosis is more common than has hitherto been appreciated [13].

Cryptococcosis has been reported uncommonly in Britain; only 22 cases had been recorded by 1962 [89]. *C. neoformans* is world-wide in its distribution, however, and the incidence of infection may be much higher than published cases indicate because of failure to recognize the condition or to report sporadic cases.

For reasons already stated, candidiasis, cryptococcosis and histoplasmosis may become increasingly important in Britain.

PATHOLOGY AND LABORATORY DIAGNOSIS OF PULMONARY MYCOSES

All fungal infections are capable of causing a variety of inflammatory reactions. Reactions in the lung may include one or more of the following: epithelial hyperplasia, histiocytic granuloma, thrombotic arteritis, a mixed pyogenic and granulomatous picture, caseating granuloma, fibrosis and calcification. The fungi causing pulmonary mycoses can usually be detected in tissue sections when it is feasible to obtain these. Much more commonly the diagnosis rests on isolation of the organism from sputum by appropriate techniques and less frequently on detection of antibodies in the serum.

For detailed information regarding the collection of specimens and their examination the reader is referred to Broadsheet No. 43 of the Association of Clinical Pathology [85].

ASPERGILLOSIS

In Britain aspergillosis is the most common, and therefore the most important, fungal disease affecting the lungs. The fungi of the genus *Aspergillus* are ubiquitous saprophytes in nature and produce airborne spores throughout the year. The organism thrives on decaying vegetation in warm, humid conditions and releases spores, particularly through the winter months. Noble and Clayton [76] have shown that there is approximately 100-fold increase in the air count of *A. fumigatus* spores in London in the months of October to February. *A. fumigatus* has been shown to produce an endotoxin which is highly lethal for mice and haemolytic for human and other animal erythrocytes [19]. These qualities may explain why *A. fumigatus* is the most common species responsible for aspergillosis in man. Other forms such as *A. niger* [112], *A. flavus* [41 & 74] and *A. nidulans* can cause disease similar to that produced by *A. fumigatus*; the rôle of *A. clavatus* in causing one type of extrinsic allergic alveolitis is mentioned elsewhere (p. 504).

Aspergilli are common laboratory contaminants and culture of the organism, unless repeated, is insufficient for diagnosis. Clinical, radiological, immunological and, when possible, histological confirmation should be sought.

Rarely aspergillosis affects apparently normal subjects; it is much more common in debilitated individuals.

There are 3 types of bronchopulmonary aspergillosis and the lungs may also be secondarily affected in the disseminated form of the disease.

The 4 varieties are:

(1) bronchial infection with allergic manifestations (p. 428)
(2) aspergilloma (p. 287)
(3) aspergillosis associated with pulmonary necrosis
(4) disseminated aspergillosis.

These forms of infection are distinct from the mild temporary acute tracheobronchitis [109] which may occur when compost or mouldy hay is being handled and large numbers of aspergillus spores inhaled.

1. BRONCHIAL ASPERGILLOSIS WITH ALLERGIC MANIFESTATIONS (p. 429)

This is characterized by the development of transient pulmonary infiltrates and associated with fever, wheezing and eosinophilia. Bronchial casts, often brown in colour, may be coughed up from which *A. fumigatus* can be cultured. Immediate type skin hypersensitivity to aspergillin is usually found in patients in this group. Serum precipitins are found in only 70% of patients with allergic aspergillosis [13 & 78].

Obstruction of bronchi by mycelium can result in collapse of a segment, lobe, or rarely a lung [34].

A. fumigatus infection resulting in pulmonary infiltration and eosinophilia has been reported as a complication of fibrocystic disease [121].

2. ASPERGILLOMA

Colonization of lung tissue previously damaged by disease has been increasingly recognized since the phenomenon of open healing of tuberculous cavities (p. 232). The localization of aspergillomata to the upper zones is well known [13]. The typical aspergilloma is a mass of mycelium lying free within a pulmonary cavity partially lined by a modified bronchial epithelium which grows into the cavity. There is usually little or no surrounding inflammatory reaction. The development of aspergillomata may be asymptomatic but mild haemoptysis is common and other features, such as weight loss and occasionally severe cachexia, may be added. Radiographically the condition is recognized by a dense opacity separated from the wall of the cavity by a halo shadow of air. The opacity may move with different positions of the patient. The cavities in which an aspergilloma may develop are not always due to tuberculosis though they most commonly are. Less frequent causes are slowly resolving pneumonia, bronchial cysts, bronchiectasis, lung abscess, sarcoidosis, pulmonary infarction, pulmonary neoplasia, pneumoconiosis and histoplasmosis [1, 6, 10, 22, 26, 44, 47, 48, 64, 78, 84, 90, 101, 106 & 116]. Serum precipitins are almost invariably present in patients with aspergillomata [13]. When skin hypersensitivity is present in a patient with aspergilloma this suggests coexisting allergic aspergillosis.

As time goes on the mass increases in size and may finally almost completely fill the cavity. During this time there may be remittent fever and progressive deterioration of health. In one of our patients with open cavity healing and an aspergilloma, infection of the mass resulted in gradual extrusion of the contents of the cavity over a period of about 18 months. During this time the clinical picture was that of chronic suppurative pneumonia.

Multiple bilateral pulmonary aspergillomata have been described [81].

3. ASPERGILLUS INFECTION ASSOCIATED WITH PULMONARY NECROSIS

Usually this occurs in debilitated subjects and the most recent case we have had was a chronic alcoholic. In this patient a middle lobe consolidation went on to cavitation and treatment had to include surgical resection, always a risk in these patients because of the possibility of bronchopleural fistula or *A. fumigatus* empyema. Both skin hypersensitivity and precipitin formation are variable in this form of the disease.

4. DISSEMINATED ASPERGILLOSIS

Usually this follows severe underlying disease such as carcinoma, leukaemia, reticuloses or the use of corticosteroid, radiomimetic or antibiotic therapy [46]. Many organs may be involved including the brain, meninges [16], kidney, heart, lymph glands and skin.

TREATMENT

Treatment of the allergic form of bronchial aspergillosis consists of repeated aerosols of the tetraene antifungal, natamycin, to which oral or inhaled nystatin or inhalations of brilliant green or 2-hydroxystilbamidine are added according to the severity. Natamycin is given 2–3 times daily in doses of 2·5 mg in a 2·5% suspension diluted with an alkaline agent. The polypeptide antibiotic X-5079 C (p. 296) is under trial [94].

Allergic bronchial aspergillosis may persist for many years with episodes of wheeze, fever, eosinophilia and radiographic evidence of transient consolidation and collapse. Some patients recover spontaneously; others worsen and develop severe chronic asthma for which corticosteroid therapy is necessary.

Amphotericin B (p. 295) is indicated in severe bronchopulmonary infection and in the disseminated type.

Sometimes an aspergilloma may be removed with the associated devitalized lung but commonly impaired pulmonary function prevents this. The type associated with pulmonary necrosis may be treated initially by the measures indicated above but usually requires resection if the clinical condition permits.

CANDIDIASIS (Moniliasis)

Winner and Hurley [120] list the following conditions which predispose to local and systemic candidiasis:

(1) Physiological: pregnancy, infancy.
(2) Local trauma: maceration, allergy of skin.
(3) Disorders of the endocrine system: diabetes mellitus, hypoparathyroidism, Addison's disease, pancreatitis, hypothyroidism.
(4) Malnutrition.
(5) Malabsorption syndrome.
(6) Antibiotic and corticosteroid therapy.
(7) Blood dyscrasias, in particular, acute leukaemia, agranulocytosis and aplastic anaemia.
(8) Postoperative states.
(9) Malignant disease.

Bronchopulmonary candidiasis is rare. Pneumonia due to *C. albicans* has been reported in debilitated patients and its rare existence has been accepted. Whether or not hypersensitivity reactions may occur in the bronchi or lungs is much more debatable and there is no good evidence for this at the moment.

Two forms of thoracic candidiasis are described:

1. BRONCHIAL CANDIDIASIS

The bronchi are coated with plaques similar to those seen in the throat and mouth in oral candidiasis and symptoms include distressing cough, sputum which is scanty or mucoid and sometimes milky in appearance [86]. The fungus may be detected in the bronchial secretions but it should be remembered that *C. albicans* is a normal inhabitant of the respiratory tract and may be recovered in sputum culture in over 50% of patients with pulmonary tuberculosis, in about a quarter of patients in hospital with other conditions, and in over 10% of healthy individuals. Repeated and heavy growths are, of course, more significant than a single isolation.

The *chest x-ray* in bronchial candidiasis is usually normal but sometimes streaky opacities may be seen, particularly in the mid and lower zones.

2. PULMONARY CANDIDIASIS

The patient is more ill and usually fevered, with rapid pulse and respiration. Cough, sputum which may be bloodstained, dyspnoea and chest pain may all occur. The chest x-ray may show ill-defined, patchy opacities, mainly in the lower halves of the lungs, denser lesions, or, less frequently, pleural effusion.

The *diagnosis* of thoracic candidiasis depends on the demonstration of budding yeast cells and filaments of *Candida* in the sputum and the repeated isolation of the organism on Sabouraud's medium.

Treatment has to take into account the predisposing factors. For example, when wide spectrum antibiotics and corticosteroids are associated these should be withdrawn if at all possible. In malignant disease treatment may only be meddlesome. The most valuable therapeutic measure appears to be nystatin given in an aerosol at 4–6-hourly intervals combined with intravenous amphotericin B (p. 295) [94].

ACTINOMYCOSIS

AETIOLOGY

The actinomycoses affecting man are due to *Actinomyces israelii* or *Nocardia asteroides*.

Although the 2 organisms may cause a very similar clinical condition they have a number of contrasting features. *A. israelii* is anaerobic or microaerophilic, is distributed widely through the world and infection is endogenous in origin. By contrast *N. asteroides* is an aerobe, geographically limited and, therefore, less commonly the cause of infection, which is exogenous in origin, contracted from soil [27]. Only about 10% of infections caused by actinomycetes are due to *N. asteroides*. Until 1960, 179 cases of infection by *N. asteroides* had been described in the world literature. Eighteen cases of pulmonary nocardiosis in children were reported up to 1967 [51].

CLINICAL FEATURES

Patients infected with actinomycetes usually have an ill-kept mouth and carious teeth from which the organism can often be isolated. Infection may affect the cervicofacial area, the lung or the abdomen, the saprophyte becoming pathogenic owing to such factors as dental extraction, or even biting, or the inhalation or swallowing of the organisms in sufficient numbers. The cervicofacial area is most commonly affected and the abdomen the least. The lungs are involved in less than a quarter of cases. We are here concerned only with the pulmonary form of the disease.

The lungs may be involved as a primary phenomenon, by aspiration, secondarily due to extension from abdominal or cervicofacial actinomycosis or, rarely, by metastasis from disseminated disease. The condition is often unilateral initially but may become bilateral. From an insidious onset it progresses with irregular fever to cough, mucopurulent or bloodstained sputum, pleuritic pain and increasing severity of systemic upset. The clinical picture may be that of severe pneumonia, lung abscess or empyema. Tuberculosis may be simulated and may actually coexist. A characteristic of the infection is the tendency to transgress fascial planes and eventually to produce abscesses and sinuses in the chest wall. Secondary involvement of the spine has been recorded [121]. Cerebral abscess from haematogenous dissemination is a rare complication.

Nocardia produces a very similar disease. Since it is due to a soil organism, infection is much more commonly found in agricultural workers. Also like other 'opportunistic' fungal infections nocardiosis may complicate disease which impair immune mechanisms [50]. These include lymphomata, leukaemia, diabetes mellitus, alveolar proteinosis [105], Cushing's syndrome and the use of wide spectrum antibiotics, corticosteroids and antimitotic agents.

In general nocardiosis is a more serious condition than the infection caused by *A. israelii*. It is said that the tendency to dissemination, with cerebral metastases, is greater [117] and that thoracic sinuses occur less frequently.

RADIOLOGY

The chest x-ray shows irregular opacities in one or both lungs with a predilection for the mid and lower zones; pleural effusion may be present. The opacities may be of any size from miliary lesions to large areas of consolidation, which may cavitate. Periostial reaction may result in a characteristic x-ray appearance of new bone formation on the under surface of adjacent ribs or vertebrae. This may result in the ribs becoming markedly thickened. Collapse of vertebrae may occur but the intervertebral discs are usually not involved.

DIAGNOSIS

Diagnosis depends on the demonstration of the organism on film or culture. The 'sulphur granules' of actinomycosis are actually colonies of the organism in which peripheral 'clubs' can be distinguished by Ziehl–Neelsen's staining. These may be found in the discharge from an actinomycotic empyema. In sputum the organism more frequently occurs as gram positive branching filaments. If it is possible to obtain a specimen of the wall of a sinus or of an empyema a histological diagnosis can usually be made from tissue sections stained by Gram's method. Nocardia cannot be distinguished by staining techniques and differentiation depends on its

ability to grow under aerobic conditions. Reliable skin tests are not yet available [29].

TREATMENT

Penicillin is the drug of choice for actinomycosis and should be given in high doses (10–12 mega units per day). Treatment requires to be prolonged and in some cases may have to be given for 6–8 months. In the later stages of treatment lower dosage or even oral treatment may suffice. Pleural effusion may require repeated aspiration and rib resection may be necessary for an established empyema [107]. When extensive infection leaves fibrotic, bronchiectatic lung, liable to secondary infection, resection may prove necessary at a later date.

The distinction of actinomycosis from nocardiosis has practical implications since sulphonamides are superior to penicillin in nocardiosis [93]. Most commonly, however, combined therapy with another antibiotic is given, based on sensitivity tests. Chemotherapy is continued for the same period as for actinomycosis. Again, surgical treatment may be indicated for empyema or residual destroyed lung predisposing to repeated infections.

CRYPTOCOCCOSIS (Torulosis)

This also is usually an 'opportunistic' infection. The disease is a subacute or chronic infection which may involve the lungs, skin or bones but has a marked predilection for the brain and meninges [21]. Cryptococcal meningitis is the most frequent manifestation and may resemble tuberculous meningitis both in its presentation and course. The outlook is grave and death is usual within a year or so of the onset of the disease. Chronic cryptococcal meningitis has been described associated with progressive dementia. Rarely cerebral cryptococcosis presents with the features of cerebral tumour [115].

Pulmonary cryptococcosis may be relatively asymptomatic or may present with fever and chest pain, cough and sputum which is sometimes bloodstained. The x-ray may show any of a variety of appearances including infiltration resembling tuberculosis, solid lesions simulating neoplasms, and lung abscess or diffuse miliary mottling. Although the condition can occur at any age it is more frequent in adults and commoner in males.

The *diagnosis* is made by finding the organism in the sputum by smear and culture. Serological diagnosis has not been considered reliable but a recent report by Walter and Jones indicates that serodiagnosis (particularly the demonstration of complement-fixing antibodies) may be valuable [113].

Treatment of pulmonary cryptococcosis has been difficult to evaluate because of the tendency to spontaneous remission in some cases. The only drug known to be of value is amphotericin B (p. 295) and this may be life-saving in cases complicated by meningitis when the drug may require to be given intrathecally as well as intravenously. Usually it is necessary to continue treatment for several months.

COCCIDIOIDOMYCOSIS

Infection with *C. immitis* results from inhalation of dustborne spores about $2 \times 5 \mu$ in size. In the lungs the spores become thick-walled, spherical structures, $20-80 \mu$ in diameter, known as sporangia or spherules. These become filled with endospores which, when released, develop into further sporangia in the tissues.

Two forms of the disease are described— *primary* and *progressive coccidioidomycosis*. Since the primary respiratory infection is frequently asymptomatic and benign and the progressive form sometimes fatal, parallels have been drawn between this disease and tuberculosis. The disease occurs at all ages and in both sexes but progressive coccidioidomycosis is much commoner in males and affects more frequently and most severely the darker skinned races, such as the Negro, Mexican or Indian [40, 42 & 79].

PRIMARY COCCIDIOIDOMYCOSIS
CLINICAL FEATURES
Primary infection occurs 10–18 days after exposure and in most cases is asymptomatic

[94]. Symptomatic primary coccidioidomycosis is associated with an 'influenza-like' illness with chest pain, headache, low grade fever, joint pains and sore throat. Haemoptysis may rarely occur. In about 5% of cases erythema nodosum or erythema multiforme may develop 1–3 weeks after primary infection. When physical signs occur these are usually those of bronchitis or patchy consolidation. Rarely pleurisy or even pleural effusion may be detected. Usually there is a leucocytosis and the ESR is raised.

RADIOGRAPHIC APPEARANCES
Radiographic abnormality may occur in the absence of symptoms [20 & 55]. X-ray changes include scattered patchy opacities, often extensive, and commonly associated with bilateral hilar adenopathy. Pleural effusion may be present. Hilar lymphadenopathy without lung changes may occur but is less common. When bronchi are partially occluded thin-walled cavitation may occur [118].

COURSE AND PROGNOSIS
Most cases of primary pulmonary coccidioidomycosis resolve with no residua within 1–2 months. Radiographic abnormality may persist longer in the form of well-defined opacities or, less commonly, as calcified lesions [7 & 54]. Sometimes a thin-walled upper lobe cavity may persist with few or no associated symptoms and tuberculosis has to be differentiated [98]. Sometimes a single dense round lesion persists, resembling a tuberculoma or a lung tumour.

PROGRESSIVE COCCIDIOIDOMYCOSIS
CLINICAL FEATURES
Only about 0·1% of cases of primary coccidioidomycosis become progressive. Progressive infection may follow the primary disease immediately or develop several months later. The clinical picture varies. Systemic upset may predominate with anorexia and weight loss and the development of signs of bronchopneumonia. Progression to *acute* miliary dissemination may result in death within 3 months [86]. More frequently

the disease is *chronic* resulting in a granulomatous reaction in the skin, lungs, bones, lymph glands, meninges [62] or brain. Multiple subcutaneous cold abscesses may occur, resembling tuberculosis.

The progressive form of coccidioidomycosis has a 60% mortality, usually within 1–2 years. Spontaneous remissions are known but are rare. The most favourable outlook appears to be in those cases in which hypersensitivity to coccidioidin is maintained [86].

RADIOGRAPHIC APPEARANCES

These include patchy or confluent opacities, bilateral hilar adenopathy, miliary shadowing and multiple thin-walled cavities.

DIAGNOSIS OF COCCIDIOIDOMYCOSIS

The *differential diagnosis* commonly includes tuberculosis and carcinoma.

The *laboratory diagnosis* depends on the finding of sporangia in sputum, bronchial aspirates or gastric washings. Sporangia can be found in both forms of the disease. A fluorescent antibody technique has been found useful experimentally and may prove helpful as a means of rapid diagnosis. So far this technique is still in the experimental stage [56]. Intraperitoneal injection of infected material into mice results in the development of sporangia after a few days and later fatal dissemination of the disease which is confirmed by tissue section.

Coccidioidin (comparable to tuberculin) gives a delayed type positive reaction when injected intradermally into patients who have developed hypersensitivity to the products of infection. The test becomes positive about a month after infection. False positives are rare, and a positive test implies past or recent infection. Coccidioidin may also be used as an antigen to detect antibody in the serum. Humoral antibodies can be detected after skin hypersensitivity has developed. As a rule they are not found in silent primary infections but are usually present in symptomatic disease. The titre of complement-fixing antibodies rises with progression and severity of the disease and has serious prognostic significance [99].

TREATMENT

Most patients need no treatment. Severe primary infection or progressive infection should be treated with intravenous amphotericin B (p. 295) [119]. Surgical treatment may be necessary for persisting localized pulmonary lesions, for complicating empyema, excision of bone lesions and drainage of cold abscesses.

HISTOPLASMOSIS

H. capsulatum is a soil organism, responsible for endemic infection in localized areas of the world (p. 285) and spread by inhalation of spores. It principally affects the reticuloendothelial system where it propagates as a yeast-like, intracellular body, 1–5 μ in diameter. It affects both sexes equally and occurs at all ages and, like coccidioidomycosis, has a primary benign form and a serious progressive form, which may be fatal. Tuberculosis may be simulated and, as in coccidioidomycosis, may coexist [67]. Children are generally more liable to progressive histoplasmosis, particularly the acute form, but since the condition may be an example of 'opportunistic' infection, old and debilitated patients are also predisposed. The lesion may be acquired in the laboratory [69].

Even transient residence in endemic areas may result in infection. It is thought that infants and children are commonly infected *via* the alimentary system which bears the brunt of the disease in them, the lungs being involved only through dissemination at a late and often preterminal stage.

PRIMARY PULMONARY HISTOPLASMOSIS

This is usually benign and asymptomatic. Infection is commonly recognized only in retrospect by characteristic x-ray appearances and a positive skin test to histoplasmin. The x-ray changes in the lungs are diffuse, miliary type opacities with hilar lymphadenopathy. The pulmonary lesions may later calcify in a characteristic way. Diffuse small calcified pulmonary opacities surrounded by a paler halo are suggestive of previous disease [43 & 49].

Symptomatic cases of primary pulmonary histoplasmosis usually present with features like influenza. Sometimes more severe symptoms occur, including malaise, anorexia, chest pain, fever, cough and haemoptysis. These may subside fairly rapidly, or persist for several months, with symptoms and signs identical with bronchitis, pneumonia or chronic pulmonary tuberculosis. Relapse after temporary improvement is not uncommon. Protracted cases of primary pulmonary histoplasmosis may show diffuse bronchopneumonic opacities with or without hilar adenopathy. Healing results in clearing of the opacities either completely or with residual fibrosis, perhaps with the later development of the characteristic calcified lesions.

The possible *differential diagnosis* is extensive but distinction is mainly necessary from miliary or chronic pulmonary tuberculosis.

PROGRESSIVE HISTOPLASMOSIS

Acute and chronic forms are recognized.

Acute progressive histoplasmosis is protean in its clinical presentation but weight loss, fever, anaemia, leucopenia, hepatosplenomegaly and mucocutaneous oral granulomata [114] are common. In children, clinical and radiographic appearances may closely resemble miliary tuberculosis. The prognosis in acute progressive histoplasmosis is grave, particularly in children, but recovery is possible [12].

Chronic progressive histoplasmosis. The clinical and radiographic features closely resemble chronic pulmonary tuberculosis and many cases have actually been found in tuberculosis hospitals in the United States. Fibrosis and cavitation are the most frequent x-ray findings. Pulmonary granulomata may occur, usually single and simulating carcinoma [52] but sometimes multiple. Solitary granulomata may also occur, particularly involving the skin, mucous membranes or lymph glands, in the absence of pulmonary lesions. Acute haematogenous spread may suddenly result in severe clinical deterioration and prove fatal.

Progressive histoplasmosis may complicate pulmonary tuberculosis, sarcoidosis [80 & 104], reticuloses [75] or leukaemia.

FUNCTIONAL ABNORMALITY

Functional studies have been recorded in only 1 case of histoplasmosis [8]. This showed a loss of diffusing surface and only minimal disturbance of air flow. It seems probable that the scattered calcified residues of histoplasmosis do not significantly affect function.

PROGNOSIS

About 0·1% of patients with histoplasmosis develop the progressive form of the disease. The disease is fatal in the vast majority of patients with acute dissemination, and in about a third of those with chronic progressive pulmonary histoplasmosis.

DIAGNOSIS

Tuberculosis (miliary or chronic fibrocaseous), lung cancer and coccidioidomycosis may require to be differentiated. The diagnosis of pulmonary histoplasmosis is made by demonstration of the organism in sputum smears and confirmed by culture. Intraperitoneal inoculation of infected material into mice results in fatal reticuloendothelial infection.

The intradermal histoplasmin test is useful as an indication of past or present infection. The test resembles the tuberculin or coccidioidin hypersensitivity tests and becomes positive 4–8 weeks after infection. Occasionally negative results are obtained during active disease.

Precipitins, agglutinins and complement-fixing antibodies develop; active disease may be confirmed by rising titres in serial specimens of serum.

TREATMENT

Symptomatic disease should be treated with intravenous amphotericin B for 7–14 days (p. 295). The drug is life-saving in the acute progressive form of the disease and results in significant clinical and radiographic improvement in the chronic progressive form with pulmonary cavitation. The favourable effects of treatment with amphotericin B have been proved by a cooperative study undertaken by the Veterans Administration of the United States Armed Forces. The effects of treatment were noted on cultures of sputum for *H. capsulatum*, x-ray appearances and antibody titres in a series of randomly selected control cases compared with randomly selected drug treated cases. The study showed conclusively that amphotericin B is the treatment of choice for chronic pulmonary histoplasmosis with active primary lesions [111].

When an isolated pulmonary granuloma cannot be distinguished from lung cancer surgical treatment is indicated.

BLASTOMYCOSIS

NORTH AMERICAN BLASTOMYCOSIS

North American blastomycosis has been known since 1894 [45]. The typical cutaneous granulomata were first described and later involvement of other organs, particularly the lungs, was recognized [45]. The condition is caused by *Blastomyces dermatitidis* and the pathological reaction is a granulomatous one. Infection is probably acquired from soil as inhaled spores. It is endemic in some southeastern regions of the United States and males are mainly affected. A cooperative study was undertaken by the Veterans Administration in the United States [110]. In this study the disease was found to be more prevalent in the middle Atlantic, south central and the Ohio–Mississippi river valley states. There was an increased incidence in persons whose occupation involved intimate contact with the soil. The most frequent sites of involvement are the skin and lungs but no organ is immune. Thus the bones, genito-urinary system and central nervous system [11] may all be involved. No symptoms are diagnostic of the disease. Cough is the most common single complaint. Skin lesions commonly cause the patient to seek attention.

The pulmonary manifestations of North American blastomycosis resemble a subacute pneumonia with low grade fever, dyspnoea, cough and purulent sputum which may be bloodstained. Chest pain and pleural involvement, rarely with effusion, may occur later. Sinus formation is also known but is less common than in actinomycosis. It is uncommon for pulmonary involvement to occur alone; usually it is only part of the systemic disease. The chest radiograph shows bronchopneumonic shadowing, hilar gland enlargement or occasionally miliary mottling. Massive opacities have been known to occur in advanced disease and these may cavitate. Tuberculosis may coexist with blastomycosis [17 & 102].

The *diagnosis* is made histologically by finding the fungus in sections of the granulomatous tissues when these are available for biopsy, e.g. skin lesions. Blastomycin gives a delayed type hypersensitivity comparable to coccidioidin, histoplasmin and tuberculin; sometimes the test is negative in severe disseminated disease.

Serodiagnostic tests are at the moment insufficiently sensitive for reliable diagnosis [110].

Treatment is by amphotericin B (p. 295).

SOUTH AMERICAN BLASTOMYCOSIS

This condition is confined to South America and is caused by *Paracoccidioides brasiliensis*. Multiple granulomata develop and spread occurs along the lymph vessels to other sites. The lesions, which may affect the mucocutaneous surfaces, are disfiguring and scarring is marked. Systemic spread is uncommon but may occur and when the lungs are involved the clinical and radiographic picture resembles miliary tuberculosis or the other forms of disseminating fungal diseases [4, 58 & 94].

Sulphadiazine suppresses the infection and amphotericin B (p. 295) is curative.

SPOROTRICHOSIS

This is due to *Sporotrichum schenckii* and affects mainly males whose occupations bring them into contact with the organism which thrives on various woods, plants and soil. The organism enters the skin through abrasion and results in the development of a subcutaneous granulomatous nodule which may ulcerate through the skin, spread along lymphatics to other areas or disseminate. When dissemination occurs the lungs, bones, central nervous system or other viscera may be affected. There is some evidence that dissemination is more likely to occur in those who have inhaled or ingested the organism, rather than from skin lesions.

Less than 20 cases of primary pulmonary sporotrichosis are well documented. It is important to recognize the condition as spontaneous cure has not been reported but cure may follow surgical treatment [25]. The sporotrichin skin test has the same significance as in most of the other fungal diseases in that it indicates present or past infection and may be negative in disseminated forms of the disease. Serodiagnosis is not reliable in sporotrichosis.

When only the skin is involved the condition responds well to potassium iodide. Local injections of amphotericin B (p. 295) or X-5079 C (p. 296) have also been used with apparent success. In disseminate disease or when the lungs are involved intravenous amphotericin B is the drug of choice.

MUCORMYCOSIS

This is a rare condition due to infection with certain species of *Mucor*, *Rhizopus* and *Absidia*, common saprophytes which in certain conditions can become pathogenic. This is another example of 'opportunistic' infection and the predisposing conditions are the same as those listed for other fungi which affect the lungs. The organism appears to be world-wide in its distribution and there is no evidence of geographical limitation or occupational predilection.

Acute pneumonia due to mucormycosis has been described [5]. Most respiratory symptoms may be encountered in this condition including pleurisy and haemoptysis. The chest radiograph shows ill-defined, diffuse opacities, frequently with cavitation. The brain, nasal sinuses, orbit and gastro-intestinal tract are other sites which may be affected by the organism.

The diagnosis is made by finding the organism on smear and culture of sputum or other exudates or in histological section.

Pulmonary mucormycosis has a poor prognosis and the best treatment appears to be amphotericin B (p. 295) [18]. Occasionally surgical treatment has been undertaken for localized pulmonary lesions, usually when the diagnosis has not been established [28 & 68].

DRUG TREATMENT OF PULMONARY MYCOSES

AMPHOTERICIN B

This drug, produced by *Streptomyces nodosus*, is active against almost all the serious pulmonary mycoses. It is poorly soluble in water and absorption from the gut is inadequate to control systemic infections. The drug should, therefore, be given intravenously in all severe cases of mycotic infections and may sometimes have to be given intrathecally in patients with cryptoccocal or coccidioidal meningitis.

The dosage of amphotericin B is still a matter of debate. A 5% aqueous glucose solution containing 50 mg of amphotericin B and 41 mg of sodium desoxycholate is suitable for both intravenous and intrathecal use. Hilldick-Smith *et al.* [50] advocate an initial dose of 10 mg of amphotericin B on the 1st day, 25 mg the 2nd day and 50 mg each day thereafter in 1000 ml of 5% glucose given over 6–8 hours. 10 mg of heparin are added to reduce the risk of local venous thrombosis. It is important to avoid salts such as sodium chloride and procaine hydrochloride since these will cause the amphoteric antibiotic to be precipitated.

Utz [108] prefers to start with a very small dose of 1 mg with daily increments of 5 mg until the optimal dose of 0·5 mg–1·5 mg/kg/day is reached.

Minimal treatment should give at least a total of 1 g of the drug over 1 month. Most adults will tolerate a total dose of up to 5 g without any evidence of renal impairment. Dosage over 5–10 g runs the risk of permanent impairment of renal function. It is important to examine the urine frequently and to estimate renal function at frequent intervals. It is also recommended that the blood count, serum potassium and liver function should be monitored weekly [94].

Common side effects of intravenous amphotericin B are nausea, anorexia, vomiting, fever, rigors, headache and malaise. It is said that chlorpromazine given shortly before the injection reduces the incidence of these side effects [94].

Oral administration of amphotericin B has been used for intestinal candidiasis.

X-5079 C

This polypeptide antifungal agent is effective in histoplasmosis, sporotrichosis, North American blastomycosis and to a lesser degree in aspergillosis. The drug is given subcutaneously at 6 hour intervals in a dosage of 3–17 mg/kg/day for periods of 7–70 days. It is potentially hepatotoxic so that liver function should be checked frequently. Information about this drug is scanty so far and it is not yet to be preferred to amphotericin B.

HAMYCIN

Hamycin is produced from *Streptomyces piprina*. It has been found to be effective against superficial fungal infections, mainly in candidiasis [95]. Experimental studies have shown a marked effect in brain infections due to *C. neoformans* [9]. Its value in systemic mycoses in man has still to be determined.

NATAMYCIN

This drug has been shown to be effective topically against a wide range of fungi. Its principal use at the moment is by inhalation in the treatment of bronchopulmonary aspergillosis [31].

OTHER DRUGS

Potassium iodide in sporotrichosis, penicillin in actinomycosis and sulphonamides in nocardiosis are the drugs of choice. 2-hydroxystilbamidine has been advocated by some workers for North American blastomycosis.

REFERENCES

[1] ABBOTT J.D., FERNANDO H.V.J., GURLING K. & MEADE B.W. (1952) Pulmonary aspergillosis following post-influenzal bronchopneumonia treated with antibiotics. *Br. med. J.* i, 523.

[2] AJELLO L. (1962) In *Fungi and Fungous Diseases*, ed. Dalldorf G., p. 69. Springfield, Ill. Thomas.

[3] AJELLO L., MANSON-BAHR P.E.C. & MOORE J.C. (1960) Amboni caves, Tanganyika; a new endemic area for *Histoplasma capsulatum*. *Am. J. trop. Med. Hyg.* 9, 633.

[4] ALMEIDA F.DE., LACAZ C. DA SILVA & NETO C.F. (1942) Dados estatisticos sôbre o granuloma Paracoccidioidico no Brasil. Importancia de seu estudo. *An. Fac. med. S. Paulo.* 18, 137.

[5] BAKER R.D. & SEVERANCE A.O. (1948) Mucormycosis, with report of acute mycotic pneumonia. *Am. J. Path.* 24, 716.

[6] BARLOW D. (1954) Aspergillosis complicating pulmonary tuberculosis. *Proc. Roy. Soc. Med.* 47, 877.

[7] BASS H.E., SCHOMER A. & BERKE R. (1948) Coccidioidomycosis. Persistence of residual pulmonary lesions. *Arch. intern. Med.* 83, 519.

[8] BATES D.V. & CHRISTIE R.V. (1964) Histoplasmosis. In *Respiratory Function in Disease*, p. 242. Philadelphia, Saunders.

[9] BENNETT J.E., WILLIAMS T.W.Jr., PIGGOTT W. & EMMONS C.W. (1964) *In vivo* activity of colloidal hamycin, an antifungal antibiotic. *Proc. Soc. exper. Biol. & Med.* 117, 166.

[10] BRUCE R.A. (1957) A case of pulmonary aspergillosis. *Tubercle (Lond.)* 38, 203.

[11] BUECHNER H.A. & CLAWSON CAROLYN M. (1967) Blastomycosis of the central nervous system. II. A report of 9 cases from the Veterans Administration cooperative study. *Am. Rev. resp. Dis.* 95, 820.

[12] BUNNELL I.L. & FURCOLOW M.L. (1948) A report on 10 proved cases of histoplasmosis. *Publ. Hlth Rep. Wash.* 63, 299.

[13] CAMPBELL M.J. & CLAYTON YVONNE M. (1964) Bronchopulmonary aspergillosis: a correlation of the clinical and laboratory findings in 272 patients investigated for bronchopulmonary aspergillosis. *Am. Rev. resp. Dis.* 89, 186.

[14] CAMPINS H., ZUBILLAGA C.Z., LOPEZ L.G. & DORANTE M. (1956) An epidemic of histoplasmosis in Venezuela. *Am. J. trop. Med.* 5, 690.

[15] CARTER H.S. & YOUNG J.L. (1950) Note on the isolation of *Cryptococcus neoformans* from a sample of milk. *J. Path. Bact.* 62, 271.

[16] CAWLEY E.P. (1947) Aspergillosis and the *Aspergilli*. Report of a unique case of the disease. *Arch. intern. Med.* 80, 423.

[17] CHERNISS E.I. & WAISBREN B.A. (1956) North American blastomycosis. *Ann. intern. Med.* 44, 105.

[18] CHICK E.W., EVANS J. & BAKER R.D. (1958) Treatment of experimental mucormycosis

(*Rhizopus oryzae* infection) in rabbits with amphotericin B. *Antibiot. Chemother.* **8**, 394.

[19] CLAYTON YVONNE M. (1960) A study of the factors which determine the pathogenicity of *Aspergillus fumigatus* for animals and an appraisal of the histological changes in animal tissue infection by this fungus. London University PhD. Thesis.

[20] COLBURN J.R. (1944) Roentgenological type of pulmonary lesions in primary coccidioidomycosis. *Am. J. Roentgenol.* **51**, 1.

[21] CONANT .N.F., SMITH D.T., BAKER R.D., CALLAWAY J.L. & MARTIN D.S. (1954) Aspergillosis. In *Manual of Clinical Mycology.* 2nd Edition, p. 204. Philadelphia, Saunders.

[22] CORPE R.F. & COPE J.A. (1956) Bronchogenic cystic disease complicated by unsuspected choleraesuis and aspergillus infestation. *Am. Rev. Tuberc.* **74**, 92.

[23] COX L.B. & TOLHURST J.C. (1946) *Human Torulosis.* Melbourne, University Press.

[24] CROFTON J. (1950) A probable case of pulmonary histoplasmosis diagnosed in England. *Thorax* **5**, 340.

[25] CRUTHIRDS T.P. & PATTERSON D.O. (1967) Primary pulmonary sporotrichosis. *Am. Rev. resp. Dis.* **95**, 845.

[26] DARKE C.S., WARRACK A.J.N. & WHITEHEAD J.E.M. (1957) Pulmonary aspergillosis—report of a case. *Br. med. J.* **i**, 984.

[27] DAVIES M.I.J. (1941) Analysis of 46 cases of actinomycosis with special reference to its etiology. *Am. J. Surg.* **52**, 447.

[28] DILLON M.L., SEALY W.C. & FETTER B.F. (1958) Mucormycosis of the bronchus successfully treated by lobectomy. *J. thorac. Surg.* **35**, 464.

[29] DYSON J.E. & SLACK J.M. (1963) Improved antigens for skin testing in nocardiosis. *Am. Rev. resp. Dis.* **88**, 80.

[30] ECKMANN B.H., SCHAEFER G.L. & HUPPERT M. (1964) Bedside interhuman transmission of coccidioidomycosis via growth on fomites. *Am. Rev. resp. Dis.* **89**, 175.

[31] EDWARDS G. & LA TOUCHE C.J.P. (1964) The treatment of bronchopulmonary mycoses with a new antibiotic—Pimaricin. *Lancet* **i**, 1349.

[32] EDWARDS PHYLLIS Q. (1958) In *Fungous Diseases and their Treatment,* ed. Riddell R.W. and Stewart G.T., p. 158. London, Butterworth.

[33] EGEBERG R.O. & ELY A.F. (1956) *Coccidioides immitis* in the soil of the Southern San Joaquin Valley. *Am. J. med. Sci.* **231**, 151.

[34] ELLIS R.H. (1965) Total collapse of the lung in aspergillosis. *Thorax* **20**, 118.

[35] EMMONS C.W. (1942) Isolation of *Coccidioides* from the soil and rodents. *Publ. Hlth Rep., Wash.* **57**, 109.

[36] EMMONS C.W. (1949) Isolation of *Histo-* *plasma capsulatum* from soil. *Publ. Hlth Rep., Wash.* **64**, 892.

[37] EMMONS C.W. (1951) Isolation of *Cryptococcus neoformans* from soil. *J. Bact.* **62**, 685.

[38] EMMONS C.W. (1955) Saprophytic sources of *Cryptococcus neoformans* associated with the pigeon (Columbia livia). *Am. J. Hyg.* **62**, 227.

[39] EMMONS C.W. (1958) Association of bats with histoplasmosis. *Publ. Hlth Rep., Wash.* **73**, 590.

[40] FIESE M.J. (1958) *Coccidioidomycosis,* p. 4, Springfield, Ill., Thomas.

[41] FINEGOLD S.M., WILL D. & MURRAY J.F. (1959) Aspergillosis: a review and report of 12 cases. *Am. J. Med.* **27**, 463.

[42] FORBUS W.D. & BESTERBREUTJE A.M. (1946) Coccidioidomycosis: a study of 95 cases of the disseminated type with special reference to the pathogenesis of the disease. *Milit. Surg.* **99**, 653.

[43] FURCOLOW M.L., MANTZ H.L. & LEWIS I. (1947) The roentgenographic appearance of persistent pulmonary infiltrates associated with sensitivity to histoplasmin. *Publ. Hlth Rep., Wash.* **62**, 1711.

[44] GERSTL B., WEIDMAN W.H. & NEWMANN A.V. (1948) Pulmonary aspergillosis. Report on 2 cases. *Ann. intern. Med.* **28**, 662.

[45] GILCHRIST T.C. & STOKES W.R. (1896) Further observations on blastomycetic dermatitis in man. *Bull. Hopkins Hosp.* **7**, 129.

[46] GOWLING N.F.C. & HAMLIN I.M.E. (1960) Tissue reactions to aspergillus in cases of Hodgkin's disease and leukaemia. *J. Clin. Path.* **13**, 396.

[47] HEPPLESTON A.G. & GLOYNE S.R. (1949) Pulmonary aspergillosis in coal workers. *Thorax* **4**, 168.

[48] HERTZOG A.J., SMITH T.S. & GOBLIN M. (1949) Acute pulmonary aspergillosis. *Pediatrics* **4**, 331.

[49] HIGH R.H., ZWERLING H.B. & FURCOLOW M.L. (1947) Disseminated pulmonary calcification. *Publ. Hlth Rep., Wash.* **62**, 20.

[50] HILLDICK-SMITH G., BLANK H. & SARKANY I. (1964) In *Fungous Diseases and their Treatment.* London, Churchill.

[51] HOLDAWAY M.D., KENNEDY J., ASHCROFT T. & KAY-BUTLER J.J. (1967) Pulmonary nocardiosis in a 3 year old child. *Thorax* **22**, 375.

[52] HUTCHINSON H.E. (1952) Laryngeal histoplasmosis simulating carcinoma. *J. Path. Bact.* **64**, 309.

[53] INNES J.R.M., SEIBOLD H.R. & ARENTZEN W.P. (1952) The pathology of bovine mastitis caused by *Cryptococcus neoformans. Am. J. Vet. Res.* **13**, 469.

[54] JAMISON H.W. (1946) A roentgen study of chronic pulmonary coccidioidomycosis. *Am. J. Roentgenol.* **55**, 396.

[55] JAMISON H.W. & CARTER R.A. (1947) The

roentgen findings in early coccidioidomycosis. *Radiology* **48**, 323.

[56] KAPLAN W. & CLIFFORD MARY K. (1964) Production of fluorescent antibody reagents specific for the tissue form of *Coccidioides immitis. Am. Rev. resp. Dis.* **89**, 651.

[57] KIER J.H., CAMPBELL C.C., AJELLO L. & SUTLIFF W.D. (1954) Acute bronchopneumonic histoplasmosis following exposure to infected garden soil. *J. Am. Med. Ass.* **155**, 1230.

[58] LACAZ C. DA SILVA (1951) Lesões pulmonares na blastomicose sul-americana. *O Hospital, Rio de Janeiro*, **39**, 405.

[59] LAZARUS A.S. & AJELLO L. (1955) Aislamiento de *Histoplasma capsulatum* del suelo de una cueva en el Peru. *Rev. med. exper. Lima.* **9**, 5.

[60] LITTMAN M.L. & ZIMMERMAN L.E. (1956) *Cryptococcosis.* New York, Grune & Stratton.

[61] LOCKET S., ATKINSON E.A. & GRIEVE W.S.M. (1953) Histoplasmosis in Great Britain. *Br. med. J.* **ii**, 857.

[62] LOCKS M.O. & HAWKINS J.A. (1963) Ventriculoatriostomy in coccidioidal meningitis. *Am. Rev. resp. Dis.* **88**, 33.

[63] LOOSLI C.G., GRAYSTON J.T., ALEXANDER E.R. & TANZI F. (1952) Epidemiological studies of pulmonary histoplasmosis in a farm family. *Am. J. Hyg.* **55**, 392.

[64] MACARTNEY J.N. (1964) Pulmonary aspergillosis: a review and a description of 3 new cases. *Thorax* **19**, 287.

[65] MADDY K.T. (1957) Ecological factors possibly relating to the geographic distribution of *Coccidioides immitis. Proc. Symp. on Coccidioidomycosis*, Phoenix, Arizona.

[66] MEARNS MARGARET, YOUNG WINIFRED & BATTEN J. (1965) Transient pulmonary infiltrations in cystic fibrosis due to allergic aspergillosis. *Thorax* **20**, 385.

[67] MELENEY H.E. (1941) Pulmonary histoplasmosis: report of 2 cases. *Am. Rev. Tuberc.* **44**, 240.

[68] MURPHY J.D. & BORNSTEIN S. (1950) Mucormycosis of the lung. *Ann. intern. Med.* **33**, 442.

[69] MURRAY J.F. & HOWARD D. (1964) Laboratory-acquired histoplasmosis. *Am. Rev. resp. Dis.* **89**, 631.

[70] MURRAY J.F., LURIE H.I., KAYE J., KOMINS C., BOROK R. & WAY M. (1957) Benign pulmonary histoplasmosis (Cave disease) in South Africa. *South Afr. med. J.* **31**, 245.

[71] MCCRACKEN B.H. (1948) Intrapulmonary calcification and histoplasmin sensitivity. *Thorax* **3**, 45.

[72] MCWHEENEY E.J., CROWE M., DUNLEVY M. & MAGAN M. (1946) A survey with histoplasmin in Dublin. *J. med. Ass. Eire* **19**, 162.

[73] NABARRO J.D.N. (1948) Primary pulmonary coccidioidomycosis: case of laboratory infection in England. *Lancet* **i**, 982.

[74] NAJI A.F. (1959) Bronchopulmonary aspergillosis. *Arch. Path. (Chicago)* **68**, 282.

[75] NELSON N.A., GOODMAN H.L. & OSTER H.L. (1957) The association of histoplasmosis with lymphoma. *Am. J. med. Sci.* **233**, 56.

[76] NOBLE W.C.N. & CLAYTON YVONNE M. (1963) Fungi in the air of hospital wards. *J. Gen. Microbiol.* **32**, 397.

[77] PARTRIDGE BETTY M. & WINNER H.I. (1965) *Cryptococcus neoformans* in bird droppings in London. *Lancet* **i**, 1060.

[78] PEPYS J., RIDDELL R.W., CITRON K.M., CLAYTON YVONNE M. & SHORT E.I. (1959) Clinical and immunological significance of *Aspergillus fumigatus* in the sputum. *Am. Rev. resp. Dis.* **80**, 167.

[79] PERRY C.B. (1950) Coccidioidomycosis. In *British Encyclopedia of Medical Practice.* 2nd Edition, Vol. 3, p. 520. London, Butterworth.

[80] PINKERTON H. & IVERSON L. (1952) Histoplasmosis. Three fatal cases with disseminated sarcoid-like lesions. *Arch. intern. Med.* **90**, 456.

[81] PLIHAL V., JEDLICKOVA Z., VIKLICKY J. & TOMANEK A. (1964) Multiple bilateral pulmonary aspergillomata. *Thorax* **19**, 104.

[82] POLES E.C. & LAVERTINE J.D.O'D. (1954) Acute disseminated histoplasmosis with a report of a case occurring in England. *Thorax* **9**, 233.

[83] POST G.W., JACKSON A., GARBER P.E. & VEACH G.E. (1958) Pulmonary sporotrichosis. *Dis. Chest* **34**, 455.

[84] PROCKNOW J.J. & LOEWEN D.F. (1960) Pulmonary aspergillosis with cavitation secondary to histoplasmosis. *Am. Rev. resp. Dis.* **82**, 101.

[85] RIDDELL R.W. (1962) Mycological techniques. Broadsheet No. 43 (New Series), Association of Clinical Pathology.

[86] RIDDELL R.W. (1963) Fungous infections of the lungs. In *Chest Diseases*, ed. Perry K.M.A. and Sellors T.H., p. 82. London, Butterworth.

[87] RIDDELL R.W. & CLAYTON YVONNE M. (1958) Pulmonary mycoses occurring in Britain. *Br. J. Tuberc.* **52**, 34.

[88] RIDGEWAY N.A., WHITCOMB F.C., ERICKSON E.E., LAW S.W. & CHOFNA I. (1961) Primary pulmonary sporotrichosis: report of 2 cases. *Trans. 20th Res. Conf. in Pulm Dis.* p. 294.

[89] ROOK A. & WOODS B. (1962) Cutaneous cryptococcosis. *Br. J. Derm.* **74**, 43.

[90] ROSS C.F. (1951) A case of pulmonary aspergillosis. *J. Path. Bact.* **63**, 409.

[91] ROTH F.J.Jr., BOYD C.C., SAGAMI S. & BLANK H. (1959) An evaluation of the fungistatic activity of serum. *J. invest. Dermat.* **32**, 549.

[92] ROTH F.J.Jr. & GOLDSTEIN M.I. (1961) Inhibition of growth of pathogenic yeasts by human serum. *J. invest. Dermat.* **36**, 383.

[93] RUNYON E.H. (1951) *Nocardia asteroides:*

studies of its pathogenicity and drug sensitivities. *J. Lab. clin. Med.* **37**, 713.

[94] SARKANY I. (1968) Systemic mycoses. In *Recent Advances in Medicine*, eds. Baron D.N., Compson N. and Dawson A.M. London, Churchill.

[95] SARKANY I. & CARON G.A. (1966) The treatment of superficial fungal infections with Hamycin and Dermostatin. *Br. J. Derm.* **78**, 232.

[96] SIEVERS M.L. (1964) Coccidioidomycosis among Southwestern American Indians. *Am. Rev. resp. Dis.* **90**, 920.

[97] SIMON J., NICHOLS R.E. & MORSE E.V. (1953) An outbreak of bovine cryptococcosis. *J. Am. vet. med. Ass.* **122**, 31.

[98] SMITH C.E., BEARD R.R. & SAITO M.T. (1948) Pathogenesis of coccidioidomycosis with special reference to pulmonary cavitation. *Ann. intern. Med.* **29**, 623.

[99] SMITH C.E., PAPAGIANIS D., LEVINE H.B. & SAITO M. (1961) Human coccidioidomycosis. *Bact. Rev.* **25**, 310.

[100] SMITH D.T. & HARRELL E.R. (1948) Fatal coccidioidomycosis: a case of laboratory infection. *Am. Rev. Tuberc.* **57**, 368.

[101] SOCHOCKY S. (1959) Infection of pneumonectomy space with *Aspergillus fumigatus* treated by 'Nystatin'. *Dis. Chest* **36**, 554.

[102] STILLIANS A.W. & KLEMPTNER H.E. (1953) Blastomycosis in tuberculous patients. *J. Am. med. Ass.* **153**, 558.

[103] SULKIN S.E. & PIKE R.M. (1951) Laboratory-acquired infections. *J. Am. med. Ass.* **147**, 1740.

[104] SYMMERS W.St.C. (1956) Histoplasmosis contracted in Britain. A case of histoplasmic lymphadenitis following clinical recovery from sarcoidosis. *Br. med. J.* **ii**, 786.

[105] TALEGHANI-FAR M., BARBER J.B., SAMPSON C. & HARDEN K.A. (1964) Cerebral nocardiosis and alveolar proteinosis. *Am. Rev. resp. Dis.* **89**, 561.

[106] TOIGO A. (1960) Pulmonary aspergillosis. *Am. Rev. resp. Dis.* **81**, 392.

[107] TUBBS O.S. (1958) Treatment of actinomycosis. In *Fungous Diseases and their Treatment*, ed. Riddell R.W. and Stewart G.T., p. 231. London, Butterworth.

[108] UTZ J.P. (1965) Antimicrobial therapy in systemic fungal infections. *Am. J. Med.* **39**, 826.

[109] VAN ORDSTRAND H.S. (1940) Pulmonary aspergillosis with report of a case. *Cleveland clin. Quart.* **7**, 66.

[110] VETERANS ADMINISTRATION — COOPERATIVE STUDY ON BLASTOMYCOSIS (1964) Blastomycosis: a review of 198 collected cases in Veterans Administration Hospitals. *Am. Rev. resp. Dis.* **89**, 659.

[111] VETERANS ADMINISTRATION—COOPERATIVE STUDY ON HISTOPLASMOSIS (1964) Histoplasmosis: II chronic pulmonary histoplasmosis treated with and without amphotericin B. *Am. Rev. resp. Dis.* **89**, 641.

[112] VILLAR T.G., PIMENTEL J.C., FREITAS E. & COSTA M. (1962) The tumour-like forms of aspergillosis of the lung (pulmonary aspergilloma). *Thorax* **17**, 22.

[113] WALTER J.E. & JONES R.D. (1968) Serodiagnosis of clinical cryptococcosis. *Am. Rev. resp. Dis.* **97**, 275.

[114] WEED L.A. & PARKHILL E.M. (1948) The diagnosis of histoplasmosis in ulcerative disease of the mouth and pharynx. *Am. J. clin. Path.* **18**, 130.

[115] WERNER W.A. (1965) Pulmonary and cerebral cryptococcosis without meningitis. *Am. Rev. resp. Dis.* **92**, 476.

[116] WHEATON S.W. (1890) Case primarily of tubercle, in which a fungus (aspergillus) grew in the bronchi and lung, simulating actinomycosis. *Trans. path. Soc. Lond.* **41**, 34.

[117] WICHELHAUSEN R.H., ROBINSON L.B., MAZZARA J.R. & EVERDING C.J. (1954) Nocardiosis. Report of fatal case. *Am. J. Med.* **16**, 295.

[118] WINN W.A. (1941) Pulmonary cavitation associated with coccidioidal infection. *Arch. intern. Med.* **68**, 1179.

[119] WINN W.A. (1962) In *Fungi and Fungous Diseases*. Ed. DALLDORF G. p. 315. Springfield, Ill., Thomas.

[120] WINNER H.I. & HURLEY ROSALINDE (1964) *Candida Albicans*. London, Churchill.

[121] YOUNG W.B. (1960) Actinomycosis with involvement of the vertebral column: case report and review of the literature. *Clin. Radiol. (Lond.)* **11**, 175.

CHAPTER 18

Chronic Bronchitis and Emphysema

DEFINITIONS

A patient with advanced chronic bronchitis, now a respiratory invalid with severe dyspnoea and distressing cough, at one time suffered only a slight morning cough associated with smoking. The symptoms had gradually progressed through the years until they seriously began to interfere with his normal life. At what stage in this deterioration the condition should be called chronic bronchitis is bound to be somewhat arbitrary. In general the term is applied to patients who have coughed up sputum on most days during at least 3 consecutive months for more than 2 successive years [94], other causes, such as tuberculosis or bronchiectasis having been excluded. 'Simple chronic bronchitis' is the term used when the sputum is mucoid, 'chronic' or 'recurrent mucopurulent bronchitis' when the sputum is persistently or intermittently mucopurulent in the absence of localized bronchopulmonary disease [94]. An additional criterion used in some surveys is the occurrence of attacks of cough and sputum in the previous 2 years which have prevented the patient from working for a total of at least 3 weeks.

Such definitions are easy to apply to the typical case but at the extremes the condition of chronic bronchitis merges into that of 'primary emphysema' [123] in which there is little cough and sputum but gross breathlessness; into asthma, in which wheeze is predominant and may, at least in the early stages, be completely reversible; and into bronchiectasis, in some cases of which there may be relatively slight evidence of widening of the bronchi but much greater evidence of bronchial distortion. Clinically it must be realized that the term 'chronic bronchitis' is a convenience rather than a straitjacket, but when the diagnosis is used for scientific purposes, as in a controlled trial or a prevalence survey, a strict definition, such as that given at the end of the last paragraph, must be both used and stated in any report.

The term 'emphysema' is primarily a morbid anatomical one and is defined in the pathological section of this chapter (see p. 310). Its diagnosis by clinical, radiological or laboratory means is less simple than was at one time supposed.

MORTALITY AND PREVALENCE

MORTALITY

There are very great *international variations* in mortality rates for bronchitis. Some comparative figures are given in fig. 18.1, the countries being shown in the order of their bronchitis mortality. England and Wales have the highest mortality from this disease. Some of the international differences, particularly those between Britain and the United States, can be partly explained by differences in diagnostic habits. Nevertheless there seems little doubt, both from clinical impression and also from some of the comparative prevalence surveys discussed below, that this disease is a much bigger problem in Britain than elsewhere. On the other hand, the interest in the disease in Britain has aroused interest elsewhere and in many countries the problem is being found to be greater than was originally suspected. In the United States death rates for emphysema in men have increased from 1·3 per 100,000 in 1950 to 12·6 in 1964; death rates from chronic bronchitis have doubled during the same period. It is uncertain how far this increase reflects better diagnosis [142], but the fact that the increase is mainly in males suggests that it is genuine.

The *trends of mortality* in England and Wales, and in Scotland, standardized for age, are shown for males in fig. 18.2 and for

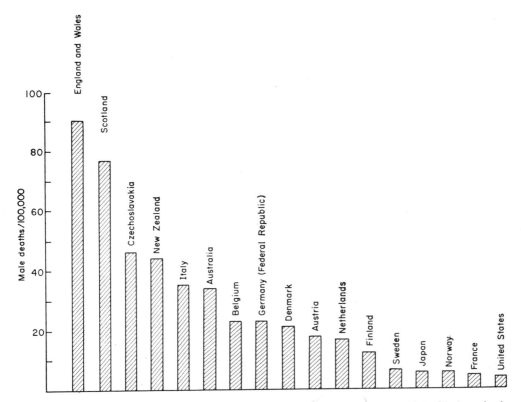

FIG. 18.1. International comparison of male mortality from bronchitis in 1964 (World Health Organisation figures).

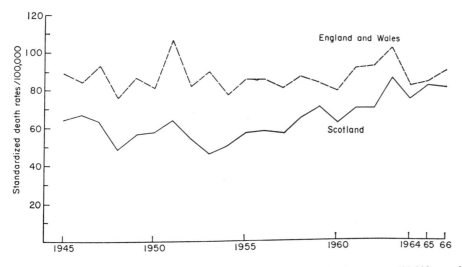

FIG. 18.2. Trends of male bronchitis mortality in Britain. Standardized death rates per 100,000 population for England and Wales and for Scotland 1945–66. (Figures calculated from Registrar-Generals' Reports.)

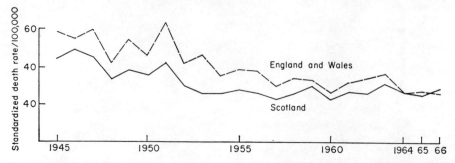

FIG. 18.3. Trends of female bronchitis mortality in Britain. Standardized death rates per 100,000 population for England and Wales and for Scotland 1945–66. (Figures calculated from Registrar Generals' Reports.)

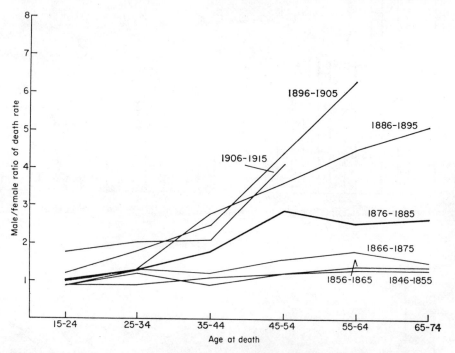

FIG. 18.4. Male–female ratio of bronchitis mortality by age in England and Wales for 10 year cohorts born between 1846 and 1905. (After Crofton and Crofton [32].)

females in fig. 18.3. For some years there has been little change in the English rates or in the rates for Scottish females but the male rates for Scotland have recently started to rise. Some of the differences between the rates for the two countries may be due to differences in diagnostic habit [33].

AGE AND SEX

In almost all countries from which figures

have been published, the male mortality rate is very much higher than the female; the male rate in England and Wales at age 55–64 in recent years is almost 6 times the female. A study has been made of the ratio between male and female deaths at different ages in persons born at specific periods. Such a group born in a specific year, or a specific period of years, is known as a 'cohort'. It has been found, both in England and Wales and in

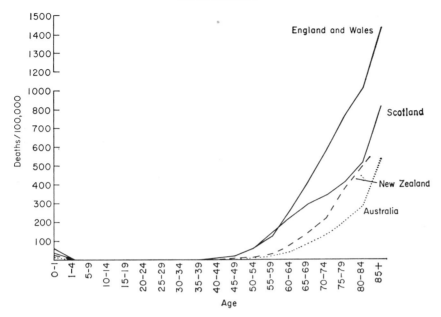

Fig. 18.5. Male bronchitis mortality by age, 1954–58, for England and Wales, Scotland, Australia and New Zealand. (Figures from Registrar-Generals' Reports and World Health Organisation.)

Scotland, that, in successive cohorts since the 19th century the male/female ratio has shown a steady increase and that, within each cohort, the male excess increases with advancing age (fig. 18.4). A similar trend is found with other diseases associated with cigarette smoking. The increase in cigarette smoking during this century, predominantly in males until 1940–50, seems the most likely explanation for these findings [32].

In Britain there is some mortality from bronchitis in infancy, mainly acute viral or bacterial disease. With advancing age the rate at first drops but after the age of 50 begins to rise steeply. In countries such as Australia and New Zealand, where the population is ethnically similar to that of Britain and where cigarette consumption is much the same, but where there is little atmospheric pollution, the rise of mortality with age occurs about 10 years later (fig. 18.5).

THE EFFECT OF URBANIZATION

In Britain there is a steady increase in mortality with increasing urbanization (fig. 18.6).

SEASONAL VARIATION

The highest mortality is in the winter. In 1954–63 in Scotland about 45% of the deaths from bronchitis occurred in the first 3 months of the year.

SOCIAL CLASS AND OCCUPATION

There is a steady increase in mortality with descending socioeconomic class, as defined by the Registrar Generals in Britain. In England and Wales in 1949–53 the standardized mortality ratio (SMR) for males aged 20–65 was 34 for social class I compared to 101 and 171 for social classes IV and V respectively [129]. The similar trend with social class in married women has been held to suggest that environment rather than occupation is the important factor [96]. But subsequent criticism [85] has suggested that this analysis, while highlighting the influence of environment on the mortality from bronchitis in workers and their wives, has failed to indicate the very big difference in mortality between workers in dusty occupations and their wives as compared with the much smaller difference between the mortality of

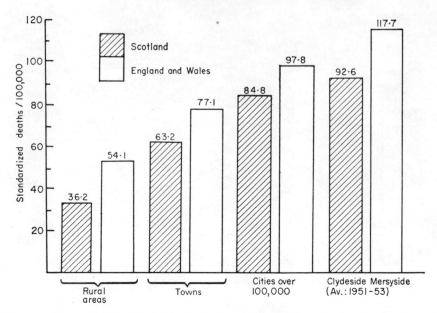

FIG. 18.6. Bronchitis mortality and urbanization. Average standardized death rates from bronchitis in males in England and Wales and in Scotland 1950–53.

men working in nondusty occupations and their wives (p. 309).

PREVALENCE

The best general indication of the prevalence of chronic bronchitis in Britain is derived from the study by the College of General Practitioners [29] which conducted a survey in sample practices throughout Britain, concentrating in both sexes on the age group 40–64. The notification was based on a questionary regarding symptoms and on a simple pulmonary function test. Taking the practitioners' diagnosis of chronic bronchitis the prevalence in this age group in men was 17% and in women 8%. In addition to the practitioners' diagnosis stricter criteria were also applied to the data, which selected a group with disabling chronic bronchitis. For this purpose chronic bronchitis was defined as including morning phlegm in the winter, attacks of cough and phlegm lasting at least 3 weeks over the previous 2 years and breathlessness on the level. Using these criteria the overall prevalence was 8% in men and 3% in women. The male excess rose steadily with age

but the ratio between males and females was lower than other surveys of hospital admissions and deaths. It was thought that the sex differences could be largely explained by smoking habits but the lower male/female ratio in this survey than in hospital surveys and in deaths suggested that bronchitis is a less severe disease in women. The survey also gave a number of pointers to aetiological factors which will be discussed below. The results of this nationwide survey are in broad agreement with previous sample surveys covering more limited areas. These have shown prevalence in men aged 55–64 in the region of 6–7% in rural areas and 10–15% in urban areas. The subject is well reviewed by the Scottish Subcommittee [129].

Much lower figures have been described from a rural area in Denmark [105]. It was concluded that this probably reflected a much lower prevalence of cigarette smoking.

AETIOLOGY

Although the causes of chronic bronchitis cannot yet be said to have been completely elucidated, it is becoming clear that there are 3 important aetiological factors: cigarette smoking, atmospheric pollution and infection. At present it is thought that the initial stimuli to increased mucus production in the respiratory tract, giving rise to chronic cough and sputum, are most often cigarette smoking and pollution of the atmosphere by smoke. It seems possible that where the individual is exposed both to cigarette smoking and to atmospheric pollution these 2 factors may act synergistically to produce a particularly severe effect. It may be that other industrial fumes and dusts act in a similar manner. It is thought that infection is seldom an initiating factor but that, once smoking or atmospheric pollution have induced the chronic cough and sputum, the patient's bronchial tree more readily becomes infected, at first in acute exacerbations and later perhaps chronically. It is probably infection which causes the major destruction in the lung tissue. It was also thought to be responsible for the steady deterioration in lung function over the years, but this is now less certain. It is possible that there is an underlying genetic factor which influences the development of symptoms in individuals with similar exposure to smoking and pollution, but the latter are of such overwhelming importance that a genetic factor is difficult to demonstrate. Some of the evidence on which these statements are based will now be briefly reviewed.

TOBACCO SMOKING

The most important evidence associating smoking and *mortality* from chronic bronchitis is that of Doll and Hill [38]. In a study, mainly aimed at determining the aetiology of lung cancer, 40,000 medical practitioners in Britain recorded their smoking habits, the cause of death being later determined in those who died during the follow-up period. It was found that the death rate for chronic bronchitis was significantly higher in cigarette smokers than in nonsmokers and increased with the amount smoked (fig. 18.7). In those who stopped smoking, which would include many who stopped for medical reasons, the mortality at first rose but by 10 years was well

below that for all smokers. There have been two other large scale prospective studies in the United States, and one in Canada, all of which have given similar results to the British study [142]. In only 1 of the studies were there sufficient women for reliable assessment; the relation of mortality to smoking was similar to that in men. The association of pipe and

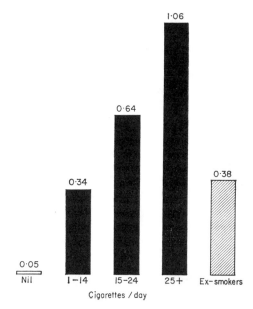

FIG. 18.7 Bronchitis death rates in British doctors, per 1000 persons per year, according to previous smoking habit (adapted from Doll and Hill [38].)

cigar smoking with mortality varied slightly in the different studies. In one there was no excess mortality; in the others the excess was relatively slight compared with cigarette smoking [142]. In a study of mortality of chronic bronchitis in Northern Ireland Wicken [145] has calculated that male mortality from the disease would have been reduced to 45% if there had been no smoking among the population.

Sample surveys of respiratory symptoms in the population have shown a much higher *prevalence* of cough and sputum among smokers than among nonsmokers. In such surveys chronic bronchitis, whatever the definition used, has been almost confined to smokers. For instance Higgins [60], in a sample survey in urban and rural populations in Britain, found that in males aged 55–64 the prevalence of chronic bronchitis was 17·6% among heavy smokers, 13·9% among light smokers, 4·4% among exsmokers and nil among nonsmokers. Similar differences were found in the College of General Practitioners Survey [29], carried out throughout Britain. Some international differences may also be due to differences in smoking habits. In a Danish island Olsen and Gilson [105], as already mentioned, found a much lower prevalence both of cigarette smoking and of bronchitis than in similar surveys in Britain. Lesser, but important, differences between urban and rural areas have been found in Britain [59]. In Finland, where there is much smoking, cough and sputum is significantly more frequent among smokers [68 & 70]. A number of these surveys have included simple tests of respiratory function, such as FEV or PEFR. On the whole the tests indicated poorer function in smokers than in nonsmokers [142].

The method of smoking is also important. Chronic bronchitis has been shown to be mainly related to cigarette smoking. Pipe and cigar smokers have a lower prevalence of the disease and less impairment of function [60 & 105]. The effects may start very early. It has been found that smoking schoolchildren have more cough and more chest illnesses than nonsmokers [66].

Several authors have studied *changes* in *respiratory function* after smoking 1 or more cigarettes. Some, such as Rothfield *et al.* [126] have been able to show little effect, but this was probably due to the technique used. Attinger *et al.* [7] found no change in normals after smoking cigarettes but a definite increase in airways resistance in bronchitic patients. Reanalysis of their results in normals in the light of later technical knowledge has shown a highly significant increase in resistance [100]. Using the body plethysmograph Nadel and Comroe [102] were able to show a significant increase in airways resistance following cigarette smoking in those with respiratory disease, in smokers without respiratory disease and in nonsmokers. After removing

most of the nicotine and volatile components from the smoke they still found raised airways resistance and concluded that it was probably due to the residual submicronic particles of the smoke causing bronchiolar constriction. A similar effect can be induced by inert carbon particles in man and animals [146]. In experimental animals there is a corresponding rise in vagal activity and both this and the constriction can be abolished by vagal cooling or atropine. Atropine also abolishes the bronchoconstrictor effect of cigarette smoke in man [135]. Miller and Sproule [100] have confirmed the rise in airways resistance in adult healthy men after cigarette smoking and could demonstrate it during normal as well as during rapid shallow breathing. They also found dynamic compliance reduced and attributed this to uneven ventilation. Significant improvement in pulmonary function has been found in young physicians 6 weeks after stopping smoking [74].

Some of the *pathological changes* in *bronchi* associated with smoking are outlined in the section dealing with bronchial carcinoma (p. 521). An increased autopsy prevalence of emphysema has been found in smokers compared with nonsmokers [4 & 110]. Megahed *et al.* [98] carried out bronchial biopsy and bronchial culture in 50 patients with chronic bronchitis. They found a close relationship between increased smoking and hypertrophy of the bronchial mucous glands: the latter was not demonstrably related to bronchial infection as measured by positive bronchial culture. An association between mucous gland hypertrophy and smoking has also been found in autopsy studies [110].

Experimental exposure of *animals* to cigarette smoke has not resulted in pathological changes entirely comparable to those of chronic bronchitis in man, but Auerbach *et al.* [8] have produced emphysema and fibrosis in dogs and other workers have noted changes similar to some of those seen in human smokers [142].

Numerous reports attest the *inhibition* of *bronchial ciliary action* by tobacco smoke [49 & 142]. There appear to be a number of ciliatoxic substances in the smoke and they may act by interfering with oxidative enzymes. Ciliary inhibition is, of course, likely to interfere with the drainage of the respiratory tract, including the clearance of smoke particles, and to encourage infection. Cigarette smoke also depresses the antibacterial activity of *alveolar macrophages* [55].

In vitro experiments on *surfactant* obtained from animal lungs have shown that cigarette smoke interferes with its action. This might, in life, favour the development of emphysema by allowing greater distension of dilated alveoli [54 & 144]. When guinea pigs were exposed to cigarette smoke for 3 hours daily for 3 weeks, surfactant extracted subsequently from their lungs was also found to have a decreased maximal surface tension, a change which would favour alveolar overdistension [54].

An association between *emphysema* and *peptic ulcer* in autopsy material has been frequently reported [52]. Peptic ulcer is claimed to be particularly prevalent in patients who have had *cor pulmonale*. No significant association was found in one series of cases admitted for acute perforation or bleeding, though the males had a higher cigarette consumption than controls [2]. It seems likely that the association between chronic bronchitis and peptic ulcer is due to a common smoking factor.

ATMOSPHERIC POLLUTION

The evidence incriminating atmospheric pollution as an aetiological factor in chronic bronchitis consists of

(1) a demonstration in Britain of increasing mortality [36, 116 & 119] and prevalence [29, 64 & 65] with increasing urbanization,

(2) a close correlation between atmospheric pollution and mortality from the disease [36, 136, 144 & 145],

(3) the demonstration that the seasonal peaks of mortality correspond with seasonal peaks of fog [119], and

(4) the demonstration that post office employees in foggy areas show a much higher rate of invalidism than those working in less foggy areas [48].

Studies by Lawther [78] have shown that,

11—R.D.

in patients with bronchitis, exacerbations are closely correlated with increases of sulphur dioxide and smoke in the atmosphere. Cornwall and Raffle [30] have found a correlation between foggy years and bronchitis incidence in London transport workers. Martin [91] found that changes in daily mortality and morbidity were correlated with changes in pollution. Martin [90] calculated that the number of additional deaths resulting from important fogs in London between 1948 and 1959 was nearly 7000, including 4000 deaths from the severe fog of 1952. In local areas in England and Wales Stocks [136] showed a highly significant correlation between mortality from bronchitis and atmospheric pollution. Fairbairn and Reid [48], in a study of postmen working out of doors in Britain, showed that absence from work owing to bronchitis, rate of invaliding with this disease, and mortality from bronchitis were closely correlated with the frequency of fog in different areas. Holland and Reid [64], in a further study of Post Office employees, found both a higher prevalence and a greater severity of bronchitis in those working in London, with a high atmospheric pollution, compared with those in relatively small and less polluted country towns. A similar gradient of severity between London on the one hand, and English country towns and the eastern United States on the other, has been found by Holland et al. [65]. An excess of bronchitis morbidity has been found in postmen [117] and in bus crews [30] working in northeast London where pollution is heaviest. Holland et al. [63] have demonstrated a correlation between atmospheric pollution, independently from temperature, and admissions to London hospitals for respiratory disease.

The precise factor in atmospheric pollution which is responsible for the adverse effect is uncertain. There is some evidence that smoke may be the most important. Two great smogs occurred in London in 1952 and 1962, both associated with rise in bronchitis mortality, much higher in 1952 than 1962. Both had similar SO_2 concentrations but in 1962 the smoke concentration was much less and so was the associated respiratory mortality [119].

It is possible that attachment of SO_2 and H_2SO_4 to smoke particles enhances their toxic effect [79].

An acute form of respiratory distress resembling acute bronchitis, and often continuing into a chronic form with predominant wheeze, has been described in individuals experiencing severe atmospheric pollution in Japan [111].

Studies in Canada and the United States have confirmed the relationship between atmospheric pollution and bronchitis [142]. Studies on twins in Sweden [25] concluded that pollution was a very much less important factor than smoking.

INFECTION

There is little direct evidence that the process of chronic bronchitis is itself initiated by infection. On the whole, such evidence as there is suggests that children who get recurrent attacks of bronchitis do not necessarily develop chronic bronchitis in later life and do not have any greater predisposition than children who are free of such infections. However, it must be admitted that the evidence is incomplete and long term prospective studies would be necessary to settle the question with certainty. Such studies would have to be continued for 30 or 40 years so there seems little likelihood that the matter will be clarified in the near future.

A number of individual patients date their chronic bronchitis from some acute respiratory episode. It is probable that such exacerbations have not really initiated the bronchitis but have only accelerated a gradual process of deterioration already occurring before the exacerbation.

Exacerbations associated with *infection* are characteristic of the stage of the disease which first brings the patient to the doctor. Almost all members of the population develop one or more upper respiratory infections during the course of the winter. In the bronchitic patient these infections almost always descend into the lower respiratory tract, resulting in exacerbations of cough, purulent sputum and often of wheeze. Such exacerbations become worse over the years and tend to last for

longer and longer periods. Pathological evidence [120] had suggested that each of these exacerbations produced a little further lung damage and effected a little more permanent deterioration in respiratory function. This was certainly a reasonable hypothesis but subsequent prospective studies on groups of bronchitics have not been able to show a correlation between chronic or recurrent infection and long term deterioration in lung function [51] though there is a temporary deterioration during an exacerbation.

The place of *viral infection* in initiating exacerbations has begun to be elucidated in recent years. So far systematic surveys have shown viruses to be important in a proportion of exacerbations which has varied from 4% to 52%, but is usually nearer the lower figure. Most of these studies did not include a search for rhinoviruses. The evidence is reviewed by Grist [57]. The viruses concerned were those causing respiratory infection in the general population and included influenza, parainfluenza and respiratory syncytial viruses. Infection with *Mycoplasma pneumoniae* (not a virus) was associated with some exacerbations in Washington [24] but has contributed little elsewhere. When a common cold illness was associated with an exacerbation of chronic bronchitis rhinovirus has been isolated in 48% of a small series in Glasgow [45] (though the group may have been somewhat atypical since it included a proportion of females with young children). Most of those from whom virus was isolated also showed a rise in antibody titre [57]. However, the overall isolation rate, including those without initiating colds, was only about 12% of all exacerbations. In Sheffield Stenhouse [134] isolated rhinovirus in 14% of 56 exacerbations. One may conclude, on present evidence, that viruses only account for a fairly small minority of exacerbations, at least as determined by present techniques of isolation and serology.

There is good evidence that *bacterial infection* with noncapsulated strains of *Haemophilus influenzae* [141] or with *Streptococcus pneumoniae* plays a major part in exacerbations of chronic bronchitis associated with pus in the sputum, though this infection may only be a complication of an exacerbation initiated by viral infection or by the physical irritation of a severe fog. The greater frequency of isolation of these bacteria from mucopurulent than from mucoid sputum in chronic bronchitics has been repeatedly demonstrated [21 & 129]. They also tend to disappear from the sputum as the pus disappears under the influence of chemotherapy. H. influenzae and pneumococci are frequently present in the nasopharynx of normal people but tend to spread into the lower respiratory tract in the winter and after colds. Direct culture of bronchial secretions in chronic bronchitis, as opposed to sputum, has in several studies demonstrated the presence of chronic infection of the bronchi by these 2 species [17, 18, 77 & 81]. The relative frequency of pneumococci and H. influenzae may vary from season to season but depends also on the techniques used for isolation. It seems possible that H. influenzae is the more important; it is certainly the more difficult to eliminate.

Burns and May [19] found serum precipitins to H. influenzae common in controls as well as in bronchitics but have claimed that a particular antibody H_1, demonstrable by double diffusion agar-gel precipitation, is more specific and is much commoner in mucopurulent and obstructive bronchitis, and in bronchiectasis, than in simple bronchitis or controls. Others have found precipitins or agglutinins in chronic bronchitics with purulent sputum and not in nonbronchitics [46]. It would be fair to say that the specificity and significance of H. influenzae antibodies in the serum has not yet been completely elucidated.

It is not necessarily the case that all exacerbations of chronic bronchitis are infectious in origin. The well documented occurrence of exacerbations during severe fog suggests that some may be largely chemical or irritative in origin, even though secondary infection is common. Exacerbations are also common during epidemics of influenza. Nevertheless it is probable that secondary bacterial infection is the main factor in producing bronchitic symptoms and lung damage even in exacerbations initiated by viral infection or fog.

OCCUPATION

The rise of mortality with descending socioeconomic class has already been mentioned (p. 303). Within each lower socioeconomic class both prevalence and mortality are higher in those exposed to industrial gases and dusts [61, 85 & 137]. It has been shown that the standardized mortality ratio (SMR) for the wives of these men is also high compared to that of other women and it has therefore been suggested [96] that it is the social environment, rather than the occupation, which is important. But Lowe [85] has pointed out that if one compares the bronchitis mortality of husbands in different occupations and in their wives, men in dusty occupations such as coalmining have a very much higher mortality than their wives in comparison with men in nondusty occupations, suggesting an important additional occupational factor. Wives of all below ground coalworkers have twice the mortality of all married women, but there is no difference between that of the wives of different types of underground worker. On the other hand the husbands working at the coal face have a mortality twice that of those working in less dusty occupations below ground. Nevertheless it has not been possible to demonstrate, in prevalence studies in coalminers, a clear relation between amount of dust exposure and amount of respiratory symptoms, perhaps because of the great importance of smoking [85]. Studies in steelworkers have shown a correlation between degree of dust exposure and bronchitis [85]. The relationship was more obvious in smokers than nonsmokers, suggesting the sort of synergism between the 2 factors which has been already noted in the case of atmospheric pollution.

In the flax industry, after standardizing for age, sex, smoking and atmospheric pollution, Pemberton and his colleagues [108] have demonstrated a clear relationship between bronchitis and degree of dust exposure.

It may be concluded that, though living

conditions, atmospheric pollution and smoking often confuse the issue, carefully designed investigations and analyses are beginning to find reliable evidence to support the clinical impression that occupations involving exposure to dust or fumes do carry an additional hazard of chronic bronchitis.

GENETIC FACTORS

There is no firm evidence of a hereditary factor [75], though there are one or two scraps of evidence which suggest this possibility. It must be remembered that parents who smoke tend to have children who smoke and the change in male/female ratio in mortality in Britain suggests a predominant environmental factor (smoking) affecting the male in particular (p. 306). The sisters of bronchitic men tend to have a higher prevalence of bronchitis than have their wives [80], but this might be due to common smoking habits. It may be, of course, that with equal exposure to smoking and atmospheric pollution there is a variable, genetically conditioned, predisposition to develop the disease. Very high prevalence rates have been reported in smokers in a few families [62 & 76]. In a study of monozygous twins, only 1 of whom smoked, Cederlof et al. [26] found that, if the nonsmoking twin had a cough, the smoking twin was more likely to have one than were other smokers whose nonsmoking twins had no cough. This suggested a possible genetic predisposing factor which might have aggravated the effect of smoking. However, the study as a whole showed the usual association between smoking and cough; the genetic factor, if any, was regarded as minimal. Eriksson [47] has described the development of emphysema at an early age in 3 members of a family, all of whom had a dysproteinaemia with a marked reduction of α_1-antitrypsin. He found evidence of a recessive inheritance. It seems possible that some such genetic factor might be responsible for certain cases with predominant emphysema not obviously related to smoking.

In view of the known predisposition to respiratory infection of children with cystic fibrosis (p. 592), it has been suggested that a milder form of the disorder, or the heterozygous state, might be a factor in at least some cases of chronic bronchitis [28 & 73]. In one series in Britain [73] the raised sweat chloride typical of cystic fibrosis was found in an important proportion of chronic bronchitics. Subsequent investigation has shown the wide variation which may occur in normals [101], the influence of dietary chloride intake [28], the lack of any significant number of chronic bronchitics with high sweat chloride levels [101] and the absence of an excess of chronic bronchitis in heterozygous parents of children with cystic fibrosis [12]. It seems therefore that cryptic cystic fibrosis does not, in fact, make a significant contribution to the prevalence of chronic bronchitis.

PATHOLOGY

Study of the pathology of chronic bronchitis has gained in recent years not only from the increased interest in the disease, but also from the possibility of examining lungs removed at operation—and therefore likely to be in a less advanced stage than those obtained at autopsy—and from the technique of inflating the lungs before fixation. Whole lung sections have been useful and fume fixation with thick lung sections has allowed a greater appreciation of changes in the three-dimensional architecture of the lungs.

BRONCHI

In accordance with the clinical evidence of increased mucus secretions, the most consistent finding in chronic bronchitis is hypertrophy of the mucus-secreting glands of the bronchial tree, which appears to be related to cigarette smoking rather than to infection [98]. This hypertrophy is relatively easy to establish by measuring the thickness of the gland layer in histological sections and comparing it to that of the bronchial wall ('Reid index' [123]). There is an increase in secretion-containing cells in the gland wall and a decrease of the granule-containing cells. There is some evidence that there may be a qualitative change in the mucus secreted in chronic bronchitis. Reid and her colleagues [124] have found an increase in the volume of mucous glands secreting a neuraminidase-resistant acid mucopolysaccharide, though further work is required before this can be regarded as specific. The hypertrophy of mucous glands is mainly in the larger bronchi and is evenly distributed throughout the lung [56 & 140].

The mucus-secreting goblet cells are often increased in number both in the larger bronchi and in the bronchioli, but this is less consistent than the hypertrophy of the glands. Bronchioli are readily blocked by this secretion. Macroscopically there may be some exaggeration of the normal longitudinal folds of mucous membrane in the larger bronchi and a development of transverse folds in the more peripheral bronchi which may show on the bronchogram. Smaller peripheral bronchi may be thickened and distorted by scar tissue.

When there is superadded acute infection the walls of the bronchi may macroscopically be obviously inflamed and pus or mucopus may lie in the lumen. Microscopically there may be infiltration with acute or chronic inflammatory cells, oedema and dilatation of capillaries. The mucous membrane may become ulcerated and, when the ulcers heal, squamous epithelium may replace columnar, though seldom over an extensive area.

BRONCHIOLES AND ALVEOLI

The more peripheral changes, in the bronchioles and alveoli, probably depend largely on infection, obstruction or both. In an advanced case foci of collapse, inflammation or scarring may be scattered irregularly throughout the lungs, especially in the subpleural areas, with intervening emphysema. It is probable that these areas mount in number over the years, as successive infections take their toll of the lung tissue.

In chronic bronchitis Reid [121 & 123], on whose work most of the preceding account is based, has described 'microabscesses' which may be responsible for progressive lung damage. The scarring, nodules, alveolar destruction and local areas of emphysema result from such areas of focal inflammation, usually too small to be visible radiologically.

EMPHYSEMA

The term is applied to a histological impression of increased air in the lung. It is commonly, but not invariably, present at autopsy in chronic bronchitis. A Ciba Symposium [27] defined emphysema as 'a condition of the lung characterized by increase beyond the normal in the size of air spaces distal to the terminal bronchiole, either from dilatation or from destruction of their walls'. A classification was suggested as follows:

(1) Dilatation alone.
(a) Unselective distribution (compensatory emphysema and emphysema due to partial main bronchus destruction).
(b) Selective distribution predominantly affecting respiratory bronchioles (e.g. focal emphysema due to dust).
(2) Destruction of the walls of air spaces.
(a) Unselective distribution (panacinar destructive emphysema).
(b) Selective distribution predominantly affecting respiratory bronchioles (centrilobular emphysema).
(c) Irregular distribution (irregular emphysema).

Leopold and Gough [82] divide emphysema pathologically into 2 types, generalized emphysema (now called 'panacinar') and centrilobular (now often called 'centriacinar') emphysema. The latter consists of dilatation of respiratory bronchioles in the centre of the lobule and is associated with chronic bronchiolitis, which gives rise both to destruction of alveolar walls and distension from air trapping. Either or both types of emphysema may be present in bronchitis and panacinar emphysema may merely be an advanced form of centriacinar [58]. Distended, irregular and unsupported airways and alveoli may give rise to airways obstruction and flap valve effects resulting in air trapping [123].

In autopsy studies the frequent relationship of emphysema to chronic bronchitis is shown by the correlation between the finding of emphysema and the Reid index of mucous gland hypertrophy [56, 138 & 139]. Milder emphysema is often confined to the upper lobes, and the severe form is usually distributed throughout the lung [56]. Both chronic bronchitis, as indicated by mucous gland hypertrophy, and emphysema can, nevertheless, sometimes occur independently [138]. Some patients dying with chronic bronchitis have little emphysema at postmortem. These patients are particularly liable to have polycythaemia and *cor pulmonale* [20A, 50A & 123].

American workers [104] have described the destruction of alveolar walls by enlargement of fenestrae—windows—in the walls of the air sac. The precise mechanism of this process of 'fenestration' is still uncertain. It may be most important in the type of patient in whom progressive breathlessness and emphysema outweigh the inflammatory and obstructive elements (primary emphysema). There may be little cough or wheeze and little hypertrophy of mucous glands. This type of patient is relatively uncommon in Britain but seems clinically more common in the United States. Possibly an extreme form is that seen in a few patients who have ruthlessly progressive emphysematous bullae, whose alveolar walls seem to disintegrate over a relatively short period, and who die in respiratory insufficiency in spite of relatively little cough or evidence of respiratory infection. This has been called 'vanishing lung' [125] as well as 'primary emphysema'. In contradistinction to the emphysema associated with chronic bronchitis, it may occur in nonsmokers. Often emphysematous bullae are confined to one area of the lung and fail to progress. Whether this is merely quantitatively different, or has indeed a different aetiology is not yet known (p. 329).

Certain other forms of emphysema are considered on p. 326.

BLOOD VESSELS

In chronic bronchitis the capillary bed may be thinned and atrophied by destruction or distension of alveolar walls. Arterioles may also be destroyed. In response to rising pressure in the pulmonary circulation, the pulmonary arteries may become distended, thickened and atheromatous [58A]. Normally venous blood from the peripheral bronchi is returned to the left atrium by the pulmonary veins, whereas the bronchial veins drain the larger proximal bronchi into the right atrium. Liebow [84] has shown that the bronchial veins are distended in emphysema and carry more returning blood than in normals.

FUNCTIONAL ABNORMALITY

AIRWAYS OBSTRUCTION

The most important disturbance of respiratory function in chronic bronchitis is generalized airways obstruction. There are 5 factors which may contribute to the obstruction, the importance of each probably varying in different patients, though knowledge is still very incomplete. These 5 factors are:

(1) mucus in the bronchial lumen,
(2) thickening of the bronchial mucous membrane by hypertrophy of the mucous glands and by oedema and inflammatory products,
(3) increase in tone of bronchial muscle,
(4) distortion of the peripheral airways by lung destruction, fibrosis and emphysema and
(5) invagination of the soft posterior wall of the larger bronchi and trachea on expiration by a steep gradient between the extrabronchial and the intraluminal pressure.

These factors will now be considered individually.

Intraluminal mucus must clearly be important. It is most likely to block small bronchi and probably different bronchi from time to time. It is easy to imagine how such a temporary block might contribute to ventilation/perfusion ($\dot{V}/\dot{Q}$) inequality as there may be a latent period before the pulmonary arterial supply to the affected portion of lung is reduced (p. 37).

Thickening of the *bronchial mucous membrane* by hypertrophied bronchial glands probably makes some contribution to diminishing the bronchial lumen. During exacerbations inflammatory exudate and oedema of bronchial walls are perhaps also important and may contribute to temporary $\dot{V}/\dot{Q}$

inequalities by favouring obstruction by mucus of the narrowed lumen.

Evidence for *increased tone* of *bronchial muscle* is largely indirect and our knowledge is far from perfect. By measuring endomural bronchial pressure with a balloon in a segmental bronchus, and at the same time following its relationship to 'pleural pressure', as measured by an oesophageal balloon, we ourselves have found evidence of increased tone of bronchial muscle at least on expiration in some wheezy bronchitics [40]. We have also demonstrated its relaxation by adrenaline [41]. Adrenaline, isoprenaline and atropine usually reduce airways obstruction to some extent in chronic bronchitics, as shown by improvement in FEV, though the improvement is less impressive than in asthma [35]. It may be that this effect is mainly on the bronchial muscle, though one cannot exclude an influence on mucous membrane oedema or mucous secretions. In bronchitis atropine often produces a reversal of airways obstruction similar to that of adrenaline, though in asthmatics it may be less effective than adrenaline [35]. It is probable that the effect in bronchitis is at least partly on mucous secretion which is reduced by atropine.

Distortion of the peripheral airways, with airways pursuing a tortuous course owing to fibrosis or emphysema, must increase airways resistance, though it is now considered (p. 15) that the peripheral airways only contribute a small proportion of the total resistance. It has been suggested [123] that a small airway with thin walls traversing an emphysematous area is likely to close on expiration, as the tenuous walls will readily be collapsed by a relatively small pressure gradient between the surrounding alveoli and the lumen. Some patients with chronic bronchitis and emphysema find it easier to breathe with their lips pursed and it was suggested that the resultant back pressure prevented the collapse of the walls. If the pressure gradient in these small bronchi is in fact less than was at one time thought (p. 13) it may be that the back pressure due to pursed lips is more important in preventing the air trapping effect

caused by obstruction of large bronchi described in the next paragraph, but it must be noted that in experiments on emphysematous lungs obtained at autopsy Petty *et al.* [109] found expiratory collapse to occur mainly in intraparenchymal airways at least down to 2 mm diameter.

Air trapping by closure of the large bronchi or trachea on expiration has been shown in some bronchitics, especially the emphysematous, by following the pattern of the spirogram on forced expiration. At a certain point there is an abrupt diminution of flow as the difference between the extra- and intrabronchial pressure becomes sufficient to invaginate the soft posterior wall of major bronchi or trachea. This has also been shown radiographically [89]. We have been able to detect the same sudden cessation of airflow in an emphysematous patient when flow was monitored during exercise.

It is uncertain which of these factors is most important. Patients with bronchitic symptoms have been shown, using the body plethysmograph, to develop a greater degree of airways resistance after smoking a cigarette than those without such symptoms, suggesting a tendency to develop increased tone of bronchial muscle after smoking. Yet long term deterioration in FEV is not significantly greater in those showing most reactivity to smoking [51]. Chronic bronchitics do not usually show the marked diminution in FEV after histamine inhalation which characterizes asthmatics (p. 401) [51].

The most useful test for respiratory obstruction is the FEV_1. This is usually diminished absolutely and also as proportion of the FVC. Normally 70–80% of the FVC is expired within one second. Other convenient measures are the Peak Expiratory Flow Rate (PEFR) and the Forced Expiratory Time.

Tests for reversibility of airways obstruction
The FEV is a convenient measurement for following a patient's progress and for determining the degree of reversibility of his disability. The technique of these tests is described in the section on asthma (p. 409). Although true bronchitics probably do not

respond to corticosteroid drugs, in a patient with severe disease admitted to hospital a trial is worth carrying out as occasionally relief may be obtained (p. 322), though some would then classify the case as one of asthma.

OVERINFLATION OF THE LUNGS

In chronic bronchitis, with or without emphysema, overinflation of the lungs is usual. This is often obvious clinically and radiologically and may be demonstrated by determining the RV and the RV/TLC ratio. The RV is often increased absolutely, as compared with the predicted value, and also as a percentage of the TLC; figures of 60% or more are not uncommon in severe disease. There are several factors responsible for the overinflation, the contribution of each probably varying in different patients. These include:

(1) loss of elasticity with overstretching of the lung tissue, especially when there is emphysema,

(2) a reflex reaction by which the patient breathes at higher FRC which assists in maintaining the patency of the narrowed airways,

(3) air trapping, at least in some areas, if the patency of the airways cannot be maintained. The poorly ventilated areas of the lungs increase, of course, the physiological dead space.

THE DIFFUSING CAPACITY (TRANSFER FACTOR)

This is often well preserved in spite of severe airways obstruction and overinflation [11, 42 & 131], though it may be reduced. Theoretically the techniques for measuring transfer of O_2 or CO should give a measure of loss of effective surface for diffusion within the lung, but there are a number of technical problems which are well discussed by Bates and Christie [11]. The steady state technique during exercise appears to give the best relation to clinical data. It tends to show diminution in patients with emphysema. Nevertheless, because of the complexities and of the difficulties in interpretation, CO or O_2 transfer measurement is not commonly used in the assessment of chronic bronchitis or emphysema.

BLOOD GASES

The disease often progresses sufficiently to interfere with alveolar ventilation to an extent which results in retention of CO_2 and the Pa,co_2 rises. The Pa,o_2 diminishes, and if sufficiently low there is diminution in Sa,o_2. These abnormalities will first be detectable when an exacerbation has further diminished the respiratory reserve, but later there will be continuous abnormality which worsens further in exacerbations. Normally CO_2 and H^+ form the main stimuli to the respiratory centre but with a constantly raised Pa,co_2 the centre gradually loses its sensitivity to CO_2, and hypoxaemia provides the bulk of the respiratory drive. In these circumstances the abolition of hypoxaemia by administration of high concentrations of O_2 during an exacerbation may result in the inhibition of respiration and a dramatic rise in Pa,co_2 resulting in coma and even in death. The true situation may be rather more complex than this simple explanation but the concept is a reasonable one as a guide to clinical action (p. 324).

When the pathology is considered it is quite understandable that airways obstruction may interfere with alveolar ventilation. In addition areas of alveolar collapse, fibrosis and pneumonia may lead to the shunting of hypoxaemic blood which is denied the possibility of gas exchange. Patients of this type are likely to become cyanosed. The hypoxaemia leads to contraction of pulmonary arterioles, which, in addition to loss of vascular bed, in due course causes a rise in pulmonary artery pressure and *cor pulmonale* [115]. There is some evidence to suggest that hypoxaemia also leads to increased airways obstruction, possibly by increased tone of bronchial muscle [6]. This is the type of case which has been somewhat ignominiously dubbed 'the blue bloater', because of his cyanosis and tendency to cardiac failure [50]. At autopsy there may be little emphysema.

In contradistinction to the 'blue bloater' is the 'pink puffer' at the other end of the spectrum. In this type of patient the predominant lesion is emphysema. By major effort the patient is able to ventilate sufficient alveoli to keep his blood gases normal, so that he appears pink, and the absence of hypoxaemia tends to preserve a normal pulmonary artery pressure and spares him from cardiac failure. He dies more often from respiratory failure [20 & 50].

Radioactive xenon scanning techniques have shown variable changes in patients with chronic bronchitis. It is common to find an excess of ventilation and blood flow in the upper parts of the lungs, compared with the normal, but in the individual patient the deviation upwards of ventilation and blood flow are not necessarily correlated and there may be gross mismatching [107]. When the variations in lung destruction, emphysema and local pneumonic areas are considered, and also the tendency for any rise in pulmonary artery pressure to deviate blood upwards by neutralizing the hydrostatic pressure effect, these mismatchings are entirely comprehensible.

BLOOD AMMONIA

The blood ammonia has been found to be raised in patients with chronic bronchitis and retention of CO_2 [43]. Clinically it may perhaps contribute to the flapping tremor sometimes seen in such patients, as such tremor also occurs in patients with raised ammonia levels associated with liver failure. In bronchitic patients with raised ammonia levels, other liver function tests may be normal. The cause of the rise is uncertain but may be connected with hypoxia. The estimation of blood ammonia has not become routine clinical practice, since its degree often parallels the Pa,CO_2.

ELECTROCARDIOGRAM

The commonest finding in the electrocardiogram in chronic bronchitis and emphysema is evidence of clockwise rotation of the heart about the anteroposterior and horizontal axes. This is shown by right axis deviation in the standard leads, an RS pattern in the chest leads extending to the left as far as $V5$ or even $V6$, together with an RS pattern in VL and a QR pattern in VF. If the heart is very long and thin VR and VL may be indistinguishable. In *cor pulmonale* the P wave may be spear-shaped and higher than normal (pulmonary P wave), especially in lead II and V_1 and V_2, the S wave may be prominent in all leads, the R wave may be prominent in V_1, T may be inverted from V_1 to V_3, or there may be right bundle branch block or low voltage tracings in the standard leads. Even in some severe cases none of these abnormalities may be present.

CLINICAL FEATURES

SYMPTOMS

EVOLUTION OF CHRONIC BRONCHITIS

The characteristic symptoms of chronic bronchitis are cough, sputum, wheeze and breathlessness. The patient himself will often date the onset of his illness from some acute exacerbation of *cough* and sputum which left him with a degree of disability which began seriously to interfere with his daily life. Nevertheless close questioning will usually reveal that he has had a smoker's cough for many years. Indeed, sample surveys have shown that a relatively high proportion of the male population over the age of 40 have winter cough and sputum (p. 305). This is almost confined to smokers and is much more common in men than in women. In most of these people the symptoms are too slight to take them to their doctors. Sometimes the individual has become so used to his cough that he denies its existence even when the questioner has himself observed him coughing during the interview.

In the patient developing chronic bronchitis, the cough gradually becomes more continuous; it then occurs during the day as well as in the morning and may keep him awake at night. A bout of coughing is frequent when he lies down, perhaps due to movement of sputum out of the bronchi when he takes up the horizontal position, but possibly due to some reflex action from cold sheets, for this may sometimes be prevented by warming the bed before the patient gets into it. Upper respiratory infections, which attack almost everyone during the winter, begin to 'go down to the chest', causing the sputum to become green or yellow and increasing its volume. At first these *exacerbations* may be so mild that the patient does not stay off work and the cough subsides to its usual level in the course of a week or two. Later he may be febrile during the attacks and may develop *wheeze* and dyspnoea. The exacerbations last for longer and longer periods and he may have to be off work for many weeks, or even months during the winter.

At a relatively early stage the patient's cough is usually susceptible to fog, and cough, wheeze and dyspnoea are worse during foggy periods. The patient with advanced disease may be unable to leave the house during foggy weather. Wheeze, which was probably originally confined to the acute attacks, may become chronic throughout the winter, beginning with his first acute exacerbation. Later, wheeze and dyspnoea may persist throughout the year.

The *sputum* is at first usually described by the patient as 'white' or 'grey', sometimes as 'black'. Between the attacks it is indeed usually mucoid, the grey or black colour being due to residue of cigarette smoking or to atmospheric pollution. Miners often have 'black' sputum. Later on the sputum may be purulent or mucopurulent between attacks. It is unwise to take the patient's word for the colour of his sputum and it is usual to ask him to bring up a specimen at each attendance so that the observer may check for himself.

There is considerable variation in different individuals in the amount of disability contributed by cough, sputum, wheeze and dyspnoea, and it may be that these differences represent variations in anatomical and physiological disorder. There are a few patients in whom emphysema is the major cause of breathlessness, whereas in others there may be relatively little emphysema, much of the breathlessness being due to diffuse airways obstruction and $\dot{V}/\dot{Q}$ inequalities (p. 37). In many all 3 factors operate.

DIFFUSE AIRWAYS OBSTRUCTION AND WHEEZE

At one extreme of the spectrum are patients in whom potentially reversible respiratory obstruction seems to be the most important factor in the disability. Sometimes these patients are overtly asthmatic in so far as corticosteroid drugs may initially result in restoration of normal function and the function may be quite normal between exacerbations. Such patients may more appropriately be diagnosed as having asthma. More frequently the reversibility to adrenaline and atropine is only partial, with perhaps 10–20% improvement in FEV, and there is little to corticosteroid drugs. Other patients, in whom perhaps emphysema is the dominant disability, have little wheeze and little reversibility of airways obstruction.

EMPHYSEMA

At the 'pure emphysema' end of the spectrum is a group of patients in whom cough, sputum and wheeze appear to be relatively unimportant and whose major disability is breathlessness. The history here is often of progressive severe dyspnoea, sometimes starting after some apparently mild respiratory infection. Within a short time the patient becomes a respiratory invalid and may die within a few years, usually from respiratory failure without *cor pulmonale*. Some of these patients are able to maintain their Sa,O_2 by hyperventilation, and also to keep the Pa,CO_2 within normal limits, up to a late stage. These are the 'pink puffers'. In some of them the patient's alveolar walls seem to 'vanish' steadily into emphysematous bullae [125], perhaps by progressive 'fenestration' of the walls of the air sac, as described above. This type of patient is apparently commoner in North America than in Britain. Most of them, but not all, are cigarette smokers; the causal rôle of tobacco is much less certain than in classical chronic bronchitis and, because of the geographical distribution of the disease, atmospheric pollution is probably unimportant.

Much more common in Britain, both clinically and pathologically, is the patient who has evidence both of diffuse airways obstruction, partially reversible, and perhaps of some emphysema, and in whom cough and sputum are prominent features.

COR PULMONALE

In the later stages of chronic bronchitis, when the patient is already dyspnoeic, he is liable to develop right sided heart failure, during respiratory exacerbations. The exacerbation may start with an upper respiratory tract infection, following which the sputum becomes purulent if it is not purulent already. The dyspnoea becomes more severe and may be accompanied by marked wheeze. Radiologically there may be evidence of pneumonia. Cyanosis increases owing to the increased difficulty of ventilation in an already damaged respiratory tract. It is thought probable that the right sided heart failure may be at least partly due to active constriction of the pulmonary vessels, but the exact factors responsible are still uncertain.

When there are full facilities for treating the condition by appropriate control of infection and hypoxia, the patient usually recovers from the particular incident, but in some later incident, after further deterioration, he will probably die, sometimes before he reaches hospital care.

PHYSICAL SIGNS

GENERAL CONDITION

In the early stages of the disease the general condition may be good. Patients with moderate bronchitis are sometimes overweight but those with advanced disease may become emaciated. In the later stages the patient may be cyanosed, even between exacerbations, though some of those with 'pure' emphysema may not be cyanosed, even though very dyspnoeic.

CLUBBING

Clubbing is unusual. Its presence suggests the possibility of a complicating bronchial neoplasm, or of bronchiectasis, though we have the impression that it is commoner in bronchitics with polycythaemia.

THE CHEST

In the later stages of the disease the chest is often barrel-shaped, with kyphosis, increased antero-posterior diameter, horizontal ribs, prominent sternal angle and wide subcostal angle. Although this is the classical appearance of emphysema, it may be due to reversible airways obstruction or lung distension by air trapping. In bronchitis it is seldom that this appearance, once established, reverses. On the other hand some bronchitics have long thin chests.

Movement of the chest wall is restricted and may largely be confined to the upper thorax. The patient may have to use his accessory muscles of respiration. In the advanced stages the costal margin may even, paradoxically, be drawn inwards on inspiration, owing to the pull of the low flattened diaphragms.

The most important finding on percussion is the decrease of hepatic and cardiac dullness, indicating inflated lungs or emphysema. Elsewhere the note may be hyperresonant.

When there is emphysema the breath sounds are usually decreased. In cases of 'pure' emphysema there may be no added sounds, but the most frequent physical finding in bronchitis is the presence of rhonchi, most often expiratory but often inspiratory as well. Rhonchi are normally widespread but may be most marked at the bases of the lungs. In mild cases they may only be present on forced expiration. Often there are no crepitations, but there may be fine or medium crepitations, especially at the bases, particularly in those with cyanosis.

THE HEART

If there is much emphysema or hyperinflation of the lung the apex beat may be difficult to identify and the cardiac dullness may be lost. The characteristic heave of right ventricular hypertrophy may be palpable to the left of the lower sternum or in the subcostal angle on the left side but is often obscured by lung inflation. Because of the inflated overlying lung it may also be difficult to hear the heart sounds. The second sound may be exaggerated, especially in the 2nd and 3rd left intercostal space, when the pulmonary arterial pressure is raised, but may be soft or absent in emphysema [147]. There may be right sided summation gallop, due to coincidence of atrial systole with the third heart sound, audible in the 4th intercostal space to the left of the sternum, or in the epigastrium. With the cardiac failure of *cor pulmonale* there may be evidence of functional tricuspid incompetence and diastolic gallop rhythm. There may be evidence of a hyperkinetic state, with warm hands, dilatation of forearm veins and increased pulse pressure, due to peripheral vasodilatation by hypercapnia. If the pulmonary vascular resistance is sufficiently high, the cardiac output is low, the hands are cold and blue and the forearm veins constricted; there may be a giant *a* wave in the jugular pulse and presystolic gallop rhythm [147].

ABDOMEN

Owing to low diaphragms the liver, though unaltered in actual size, may be palpable, sometimes extending several finger-breadths below the right costal margin. If there is cardiac failure there may be true enlargement of the liver, which may be tender.

JUGULAR VENOUS PRESSURE

This requires careful observation. If there is much airways obstruction the patient may have to raise his intrathoracic pressure well above atmospheric in order to achieve expiration. This will be reflected in a raised jugular venous pressure on expiration, but the level will drop below the level of the sternal angle on inspiration. If the jugular venous pressure remains raised more than 5 cm or so above the sternal angle on inspiration cardiac failure is probably present. Sometimes, if the patient is using his accessory muscles of respiration, the external jugular venous pressure may apparently be raised on inspiration owing to obstruction of the venous return by the sternomastoid muscle. Careful observation will show that the vein has emptied below the level of the muscle. The internal jugular pressure will not be affected by this factor and is therefore more reliable.

OEDEMA

Oedema will only be present if there is right sided cardiac failure or coincident venous thrombosis.

OPTIC DISCS

Venous engorgement may be observed when there is severe right sided failure. Gross retention of carbon dioxide may occasionally lead to a rise in pressure of the cerebrospinal fluid and so to papilloedema.

RADIOLOGY (see Simon [132])

The straight postero-anterior chest film may show no obvious abnormality, even in patients with very appreciable disability. More frequently the distension of the lung results in low, flattened *diaphragms* above which the posterior portions of the 11th or even 12th ribs may be visible. The *heart*, 'drawn out' by the depressed diaphragms, often appears long and thin. The *hilar vessels* may be conspicuous, with enlargement of the proximal parts of the pulmonary arteries. On the other hand the peripheral vascular shadows may be thinned, straightened or lost as vessels are damaged or destroyed by the advancing disease [20A, 50A].

Sometimes there are *bullae*, identified by fine hair-like margins and lack of vascular shadow. In some patients there may be a localized bulla at one apex, perhaps 5 cm or more in diameter, which may be discovered on routine radiology and may not be progressive; respiratory function tests may be quite normal. In others, bullae, at the base or elsewhere, may form part of the general bronchitic picture. In yet others the original bulla may progressively enlarge, bullae may appear elsewhere in the lung and the alveolar walls may gradually disintegrate to form large air spaces, a form of lung atrophy which has been referred to as 'vanishing lung' (see p. 312).

Although it is probable that in many cases of chronic bronchitis the lung function is gradually destroyed by small recurrent foci of collapse and pneumonia, these areas are usually only identified on histology and may not be obvious radiologically. Nevertheless sometimes patients with chronic bronchitis have x-rays showing persistent diffuse irregular patchy shadowing, presumably areas of fibrosis and destruction due to repeated infections. Should bronchopneumonia supervene there will be transient patchy basal shadows. Of course the heart will enlarge if the right ventricle fails.

On *fluoroscopy* the main findings are the low flat diaphragms and the diminished diaphragmatic movement. Whereas the range of movement of normal diaphragms with full respiration may be 6 or 8 cm and is always at least 3 cm, in severe bronchitis and emphysema movement may be only a centimetre or so; sometimes, owing to the upward drag of the costal margins on inspiration, the flattened diaphragm may be drawn paradoxically upwards on inspiration. This, of course, is different from true paradoxical movement due to paralysis of the phrenic nerve. In the latter condition inspiratory sniffing gives rise to a sharp upward movement of the convex diaphragm quite different from the slight upward movement of the flattened diaphragm in advanced bronchitis. On screening it may also be possible to detect enlargement of the pulmonary outflow track and of the right ventricle. The lung fields may fail to darken normally on expiration.

Bronchography may reveal irregular, narrowed, or distorted bronchi. There is often irregularity in peripheral filling of the bronchi and the opaque material may show pooling in dilated bronchioles. There may be diminution in the number of side branches of bronchi. There may also be apparent diverticula in the larger bronchi, owing to opaque material entering the mouths of hypertrophied mucous glands. These findings are of interest, but there is no necessity for routine bronchography in chronic bronchitis.

SPUTUM

The sputum in chronic bronchitis is very variable. In the early stages it is often mucoid and may contain froth. In acute exacerbations it usually contains more or less pus. Later it may be mucopurulent almost continuously. There may be considerable variation in volume and type from time to time. In some patients, in whom wheeze is a major factor, it may be found that most of the pus cells are

eosinophils. Such patients are more likely to respond to corticosteroid therapy. In general the presence of pus cells is thought to suggest infection of the lower respiratory tract; apparently the cells can reach the lumen of the bronchus by diapedesis without obvious bronchial ulceration. As already mentioned, the organisms most likely to be cultured from the sputum are *Str. pneumoniae* or *H. influenzae*.

HAEMATOLOGICAL FINDINGS

The white cell count may be raised in acute exacerbations, especially if there is bronchopneumonia. Occasionally there is an eosinophilia, most often when the picture is dominated by paroxysmal wheeze, but sometimes eosinophilia is an unexpected finding. Such patients are more likely to have reversible airways obstruction and to respond to corticosteroid therapy. Perhaps surprisingly, polycythaemia, as usually measured, is relatively uncommon. It has been suggested that in many of the cases without overt polycythaemia the red cell mass is in fact increased but that this increase is concealed by a simultaneous increase in blood volume [130], a finding which is commoner in patients who have had episodes of cardiac failure. The controls in this investigation might be criticized and later work has shown that polycythaemia is closely related to the degree of chronic hypoxaemia between exacerbations [69].

PREVENTION

From what has been said under the heading of Aetiology (p. 304) it must be clear that a great deal of chronic bronchitis is theoretically preventable. The 2 main measures are the prevention of atmospheric pollution and the prevention of cigarette smoking. In Britain at the time of writing a very small beginning has been made in the prevention of atmospheric pollution by the development of smokeless zones and the use of more efficient methods of fuel burning. In some areas an attempt has been made to inform schoolchildren about the dangers of cigarette smoking. There is evidence that this has increased their knowledge but has had little effect on smoking habits [92]. Of course the money and effort have been vastly less than those expended on tobacco advertising. Intellectual appreciation of the risks has reduced smoking among doctors [127] and perhaps among university graduates [86] and probably accounts for the small reduction in tobacco consumption in Britain over the last few years (p. 305), but a very much greater reduction will be required to have any significant effect on the prevalence of chronic bronchitis. Wicken [145] has calculated that, if there were no smoking, the mortality from bronchitis in Northern Ireland would be more than halved.

TREATMENT

The treatment of chronic bronchitis can be considered under the headings of the long term management of the patient and the short term management of exacerbations.

LONG TERM MANAGEMENT

SMOKING

The most important step which can be taken to prevent the progression of bronchitis in the individual patient is for him to give up smoking. The evidence for the aetiological rôle of smoking in the disease, and the evidence for its effect in interfering with lung function, have already been outlined. It is rational to suppose that stopping smoking will reduce the rate of progression. This conclusion is also supported by clinical impressions, although so far not by the evidence of a carefully controlled long term prospective trial. Indeed, it is doubtful whether such a trial would be ethically justifiable. The decrease in mortality in doctors who have stopped smoking has already been mentioned (p. 305).

It is often not easy to persuade the patient to stop smoking. As he usually presents himself for the first time during an acute exacerbation of his bronchitis, it is wise for the doctor to attempt straight away to stop him smoking. This may be easier at a time when he is not feeling well, when the addiction is less delectable and when he is probably anxious about his health. It may be much more difficult when he has recovered from the exacerbation. If a patient is ill enough to be admitted to hospital and he comes into a ward where smoking is forbidden, the moral support of other patients may make it easier for him to give up the habit [128]. Drugs such as lobeline have been advocated during the withdrawal period, but a carefully controlled trial has shown that lobeline has no advantage over a placebo [16]. However, the placebo effect is not to be neglected and for this purpose a simple barbiturate or a tranquillizer, such as chlorpromazine (tablets BP 25 mg 3 times daily) may be prescribed.

Antismoking clinics have been tried, using individual interviews, group therapy and medication [10 & 71]. In general their success seems hardly commensurate with the medical effort, and most have been ultimately abandoned. It must be acknowledged that so far no really effective technique or method has been evolved, though it must be hoped that in due course either a psychological or a pharmacological method will be found which will allow the addiction to be broken relatively painlessly.

ATMOSPHERIC POLLUTION

Although it is probable that the patient with chronic bronchitis would be very much better in a climate without atmospheric pollution, a change to such a climate is usually impracticable. The exceptional patient may be able to move for the winter, or permanently, to such a climate as the south of France, North Africa, Australia or New Zealand. Within Britain it may sometimes be feasible to move from a heavily polluted area of the town to a place of residence which is less dangerous. Occasionally it may be possible to obtain suitable work in a rural area away from smoke. 'Smog masks' have been advocated but have proved too uncomfortable for general adoption, but the patient may be advised to stay indoors in foggy weather and to sleep with closed windows. If the patient's job entails contact with dust or fumes he may be able to change it, although the financial and social implications of such advice must be carefully weighed.

CHEMOTHERAPY

There have been a number of double-blind controlled trials of long term preventive chemotherapy in chronic bronchitis. The earlier trials have been reviewed by a Scottish Subcommittee [129] and by Johnston [72]. The most practicable drug for this purpose is tetracycline. When this has been given in a daily dose of 1 g, either as 0·25 g 4 times daily, or 0·5 g twice daily, most trials have shown a statistically significant advantage over placebo tablets, sometimes in reducing the number of exacerbations, more often in curtailing them. When the dose has been lowered to 0·5 g daily an advantage has been demonstrated in some trials but not in others. This may depend on the relative frequency of the highly susceptible pneumococcus or the less susceptible *H. influenzae*. Unfortunately there is no evidence that decreasing exacerbations reduces the deterioration in pulmonary function [95].

Certain investigations have shown that oral penicillin has a marginal advantage over placebo tablets, somewhat similar to that of 0·5 g tetracycline daily. Erythromycin may be equivalent to tetracycline [53]. Most trials have indicated that sulphonamides are ineffective. A new long-acting sulphonamide (sulphormethoxine) has been effective in a preliminary trial, given once weekly, but skin rashes may be a problem and we would not at present recommend it [112]. The effect of ampicillin seems to be similar to that of tetracycline [1 & 99] but it is more expensive. There are now a number of other tetracycline derivatives on the market; they are more expensive and have no advantages in practice.

Long term tetracycline therapy is usually free from side effects, although patients occasionally develop abdominal discomfort, *pruritus ani* or diarrhoea, and some are quite unable to take the drug. Sometimes oxytetracycline or chlortetracycline is better tolerated; at the time of writing the former is cheaper and therefore the tetracycline of choice. Hypersensitive reactions, with fever or rash, are rare. Fungal infections or vitamin deficiencies are most unusual in bronchitic patients treated with tetracycline drugs and it is certainly unjustifiable to give fungicides or vitamins as a routine when using this treatment.

The problem of selection of patients for long term chemotherapy is a difficult one. The treatment is still very expensive and should not be lightly prescribed. It would seem justifiable if the patient is still employed but has had to miss considerable periods of work because of exacerbations of bronchitis. Whether it is justified if the patient is not prepared to help himself by giving up smoking is more debatable. Every patient calls for individual judgement, and humanitarian will usually outweigh economic considerations. Chemoprophylaxis may prevent the need for much more costly hospital treatment.

A less expensive method is to treat exacerbations as soon as they begin. The patient is provided with a small supply of tetracycline and is told to take 0·25 to 0·5 g 4 times daily at once if there is any exacerbation of his cough or if pus appears in the sputum. It seems to be easier to control the infection at this stage, perhaps because of a lower bacterial population, but unfortunately it is often very difficult to train patients to begin treatment sufficiently early and controlled trials have usually shown poorer results than with daily prophylaxis [15].

BRONCHODILATOR DRUGS

The degree of reversibility of airways obstruction varies a good deal from patient to patient. This can be measured if there are facilities to carry out tests for reversibility (p. 409). It must be remembered that in a patient with very considerable disability an increase of 150 or 200 ml in FEV may represent a 25% gain and result in important subjective improvement. If objective tests are not feasible the clinician must depend on the patient's subjective impressions, notoriously unreliable, or on the number of rhonchi.

The use of bronchodilator drugs is discussed in the chapter on asthma (p. 414). In bronchitis the results of their use are usually less impressive than in asthma and often only a relatively small proportion of the patient's respiratory disability is reversible. Paroxysms of 'bronchospasm' are much less frequent than in asthma so that bronchodilator drugs by injection are less often required except sometimes in acute exacerbations. For a short term effect bronchodilators by inhalation are of value in wheezy patients. Most patients obtain some benefit from the oral bronchodilators, the most appropriate for the individual patient being found by trial and error. As in asthma it should be remembered that the effects are relatively short-lived and the drugs should be repeated every 2–3 hours or before particular effort. Dosage should be adjusted so as to obtain maximal therapeutic effect with minimal side effects. If tolerated, ephedrine is often the best drug, but it is thought, probably correctly, that in some patients it becomes less effective with continued use. In that case some other drug should be used for a few days, returning to ephedrine later.

CORTICOSTEROID DRUGS

On the whole corticosteroid drugs tend to be unhelpful in bronchitis, but may have a dramatic effect in the occasional case. Some workers have suggested that if there is a response to corticosteroid drugs the case should be regarded as one of asthma. The presence of eosinophils in the sputum is a useful indication of a probable effect. Naturally corticosteroids are more likely to be effective in a patient in whom wheeze is a prominent feature. Our experience is that one cannot be certain in advance which patient will respond and that in any patient with severe disability it is worth while giving prednisolone or prednisone 30–40 mg daily for a week, with daily measurement of FEV, in order to determine whether corticosteroids are effective. In only a very few will they be found to be of value. In these patients they may certainly be used in exacerbations, with appropriate chemotherapeutic cover. In deciding whether long term treatment is justifiable the risks must be balanced against the probable benefit. In some patients corticosteroid treatment may make all the difference between working and being unable to work. The complications of treatment, and their prevention, are considered on p. 417.

PHYSIOTHERAPY

The value of breathing exercises is controversial. It is understandable that, when taught by a passionate devotee, the placebo value is considerable. It is more difficult to demonstrate an objective benefit [22]. A resort to his exercises in moments of crisis or panic may help to calm the patient and give him self-confidence and it is possible that some patients learn to breathe more effectively. Postural drainage may be of value in certain patients with a good deal of sputum and may be useful in the morning to clear the bronchi.

EXPECTORANTS AND MUCOLYTIC AGENTS

Traditional expectorants have nearly always failed to show an effect when used in controlled trials, though patients sometimes seem to value them. Any simple expectorant, or any hot drink first thing in the morning, may help the patient to clear his bronchi, though the inhalation of a bronchodilator is often more effective. New mucolytic agents with exciting claims frequently shoot like well advertised comets across the therapeutic sky and disappear with equal speed. None has yet established itself as a valuable measure in treatment.

ANTIDEPRESSANTS

In a patient with severe chronic dyspnoea who is a respiratory cripple, antidepressant drugs such as imipramine may help to alleviate distress.

SOCIAL ASPECTS

Chronic bronchitis often severely interferes with employment and social life, especially in unskilled workers [23 & 103]. Difficulties of getting to work, the number of stairs to be climbed to a home in a tenement or flat, unsuitability of work, loneliness and isolation in the respiratory invalid living alone, all contribute to the sum of suffering. Some of these difficulties can be remedied by social action. The medical social worker should be used to the full and every attempt made to keep the patient at work, or find him suitable work, and to obtain appropriate housing. Some possible community approaches to a grave problem have been outlined in a report by Nielson and Crofton [103].

THE MANAGEMENT OF ACUTE EXACERBATIONS

Acute exacerbations of bronchitis vary from a mild increase of cough and sputum, without general upset or much increase in dyspnoea, to a severe and prostrating exacerbation, perhaps with accompanying bronchopneumonia and cardiac failure. Although some exacerbations may be initiated by an increase in atmospheric pollution, infection is usually a very important part of the condition and its treatment dominates the patient's recovery. Theoretically effective treatment may also minimize the amount of residual lung damage, though this has not been convincingly demonstrated (p. 308). A mild cold may not require treatment, beyond staying indoors for a day or two, but any exacerbation which results in pus in the sputum, especially if the patient already has impaired respiratory function, should be treated with chemotherapy. Bronchodilators may also be necessary to relieve dyspnoea. Although some moderately severe attacks may be treated adequately at home, these patients will often require oxygen and are best admitted to hospital. It is surprising how rapidly a patient may respond to treatment in hospital when a week or more of chemotherapy at home has been unsuccessful. Perhaps the stable warm atmosphere and more intensive chemotherapy are the principal reasons.

In a severe exacerbation the most important therapeutic considerations are the treatment of infection and the administration of oxygen. The maintenance of an adequate airway is an essential part of oxygen therapy. In the treatment of *cor pulmonale* these two factors are still the most important, digitalis and diuretics being no more than secondary adjuvants. The principal therapeutic measures will now be dealt with in more detail.

CHEMOTHERAPY

In the absence of clinical or radiological evidence of pneumonia *H. influenzae* and *Str. pneumoniae* are the most important causes of exacerbations. Both organisms quite frequently occur together. In a small proportion of patients, in whom pneumonia is present, staphylococci may be responsible; *Klebsiella pneumoniae* infection is even rarer. In attacks mild enough to be treated at home it is best to assume that *H. influenzae* or the pneumococcus is the responsible organism. Little help is usually obtained from routine bacteriological investigation. In a very severe case admitted to hospital it is worth while having a direct smear of the sputum examined in order to exclude the possibility that staphylococci or *K. pneumoniae* are responsible (p. 137). If either of the latter organisms is found chemotherapy should be on the appropriate lines (p. 137). The following passages refer to patients in whom neither of these organisms is isolated.

Earlier trials of the chemotherapy of exacerbations have been reviewed by the Scottish Subcommittee [129] and by Johnston [72]. It is probable that any of the chemotherapeutic agents recommended will be effective if the infection is due to the pneumococcus, but *H. influenzae* is less susceptible to chemotherapy and in consequence more difficult to control. Present evidence suggests that the most powerful agents are benzylpenicillin *plus* streptomycin, and chloramphenicol. Very high doses of benzylpenicillin alone (3 mega units twice daily) may give results equivalent to streptomycin *plus* penicillin in conventional doses [83]. The tetracycline group of drugs is probably a little inferior to those so far mentioned, although a direct controlled comparison has not been carried out. Ampicillin, in a dose of 0·25–0·5 g 4 times daily, is probably equivalent to tetracycline [1, 9 & 93]. In a dose of 1 g 6 hourly it is claimed to eliminate *H. influenzae* more completely and to render the patient free from relapse for many weeks subsequently [93], but this was not a controlled trial. The oral penicillins, other than ampicillin, are inferior and are best avoided for exacerbations. Cephaloridine is only superior to penicillin *plus* streptomycin when given intramuscularly in a dose of 6 g daily and this dose may give rise to nephrotoxic effects [114]. In any case the wide use of this drug may result in the development of resistant strains of staphylococci in the environment and these may show cross resistance with methicillin and cloxacillin, which would be highly undesirable (p. 88). Gentamicin and colistin have not been successful in patients superinfected with *Pseudomonas pyocyanea* or *Klebsiella pneumoniae* [113].

The patient with a mild exacerbation at home may be treated with tetracycline 0·5 g 4–6 times daily. The dose can be halved when the sputum has been mucoid for 2–3 days. Treatment should be continued for 7–14 days. In the patient on long term preventive tetracycline therapy it will often be sufficient for him to double the dose of tetracycline if cough and sputum increase or if the sputum becomes purulent. Patients should be trained to observe their sputum for pus and any patient under regular observation should bring up a specimen of sputum with him when he attends the doctor. More severe infections at home are also often satisfactorily treated with tetracycline.

Although chloramphenicol is more powerful it carries the risk of blood dyscrasia. This is rare, but it may be fatal in up to 50% of patients, so that chloramphenicol is not justifiable unless there is good reason to accept the risk involved. It seems that the risk is smaller in patients of bronchitic age than in younger people. If given, the dose of chloramphenicol should be 0·5 g 4 times daily, reducing the dose to half when the sputum becomes mucoid. The course should normally not be continued for more than 7 days, the total dose should never exceed 25 g and the course should not be repeated within 3 months.

For a severe attack, either in hospital or at home, it is best to use either penicillin *plus* streptomycin or high dosage penicillin. Penicillin 1 mega unit *plus* streptomycin

0·5 g twice daily is usually sufficient, but for a very bad case the same doses may be given 6 hourly until the patient's clinical condition improves. It is wise not to continue the streptomycin for more than 5–7 days and it is best avoided in the very old, the deaf, those with poor sight or those with any evidence of renal impairment. Benzylpenicillin 3 mega units twice daily has been shown to be at least as effective as benzylpenicillin 1 mega unit *plus* streptomycin 0·5 g twice daily [83]. High dosage penicillin by intramuscular injection is painful. It is best to administer 0·5 ml of 0·5% procaine first and then to give the penicillin through the same needle. If penicillin *plus* streptomycin is being used and there is any possibility of the patient having tuberculosis, or if he has a history of tuberculosis, it is undesirable to give streptomycin without an accompanying antituberculosis drug. In that case isoniazid 100 mg twice daily may be added in order to avoid any risk of the tubercle bacilli developing streptomycin resistance (p. 87). If the patient is desperately ill it is reasonable to give the high dosage penicillin 6 hourly initially.

OXYGEN THERAPY

In any severe exacerbation of bronchitis the attainment of adequate oxygenation is one of the first aims of therapy. This depends on maintaining an adequate airway and providing an adequate supply of oxygen. But in some patients with hypercapnia the respiratory centre has lost its normal sensitivity to CO_2 and has become dependent on the drive of hypoxia to maintain respiration. Particular care is therefore required. Sedatives, and especially morphia, are highly dangerous. This subject, and the techniques of controlled oxygen therapy are dealt with in the section on respiratory failure (p. 345).

PHYSIOTHERAPY

Physiotherapy is of much less importance than oxygen therapy and chemotherapy. In fact a controlled trial of assisted coughing, postural draining and breathing exercises was unable to detect any advantage from these measures [5], though we feel that assisted coughing can be of value in patients who are too drowsy to cough up loose sputum without rousing and assistance.

TREATMENT OF *COR PULMONALE*

The most important measures in the treatment of *cor pulmonale* resulting from acute exacerbations of bronchitis are those used in the treatment of the exacerbation itself, that is to say, oxygen and chemotherapy. No other measures may be necessary, but if there is considerable oedema diuretics are often of value. For a number of years there was controversy as to whether digitalis was positively harmful. It may indeed cause cardiac irregularity if there is hypoxia and low serum potassium resulting from diuretic therapy, or coincident cardiac ischaemia. It is uncertain whether digitalis makes a definite contribution to the control of cardiac failure. Nevertheless, if there is any notable degree of failure it is reasonable to give digitalis because of its cardiotonic action but watching carefully for toxic effects.

BRONCHODILATOR DRUGS

Bronchodilators may be of value in acute exacerbations of bronchitis. If the patient is very wheezy aminophylline 0·25–0·5 g given slowly intravenously over 2–10 minutes is often useful, not only in helping to relax bronchial muscle but in acting as a respiratory stimulant and thus assisting clearance of the respiratory tract. Inhalation of 2% isoprenaline, either with a positive pressure machine or with a Wright's nebulizer, may also be of value. Ephedrine 30–60 mg may then be given orally. The place of corticosteroids in the treatment of acute exacerbations is at present uncertain and they are not generally given.

The value of oxygen and of chemotherapy in exacerbations, whether or not complicated by *cor pulmonale*, seems undoubted. It is difficult to be certain of the value of other measures, since the patient who is receiving adequate oxygen and chemotherapy will tend to get better anyway and the part played by other drugs is difficult to measure without a carefully controlled trial.

PROGNOSIS

PROGNOSIS OF ACUTE EXACERBATIONS

For patients treated in hospital the prognosis for an acute exacerbation of bronchitis, even in those desperately ill, is surprisingly good, though at some stage, either at home or in hospital the respiratory reserve is finally eroded and death occurs. Every attack does further damage to the lungs and sooner or later the patient is overwhelmed by an exacerbation.

LONG TERM PROGNOSIS OF CHRONIC BRONCHITIS

Present evidence suggests that by the time a patient has sufficient disability to come to medical attention because of breathlessness or because of repeated absences from work with bronchitis, the disease is already so advanced that the prognosis in most cases is poor. Nevertheless, a proportion of patients will improve. Whether this proportion can be increased by appropriate treatment remains to be determined.

In a 5 year [97] and 10 year [106] follow-up of 327 civil servants who were investigated because of having had at least 3 illnesses due to bronchitis during a year, or 2 illnesses which lasted more than a fortnight, Oswald *et al.* [106] found that the overall death rate in the males at 5 years was 4·2 times, and at 10 years 2·6 times greater than that predicted for a group, comparable for age and sex, in the general population; the ratio was higher in the younger groups. The excess of deaths was almost entirely due to increased mortality from respiratory causes. Prognosis was closely related to the degree of breathlessness. 50% of those with severe breathlessness were dead within 5 years and 50% of those with moderate breathlessness within 8 years. Of the men less than 50 years of age who at the beginning of the investigation were capable of sedentary work but were breathless on walking at moderate speed on the flat or on climbing 12 stairs, 38% were dead within 5 years. Neither age at onset nor duration of bronchitis were useful guides to prognosis. At the initial examination emphysema was diagnosed on the basis of flattened diaphragms, narrow heart and enlarged proximal pulmonary vasculature with narrowed vessels peripherally. 53% of patients with such a radiological pattern had died within 5 years; if obvious bullae were also present at the initial investigation the 5 year death rate rose to 70% [133]. Very similar figures for overall mortality were found by Reid and Fairbairn [118] in their study of bronchitic postmen.

Jones and his colleagues [72A] have shown that later mortality is closely related to Pa, CO_2.

In considering the progress of symptoms in Medvei and Oswald's study, the majority of men under 50 years of age with mild breathlessness at the initial interview considered themselves better 5 years later. Nearly 60% of those with moderate breathlessness had also improved, although 42% were worse or dead. Of those over the age of 50 years at the first interview, however mild the initial degree of breathlessness, more than 50% were either worse or dead 5 years later.

OTHER FORMS OF EMPHYSEMA [123]

Certain forms of emphysema occur without air trapping and are therefore less important clinically. These include the atrophic emphysema of aged lung (*senile emphysema*); *paraseptal emphysema* along lobular boundaries; and *compensatory emphysema*, merely consisting of overinflation of normal lung tissue to fill space resulting from shrinkage or removal of abnormal lung. *Centriacinar emphysema* (centrilobular emphysema) occurs in the early stages of chronic bronchitis (p. 311) and also in coalminers' pneumoconiosis (p. 473).

There are also other types of emphysema associated with airways obstruction but not necessarily with chronic bronchitis. *Primary emphysema* has already been discussed (p. 316). Emphysema is common in the neighbourhood of pulmonary scars from any cause, presumably owing to damage to alveolar walls by the original cause of the scar, either directly from inflammatory ulceration or indirectly by injury to blood vessels. *Local obstructive emphysema* may occur if there is a ball valve obstruction in a large bronchus, as in primary pulmonary tuberculosis (p. 203). *Infantile lobar emphysema* and *emphysema with bronchial atresia* are due to congenital abnormalities, but hypoplasia of lung and over-inflation can also occur as a result of *bronchiolitis obliterans* or bronchitis in childhood.

Some of these conditions will now be considered.

SENILE EMPHYSEMA

In the aged lung the alveoli and the respiratory ducts may be enlarged but no reduction in blood vessels or capillaries has been found. Although there is steady decrease of FEV with age, this is less in nonsmokers than in smokers. The FRC and RV may be somewhat increased, as also the lung compliance, compared with younger individuals. These changes are regarded as atrophic and part of the ageing process.

PARASEPTAL EMPHYSEMA

This type of emphysema does not usually give rise to symptoms or signs. It is found mainly in the alveolar areas which lie against connective tissue septa, especially at the sharp edges of the lung, such as the anterior edge of the upper or middle lobe and the lingula and the costodiaphragmatic rim, and around large bronchi and blood vessels. It is thought that the cause may be atrophic as the bullae lie mainly at the termination of the pulmonary vessels where there is also less supporting elastic tissue. Although usually causing no symptoms a bulla may rupture, resulting in spontaneous pneumothorax, or may occasionally enlarge sufficiently to compress neighbouring lung and impair function. Larger bullae may be visible radiologically.

INFANTILE LOBAR EMPHYSEMA

DEFINITION

Infantile lobar emphysema is an apparent obstructive distension of one lobe in an infant, often giving rise to severe dyspnoea and necessitating surgical removal.

PATHOLOGY AND PATHOGENESIS
[14 & 123]

An upper lobe, especially the left, or the middle lobe, is most often affected. The lobe, or occasionally part of it, is grossly distended, with thin atrophic alveoli, and impinges on the neighbouring lung often causing collapse. Its artery may be small and the blood supply reduced. It is thought that in some patients there is atresia of bronchial cartilage causing ball valve obstruction. In others the obstruction may be inflammatory or due to mucus or to a flap of mucous membrane. Bolande *et al.* [14] found increased deposit of collagenous connective tissue in the alveolar walls, but no bronchial lesions, in all of 7 cases. In a number of patients the cause is obscure.

CLINICAL FEATURES [31]

Most infants with this condition develop symptoms when less than 6 weeks old, the chief manifestation being dyspnoea which can prove fatal. The rest of the lung, heart, mediastinum, diaphragm and even chest wall may be displaced or bulged by the distended lobe. Cough and stridor may occur. A few patients have less distension and milder symptoms which allow surgery to be withheld, at least for several years. There may be accompanying congenital abnormalities of the heart.

TREATMENT

Most of the acute cases require surgery. As the cause of the obstruction can seldom be identified, the lobe usually has to be removed.

LOBAR EMPHYSEMA WITH BRONCHIAL ATRESIA

This appears to be a rare variant of the above [123]. There is complete atresia of the proximal bronchus, which is blind on its hilar side but may be patent peripherally. The left upper lobe is transradiant and hypoplastic, being aerated by cross ventilation. Most patients have been diagnosed in young adult life and have been symptom free, a transradiant left upper zone on the radiograph having drawn attention to the anomaly.

UNILATERAL EMPHYSEMA OF A LUNG OR LOBE DUE TO LOCALIZED BRONCHIOLITIS OR BRONCHITIS
(Macleod's syndrome)

Macleod [88] drew attention to patients whose chest x-ray showed unilateral hypertransradiancy. This appearance has aroused considerable interest. It was found that the pulmonary artery on the affected side was often small and angiograms showed a poor blood supply. Study of a number of resected specimens [122] usually revealed evidence of previous widespread patchy bronchiolitis or sometimes bronchitis. It seems likely that this dated from childhood. Some cases have probably been secondary to tuberculosis in childhood.

PATHOLOGY [123]

The affected lung is usually normal or subnormal in size. When it has been removed at operation it has been found, on opening the chest, that it does not deflate. Carbon distribution in the lung is patchy, probably indicating that carbon is deposited where the bronchial supply is normal but that, where the alveoli are aerated by collateral drift, the dust is deposited before it reaches the affected alveoli. There is panacinar emphysema but there is evidence that the number of alveoli is less than the normal. As the bronchi appear to have a full complement of branches, it is thought that the causal condition must occur between birth and the age of 8 when the alveolar numbers normally reach the adult figure. There is usually evidence of patchily distributed obstruction and obliteration of the bronchioles and small bronchi, but sometimes of larger bronchi. The pulmonary artery is often less hypoplastic than might be expected from the preceding angiogram, suggesting that the latter appearance may be functional and a response to the decreased oxygenation of the lung. Nevertheless there is often hypertrophy of pulmonary artery walls and decrease in the number of branches.

FUNCTIONAL ABNORMALITY

There is usually some evidence of airways obstruction and an increase in RV. The figures may be intermediate between those of normal people and those of patients with obvious chronic bronchitis. Bronchospirometry has shown a diminished oxygen uptake from the affected lung, which may be only 5 or 10% of the total for both lungs. Uptake is usually not increased by voluntary hyperventilation. Studies with radioactive gases [44] show little ventilation or blood flow in the affected lung. In some of these patients the main bronchus may be seen bronchoscopically to collapse on expiration but in at least one case repair and support of the bronchus has not remedied the condition, indicating that there was also peripheral damage of bronchi [123].

CLINICAL FEATURES

Many patients are unable to recall a childhood incident which might have been responsible for the condition but unilateral hypertransradiancy has been shown to develop, in patients with previously normal radiographs, after primary tuberculosis or measles. It seems likely that other forms of bronchiolitis in infancy may also be responsible. Most patients have been diagnosed at mass radiography and are often quite free from symptoms. In older patients there is sometimes accompanying chronic bronchitis, which may be coincidental. However, when the patchy obstructions are in larger bronchi, secondary infection seems to be commoner; the bronchi are often bronchiectatic and bronchial infection may be chronic. In many of these patients the em-

physema may be indicated by an increased resonance of the percussion note and by decreased breath sounds over the affected area.

RADIOLOGY

X-ray of the chest shows unilateral hypertransradiancy with decrease in the shadows of the blood vessels both at the hilum and in the lung. The mediastinum may be deviated to the affected side. The diaphragm may be normal in position or low. Screening of the chest or films taken on inspiration and expiration usually show air trapping with the mediastinum deviated to the contralateral side on expiration and failure of the affected side to darken on expiration. On angiography the pulmonary artery is small and there is poor peripheral filling. Bronchograms show poor peripheral filling and dilatation of the bronchi, with absence of the normal narrowing peripherally or with frank bronchiectasis. The endings of the bronchi are usually irregular, terminating either in an irregular tapering shadow, in a bulbar shadow or in a pool [123].

DIFFERENTIAL DIAGNOSIS

Unilateral changes in soft tissue cover, such as paralysed muscles, congenital absence of the pectoral muscles or mastectomy may give an appearance of unilateral hypertransradiancy but the differentiation is easily made by examining the patient. In compensatory emphysema the collapsed lobe can usually be visualized and the vessels in the emphysematous lobe are fanned out. It may be a little more difficult to differentiate the condition from a local accentuation of generalized emphysema but in this condition the heart is often long and narrow and hilar vessels on both sides tend to be accentuated rather than diminished. The diaphragms are likely to be low and a lateral film would show the enlarged retrosternal zone in generalized emphysema whereas in unilateral hypertransradiancy due to bronchiolitis in childhood the lung is normal or decreased in size. Occasionally one pulmonary artery is congenitally absent and in congenital heart disease the blood flow is sometimes very much decreased to one lung. In both of these there will be no evidence of air trapping. Occasionally hypoplasia of one lung may occur without hypertransradiancy but with a small and shrunken lung [123].

PROGNOSIS AND TREATMENT

In the majority of patients there are no symptoms and there is adequate respiratory reserve in the normal lung. The patient is, of course, at increased risk and pneumonia in the unaffected lung will be more serious than in a normal person. Patients with other respiratory disease obviously suffer by having a decreased respiratory reserve. Occasionally secondary infection and bronchiectasis in the affected lobe or lung is sufficient to justify resection.

LARGE EMPHYSEMATOUS BULLAE

A bulla has been arbitrarily defined as an emphysematous space greater than 1 cm in diameter [27]. Smaller bullae are only important in so far as they may give rise to spontaneous pneumothorax (p. 442) or because the radiological detection of their presence may be additional evidence that there is widespread pulmonary emphysema.

PATHOLOGY

Bullae may occur with a number of different types of emphysema. They are commonly found with paraseptal emphysema and in emphysema associated with scars. These two types may account for a high proportion of the relatively common apical bullae which may be detected radiologically. Bullae, sometimes large, may be seen in the late stages of fibrotic sarcoidosis or pneumoconiosis. They are sometimes associated with the lobar emphysema of infancy (p. 327). Clinically the most important types are those accompanying panacinar emphysema, either primary or, more often, with chronic bronchitis. Morphologically Reid [123] classifies bullae into 3 types:

Type 1: Narrow-necked bulla which protrudes on the surface of the lung and is attached to it by a pedicle. This represents the distension of a relatively small portion of original lung tissue. Such bullae are commonly found in the lung apex and where septa are numerous. They are particularly appropriate for surgical removal if they are making an important contribution to symptoms.

Type 2: Superficial broad-based bulla which is limited externally by the pleura and internally by a region of emphysematous lung. It represents an inflation of a superficial layer of lung and the bulla is usually crossed by blood vessels. These bullae may be found anywhere throughout the lung.

Type 3: Broad-based and deep bulla. This is similar to Type 2 except that a greater depth of lung is involved and the bulla may extend almost to the hilum. A large amount of lung tends to be involved and to be relatively little overinflated. The bulla is usually limited by emphysematous lung on all its surfaces. Any lobe may be affected.

PATHOGENESIS

The pathogenesis is not completely certain. It is probable that in general it consists in an exaggeration of the mechanisms which give rise to emphysema (p. 331). Particularly in Type 1 there may be a scar at the neck of the bulla. This may result in obliteration of a bronchus and inflation of the bulla by collateral ventilation so that air enters on deep inspiration but escapes with difficulty. It is possible that in some cases there is a valve mechanism in draining bronchi and this may even arise secondarily as the bulla stretches and narrows neighbouring bronchi or bronchioles [87].

RADIOLOGY [123]

In individuals without important respiratory symptoms bullae are radiologically more commonly seen at the apices. In a series of patients with widespread emphysema [123] bullae were seen in the upper zone in approximately one third, in the lower zone in rather less than a third, in the upper and lower zone in 16%, while in the remainder the distribution was uncertain. Whether a bulla is detected in the x-ray will depend on its size and the degree to which it is obscured by overlying lung. Some bullae may be obvious in a lateral film whereas in a posteroanterior they are obscured. The bulla is seen as an area of hypertransradiancy which is particularly well marked in Type 1. In Type 2 the wall of the bulla may be seen as a fine line, though the outer wall will be merged with the pleura. In Types 2 and 3 the identification of the wall is usually only partial but a thin line of compressed lung may be detectable. Sometimes the wall is partly formed by a connective tissue septum or by infolded pleura. If there is marked compression of the lung this may also be obvious. Bullae may depress the diaphragm. This depression is sometimes localized, the upper surface of the diaphragm showing a slight convexity downwards. The fine line of the bulla wall may be detectable at the lateral edges of the convexity. Bullae rarely displace the heart or trachea though sometimes they extend across the retrosternal space to show a fine convex line in the opposite lung. Fluoroscopy of a large bulla may show, on expiration, deviation of the mediastinum to the opposite side, due to air trapping, and failure of the bullous area to darken. A bronchogram may define a bulla more precisely than the straight film and may give an indication of the amount of lung involved in the bulla. Tomography may also, by outlining the blood vessels, indicate how much lung is involved. Bullae occasionally become infected in which case there may be a fluid level, sometimes with surrounding lung shadowing. Such an infection may result in the closure of the bronchial connections and shrinking or even obliteration of the bulla [39].

FUNCTIONAL ABNORMALITY

Respiratory function tests usually show evidence of widespread airways obstruction due to bronchitis or emphysema, at least when the patient has dyspnoea (p. 317). When the remainder of the lung is normal the large bulla may or may not be taking part in ventilation. If it is, the RV will be increased and of course regional function studies, by radioactive gases (p. 48) or by lobar and segmental gas analysis

with a mass spectrometer (p. 49), will confirm the inactivity of the bullous area. The spirogram may have a double form or notch on expiration showing the slow emptying of the bullous area (p. 42). The clinician, in considering surgery, will have to make a judgement whether the patient's symptoms are greater than would be accounted for by his general lung function and whether, therefore, the bulla is making an important contribution to the symptoms. This judgement is a difficult one. Naturally if large bullae are removed from patients with minimal symptoms and relatively normal remaining lung the result of operation may be graded as excellent, even though the patient is not necessarily much better off than he was before. On the other hand, if a bulla is removed from a patient with very considerable symptoms he may sometimes, if judgement has been good, be temporarily improved. Unfortunately there is later deterioration as the function of the remaining lung diminishes or bullae elsewhere enlarge.

CLINICAL FEATURES

If the remaining lung, or most of the remaining lung, is normal the patient is unlikely to have symptoms. In a recent review Davies et al. [37] in a study of 40 resection cases found that all patients with dyspnoea suffered from chronic bronchitis, widespread emphysema or other disease. Apical bullae are frequently found on routine radiography. If the patient is free from symptoms no action should be taken. Intense medical interest is merely likely to result in arousing the patient's anxiety unnecessarily. The only exception to this rule is a giant bulla in a young infant which may give rise to severe dyspnoea. Such a bulla will only be discovered if the infant has developed symptoms. The clinical and therapeutic problems are similar to those of lobar emphysema (p. 327).

Occasionally an adult with a large bulla may have local discomfort or pain, perhaps related to effort; discomfort may be present before the patient knows that he has a bulla [3]. Such symptoms have been relieved by obliteration or removal of the bulla.

The main clinical problem arises when a patient with primary emphysema or chronic bronchitis has one or more large bullae. The clinician has to decide whether the bulla is making a major contribution to the patient's disability and whether his symptoms could be improved by its obliteration. As already mentioned, symptoms are unlikely to arise unless the patient's respiratory reserve is already fairly severely impaired. In many cases of chronic bronchitis the severity of cough and sputum, the frequency of exacerbations and the widespread bilateral physical signs will indicate that any contribution by the bulla or bullae to the disability is relatively slight. Davies *et al.* [37] found that even displacement or compression of lung adjacent to the bulla did not improve the chance that operation would benefit the patient. In patients without significant bronchitis but with primary emphysema there is often evidence of multiple bilateral bullae. It may occasionally be justifiable in such cases to remove a single very large bulla causing major compression of the remaining lung, though it is usually only a matter of time before the patient again deteriorates.

TREATMENT

The only treatment to be considered for large bullae is surgical obliteration. Surgical technique has been varied. Excision, plication, lung resection or two-stage decompression have been employed. Some surgeons consider it is of value to carry out pleurectomy following the removal of the cyst in order to ensure against pneumothorax due to leaking lung.

Belcher [13] reported on 90 patients who had bullae or epithelial cysts operated on with follow-up up to 10 years. Operative mortality was 12%. 35% had died since operation, mostly from respiratory failure, but more than half the survivors had good subjective results. Adverse factors were advancing age, the necessity of a lobectomy rather than local surgery and severe residual emphysema. Bilateral disease had a less adverse effect than might have been expected. In general the bigger the bulla the better the result. Hugh-Jones [67] found dramatic benefit by surgery

in 20% and improvement in 50%. The operative mortality was 10% and he was in some doubt whether operation was often justified.

PATHOGENESIS OF EMPHYSEMA

It will be obvious from much of the above that in man there are 4 basic processes which may be responsible for emphysema:

(1) hypoplasia,
(2) atrophy,
(3) overinflation and
(4) destruction [123].

The destruction may be either direct destruction of the alveolar wall, usually by infection, or indirect destruction by interfering with its blood supply. Local abnormalities or the influence of smoking on surfactant (p. 11) may contribute to overinflation. Reid [123] reviews attempts to produce emphysema experimentally. She says that there are no experiments which have reproduced emphysema by hypoplasia or atrophy but there are a number of experiments in which emphysema has been produced by overinflation or destruction. The reader is referred to Reid's review for details. One's impression is that experimental work has not yet thrown any startling light on the development of emphysema in man.

REFERENCES

[1] ALLAN G.W., FALLON R.J., LEES A.W., SMITH J. & TYRRELL W.F. (1966) A comparison between ampicillin and tetracycline in purulent chronic bronchitis. *Br. J. Dis. Chest* **60**, 40.

[2] ALLIBONE A. & FLINT F.J. (1958) Bronchitis, aspirin, smoking, and other factors in the aetiology of peptic ulcer. *Lancet* ii, 179.

[3] ALLISON P.R. (1947) Giant bullous cysts of the lung. *Thorax* **2**, 169.

[4] ANDERSON A.E.Jr., HERNANDEZ J.A., HOLMES W.L. & FORAKER A.G. (1966) Pulmonary emphysema. Prevalence, severity and anatomical patterns in macrosections, with respect to smoking habits. *Arch. environm. Hlth* **12**, 569.

[5] ANTHONISEN P., RIIS P. & SØGAARD-ANDERSEN T. (1964) The value of lung physiotherapy

in the treatment of acute exacerbation in chronic bronchitis. *Acta med. scand.* **175**, 715.

[6] ASTIN T.W. & PENMAN R.W.B. (1967) Airway obstruction due to hypoxemia in patients with chronic lung disease. *Am. Rev. resp. Dis.* **95**, 567.

[7] ATTINGER E.O. GOLDSTEIN M.M. & SEGAL M.S. (1958) Effects of smoking upon the mechanics of breathing. *Am. Rev. Tuberc.* **77**, 1.

[8] AUERBACH O., HAMMOND E.C., KIRMAN D. & GARFINKEL L. (1967) Emphysema produced in dogs by cigarette smoking. *J. Am. med. Ass.* **199**, 241.

[9] AYLIFFE G.A.J. & PRIDE N.B. (1962) Treatment of exacerbations of chronic bronchitis with ampicillin. *Br. med. J.* **ii**, 1641.

[10] BALL K.P., KIRBY B.J. & BOGEN CONNIE (1965) First year's experience in an antismoking clinic. *Br. med. J.* **i**, 1651.

[11] BATES D.V. & CHRISTIE R.V. (1964) *Respiratory Function in Disease. An Introduction to the Integrated Study of the Lung.* Philadelphia, Saunders.

[12] BATTEN J., MUIR D., SIMON G. & CARTER C. (1963) The prevalence of respiratory disease in heterozygotes for the gene for fibrocystic disease of the pancreas. *Lancet* **i**, 1348.

[13] BELCHER J. (1967) Emphysematous bullae: Surgical follow up. In Proceedings of the Thoracic Society. *Thorax.* **22**, 287.

[14] BOLANDE R.B., SCHNEIDER A.F. & BOGGS J.D. (1956) Infantile lobar emphysema. An etiological concept. *Arch. Path.* **61**, 289.

[15] BRITISH TUBERCULOSIS ASSOCIATION (1961) Chemotherapy of bronchitis. Influence of penicillin or tetracycline administered daily, or intermittently for exacerbations. A report to the Research Committee of the British Tuberculosis Association by its Bronchitis Subcommittee. *Br. med. J.* **ii**, 979.

[16] BRITISH TUBERCULOSIS ASSOCIATION (1963) Smoking deterrent study. A report from the Research Committee of the British Tuberculosis Association. *Br. med. J.* **ii**, 486.

[17] BROWN C.C.Jr., COLEMAN M.B., ALLEY R.D., STRANAHAN A. & STUART-HARRIS C.H. (1954) Chronic bronchitis and emphysema. Significance of the bacterial flora in the sputum. *Am. J. Med.* **17**, 478.

[18] BRUMFITT W., WILLOUGHBY M.L.N. & BROMLEY L.L. (1957) An evaluation of sputum examination in chronic bronchitis. *Lancet* **ii**, 1306.

[19] BURNS M.W. & MAY J.R. (1967) *Haemophilus influenzae* precipitins in the serum of patients with chronic bronchial disorders. *Lancet* **i**, 354.

[20] BURROWS B., NIDEN A.H., FLETCHER C.M. & JONES N.L. (1964) Clinical types of chronic obstructive lung disease in London and in Chicago. *Am. Rev. resp. Dis.* **90**, 14.

[20A] BURROWS B., FLETCHER C.M., HEARD B.E., JONES N.L. and WOOTLIFF J.S. (1966). The emphysematous and bronchial types of chronic airways obstruction. A clinicopathological study of patients in London and Chicago, Lancet **i** 830.

[21] CALDER MARGARET A., LUTZ W. & SCHONELL M.E. (1968) A 5 year study of bacteriology and prophylactic chemotherapy in patients with chronic bronchitis. *Br. J. Dis. Chest* **62**, 93.

[22] CAMPBELL E.J.M. & FRIEND J. (1955) Action of breathing exercises in pulmonary emphysema. *Lancet* **i**, 325.

[23] CAPLIN M., CAPEL L.H. & WHEELER W.F. (1964) A bronchitis registry in east London. A report on the first year's work. Part II. Social findings. *Br. J. Dis. Chest* **58**, 112.

[24] CARILLI A.D., GOHD R.S. & GORDON W. (1964) A virological study of chronic bronchitis *New Engl. J. Med.* **270**, 123.

[25] CEDERLOF R. (1966) Urban factor and prevalence of respiratory symptoms and 'angina pectoris'. A study of 9168 twin pairs with the aid of mailed questionnaires. *Arch. environm. Hlth* **13**, 743.

[26] CEDERLOF R., FRIBERG L., JONSSON E. & KAIJ L. (1966) Respiratory symptoms and 'angina pectoris' in twins with reference to smoking habits. *Arch. environm. Hlth* **13**, 726.

[27] CIBA SYMPOSIUM (1959) Terminology, definitions and classification of chronic pulmonary emphysema and related conditions. *Thorax* **14**, 286.

[28] COATES E.O.Jr. & BRINKMAN G.L. (1963) Sweat chlorides in patients with chronic bronchial disease and its relation to muco-viscidosis (cystic fibrosis). *Am. Rev. resp. Dis.* **87**, 673.

[29] COLLEGE OF GENERAL PRACTITIONERS (1961) Chronic bronchitis in Great Britain. *Br. med. J.* **ii**, 973.

[30] CORNWALL C.J. & RAFFLE P.A.B. (1961) Bronchitis—sickness absence in London transport. *Br. J. industr. Med.* **18**, 24.

[31] COTTOM D.G. & MYERS N.A. (1957) Congenital lobar emphysema. *Br. med. J.* **i**, 1394.

[32] CROFTON EILEEN & CROFTON J. (1963) Influence of smoking on mortality from various diseases in Scotland and in England and Wales. An analysis by cohorts. *Br. med. J.* **ii**, 1161.

[33] CROFTON EILEEN (1965) A comparison of the mortality from bronchitis in Scotland and in England and Wales. *Br. med. J.* **i**, 1635.

[34] CROFTON J., DOUGLAS A., SIMPSON D. & MERCHANT SYLVIA (1963) The measurement of bronchial endomural or 'squeeze' pressure. *Thorax* **18**, 68.

[35] CROMPTON G.K. (1968) A comparison of responses to bronchodilator drugs in chronic bronchitis and chronic asthma. *Thorax* **23**, 46.

[36] DALY C. (1959) Air pollution and causes of death. *Br. J. prev. soc. Med.* **13**, 14.

[37] DAVIES G., SIMON G. & REID L. (1967) Quoted Reid (1967) *op. cit.*

[38] DOLL R. & HILL A.B. (1964) Mortality in relation to smoking: 10 years' observations of British doctors. *Br. med. J.* **i**, 1399, 1460.

[39] DOUGLAS A.C. & GRANT I.W.B. (1957) Spontaneous closure of large pulmonary bullae. A report on 3 cases. *Br. J. Tuberc. Dis. Chest.* **51**, 335.

[40] DOUGLAS A., SIMPSON D., MERCHANT SYLVIA, CROMPTON G. & CROFTON J. (1966a). The measurement of endomural bronchial (or 'squeeze') pressures in bronchitis and asthma. *Am. Rev. resp. Dis.* **93**, 693.

[41] DOUGLAS A., SIMPSON D., MERCHANT SYLVIA, CROMPTON G. & CROFTON J. (1966b) The effect of antispasmodic drugs on the endomural bronchial (or 'squeeze') pressures in bronchitis and asthma. *Am. Rev. resp. Dis.* **93**, 703.

[42] DUBOIS A.B. (1962) Industrial bronchitis and the function of the lungs. *Arch. environm. Hlth* **4**, 128.

[43] DUTTON R.Jr., NICHOLAS W., FISHER C.J. & RENZETTI A.D.Jr. (1959) Blood ammonia in chronic pulmonary emphysema. *New Engl. J. Med.* **261**, 1369.

[44] DYSON N.A., HUGH-JONES P., NEWBERY G.R., SINCLAIR J.D. & WEST J.B. (1960) Studies of regional lung function using radioactive oxygen. *Br. med. J.* **i**, 231.

[45] EADIE M.B., STOTT E.J. & GRIST N.R. (1966) Virological studies in chronic bronchitis. *Br. med. J.* **ii**, 671.

[46] EDITORIAL (1965) *Haemophilus influenzae* and chronic bronchitis. *Lancet* **ii**, 776.

[47] ERIKSSON S. (1964) Pulmonary emphysema and α_1-antitrypsin deficiency. *Acta med. scand.* **175**, 197.

[48] FAIRBAIRN A.S. & REID D.D. (1958) Air pollution and other local factors in respiratory disease. *Br. J. prev. soc. Med.* **12**, 94.

[49] FALK H.L., TREMER HERTA M. & KOTIN P. (1959) Effect of cigarette smoke and its constituents on ciliated mucus-secreting epithelium. *J. nat. Cancer Inst.* **23**, 999.

[50] FLETCHER C.M., HUGH-JONES P., McNICOL M.W. & PRIDE N.B. (1963) The diagnosis of pulmonary emphysema in the presence of chronic bronchitis. *Quart. J. Med.* **32**, 33.

[50A] FLETCHER C.M. (1968). Some observations on the bronchial and emphyscmatous types of patient with severe generalized airways obstruction. In *Form and Function in the Human Lung*, ed. CUMMING G. and HUNT L.B. p. 230. Edinburgh, Livingstone.

[51] FLETCHER C.M. (1968) Bronchial infection and reactivity in chronic bronchitis. *J. roy. Coll. Physcns Lond.* **2**, 183.

[52] FLINT F.J. & WARRACK A.J.N. (1958) Acute peptic ulceration in emphysema. *Lancet* **ii**, 178.

[53] FRANCIS R.S., MAY J.R. & SPICER C.C. (1964) Influence of daily penicillin, tetracycline, erythromycin and sulphamethoxypyridazine on exacerbations of bronchitis. A report to the Research Committee of the British Tuberculosis Association. *Br. med. J.* **i**, 728.

[54] GIAMMONA S.T. (1967) Effects of cigarette smoke and plant smoke on pulmonary surfactant. *Am. Rev. resp. Dis.* **96**, 539.

[55] GREEN G.M. & CAROLIN D. (1967) The depressant effect of cigarette smoke on the *in vitro* antibacterial activity of alveolar macrophages. *New Engl. J. Med.* **276**, 421.

[56] GREENBERG S.D., BONSHY S.F. & JENKINS D.E. (1967) Chronic bronchitis and emphysema: correlation of pathologic findings. *Am. Rev. resp. Dis.* **96**, 918.

[57] GRIST N.R. (1967) Viruses and chronic bronchitis. *Scot. med. J.* **12**, 408.

[58] HEARD B.E. (1959) Further observations on the pathology of pulmonary emphysema in chronic bronchitis. *Thorax* **14**, 58.

[58A] HEATH D. (1968). Hypertensive pulmonary vascular disease in emphysema and states of chronic hypoxia. In *Form and Function of the Human Lung*, ed. CUMMING G. and HUNT L.B. p. 163. Edinburgh, Livingstone.

[59] HIGGINS I.T.T. & COCHRAN J.B. (1958) Respiratory symptoms, bronchitis and disability in a random sample of an agricultural community in Dumfriesshire. *Tubercle, Lond.* **39**, 296.

[60] HIGGINS I.T.T. (1959) Tobacco smoking, respiratory symptoms and ventilatory capacity: studies in random samples of the population. *Br. med. J.* **i**, 325,

[61] HIGGINS I.T.T. (1961) The rôle of occupation in chronic bronchitis. In *Bronchitis: An International Symposium*, ed. Orie N.G.M. and Sluiter H.J. Assen, Netherlands, Royal Van Gorcum Ltd.

[62] HOLE B.V. & WASSERMAN K. (1965) Familial emphysema. *Ann. intern. Med.* **63**, 1009.

[63] HOLLAND W.W., SPICER C.C. & WILSON J.M.G. (1961) Influence of the weather on respiratory and heart disease. *Lancet* **ii**, 338.

[64] HOLLAND W.W. & REID D.D. (1965) The urban factor in chronic bronchitis. *Lancet* **i**, 444.

[65] HOLLAND W.W., REID D.D., SELTSER R. & STONE R.W. (1965) Respiratory disease in England and the United States. Studies in comparative prevalence. *Arch. environm. Hlth* **10**, 338.

[66] HOLLAND W.W. & ELLIOTT A. (1960) Cigarette smoking, respiratory symptoms and anti-smoking propaganda. An experiment. *Lancet* **i**, 41.

[67] HUGH-JONES P. (1967) Address at meeting of Thoracic Society.

[68] HUHTI E. (1965) Prevalence of respiratory symptoms, chronic bronchitis and pulmonary emphysema in a Finnish rural population. Field survey of age 40–64 in the Harjavalta area. *Acta tuberc. pneumonol. scand., Suppl.* **61**.

[69] HUME R. (1968) Blood volume changes in chronic bronchitis and emphysema. *Br. J. Haematol.* **15**, 131.

[70] JÄRVINEN K.A.J., PÄTIÄLÄ J. & THOMANDER K. (1960) The rôle of chronic smoking in the etiology of obstructive pulmonary emphysema. A study of 3375 persons. *Ann. med. intern. fenn.* **149**, 307.

[71] JOHNSTON G. (1963) An antismoking clinic. *Hlth Bull. (Scotland)* **21**, 41.

[72] JOHNSTON R.N. (1963) Antibiotics in chronic bronchitis. In *Chronic Respiratory Disorders: a Symposium*. Edinburgh, Royal College of Physicians.

[72A] JONES N.L., BURROWS B. and FLETCHER C.M. (1967) Serial studies of 100 patients with chronic airways obstruction in London and Chicago. *Thorax* **22**, 327.

[73] KARLISH A.J. & TARNOKY A.L. (1960) Mucoviscidosis as a factor in chronic lung disease in adults. *Lancet* **ii**, 514.

[74] KRUMHOLZ R.A., CHEVALIER R.B. & ROSS J.C. (1965) Changes in cardiopulmonary functions related to abstinence from smoking. Studies in young cigarette smokers at rest and exercise at 3 and 6 weeks of abstinence. *Ann. intern. Med.* **62**, 197.

[75] KUENSSBERG E.V. (1962) Are duodenal ulcer and chronic bronchitis family diseases? *Proc. roy. Soc. Med.* **55**, 299.

[76] LARSON R.K. & BARMAN M.L. (1965) The familial occurrence of chronic obstructive pulmonary disease. *Ann. intern. Med.* **63**, 1001.

[77] LAURENZI G.A., POTTER R.T. & KASS E.H. (1961) Bacteriologic flora of the lower respiratory tract. *New Engl. J. Med.* **265**, 1273.

[78] LAWTHER P.J. (1958) Climate, air pollution and chronic bronchitis. *Proc. roy. Soc. med.* **51**, 262.

[79] LAWTHER P.J. (1965) Quoted Stuart-Harris (1965) *op. cit.*

[80] LAYLAND W.R. (1964) An occupational and familial study of the symptoms of chronic bronchitis. M.D. Thesis. University of Sheffield, Quoted Stuart-Harris C.H. (1965). The pathogenesis of chronic bronchitis and emphysema. *Scot. med. J.* **10**, 93.

[81] LEES A.W. & McNAUGHT W. (1959) Bacteriology of lower respiratory tract secretions, sputum and upper respiratory tract secretions in 'normals' and chronic bronchitics. *Lancet* **ii**, 1112.

[82] LEOPOLD J.G. & GOUGH J. (1957) The centrilobular form of hypertrophic emphysema and its relation to chronic bronchitis. *Thorax* **12**, 219.

[83] LEWIS D.O. & PINES A. (1965) Treatment of exacerbations of bronchitis with high dosage penicillin and with penicillin plus streptomycin. *Br. J. Dis. Chest* **59**, 177.

[84] LIEBOW A.A. (1953) The bronchopulmonary venous collateral circulation with special reference to emphysema. *Am. J. Path.* **29**, 251.

[85] LOWE C.R. (1968) Chronic bronchitis and occupation. *Proc. roy. Soc. Med.* **61**, 98.

[86] LYNCH G.W. (1963) Smoking habits of medical and nonmedical university staff. Changes since R.C.P. report. *Br. med. J.* **i**, 852.

[87] McLEAN K.H. (1957) The histology of localized emphysema. *Austr. Ann. Med.* **6**, 282.

[88] MACLEOD W.M. (1954) Abnormal transradiancy of one lung. *Thorax* **9**, 147.

[89] MACKLEM P.T., FRASER R.G. & BATES D.V. (1963) Bronchial pressure and dimensions in health and obstructive airway disease. *J. appl. Physiol.* **18**, 699.

[90] MARTIN A.E. (1961) Epidemiological studies of atmospheric pollution: a review of British methodology. *Monthly Bull. Minist. Hlth Lab. Serv.* **20**, 42.

[91] MARTIN A.E. (1964) Mortality and morbidity statistics and air pollution. *Proc. roy. Soc. Med.* **57**, 969.

[92] MARTIN F.M. & STANLEY GILLIAN R. (1965) Experiments in dissuasion. An assessment of 2 antismoking campaigns. *Health Bull. (Scotland)* **23**, 1, **24**, 13.

[93] MAY J.R. & DELVES DOREEN M. (1964) Ampicillin in the treatment of *Haemophilus influenzae* infections of the respiratory tract. *Thorax* **19**, 298.

[94] MEDICAL RESEARCH COUNCIL (1965) Definition—Classification of chronic bronchitis for clinical and epidemiological purposes. *Lancet* **i**, 776.

[95] MEDICAL RESEARCH COUNCIL (1966a) Value of chemoprophylaxis and chemotherapy in early chronic bronchitis. A report to the Medical Research Council by their working party on trials of chemotherapy. *Br. med. J.* **i**, 1317.

[96] MEDICAL RESEARCH COUNCIL (1966b) Chronic bronchitis and occupation. *Br. med. J.* **i**, 101.

[97] MEDVEI V.C. & OSWALD N.C. (1962) Chronic bronchitis: a 5 year follow up. *Thorax* **17**, 1.

[98] MEGAHED G.E., SENNA G.A., EISSA M.H., SALEH S.Z. & EISSA H.A. (1967) Smoking versus infection as the aetiology of bronchial mucous gland hypertrophy in chronic bronchitis. *Thorax* **22**, 271.

[99] MILLARD F.J.C. & BATTEN J.C. (1963) Comparison of ampicillin and tetracycline in chronic bronchitis. *Br. med. J.* **i**, 644.

[100] MILLER J.M. & SPROULE B.J. (1966) Acute effects of inhalation of cigarette smoke on

mechanical properties of the lungs. *Am. Rev. resp. Dis.* **94**, 721.

[100A] MITCHELL R.S., VINCENT T.W., RYAN S. and FILLEY G.F. (1964) Chronic obstructive bronchopulmonary disease. IV. The clinical and physiological differentiation of chronic bronchitis and emphysema. *Am. J. med. Sci.* **247**, 513.

[101] MUIR D., BATTEN J. & SIMON G. (1962) Mucoviscidosis and adult chronic bronchitis. Their possible relationship. *Lancet* i, 181.

[102] NADEL J.A. & COMROE J.H. (1961) Acute effects of inhalation of cigarette smoke on airway conductance. *J. appl. Physiol.* **16**, 713.

[103] NEILSON MARY G.C. & CROFTON EILEEN (1965) *The Social Effects of Chronic Bronchitis: a Scottish Study.* London, The Chest and Heart Association.

[104] ODERR C.P., PIZZOLATO P. & ZISKIND J. (1959) Microradiographic techniques for study of emphysema. *Am. Rev. resp. Dis.* **80**, *Suppl.*, p. 104.

[105] OLSEN H.C. & GILSON J.C. (1960) Respiratory symptoms, bronchitis and ventilatory capacity in men: an Anglo-Danish comparison, with special reference to differences in social habits. *Br. med. J.* i, 450.

[106] OSWALD N.C., MEDVEI V.C. & WALLER R.E. (1967) Chronic bronchitis: a 10 year follow up. *Thorax* **22**, 279.

[107] PAIN M.C.F., GLAZIER J.B., SIMON H. & WEST J.B. (1967) Regional and overall inequality of ventilation and blood flow in patients with chronic airflow obstruction. *Thorax* **22**, 453.

[108] PEMBERTON J. (1968) Occupational factors in chronic bronchitis. *Proc. roy. Soc. Med.* **61**, 95.

[109] PETTY T.L., MIERCORT R., RYAN S., VINCENT T., FILLEY G.F. & MITCHELL R.S. (1965) The functional and radiographic evaluation of postmortem human lungs. Clinical, physiologic, roentgenologic, and pathologic correlations in normal subjects and patients with emphysema and chronic bronchitis. *Am. Rev. resp. Dis.* **92**, 450.

[110] PETTY T.L., RYAN S.F. & MITCHELL R.S. (1967) Cigarette smoking and the lungs. Relation to postmortem evidence of emphysema, chronic bronchitis and black lung pigmentation. *Arch. environm. Hlth* **14**, 172.

[111] PHELPS H.W. & KOIKE S. (1962) 'Tokyo-Yokohama asthma'. The rapid development of respiratory distress presumably due to air pollution. *Am. Rev. resp. Dis.* **86**, 55.

[112] PINES A. (1967) Controlled trials of a sulphonamide given weekly to prevent exacerbations of chronic bronchitis. *Br. med. J.* ii, 202.

[113] PINES A., RAAFAT H. & PLUCINSKY K. (1967) Gentamycin and colistin in chronic purulent bronchial infections. *Br. med. J.* i, 543.

[114] PINES A., RAAFAT H., PLUCINSKY K., GREENFIELD J.S.B. & LINSELL W.D. (1967) Cephaloridine compared with penicillin and streptomycin in chronic purulent bronchitis. Controlled trials of increasing dosage of cephaloridine. *Br. J. Dis. Chest* **61**, 101.

[115] PLATTS MARGARET M., HAMMOND J.D.S. & STUART-HARRIS C.H. (1959) A study of cor pulmonale in patients with chronic bronchitis. *Quart. J. Med., N.S.* **29**, 559.

[116] REGISTRAR GENERAL (1958) Statistical Review of England and Wales for the year 1958. Part III. Commentary, p. 58.

[117] REID D.D. (1956) General epidemiology of chronic bronchitis. *Proc. roy. Soc. Med.* **49**, 767.

[118] REID D.D. & FAIRBAIRN A.S. (1958) The natural history of chronic bronchitis. *Lancet* i, 1147.

[119] REID D.D. (1964) Air pollution as a cause of chronic bronchitis. *Proc. roy. Soc. Med.* **57**, 965.

[120] REID LYNNE (1958) The pathology of chronic bronchitis. In *Recent Trends in Chronic Bronchitis,* ed. Oswald N.C. London, Lloyd-Luke (Medical Books).

[121] REID LYNNE (1961) The pathology of chronic bronchitis. *Br. J. clin. Pract.* **15**, 409.

[122] REID LYNNE & SIMON G. (1962) Unilateral lung transradiancy. *Thorax* **17**, 230.

[123] REID LYNNE (1967) *The Pathology of Emphysema.* London, Lloyd-Luke (Medical Books).

[124] REID LYNNE (1968) Mucus in chronic bronchitis. *J. roy. Coll. Phycns Lond.* **2**, 173.

[125] RICHARDS D.W. (1956) The ageing lung. *Bull. N.Y. Acad. Med.* **32**, 407.

[126] ROTHFIELD E.L., BIBER D. & BERNSTEIN A. (1961) Acute effect of cigarette smoking on pulmonary function studies. *Dis. Chest* **40**, 284.

[127] ROYAL COLLEGE OF PHYSICIANS OF LONDON (1962) *Smoking and Health.* London, Pitman.

[128] SANGSTER J.F. (1967) A no-smoking ward. *Lancet* ii, 765.

[129] SCOTTISH SUB-COMMITTEE (1963) *Bronchitis: A Report to the Scottish Standing Medical Advisory Committee.* H.M. Stationery Office, Edinburgh.

[130] SHAW D.B. & SIMPSON T. (1961) Polycythaemia in emphysema. *Quart. J. Med.* **30**, 135.

[131] SHEPARD R.H., COHN J.E., COHEN G., ARMSTRONG B.W., CARROLL D.G., DONOSO H. & RILEY R.L. (1955) The maximum diffusing capacity of the lung in chronic obstructive disease of the airways. *Am. Rev. Tuberc.* **71**, 249.

[132] SIMON G. (1958) Radiological appearances. In *Recent Trends in Chronic Bronchitis,* ed. Oswald N.C. London, Lloyd-Luke (Medical Books).

[133] SIMON G. & MEDVEI V.C. (1962) Chronic

bronchitis: radiological aspects of a 5 year follow up. *Thorax* **17**, 5.

[134] STENHOUSE A.C. (1967) Rhinovirus infection in acute exacerbations of chronic bronchitis: a controlled prospective study. *Br. med. J.* **ii**, 461.

[135] STERLING G.M. (1967) Mechanism of bronchoconstriction caused by cigarette smoking. *Br. med. J.* **ii**, 275.

[136] STOCKS P.C. (1959) Cancer and bronchitis mortality in relation to atmospheric deposit and smoke. *Br. med. J.* **i**, 74.

[137] STUART-HARRIS C.H. (1965) The pathogenesis of chronic bronchitis and emphysema. *Scot. med. J.* **10**, 93.

[138] THURLBECK W.M. & ANGUS G. ELSPETH (1963) The relationship between emphysema and chronic bronchitis as assessed morphologically. *Am. Rev. resp. Dis.* **87**, 815.

[139] THURLBECK W.M. & ANGUS G. ELSPETH (1964) A distribution curve for chronic bronchitis. *Thorax* **19**, 436.

[140] THURLBECK W.M. & ANGUS G. ELSPETH (1967) The variation of Reid index measurements within the major bronchial tree. *Am. Rev. resp. Dis.* **95**, 551.

[141] TURK D.C. & MAY J.R. (1967) *Haemophilus influenzae. Its clinical importance.* London, The English Universities Press.

[142] UNITED STATES PUBLIC HEALTH SERVICE (1967) *The Health Consequences of Smoking. A Public Health Service Review.* Washington, U.S. Department of Health, Education and Welfare.

[143] WEBB W.R., COOK W.A., LANIUS J.W. & SHAW R.R. (1967) Cigarette smoke and surfactant. *Am. Rev. resp. Dis.* **95**, 244.

[144] WICKEN A.J. & BUCK S.F. (1964) Report on a study of environmental factors associated with lung cancer and bronchitis mortality in areas of North-east England. London, Tobacco Research Council Research Paper 8.

[145] WICKEN A.J. (1966) Environmental and personal factors in lung cancer and bronchitis mortality in Northern Ireland, 1960–62. London, Tobacco Research Council Research Paper 9.

[146] WIDDICOMBE J.G., KENT D.C. & NADEL J.A. (1962) Mechanism of bronchoconstriction during inhalation of dust. *J. appl. Physiol.* **17**, 613.

[147] WOOD P. (1956) *Diseases of the Heart and Circulation,* 2nd Edition. London, Eyre and Spottiswoode.

CHAPTER 19

Respiratory Failure

When the lungs cannot fulfil their primary function of adequate gas exchange at rest and on exercise respiratory insufficiency or respiratory failure is said to exist. In essential this means a fall in Pa,o_2 with or without a rise in Pa,co_2, usually due to lung disease but not always so. In terms of actual figures Campbell [1] has suggested that a Pa,o_2 at rest below 60 mm Hg or a Pa,co_2 above 49 mm Hg should be used to define respiratory failure. Blood gas abnormality may, of course, occur in conditions not associated with respiratory insufficiency. An example of this is the low Pa,o_2 of anatomical right to left intracardiac shunts.

As in heart failure respiratory failure is first in evidence on exercise; later it occurs at rest. Although dyspnoea is a common feature of the diseases causing respiratory failure it must not be thought to be a necessary accompaniment. A patient with primary alveolar hypoventilation with respiratory failure may have no complaint of dyspnoea. Conversely many patients can achieve adequate alveolar ventilation by virtue of increased pulmonary work so that they maintain normal blood gases. They do not, by definition, have respiratory failure yet they may be very dyspnoeic, e.g. 'pure' panacinar emphysema (until late in the disease (p. 316)), early restrictive lung disease.

There are all grades of respiratory failure and the condition may be *acute* (and possibly remittent) or *chronic*. To restrict the term 'chronic respiratory failure' to patients with abnormal blood gases *at rest* is to exclude a large number who are severely disabled on minor exercise. The wider view that chronic respiratory failure implies chronic disturbance of respiratory function with blood gas disturbance and associated symptoms is to be preferred. There are 2 primary causes of respiratory failure and 2 broadly classifiable types. The causes are *inadequate alveolar ventilation* and *imbalance of ventilation and perfusion* $(\dot{V}/\dot{Q})$. Often both factors are present but in varying degrees. The types are based on blood gas studies—each has a low Pa,o_2 but in the first there is a raised Pa,co_2 and the second a normal or low Pa,co_2. The first is by far the most common as a clinical problem. $\dot{V}/\dot{Q}$ imbalance is common to both. In one, alveolar underventilation is present and the Pa,co_2 rises; in the other enough alveoli are ventilated to keep the Pa,co_2 normal or even low, but the shunt of blood through other inadequately ventilated alveoli results in a low Pa,o_2 (p. 37).

RESPIRATORY FAILURE WITH LOW Pa,o_2 AND NORMAL OR LOW Pa,co_2

This is the respiratory insufficiency associated with those conditions affecting the alveolar wall and interstitium of the lung resulting in lowered values for CO transfer factor and a restrictive pattern of ventilatory abnormality, e.g. sarcoidosis, lymphatic carcinomatosis, interstitial pulmonary fibrosis, pulmonary oedema etc., but also including pneumonia and major pulmonary collapse. Effective alveolar membrane for gas transfer is also reduced in 'pure' emphysema. In all of these conditions $\dot{V}/\dot{Q}$ imbalance is marked (p. 37). $\dot{V}/\dot{Q}$ imbalance results either in increased dead space and wasted ventilation, or venous admixture (p. 37). The former never occurs as an isolated phenomenon but if it did it would not affect the blood gases; the latter results in a return to the pulmonary veins of blood with a high Pa,co_2 and a low Pa,o_2. The homeostatic control of respiration will result in increased ventilation in response to the raised Pa,co_2 so that excess CO_2 is excreted by the normal areas of the lung

= Alveolar hypoventilation.

facilitated by the shape of the CO_2 dissociation curve (p. 34). This requires that the central control of respiration is intact and that the lungs are mechanically able to respond to increased Pa,CO_2 drive. It has already been seen that hyperventilation cannot cause much more O_2 to be taken up in the normal areas of the lung since the blood there is already fully oxygenated (p. 34). In lobar pneumonia, therefore, where $\dot{V}/\dot{Q}$ imbalance occurs but the lung can normally respond to Pa,CO_2 increase by alveolar hyperventilation there is hypoxia but a normal Pa,CO_2. In the other restrictive ventilatory disorders the ability to ventilate to the extent to maintain a normal or low Pa,CO_2 is preserved until late in the disease.

Oxygen therapy is of paramount importance in management and may be given with impunity in this group since there is no hypercapnia.

RESPIRATORY FAILURE WITH LOW Pa,O_2 AND RAISED Pa,CO_2 (fig. 19.1).

It is with this type of respiratory insufficiency that the rest of this chapter will mainly be concerned.

When the Pa,CO_2 rises due to reduced alveolar (effective) ventilation the Pa,O_2 must fall; knowing one of these values the other may be predicted (see alveolar gas equation (p. 32) and O_2–CO_2 diagram (p. 33)). It is very unusual for CO_2 retention to occur with an FEV_1 over 1·2 litres [3]. The causes of alveolar underventilation have been mentioned on p. 34. The commonest of all is chronic bronchitis which may result in chronic respiratory failure with superimposed acute exacerbations, usually due to infection. The chronic bronchitic with an infective exacerbation may have bronchopneumonia with scattered areas of lung where the $\dot{V}/\dot{Q}$ is low and in addition there is an inability to in-

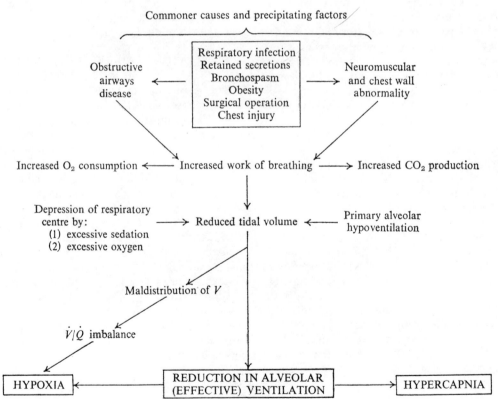

FIG. 19.1. Interrelated factors in hypercapnic respiratory failure.

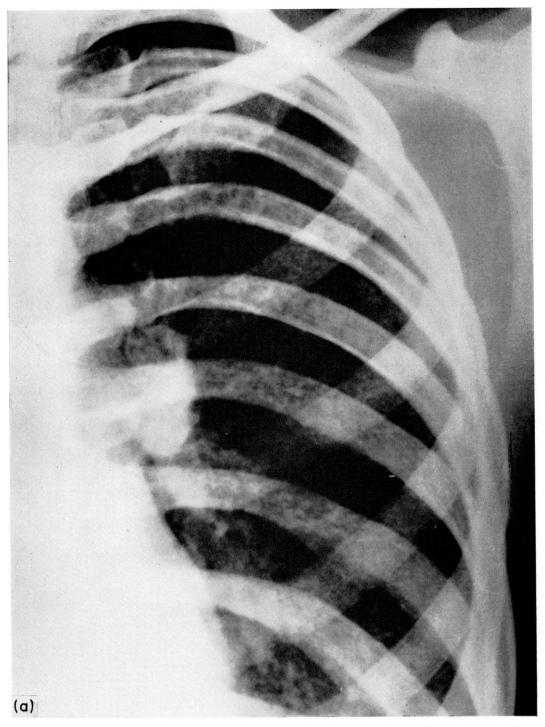

(a)

PLATE 12.1. (a). Part of the left upper zone of an x-ray of the chest of a 15-year-old-girl admitted with tuberculous meningitis and miliary tuberculosis. The faintly mottled shadows in the interspaces are just visible. There is an enlarged hilar lymph node. This contrasts with a film (b) taken 4 months later after the lesions have largely cleared under chemotherapy.

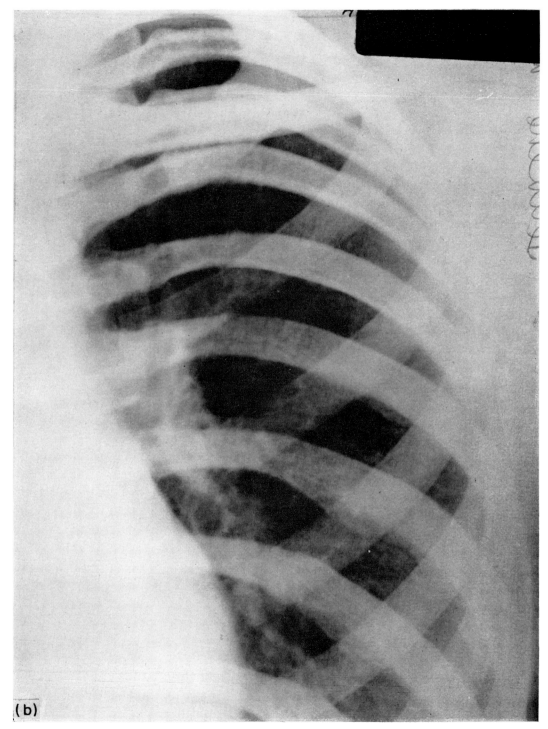

(b)

Plate 12.1.

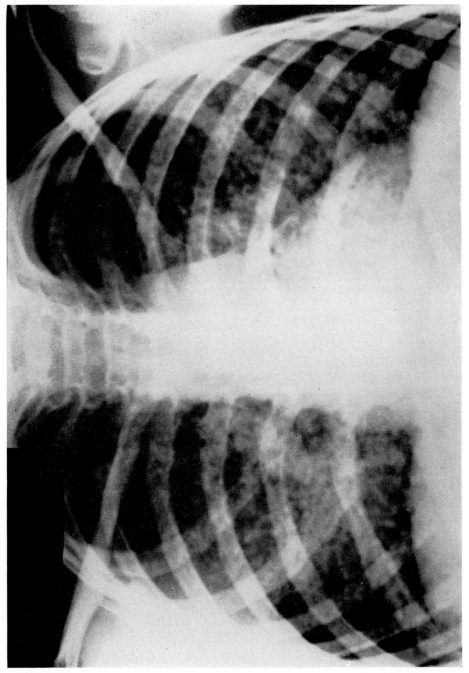

PLATE 12.2. Coarse diffuse miliary tuberculosis in a 7-year-old-girl. Temperature 105°F. Complicated by thrombocytopenic purpura. Recovery under chemotherapy.

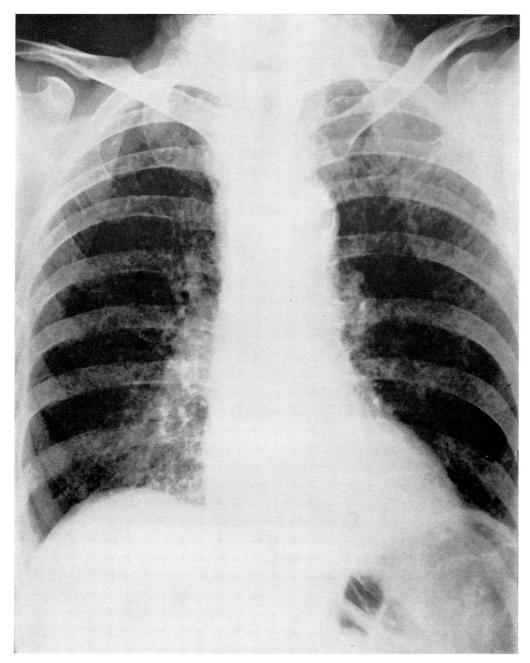

PLATE 12.3. Fine diffuse miliary tuberculosis in a 74-year-old-woman presenting with pyrexia. Complicated by severe hypokalaemia during 3rd month of treatment. Eventual recovery.

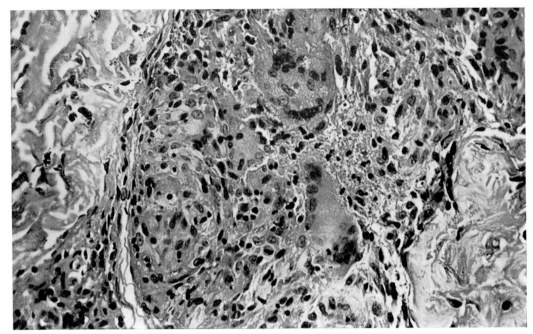

PLATE 23.1. Histology of sarcoid follicle.

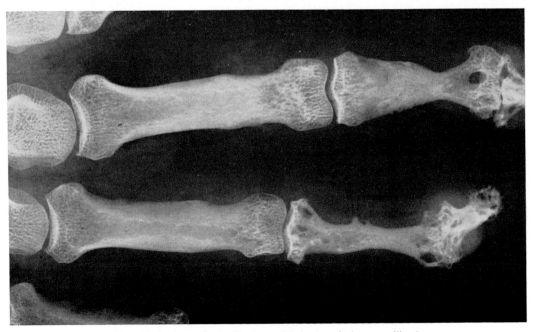

PLATE 23.2. Sarcoidosis. Cystic osteitis (note soft tissue swelling.)

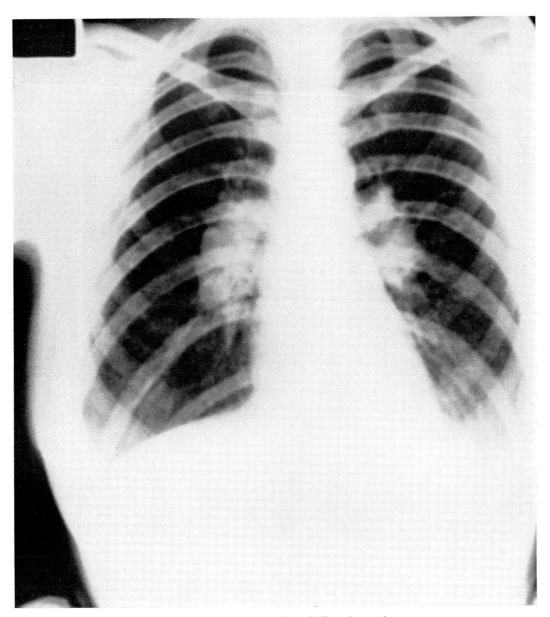

PLATE 23.3. Sarcoidosis. Bilateral hilar adenopathy.

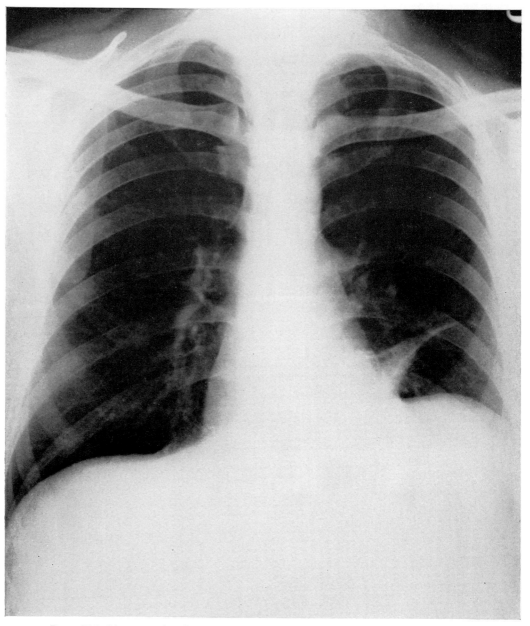

PLATE 27.1. Linear opacity of pulmonary infarction. Note elevation of left hemidiaphragm.

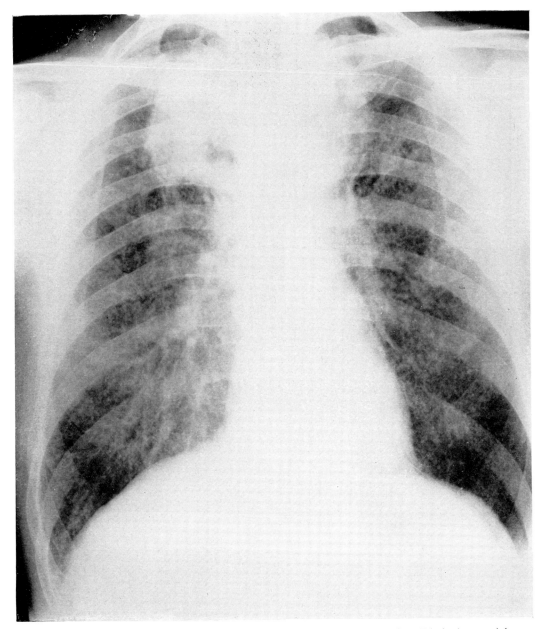

PLATE 28.1. Complicated coalworkers' pneumoconiosis. Note fibrotic masses of PMF in both upper lobes.

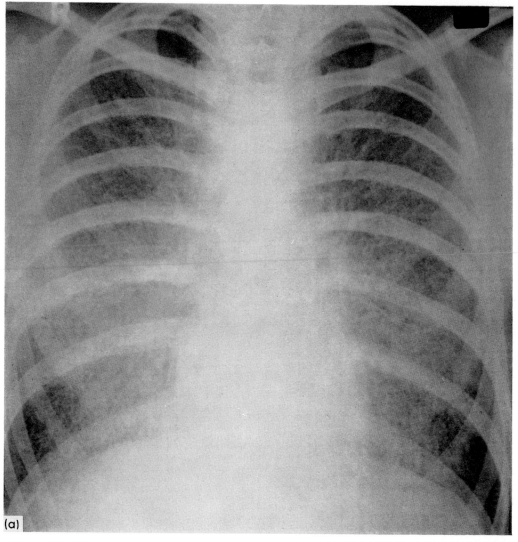

PLATE 37.1. Pulmonary alveolar microlithiasis: (a) Chest film to show diffuse distribution, (b) detail to show fine dense shadows. (By courtesy of Dr. T.A.C. McQuiston)

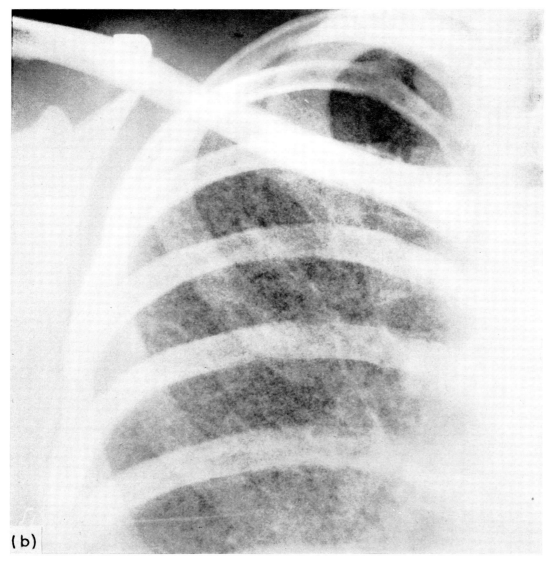

(b)

PLATE 37.1.

crease the alveolar ventilation. Thus there is a combination of $\dot{V}/\dot{Q}$ imbalance and inadequate alveolar ventilation. This results in a lowered Pa,O_2 which in this instance is usually proportionately more marked than the rise in Pa,CO_2.

Acute respiratory failure due purely to alveolar underventilation can occur in such conditions as poliomyelitis, polyneuritis, myasthenia gravis, drugs and poisons affecting the respiratory centre (e.g. morphine), cerebrovascular accidents, chest injury and acute oedema of the larynx. Later in these conditions the development of alveolar collapse may add a venous admixture effect.

When respiratory failure is of sudden onset the Pa,CO_2 increase is associated with only a slight rise in HCO_3^-. This may be insufficient to prevent a fall in blood pH. Slowly developing respiratory failure allows time for renal compensatory changes to occur so that there is often quite marked increase in HCO_3^-, and usually a normal or near normal pH. The clinical findings in CO_2 retention depend on the acuteness of its development and its severity (p. 46). Suspicion of respiratory failure should immediately demand precise assessment of the state of the blood gases, particularly the Pa,CO_2. The rebreathing method for Pa,CO_2 (p. 45) has a major rôle in this context.

The *consequences of pulmonary insufficiency* are those due to hypoxia or hypercapnia, or a combination of both. The effects involve many organs and the secondary phenomena which result may have further deleterious effects on respiratory function. The treatment of these secondary phenomena may, therefore, be important.

The effects of *hypoxia* depend on the degree, the duration and the speed with which the O_2 depletion has occurred. Those tissues which are highly sensitive to O_2 lack are principally affected—the brain, the heart, the pulmonary vessels and the liver. The *brain*, which consumes about 3 ml per 100 g of brain tissue per minute, shows the effects of O_2 deprivation in the EEG (abnormal slow waves) within seconds. Total O_2 deprivation even for short periods can result in irreversible brain damage and severe hypoxia can lead to

CNS depression with visual disturbances, dysarthria, incoordination, coma and death. Even brief hypoxia causes increased permeability of the brain capillaries which may result in cerebral oedema. In general, moderate hypoxia results in irritability of the CNS as opposed to the depressant effect of hypercapnia. Thus acute hypoxia of moderate degree results in increased mental and nervous irritability and perhaps delirium; chronic hypoxia of similar severity may cause impaired judgement, psychological disturbances and increased neuromuscular irritability.

The *heart* consumes about 10 ml of oxygen per 100 g of heart tissue per minute, two thirds concerned with muscular contraction and one third with other metabolic activities. A moderate degree of hypoxia appears to be well tolerated in that the crude histology is not effected but when coronary flow is less than 25% fatty degeneration, tissue necrosis and focal haemorrhage develop. Prolonged anoxia at this level results in irreversible cardiac damage. The hypoxic heart is liable to be irritable due to the particular susceptibility of the conducting tissue. Arrhythmias may, therefore, occur. The tendency to arrhythmia may be exaggerated by digitalis therapy and may even be further exaggerated when there has been potassium loss associated with diuresis. Long sustained hypoxia results in myocardial fibrosis.

Hypoxia, particularly in the chronic state, is known to *increase cardiac rate and output* and to *dilate peripheral blood vessels* (witness the bounding pulse and peripheral vasodilatation in *cor pulmonale*).

The *pulmonary arteries* respond to hypoxia by vasoconstriction (p. 36) resulting in increase in pulmonary vascular resistance and pulmonary hypertension which in time lead to *cor pulmonale*. It is possible that hypercapnia may play some part in the active pulmonary vascular constriction but its rôle is not at present clear.

Although pulmonary attrition with loss of vasculature must play some part in the development of increased pulmonary vascular resistance in chronic obstructive airways disease it is probably less important than the vasoconstrictor effect due to anoxia. Gross lung destruction from tuberculosis or panacinar emphysema only rarely results in *cor pulmonale*. There is no doubt, however, that massive destruction of the vascular bed, e.g. from recurrent pulmonary microembolism (p. 463) does result in pulmonary hypertension and right ventricular failure. But in the common situation where a patient with chronic bronchitis develops an exacerbation the factor of increased anoxia is undoubtedly the most important one in causing increase in the pulmonary vascular resistance which may reach the stage when right sided heart failure occurs. The treatment of this hypoxia is an urgent priority but, unlike the respiratory failure associated with a low or normal Pa,co_2, oxygen must be given with caution (p. 26).

The rôle of hypoxia in the control of ventilation has already been mentioned (p. 25). Usually the Pa,o_2 has to fall below 60 mm Hg before stimulation of respiration becomes appreciable. Hypercapnia normally enhances the effect of hypoxia on respiration. In some patients with chronic obstructive airways and hypercapnic respiratory failure the principal drive to respiration may be hypoxia. To what extent the dyspnoea of chronic hypercapnic respiratory failure is due to the hypoxic drive is not known but oxygen therapy in some patients seems to improve effort tolerance and relieve dyspnoea to some extent.

The *liver* may be damaged by hypoxia but, because of its large functional reserve and capacity to regenerate, any effect of single insults of oxygen deprivation may be difficult or impossible to detect; certainly liver function tests show no abnormality. The distribution of blood flow in the liver ensures that the peripheral cells in the lobule are perfused earlier than those in the centre. Severe hypoxia or marked decrease in perfusion affecting the liver will, therefore, result in proportionately greater damage to the centrilobar cells. When hypoxia is acute and severe, hepatic oedema or necrosis may occur. A more chronic state of hypoxia results in a slower process of cell death and fibrous tissue replacement.

Secondary polycythaemia is another consequence of persistent hypoxia. It is not known why it is not always present in those patients presenting with respiratory failure. It may be that only those patients with a persistently low Pa,o_2 show this phenomenon (p. 319) whereas those who intermittently develop marked hypoxia as a result of respiratory infection, but in the interval can maintain a reasonable Pa,o_2, are less liable.

The polycythaemia results from increased production of erythropoietin which increases the red cell mass. There is also increase in extracellular fluid and plasma volume which may mask the increase in red cell mass so that the haematocrit value may be normal (but see p. 319). Secondary polycythaemia may best be differentiated from the primary form by the absence of splenomegaly, leucocytosis and platelet increase. The previous view that a lowered So_2 suggested primary polycythaemia as opposed to the polycythaemia secondary to cardiac or pulmonary disease has been shown to be erroneous. It is possible that hypoxia in patients with primary polycythaemia who have no overt heart or lung disease may be due to the occurrence of unrecognized pulmonary thromboembolism. Thrombotic complications are common in primary polycythaemia but uncommon in the secondary type, perhaps due to platelet increase in the former. It is not known whether secondary polycythaemia in chronic respiratory failure is a favourable feature (by increasing the capacity for O_2 transport) or an adverse one (by increasing viscosity of the blood and therefore increasing the cardiac work). Frequently this creates a dilemma for the clinician faced with the problem of a patient with increasing chronic respiratory and/or cardiac failure.

It is difficult to distinguish the effects of *hypercapnia* from those of hypoxia and of the respiratory acidosis which frequently follows hypercapnia. Increase in Pa,co_2 is, however, known to have definite effects on at least 4 systems—the CNS, the kidney and the pulmonary and systemic circulations. In general the effects of hypercapnia develop more slowly and are less serious than those of hypoxia.

Acute rise in Pa,co_2 normally results in a rapid increase in ventilation (p. 47) which restores the blood gases to normal. Chronic hypercapnia may, however, lead to diminishing responses to incremental rise in Pa,co_2 (p. 26) so that the hypoxic drive to respiration becomes the more important.

The *CNS effects* of hypercapnia are variable from patient to patient and there appears to be a poor correlation between the Pa,co_2 and the development of these effects, because change in Pa,co_2 may be more important than the actual level. The precise rôle of CO_2 in their development is, therefore, difficult to evaluate. Rise in Pa,co_2 results in dilatation of cerebral blood vessels, increase in cerebral blood flow and increase in CSF pressure. The CNS features usually attributed to excess CO_2 include drowsiness in some patients, flapping tremor, coma (not found with a Pa,co_2 less than 80 mm Hg but nearly always with a Pa,co_2 more than 120 mm Hg), cerebral oedema, papilloedema and abnormalities in the EEG. Muscle twitching is also usually grouped with these but as this is a manifestation of neuromuscular irritability it is possible that the dominant factor in its production is hypoxia. Headache on waking is common in chronic hypercapnia, presumably due to progressive increase in CO_2 retention during sleep. Headache may sometimes be relieved by giving oxygen and in these cases presumably is due primarily to hypoxia.

The importance of the *kidney* in minimizing the changes in blood pH due to hypercapnia has already been mentioned (p. 47). When severe hypercapnia results in marked acidosis this may be due to renal failure. It has been suggested that the fluid retention in the chronically hypoxic and hypercapnic patient (blue and bloated (p. 314)) in the absence of heart failure may be due to reabsorption of HCO_3^- and Na^+ which increases the fluid in the extracellular space.

Pulmonary arterial vasoconstriction and its possible association with a raised Pa,co_2 level has already been mentioned (p. 339). This effect may be due to the accompanying acidosis.

Hypercapnia tends to dilate the vessels of the *peripheral circulation* by a direct effect on vascular muscle but also produces vasoconstriction by sympathetic stimulation. The actual effect in the individual patient depends on the balance of the two and is variable. Sympathetic stimulation is also responsible for tachycardia and sweating. In marked hypercapnia generalized vasodilatation may be associated with hypotension. Fall in blood pressure may also result when severe hypercapnia is allowed to occur during anaesthesia.

Other features occasionally encountered in pulmonary insufficiency, usually when well established and severe, are *gastric dilatation* and *paralytic ileus*.

The *diagnosis* of respiratory failure and the measurement of its *severity* depend on the demonstration of abnormality of the arterial blood gases at rest and perhaps also during and after exercise. This is because quite marked abnormality may have to be present before the clinical features become apparent and even then the features are largely non-specific. There is, of course, little difficulty in making the diagnosis on clinical grounds if the patient is known to have had longstanding pulmonary disease and is then found to have cyanosis and obvious difficulty in breathing. On the other hand in conditions such as polyneuritis affecting the respiratory muscles the development of respiratory failure may be insidious and may remain unsuspected until it is relatively far advanced unless serial measurements are made of the blood gases.

THE MANAGEMENT OF ACUTE RESPIRATORY FAILURE

The priorities in the management of acute respiratory failure vary according to the aetiology but the primary aims of treatment are the same in all cases, namely to maintain clear airways and to ensure adequate alveolar ventilation while treating, if possible, the primary condition. In the failure associated with a normal or low Pa,co_2 these considerations usually present little difficulty and treatment of the primary cause, e.g. antibiotics for lobar pneumonia, corticosteroids for diffuse interstitial pulmonary disease, may be all that is required apart from the use of oxygen. The same may apply to such conditions as acute laryngeal oedema where adrenaline (0·2 ml of 1:1000 solution intramuscularly) is usually the first measure in treatment; or to status asthmaticus (p. 418) where corticosteroid and bronchodilator drugs are urgent priorities. When there is an acute failure of ventilatory effort, from neuromuscular disease or from the acute effect of drugs on the respiratory centre, the institution of assisted ventilation at the earliest possible moment is the first line of treatment. The maintenance of a clear airway poses problems of variable urgency in each of these instances. A chest radiograph is essential to exclude coincidental disease such as pneumonia or pneumothorax, and any sputum should be sent for culture.

In Britain far the commonest type of respiratory failure is hypercapnic and hypoxic failure associated with exacerbations of chronic bronchitis. 'Respiratory failure' is frequently regarded as synonymous with this. The main associated factors and the effects of this type of respiratory failure are represented diagrammatically in fig. 19.1 and the salient features of its management are listed in table 19.1.

THE TREATMENT OF ACUTE HYPERCAPNIC RESPIRATORY FAILURE
(table 19.1)

The precipitating factor is most commonly infection and infection should be presumed even though there may be little clinical evidence of it. Appropriate antibiotic therapy (p. 323) must be started as soon as possible. But the first priority is to secure a free airway, appropriate ventilation and adequate oxygenation. *Supervised coughing* and changing the patient's position frequently from side to side (formal postural drainage is seldom possible), may suffice to clear the airways. When physiotherapists are not available this may need to be a duty of the doctor or the nurse. Cough may be limited by the patient's exhaustion, by muscular weakness, by air trapping, or by pain due to rib fracture or pleurisy. If chest pain is sufficiently severe to require some form of sedation great caution

TABLE 19.1

Treatment of Hypercapnic Respiratory Failure

Priority	Problem	Treatment
1	Retained secretions (ineffective cough)	Supervised coughing, Bronchoscopic aspiration, Aspiration via endotracheal tube, Tracheostomy
2	Hypoxaemia	Graduated oxygen therapy
3	Alveolar hypoventilation (may improve with improvement of 1 and 2)	Respiratory stimulants Artificial ventilation via (1) endotracheal tube, (2) tracheostomy
4	Respiratory infection	Antibiotics
5	'Bronchospasm'	Isoprenaline aerosol, I.V. Aminophylline, Corticosteroid drugs
6	Cardiac failure	Diuretics, ?Digoxin

is necessary lest the already failing respiratory centre be further depressed. If there appears to be an associated reversible component of airways obstruction bronchodilator drugs (e.g. isoprenaline aerosol; intravenous aminophylline) are indicated. If cough is ineffective the airways may require to be cleared by *bronchoscopic aspiration*. When there is impaired consciousness and consequent inability to clear secretions the use of *respiratory stimulants* may be beneficial. Nikethamide (2–4 ml of a 25% solution intravenously) is commonly used but its effect is transient. Intermittent intravenous injection of nikethamide via an indwelling Gordh needle may be necessary. Vanillic acid diethylamide ('Vandid' or 'Ethamivan') by intravenous drip (3·24 g in 540 ml) may give more prolonged respiratory stimulation, the drip rate being scaled to the response desired. Respiratory stimulants should always be looked on as a short term measure. Some clinicians believe that they have little part to play and may even be harmful in the respiratory failure of chronic obstructive airways disease since they stimulate nonrespiratory as well as respiratory muscles, using oxygen which the patient so desperately needs and increasing unnecessarily the production of carbon dioxide which he cannot eliminate efficiently. The end result may be a worsening of the respiratory acidosis. Nevertheless respiratory stimulants may literally allow a breathing space while evaluation of the case and preparation for other treatment measures are proceeding. The general consensus of opinion favours their use, with reservation regarding their place in prolonged hypercapnic failure. Certainly in the acute situation they arouse the patient, stimulate him to clear his secretions and help to prevent serious cerebral anoxia.

These early measures may require to be continued and bronchoscopy may need to be repeated once or even twice over the first few hours or so while other treatment, principally *antibiotics* and *controlled oxygen therapy*, are altering the situation for the better. But if it is obvious that secretions are re-accumulating rapidly or if aspiration from the oesophagus or upper respiratory tract seems likely (as in bulbar palsy or the coma of barbiturate poisoning) a *cuffed endotracheal tube* should be passed and repeated aspiration continued by this route. It is always desirable to give this method a trial before considering the ultimate measure of *tracheostomy* which has a number of disadvantages, although it may be life-saving. Tracheostomy allows ready access to the bronchial tree for the purposes of clearing secretions; unfortunately it also allows ready access of infection resistant to the antibiotics employed, and in the hospital context this may mean superinfection with resistant staphylococci. This risk, coupled with the facts that it is painful and uncomfortable, that it reduces the expulsive force of coughing and can be later complicated by tracheal stenosis (mainly owing to removal of the support from the cartilaginous rings) should make the clinician hesitate before embarking on tracheostomy. On the positive side, in addition to facilitating clearing of secretions, tracheostomy reduces the dead space by about 60 ml and permits *prolonged*

assisted respiration. It is important to remember that, for obvious reasons, it is often not humane to perform tracheostomy in the gravely crippled bronchitic (p. 343). It is important, therefore, to determine the degree of disability existing before the onset of failure, either from the patient or his relatives, or preferably from both.

If adequate respiratory effort cannot be maintained by the measures mentioned and alveolar hypoventilation (as judged by a persistently high or rising Pa,CO_2) becomes the critical factor for survival, the use of *mechanical ventilation* becomes compulsory if the patient's state prior to the onset of respiratory failure makes this ethically justifiable. Initially this may be given via an endotracheal tube even when the patient is conscious, usually by the judicious use of sedation. This is the optimum method in the first instance. Endotracheal tubes can certainly be tolerated for 48 hours (by which time the crisis may be past) and sometimes even for periods up to a week. Assisted ventilation may be given manually in the emergency situation employing the Ambu Resuscitator, and later by one of a number of intermittent positive pressure ventilators. Volume-cycled machines (Cape, Smith-Clarke, Radcliffe etc.) are to be preferred to pressure-cycled machines since the latter cut out when a certain pressure is reached and this may be achieved by a kinked endotracheal or tracheostomy tube, or by secretions, or by resistive airways so that little or no effective ventilation is being given. The minute volume aimed at is between 6 and 8 l/min as a rule and this should be frequently monitored by a gas meter at the expiratory end of the machine. The rate should be below 20 per minute. Overinflation must be avoided since this impedes venous return and results in a falling blood pressure. Negative phases on expiration have been advocated to assist deflation and also to maintain adequate pulmonary blood flow in respiratory failure where the elastic lung recoil is likely to be impaired. There is, in fact, no profit as a rule from having a negative phase on expiration and it may be positively disadvantageous in emphysema since it assists collapse of airways and promotes further air trapping. Synchronization of the patient's ventilatory effort with the selected rate and stroke volume of the machine may be difficult at first. If this problem occurs the best course is to ablate the effect of the respiratory centre altogether by intramuscular morphine (10 mg) or pethidine (50 mg), as a temporary expedient. Often a single dose of morphine or pethidine is enough and thereafter the patient's respiratory effort becomes synchronous with the action of the machine. It is important to remember that the *humidifying* action of the upper respiratory tract is no longer available, so that the gas delivered by intermittent positive ventilation must be humidified, ideally with a temperature-controlled heated humidifier.

Distinction has been made between *controlled ventilation* and *assisted ventilation* and although this is to some extent a play on words it serves to remind one of the different modes of artificial ventilation which are possible by machine respirators. Controlled ventilation is taken to imply automatic cycling with the machine delivering a preset volume at a preset rate independent of any spontaneous respiration by the patient. Assisted respiration is positive pressure reinforcement of tidal volume initiated by the patient's inspiratory effort, the negative pressure produced by the start of inspiration triggering the machine. Obviously, controlled ventilation requires either synchronization of the patient's spontaneous effort with the action of the machine or sufficient damping of spontaneous breathing either centrally (e.g. morphine effect on respiratory centre) or peripherally (e.g. effect of scoline on thoracic muscles). Indications for controlled as opposed to assisted ventilation are flail chest due to trauma (with appropriate depression of the respiratory centre), paralysis of the muscles of respiration, and when the viscous work of breathing is greatly increased as in chronic bronchitis. In the latter case controlled ventilation with slower and deeper inflations results in more even distribution of gas. Also the very poor spontaneous respiratory effort may mean that there is insufficient negative

pressure to trigger the machine when assisted ventilation is used in this type of case.

Assisted ventilation with patient triggering is preferred to controlled ventilation when the drive to respiration is relatively strong (e.g. if there is associated pneumonia or atelectasis), when chronic hypercapnia is not associated with chronic obstructive airways disease so that too rapid reduction in Pa, CO_2 might occur (since this may induce cardiac arrhythmia and arrest) and during the process of weaning a patient from mechanical ventilation.

The important factor in the effective use of a positive pressure ventilator is complete familiarity by all members of the team with its working. So far as the efficiency of artificial ventilation is concerned this is more important than technical variations between machines.

Routine observation of a patient having intermittent positive pressure ventilation should include clinical assessment (e.g. cyanosis etc.), pulse rate, blood pressure, minute volume, blood gases, bacteriology of tracheostomy wound and aspirated secretions, fluid intake and urine output. A standard chart of the various observations is valuable for assessing progress.

Prolonged inflation of a cuffed endotracheal or tracheostomy tube may lead to pressure necrosis of the trachea unless the cuff is intermittently released for a brief period every 2 hours. It is important, however, to ensure that the tube has not been displaced during the period of deflation. Strict asepsis should be observed whenever suction is performed or the tube replaced. In general antibiotic treatment (p. 84) should be used with the view that the least embracing of the drugs is to be preferred to those which create an ecological vacuum and so enhance superinfection by resistant organisms (e.g. *Staphylococcus pyogenes* and *Pseudomonas pyocyanea*) which is the commonest cause of death in prolonged mechanical respiration.

Weaning from the machine usually requires to be a graduated process. In general, the longer the patient has needed mechanical ventilation the longer the weaning process.

Apart from the state of recovery from the primary condition there are 2 phenomena which may influence the pattern and duration of the weaning process. Firstly prolonged mechanical ventilation may accustom the respiratory centre to a relatively low Pa,co_2 so that dyspnoea may occur on stopping controlled or assisted ventilation even though the Pa,co_2 is normal or even low (p. 25). Secondly, it seems probable that the stretch receptors in the lung and chest wall become attuned to deep inflation. The sudden loss of this sensation may result in dyspnoea.

Attempts at weaning should be begun during the day time when the efficacy of spontaneous breathing can be most conveniently and precisely determined. If there is doubt about return of adequate spontaneous breathing mechanical ventilation is resumed and commonly it is safer to put the patient back on the machine for the first night or two of the weaning process. Progressive tachycardia, tachypnoea or dyspnoea, reduction in tidal volume (assessed by the Wright Ventilation Meter), and, particularly, reduction in vital capacity indicate that mechanical ventilation should be resumed. It has been shown in this context that serial tests of vital capacity are more accurate indicators of respiratory efficiency than tidal volume or respiratory rate since the ability to perform periodic sighing which is necessary to avoid atelectasis has a closer correlation with vital capacity. Serial blood gas and pH estimations are, of course, the most precise indications of the returning efficiency of the respiratory system and are essential investigations when weaning from mechanical ventilation is being undertaken.

OXYGEN THERAPY IN ACUTE
HYPERCAPNIC RESPIRATORY FAILURE

Hypoxia always demands oxygen therapy but in some patients with hypercapnic failure the free use of oxygen may worsen alveolar ventilation by removing the sole remaining ventilatory drive. This is not universal, however, and greater harm is more frequently done by withholding oxygen than by using it relatively freely. Also oxygen therapy must be continuous and not intermittent since any

underventilation induced may continue when oxygen is withdrawn, worsening the hypoxia even further since the patient is now breathing only atmospheric air. A logical approach to the problem of hypoxia is to push oxygen to the reasonable limit, being prepared to deal with any underventilation it may cause, either by respiratory stimulants or by intermittent positive pressure ventilation. The safe method of oxygenation in the patient who is ventilating reasonably well is the use of masks (Ventimask, Edinburgh mask) which provide graduated concentrations of oxygen while preventing carbon dioxide rebreathing. Frequent observation of the clinical state and repeated Pa,co_2 measurements (by rebreathing technique if possible or by arterial puncture if necessary) will indicate whether it is safe or not to increase the percentage oxygen supplied. The Ventimask which comes in 3 kinds, supplying oxygen at a concentration of 24% or 28% with a 4 l/min flow or at 35% with an 8 l/min flow, is popular because of the blast of cool air on the face which is comforting to the dyspnoeic patient. For this reason it is generally preferred by the patient to the Edinburgh mask although the latter allows more precise incremental increase in oxygen concentration and is cheaper. When there is severe CO_2 retention it is safer to use the 24% mask initially. A head tent which allows controlled oxygen therapy is available for those patients who do not tolerate a mask. Desirable aims with graduated oxygen therapy are a Pa,o_2 of at least 50 mm Hg and a pH above 7·25 [2]. In the absence of appropriate masks intranasal catheters may be used as a second best.

When intermittent positive pressure is used oxygen may be given freely since there is no concern about the result of high oxygen concentrations on the ventilatory drive; indeed the more the respiratory centre and the rest of the body is oxygenated the better.

TREATMENT OF THE COMPLICATIONS OF
ACUTE HYPERCAPNIC RESPIRATORY
FAILURE

Energetic treatment of respiratory failure along the lines already described usually results in improvement in the *complications*, the most important being *cor pulmonale* with congestive cardiac failure and *acidosis*. Diuretics are useful if oedema is present. Digoxin may be given if there are no contra-indications such as incidental ventricular arrhythmias. The hypokalaemia resulting from potent diuretics may make the use of digoxin positively dangerous. The effect of digoxin in any case is not impressive since the heart failure is a secondary phenomenon and improvement mostly depends on effective treatment of the respiratory failure. Similarly the acidosis accompanying respiratory failure usually improves with treatment of the primary condition.

In summary acute hypercapnic failure requires treatment with antibiotics and graduated oxygen in every case and also physiotherapy according to the patient's ability to cooperate. Some need respiratory stimulants, some require bronchoscopy to clear secretions or intermittent suction through a cuffed endotracheal tube; a few need intermittent positive pressure respiration via the endotracheal tube; and a relatively small percentage of the total need prolonged mechanical ventilation along with tracheostomy. Digoxin, diuretics and bronchodilators (including corticosteroid drugs) are additional measures which may be required in the individual case. Lastly, on recovery from acute respiratory failure the patient should be fully assessed with regard to respiratory and cardiac function so that base lines can be obtained which will be of value in future management and so that any preventive measures (e.g. chemoprophylaxis, bronchodilator therapy) may be implemented.

PROGNOSIS OF ACUTE RESPIRATORY FAILURE

The more advanced the primary disease and the older the patient the poorer the prognosis. In general the more energetic the treatment the better the immediate prognosis. A mortality of 28% in 80 patients with a Pa,CO_2 over 55 mm Hg has been recorded by McNicol [4]. Prognosis does not correlate with the initial biochemical severity of the illness [4].

CHRONIC RESPIRATORY FAILURE

As in acute respiratory failure the commonest cause of chronic failure is chronic bronchitis with or without emphysema. Full assessment of the case will indicate which factors are amenable to treatment, e.g. stopping smoking, prophylactic antibiotics, bronchodilators etc. Sometimes, though rarely, reduction of polycythaemia is indicated after thorough assessment. Dichlorphenamide, a carbonic anhydrase inhibitor which gives a metabolic acidaemia and results in a fall in Pa,CO_2 in some patients, had a vogue which has passed in most centres where studies have shown that the side effects of nausea, headache and paraesthesiae usually outweigh any benefit it produces. Nevertheless it may be worth trying if the respiratory chemostat is stuck at a high Pa,CO_2 when acute failure has been overcome.

In selected cases the use of portable oxygen by means of a lightweight cylinder and a mask may allow a patient to lead a more comfortable existence in his home, e.g. relief of dyspnoea after climbing stairs, eating, going to the bathroom, etc.

In those cases with emphysematous bullae which are taking little or no part in gas exchange and are compressing normal lung surgical treatment after appropriate assessment, including anatomical and topographical studies of function (p. 48), may result in considerable improvement in ventilatory function. Only very few patients come into this category.

FURTHER READING

Safar P., Ed. (1965) *Clinical Anaesthesia, Respiratory Therapy*. Oxford, Blackwell Scientific Publications.

REFERENCES

[1] Campbell E.J.M. (1965) Respiratory failure. *Br. med. J.* i, 1451.
[2] Hutchison D.C.W., Flenley D.C. & Donald K.W. (1964) Controlled oxygen therapy in respiratory failure. *Br. med. J.* ii, 1159.
[3] McNicol M.W. & Pride N.B. (1965) Unexplained underventilation of the lung. *Thorax* 20, 53.
[4] McNicol M.W. (1967) The management of respiratory failure. *Hosp. Med.* 1, 601.

CHAPTER 20

Bronchiectasis

DEFINITION

The term bronchiectasis is primarily a morbid anatomical one. It is used to indicate chronically dilated bronchi, as demonstrated by bronchography or by morbid anatomical examination. Clinically bronchiectasis is only important if there is bronchial infection or if it gives rise to haemorrhage.

PREVALENCE

The prevalence of bronchiectasis in a population could only be accurately estimated if bronchograms were carried out on a random sample. Failing this, perhaps the best available estimate is that of Wynn-Williams [51] who computed the prevalence in Bedford, a town of 150,000 inhabitants in Southern England, as approximately 1·3 per 1000 population. The estimated prevalence in 3,617,550 examinations by miniature radiography in England and Wales in 1956 was 1·15 per 1000 as compared to 1·9 per 1000 for pulmonary tuberculosis. The prevalence in 1946 was 0·77 per 1000, so that there is certainly no suggestion of a fall between 1946 and 1956 (figures calculated from Chief Medical Officer's Reports, England and Wales [11]). In the Aberdeen area of Scotland Clark [12] reported that the 'average annual incidence of discovered bronchiectasis' in 1946–55 inclusive was 10·6 per 100,000 child population, which might give a cumulative prevalence in agreement with the figures quoted above.

AETIOLOGY AND PATHOGENESIS

The aetiology of bronchiectasis is still uncertain and different factors may well be involved in different patients.

CONGENITAL FACTORS

At one time it was thought that most cases of bronchiectasis were congenital. The best evidence that some cases may in fact be of congenital origin is the occurrence of bronchiectasis in about 20% of patients with dextrocardia, an association originally pointed out by Kartagener [27] and confirmed by others [1 & 38]. The patients usually have sinusitis or absent frontal sinuses. It seems unlikely that the bronchiectasis is due to pressure on a bronchus by the abnormal heart or blood vessels, for there is no consistency in the anatomical distribution of the changes.

Spencer [43], as a pathologist, considers congenital bronchiectasis not uncommon, basing his views on the absence of any evidence of lung tissue in certain cases. He thinks there is failure of the alveoli and peripheral bronchi to develop.

Bronchiectasis is usually present in *sequestrated lung* (p. 7), which of course is a congenital abnormality [6 & 8], and often in *unilateral pulmonary emphysema* (p. 327).

Bronchiectasis may complicate cystic fibrosis (mucoviscidosis), but in this disease the primary abnormality is probably in the mucus and the bronchiectasis is due to bronchial blockage and secondary infection [3]. Bronchiectasis may also be associated with congenital *hypogammaglobulinaemia*, but in this instance the bronchiectasis is acquired because of the patient's reduced capacity to resist bacterial infection [19]. Bronchiectasis may also occur in acquired hypogammaglobulinaemia [44].

OBSTRUCTION AND INFECTION

It seems that in the great majority of patients bronchiectasis is acquired, usually in childhood. In most cases both the factors of

347

obstruction and of infection are probably necessary.

OBSTRUCTION

Obstruction may cause bronchiectasis in 1 of 2 ways:

(1) Obstruction of many small bronchi.
(2) Obstruction of a single large bronchus.

(1) During an acute respiratory infection mucus may be aspirated into the small peripheral bronchi, obstructing their lumina and causing collapse of the lung beyond. The collapse results in a more negative intrapleural tension which, because of the collapsed alveoli, results in a greater transmural pressure in the bronchi proximal to the obstruction. These bronchi are still in communication with the atmosphere and the difference between the atmospheric pressure and the greater intrapleural negative tension causes them to expand [28]. If the walls of these larger bronchi become infected, and their muscular and elastic tissue damaged, then, even if the lung subsequently re-expands, the bronchi may be unable to return to their former size. More important, they may lose their ability to contract on expiration, which is probably one of the most important factors in clearing the bronchus of secretion. Further secondary infection is therefore more likely to occur and a vicious circle is set up. If there is no damage to the bronchial wall, the bronchi may return to their former size after re-expansion of the lung [5, 29 & 35]. By routine bronchography in pneumonia it has been found that bronchial abnormalities, including dilatation, are common, but in most patients revert to normal in due course [5]. When dilatation occurs without obvious pulmonary collapse it may be that the pneumonia causes temporary decrease in the tone of bronchial muscle. Permanent bronchiectasis follows only if there is irreversible damage to the bronchial wall. This is more likely to follow pneumonia in childhood, particularly that complicating *measles* and *whooping cough* [4 & 40] and particularly if treatment is inadequate.

(2) Bronchial obstruction may contribute to bronchiectasis in another way. One of the larger bronchi may become obstructed, for instance by a *foreign body* or an *adenoma*. If no infection occurs beyond the obstruction, the lung and bronchi may merely collapse. If infection occurs beyond the obstruction then the bronchi can become grossly dilated by the outpouring of infected secretion, unable to escape. This conclusion is based both on clinical experience and on experimental work in rabbits [45].

INFECTION

Besides its importance in association with obstruction it is possible that infection can produce bronchiectasis by damage to the bronchial wall without actual collapse. When bronchograms are done in *postprimary pulmonary tuberculosis* bronchiectasis is almost universal [10 & 17]. Because the bronchiectasis is usually in the better drained upper lobes, secondary infection is relatively unusual and clinical symptoms of bronchiectasis rarely develop.

Bronchiectasis is associated with about 15% of cases of *primary pulmonary tuberculosis* in which a lobar or segmental shadow is detected on the x-ray. Such anatomical bronchiectasis seldom gives rise to symptoms unless all the basal segments of one of the lower lobes are affected, when symptoms are common. Symptoms also occur in some cases of middle lobe disease [7]. Presumably the important factor is that the lower and middle lobes are less well drained than the upper lobes, which are more commonly affected by 'epituberculosis'. The factors involved are discussed on p. 203. Wynn-Williams [51] thought that 7% of 155 cases in Bedford were associated with old primary tuberculosis.

It seems possible that bronchiectasis may also follow *bronchiolitis* in infants. Williams and O'Reilly [49], in a study of bronchiectasis in 241 children, differentiated two main types of the acquired disease. They described 'subacute pyogenic pulmonary collapse' complicating an acute bacterial infection and usually occurring between the ages of 2 and 6, with no overt evidence of a familial predisposition to respiratory disease. The pathogenesis of this type is similar to that already described.

The second type usually began with bronchiolitis occurring under the age of 3. The onset was insidious. The infant had a chronic upper respiratory infection. No pyogenic organisms were detectable in the earlier stages. The bronchiectasis affected mainly the peripheral bronchi and was often generalized and cystic in type. In 38% there was a family history of chronic respiratory disease and in 14% of bronchiectasis, though the investigation was carried out in Melbourne, where chronic respiratory disease in adults is not as common as in Britain. It seems possible that this type of bronchiectasis might be associated with, or at least initiated by, a viral infection, though it is likely that major bronchial damage is due to bacteria. The nature of the infecting agents is discussed below. The high incidence of cystic bronchiectasis in Maoris, reported by Hinds [24], might be due to a racial or familial susceptibility to respiratory infection or to inadequate treatment of such infection.

BRONCHIECTASIS IN ASTHMATIC PULMONARY EOSINOPHILIA [14]

Bronchiectasis is relatively common at sites of recurrent shadows in pulmonary eosinophilia with asthma. It occurs particularly in patients who cough up plugs or casts. At least in some of these patients the asthma is associated with hypersensitivity to *Aspergillus fumigatus* (p. 429).

FIBROSIS

At one time bronchiectasis was thought to be due to the drag of fibrous tissue on the wall of a bronchus. It is true that bronchiectasis may be associated with almost any condition which gives rise to severe lung fibrosis. In many of these conditions the principal factor is probably the damage to the bronchial wall by infection. Bronchiectasis can, for instance, occur in sarcoidosis but usually only in the advanced chronic stage when there is considerable lung fibrosis and secondary infection.

AGE AND SEX

Bronchiectasis most commonly begins in childhood [4 & 32]. This is possibly because the small lumen of the child's bronchus makes obstruction more likely; possibly because the child's interalveolar pores are ill-developed, collateral ventilation more difficult [43] and lung collapse more likely; or possibly because the wall of the child's bronchus is softer and more easily damaged. The relative prevalence of bronchiectasis in the two sexes is uncertain. In Bedford, England, Wynn-Williams [51] found a slightly higher prevalence of bronchographically proved bronchiectasis in males. Figures derived from mass radiography indicate twice as high a prevalence in males, though the male preponderance is mainly over the age of 45 [11]; the criteria for diagnosis in these cases is less certain. On the other hand Davis *et al.* [16] in hospital cases in the United States found twice as many cases in females and state that this is the usual proportion. Much may depend on the selection of patients.

PATHOLOGY [32 & 43]

The bronchi may be lined with squamous or columnar epithelium, or the epithelium may be ulcerated. There may be a variable degree of destruction of the wall, which sometimes is only represented by occasional pieces of cartilage or muscle. Both the wall and the lumen of the bronchus are infiltrated with neutrophils. In severe cases combined radiological and morbid anatomical studies indicate obliteration of side branches, witnessing to the amount of bronchial damage which has occurred [41]. In cylindrical bronchiectasis, the milder type, reduction of side branches in the bronchogram may be merely due to blocking by secretion. There may be a variable amount of fibrosis, collapse or pneumonia in the surrounding lung. Peribronchial fibrosis is common. There is evidence that in bronchiectasis the pulmonary arteries accompanying the affected bronchi may be initially thrombosed and perhaps later recanalized. The vascular supply of the area is mainly derived from the bronchial arteries which are much hypertrophied. Anastomoses between the bronchial and pulmonary arteries are frequent [13 & 33].

Whitwell [48] described a type of bronchiectasis which he termed 'follicular' bronchiectasis. This is seen in children and symptoms usually start before the age of 7. It is characterized pathologically by hypertrophy of lymphoid tissue within the lung and at the hilum, and by lymphocytic infiltration of the bronchial walls. It most often affects the left lower lobe and most cases follow measles or whooping cough. It is possible that this type of bronchiectasis may be associated with viral infection, as suggested by MacFarlane and Sommerville [30].

BACTERIOLOGY AND VIROLOGY

BACTERIA

The bacteria causing the original bronchial damage are likely to be those causing the pneumonia. In the past, streptococcal pneumonias were particularly damaging [5]. In established bronchiectasis the damaged and flaccid bronchi are invaded by other bacteria. Prior to the introduction of antibiotics infection with anaerobic bacteria was common. This was responsible for the distressing, foul-smelling sputum. The anaerobes were usually either Vincent's organisms (*Fusiformis fusiformis* together with *Treponema vincenti*) or anaerobic streptococci (a somewhat ill-defined group: see Wilson and Miles [50]). Fortunately anaerobic bacteria respond well to treatment with antibiotics so that anaerobic infection and foul sputum are now seldom seen. Investigations over recent years incriminate *Haemophilus influenzae* [2, 21, 36, 37 & 46] as the most common complicating organism, although in patients with cystic fibrosis (mucoviscidosis) staphylococci are most frequently found.

VIRUSES

MacFarlane and Sommerville [30] in Glasgow found raised antibody titres to adenoviruses in 11 of 18 children with bronchiectasis. It is of interest that in 137 bronchiectatic patients in the U.S. Navy a much higher rate of raised antibody titres to adenoviruses was also found than in patients with bronchopneu-

monia, bronchitis or other conditions [42]. Apart from influenza B from 2 cases no viruses were isolated from the bronchi. Anaerobic mycoplasmata were isolated from nearly a third of those with bronchiectasis, compared to a sixth of those with bronchopneumonia, but the significance of this is uncertain; no serological studies were done. Adenovirus infection is, of course, common in childhood but is usually mild or symptomless. More impressive evidence would be required before accepting its aetiological rôle in bronchiectasis.

Bronchiectasis following measles is probably associated with complicating bacterial infection. It may be concluded that, though pneumonias responsible for later bronchiectasis may sometimes be initiated by viral infection, it is likely that the major damage to the bronchial wall is bacterial.

FUNCTIONAL ABNORMALITY

The overall functional abnormality in bronchiectasis will depend on the extent of the lung damage and the extent of complicating chronic bronchitis. Bronchiectasis confined to the middle lobe, for instance, may cause little demonstrable impairment of lung function. Severe unilateral bronchiectasis, with virtual destruction of one lung, may result in less than 10% of the O_2 uptake occurring in that lung, though it may receive a third of the ventilation [6]. There is evidence that in bronchiectasis quite extensive shunts may occur from the systemic to the pulmonary circulation by means of the hypertrophied bronchial arteries and bronchopulmonary anastomoses. The evidence consists of (1) a higher Sa,O_2 in blood from the pulmonary artery supplying affected segments, (2) higher pressures in the pulmonary vessels of the affected segment, as measured by a wedged catheter and (3) an excess of left over right ventricular output in some patients with bronchiectasis [6]. The substitution of systemic for pulmonary vascular supply to the affected lung may account for a greater reduction of O_2 uptake than of ventilation.

Regional functional studies have not been

extensively made in bronchiectasis, but without them the contribution of an affected segment to lung function may be difficult to assess with certainty. If the affected lung is poorly ventilated and poorly perfused with pulmonary artery blood it may make little contribution, as has been shown in a few cases by radioactive xenon studies [6]. In some cases with marginal overall function such studies, or bronchospirometry, may have to be carried out before contemplating surgery. Nonfunctioning lung which is making a major contribution to sputum production might be best removed, though the change in position of the residual bronchi (e.g. the lingular), and the possible strain on their partially damaged walls must be remembered; overt bronchiectasis in such cases may manifest itself only postoperatively.

When there is generalized bronchitis, as shown by widespread rhonchi, wheeze and the typical bronchographic changes, the functional effects of bronchitis (p. 312) will be added to those of bronchiectasis.

The efficiency of cough depends largely on the ratio of tube diameter to particle size [6]. Cinefluorographic studies, including in some cases measurement of intrabronchial pressure [22], have shown that in cylindrical bronchiectasis the cough function may be normal but that in some cases of cystic and saccular bronchiectasis the proximal part of the affected bronchi may collapse completely with cough, trapping the sputum in the bronchiectatic segments which, instead of the normal marked narrowing with cough, maintain an almost inspiratory calibre. This abnormality is an exaggeration of the inadequate movement of the damaged bronchi in ordinary breathing which contributes to the poor bronchial drainage.

It has been shown that, if surgery is carried out judiciously and in suitable patients, it can result in little impairment, and even in gradual improvement, of lung function. It seems that, when the residual lung is normal, it can take up the residual space without loss of function [26]. This of course will not be true if the residual lung is abnormal in any way or if there is bronchitis.

CLINICAL FEATURES
SYMPTOMS
Cough and *purulent sputum* are the classical symptoms of bronchiectasis. There is great variation from patient to patient in the severity of cough and the quantity of sputum. Patients with the mildest disease may only have cough and sputum for a week or two after a cold or none at all; patients with the severest form of disease may cough up 200 or 300 ml of purulent sputum a day throughout the year. Most untreated cases of bronchiectasis have some cough and sputum throughout the year, increasing after upper respiratory infections. The history of cough usually goes back to childhood.

Haemoptysis is not infrequent in bronchiectasis. It usually consists merely of streaks of blood in the sputum but occasionally is very severe. Oddly enough, the most severe haemoptysis may occur in patients with relatively little previous history of chronic cough and sputum and sometimes with very limited bronchiectasis. The severity may be due to the hypertrophy of the bronchial arteries and, in consequence, bleeding from the systemic circulation. The middle lobe bronchus is the most common site of severe bleeding, which may follow the erosion of an artery by a 'broncholith', a nodule of calcium derived from a lymph gland remaining from a primary tuberculous complex. In so-called 'dry bronchiectasis' haemoptysis may be the only symptom. Bronchiectasis, therefore, always comes into the differential diagnosis of any unexplained haemoptysis.

The amount of *dyspnoea* and *wheeze* of which a patient complains will depend on the amount of generalized bronchitis and on the amount of lung collapse and destruction which has resulted from the original, or from repeated, pneumonias. Recurrent exacerbations of respiratory infection are usual, often initiated by upper respiratory infections, such as the common cold. Chronic bronchitis is a common sequel.

PHYSICAL SIGNS
The *general condition* of the patient may be very good or, in patients who have severe

longstanding disease, may be very poor. Nevertheless, it is rare nowadays to see the emaciated chronic invalids with bronchiectasis who at one time were relatively common in chest hospitals. In the more severe cases there may be *clubbing* of the fingers, apparently in some way associated with hypertrophy of the bronchial arteries [47].

In the chest the most important physical sign is the presence of medium or coarse *crepitations*. The presence of such crepitations in the same area of the chest at repeated examinations over a period of months is suggestive of bronchiectasis in a patient who has a consistent history. In addition there may be signs of collapse, fibrosis or pneumonia, either as residua of the original infection or as a result of later complications.

RADIOLOGY

There is no entirely characteristic radiographic appearance on the straight film. Occasionally cystic spaces, sometimes with a fluid level, may be seen, although it is not possible on a straight x-ray to be sure that the cysts are bronchial. In one large series [23] cystic appearances were seen in only 13%. There are often the radiological appearances of collapse, fibrosis or patchy pneumonia. But in some patients, 7% of one series [23], the straight film may appear to be normal.

Diagnosis can only be made with certainty by bronchography. When the more peripheral bronchi are affected, the bronchiectatic spaces are often cystic. When the larger bronchi are affected, they may be fusiform or saccular. The term 'saccular' is used to indicate a steady increase in calibre in the peripheral part of a bronchus and occurs with the most severe damage. These terms are purely descriptive and there is little to be said for using them as a basis for classification, especially as a mixture of types is not uncommon. Sometimes bronchi are distorted and obviously abnormal but not clearly dilated. Such cases will be classed as purulent bronchitis, although the distinction is a somewhat artificial one. It is common to find distorted bronchi in one area and dilated bronchi in others.

In most reported series the left side, especially the lower lobe, is more often affected than the right. The lingular segment of the left upper lobe is often affected in patients who have bronchiectasis of the left lower lobe. In about a third of cases the bronchiectasis is bilateral and even higher figures have been recorded [6].

DIAGNOSIS

A certain diagnosis of bronchiectasis can only be made by bronchography. A history of persistent or recurrent cough, particularly with purulent sputum and extending back to childhood, may be very suggestive and is reinforced if coarse or medium crepitations are found in a particular area of the chest at repeated examination over a period of months or years. This impression will of course be reinforced if clubbing is present and if there are consistent findings on straight x-ray. In examining the radiograph it is well to remember that a collapsed left lower lobe may easily be concealed behind the heart. A penetrating or a lateral film should be carried out in a case where symptoms and physical signs are suggestive.

In childhood recurrent bronchitis is very much commoner than bronchiectasis. In bronchitis the signs are usually of generalized rhonchi rather than localized crepitations. Adults with uncomplicated chronic bronchitis seldom give a history which goes back to childhood; symptoms usually begin in the fourth or fifth decade. Many patients with bronchiectasis, however, also have generalized bronchitis.

When the presenting symptom is haemoptysis bronchiectasis has, of course, to be differentiated from other causes of haemoptysis such as pulmonary tuberculosis, lung abscess, carcinoma of the bronchus, adenoma, mitral stenosis, etc. If there is doubt after radiographic examination the crucial investigation is the bronchogram.

The decision as to when to do a bronchogram is not always a simple one. In young children a bronchogram involves a general anaesthetic and should not be undertaken lightly. The diagnosis may be probable on the history and physical signs and becomes more probable if the physical signs remain constant over a number of months or years. A bronchogram is of course indicated if surgery is in question, so that the extent of the disease may be defined. Surgery should seldom be contemplated until the effect of conservative measures has been observed for a year.

COMPLICATIONS

PNEUMONIA

The recurrent exacerbations, usually secondary to upper respiratory tract infection, which are so common in bronchiectasis, frequently give rise to patchy pneumonia in the region of the abnormal bronchi. These patches are often multiple and usually 0·5–2 cm in diameter on the x-ray. The severity of the accompanying symptoms is variable but frequently comparatively slight.

PLEURISY

Pleuritic pain, perhaps accompanied by a rub, may accompany the episodes of pneumonia. Bronchiectasis is probably the commonest cause of recurrent dry pleurisy in the same site, usually complicating successive upper respiratory tract infections. There may be no chronic cough and sputum to suggest the nature of the underlying disease and no local crepitations, except perhaps during the exacerbation itself.

PLEURAL EFFUSION OR EMPYEMA

Pleural effusion or empyema is a relatively rare accompaniment of previously diagnosed bronchiectasis. Underlying bronchiectasis is, however, not uncommon in chronic empyema. Presumably the original infected collapse had given rise to both.

SINUSITIS

Sinusitis is a common complication of bronchiectasis and almost universal in severe cases. Infection in these cases seems to occur in the respiratory tract as a whole. There is little point in attempting radical operative treatment of the sinusitis if the bronchiectasis is not being dealt with at the same time. If the bronchiectasis can be controlled, either by surgical or by medical means, then surgery may be justifiable for the sinusitis if this has not also come under control.

HAEMOPTYSIS

As mentioned above, severe haemoptysis occasionally occurs in bronchiectasis, and mild haemoptysis is common. Very occasionally severe and uncontrollable haemoptysis may be an indication for emergency resection of the part of the lung affected. Milder, but less threatening, haemoptysis is sometimes a reason for a more deliberate surgical attack. Severe haemoptysis may be an occasional cause of death in bronchiectasis, but this should not occur if the patient is admitted promptly to a thoracic surgical unit. Sometimes the localization of the site of the haemoptysis may prove a problem.

BRAIN ABSCESS

Brain abscess is a classical complication of bronchiectasis and in the past one of the notorious causes of death in this condition. We have seen it complicating very limited bronchiectasis. The absence of abscesses elsewhere suggests that the infection reaches the brain by means of the vertebral veins.

AMYLOIDOSIS

Although a classical complication of bronchiectasis, amyloidosis is in fact rare. Nevertheless this possibility should be borne in mind. The urine should be tested for protein from time to time and the abdomen, as well as the chest, examined. If there is enlargement of the liver or spleen, the possibility of amyloidosis should immediately come to mind.

PREVENTION

The prompt and thorough treatment of respiratory infection, together with physiotherapy designed to secure re-expansion of the lung, should reduce the attack rate of bronchiectasis. Though at present there is no more than an impression that a reduction has occurred in the community as a whole, the absence of any bronchiectasis in a follow-up study of a series of children in whom bronchopneumonia complicated whooping cough, but who had full hospital treatment [25], suggests that good treatment of severe lower respiratory infections in childhood can indeed prevent the disease. After any severe respiratory infection it is wise to have the patient x-rayed to ensure that the lungs have returned to normal. Any residual lesions should be intensively treated.

TREATMENT

Medical treatment aims to relieve or mitigate the symptoms of bronchiectasis, surgical treatment to eliminate the disease itself. The latter is obviously preferable, but it is doubtful how often it is practicable. Medical treatment consists of chemotherapy and postural drainage, surgical treatment of resection.

CHEMOTHERAPY

Chemotherapy may be used for the continuous control of bronchial infection or for the treatment of exacerbations, or for both. The problem is very similar to that of the chemotherapy of chronic bronchitis, into which there has been much more careful investigation (p. 321). Most of the conclusions from research on the chemotherapy of chronic bronchitis are applicable to the chemotherapy of bronchiectasis. Bacteriological investigation is of little value unless there is close liaison between the clinician and the bacteriologist and the standard of both the collection and the culture of specimens rises above routine level. Failing such close liaison the clinician should treat on empirical grounds. As mentioned above (p. 350), if the patient has foul sputum the responsible bacteria are probably anaerobes. But foul sputum is now relatively rare and *Haemophilus influenzae* is the most common organism found when careful bacteriological studies are carried out. The pneumococcus may also play a part in some cases, at least in exacerbations.

CHEMOTHERAPY OF EXACERBATIONS

The principles of the chemotherapy of exacerbations are the same as those for exacerbations of chronic bronchitis (p. 323). Occasionally the sputum fails to convert to mucoid in spite of the successive use of antibiotics. Surprisingly enough, intensive treatment with several drugs, for instance penicillin, streptomycin, oxytetracycline and ampicillin (which is safer than chloramphenicol) may be successful, but clearly such polypharmacy must only be a last resort and is rarely necessary. As soon as the sputum has become mucoid the patient should be discharged home, in case he picks up a hospital infection.

SUPPRESSIVE CHEMOTHERAPY

Suppressive chemotherapy is used to control chronic bronchial infection and to prevent exacerbations. Although there have been a large number of controlled trials in the preventive chemotherapy of chronic bronchitis there have been few in bronchiectasis. The results in bronchitis (p. 321) are probably applicable to bronchiectasis. The Medical Research Council trial of chemotherapy in bronchiectasis [34] showed that tetracycline, in a dose of 0·5 g 4 times daily, given on 2 days a week such as Wednesdays and Sundays, significantly reduced sputum quantity, cough and work loss, compared to controls treated with placebo tablets. Although there has been no direct comparison, later work on chronic bronchitis (p. 321) suggests that at present tetracycline 0·5 g twice daily is the most practical and effective long term suppressive treatment. Tetracycline in a dose of 2 g/day has also been found effective in patients with bronchiectasis and acquired hypogammaglobulinaemia [44]. The effect of ampicillin is probably similar to that of tetracycline but ampicillin is more expensive.

Patients with mild bronchiectasis, who develop symptoms solely after an upper respiratory infection, may require preventive treatment only when the upper respiratory infection starts. More severe cases may require treatment throughout the winter months, the most severe throughout the entire year. With moderate or severe cases it is seldom possible to keep the patient entirely free from sputum, but it is usually possible to maintain his symptoms within reasonable bounds, to enable him to be socially acceptable and to keep him at work, provided his respiratory reserve is sufficient to cope both with his job and with the necessary travelling. A patient with severe disease is often helped by a short admission to hospital for intensive chemotherapy and postural drainage, after which the benefit can be maintained by long term treatment with a tetracycline.

POSTURAL DRAINAGE

The bronchiectatic bronchus has lost its elasticity and its bronchomuscular tone, both of which are important factors in clearing the normal bronchus of secretion. If the mucous membrane has become squamous, or if there is surface ulceration, there will be no cilia. Even when cilia survive, the excessive secretion may drown the mucus blanket and the cilia will beat ineffectively. The bronchus has therefore lost its main clearing mechanisms and, if in the lower part of the lung, forms a sump of infected secretions, a perpetual threat to other parts of the bronchial tree and a source of toxicity to the patient. Gravity has to be used to keep the sump empty and thereby reduce the secondary infection and the toxicity of retained secretions.

The position the patient should adopt for postural drainage depends, of course, on the site of the affected bronchi. If it is remembered that the object is to move the sputum, with the aid of gravity, towards the hilum, it should be obvious enough from the bronchogram what position or positions are optimal in the individual case. To empty basal bronchi a young relatively fit patient can lean over the side of the bed with his head on his folded arms and his thorax vertical. For less fit patients the foot of the bed may be elevated on a couple of chairs. Special beds are available for postural drainage. In the home, a carpenter can construct a light A-shaped folding frame of wood and canvas strips which can be padded with cushions or pillows. It is important to remember that a patient with bronchiectasis of the middle lobe or lingula must lie on his back, with the bed elevated head downwards and with a pillow under the affected side.

Having adopted the appropriate position the patient should take deep breaths to aid the emptying of the segmental bronchi into the main bronchi and trachea, and then cough to clear the larger air passages. If possible he should be instructed in the procedure by a physiotherapist who may help to dislodge the sputum by light pummelling of the thorax. Sometimes most sputum is produced after resuming the upright position.

When a patient is admitted to hospital with an exacerbation, and especially if he has much sputum, postural drainage should be done several times a day and should continue on each occasion until no further sputum is brought up. At home he should get rid of the night's secretions first thing in the morning and repeat the process last thing at night to avoid the fit of coughing which may occur when he lies down and sputum overflows into the larger bronchi.

Postural drainage is tedious and embarrassing to the patient. It must, at home, be carried out in privacy. When there is much secretion he should be strongly encouraged to persist. When there is very little, he should be relieved of this troublesome routine, but be told to resume it at any time if he develops a cold.

SURGERY

At a time when the prognosis of bronchiectasis was regarded as very poor and thoracic surgery was beginning to prove safe and successful in a number of conditions there was an obvious attraction in the idea of resecting the affected segments of bronchiectatic lung, and very large numbers of patients were operated on. Many successful series were reported. After a period of great surgical activity, enthusiasm for surgery among physicians has somewhat waned, partly because of the evidence of improved prognosis and control since the introduction of chemotherapy, partly perhaps because physicians see the surgeons' less successful cases [15].

Most will agree that surgical treatment is highly successful in patients with moderate or severe symptoms, whose bronchiectasis is localized to a single lobe or segment, without clinical or bronchographic evidence of bronchiectasis or bronchitis affecting other parts of the lung. Unfortunately such cases are rare. When there is generalized bronchitis, or when any bronchographically abnormal bronchi are left behind after operation, even though the residual bronchi are not initially strictly bronchiectatic, the results may be disappointing. Any important impairment of respiratory function may make operation inadvisable unless it can be shown (p. 351) that the bronchiectatic area of the lung makes only a very small contribution to function. In general, the results are unimpressive after the age of 40 and are best in older children and young people [15].

A decision regarding surgery is therefore difficult. Many patients have such extensive bilateral disease that surgery is out of the question. In others, symptoms are so mild and so easily controlled medically that the discomfort and slight risk of resection seem hardly justifiable. Between these extremes are many patients in whom the balance of decision is more even. In these patients the state of the other bronchi, the amount of bronchitis, the respiratory function, the age, the mental outlook, the quality of surgical skill available and the response to medical control will all have to be carefully assessed. In general we believe that surgical treatment should not be advised until medical treatment has been given at least a year's trial.

Surgery has also to be considered in relation to some of the less usual presentations of the disease. If a relatively fit patient has had moderate or severe haemoptysis due to a localized area of bronchiectasis, especially if the haemoptysis has occurred more than once, he should be seriously considered for resection, which would usually be indicated. Recurrent pleurisy or recurrent pneumonia in cases with strictly localized disease may again justify surgery. In cases with bronchiectasis distal to a bronchial adenoma, a foreign body in the bronchus or a bronchial carcinoma, resection would usually be indicated if it is feasible.

It is somewhat difficult to assess the results of published series of cases treated surgically. Gudbjerg [23] reviewed published surgical results up to 10 years ago. He found that 50–75% were symptom free or clinically improved but that residual bronchiectasis, or bronchiectasis that later became overt, occurred in 10–40% of operated cases. Clark [12] reviewed all the cases of bronchiectasis in childhood diagnosed in Aberdeen, Scotland, over a 10 year period. Surgery was carried out in 75%. In a follow-up varying between 6 months and 12 years after operation 55% were classed as completely recovered and a further 16% as much improved, a total of 71% with what he regarded as very satisfactory results. Against this there was an operative mortality of 1·9% and a case mortality of 2·5%. He agrees that a period of watching under medical treatment is usually advisable, especially as there is a high rate of postoperative complication in young children following lobar or segmental resection. However, he considers that if there is severe bronchiectasis involving the whole of one lung early pneumonectomy may be advisable to prevent spread and to improve the general condition. Reviewing previous surgical series, amounting to over 500 children in all, he found that 67% had been classed as 'cured' or 'much improved'. He concludes that surgery is the treatment of choice for bronchiectasis in children but that operation should, where possible, be deferred to later childhood. Borrie and Lichter [9] also obtained excellent results in recent years. They reported on 125 patients operated on in the 10 years 1952–62. Most of the patients were aged 10–40. Postoperative complications were common but temporary. There was only 1 operative death. Complete absence of symptoms was achieved in 55% of unilateral cases; an additional 42% were said to have full physical capacity but occasional cough or clear sputum. 34 patients had bilateral resections. 31% of these were symptom free and a further 53% had only minimal symptoms. All the cases were said to have been referred because of 'failure of medical treatment' but of course it would have been of considerable value to know the details of selection. It is clear, however, that excellent results can be obtained in properly selected cases.

These last 2 series in particular might encourage physicians to have a more enthusiastic view of surgery, though we would advise careful consideration of all the factors outlined in previous paragraphs.

PROGNOSIS

In the period before the use of modern chemotherapy the published prognosis of bronchiectasis was bad. In 5 studies published between 1931 and 1941, covering 789 cases followed up for 2–14 years, the overall mortality was 27·5% [18]. On the whole at that time only severe bronchiectasis was diagnosed. On the other hand McKim [31] reported that 41 of 49 patients, treated as outpatients and followed up for 9–20 years, were alive; only 3 were worse and more than half were better than at the time of diagnosis. Fine and Steinhausen [20] reported that 75% of 26 patients diagnosed at radiography had few or no symptoms 2 years later. In a survey of all known cases in a population Wynn-Williams [51] found that 20% were symptom free and almost all led a relatively normal life. In a series of 66 children, mostly treated surgically, more than three quarters were improved or well at follow-up, but the same was true of a smaller group treated medically [4]. Some results of surgical treatment have already been outlined.

One can perhaps summarize the position on prognosis by saying that with modern treatment, medical or surgical, the prognosis for survival is good. Long term survival depends mainly on the amount of lung destruction and the amount of generalized bronchitis at the time of diagnosis. Some patients with strictly localized bronchiectasis may be made permanently symptom free by surgery. In the remainder the symptoms may be reasonably well controlled by medical treatment, but usually not abolished. However, most of these patients are enabled to lead a relatively normal life, even if they suffer from some chronic cough and sputum and have more frequent respiratory exacerbations than normal people.

REFERENCES

[1] ADAMS R. & CHURCHILL E.D. (1938) Situs inversus, sinusitis, bronchiectasis. *J. thorac. Surg.* 7, 206.

[2] ALLISON P.R., GORDON J. & ZINNEMANN K. (1943) The incidence and significance of *H. influenzae* in chronic bronchiectasis. *J. Path. Bact.* 55, 465.

[3] ANDERSEN DOROTHY H. (1958) Cystic fibrosis of the pancreas. *J. chron. Dis.* 7, 58.

[4] AVERY M.E., RILEY M.C. & WEISS A. (1961) The course of bronchiectasis in childhood. *Bull. Johns Hopkins Hosp.* 109, 20.

[5] BACHMAN A.L., HEWITT W.R. & BEEKLEY H.C. (1953) Bronchiectasis. A bronchographic study of 60 cases of pneumonia. *Arch. intern. Med.* 91, 78.

[6] BATES D.V. & CHRISTIE R.V. (1964) *Respiratory Function in Disease. An Introduction to the Integrated Study of the Lung.* Philadelphia, Saunders.

[7] BENTLEY F.J., GRZYBOWSKI S. & BENJAMIN B. (1954) *Tuberculosis in Childhood and Adolescence.* London, The National Association for the Prevention of Tuberculosis.

[8] BLESOVSKY A. (1967) Pulmonary sequestration. A report of an unusual case and a review of the literature. *Thorax* 22, 351.

[9] BORRIE J. & LICHTER I. (1965) Surgical treatment of bronchiectasis; ten year survey. *Br. med. J.* ii, 908.

[10] BOYER L.B. (1946) Bronchography in tuberculosis: a clinical study. *Am. Rev. Tuberc.* 54, 111.

[11] CHIEF MEDICAL OFFICER REPORTS (1947 and 1957). Ministry of Health, London, Her Majesty's Stationery Office.

[12] CLARK N.S. (1963) Bronchiectasis in childhood. *Br. med. J.* i, 80.

[13] COCKETT F.B. & VASS C.C.N. (1951). A comparison of the rôle of bronchial arteries in bronchiectasis and in experimental ligation of the pulmonary artery. *Thorax* 6, 268.

[14] CROFTON J.W., LIVINGSTONE J.L., OSWALD N.C. & ROBERTS A.T.M. (1952) Pulmonary eosinophilia. *Thorax* 7, 1.

[15] CROFTON J. (1966) Bronchiectasis. II. Treatment and prevention. *Br. med. J.*, i, 783.

[16] DAVIS M.B., HOPKINS W.A. & WANSKER W.C. (1962) The present status of the treatment of bronchiectasis. *Am. Rev. resp. Dis.* 85, 816.

[17] DORMER B.A., FRIEDLANDER J. & WILES F.J. (1944 and 1945) Bronchography in pulmonary tuberculosis. *Am. Rev. Tuberc.* 50, 283, 287; 51, 455, 519.

[18] EDITORIAL (1949) Bronchiectasis. *Br. med. J.* **ii,** 970.

[19] EDITORIAL (1961) Hypogammaglobulinaemia. *Lancet* **i,** 151.

[20] FINE A. & STEINHAUSEN T.B. (1946) Nondisabling bronchiectasis. *Radiology* **46,** 237.

[21] FRANKLIN A.W. & GARROD L.P. (1953) Chloramphenicol treatment of bronchiectasis in children. *Br. med. J.* **ii,** 1067.

[22] FRASER R.G., MACKLEM P.T. & BROWN W.G. (1965) Airway dynamics in bronchiectasis. A combined cinefluorographic-manometric study. *Am. J. Roentgenol.* **93,** 821.

[23] GUDBJERG C.E. (1957) Radiological diagnosis of bronchiectasis and prognosis after operative treatment. *Acta radiol. Stockh. Suppl.* 143.

[24] HINDS J.R. (1958) Bronchiectasis in the Maori. *N.Z. med. J.* **57,** 328.

[25] JERNELIUS H. (1964) Pertussis with pulmonary complications. A follow up study. *Acta paediat.* (*Stockholm*) **53,** 247.

[26] KAMENER R., BECKLAKE MARGARET R., GOLDMAN H. & McGREGOR M. (1958) Respiratory function following segmental resection of the lung for bronchiectasis. *Am. Rev. Tuberc.* **77,** 209.

[27] KARTAGENER M. (1933) Zur Pathogenese der Bronchiektasien: I. Bronchiektasien bei Situs viscerum inversus. *Beitr. Klin. Tuberk.* **83,** 489.

[28] LANDER F.P.L. (1946) Bronchiectasis and atelectasis. Temporary and permanent changes. *Thorax* **1,** 198.

[29] LEES A.W. (1950) Atelectasis and bronchiectasis in pertussis. *Br. med. J.* **ii,** 1138.

[30] MACFARLANE P.S. & SOMMERVILLE R.G. (1957) Nontuberculous juvenile bronchiectasis: a virus disease? *Lancet* **i,** 770.

[31] McKIM A. (1952) Bronchiectasis as seen in an ambulant clinic service. *Am. Rev. Tuberc.* **66,** 457.

[32] McNEIL C., MACGREGOR A.R. & ALEXANDER W.A. (1929) Studies of pneumonia in childhood. IV. Bronchiectasis and fibrosis of the lung. *Arch. Dis. Childh.* **4,** 170.

[33] MARCHAND P., GILROY J.C. & WILSON V.H. (1950) An anatomical study of the bronchial vascular system and its variations in disease. *Thorax* **5,** 207.

[34] MEDICAL RESEARCH COUNCIL (1957) Prolonged antibiotic treatment of severe bronchiectasis. *Br. med. J.* **ii,** 255.

[35] MORLE K.D.F. & ROBERTSON P.W. (1953) Segmental aspiration pneumonia and bronchiectasis. *Br. med. J.* **i,** 130.

[36] MULDER J. (1938) *Haemophilus influenzae* (Pfeiffer) as an ubiquitous cause of common acute and chronic purulent bronchitis. *Acta med. scand.* **94,** 98.

[37] MULDER J., GOSLINGS W.R.O., VAN DER PLAS M.C. & CARDOZO P.L. (1952) Studies in the treatment with antibacterial drugs of acute and chronic mucopurulent bronchitis caused by *Haemophilus influenzae*. *Acta med. scand.* **143,** 32.

[38] OLSEN A.M. (1943) Bronchiectasis and dextrocardia. *Am. Rev. Tuberc.* **47,** 435.

[39] PATERSON J.F. (1952) The disappointing results of pulmonary resection for bronchiectasis. *Canad. med. Ass. J.* **66,** 433.

[40] PERRY K.M.A. & KINGS D.S. (1940) Bronchiectasis. A study of prognosis based on a follow up of 1400 patients. *Am. Rev. Tuberc.* **41,** 531.

[41] REID LYNNE McA. (1950) Reduction in bronchial subdivision in bronchiectasis. *Thorax* **5,** 233.

[42] RYTEL M.W., CONNER G.H., WELCH C.C., KRAYBILL W.H., EDWARDS E.A., ROSENBAUM M.J., FRANK P.F. & MILLER L.F. (1964) Infectious agents associated with cylindrical bronchiectasis. *Dis. Chest* **46,** 23.

[43] SPENCER H. (1962) *Pathology of the Lung.* Oxford, Pergamon Press.

[44] SUHS R.H., DOWLING H.F. & JACKSON G.C. (1965) Hypogammaglobulinaemia with chronic bronchitis or bronchiectasis: treatment of five patients with longterm antibiotic therapy. *Arch. intern. Med.* **116,** 29.

[45] TANNENBERG J. & PINNER M. (1942) Atelectasis and bronchiectasis: an experimental study concerning their relationship. *J. thorac. Surg.* **11,** 571.

[46] TURK D.C. & MAY J.R. (1967) *Haemophilus influenzae. Its Clinical Importance.* London, English Universities Press.

[47] TURNER-WARWICK MARGARET (1963) Systemic arterial patterns in the lung and clubbing of the fingers. *Thorax* **18,** 238.

[48] WHITWELL F. (1952) A study of the pathology and pathogenesis of bronchiectasis. *Thorax* **7,** 213.

[49] WILLIAMS H. & O'REILLY R.N. (1959) Bronchiectasis in children: its multiple clinical and pathological aspects. *Arch. Dis. Childh.* **34,** 192.

[50] WILSON G.S. & MILES A.A. (1955) Anaerobic streptococci. In *Topley & Wilson's Principles of Bacteriology and Immunity*, Vol. 1, 4th Edition. London, Arnold.

[51] WYNN-WILLIAMS N. (1953) Bronchiectasis: a study centred in Bedford and its environs. *Br. med. J.* **i,** 1194.

CHAPTER 21

Pulmonary Syphilis

When syphilis was a common disease thoracic involvement was rare. Now it is an extreme rarity. Usually it is congenital, affecting principally the lung parenchyma. The less common acquired disease in adults may affect the trachea, bronchi and lungs. Very rarely the ribs may be involved (p. 623).

CONGENITAL PULMONARY SYPHILIS

This is usually found in babies who are stillborn or die a few days after birth. The lung shows diffuse consolidation and its pale grey colour is responsible for the name 'pneumonia alba'. The pathological appearances are essentially those of an interstitial pneumonia with fibrous tissue formation and maldevelopment of alveoli which are lined by cuboidal epithelium, giving a glandular appearance [5 & 6]. The lung swarms with treponemata. Uncommonly, nodular lesions resembling gummata are seen in grossly affected lungs.

ACQUIRED PULMONARY SYPHILIS

Three forms are described [1, 2, 3 & 4].

1. BRONCHIAL INVOLVEMENT

During the secondary stage of syphilis bronchial hyperaemia may result in cough and sputum. This is rarely recognized. Gummatous ulceration of the trachea or bronchi during the tertiary phase may result in cough, bloodstained sputum and retrosternal discomfort. Fibrosis may occur leading to bronchial stenosis with, perhaps, stridor. The features may closely simulate lung cancer, particularly when bronchial narrowing results in collapse of a segment or lobe.

2. GUMMATA OF THE LUNG

These may be single or multiple, small or large. Large gummata are usually single and may necrose, giving the clinical and radiographic appearances of lung abscess. Multiple gummata are commonly smaller and frequently asymptomatic.

3. DIFFUSE PULMONARY FIBROSIS

This is the least common variety of thoracic syphilis.

Involvement of other organs may coexist with any of the forms of acquired thoracic syphilis.

DIAGNOSIS

Acquired thoracic syphilis may be diagnosed by a combination of suggestive bronchial or pulmonary lesions and a positive Wassermann reaction. Nevertheless in such a rare disease, histological evidence is also required if the diagnosis is to be unequivocal. The results of treatment may also support the diagnosis.

The Wassermann is always positive but clinical and radiographic signs in the lungs are nonspecific. Occasionally tracheal or bronchial lesions are confirmed by biopsy at bronchoscopy. A solid lesion may be resected in the belief that it is a cancer and so give the diagnosis. When the case presents as a lung abscess the diagnosis is more difficult; antibiotic treatment results in cure with only trivial residual fibrosis but the association with syphilis can only be inferred from the effect on the serological tests. The only clue to the rare form of diffuse pulmonary fibrosis may be the serology and the effect of treatment on this, since radiographic clearing with treatment may not be impressive.

TREATMENT

Treponema pallida shares with the Group A beta haemolytic streptococcus and the pneumococcus the genetic incapability of developing resistance to penicillin and this is the drug of choice. One to 4 mega units per day for 1 month will certainly achieve bacteriological cure. Sometimes surgical excision of destroyed lung is later required because of repeated secondary infection.

REFERENCES

[1] DANEMANN H.A., COHEN D.B. & SNIDER G.L. (1961) Syphilitic gumma of the lung. *Arch. intern. Med.* **108,** 897.

[2] DORMER B.A., FREIDLANDER J. & WISE F.J. (1945) Syphilis of the lung in Bantus. *Br. J. Tuberc.* **39,** 85.

[3] HARTUNG A. & FRIEDMAN J. (1932) Pulmonary syphilis: a report of 3 cases of acquired lung syphilis in adults with particular reference to roentgen aspects. *J. Am. med. Ass.* **98,** 1969.

[4] MORGAN A.D., LLOYD W.E. & PRICE THOMAS C. (1952) Tertiary syphilis of the lung and its diagnosis. *Thorax* **7,** 125.

[5] McINTYRE M.C. (1931) Pulmonary syphilis. *Arch. Path.* **11,** 258.

[6] O'LEARY O.A. & ACKERLY O.E. (1945) Syphilis of the lung. *Lancet* **65,** 154.

CHAPTER 22

Parasitic Diseases of the Lung

Parasitic lung disease [15, 23 & 32] may be caused by protozoa (amoebiasis, toxoplasmosis, Pneumocystis carinii pneumonia (p. 141), helminths (trematodes—paragonimiasis, schistosomiasis; cestodes—hydatid disease; nematodes—ascariasis, ancylostomiasis, filariasis) and pentastomes—pentastomiasis.

THORACIC AMOEBIASIS

Amoebiasis is due to Entamoeba histolytica which primarily affects the large intestine. Thoracic amoebiasis is usually a complication of an amoebic abscess of the liver.

MODE OF INFECTION AND PATHOGENESIS

Infection is from man to man. E. histolytica is infective only in its cystic form since the vegetative amoeba passed in the stools of patients with acute amoebic dysentery cannot survive for any length of time outside the host and furthermore is destroyed by gastric juice. Cysts swallowed in food or water are digested by alimentary enzymes which free vegetative amoebae. These grow and invade the colonic mucosa giving rise to ulceration and the symptoms of intestinal amoebiasis. Some penetrate intestinal veins and reach the liver where they multiply and produce foci of necrosis (hepatic amoebiasis) which may coalesce to form an abscess, most commonly in the upper part of the right lobe. The abscess wall swarms with amoebae but they are uncommonly found in the classical 'anchovy sauce' pus.

Rarely primary involvement of the lung may occur without evidence of infection of the liver. A liver abscess may rupture into the pleura (p. 161) or lung (the commonest way in which thoracic amoebiasis occurs), or into the pericardium, bowel or peritoneum.

CLINICAL FEATURES

A previous history of intestinal amoebiasis is present in only about one half of cases and there may be a long latent period before hepatic amoebiasis develops (30 years or more) [15]. Symptoms may be vague but the most usual features are fever (sometimes with rigors), painful enlargement of the liver, weight loss which may be extreme and, when the thorax is involved, pain in the right lower chest and the right shoulder. When abscess affects the left lobe of the liver there may be left shoulder pain. A moderate neutrophil leucocytosis, mild anaemia and a raised ESR are present except occasionally in a chronic abscess. Extension of infection through the diaphragm may result in fibrinous pleurisy, pleural effusion (p. 273), or basal pneumonia [5]. Empyema may also occur but pleurodesis between diaphragmatic and visceral pleura frequently prevents this so that the abscess ruptures into the lower or middle lobe of the right lung. Communication with a bronchus may then occur and is followed by coughing up of the typical brownish-red 'anchovy sauce' pus in which amoebae may be found. Bile staining of sputum may occur after pus is coughed up. Pleural or pulmonary involvement carries a serious prognosis unless promptly treated [21]. Secondary bacterial infection may further complicate hepatic/or thoracic amoebiasis.

RADIOGRAPHIC APPEARANCES

Liver involvement results in a smooth, sometimes localized elevation of the right hemidiaphragm, best seen in the lateral view. Obliteration of the costophrenic angle by a small effusion may occur before penetration of the diaphragm. Screening may show an immobile diaphragm or paradoxical movement.

Lung abscess, effusion or empyema add their distinctive appearances. When an abscess has eroded a bronchus, streaky opacities may outline the path of infection from the lung base to the hilum.

TREATMENT

The rare primary pulmonary amoebiasis can be treated by a course of injections of emetine hydrochloride. In the vast majority of cases, however, treatment of the pulmonary infection requires treatment of the coexisting abscess of the liver, which, in addition, may need to be aspirated or drained surgically.

The specific effect of subcutaneous emetine hydrochloride in amoebiasis is so certain that a case of unexplained pyrexia in patients in or from the tropics should be given a therapeutic trial of the drug. The standard treatment for amoebic abscess of the liver is 60 mg daily for 10–12 days. Results are evident within a few days. A shorter course followed by chloroquine is to be preferred if there is any indication of cardiac disease [26 & 30]. Antibacterial chemotherapeutic agents are indicated only if secondary bacterial infection complicates rupture of a liver abscess.

An effusion or empyema should be aspirated as frequently as necessary. Thoracic surgical treatment is indicated if an empyema persists (commonly associated with secondary infection), if communication persists between the bile ducts and bronchi or if the residual damage from a pulmonary abscess results in recurrent bacterial infection. Surgical treatment may, therefore, involve drainage of an empyema or pulmonary resection.

Following treatment for hepatic amoebiasis it is essential to eradicate amoebae from the bowel with emetine bismuth iodide or diloxanide furoate to prevent reinfection of the liver.

TOXOPLASMOSIS

Infection with the sporozoon *Toxoplasma gondii* is world-wide and, although infrequently recognized and reported in Britain, is in fact relatively common. In most cases it is a mild or even asymptomatic, self-limiting disease. Acute forms with serious manifestations and sometimes a fatal outcome may, however, occur. Chronic forms with protean manifestations comprise a third group. The disease may be congenital or acquired.

PREVALENCE

The Sabin-Feldman dye test (p. 363) which becomes positive early and persists for years gives an index of prevalence which varies greatly in different parts of the world, from 4% in the Navajo Indians to 29% in Britain and 94% in Guatemala [15].

MODE OF INFECTION

Although domestic animals and rabbits, rats, pigs, sheep and cattle are known to be potential reservoirs of infection, it is not known precisely how man is infected, with the exception of the congenital form when the foetus is infected through the placenta. Ingestion and droplet infection are possibilities and the suggestion of an arthropod vector has been made. *T. gondii* can penetrate unbroken skin [15]. Infection acquired in the laboratory is usually severe.

PATHOLOGY

Inflammation with necrosis characterizes the pathological response to infection. The inflammatory lesion takes the form of a granulomatous reaction with central necrosis, surrounded by lymphocytes and plasma cells. The granuloma may later calcify. Lesions are widespread in the congenital form of the disease, predominantly affecting the central nervous system and the eyes. The heart, lungs, adrenals, spleen, lymph glands and muscles are also involved but usually only transiently. Death normally occurs from progression of central nervous system infection and autopsy shows large necrotic areas in the brain and persisting chorioretinitis. Should the child survive, the brain may later show cystic formation and patchy calcification, seen in the x-ray outlining the ventricles. The cerebral changes are mainly in the subependymal areas and shedding of necrotic tissue into the ventricles may cause internal hydrocephalus.

Pulmonary toxoplasmosis is an acquired

disease in adults and takes the form of an interstitial pneumonia.

CLINICAL AND RADIOGRAPHIC FEATURES

Congenital infection may show all degrees of severity, principally affecting the central nervous system. Convulsions, microphthalmos, endophthalmos, nystagmus, tremors, muscle palsies and chorioretinitis are all common. Hepatosplenomegaly, jaundice and purpura are less common. The disease is frequently fatal and survival always leaves severe neurological residua.

Acquired disease is acute or chronic; the latter is the more frequent. Acute acquired disease, which is often fatal, affects children more commonly than adults and, like the congenital form, predominantly affects the central nervous system, resulting in encephalomyelitis. Sometimes acute disease is associated with a typhus-like rash.

Acquired pulmonary toxoplasmosis may be acute or chronic. It may be so slight as to be unsuspected. *Acute manifestations* include influenza-like symptoms with headache, muscle pains, fever, cough, conjunctivitis and a maculopapular rash. Superficial lymphadenopathy may be present and crepitations may be heard in the lungs. The chest x-ray shows patchy consolidation. Associated myocarditis may result in pericardial effusion.

Chronic acquired toxoplasmosis mainly presents as generalized lymphadenopathy which may or may not be associated with fever. It has many features resembling glandular fever but the Paul-Bunnell test is negative. Pulmonary manifestations are slight or nonexistent; when present the features are nonspecific.

Chorioretinitis may occur in all forms of the disease.

DIAGNOSIS

Definitive diagnosis depends on isolating the organism. This is seldom achieved from human tissues but biopsy material from bone marrow, lymph glands or muscle may reveal the organism when inoculated intracerebrally into mice or guinea pigs. Usually an absolute lymphocytosis is present. The negative Paul-Bunnell test is evidence against glandular fever.

The Sabin-Feldman dye test which depends on the observation that the sporozoon fails to stain with methylene blue in the presence of serum containing antibody is much used and is more reliable and becomes positive earlier than the complement fixation test. Positive dye tests with serum dilutions of 1/16 upwards are considered diagnostic. The test may remain positive in low dilution for years. In the acute disease positive tests may be obtained with serum dilutions up to 1/4000 [15]. As in viral infections a rising titre is highly suggestive of recent infection.

TREATMENT

Treatment is by a combination of a sulphonamide (1 g 6 hourly) and pyrimethamine (25 mg daily), given for 2 weeks. Corticosteroid therapy has occasionally been used but its true place in therapy has not been accurately evaluated.

PARAGONIMIASIS
(Endemic Haemoptysis)

Paragonimiasis is caused by infection with lung flukes of which *Paragonimus westermani* is the most common (first described in a tiger in Amsterdam Zoo by Westerman in 1877). The disease is found most commonly in the Far East but endemic foci have been reported in South America, Africa (principally the Cameroons) and India. Infection occurs by eating inadequately cooked fresh water crustacea.

Life cycle of Paragonimus

The adult worm lives in the lungs of man, dogs, cats and wild animals. Ova coughed up in sputum, or swallowed and passed in the stool liberate larvae (miracidia) in water. These are ingested by the snail *Melania*, in which further development occurs into cercariae which are discharged to enter the second intermediate host, a crustacean, usually a freshwater crab or crayfish. Metacercariae formed in the muscles of the crustacean infect man when ingested. Digestion of the cyst wall of metacercariae frees the embryo which penetrates the gut wall and passes through the peritoneum, diaphragm and pleura to reach the lung where maturation to the adult worm occurs.

PATHOLOGY

The pulmonary reaction to *P. westermani* infection is cyst formation, produced by the worm burrowing into the lung. It finally comes to lie in a cyst containing reddish-brown material surrounded by fibrosis. Heavy infections may result in cysts being more widespread, involving the peritoneum, intestine, pleura, brain, liver, spleen or lymph nodes.

CLINICAL AND RADIOGRAPHIC FEATURES

A gradual onset is the rule. Early in the infection epigastric pain may occur as the larvae pass through the peritoneal cavity. The main symptoms are, however, respiratory and consist of chest discomfort or actual pleuritic pain, chronic cough and copious sputum which is initially rusty in colour resembling that of pneumococcal pneumonia. Later there is frank haemoptysis which may be severe. Pleural effusion and empyema have been recorded [25]. The parasite may provoke a bronchopneumonic reaction but this differs from the usual form by the relative absence of fever. Finger clubbing is common. There may be few or no abnormal physical signs in the lungs unless pneumonia occurs or the pleura is involved.

The classical *x-ray appearances* are of *multiple air-containing cysts* (up to 1–2 cm in diameter with a thick base). Bronchopneumonic shadows and/or the appearances of pleural effusion may also occur. Flukes may die after many years (sometimes 20 or more) and become calcified. Coexisting tuberculosis may be difficult to distinguish on radiographic grounds.

Diffuse disease may result in such features as diarrhoea, abdominal pain, hepatospleno-megaly, superficial lymphadenitis, prostatitis, epididymitis, Jacksonian epilepsy, headache,

hemiplegia and cutaneous ulcers. Paragonimiasis usually follows a chronic course.

DIAGNOSIS

Absolute diagnosis depends on finding ova in the sputum or stool. They are better seen by adding 0·1% sulphuric acid. The cystic lung changes have to be distinguished principally from pulmonary tuberculosis but a variety of conditions, including Caplan's syndrome, rheumatoid lung, polyarteritis nodosa, Wegener's granulomatosis and Hodgkin's disease, have all been known to simulate the x-ray appearances of paragonimiasis.

PREVENTION

The disease can be controlled by avoiding eating inadequately cooked crustacea in endemic areas. 'Drunken crab', a Chinese delicacy made from raw crab meat soaked in alcohol, is not safe [15].

TREATMENT

The most useful drug is bithionol (2, 2-thiobis-4,6-dichlorphenol). Recommended treatment varies from a single daily dose of 30 mg/kg body weight orally [15] to a dose of 5 mg/kg in 3 divided doses [32] on alternate days over a period of 10–15 days. Total elimination of the parasite is difficult. Potassium iodide 1·3 g 3 times daily is said to be of value. Emetine, chloroquine and sulphonamides have all been tried with varying success.

Antibiotic therapy for secondary infection is indicated when this occurs.

SCHISTOSOMIASIS [15]
(Bilharziasis)

The helminth responsible is usually either *Schistosoma haematobium* or *Schistosoma mansoni*. Pulmonary lesions are always secondary to urinary or intestinal infection. Schistosomiasis ranks with tuberculosis among the outstanding problems facing the World Health Organization today. The disease is very widespread in the tropics but pulmonary complications are only seen in areas of extremely high infection, principally Egypt. The causative organism was first discovered by Bilharz in Egypt in 1851 and most reports deal with the disease in that country [2, 4, 8, 16, 18, 19, 20, 24 & 28].

In all areas except China, Japan, Taiwan and the Phillipines *S. haematobium* and *S. mansoni* are the infecting organisms; in these exceptions it is *S. japonicum*.

Life cycle of Schistosoma [32]

The parasite infects man by the passage of cercariae, derived from the intermediate host, a freshwater snail, through the skin when bathing, or the buccal mucous membrane when drinking infected water. The larvae enter the blood stream and reach the heart and lungs. They may cause haemoptysis in their passage through the lungs to the systemic circulation. When the larvae reach the venous system they develop into adult worms. Deposition of ova begins about $2\frac{1}{2}$ months after infection. Infection which does not seriously affect vital organs may persist in man for up to 30 years [15].

The ova are the usual cause of the pulmonary disease but sometimes the worms themselves reach the lung.

PATHOLOGY

The ova of *S. haematobium* are laid mainly in the walls of the genitourinary tract. Those of *S. mansoni* and *S. japonicum* are deposited mainly in the lower bowel, but may enter the systemic or mesenteric veins and pass through the heart to become blocked in pulmonary arterioles. They may also affect many other systems. The ova of *S. haematobium* reach the inferior vena cava from vesical, ureteric, prostatic and uterine venous plexuses; the ova of *S. mansoni* and *S. japonicum* can reach the vena cava from the portal venous system through dilated portocaval anastomoses due to accompanying cirrhosis of the liver which may also be an important route for *S. haematobium* in patients with dual infection when hepatic cirrhosis is due to *S. mansoni*. It is almost a rule that the affected agricultural workers in the Nile delta have hepatosplenomegaly as well as their urinary or intestinal schistosomiasis.

Impaction of ova in a pulmonary arteriole results in an arteriolitis which destroys the media of the vessel and provokes a distinctive reaction round the ovum after it penetrates the vessel wall ('bilharzial tubercles'). In the early stages the reaction consists of eosinophils, epithelioid cells, giant cells and, later, lymphocytes. When the cellular reaction subsides it leaves a nodular scar containing the disintegrated ovum which may be calcified. The affected arteriole becomes occluded by intimal thickening but some degree of recanalization may later occur. Other sequelae to necrotizing arteriolitis are 'angiomatoid' formation without thrombus formation and, less commonly, pseudoaneurysms [17].

Repeated embolization results in arterial obliteration, pulmonary hypertension, *cor pulmonale* and finally right-sided cardiac failure. The main pulmonary artery and its branches may be grossly dilated, thickened, atheromatous, calcified or even thrombosed. In the common form of the disease the pulmonary lesion primarily affects the vessels. Deposition of ova may also occur in the lung tissue but this is of less pathological importance. The lungs are never affected by fibrosis to any extent.

When the worms themselves reach the lungs and form emboli, arterial thrombosis is accompanied by a focal pneumonia [8]. The inflammatory reaction subsides in time and the worm dies, becomes calcified and surrounded by a fibrous capsule.

FUNCTIONAL ABNORMALITY

When the disease involves pulmonary arterioles only, pulmonary hypertension occurs with raised pulmonary vascular resistance and normal or slightly reduced cardiac output [7]. The arterial oxygen saturation is normal or only slightly reduced [1, 3 & 27] until the late stages of the disease when arterial undersaturation can become marked. Ventilatory capacity is usually normal or only slightly impaired [7 & 11]. No function tests appear to have been made in the form involving the lung parenchyma.

CLINICAL FEATURES

In the early stages asthmatic or bronchitic

symptoms may lead to routine radiography of the chest and early detection of the disease [9, 19 & 20]. More commonly pulmonary involvement is not recognized until pulmonary hypertension and *cor pulmonale* have developed. Cyanosis is rare until heart failure occurs and finger clubbing is not usually a feature. In Brazil where infection is limited to *S. mansoni* a variant of the disease has been described with cyanosis, finger clubbing but no significant pulmonary hypertension [10]. This has been attributed to pulmonary arteriovenous shunts [17].

The clinical picture mainly relates to the stage at which the disease is recognized. The early asthmatic and bronchitic features have been mentioned. Sometimes treatment with antimony early in the disease results in an acute bronchopneumonic reaction in the lungs. The commonest clinical pattern is, however, increasing dyspnoea, sometimes with cough and haemoptysis and the gradual development of *cor pulmonale* and congestive cardiac failure [14]. As with *cor pulmonale* from other conditions the heart is usually in sinus rhythm and arrythmias are uncommon.

RADIOGRAPHIC APPEARANCES

Early manifestations of established disease are diffuse miliary mottling very like miliary tuberculosis [9, 19 & 20]. It is believed that the miliary changes are due to bilharzial tubercles.

When *cor pulmonale* occurs cardiomegaly with enlargement of the right ventricle and distension of the main pulmonary artery and its branches develop. Sometimes the pulmonary artery shows aneurysmal dilatation.

DIAGNOSIS

Diagnosis of the early case of pulmonary schistosomiasis is suggested by diffuse, transient miliary changes in the lung fields associated with fever and eosinophilia and a positive schistosomal complement fixation test. Hepatosplenomegaly may or may not be present. Absolute diagnosis is made by finding the ova in the urine, stool or rectal snip. Only rarely can they be found in the sputum.

When pulmonary hypertension develops, other causes, mainly mitral stenosis and recurrent microembolism, have to be excluded on historical and clinical grounds.

PREVENTION AND CONTROL

Prevention consists of avoiding water suspected of contamination. Those who develop 'swimmer's itch' in an endemic area (actually a cercarial dermatitis) should be treated with specific drugs to abort the disease at the larval phase.

Control involves promoting public awareness of the risks of contamination of water by urine and faeces, and attempts to destroy the intermediate snail hosts by methods which include copper sulphate, the more effective sodium pentachlorphenate and dinitro-*o*-cycle-hexylphenol (DCHP), and the siluroid catfish *H. fossilis* which feeds on snails.

TREATMENT [15 & 32]

When the stage of pulmonary hypertension is reached therapy is of little value. The primary aim is prevention. Urinary or intestinal infections should be treated vigorously with antimonial compounds, the most effective being intravenous sodium antimonyl tartrate. In the early stages of lung involvement treatment may result in an acute allergic reaction which can endanger life [9].

When heart failure is present it is too late to apply antiparasitic treatment since in addition to the possibility of lung reactions the already strained myocardium may suffer from the toxic action of antimony. Treatment then is that of congestive cardiac failure. When failure develops this means the heart has compensated to the full and death usually occurs within a few months.

THORACIC HYDATID DISEASE

Hydatid disease is due to the cestode *Echinococcus granulosus* and occurs in nearly all parts of the world. Highly endemic areas include the Middle East, India and South America. Preventive measures have greatly reduced the incidence in Iceland, Australia and New Zealand. In Britain areas such as

Wales and Sutherland continue to yield cases sporadically.

Life cycle of E. granulosus.

The minute adult worms inhabit the small intestine of the dog and other canines and ova are excreted in the faeces. The ova may gain entry to the alimentary tract of a secondary host which may be sheep, cattle, pigs, camels or man. Man is nearly always infected through handling dogs. In the secondary host the embryo is freed and penetrates the intestinal wall to enter the portal circulation. Since the embryo is about 20 µ in length it can block a capillary in many sites. The liver is the first hurdle for the embryo and many become lodged there but about 10–20% pass through the liver and finally obstruct vessels in the lung. It is rare for the embryo to pass both barriers and reach other organs.

When the embryo lodges in a capillary it begins to form a cyst which has 2 walls, an outer laminated ectocyst and an inner germinal endocyst. The cyst stimulates a reaction in the host which results in a surrounding fibrous adventitial coat. The germinal layer is concerned with reproduction and forms sacs, known as 'brood capsules', from the inner wall of which the scolex (or head) develops and finally forms a miniature worm, about 160 µ in length, consisting of the scolex, a number of hooklets and a minute body. Brood capsules can be seen on macroscopic examination of hydatid fluid; microscopic examination shows scolices and hooklets. The dog is infected by eating diseased organs, principally the liver. Jackals, wolves, foxes, cats and other carnivora are less common primary hosts; moose, caribou and reindeer are less common intermediate hosts [31].

PATHOLOGY

Apart from the formation of the adventitial layer a pulmonary hydatid cyst causes little reaction and its principal effects are compression and collapse of adjacent lung. Since the adventitial layer is thin and yielding, the cyst may enlarge freely to erode bronchi, blood vessels, mediastinal structures or even the chest wall. Rarely primary hydatid cysts of the heart may occur. These are usually solitary and pose difficult diagnostic problems [13].

Pulmonary hydatid cysts may be simple or complicated, unilateral or bilateral. The complications are principally rupture, or infection, or both. About 20% of pulmonary cysts are bilateral [22], due to multiple primary infection. At least 10% of pulmonary hydatids have coexisting hepatic cysts.

Pulmonary cysts may grow to a very large size and almost fill a hemithorax. Finally rupture into a bronchus usually occurs and the contents are coughed up. In a few cases this results in spontaneous cure; much more commonly complicating infection results in the features of lung abscess. Sometimes the laminated membrane, having been breached, lies free in the adventitious capsule. The x-ray then shows what is referred to as the 'water lily' sign due to the curled-up membrane floating on fluid. When this occurs infection is a very common complication. Occasionally a cyst ceases to enlarge because the parasites have died. Calcification of the wall may then become complete.

So-called *secondary hydatid disease* of the thorax results from rupture of a primary lung or hepatic cyst. Rupture of a pulmonary cyst may occur spontaneously or result from attempts at diagnostic aspiration, or as a complication of surgical removal. The pleural cavity and lungs are strewn with scolices and brood capsules which in time (sometimes years) become cysts. These may fill the hemithorax and destroy the lung, enter the mediastinum and sometimes compress the spinal cord, or erode the diaphragm. Radical removal is extremely difficult but has sometimes been accomplished by pleuropneumonectomy.

Secondary pulmonary hydatid disease may also occur from invasion of the diaphragm by hepatic cysts which rupture into the lung. If the cyst contains live daughter cysts, pleuropulmonary seeding occurs. More frequently infection of the primary cyst kills its contents and thoracic manifestations are those of pulmonary infection and empyema. When communication occurs with a bronchus, bile is present in the sputum.

CLINICAL FEATURES

According to its size a hydatid cyst may be symptomless or result in lung compression, bronchial or pleural involvement, or mediastinal compression. Thus the features may include dyspnoea, cough with purulent sputum, pleuritic pain or effusion, dysphagia and phrenic paralysis. Much the most common cause of symptoms is impending or actual rupture of the cyst into a bronchus.

When a cyst is about to erupt, haemoptysis is common, the amount varying from a trace to quite severe bleeding. Allergic reactions to the contents of the cyst may occur, including pruritus, urticaria and wheezy attacks. The blood may show an eosinophilia.

When intrabronchial rupture actually occurs symptoms depend on the amount of leak. A small leak may result in cough and the production of a little watery or bloodstained fluid which has a salty taste. Sometimes pieces of laminated membrane are found in the sputum. Allergic phenomena are common and marked blood eosinophilia is the rule. Fatal anaphylactic shock has been known to occur after rupture into a large vein or the heart [15]. When the cyst erodes a large area of bronchus sudden coughing occurs with a gush of bloodstained, salty fluid which may contain pieces of membrane, sometimes large enough to occlude the bronchi or trachea and result in cyanosis or even death.

If the evacuated cyst does not become infected the condition may be spontaneously cured leaving only trivial linear fibrosis at the site of the original cyst. Infection is a more frequent sequel, however, and the clinical picture then becomes that of lung abscess (p. 159). Incomplete evacuation of the cyst always results in infection.

When assessing cure the frequency of multiple infection should always be kept in mind.

DIAGNOSIS

Hydatid infection should always be included in the differential diagnosis of any obscure pulmonary lesion in areas where the condition is endemic. It is particularly important to remember that aspiration of a cyst in the mistaken belief that it is an encysted effusion may result in dissemination in the thorax. The important aspects of diagnosis include radiology, immunological testing and cytological examination of the sputum. A rounded or oval homogeneous opacity with a 'hair-line' edge is common. The 'water lily' appearance is diagnostic. Air may leak into the space between the laminated membrane and the adventitial capsule prior to rupture giving rise to a halo appearance above the pulmonary mass. A cyst in the liver may elevate the right hemidiaphragm.

The immunological tests are the Casoni test and complement fixation test. When fresh active hydatid fluid is injected intradermally in a patient with a hydatid cyst a wheal with surrounding erythema develops within 20 minutes and is followed by an indurated area which persists for 1–2 days. The test is positive in 90% of infected patients and may persist for several years after cure. It does not, therefore, signify the presence of residual cysts; also, reinfection can only be inferred if a negative Casoni test was recorded after the initial incident. The complement fixation test is positive in about 75% of cases [12]. If the cyst is well walled off the complement fixation test may be negative. When cysts become inactive the test also becomes negative.

When a cyst leaks into a bronchus hooklets and scolices may be detected in the sputum.

Wilson *et al.* have reported a large series of cystic hydatid disease in Alaska [31]. In their experience the disease differs from the European variety in severity and prognosis to the extent that 2 distinct forms of *E. granulosus* have been postulated, the 'classical' form with a domestic animal cycle and a less virulent 'sylvatic' form which has a wild animal cycle (definitive host the wolf; moose, reindeer or caribou the intermediate host). The clinical differences are so marked that conservative management is advocated for the sylvatic form as opposed to the urgent surgical treatment necessary for the classical type of the disease.

TREATMENT

This involves surgical removal of the cyst or cysts. At operation it is important to protect the pleura from being contaminated if the cysts should rupture. Simple cysts may be removed along with the adventitial membrane but complicated cysts require pulmonary resection since the surrounding lung is invariably involved. Sometimes it is necessary to deal with hepatic cysts at the same time by incision through the diaphragm. A complicated hepatic cyst which has involved the lung and pleura is a formidable surgical challenge.

THORACIC INFESTATIONS BY NEMATODES

AETIOLOGY AND PATHOGENESIS

The larvae of hookworm (*Ancylostomum*) and *Strongyloides* penetrate the skin from warm, moist soil and enter the blood vessels, finally reaching the heart and lungs. Man becomes infected with *Ascaris* and *Oxyuris* by swallowing ova which penetrate the intestinal wall and migrate in blood vessels towards the lungs. All of the members of this group finally reach the intestine via the trachea, oesophagus and stomach.

CLINICAL AND RADIOGRAPHIC FEATURES

Passage through the lungs of the larvae results in blockage of pulmonary arterioles and small pulmonary infarcts. Pulmonary manifestations rarely occur except in heavy infections with *Ascaris lumbricoides* in children. Symptoms and signs may include episodes of fever, cough, haemoptysis and dyspnoea, associated with eosinophilia. Physical examination of the lungs is usually not helpful. The x-ray shows transient pulmonary opacities. *Oxyuris* has been recorded as causing a diffuse pulmonary fibrosis [6].

In filariasis, adult *Wuchereria bancrofti* in long continued, heavy infections may occasionally block the thoracic duct and result in chylothorax.

Tropical pulmonary eosinophilia (p. 432) is probably due to the death of microfilariae of a species of filaria which cannot develop further in man.

PROPHYLAXIS AND TREATMENT

Prevention includes proper sanitation, protection of the feet in the case of hookworm and *Strongyloides* and treatment of known carriers. The adult *Ascaris* can be expelled by administering piperazine which is also effective for *Oxyuris*. The larvae are unaffected by any anthelminthics. Radical cure of *Strongyloides* is difficult but may follow the use of dithiazinine iodide or thiabendazole. Tetrachloroethylene followed by a saline purgative is the treatment for adult hookworm. Control of filariasis depends on the abolition of infected mosquitoes. Diethylcarbamazine is effective in tropical pulmonary eosinophilia but only in the early stages of infection by *W. bancrofti*.

PULMONARY PENTASTOMIASIS

The arachnids, *Linguatula serrata* and *Armillifer armillatus* inhabit the nostrils of birds, snakes and several mammals. Man may be infected by the larval stage, probably most commonly from dogs, and the parasite can reach the lungs. Man may also be infected by eating snakes or vegetation contaminated by snakes' ejecta. If the second larval stage dies in the lungs of man an acute or chronic inflammatory reaction results.

The condition is widespread in Europe, Africa and South America. Its occurrence has been reported in Britain and the surprisingly high incidence of 27% in all autopsies over the age of 10 has been recorded in Amsterdam [29]. Calcified larvae may be detected in the chest x-ray.

REFERENCES

[1] ASHBA J.K. (1959) Pulmonary functions in cardiopulmonary schistosomiasis. Thesis for M.D. Alexandría.

[2] AZMY S. (1932) Pulmonary arteriosclerosis of bilharzial nature. *J. Egypt med. Ass.* **15**, 87.

[3] BARBATO E., LIMA E.P., MERLINO G., COTRIM E. & DANTAS O.M. (1951) Aspectos particulares

da arteria pulmonar na esquistossomose mansoni. *Arquiv. Brasil Cardiol.* **4**, 233.

[4] BEDFORD D.E., AIDARAS S.M. & GIRGIS B. (1946) Bilharzial heart disease in Egypt. Cor pulmonale due to bilharzial pulmonary endarteritis. *Br. Heart J.* **8**, 87.

[5] BOOKLESS A.S. (1950) Thoracic amoebiasis. *J.R. Army med. Crps.* **94**, 52.

[6] BRANDT M. (1949) Parasitic pulmonary fibrosis due to *Oxyuris vermicularis. Tuberk. Artz.* 3, 655.

[7] CORTES F.M. & WINTERS W.L. (1961) Schistosomiasis cor pulmonale. *Am. J. Med.* **31**, 808.

[8] DAY H.B. (1937) Pulmonary bilharziasis. *Trans. R. Soc. trop. Med. Hyg.* **30**, 575.

[9] ERFAN M., ERFAN H., MOUSA A.H. & DEEB A.A. (1949) Chronic pulmonary schistosomiasis. A clinical and radiological study. *Trans. R. Soc. trop. Med. Hyg.* **42**, 477.

[10] FARIA J.L. DE, BARBAS J.V., FUJIOKA T., LION M.F., DE ANDRADRE E SILVA U. & DECOURT L.V. (1959) Pulmonary schistosomatic arteriovenous fistulas producing a new cyanotic syndrome in Manson's schistosomiasis. *Am. Heart J.* **58**, 556.

[11] FARID Z., GREER J.W., ISHAK D.G., EINAGAH A.M., LeFOLVAN P.C. & MOUSA A.H. (1959) Chronic pulmonary schistosomiasis. *Am. Rev. Tuberc.* **79**, 119.

[12] FAIRLEY N.H. (1922) Researches on the complement fixation reaction in hydatid disease. *Quart. J. Med.* **15**, 224.

[13] GIBSON D.S. (1964) Cardiac hydatid cysts. *Thorax* **19**, 151.

[14] GIRGIS B. (1952) Pulmonary heart disease due to bilharzia; the bilharzial *cor pulmonale.* A clinical study of 20 cases. *Am. Heart J.* **43**, 606.

[15] HARGREAVES W.H. & MORRISON R.J.G. (1965) *The Practice of Tropical Medicine.* London, Staples Press.

[16] IBRAHIM M. & GIRGIS B. (1960) Bilharzial cor pulmonale. Clinicopathological report of 50 cases. *J. trop. Med.* **63**, 55.

[17] JAWAHIRY K.I. & KARPAS C.M. (1963) Pulmonary schistosomiasis: a detailed clinicopathologic study. *Am. Rev. resp. Dis.* **88**, 517.

[18] KENAWY M.R. (1950) The syndrome of cardiopulmonary schistosomiasis (Cor Pulmonale). *Am. Heart J.* 39, 678.

[19] MAINZER F. (1935) Sur la bilharziose pulmonaire, maladie des poumons simulant la tuberculose. *Acta med. scand.* **85**, 538.

[20] MAINZER F. (1938) Clinical aspects of pulmonary diseases induced by *Schistosoma haematobium* and *mansoni. J. Egypt med. Ass.* **21**, 762.

[21] OCHSNER A. & DEBAKEY M. (1943) Amoebic hepatitis and hepatic abscess: analysis of 181 cases with review of the literature. *Surgery* **13**, 460.

[22] OFFICER BROWN C.J. (1958) Surgical pathology of hydatid cysts of the lung. *Postgrad. med. J.* **34**. 195.

[23] PERRY K.M.A. & HOLMES SELLORS T. (1963) *Chest Diseases.* London, Butterworth.

[24] SHAW A.F.B. & GHAREEB A.A. (1938) The pathogenesis of pulmonary schistosomiasis in Egypt with special reference to Ayerza's disease. *J. Path. Bact.* **46**, 401.

[25] SHU-NGOEH K. & DJE-DI W. (1949) Pleural paragonimiasis complicated by empyema thoracis. *Chin. med. J.* **67**, 211.

[26] SODEMAN W.A. & LEWIS B.D. (1945) Amoebic hepatitis. *J. Am. med. Ass.* **129**, 99.

[27] SOLIMAN H.S. (1950) Cardiac catheterization in pulmonary bilharziasis. Thesis for M.D. Cairo.

[28] SOROUR M.F. (1932) The pathology and morbid histology of bilharzial lesions in various parts of the body. *C. R. Congrés int. Méd. trop. et Hyg., Cairo,* 1928, Vol. 4, p. 321.

[29] STRAUB M. (1936) Infestation with *Pentastomum denticulatum* among inhabitants of Amsterdam. *Ned. T. Genesk.* **80**, 1468.

[30] WEBSTER B.H. (1960) Pleuropulmonary amoebiasis. *Am. Rev. resp. Dis.* **81**, 683.

[31] WILSON J.F., DIDDAMS A.C. & RAUSCH R.L. (1968) Cystic hydatid disease in Alaska. *Am. Rev. resp. Dis.* **98**, 1.

[32] WRIGHT F.J. & BAIRD J.P. (1968) *Tropical Diseases,* 3rd Edition. London, Livingstone.

CHAPTER 23

Sarcoidosis

In the years since the 1939–45 war sarcoidosis, which was originally regarded as a rarity and of interest only to the dermatologist, has been increasingly recognized as a relatively common condition with protean manifestations which bring it within the scope of almost every branch of medicine [121, 122, 123, 130 & 152]. Concepts of sarcoidosis have changed considerably since it was first described almost a century ago. It is now known to be a disease of world wide distribution which most frequently affects the hilar lymph nodes and the lungs. Intrathoracic involvement is also the most common accompaniment of sarcoidosis affecting other systems. This shift in emphasis stemmed from the recognition in the early 1940's that bilateral hilar adenopathy, with or without erythema nodosum, was an early stage of the disease and that in this form it was essentially benign and self-limiting [91 & 92].

DEFINITION

Until the precise cause of sarcoidosis is known the following descriptive paragraph prepared by the Second International Conference will continue to be useful in place of a definition—
'Sarcoidosis is a systemic granulomatous disease of undetermined aetiology and pathogenesis. Mediastinal and peripheral lymph nodes, lungs, liver, spleen, skin, eyes, phalangeal bones and parotid glands are most often involved, but other organs or tissues may be affected. The Kveim reaction (p. 379) is frequently positive and tuberculin-type hypersensitivities are frequently depressed. Other important laboratory findings are hypercalciuria and increased serum globulins. The characteristic histological appearance of epithelioid tubercles with little or no necrosis is not pathognomonic and

tuberculosis, fungal infections, beryllium disease and local sarcoid reactions must be excluded. The diagnosis should be regarded as established for clinical purposes in patients who have consistent clinical features together with biopsy evidence of epithelioid tubercles or a positive Kveim test'.

HISTORICAL BACKGROUND
(Table 23.1)

The history of sarcoidosis has been bedevilled by semantic argument since the start. It still is. There have been 3 phases:
(1) Until recently it was generally agreed that the first recorded reference to a case of sarcoidosis was Jonathan Hutchinson's description in 1869 of a patient with 'anomalous disease of the fingers' to which he gave the term 'papillary psoriasis'. Hutchinson did not identify this with what he was to describe later as skin lesions which were undoubtedly due to sarcoidosis and it now seems that any claims to priority are dubious, resting only on clinical description [130]. Besnier in 1889 gave a detailed account of a patient with the clinical features of lupus pernio but did not study the histopathology. Within 3 years Tenneson described a similar case in which the histology was studied and the typical granulomatous lesion found [148]. In 1898 Hutchinson described skin lesions which principally affected the face, arms and hands and were referred to for a long time as 'Mortimer's Malady', a tribute to the lady who was the first of a series of patients with these manifestations. In his comment on 4 cases Hutchinson showed remarkable foresight when he wrote 'the truth is probably that the various pathogenetic influences are capable of the most various combinations and that we have, on all sides, connecting links between maladies

TABLE 23.1

Historical Background of Sarcoidosis

Date	Author	Description
1869	Hutchinson [59]	'Anomalous disease of skin of fingers' (Papillary psoriasis)
1889	Besnier [9]	Lupus pernio
1898	Hutchinson [60]	Lupus vulgaris multiplex non-ulcerans ('Mortimer's Malady')
1899	Boeck [10]	Multiple benign sarcoid
1904	Kreibich [86]	Bone changes ('chronic osteomyelitis') in cases of lupus pernio
1905	Boeck [11]	Benign miliary lupoid
1906	Darier and Roussy [28]	Subcutaneous sarcoids
1909	Heerfordt [50]	Uveo-parotid fever
1914	Schaumann [132]	'Sur le lupus pernio'
1917	Schaumann [131]	Benign lymphogranuloma
1920	Jungling [80]	Osteitis tuberculosa multiplex cystica
1940+		Universal acceptance of term 'sarcoidosis'

which have gained distinctive names'. Over the next few years Boeck, Heerfordt and Jungling, unaware of the unitary nature of the disease, described clinical pictures which were regarded as disease entities and given eponymous designations (Table 23.1). The name 'sarcoid' was introduced by Boeck because of a superficial resemblance of a skin lesion to sarcoma (i.e. sarcoma-like).

(2) In 1914 Schaumann recognized the relation between the various recorded presentations and in an essay entitled 'Sur le lupus pernio' emphasized the systemic nature of the disease. (For some reason the essay was not published until 1934.) In 1917 he suggested the term 'lymphogranuloma benigna'. This was something of a euphemism considering that Schaumann himself [133] stated in 1936 'the most usual course is that a classical tuberculosis manifests itself in the lungs, peritoneum, etc. causing death'. It is clear that he favoured a tuberculous aetiology. He stated that the 'benignity indicated in the name should be regarded as only relative and referring to the protracted course of the disease and, for a long time, its insignificant effect on general condition'. Apart from tuberculosis, death frequently occurred from 'debility, usually combined with severe dyspnoea and cardiac weakness'. It should, of course, be remembered that it was mainly the chronic form of the disease which was being recognized and that many cases were erroneously treated in tuberculosis sanatoria, with inevitable exposure to infection.

(3) Progress in the study of sarcoidosis was greatly stimulated by the introduction of mass miniature radiography during the 1939–45 war. It soon became apparent that the hilar glands and the lungs were most commonly affected and that very many cases were asymptomatic. The essentially benign nature of the vast majority of the cases disclosed by mass radiography was increasingly appreciated when spontaneous resolution of the thoracic manifestations of sarcoidosis, particularly hilar lymphadenopathy, was found to be the rule. It also became obvious that many patients with sarcoidosis had previously been wrongly classified as tuberculous.

'Sarcoidosis' is now accepted internationally as the name of the condition.

In the last 20 years a series of international conferences have made important contributions to the knowledge of sarcoidosis and have encouraged investigations on a wide front into the epidemiology, pathology and treatment of the disorder. It is now recognized that sarcoidosis occurs in all races and in almost every country [62]. It is true to say that wherever physicians have become aware of the disease the diagnosis has been increasingly made [120].

A 4th phase in the history of sarcoidosis will begin when the aetiology is known.

EPIDEMIOLOGY

Extensive reference has been made to the epidemiology of sarcoidosis in the Second, Third and Fourth International Conferences on Sarcoidosis [121, 122 & 123].

PREVALENCE

RACE AND GEOGRAPHICAL FACTORS

Information regarding the prevalence of sarcoidosis in different parts of the world is patchy; valid statistics on attack rates are lacking even in the most developed countries.

Much of the available data relates to selected populations. Only in those parts of the world where intensive MMR studies have been made are the figures reasonably comparable; in general it is in these areas that there has also been a high degree of awareness of sarcoidosis. The results of an international study of pulmonary sarcoidosis detected by mass miniature radiography were reported in the Proceedings of the Third International Conference on Sarcoidosis (1963) [122] and are given in Table 23.2. It will be seen that there is considerable disparity in prevalence in the figures given for the various countries. This disparity might indicate a distinctive geographical pattern for the disease and might suggest that sarcoidosis is an entity determined by a specific environmental factor, or factors. But a possible variation in awareness of the disease must be borne in mind. Sarcoidosis appears to be much less frequent in tropical than in temperate areas. It seems rare among Chinese [120], among Indians and among Africans resident in Africa. In contrast sarcoidosis is particularly prevalent among negroes in the United States of America. This may not be related to genetic factors but to social, economic and geographical influences [63]. So far as is known no comparable difference between ethnic groups has been found in other countries, though Irish immigrants in London appear to have a much higher prevalence of sarcoidosis than the indigenous population. This is particularly marked in women in the 20–40 range [4].

It has been suggested that the abnormality in sarcoidosis may lie in the host who may respond with a sarcoid reaction to a variety of external agents [108]. This 'sarcoid diathesis' might be affected by genetic factors, including race. This concept, so far it relates to a possible tuberculous aetiology, is discussed below.

URBAN AND RURAL DISTRIBUTION

There is an impression that sarcoidosis occurs more commonly in rural than in urban areas. There is limited evidence in favour of this [55 & 94], but precise knowledge of prevalence of the disease in particular areas of any country is lacking and the impression remains no more than an impression.

AGE AND SEX INCIDENCE

Most studies have shown the highest incidence in the 3rd and 4th decades [31, 36 & 93], with a variable female preponderance [31, 34 & 63]. Children and the aged are not immune [109] but the disease is rare at the extremes of life. In an Edinburgh series of more than 450 cases those under 20 and those over 70 together comprised less than 5% of the total [36]. The youngest in this series was a girl of 14 with pulmonary opacities and the oldest a woman of 76 presenting with iridocyclitis.

AETIOLOGY

The cause of sarcoidosis remains unknown. The following possibilities have been suggested:

(1) Tuberculosis,
(2) Pine pollen,
(3) Atypical mycobacteria or fungi,
(4) Occupational or social factors.

These will now be reviewed briefly.

POSSIBLE ASSOCIATION WITH TUBERCULOSIS

In reporting 'Mortimer's Malady' Jonathan Hutchinson stated: 'I have to describe a form of skin disease which has, I believe, hitherto escaped special recognition. It may not improbably be a tuberculous affection and one of

TABLE 23.2

Prevalence of Pulmonary Sarcoidosis. [From Proceedings of the Third International Conference on Sarcoidosis 1963 (1964) *Acta med. scand.*, Suppl. 425.]

Country	Reporter	No. of examined (in thousands)	No. of sarcoidosis cases			
			Total	Males	Females	Prevalence per 100,000
Scandinavia						
Finland	Pätiälä	1430	111			8·1
	Riska & Selroos	155	8			5·1
Norway	Riddervold	1448	387	181	206	26·7
Sweden	Bauer & Wijkström I	1873	1023	453	570	55[1]
	Bauer & Wijkström II	1351	867	396	471	64
Great Britain and Eire						
London	James	868	160	87	73	19
Scotland	Douglas	1709	141	59	82	8·2 (6·5 – 18)
N. Ireland	Milliken	1448	149	60	89	10·3
Eire	Logan	383				33·3
European Continent						
Czechoslovakia	Levinský & Altmann	3436	118	53	65	3·4
France	Turiaf	207	20			c.10
Germany						
W. Berlin	Fried	(2200[2])	319	114	205	14·5
Leipzig	Lindig	1017	134	48	86	13·3
Hungary	Mándi & Kelemen	c. 91	5			5
Italy	Muratore	17	2			(11·6)
The Netherlands	Orie & Brugge	4591	994	370	624	21·6
Poland	Jaroszewicz	93	10			10·7
Portugal	Villar	c. 3500	6			0·2
Switzerland	Sommer	3161	515			16·3
Yugoslavia	La Grasta	277	33	6	27	11·9
America						
Canada	Pollak	c. 77	≧8			≧10·5
Argentine	Rey	340[3]	17			5·0
	Castells	695	7			1·0
Brazil	Certain & de Paula	1810	4			0·2
Uruguay	Purriel	1839	8			0·4
Asia						
Israel	Rakower	422	7	6	1	1·6
Japan	Hosoda & Nobechi	193	11			5·6
Australia and New Zealand						
Australia	Marshman	1571	145	66	79	9·2
New Zealand	Reid	1081	171	88	83	16 (6·1– 24·3)

[1] I, II: two surveys.   [2] Population.   [3] University students.

the Lupus family, but if so it differs widely from all other forms of lupus both in its features and its course.' Thus tuberculosis as a possible cause of sarcoidosis was in the field from the start. Boeck in describing 'benign miliary lupoid' inclined to a tuberculous aetiology as did Jungling in his description of bone lesions. A tuberculous aetiology was suggested by the histological appearance and, at one time, by the relatively frequent complication of sarcoidosis by overt tuberculosis. Enthusiasm for a causal relationship between the two diseases has waned with the years and proponents of the theory are now very much in a minority [56, 95 & 96]. Those who supported a tuberculosis aetiology had to account for a number of paradoxical features. The facts that tubercle bacilli were seldom, if ever, found in sarcoid lesions and that tuberculin hypersensitivity was either reduced or absent were explained on the basis that the reactivity of the host was changed (p. 373) or that the property of the tubercle bacillus was altered.

Several observations suggest that sarcoidosis is aetiologically independent of tuberculosis [96]:

(1) The clinical picture of sarcoidosis bears only a superficial resemblance to that of classical tuberculosis. For example the predilection of the two diseases for specific organs is different. Whereas the uveal tract, the salivary and lachrymal glands and skeletal muscle are not uncommonly involved in sarcoidosis this is seldom the case in tuberculosis. On the other hand the serous membranes are involved very rarely in sarcoidosis, and the adrenals not at all, whereas both are commonly affected by tuberculosis.

(2) Though histologically sarcoidosis closely resembles non-caseating tuberculosis, other agents, such as beryllium, give rise to an identical reaction.

(3) Tuberculin anergy is often used by adherents to suggest an abnormal host reaction to the tubercle bacillus, but it would be surprising that tuberculin anergy in sarcoidosis should frequently coexist with erythema nodosum which is a hyperergic phenomenon. In addition, we have seen patients with anergic

sarcoidosis who have developed complicating tuberculosis with coincident conversion to a strongly positive tuberculin test, indicating their capacity to react normally to the tubercle bacillus. We have also seen patients with previous overt tuberculosis, and a positive tuberculin test, become anergic to tuberculin when they later developed sarcoidosis. It seems more likely that the anergy is the result rather than the cause of sarcoidosis and this is supported by the fact that patients may also be anergic to other antigens (p. 377).

(4) There is a different age distribution. Sarcoidosis was apparently rare in young children at a period when childhood tuberculosis was common.

(5) Studies in various parts of the world have shown a divergent incidence of tuberculosis and sarcoidosis. In economically developed countries the prevalence of sarcoidosis has remained steady or actually increased while that of tuberculosis has dramatically decreased.

(6) Antituberculosis drugs have no effect on sarcoidosis. Corticosteroid therapy is used successfully in sarcoidosis usually without the protection of antituberculosis chemotherapy.

(7) Poor social conditions, which are so important in the epidemiology of tuberculosis, do not appear to be of significance in that of sarcoidosis.

Nevertheless most large series of sarcoidosis have shown an incidence of complicating tuberculosis higher than would be expected. This is particularly true of the earlier reports. In the first 100 cases studied in Edinburgh from 1952 onwards the rate of complicating tuberculosis was 3%, but tuberculosis has not occurred in any of more than 350 subsequent cases, during a period when tuberculosis in the area has declined dramatically. The theory that sarcoidosis reduces the patient's resistance to tuberculosis has to take into account the fact that immunological capacity as a whole remains very good in sarcoidosis (p. 378). The higher incidence of tuberculosis seems more likely to be due to the fact that the earlier studies of pulmonary sarcoidosis were mainly concerned with chronic cases, which were often misdiagnosed and treated in tuberculosis sanatoria. The pool of infection in the population at large was also high; in our first 100 cases there was evidence of previous tuberculous infection in 14%. We have not encountered any case of pulmonary sarcoidosis developing pulmonary tuberculosis under observation, even in those treated with corticosteroid drugs. Those who did develop tuberculous manifestations had lesions affecting intercostal glands or the kidney.

POSSIBLE ASSOCIATION WITH PINE POLLEN

The predominance of sarcoidosis in the United States among patients born in the southeastern states led to a study of environmental factors and pine pollen came under scrutiny as a possible cause of the condition. Acid-fast lipid components of the pollen were found to be capable of producing atypical localized epithelioid granulomata in animals [90] but inhalation and ingestion experiments failed to produce sarcoid lesions [13] and world figures for prevalence of sarcoidosis in relation to the concentration of pine forests have failed to show any constant association [26 & 31]. Ingenious and attractive though the pine pollen theory is, there is insufficient epidemiological or laboratory evidence to support it at present.

POSSIBLE RÔLE OF ATYPICAL MYCOBACTERIA OR FUNGI

The possible rôle of antigens derived from atypical mycobacteria is being studied [15], but at the moment there is no definite evidence linking sarcoidosis with infection by these organisms [16]. In a study of the occurrence of intrathoracic calcification in sarcoidosis Israel *et al.* [65] concluded that the infrequency with which calcification occurs as a sequel to sarcoidosis in the United States suggested that mycobacteria and fungi are rarely related to sarcoidosis, either as a cause or as a secondary invader. Infection of any kind appears to be unlikely as a cause since the condition is rare in family contacts

although a few cases have been reported [118]. In our own series there has been only one instance of a mother and son developing sarcoidosis simultaneously; erythema nodosum and bilateral hilar adenopathy occurred in both.

POSSIBLE OCCUPATIONAL OR SOCIAL FACTORS

In the Edinburgh series an attempt was made by questionnaire to determine if any relationship existed between sarcoidosis and occupation, social class and the patient's geographical location from birth onwards. There was no discernible predilection for any social group or for any geographical location; patients' occupations varied from chartered accountant to chicken sexer, from barrister to barman [32].

GENERAL CONCLUSIONS REGARDING AETIOLOGY

There is much to support the view that sarcoidosis is a disease entity with a common provoking agent. Kveim test material from one source (spleen of a New York patient) has served as an effective test agent throughout the world (p. 379). This would support the concept of a common primary cause of the condition. Clinical features, laboratory findings and natural history as observed in Britain, Sweden and U.S.A. are virtually identical, with a few exceptions. The only notable differences are the greater frequency of erythema nodosum and the more benign course of the hilar adenopathy syndrome in European patients, and a greater frequency of pulmonary fibrosis in American patients. These variations need not imply differences in aetiology. The incidence of pulmonary fibrosis may, to some extent, reflect the varied use of corticosteroid therapy.

The lungs would appear to be the common portal of entry for the agent or agents responsible for sarcoidosis but so far there is insufficient evidence to implicate any known bacterial, viral, fungal or chemical agent. A major stumbling block is the failure to reproduce the disease in experimental animals.

IMMUNOLOGY [63 & 130]

DEPRESSION OF TUBERCULIN REACTION

It was early appreciated that the immunological responses of patients with sarcoidosis were abnormal. The earliest observation was that patients with sarcoidosis have depressed reactivity to delayed type hypersensitivity. It is not surprising that tuberculin was first used and both Boeck in 1916 and Schaumann in 1917 described low tuberculin reactivity in sarcoid patients. Numerous studies since then have shown that approximately two-thirds of patients with active sarcoidosis fail to react to 100 TU. About a quarter do react to 100 TU, less than a tenth to 10 TU and less than 1 in 20 to 1 TU. Depressed tuberculin hypersensitivity may persist for years after all evidence of activity has waned [64]. In general early sarcoidosis is associated with a lower incidence of negative reactors than the more chronic form.

The initial observation regarding tuberculin hypersensitivity was made at a time when tuberculosis was rife and ingenious efforts were necessary to explain it. Jadassohn [67 & 128] suggested that patients with sarcoidosis could deal with tuberculin so rapidly that only a weak or no skin reaction was obtained. The presence of circulating antibodies was suggested by Martenstein and Pinner [104 & 116] who based their belief in the 'anergic state' on the production of 'anticutins' which counteracted the tuberculin reaction. This theory was later discarded when Pinner et al. [117] were unable to repeat the earlier experiments supporting the presence of anticutins.

Further evidence of immunological incompetence has been obtained by studies of the effect of BCG vaccination in patients with sarcoidosis. Only one third showed tuberculin conversion, and this transiently [66]. The theory that BCG organisms are destroyed rapidly in sarcoidosis patients has been disproved. Biopsy from BCG vaccination sites has shown that the organisms do persist at the site of injection and in the axillary lymph nodes despite absence of tuberculin hypersensitivity [58 & 63]. Radioactive labelled BCG vaccine has confirmed these findings [101].

DEPRESSION OF OTHER DELAYED TYPE HYPERSENSITIVITY

It was also shown that the altered immunological reaction to tuberculin simply represented lack of response to delayed type hypersensitivity in general. Thus reactions to mumps virus antigen [44], to Candida albicans antigen, to trichophytin [18, 45 & 142] and to PPD from atypical mycobacteria [65] have all been shown to be depressed in patients with sarcoidosis. With the introduction of BCG and the declining pool of tuberculous infection an alternative to tuberculin may become necessary as an indicator of depressed delayed type hypersensitivity. In Britain Citron found that 90% of control subjects reacted to an antigen prepared from Candida albicans and this may prove a satisfactory alternative to tuberculin [18].

Oil emulsions of tuberculin enhance the tuberculin reaction both in tuberculin positive and tuberculin negative patients with sarcoidosis suggesting that some residual hypersensitivity persists [73 & 135]. Enhancement of tuberculin reactivity has also been shown by the use of local or systemic corticosteroid drugs [20].

Studies with tuberculin cannot, therefore, be considered as evidence supporting a tuberculous aetiology (p. 373). They no more link tuberculosis to sarcoidosis than to other conditions, such as lymphadenoma, in which depression of delayed type hypersensitivity has been demonstrated.

OTHER TYPES OF HYPERSENSITIVITY

Certain chemicals are known to be contact sensitizers. The most potent is pentadecyl catechol, a constituent of poison ivy. Skin sensitivity to the poison ivy allergen is the same in sarcoidosis patients and controls [39].

NATURE OF SARCOID ANERGY

Urbach, Sones and Israel [151] injected intradermally into tuberculin negative sarcoidosis patients and controls centrifuged white blood cells from tuberculin positive individuals.

Tuberculin subsequently injected at these sites gave equal reactions in both groups, as occurs in normal tuberculin negative individuals [87]. This indicates that no neutralizing substance or anticutins can be responsible for the low degree of tuberculin hypersensitivity and that there is no intrinsic lack of reactivity of the skin in sarcoidosis. These workers concluded that the immunological deficit must be due to diminished antibody production or transport.

So far as circulating antibody is concerned this is not affected in sarcoidosis [14, 48 & 142]. The defect appears to be due to impaired ability to form the cell borne antibodies thought to be responsible for delayed type hypersensitivity. This has received support from the work of Citron [19] who studied the cytotoxic effect of tuberculin on human white cells in tissue culture. Cytotoxic effect was estimated by the inhibition of normal migration of white cells from a central clot into the surrounding culture medium. Inhibition was shown in tuberculin positive individuals but not in sarcoid patients with depressed tuberculin reactivity. Thus the white cells of tuberculin negative sarcoid subjects did not carry the antibody responsible for tuberculin hypersensitivity. A number of the patients showed radiographic evidence of previous tuberculosis, suggesting deficient production of cell borne antibodies.

ALTERED SERUM PROTEINS

Other features relating to the immunology of sarcoidosis are the presence of hyperglobulinaemia and alteration in the serum electrophoretic pattern in many cases, mainly in the form of increased gammaglobulin [41 & 136]. These are most commonly found in active extensive sarcoidosis and are probably related to activity of immunological processes.

Despite all these investigations the nature of the immunological defect in sarcoidosis remains a mystery.

PATHOLOGY

The histological reaction in active sarcoidosis consists essentially of nodular collections of large, closely packed, pale staining histiocytes ('*epithelioid*' *cells*). In early lesions the nodules are all characteristically at the same stage of development. A few *multinucleated giant cells* are usually seen among the histiocytes and some lymphocytes are often present at the periphery of the nodule (Plate 23.1). In addition *inclusion bodies* of various kinds sometimes occur in the cytoplasm of the giant cells. There are 3 types:

(1) The *Schaumann bodies* which are round or oval and vary in size from that of a leucocyte to about 100 μ in diameter. The larger of these bodies (sometimes referred to as conchoid bodies) seem to be formed of basophilic, concentric lamellae which appear to contain calcium and iron.

(2) *Doubly refractile crystalline* inclusion bodies which may contain calcium and iron have been described.

(3) *Asteroid bodies* whose name is self-explanatory.

Necrosis does not occur in the sarcoid nodule, or is only minimal. In consequence the reticulin between the histiocytes and around the nodules remains intact. When present this is an important point of distinction from the tuberculous follicular reaction. No acidfast bacilli are found in the sections or can be cultured from them, with rare exceptions which may be explained by pre-existing coexisting or consequential independent infection.

Nevertheless the sarcoid lesion is not specific and may occur in tuberculosis as well as in such varied conditions as leprosy [72 & 84], tertiary syphilis, fungal infection (e.g. histoplasmosis) and berylliosis [79, 140 and p. 500]. A localized sarcoid reaction of the same histological pattern is sometimes observed in the vicinity of lesions due to carcinoma (often in the regional lymph nodes), lymphomata, fungal infections [102], trauma and chemical injury. Examples of the last named include necrobiosis lipoidica and zirconium granuloma. Zirconium, a constituent of deodorant sticks, has been shown to cause a chronic axillary dermatosis through the development of a specific hypersensitivity reaction. These 'local sarcoid tissue reactions' [74] can be distinguished from systemic sarcoidosis since patients with local reactions may fail to show depressed or negative tuberculin type hypersensitivity reactions (p. 377) (with the possible exception of lyphomata) and the Kveim test (p. 379) is negative. Lack of any evidence of sarcoid lesions in other tissues or organs is an additional distinguishing feature.

Sarcoid follicles may resolve completely. When healing occurs in longstanding cases the cellular nodules become replaced by fibrous tissue. In *chronic sarcoidosis* follicles with the characteristic appearance may exist among masses of avascular fibrous tissue. Sclerosis of a follicle usually begins at the periphery with the formation of discrete hyaline clumps which fuse to girdle the nodule, and hyalinosis proceeds in a centripetal fashion until the follicle is wholly involved [150].

Several *electron microscopic studies* have been made of Kveim and sarcoid lesions [6, 35, 51, 81 & 155]. Seen by the electron microscope the epithelioid cells in the sarcoid lesions are closely packed. At their margins there is much plication and interdigitation of the various cells [35]. All the cells have large numbers of mitochondria, indicating high metabolic activity. Certain cells show small dark bodies which are some kind of granule and may include large, pale vacuole-like bodies which probably contain protein. Very dark fibrillar material between the cells has the appearance of collagen. The giant cells show irregular peripheral nuclei. It is commonly thought that giant cells are sluggish and of low metabolic activity, but mitochondria are very numerous suggesting that the cell is, in fact, highly active metabolically.

The *Kveim reaction* (see below) shares with the sarcoid lesion the complicated interdigitation of epithelioid cell membranes and the feature of numerous mitochondria. Protein-containing intracytoplasmic vacuoles which may be seen in sarcoid glands have not so far been found in our own studies of Kveim lesions. Intercellular collagen is a feature common to both; in the Kveim lesion there is a suggestion that collagen is actually being taken into the cell substance by the villous cytoplasmic processes at the periphery of the epithelioid cells [35].

THE KVEIM TEST [123]

VALUE OF THE TEST

Following Kveim's description of his method of skin testing in sarcoidosis in 1941 his test has been widely used and is now generally accepted as a useful and reliable confirmatory diagnostic aid [139]. False positive reactions are rare, only 1–2% [138], and a positive test can be regarded as virtual proof of active sarcoidosis. The more active the disease the greater the likelihood of the test being positive. Its highly specific nature makes it an invaluable tool in the elucidation of atypical cases and often obviates the need for more traumatic forms of biopsy. Unfortunately, even with the best test substances at present available, positive results are obtained in only 3 out of 4 cases with clinical evidence of the disease [33 & 63].

NATURE OF THE TEST SUBSTANCE

The Kveim test substance is remarkably stable; its activity is destroyed only by autoclaving or exposure to alkali. It can stand boiling for 30 minutes [110]. Freeze dried test material kept for several months at room temperature will still retain its potency and specificity [33 & 83]. The active principle is particulate. It is not water soluble and is not contained in the nucleoprotein or the lipid fraction of the material [17 & 127]. Its precise nature is still unknown. Other substances can produce local sarcoid reactions in systemic sarcoidosis (e.g. killed tubercle bacilli) but none so reliably as sarcoid tissue.

METHOD OF TESTING

The test is performed by injecting intradermally 0·1–0·2 ml of a saline suspension of human sarcoid tissue, usually obtained from cervical glands. Rarely a spleen affected by sarcoidosis has been removed and has given large quantities of test substance. Within 2–3 weeks a positive test will show a purplish-red nodule at the site of injection. Biopsy at 4–6 weeks reveals sarcoid tissue on histological examination. It is important to remember that a tissue may show classical sarcoid granulomata but may be inactive as a test substance. Conversely tissue which has been the site of longstanding sarcoidosis and is largely fibrotic may sometimes prove highly effective.

The forearm is usually used as the site of injection. Biopsy is ideally made with a high speed or Hayes-Martin drill which can remove a small core of skin without leaving an important scar. If such a tool is not available a good case can be made for using the upper and outer thigh, since formal biopsy can leave unsightly scarring.

Coincident corticosteroid therapy depresses the reaction. If possible, therefore, treatment should not be given until the test is read.

FUNCTIONAL ABNORMALITY

There have been numerous studies of abnormalities of respiratory function associated with the various stages of intrathoracic sarcoidosis, from bilateral hilar adenopathy through pulmonary infiltration without fibrosis to established fibrosis [12, 103, 137, 145 & 157]. Functional impairment cannot be predicted from the radiographic appearances. A patient whose x-ray has become normal may still have significant pulmonary sarcoidosis as judged by reduction in static lung volumes, decreased pulmonary compliance and a reduction in CO transfer factor [7]. Conversely extensive shadowing may sometimes be associated with little impairment of function. The most subtle indication of functional abnormality seems to be decrease in the *CO transfer factor* which may be evident only in exercise studies. Reduced Tco has been demonstrated in patients whose x-ray shows only hilar adenopathy.

There is usually no evidence of airways obstruction. Obstructive airways disease, if it occurs, is most frequently due to complicating chronic bronchitis, but very occasionally to multiple bronchial stenoses due to sarcoidosis.

The value of corticosteroid therapy in preventing functional impairment in pulmonary sarcoidosis has not been proved conclusively. Only a controlled clinical trial continued for at least 5 years will answer this problem; Scadding [130] has pointed out the ethical and practical difficulties this would involve.

CLINICAL FEATURES [107 & 130]

The diversity of the possible clinical manifestations of sarcoidosis is such that a practitioner in almost any branch of medicine may be called upon to make the diagnosis. All kinds of combinations of organ involvement are possible (Table 23.3). Only the serous membranes and the adrenals appear to be sacrosanct (p. 375). Three cases only of pleural sarcoidosis [85] are on record. No authenticated adrenal involvement has been reported apart from a suggestive but unproved case in Maycock's series [107].

Sarcoidosis would be relatively unimportant were it not for the fact that it can affect vital organs (eyes, heart, lungs and kidneys) in a chronic fashion with the development of irreversible fibrosis resulting in variable functional impairment. Affection of the eyes can lead to blindness. Death can occur from cardiac, respiratory or renal failure.

THORACIC SARCOIDOSIS

The *hilar glands* and the *lungs* are the organs most commonly affected in sarcoidosis. Intrathoracic involvement is the most frequent accompaniment of sarcoidosis affecting other organs [63].

HILAR LYMPHADENOPATHY

Enlargement of hilar lymph glands, with or without associated paratracheal involvement, is the commonest manifestation of sarcoidosis (Plate 23.2). Usually the glands are bilaterally and symmetrically involved. In a few, hilar enlargement may appear unilateral [156] and the diagnosis in these is sometimes made at exploratory thoracotomy. Undoubtedly many cases of hilar adenopathy due to sarcoidosis go unrecognized because of the absence of symptoms.

TABLE 23.3

Possible Presentations of Sarcoidosis (after James [68])

Chest physician
  Hilar glands
  Diffuse pulmonary opacities
  Breathlessness

Ophthalmologist
  Conjunctivitis—non-specific
              —phlyctenular
  Keratoconjunctivitis
  Uveitis—anterior and posterior
  Enlarged lachrymal glands
  Sjögren-like syndrome (when salivary glands
    involved)
  Glaucoma

Neurologist
  Eye changes
  Meningitis
  Isolated cranial nerve lesions
  Space-occupying lesions
  Pituitary involvement (usually posterior)

Rheumatologist
  Subcutaneous tissue swellings
  Polyarthralgia
  Bone cysts

Gastroenterologist
  Hepatomegaly
  Splenomegaly

Dermatologist
  Erythema nodosum
  Nodules
  Papules
  Plaques
  Scars
  Lupus pernio

Cardiologist
  Pulmonary heart disease
  Myocarditis and congestive cardiac failure
  Conduction disorders

Surgeon
  Diagnostic lymph node biopsy
E.N.T. Surgeon
  Nasal granuloma
  Laryngeal plaques

General Physician
  All above for 'sorting out'
  Atypical mumps
  Hypercalcaemia
  Renal calculi
  Impaired renal function

In Britain the commonest association which may suggest the diagnosis is *erythema nodosum* [70] which occurred in 39% of patients with enlarged hilar glands in the Edinburgh series and in 17% of patients presenting with pulmonary opacities. The female to male ratio was 3:1 in this series. Sarcoidosis is now the commonest cause of erythema nodosum in the 20–40 age group in Britain. Its occurrence should always prompt further investigation by a chest x-ray.

The association of erythema nodosum with sarcoidosis would appear to vary quite importantly in different parts of the world. Common in Scandinavia [97] and Britain, erythema nodosum is an unusual manifestation of sarcoidosis in the United States; this applies to the white as well as to the coloured population. In North America a generation ago erythema nodosum was apparently equally uncommon as a complication of primary tuberculosis [143].

Polyarthralgia affecting principally the knees, ankles, wrists and elbows is a frequent accompaniment of erythema nodosum and may precede the skin rash. The joint symptoms commonly subside in 3–6 weeks; associated joint effusions are uncommon.

Other presenting symptoms may include cough, dyspnoea, chest pain [2], loss of weight, malaise or excessive fatigue.

COURSE OF HILAR ADENOPATHY

The hilar lymphadenopathy syndrome, with or without erythema nodosum, is most commonly a benign manifestation. Some 80% will resolve spontaneously in the 1st year and a further 10% show spontaneous regression in the 2nd year. The average time for the chest x-ray to become normal is about 8 months [34]. About 1 in 10 cases of hilar lymphadenopathy will become chronic, with or without the development of further manifestations such as pulmonary opacities. In general, the older the age at onset the greater the chance of chronicity. In a few of the cases which resolve spontaneously transient pulmonary opacities may develop when the glands begin to regress and clear spontaneously by the time they completely resolve. Plaque-like *calcification* or sometimes eggshell calcification may rarely develop in persistently enlarged hilar and mediastinal lymph glands [65]. This has occurred only once in our series, in a patient with coincident lupus pernio.

PULMONARY MANIFESTATIONS

Pulmonary opacities may coincide with hilar glandular enlargement or may develop as the glands are resolving. There are often no symptoms but there may be those already outlined for hilar adenopathy. Rarely the patient is first seen with *chronic progressive dyspnoea* complicating longstanding pulmonary disease with fibrosis.

The types of pulmonary involvement may be classified as follows:

(1) Disseminated miliary lesions.
(2) Disseminated nodular lesions.
(3) Linear type of infiltration extending fanwise from the hilum.
(4) Diffuse and confluent patchy shadows.
(5) Diffuse fibrosis.
(6) Diffuse fibrosis with cavitation [98].
(7) Changes similar to chronic tuberculosis as regards location and distribution.
(8) Bilateral confluent massive opacities resembling areas of pneumonia.
(9) Atelectasis.

Of the varieties of pulmonary change cavitation and atelectasis are the least common. It is probable that many cases of so-called cavitation are, in fact, due to emphysematous bullae. Aspergillomata may rarely develop in persisting cavities.

60% of pulmonary opacities in the Edinburgh series showed spontaneous clearing. Half of these had cleared within 1 year, 80% within 2 years and the remaining 20% in periods from 3 to 7 years. Excluding those cases taking more than 2 years to clear, the average time for spontaneous resolution of pulmonary opacities was around 11 months.

Of patients with pulmonary opacities in which corticosteroid therapy was considered necessary (p. 387) some 50% showed clearing without any 'rebound' phenomena after the withdrawal of treatment so that, in all, over 80% of pulmonary opacities cleared either spontaneously or with corticosteroids and did not recur. These patients obviously belong to the subacute transient group of sarcoidosis and the duration of corticosteroid therapy must have coincided with the period of waning activity of the disease. A few patients who, for a variety of reasons, were not treated with corticosteroids early in the disease now have serious respiratory disability from pulmonary fibrosis. These patients have also developed the features of chronic bronchitis over the years.

As in the hilar gland group about 1 in 10 Edinburgh cases with pulmonary involvement proved to have chronic disease. Males fared worse than females as far as the tendency to chronicity was concerned, but fortunately the use of long-term corticosteroid therapy would seem to have prevented important disability.

The *bronchi* may be involved in sarcoidosis through external compression by glands resulting in *atelectasis* in a very few cases, or sarcoid lesions may actually be present in the bronchi [21 & 30]. Reports would seem to suggest that the more often bronchial mucosal lesions are sought the more commonly they are found. Bronchostenoses [21, 30 & 53] due to sarcoidosis are known to occur.

In the upper respiratory tract sarcoidosis may be encountered in the form of *nasal granulomata* giving rise to varying degrees of blockage of the nasal airways, or as *laryngeal plaques*.

SARCOIDOSIS IN OTHER ORGANS AND TISSUES

LYMPHATIC SYSTEM

The lymph glands most frequently affected in sarcoidosis are those of the hilar and paratracheal groups (p. 380). Of the superficial lymph glands those of the right scalene group are most commonly affected, but enlargement of any of the superficial glands (e.g. epitrochlear) may be found. The involvement of superficial lymph glands provides readily accessible tissue for biopsy.

EYES

Ocular manifestations have been reported in as high a proportion as 25% of patients with sarcoidosis [1, 24, 63, 69, 107 & 111]. The eyes should be examined routinely, preferably with a slit lamp, in all cases of sarcoidosis since mild asymptomatic eye involvement may be commoner than is suspected. *Uveitis* is the most frequent manifestation of eye involvement causing symptoms. It develops acutely with pain in the eyes and misty vision in about one third of the cases while the remainder show the chronic form which develops insidiously. *Conjunctivitis* may occur, sometimes of the phlyctenular type, particularly in early sarcoidosis. If this is associated with follicle formation, conjunctival biopsy may provide histological proof of the diagnosis. *Retinal lesions* have been recognized recently. *Keratoconjunctivitis sicca* results in dryness of the eyes; a Sjögren-like syndrome may be encountered if the salivary glands are also involved. The *lachrymal glands* may be enlarged.

SKIN

The commonest skin manifestation in sarcoidosis is *erythema nodosum* (p. 381) which in severe cases may be accompanied by prolonged pyrexia [112]. *Maculopapular eruptions*, *subcutaneous nodules*, *plaques* and *lupus pernio* are other lesions which may be found. Occasionally old *scars* may become infiltrated with sarcoid tissue. The clinical examination of a case of suspected sarcoidosis should include inspection of previous traumatic, operation and vaccination scars for the development of lividity which suggests infiltration. Women appear to be more prone to chronic skin lesions. Rarely the site of a previous Mantoux test may become infiltrated with sarcoid tissue.

ALIMENTARY SYSTEM

Involvement of the *salivary glands* and *liver* is common; affection of the pancreas and the gastrointestinal tract is rare. There is no evidence that classical Crohn's disease is a manifestation of sarcoidosis [42 & 115]. The Kveim test has been shown to be negative in a series of cases which fulfilled the criteria of Crohn's disease [138]. The small and large bowel and stomach appear to be very rarely involved. One of our cases, presenting with a mass in the right iliac fossa proved to have a granulomatous condition affecting the terminal ileum and ascending colon and a positive Kveim test was obtained to 2 different test substances. A second case had mesenteric lymphadenopathy, other evidence of multisystem involvement and a positive Kveim test.

Liver involvement, though frequent as judged by the results of biopsy, does not usually cause symptoms. Abdominal discomfort may occur to a greater or lesser degree when the organ is grossly enlarged. Serious effects from involvement of the liver with sarcoidosis appear to be unusual.

UVEOPAROTID FEVER

Uveoparotid fever was described by Heerfordt in 1909 as a febrile illness characterized by uveitis and swelling of the parotids, accompanied frequently by *facial palsy*. At first thought to be a mild form of tuberculosis, uveoparotid fever is now recognized as one of the curious combinations of organ involvement which may occur in sarcoidosis. *Parotid enlargement* is bilateral in more than half the cases [47] and may be mistaken for mumps. Unlike mumps, however, the swollen parotids are not painful. Enlargement of the *lachrymal* and other salivary glands may sometimes accompany the uveoparotid syndrome.

HAEMOPOIETIC SYSTEM

Enlargement of the *spleen* is a relatively common finding in sarcoidosis and usually is symptomless. Gross enlargement may give rise to abdominal discomfort. Spontaneous rupture of the spleen has been recorded [126]. Hypersplenism associated with splenic enlargement is relatively rare [126]. Haemolytic anaemia has been described [52 & 126].

NERVOUS AND ENDOCRINE SYSTEMS
[5, 23, 27, 29, 40, 46, 54, 76, 77, 78, 106, 113, 134, 149 & 153]

Sarcoidosis affecting the nervous system by infiltration or sarcoid deposits may result in a variety of clinical pictures. These include peripheral neuropathy, meningitis, meningo-encephalitis, space-occupying lesions and pituitary involvement. Transverse myelitis, due to adhesive arachnoiditis or to localized deposits, is the least common of the cerebrospinal manifestations. Although the number of reported cases of involvement of the nervous system with sarcoidosis is few it would appear that response to treatment is unpredictable and often disappointing. We have had 2 cases with meningoencephalitis in which death occurred despite high dosage of corticosteroid and in which early granulomata were still present at autopsy. On the other hand, a case with marked meningeal involvement recovered from a comatose state when treated with prednisolone and has remained well on a maintenance dosage.

Sarcoid invasion of the posterior pituitary or hypothalamus may result in *diabetes insipidus*. It is rare for sarcoidosis to involve the anterior pituitary or any of the other endocrine glands sufficiently to disturb function.

SKELETAL SYSTEM

Bone involvement in sarcoidosis most commonly affects the terminal phalanges of the hands and feet, although the proximal limb bones are occasionally involved in severe cases. Radiologically the punched-out *bone cysts* (Plate 23.3) initially noted by Kreibich (1904) [86] and later studied in detail by Jungling [80] are the most typical of the skeletal changes, but diffuse infiltration of the phalangeal shaft and destruction of cortical and medullary bone are occasionally seen. The bone lesions are not affected by treatment with corticosteroids [75]. They were only present in 3% of the Edinburgh series.

Subcutaneous tissue swellings affecting several of the fingers or toes are frequently associated with bone involvement and add to the disability resulting from progressive disorganization of the terminal phalanges. It is unusual to find radiographic bone changes without clinical evidence of abnormality in the digits. Unlike the bone cysts the subcutaneous swellings are usually improved by corticosteroid therapy. Skin sarcoids commonly coexist.

There is no connection, as a rule, between the disorder of calcium metabolism found in some cases of sarcoidosis and the frequency of bone lesions in the disease [105].

Sarcoid granulomata may occur in *skeletal muscle*, most commonly affecting the pectoral, shoulder, arm and calf muscles [25, 37, 49, 119, 125, 141 & 154]. The muscle foci are usually symptomless, but exceptionally there may be pain, weakness, atrophy or even pseudohypertrophy. Only very rarely can nodules be palpated in muscles; they can be more often detected in tendon sheaths.

'*Sarcoid arthritis*', independent of erythema nodosum, has been described [82]. In the vast majority of cases, however, the polyarthralgia of sarcoidosis is simply a feature of the erythema nodosum syndrome.

GENITOURINARY SYSTEM
[8, 22, 99 & 100]

Sarcoidosis may affect the kidneys in two ways, both of which can cause varying degrees of functional impairment. There may either be invasion of the organ by sarcoid granuloma or deposition of calcium in and around the renal tubules (nephrocalcinosis) secondary to *hypercalcaemia*, or, more commonly, *hypercalciuria* [38 & 89]. The disturbance of calcium metabolism in sarcoidosis is due to an unexplained increase in sensitivity to vitamin D which results in an increased absorption of calcium from the gut. The value of corticosteroid drugs in preventing (or reversing) this effect is well established. It is a sobering thought that in the relatively recent past a popular remedy employed in the treatment of sarcoidosis was vitamin D in high dosage. It has been shown that exposure to sunlight increases the degree of hypercalcaemia and there is an impression that hypercalcaemia associated with sarcoidosis is more common in the warmer countries with a greater amount of sunlight [147]. The symptoms include tiredness, muscular weakness, thirst, polyuria, vomiting and constipation. There may be deposition of excess calcium in the kidneys, cornea and subcutaneous tissues [147]. When direct sarcoid involvement of the kidney is suspected renal biopsy is justified [114].

CARDIOVASCULAR SYSTEM

The cardiovascular system may be affected by sarcoidosis in two ways [43]. Extensive pulmonary fibrosis can lead to *cor pulmonale* with congestive heart failure; actual *involvement of the myocardium* with sarcoid tissue may result in conduction disorders, congestive failure, or even sudden death.

COURSE OF THE DISEASE

The possible course of the disease in respiratory sarcoidosis has already been outlined (p. 381), but will be repeated briefly here. Sarcoidosis may be divided into two clinical types (subacute and chronic) which differ in mode of onset, age incidence, course and prognosis. The two types are not completely distinct. In the *subacute form* the disease undergoes spontaneous resolution, usually within 2 years as a rule, with no functional residua. Typically the subacute variety occurs in the under 30 age group and has a fairly abrupt onset; the Kveim test is usually positive. In the *chronic form* the disease commonly presents insidiously after the age of 30 and persists beyond 2 years. The resulting fibrosis imposes variable functional disability, depending on the organ involved. Chronic sarcoidosis affecting the lungs can lead to extensive fibrosis with *cor pulmonale* and congestive cardiac failure. If the eyes are affected secondary glaucoma or opacities in the anterior chamber can lead to blindness in the untreated case. The Kveim test may be negative in chronic sarcoidosis.

The hilar lymphadenopathy syndrome with or without erythema nodosum nearly always belongs to the subacute group. Most pulmonary opacities will also be found to be manifestations of subacute sarcoidosis.

Maculopapular skin eruptions are usually transient manifestations but skin plaques, keloids and lupus pernio are chronic and persistent. Bone cysts are only found in the chronic form of the disease and are frequently associated with subcutaneous tissue swellings affecting several of the fingers or toes. Chronic skin lesions and bone cysts may be associated with lung lesions which pursue a similarly chronic course. Anterior uveitis and acute conjunctivitis are usually associated with self-limiting sarcoidosis but posterior uveitis and keratoconjunctivitis sicca are chronic manifestations of the disease. Hypercalcaemia and the relatively more common hypercalciuria may occur as transient phenomena but may persist to be associated with nephrocalcinosis and renal failure. We have not found persistent hypercalcaemia or hypercalciuria in any of the cases studied in Edinburgh. Perhaps our northern situation, cloudy skies and atmospheric pollution have something to do with this.

Superficial lymphadenopathy and parotid enlargement are usually self-limiting and rarely persist.

The influence of treatment on prognosis is discussed on p. 387.

CLINICAL INVESTIGATION OF SUSPECTED SARCOIDOSIS

An *x-ray of the chest* is essential, no matter what the initial presentation of the disease, since pulmonary involvement may accompany sarcoidosis affecting other systems, and the recognition of this may determine the need for treatment. The weak or negative response to the *tuberculin test* (p. 377) is often helpful in diagnosis. The *Kveim test* (p. 379) is positive in most cases but takes up to 6 weeks to become positive.

The *serum calcium* should be estimated along with a quantitative *24-hour urine calcium*. If the latter is over 300 mg, hypercalciuria of possible sarcoid origin should be considered.

The *sputum* should be examined routinely for acidfast bacilli and cultures made.

Although much has been made of the finding of raised *serum globulins* [88] in some cases of sarcoidosis, estimation of the serum protein is of little value aetiologically, diagnostically or prognostically. Similarly, there are no findings in examination of the *peripheral blood* which are of value in the diagnosis of sarcoidosis.

In certain areas of the world (e.g. U.S.A.) skin tests, serology and sputum examination for *fungi* may be indicated.

Every physician seems to remember to obtain an x-ray of the hands and feet when investigating a suspected case of sarcoidosis, but this practice is very largely a waste of money. Cystic osteitis is encountered only in chronic cases, usually only when there is clinical abnormality of the fingers.

Biopsy is often crucial to the diagnosis. Strictly speaking an absolute diagnosis of sarcoidosis cannot be made on suggestive clinical and radiographic findings alone because of the similarity between sarcoidosis and other conditions such as tuberculosis and reticulosis. Similarly, a biopsy report describing sarcoid tissue is of itself insufficient for absolute diagnosis as this might simply represent a local sarcoid tissue reaction. When typical clinical and radiographic findings are supported by histological proof of the sarcoid granulomatous process, and tuberculosis has been excluded by the tuberculin test and by bacteriology of the sputum, the diagnosis of systemic sarcoidosis can, in Britain, be confidently made.

The desirability of histological confirmation of the disease in every case was undoubted in the years when the patterns of the disease were being evaluated, but we have now reached the stage when the quest for demonstrable sarcoid tissue must be tempered by the knowledge concerning the presentation and the behaviour of sarcoidosis which has accrued over the past 2 decades. In Britain a young woman with erythema nodosum, bilateral hilar lymphadenopathy and a negative tuberculin test has sarcoidosis for all practical purposes; we would hesitate to employ any

biopsy procedure in these circumstances. On the other hand, obscure bilateral pulmonary changes may justify biopsy, including scalene node biopsy, mediastinoscopy and even lung biopsy (preferably by high speed air drill). The more bizarre the presentation, the more the need for histological support for the diagnosis. If potent Kveim reagent is not available, the decision whether to perform diagnostic biopsy will exercise the physician's judgement. The presence of erythema nodosum is a comforting sign and makes sarcoidosis much more likely than lymphadenoma or other lymphoma.

The tissues found to be useful for biopsy in sarcoidosis have increased in number with the years (Table 23.4) and now include superficial lymph glands (most commonly the right scalene group), mediastinal glands, skin, palate, bronchus, lung, liver, conjunctiva, gastrocnemius muscle, bone marrow, old

TABLE 23.4

Results of Biopsy in Sarcoidosis (several authors)

Readily accessible abnormalities	Percentage positive (approx).
Epitrochlear lymph nodes	100
Enlarged parotid glands	100
Nasal mucosal lesions	100
Subcutaneous nodules	100
Cutaneous lesions (including livid scars)	90
Palpable scalene lymph nodes	90
Inguinal lymph nodes	90
Axillary lymph nodes	80
Enlarged tonsils	80
Bronchial mucosa (visible abnormality)	80
Conjunctival lesions	75
Less readily accessible abnormalities	
Mediastinal lymph nodes	100
Lung	100
Liver	80
Scalene fat pad	40–75
Gastrocnemius muscle	70
Palate	40
Bronchial mucosa (no visible abnormality)	30–40
Bone marrow	30

scars (operation, vaccination, etc.) which have developed a livid hue from infiltration with sarcoid tissue, and the Kveim nodule. The wide range of positivity rates given for scalene fat pad biopsy is probably explained by the fact that some authors have not distinguished between biopsy of palpable nodes and 'blind' biopsy. Carlens (Stockholm) has popularized the removal of mediastinal glands through a small incision in the suprasternal notch (mediastinoscopy). This method is almost 100% effective in obtaining proof of the diagnosis in patients with thoracic sarcoidosis and is likely to receive general acceptance as an important diagnostic aid. It is a debatable point whether a series of minor procedures with lower positivity rates are to be preferred to the single relatively major procedure of mediastinoscopy. Mediastinoscopy in practised hands is reported to be free from important risks and even the scar is less than that usually produced by scalene node biopsy.

TREATMENT

There is no known curative treatment for sarcoidosis. Nevertheless corticosteroids can, in nearly every case, suppress the manifestations of active sarcoidosis. There are 2 possible exceptions to this in our experience, namely muscle sarcoidosis with pseudo-hypertrophic features and some cases of cerebral sarcoidosis. In general corticosteroids are indicated when vital organs are involved or if there is important systemic upset. Scadding [130] discusses in detail the use of corticosteroid therapy in pulmonary sarcoidosis and takes the view, shared by Israel, Svanborg and Stone et al. [61, 144 & 146] that it has not been proved that corticosteroid therapy prevents the development of pulmonary fibrosis in every case. Stone et al. [144] rightly emphasize the fallacy of trying to appraise the course of sarcoidosis in patients followed for relatively short periods of time. Controlled clinical trials would give the answer if sufficiently prolonged but there are major ethical obstacles. It is generally agreed that the granuloma of sarcoidosis can vanish completely under corticosteroid therapy and can be continuously suppressed. If, therefore, the granuloma is the precursor of fibrosis and the granuloma is controlled it would seem reasonable to conclude that corticosteroid drugs do, in fact, influence the course of the disease [57]. If, of course, treatment is given for only a short period in the chronic form of the disease, or if fibrosis has already occurred, treatment cannot be expected to be wholly successful. So far as the prevention of pulmonary fibrosis is concerned the problem must remain *sub judice* but the indications for the use of corticosteroids are usually clear-cut.

It is a frequent finding that active sarcoid lesions show some degree of remission in later months of pregnancy, with subsequent relapse after parturition if the activity of the process has not waned by then [129]. Presumably this is due to a higher circulating level of cortisol during pregnancy.

Eye involvement always demands corticosteroid therapy. It should be emphasized that the only safe practice is to employ systemic treatment in all cases when the eyes are affected.

Treatment is indicated when there is *progressive involvement of the lung parenchyma* as shown by progression of radiographic changes, increasing dyspnoea or deteriorating respiratory function. On the basis of radiographic appearance alone, which is the commonest criterion used, a useful rule is to treat if there is progression of lesions after 3 months of observation or if the lesions remain unaltered after 6 months. Hilar glandular enlargement *per se*, even if a persistent feature, does not require treatment.

Persistent hypercalcaemia or *hypercalciuria* warrant treatment to prevent the development of nephrocalcinosis and renal failure [3].

CNS and *myocardial sarcoidosis* are indications for the use of corticosteroids. *Disfiguring skin lesions*, even if unassociated with involvement of vital organs, may also justify treatment. In longstanding lupus pernio when fibrosis has occurred the results of treatment are often disappointing but the disfiguring discoloration can be concealed by creams or powders.

Persisting or *recurring erythema nodosum* with *important systemic upset* may occasionally compel the use of suppressive corticosteroid therapy (Fig. 23.1). In such cases a short course over a few weeks usually suffices and it is rare for erythema nodosum to recur. The associated hilar glandular involvement may, of course, take several months to resolve completely.

Most cases of active sarcoidosis will respond to 10 mg prednisolone per day but usually higher dosage (20 mg) is employed initially while the manifestations are being brought under control. The level of maintenance dosage aimed at is the lowest which will suppress clinical and/or radiographic evidence of activity. Usually this is in the region of 10 mg per day. In some chronic cases control may finally be achieved with as little as 5 mg prednisolone per day.

Opinions are still divided over the need for coincident antituberculosis chemotherapy. A few physicians who prefer to remain agnostic regarding the aetiological relationships of tuberculosis and sarcoidosis continue to give antituberculosis drugs along with corticosteroids but most now consider this unnecessary. Antituberculosis chemotherapy *per se* has no effect on sarcoid lesions. Nevertheless, as in other contexts, patients who have evidence of unstable tuberculous lesions should have coincident antituberculosis chemotherapy for a sufficiently long period to ensure against relapse.

The minimum *duration* of initial corticosteroid treatment is usually 3–6 months, but the total duration of treatment necessary can only be determined after trial and error. A common practice is to treat for at least 6 months and then attempt withdrawal. In subacute sarcoidosis, when the activity of the disease has waned during the period of suppressive corticosteroid therapy, withdrawal will be possible without 'rebound' manifestations. If the process is still active relapse will occur promptly after cessation of treatment or after reduction of the dosage of corticosteroid below the effective suppressive level. Treatment will then require to be resumed for a further period. In patients with chronic sarcoidosis treatment may be necessary for several years or may even be lifelong.

Oxyphenbutazone [71] and chloroquine [124] have also been shown to have a suppressive effect on sarcoidosis but neither is to be preferred to corticosteroids. Indeed the potential toxicity of chloroquine almost proscribes the use of the drug in sarcoidosis.

PROGNOSIS

The variations in the natural course of the disease have been outlined above, both for respiratory sarcoidosis and for sarcoidosis in general. Most lesions of sarcoidosis are benign and self-limiting, but a few, because they occur in vital organs or because of chronicity and fibrosis, can lead to important functional disability or even death. If diagnosed before there is severe irreversible fibrosis the adverse effects can usually be suppressed by corticosteroid drugs though these

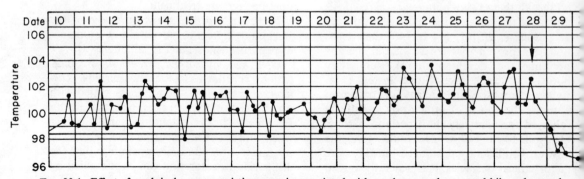

FIG. 23.1. Effect of prednisolone on persisting pyrexia associated with erythema nodosum and hilar adenopathy.

may be less effective in some cases of neurological and muscular sarcoidosis.

REFERENCES

[1] AINSLIE D. & JAMES D.G. (1956) Ocular sarcoidosis. *Br. med. J.* **i**, 954.

[2] ANDERSON J. & BOUGHTON C.R. (1957) The concept of mediastinal pain. *Br. med. J.* **i**, 1490.

[3] ANDERSON J., DENT C.E., HARPER C. & PHILPOT G.R. (1954) Effect of cortisone on calcium metabolism in sarcoidosis with hypercalcaemia: possibly antagonistic actions of cortisone and vitamin D. *Lancet* **ii**, 720.

[4] ANDERSON R., BRETT G.Z., JAMES D.G. & SILTZBACH L.E. (1963) The prevalence of intrathoracic sarcoidosis. *Med. thorac.* **20**, 152.

[5] ASZKENAZY, C.L. (1952) Sarcoidosis of the central nervous system. *J. Neuropath.* **11**, 392.

[6] BASSET F., COLLET A., CHRÉTIEN J., NORMAND-REUET C. & TURIAF J. (1967) Étude ultra-microscopique des cellules de la réaction de Kveim. In *La Sarcoidose*. Proceedings of the Fourth International Conference on Sarcoidosis 1966, ed. Turiaf J. & Chabot J., p. 89. Paris, Masson.

[7] BATES D.V. & CHRISTIE R.V. (1964) Pulmonary sarcoidosis. In *Respiratory Function in Disease*, p. 306. London, Saunders.

[8] BELL N.H., GILL J.R.Jr. & BARTTER F.C. (1961) Calcium metabolism in sarcoidosis. Proceedings of the Second International Conference on Sarcoidosis 1960. *Am. Rev. Resp. Dis.* **84**, 27.

[9] BESNIER E. (1889) Lupus pernio de la face. *Ann. Derm. Syph., Paris.* **10**, 333.

[10] BOECK C. (1899) Multiple benign sarkoid of the skin. *J. cutan. Dis.* **17**, 543.

[11] BOECK, C. (1905) Fortgesetzte Untersuchungen über das multiple benigne Sarkoid. *Arch. Derm. Syph., Wien.* **73**, 71, 301.

[12] BOUSHY S.F., KURTZMAN R.S., MARTIN N.D. & LEWIS B.M. (1965) The course of pulmonary function in sarcoidosis. *Ann. intern. Med.* **62**, 939.

[13] BRIEGER H., LaBELLE C.W., GODDARD J.W. & ISRAEL H.L. (1962) Experimental exposure to spruce and pine pollen: pulmonary changes. *Arch. environ. Hlth* **5**, 470.

[14] CARNES W.H. & RAFFEL S. (1949) Comparison of sarcoidosis and tuberculosis with respect to complement fixation with antigens derived from the tubercle bacillus. *Bull. Johns Hopk. Hosp.* **85**, 204.

[15] CHAPMAN J.S. (1961) A serological reaction associated with sarcoidosis. *Proc. Soc. exp. Biol. Med.* **107**, 321.

[16] CHAPMAN J.S., BAUM J., CLARK JEAN & SPEIGHT M. (1967) Mycobacterial antibodies in immunoglobulins IGA and IGM of patients with sarcoidosis. *Am. Rev. Resp. Dis.* **95**, 612.

[17] CHASE M.W. & SILTZBACH L.E. (1961) Further studies on the fractionation of materials used in the intracutaneous diagnostic test for sarcoidosis. *Excerpta medica* **42**, 58.

[18] CITRON K.M. (1957) Skin tests in sarcoidosis. *Tubercle, Lond.* **38**, 33.

[19] CITRON K.M. (1958) Tissue culture studies of tuberculin sensitivity in man. *Tubercle, Lond.* **39**, 65.

[20] CITRON K.M. & SCADDING J.G. (1957) The effect of cortisone upon the reaction of the skin to tuberculin in tuberculosis and in sarcoidosis. *Quart. J. Med.* **26**, 277.

[21] CITRON K.M. & SCADDING J.G. (1957) Stenosing non-caseating tuberculosis (sarcoidosis) of the bronchi. *Thorax* **12**, 10.

[22] COBURN J.W., HOBBS C., JOHNSTON G.S., RICHERT J.H., SHINABERGER J.H. & ROSEN S. (1967) Granulomatous sarcoid nephritis. *Am. J. Med.* **42**, 273.

[23] COLOVER J. (1948) Sarcoidosis with involvement of the nervous system. *Brain* **71**, 451.

[24] COWAN C.L. (1959) Ocular sarcoidosis. *J. Nat. Med. Ass.* **51**, 371.

[25] CROMPTON M.R. & MacDERMOTT V. (1961) Sarcoidosis associated with progressive muscular wasting and weakness. *Brain* **84**, 62.

[26] CUMMINGS M.M. (1964) An evaluation of the possible relationship of pine pollen to sarcoidosis (A critical summary). Proceedings of the Third International Conference on Sarcoidosis 1963. *Acta med. scand.*, Suppl. 425, p. 48.

[27] CUMMINS S.D., CLARK D.H. & GANDY T.H. (1951) Boeck's sarcoid of the thyroid gland. *Arch. Path.* **51**, 68.

[28] DARIER J. & ROUSSY G. (1906) Des sarcoïdes sous-cutanées. *Arch. med. exp.* **18**, 1.

[29] DAUM J.J., CANTER H.G. & KATZ S. (1965) Central nervous system sarcoidosis with alveolar hypoventilation. *Am. J. Med.* **38**, 893.

[30] DiBENEDETTO R.J. & RIBAUDO C. (1966) Bronchopulmonary sarcoidosis. *Am. Rev. Resp. Dis.* **94**, 952.

[31] DOUGLAS A.C. (1961) Sarcoidosis in Scotland. Proceedings of the Second International Conference on Sarcoidosis 1960. *Am. Rev. Resp. Dis.* **84**, 143.

[32] DOUGLAS A.C. (1964) Epidemiology of sarcoidosis in Scotland. Proceedings of the Third International Conference on Sarcoidosis 1963. *Acta med. scand. Suppl.* 425, p. 118.

[33] DOUGLAS A.C. (1964) Skin reactions of delayed type. Proceedings of the Third International Conference on Sarcoidosis 1963. *Acta med. scand.*, Suppl. 425, p. 189.

[34] DOUGLAS A.C. (1964) The prognosis of early sarcoidosis. Proceedings of the Third International Conference on Sarcoidosis 1963. *Acta med. scand.*, Suppl. 425, p. 284.

[35] DOUGLAS A.C. (1967) Electron microscopy of Kveim and sarcoid lesions. In *La Sarcoidose*. Proceedings of the Fourth International Conference on Sarcoidosis 1966, ed. Turiaf, J. & Chabot J., p. 117. Paris, Masson.

[36] DOUGLAS A.C. (1967) Sarcoidosis. *Proc. Roy. Soc. Med.* **60**, 983.

[37] DYKEN P.R. (1962) Sarcoidosis of the skeletal muscle: a case report and review of the literature. *Neurology (Minneap.)* **12**, 643.

[38] ELLMAN P. & PARFITT A.M. (1960) The resemblance between sarcoidosis with hypercalcaemia and hyperparathyroidism. *Br. med. J.* **ii**, 108.

[39] EPSTEIN W.L. & MAYCOCK R.L. (1957) Induction of allergic contact dermatitis in patients with sarcoidosis. *Proc. Soc. exp. Biol., N.Y.* **96**, 786.

[40] FAZLULLAH S. (1962) Sarcoidosis with involvement of the nervous system. *Dis. Chest* **4**, 685.

[41] FISHER A.M. & DAVIS B.D. (1942) The serum proteins in sarcoid: electrophoretic studies. *Bull. Johns Hopk. Hosp.* **71**, 364.

[42] FLETCHER J. & HINTON J.M. (1967) Tuberculin sensitivity in Crohn's disease. *Lancet* **ii**, 753.

[43] FORBES G. & USHER A. (1962) Fatal myocardial sarcoidosis. *Br. med. J.* **ii**, 771.

[44] FRIOU G.J. (1952) Delayed cutaneous hypersensitivity in sarcoidosis. *J. clin. Invest.* **31**, 630.

[45] FRIOU G.J. (1952) A study of the cutaneous reactions to Oidiomycin, Trichophytin, and mumps skin test antigens in patients with sarcoidosis. *Yale J. Biol. Med.* **24**, 233.

[46] GOODSON W.H.JR. (1960) Neurological manifestations of sarcoidosis. *Southern med. J.* **53**, 1111.

[47] GREENBERG G., ANDERSON R., SHARPSTONE P. & JAMES D.G. (1964) Enlargement of parotid gland due to sarcoidosis. *Br. med. J.* **ii**, 861.

[48] GREENWOOD R., SMELLIE H., BARR M. & CUNLIFFE A.C. (1958) Circulating antibodies in sarcoidosis. *Br. med. J.* **i**, 1388.

[49] HARVEY J.C. (1959) A myopathy of Boeck's sarcoid. *Am. J. Med.* **26**, 356.

[50] HEERFORDT C.F. (1909) Über eine 'Febris uveo-parotidea subchronica'. *v. Graefes Arch Ophthal.* **70**, 254.

[51] HIRSCH J.G., FEDORKO MARTHA E. & DWYER CAROL M. (1967) The ultrastructure of epithelioid and giant cells in positive Kveim test sites and sarcoid granulomata. In *La Sarcoidose*. Proceedings of the Fourth International Conference on Sarcoidosis 1966, ed. Turiaf J. & Chabot J., p. 59. Paris, Masson.

[52] HIRSCHMAN R.J. & JOHNS CAROL J. (1965) Hemoglobin studies in sarcoidosis. *Ann. intern. Med.* **62**, 129.

[53] HONEY M. & JEPSON E. (1957) Multiple bronchostenosis due to sarcoidosis. *Br. med. J.* **ii**, 1330.

[54] HOOK O. (1954) Sarcoidosis with involvement of the nervous system: report of nine cases. *AMA Arch Neurol. Psychiat. (Chicago)* **71**, 554.

[55] HORWITZ O. (1961) Geographic epidemiology of sarcoidosis in Denmark, 1954–57. *Am. Rev. Resp. Dis.* **5**, 135.

[56] HOSODA Y. & CHIBA Y. (1964) The relationship of sarcoidosis to tuberculosis. Proceedings of the Third International Conference on Sarcoidosis 1963. *Acta med. scand., Suppl.* 425, p. 271.

[57] HOYLE C., SMELLIE H. & LEAK D. (1967) Prolonged treatment of pulmonary sarcoidosis with corticosteroids. *Thorax* **22**, 519.

[58] HURLEY H.J. & SHELLEY W.B. (1959) Comparison of the granuloma producing capacity of normals and sarcoid granuloma patients: experimental analysis of the sarcoid diathesis theory. *Am. J. med. Sci.* **237**, 385.

[59] HUTCHINSON J. (1877) *Illustrations of Clinical Surgery*, p. 42. London.

[60] HUTCHINSON J. (1898) Cases of Mortimer's malady. *Arch. Surg., Lond.* **9**, 307.

[61] ISRAEL H.L. (1954) Cortisone treatment of sarcoidosis: experience with 36 cases. *J. Am. med. Ass.* **156**, 461.

[62] ISRAEL H.L. (1964) Sarcoidosis. *Postgrad. Med.* **36**, 493.

[63] ISRAEL H.L. & SONES M. (1961) Sarcoidosis. *Adv. Tuberc. Res.* **11**, 214.

[64] ISRAEL H.L. & SONES M. (1965) Immunologic defect in patients recovered from sarcoidosis. *New Engl. J. Med.* **273**, 1003.

[65] ISRAEL H.L., SONES M., ROY R.L. & STEIN G.N. (1961) The occurrence of intrathoracic calcification in sarcoidosis. *Am. Rev. Resp. Dis.* **84**, 1.

[66] ISRAEL H.L., SONES M., STEIN S.C. & ARONSON J.D. (1950) BCG vaccination in sarcoidosis. *Am. Rev. Tuberc.* **62**, 408.

[67] JADASSOHN W. (1932) Immunbiologie der Haut. In *Handbuch der Haut und Geschlechtskrankheiten*, vol. 2, p. 367. Berlin, Julius Springer.

[68] JAMES D.G. (1956) Diagnosis and treatment of sarcoidosis. *Br. med. J.* **ii**, 900.

[69] JAMES D.G. (1959) Ocular sarcoidosis. *Am. J. Med.* **26**, 331.

[70] JAMES, D.G. (1961) Erythema nodosum. *Br. med. J.* **i**, 853.

[71] JAMES D.G., CARSTAIRS L.S., TROWELL JOAN & SHARMA O.P. (1967) Treatment of sarcoidosis: report of a controlled therapeutic trial. *Lancet* **ii**, 526.

[72] JAMES D.G. & JOPLING W.H. (1961) Sarcoidosis and leprosy. *Trop. Med. & Hyg.* **64**, 42.

[73] JAMES D.G. & PEPYS J. (1956) Tuberculin in aqueous and oily solutions; skin test reactions in normal subjects and in patients with sarcoidosis. *Lancet* **i**, 602.

[74] JAMES D.G., PETERS P.M. & THOMSON A.D. (1962) Local sarcoid-tissue reactions. *Lancet* **i**, 1211.

[75] JAMES D.G. & THOMSON A.D. (1959) The course of sarcoidosis and its modification by treatment. *Lancet* **i**, 1057.

[76] JEFFERSON M. (1957) Sarcoidosis of the nervous system. *Brain* **80**, 540.

[77] JEFFERSON M. (1958) The nervous system in sarcoidosis. *Postgrad. med. J.* **34**, 259.

[78] JONASSON J.V. (1960) Sarcoidosis of the nervous system; reports of four cases with interesting signs. *Acta psychiat. scand.* **35**, 182.

[79] JORDAN J.W. & DARKE C.S. (1958) Chronic beryllium poisoning. *Thorax* **13**, 69.

[80] JUNGLING O. (1920) Ostitis tuberculosa multiplex cystica (eine eigenartige Form der Knochentuberkulose). *Fortschr. Röntgenstr.* **27**, 375.

[81] KALIFAT S.R., BOUTEILLE M. & DELARUE J. (1967) Étude ultrastructurale des altérations cellulaires et extra-cellulaires dans le granulome sarcoidosique. In *La Sarcoidose*. Proceedings of the Fourth International Conference on Sarcoidosis 1966, ed. Turiaf J. & Chabot J., p. 71. Paris, Masson.

[82] KAPLAN H. (1963) Sarcoid arthritis. *Arch. intern. Med.* **112**, 924.

[83] KENNEDY W.P.U. (1967) An evaluation of freeze-dried Kveim reagent. *Br. J. Chest* **61**, 40.

[84] KOOIJ R. (1964) Sarcoidosis or leprosy? *Br. J. Dermat.* **76**, 203.

[85] KOVNAT P.J. & DONOHUE R.F. (1965) Sarcoidosis involving the pleura. *Ann. intern. Med.* **62**, 120.

[86] KREIBICH K. (1904) Über Lupus pernio. *Arch. Derm. Syph.*, Wien. **71**, 3.

[87] LAWRENCE H.S. (1949) The cellular transfer of cutaneous hypersensitivity to tuberculin in man. *Proc. Soc. exp. Biol.* **71**, 516.

[88] LEADING ARTICLE (1957) Hyperglobulinaemia. *Br. med. J.* **i**, 875.

[89] LEADING ARTICLE (1964) Hypercalcaemia in sarcoidosis. *Br. med. J.* **ii**, 707.

[90] LINDER A., KUTKAM T., SOKATCH J. & HAMMARSTEN J.F. (1961) Experimental induction of tubercles in rats with pine pollen. XVIth International Tuberculosis Conference. Abstracts of Papers, *Excerpta Medica International Congress Series*, No. 41, p. 73.

[91] LÖFGREN S. (1946) Erythema nodosum: studies on etiology and pathogenesis. *Acta med. scund., Suppl.* 174.

[92] LÖFGREN S. (1953) Primary pulmonary sarcoidosis. *Acta med. scand.* **145**, pp. 424, 465.

[93] LÖFGREN S. (1955) Some aspects of the relationship between sarcoidosis and tuberculosis. Trans. NAPT Fourth Commonwealth Health and Tuberculosis Conference, NAPT London, 1955.

[94] LÖFGREN S. (1957) Diagnosis and incidence of sarcoidosis. *Br. J. Tuberc.* **51**, 8.

[95] LÖFGREN S. (1959) Immunological and aetiological aspects of sarcoidosis. *Acta tuberc. scand., Suppl.* 45, p. 19.

[96] LÖFGREN S. (1964) Sarcoidosis and its relationship to tuberculosis. *The Royal Netherlands Tuberculosis Association. Selected Papers*, Vol. 8, p. 12.

[97] LÖFGREN S. (1967) The concept of erythema nodosum revised. *Scand. J. resp. Dis.*, **48**, 348.

[98] LÖFGREN S. & LINDGREN A.G. (1959) Cavern formation in pulmonary sarcoidosis. *Acta chir. scand., Suppl.* 245, p. 113.

[99] LÖFGREN S. & NORBERG RENEE (1959) Metabolic aspects of sarcoidosis. *Acta tuberc. scand., Suppl.* 45, p. 40.

[100] LÖFGREN S., SNELLMAN B. & LINDGREN A.G. (1957) Renal complications in sarcoidosis. *Acta med. scand.*, **159**, 296.

[101] LÖFGREN S., STROM L. & WIDSTROM G. (1954) Tuberculosis immunity in sarcoidosis studied with the aid of radioactive BCG vaccine. *Acta paediat., Uppsala (Suppl.* 100) **43**, 160.

[102] LURIE H.I. (1963) Five unusual cases of sporotrichosis from South Africa showing lesions in muscles, bones and viscera. *Br. J. Surg.* **50**, 585.

[103] MARSHALL R., SMELLIE H.C., BAYLIS J.H., HOYLE C. & BATES D.V. (1958) Pulmonary function in sarcoidosis. *Thorax* **13**, 48.

[104] MARTENSTEIN H. (1921) Wirkung des Serums von Sarkoid-Boeck- und Lupuspernio-Kranken auf Tuberkulin. *Arch. Derm. Syph.*, *Berlin* **136**, 317.

[105] MATHER G. (1957) Calcium metabolism and bone changes in sarcoidosis. *Br. med. J.* **i**, 248.

[106] MATTHEWS W.B. (1959) Sarcoidosis of the nervous system *Br. med. J.* **i**, 267.

[107] MAYCOCK R.L., BERTRAND P., MORRISON CLAIRE E. & SCOTT J.H. (1963) Manifestations of sarcoidosis. Analysis of 145 patients, with a review of 9 series selected from the literature. *Am. J. Med.* **35**, 67.

[108] MICHAEL M.JR. (1958) Sarcoidosis: disease or syndrome. *Am. J. med. Sci.* **235**, 148.

[109] McGOVERN J.P. & MERRITT D.H. (1953) Sarcoidosis in childhood. *Adv. Pediat.* **8**, 97.

[110] NELSON C.T. (1957) The Kveim reaction in sarcoidosis. *J. chron. Dis.* **6**, 158.

[111] NIELSEN R.H. (1959) Ocular sarcoidosis. *AMA Arch. Ophthal. (Chicago)* **61**, 455.

[112] NOLAN J.P. & KLATSKIN G. (1964) The fever of sarcoidosis. *Ann. intern. Med.* **61**, 455.

[113] NORA J.R., LEVITSKY J.M. & ZIMMERMAN H.J. (1959) Sarcoidosis with panhypopituitarism and diabetes inspidus. *Ann. intern. Med.* **51**, 1400.

[114] OGILVIE R.I., KAYE M. & MOORE S. (1964) Granulomatous sarcoid disease of the kidney *Ann. intern. Med.* **61**, 711.

[115] PHEAR D.N. (1958) The relation between regional ileitis and sarcoidosis. *Lancet* ii, 1250.

[116] PINNER M. (1938) Non-caseating tuberculosis. *Am. Rev. Tuberc.* **37**, 690.

[117] PINNER M., WEISS M. & COHEN A.C. (1943) Procutins and anticutins. *Yale J. Biol. Med.* **15**, 459.

[118] PLUMMER N.S., SYMMERS W.ST.C. & WINNER H.I. (1957) Sarcoidosis in identical twins: with torulosis as a complication in one case. *Br. med. J.* ii, 599.

[119] POWELL L.W.JR. (1953) Sarcoidosis of the skeletal muscle. Report of 6 cases and review of the literature. *Am. J. Clin. Path.* **23**, 881.

[120] PRESENT D.H. & SILTZBACH L.E. (1967) Sarcoidosis among the Chinese and a review of the worldwide epidemiology of sarcoidosis. *Am. Rev. Resp. Dis.* **95**, 285.

[121] PROCEEDINGS OF THE SECOND INTERNATIONAL CONFERENCE ON SARCOIDOSIS 1960 (1961) *Am. Rev. Resp. Dis.* **84**, 5, part 2.

[122] PROCEEDINGS OF THE THIRD INTERNATIONAL CONFERENCE ON SARCOIDOSIS 1963 (1964) *Acta med. scand., Suppl.* 425.

[123] PROCEEDINGS OF THE FOURTH INTERNATIONAL CONFERENCE ON SARCOIDOSIS 1966 (1967) Ed. Turiaf J. & Chabot J. Paris, Masson.

[124] REPORT FROM THE RESEARCH COMMITTEE OF THE BRITISH TUBERCULOSIS ASSOCIATION (1967) Chloroquine in the treatment of sarcoidosis. *Tubercle* **48**, 257.

[125] RITHFELD B., FOLK E.E.III. (1962) Sarcoid myopathy. *J. Am. med. Ass.* **179**, 903.

[126] ROBERTS J.C. & RANG M.C. (1958) Sarcoidosis of liver and spleen. *Lancet* ii, 296.

[127] ROGERS F.J. & HASERICK J.R. (1954) Sarcoidosis and the Kveim reaction. *J. invest. Derm.* **23**, 389.

[128] ROSTENBERG A.JR. (1951) Etiologic and immunologic concepts concerning sarcoidosis. *Arch. Derm. Syph.* **64**, 385.

[129] RUSSELL K.P. (1951) Sarcoidosis (Boeck's sarcoid) and pregnancy. *Am. Rev. Tuberc.* **63**, 603.

[130] SCADDING J.G. (1967) *Sarcoidosis.* London, Eyre & Spottiswoode.

[131] SCHAUMANN J. (1917) Études sur le lupus pernio et ses rapports avec les sarcoides et la tuberculose. *Ann. Derm. Syph., Paris.* **5**, 357.

[132] SCHAUMANN J. (1934) Sur le lupus pernio. Mémoire présenté en Novembre 1914 à la Société française de Dermatologie et de Syphiligraphie pour le Prix Zambaco. Stockholm.

[133] SCHAUMANN J. (1936) Lymphogranulomatosis benigna in the light of prolonged clinical observations and autopsy findings. *Br. J. Dermatol.* **48**, 399.

[134] SCHONELL M.E., GILLESPIE W.J. & MALONEY A.E.J. (1968) Cerebral sarcoidosis. *Br. J. Dis. Chest* **62**, 195.

[135] SEEBERG G. (1951) Tuberculin sensitivity in lymphogranulomatosis benigna studied with depot tuberculin. *Acta derm.-venereol., Stockh.* **31**, 427.

[136] SEIBERT F.B. & NELSON J.W. (1943) Electrophoresis of serum proteins in tuberculosis and other chronic diseases. *Am. Rev. Tuberc.* **47**, 66.

[137] SHARMA O.P., COLP C. & WILLIAMS M.H. (1966) Course of pulmonary sarcoidosis with and without corticosteroid therapy as determined by pulmonary function studies. *Am. J. Med.* **41**, 541.

[138] SILTZBACH L.E. (1961) Kveim test in sarcoidosis. *J. Am. med. Ass.* **178**, 476.

[139] SILTZBACH L.E. (1967) Concepts of sarcoidosis in the light of the Kveim reaction. In *La Sarcoidose.* Proceedings of the Fourth International Conference on Sarcoidosis 1966, ed. Turiaf J. & Chabot J., p. 129. Paris, Masson.

[140] SLAVIN P. (1949) Diffuse pulmonary granulomatosis in young women following exposure to beryllium compounds in the manufacture of radio tubes. *Am. Rev. Tuberc.* **60**, 755.

[141] SNORRASON E. (1947) Myositis fibrosa progressiva. Lymphogranulomatosis benigna Boeck. (Fibrous progressive myositis in Boeck's benign lymphogranulomatosis). *Nord. Med.* **36**, 2424.

[142] SONES M. & ISRAEL H.L. (1954) Altered immunologic reactions in sarcoidosis. *Ann. intern. Med.* **40**, 260.

[143] SONES M. & ISRAEL H.L. (1960) Course and prognosis of sarcoidosis. *Am. J. Med.* **29**, 84.

[144] STONE D.J., SCHWARTZ A., FELTMAN J.A. & LOVELOCK F.J. (1953) Pulmonary function in sarcoidosis: results with cortisone therapy. *Am. J. Med.* **15**, 468.

[145] SVANBORG N. (1961) Studies on cardiopulmonary function in sarcoidosis. *Acta med. scand., Suppl.* 366.

[146] SVANBORG N. (1964) The therapy of sarcoidosis. *Acta med. scand., Suppl.* 425, p. 295.

[147] TAYLOR R.L., LYNCH H.J. & WYSOR W.G. (1963) Seasonal influence of sunlight on the hypercalcaemia of sarcoidosis. *Am. J. Med.* **34**, 221.

[148] TENNESON H. (1892) Lupus pernio. *Ann. Derm. Syph., Paris* **3**, 1142.

[149] THOMPSON J.R. (1961) Sarcoidosis of the central nervous system: report of a case simulating intracranial neoplasm. *Am. J. Med.* **31**, 927.

[150] UEHLINGER E.A. (1961) The morbid anatomy of sarcoidosis. Proceedings of the Second International Conference on Sarcoidosis 1960. *Am. Rev. Resp. Dis.* **84**, 6.

[151] URBACH F., SONES M. & ISRAEL H.L. (1952) Passive transfer of tuberculin sensitivity to patients with sarcoidosis. *New Engl. J. Med.* **247**, 794.

[152] U.S. Department of Health, Education and Welfare (1964) Bibliography on Sarcoidosis 1878–1963. Public Health Service Publication No. 1213. (Bibliography Series No. 51).

[153] Walker A.G. (1961) Sarcoidosis of the brain and spinal cord. *Postgrad. med. J.*, **37**, 431.

[154] Wallace S.L., Lattes R., Malia J.P., & Ragan C. (1958) Muscle involvement in Boeck's sarcoid. *Ann. intern. Med.* **48**, 497.

[155] Wanstrup J. (1967) On the ultrastructure of granuloma formation in sarcoidosis. In *La Sarcoidose*. Proceedings of the Fourth International Conference on Sarcoidosis 1966, ed. Turiaf, J. & Chabot J., p. 110. Paris, Masson.

[156] Williams M.J. (1961) Sarcoidosis presenting with unilateral hilar lymph node enlargement. *Scot. med. J.* **6**, 18.

[157] Young R.C.Jr., Carr Christina, Shelton T.G., Mann Marion, Ferrin Adrienne, Laurey J.R. & Harden K.A. (1967) Sarcoidosis: relationship between changes in lung structure and function. *Am. Rev. resp. Dis.* **95**, 224.

CHAPTER 24

Bronchial Asthma

DEFINITION

The term 'bronchial asthma', often used un-qualified as 'asthma', is employed to describe recurrent, generalized airways obstruction which, at least in the early stages, is paroxysmal and reversible. It must be differentiated from 'cardiac asthma' associated with left heart failure, though this term is now, very properly, falling into disuse. The most important clinical manifestations are dyspnoea and wheeze, although in severe asthma the obstruction may be so great that there is no audible wheeze. In some cases, especially among children [76], and the middle aged, it is difficult to decide whether 'asthma' or 'bronchitis' is the most appropriate diagnostic term. In these patients cough and sputum, as well as wheeze, are important manifestations, yet the airways obstruction can be to a large extent reversed by drugs such as adrenaline or corticosteroids. The choice of the label will depend on whether reversible obstruction or cough and sputum are the most prominent features. This is a reminder that all names given to diseases are merely labels for groups of phenomena and are necessarily over-simplifications.

PREVALENCE

The relative prevalence of asthma in the 2 sexes is different at different ages. In children up to the age of 15 the prevalence in boys is usually reported as between 1 and 2% with a much lower figure of 0·5–1% in girls. In both sexes there is a sharp decrease after the age of 7 [110], probably because the bronchi are becoming larger and less readily obstructed. In adults the figure given in most series from Northern Europe is about 1% and from North America about 0·5% of the population.

The overall prevalence in women seems to be slightly higher than in men. There is a marked difference between the sexes in age of onset. Williams [110] found that in males asthma started before the age of 35 in 90% and before the age of 15 in 80%. In females, on the other hand, it started before the age of 35 in 75% and in only 40% before the age of 15. In no less than 25% of women asthma began after the age of 35, compared to 10% in men. In a sample survey of general practices in England and Wales in 1955–56, 8·9 per 1000 of the population consulted their doctors for asthma during the year, with a fairly even distribution over the age range [49 & 69]. In the same period 35 per 100,000 of the population in Wales, and 31 in East Anglia, received hospital treatment for asthma.

Graham *et al.* [54], in a study in the general population, found a greater prevalence of asthma in children from the higher socio-economic groups. There is often a clinical impression that asthmatics are more intelligent, but the evidence is not conclusive (p. 399).

MORTALITY

The mortality of asthma is relatively low compared to the morbidity. Fig. 24.1 shows the marked initial fall in mortality in England and Wales after the introduction of corticosteroid drugs and the disturbing rise since 1960. The overall increase has been 42% up to 1965. In the 5–34 age group it has been 165% and in the 5–14 group 330% [31 & 93]. A similar overall rise, after a previous fall, has occurred in Scotland and probably in New Zealand [93]. Some of the rise may be due to the postponement of deaths by corticosteroid drugs but there is a possibility

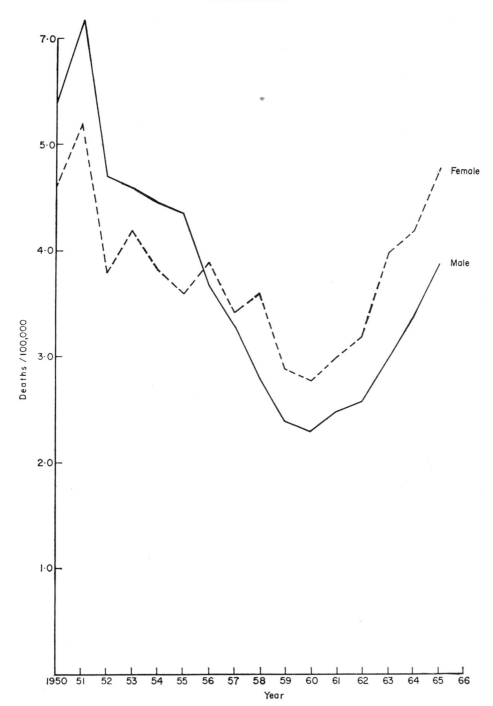

FIG. 24.1. Death rates per 100,000 population for asthma, England and Wales 1950–65. Note the decline after the introduction of corticosteroid drugs in 1951, the higher female rate since 1956 and the rise in both sexes since 1960 (see text).

Figures from the Registrar-General's Reports. Note that the method of recording changed between 1956 and 1957; up till 1957 deaths in which 'bronchitis with asthma' were recorded on the death certificate were included under 'asthma'; after that date they were excluded.

that the cardiac effect of inhaled bronchodilator drugs may play a part [94] (p. 414).

The death rates by age in 1965 are shown
in fig. 24.2. The higher female death rate in
middle age, and the overall higher female

*Per 100,000
population*

10–15	Japan, Germany.
6–7	England/Wales, Scotland, Ireland, Netherlands, Italy.
4–4·5	Denmark, Norway, Spain, Finland.
About 2	France, U.S.A. (whites and nonwhites), New Zealand, Australia, Canada.

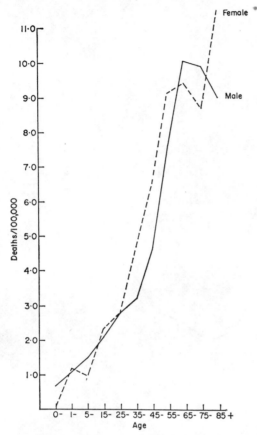

FIG. 24.2. Asthma mortality by age and sex, England and Wales 1965. Note the higher female rates in middle age. Figures from the Registrar-General's Reports.

death rates since 1956, should be noted. The
higher rates for males before 1956 may have
been due to associated bronchitis, as indicated
in the note accompanying fig. 24.1.

There is a variation in recorded mortality
in different countries, though some of the
differences may be associated with diagnostic
habits. The following table, summarized from
Williams [110], covers the period 1946–1950
before corticosteroids were available:

PATHOGENESIS

BRONCHIAL OBSTRUCTION

Three main factors probably contribute to the
bronchial obstruction which characterizes
asthma:

(1) *Contraction of bronchial muscle* or true
'bronchospasm'. Contraction of the bronchial
muscle is certainly the most important factor
in experimental asthma in guinea pigs. Contraction of bronchial muscle in response to a
specific allergen has been shown experimentally in human lungs resected from patients
with allergic asthma [90]. The bronchial
muscle is found to be hypertrophied in
patients dying from *status asthmaticus* [95].
We ourselves have been able to demonstrate
hyperactivity of bronchial muscle, by measuring the 'squeeze' pressure exerted by the
bronchi on expiration by means of a balloon
in a segmental bronchus [32].

(2) *Swelling of the mucous membrane.* The
importance of this is uncertain. At autopsy
much of the bronchial epithelium is shed,
though the basement membrane is thickened
[95].

(3) *Plugging with viscid mucus.* In cases
dying in *status asthmaticus* the characteristic
findings at autopsy are an increase in mucous
glands and goblet cells with plugging of the
peripheral bronchi by viscid mucus. It may be,
of course, that the plugging occurs because
the bronchial muscle is unable to relax and
the bronchi cannot be cleared. Local dehydration may also play a part. Replacement of
ciliated cells by goblet cells may also interfere
with the clearing mechanism.

While there is no complete certainty about the relative importance of the 3 factors, experimental and clinical evidence does suggest that contraction of the bronchial muscle is probably the most important component in the attack of paroxysmal asthma.

HYPERSENSITIVITY

Although the pathogenesis of asthma is by no means fully elucidated it is generally accepted that the bronchi of patients with asthma are 'hypersensitive', that is to say they react to certain stimuli, some specific (allergens) and some nonspecific, differently from those of the rest of the population. Cases of asthma have been divided into 2 main groups: 'extrinsic', in which an external allergen can be demonstrated, and 'intrinsic' in which it cannot. Although a convenient division, and although the groups differ broadly in other respects, the division is a provisional one, as allergic factors may in due course be demonstrated in the intrinsic group.

GENETIC FACTORS

There is often a family history of asthma or of other manifestations of hypersensitivity [68, 76, 91 & 108]. Childhood eczema seems more frequently related, both in patients and their relatives, than adult eczema. Vasomotor rhinitis, hayfever and Besnier's prurigo are also associated. Gastrointestinal allergy and migraine appear to be less common [91]. Williams and Williams [108] found that about 50% of patients gave a history of allergy in close relatives, compared to about 12% of individuals without asthma. Leigh and Marley [68] found that 43% of first degree relatives of patients with asthma developed the disease by the age of 65. Ratner and Silberman [84] found that 59% of children with atopic eczema later developed respiratory allergies. However they also made a critical examination of the literature and concluded that the evidence for a genetic factor in allergy is by no means as clearcut as is often claimed. The exact genetic factor and the mode of inheritance are uncertain. The genetic component is made even more difficult to define by the elusiveness of a precise and un-exceptionable definition of asthma itself [45 & 84]. There is evidence that many more people may be skin-test positive than have clinical allergic manifestations and that hypersensitivity may be initiated by intense exposure to an allergen; that is to say both genetic and environmental factors may contribute. The period of exposure may also be a factor. In a study of 50 bakers who developed bronchial hypersensitivity to flour Schwartz [91] found the mean period of exposure before developing asthma to be 14 years; 90% of the patients had developed vasomotor rhinitis after a mean exposure period of 10 years. Frankland [45] quotes the high rate of development of hypersensitivity in potentially atopic individuals working in laboratories in close contact with locusts which are highly allergenic. We have seen lifelong asthma appear for the first time after serum sickness, and asthma, due to specific allergy to cats, initiated by a patient waking up with a cat on her face. The mechanism may be an increased sensitivity of the shock organ to histamine and other initiating substances [45].

MENSTRUATION AND PREGNANCY

A few women, who develop asthma for the first time at puberty, may tend to have exacerbations during the 7–10 days before their periods [86]. Such patients tend to be better during pregnancy, as do patients with demonstrable allergic asthma; in other types of asthma the effect of pregnancy is unpredictable [63].

ADRENOCORTICAL DEFICIENCY

In view of the often dramatic response of asthma to corticosteroid drugs, it was natural to consider the possibility that there might be an element of adrenocortical deficiency in the pathogenesis of asthma. Although the evidence is somewhat conflicting it would be fair to say that so far there is no unequivocal or consistent support for such a theory [36].

STIMULI CAUSING ATTACKS OF ASTHMA

The stimuli responsible for attacks of asthma may be classified as follows:

(1) *Allergic factors.* Allergic factors are

particularly important in children with a history of infantile eczema and asthma, although these form only a minority of young children with asthmatic symptoms. Allergic factors are often prominent in patients whose asthma starts in later childhood, adolescence or early adult life. Very many different types of allergen have been identified in individual patients. Hypersensitivity to pollens is relatively common and many asthmatics have a history of hay fever. Sensitivity to food allergens, such as eggs, wheat, cow's milk or chocolate, is said to be particularly common in infants and children [46]. Nevertheless, food as the sole precipitating factor in asthma is rare. Chobot et al. [17] found that food as the sole identifiable allergen occurred only in 0·25% of their series, although in children under the age of 3, 15% were allergic to food as well as to other substances. Allergy to house dust and to fungi and their spores [62] is commoner in older individuals. The exact factor in house dust which is responsible for the hypersensitivity reaction was for long uncertain; it now appears that it may be an allergen derived from mites of the *Dermatophagoides* species which subsist on human skin peelings and are commoner in damp houses and in damp years [103]. House dust asthma tends to be at its worst between July and November [103]. The relevant allergen or allergens apparently form part of the mite itself but may also be produced in an external secretion. It may contaminate kapok, wool and feathers. Other common allergens are animal dander, especially from cats, dogs and horses; feathers; and orris root used in face powder. About 1% of asthmatics are said to be sensitive to aspirin; nasal polyposis is said to be commoner in these patients [10]. In many patients no hypersensitivity to specific allergens can be demonstrated, either by clinical history or by skin or inhalation tests. Others give positive reactions to tests with a wide variety of antigens.

(2) *Infection*. Infection as a precipitating factor in attacks of asthma is most important in those in whom asthma first comes on in early childhood [68] and in those, particularly women, in whom it starts in middle age. It is not usually possible to demonstrate an allergic reaction to any specific infecting agent [82] but it may be that in these patients inflammation of the bronchi from the infection starts off a chain of reactions resulting in asthma. Perhaps the later reactions in this chain are similar to those which have been more carefully studied in experimental allergic asthma. It is known that sensitizing antibodies tend to accumulate in inflamed tissues and it may be that such antibodies are responsible for the asthmatic reaction to an agent which in normal people would only produce an upper respiratory infection or at most an attack of simple bronchitis. On the other hand it may be that the infection is really a complication of a primary asthmatic condition rather than the initiating factor.

In a review of 100 patients with 'infective asthma' Swineford et al. [97] in the United States claim to have found other allergic factors in 88, which would be much higher than in our experience. They identified 'physical allergy' (the effect of cold air, etc.), 'potential bronchial reflexes', and psychogenic factors in others. We would have less quarrel with this conclusion but our different experience regarding allergic factors may reflect semantic differences or other differences in medical attitude rather than a basic difference in type of patient. They found the sinuses were often affected and lower respiratory tract infection was common.

Hajos [58] has claimed to have shown specific delayed hypersensitivity to intradermal injection of bacterial products and also bronchial hypersensitivity, but a double blind trial of autogenous vaccines has not demonstrated any therapeutic effect in 'infective asthma' [43 & 44].

(3) *Psychological*. In 2 surveys in the general population in Britain [54 & 68] it was found that psychiatric disturbance was commoner in asthmatic children than in controls, though in 1 of the surveys [54] it was not commoner than in other children with physical handicaps. There was no evidence of any specific personality type in either of these investigations. Families of asthmatics seemed to have a higher prevalence of neurosis and other

psychiatric illnesses [68]. Graham *et al.* [54] found that asthmatic children in the general population were more intelligent than controls (at a marginal level of significance), as has often been supposed, but that their educational achievements were certainly no greater. However, Rees [86], in hospital patients, found the distribution of measured intelligence the same in asthmatics and controls. Possibly a selective factor operates in hospital cases, but the frequent clinical impression of an association with intelligence may be exaggerated. Rees [86] found evidence of major psycho-social stress, of a wide variety of types, immediately preceding the onset of asthma in 35% of 800 asthmatics, a significantly higher proportion than in a control group. There is no doubt that attacks of asthma can be precipitated by psychological upset, although it is doubtful whether psychological upset alone is ever the only factor responsible for a patient having asthma. For instance, a young woman without any previous history of asthma lost her fiancé in an accident 2 weeks before they were due to be married. Following this disaster she went to stay with a friend. In the middle of the night she awoke to find a cat lying on her face. She had an acute attack of asthma and thereafter was liable to develop asthma whenever she came into contact with cats. Dekker and Groen [28] have demonstrated impairment of vital capacity developing in asthmatic subjects when presented with objects associated with their emotional problems. In one individual who had had a series of severe emotional crises as a child when her mother threw away a goldfish to which she was greatly attached, severe impairment of vital capacity was demonstrated not only when she was presented with a goldfish in a bowl but when she was presented with a toy goldfish in the bowl or even the bowl without the goldfish, while an even worse attack occurred when the doctor dropped the bowl on the floor and it was smashed. In view of the somatic components of anxiety and other emotional upsets it is not surprising that, in patients with an asthmatic tendency, emotional episodes are liable to aggravate asthma.

Sometimes, especially in children, the asthma can become a protective reaction and patients have confessed how, when they were children, they were able to 'give themselves' an attack of asthma in order to get their own way. In many this may occur without conscious motivation.

Parents of asthmatic children are often accused of being over-protective, a very understandable reaction. Rees [86] claims that this attitude often precedes the onset of asthma and that much can be done by correcting faulty outlook in the parents. Nevertheless, in the great majority of patients psychological factors seem to be secondary rather than primary.

It must be emphasized that multiple factors often operate in asthma. Williams and his colleagues [109] in a review of 487 cases considered that there was an infective factor in 88%, psychological in 70% and allergic in 64%. All 3 played a part in 38%. They thought the infective factor alone was only present in 11%, the allergic alone in 3·3% and the psychological in 1·2%. Inevitably these assessments are somewhat subjective but they serve to show the potential multiplicity of factors and our sad lack of objective, repeatable and measurable criteria in investigating the aetiology of asthma.

It has been shown [80] that guinea pigs given a conditioning stimulus at the same time as asthma was induced by exposure to an allergen could later develop asthma when given the stimulus alone. Such conditioning stimuli have occasionally been noted clinically. For instance, an asthmatic attack when the patient sees an artificial flower, knowing that he is allergic to the pollen of the real thing.

(4) *Exercise.* Exercise quite frequently induces asthma, though there is some variation between indivduals. In a few the asthma is relieved. It has been found that, after 8 minutes' excrcise, the decrease in FEV is maximal within 15 minutes and disappears over the next 30 minutes [72]. The exact mechanism is uncertain but a similar effect can be induced by voluntary hyperventilation [57].

(5) *Air pollution and 'local asthma'*. Patients with asthma tolerate atmospheric pollution or cigarette smoke badly. Outbreaks of local asthma, as in United States servicemen stationed in the Tokyo-Yokohama area and in the inhabitants of New Orleans, seem likely to have been due to atmospheric pollutants, though the evidence is incomplete and the disease induced may have been more in the bronchitic range (according to British usage) than in the asthmatic [37]. Nevertheless true asthmatics are often worse in foggy weather.

(6) *Other nonspecific factors*. Most asthmatics are unable to smoke because they find tobacco smoke irritating. Other smokes may have a similar effect, as may such things as the smell of fresh paint, strong perfume or cold air. Tiffenau [102] has shown that irritable cough and decrease in FEV is much more readily induced in asthmatics than normals by giving successive 15 second inhalations of 1, 3, 10, 30 and 100 mcg of acetylcholine. Cough, often with pricking and tickling, develops in 75% of asthmatics, at least with the larger dose, whereas it occurs with only occasional normals with 100 mcg inhalation. Decrease in FEV is even more readily induced, usually occurring with 10 mcg. He considers the initial reaction is a reflex stimulus and is prevented, or at least a mild reaction to a low dose is prevented, by an aerosol of 1% hexamethonium dibromide. Once airways obstruction has been initiated the hexamethonium has little effect, suggesting a reflex; this later effect is reversed by bronchodilator drugs and he thinks it is partly due to a direct effect of acetylcholine on bronchial muscle. Unfortunately similar effects may be produced by acetylcholine in patients with 'banal bronchitis' or even with a cold, so that the reaction probably only indicates bronchial hypersensitivity from whatever cause. Similar responses may be evoked by histamine inhalation [9], the bronchi of asthmatics being more sensitive than those of normal people.

(7) *Reflex factors* are not well established. Patients with nasal polypi are sometimes relieved of their asthma if these are removed, but not necessarily so. Asthma has been induced by inflating a balloon inserted into the maxillary sinus through an antrostomy opening [98].

THE ALLERGIC REACTION

Although our knowledge of the details of the asthmatic reaction or reactions is still very incomplete, most is known about asthma associated with demonstrable Type I allergy [45 & 80].

REAGINS

The evidence suggests that antibodies known as reagins become fixed to cells. The allergic reaction is probably precipitated by the interaction of allergens with this fixed antibody. This probably initiates a chain of enzyme-controlled reactions whose end products may affect bronchial muscle, capillaries and mucous glands (see below). The exact cell or cells concerned is still uncertain but basophil mast cells are probably involved.

Until recently there was much controversy as to the identity of the sensitizing antibodies (reagins) and it seemed possible that, in different conditions and in different individuals, the relevant reagin might belong to any of the 3 main classes of human immunoglobulin (IgG, IgA and IgM [4, 96 & 100]). But a new class of immunoglobulin, originally named IgND but now by international agreement IgE, has recently been discovered and seems likely to be identical with reaginic antibody [39 & 65]. Johansson [65] found IgE in 63% of patients with allergic asthma, compared to 5% of those with nonallergic asthma. Moreover within the allergic group the amount of IgE was much greater than in the few controls who did possess IgE. Coombs *et al.* [23] have studied a group of asthmatics hypersensitive to castor bean and have shown that the titres of IgE correlated well with clinical data and with passive cutaneous anaphylaxis (see below) carried out in baboons. They used an immunological technique by which the allergen is fixed by photooxidation to rabbit antibodies against human red cells. The antibody-allergen complex combines with human red cells without agglutinating them. The red cells will now absorb only reaginic antibody specific to the fixed allergen. The presence of the reagin may be demonstrated by exposing the cells to antihuman globulin or, more specifically, to anti-IgE globulin prepared by immunizing animals. An even more sensitive radio-immunoabsorbent technique has been evolved [39] and it seems likely that the estimation of reagins may before long be used in clinical practice.

Experimentally the allergic reaction may be blocked by circulating antibodies known as incomplete antibodies or blocking antibodies which do not cause precipitation or agglutination, although they fix complement. Such antibodies are also protective from an immunological point of view [107].

PRAUSNITZ-KÜSTNER (P–K) AND PASSIVE CUTANEOUS ANAPHYLAXIS TESTS

Reagins may be demonstrated by the capacity of serum containing them to sensitize the cells of a normal individual to the relevant allergen. In the P–K test the serum from the affected individual is injected intradermally into a normal person. The latter's cells, in the area of the injection, are rendered hypersensitive to the relevant allergen, as may be demonstrated by a subsequent skin test. Owing to the risk of transferring serum hepatitis, this test is not used in man and unfortunately the skin of animals has proved unsatisfactory. Instead, the passive cutaneous anaphylaxis test has been employed. The test serum, or dilutions of it if titration is required, is injected intradermally into an area of the animal's skin clipped free of hair. After 4–24 hours allergen, together with a dye such as Evan's blue, is injected intravenously. The sites of reaction are shown by the escape of dye from the dilated and damaged capillaries in the sensitized area of skin [22]. Both these methods remain research tools and they do not at present find a place in routine practice.

SUBSTANCES RESPONSIBLE FOR THE ASTHMATIC REACTION

(1) *Histamine.* In the guinea pig, on which most experimental work has been done, exposure of the isolated lung from a sensitized guinea pig to the specific antigen added to the perfusing fluid results in the release of histamine. There is evidence to suggest that the antigen-antibody reaction initiates a chain of enzyme-facilitated events which result in the release of histamine. The histamine is probably derived from the basophil mast cells which can be shown to discharge their histamine-containing granules during allergic reactions [12]. It seems possible that eosinophil cells may engulf these granules and possess an antihistamine action [20]. The addition of histamine to the perfusing fluid, whether the lung is from a normal or from a sensitized guinea pig, results in severe spasm of the bronchial muscle. It also causes local oedema and probably secretion of the bronchial glands [12]. In guinea pigs histamine is probably the most important factor responsible for the asthmatic reaction and much of the immediate reaction to perfusion with the allergen can be prevented by antihistamine drugs. In man, though histamine has been shown to be released by specific allergen added to resected lung from asthmatic subjects [90], the use of antihistamine drugs has proved disappointing clinically and it seems that histamine is a less important component than in the guinea pig. Patients with asthma who are hypersensitive to certain specific allergens, such as pollens, may develop an immediate asthmatic attack if they are given test inhalations containing the allergen. Herxheimer [59] has shown that such an immediate reaction can sometimes be prevented by antihistamine drugs, so that histamine must to some extent be involved at least in some types of allergic asthma.

(2) *Slow reacting substance* [11]. This substance, known as SRS-A (Slow Reacting Substance-Anaphylaxis) is clearly important in causing bronchial muscular contraction in man. It is 10 times more active in human than in guinea pig muscle. It is probably released as a result of an enzyme action on a specific substrate, this reaction being initiated by allergen-antibody interaction. The maximal effect on the bronchial muscle is reached later and lasts much longer than that due to histamine and the action is not antagonized by

antihistamine drugs. It is possibly antagonized by homochlorcyclizine [42]. Much work is now being put into the search for SRS-A antagonists which might be clinically effective.

(3) *Bradykinin*. Bradykinin is a basic nonapeptide which is readily produced by, and rapidly destroyed in, a number of processes in lung and skin. It can cause bronchoconstriction when given by aerosol to guinea pigs or man [12]. It may prove to play an important part in the asthmatic reaction.

(4) *Serotonin (5-Hydroxytryptamine or 5-HT)*. This substance is bronchoconstrictor in the guinea pig, dog and cat, but has not yet been shown definitely to affect man, nor is asthma relieved by powerful drugs antagonizing serotonin [12]. Asthma is a characteristic clinical manifestation of carcinoid tumours in man. These tumours produce large amounts of 5-HT though sometimes without resulting in asthma (p. 407). In man, therefore, the contribution of 5-HT to the asthmatic reaction is still unproven.

PATHOGENESIS OF THE INFECTIVE TYPE OF ASTHMA

The pathogenesis of this type of asthma is uncertain. Although there have been claims of demonstrable allergy to bacterial products Pepys [82] considers that no unequivocal evidence has yet been presented. Neverthless there is often eosinophilia in the sputum or blood in asthma associated with respiratory infections, suggesting a Type I allergic component [97]. The rather tenuous evidence regarding allergy to infective agents is briefly reviewed by Swineford *et al.* [97]. It is clear that no firm conclusions can yet be drawn. It may be that the chain of reactions leading to asthma is facilitated by inflammation of the bronchial mucous membrane which thereby becomes hypersensitive to nonspecific stimuli, such as cold air, smoke or coughing, though the eosinophilia suggests an atopic component at some point. Indeed such individuals often have a family history of allergic disorders [68].

EOSINOPHILIA AND BASOPHIL MAST CELLS

Eosinophilia, both in the tissues and in the blood, is characteristic of all Type I allergic reactions. In spite of a great deal of research work no clear evidence of the part played by eosinophils has yet been found, though there is some evidence that they may have an antihistamine function [20]. Mast cells, corresponding to the basophil cells of the blood, are plentiful throughout the tissues and increased numbers are present in the bronchi in asthma, although they tend to be removed by the ordinary methods of preparing tissue for pathological examination. There is no increase of mast cells in the blood. As already mentioned, the histamine which takes part in the asthmatic reaction is probably derived from the mast cells of the tissue.

PATHOLOGY

When death occurs in asthma, it is often sudden and unexpected, less frequently after prolonged *status asthmaticus* (89). The characteristic findings [7, 16, 95 & 111] are a plugging of all the smaller bronchi, especially those between 0·2 and 1 cm in diameter, with viscid yellowish plugs of mucus. The lungs are grossly distended and there is variable complicating pneumonia. Microscopically there is a great increase in the number of goblet cells, which largely replace the ciliated cells of the epithelium, an increase of mucous glands, a shedding of the more superficial layers of the epithelium, a thickening of the basement membrane and the presence of large numbers of eosinophils both in the wall of the bronchus and in the contained mucus. The bronchioli are relatively spared [111]. Areas of squamous metaplasia may occur [75] and there may be fibrosis of the bronchial wall, though some of the cases with these changes might have been classed as bronchitis in Britain. However squamous metaplasia in the medium and smaller bronchi, combined with thickening of the basement membrane, is regarded by Bohrod [7] as almost pathognomonic and he describes it in children in whom chronic bronchitis is a less likely explanation. In addition, the bronchial musculature is greatly hypertrophied and areas of pneumonia, either within the alveoli or in the interstitial tissue, may also be present and may include infiltration with eosinophils.

Studies by bronchial biopsy have shown characteristic subepithelial infiltration with eosinophils, which contrasts with the findings in bronchitis [52].

FUNCTIONAL ABNORMALITY

The main abnormality in asthma is *airways obstruction*. As the airways are normally narrower on expiration obstruction is particularly severe during this phase. FEV and FVC are reduced, as is FEV as a percentage of FVC. During an attack the FEV/FVC ratio will be well below 70%. In a number of asthmatics, but by no means all [5], breathing occurs with the lungs in a more inflated position, resulting in an increased FRC. This may be partly a reflex effect tending to keep the bronchi open, but may be merely due to trapping. As inspiratory capacity is usually reduced, the ratio of RV to TLC is increased, but sometimes a patient may have quite severe respiratory impairment without impressive changes in these values [5].

The airways obstruction is usually much more reversible than in the case of chronic bronchitis. The subcutaneous injection of adrenaline or the inhalation of isoprenaline (p. 414) usually results in an increase of FEV of more than 20% within 20 min; the increase may be as much as 100%. An even greater improvement of FEV may be obtained, especially in early or mild asthma, by giving a corticosteroid drug (p. 416) though maximal reversal of obstruction may take up to a week, sometimes longer (p. 409). In the converse reaction of increasing airways obstruction the asthmatic has been shown to be much more sensitive than normals to the inhalation of very small quantities of acetylcholine or histamine [41, 60 & 102] (p. 400).

There is much to support the view that airways obstruction in asthma is not uniform throughout the lung. In a closely reasoned analysis Campbell et al. [15] concluded that critical narrowing first occurs in the larger airways in asthma, though in the smaller airways in emphysema. The Pa,O_2 may often

14—R.D.

be decreased in moderate or severe asthma without elevation of Pa,CO_2 [87, 88 & 99], indicating disturbance of $\dot{V}/\dot{Q}$ relationships, presumably mainly due to uneven ventilation. *Non-uniformity* of *gas distribution* has also been demonstrated by nitrogen washout, helium equilibration and radioactive xenon techniques [5]. It has also been shown by a raised physiological dead space/tidal volume ratio ((V_D/V_T) and by the demonstration of a shunt effect when breathing 100% oxygen [99].

Personal observation at bronchoscopy does not suggest any crude variation in bronchoconstriction among the larger bronchi, though in susceptible subjects unilateral bronchospasm has been induced by introducing an allergen into one lung by bronchial catheter [2]; relief was obtained within 15 minutes by adrenaline suggesting a bronchospastic effect by the allergen. It is possible that random distribution of intraluminal mucus, rather than a variation in the degree of bronchospasm, may be responsible for the local variation in ventilation. In severe asthma and in status asthmaticus the Pa,CO_2 is often elevated and respiratory acidosis is common [99], particularly if the patient has been sedated. Sometimes a low pH without a gross rise in Pa,CO_2 indicates a metabolic acidosis, possibly due to the intensive effort of breathing with inadequately oxygenated muscle.

Naturally the airways obstruction causes a rise in *air flow resistance* and an increase in the *work of breathing*, which may be of the order of 5 or 10 times greater than normal [5]. In less severe asthma the DL,CO may be relatively well preserved in spite of ventilatory defect and $\dot{V}/\dot{Q}$ abnormalities, but in severe asthma the reduced surface area available for gas exchange leads to a reduction.

It has recently been shown that bronchodilator drugs may relieve both airways obstruction and the patient's symptoms without importantly affecting the Pa,O_2. Adrenaline may improve Pa,O_2 transiently by stimulating breathing but the level may then revert to the previous figure in spite of symptomatic improvement [87]. The latter is presumably due to decrease in the work of breathing and the former to persistence of $\dot{V}/\dot{Q}$ imbalance. Voluntary overbreathing tends to correct the Pa,o_2. Intravenous aminophylline has an unpredictable effect on Pa,o_2 which may even decrease, possibly due to dilatation of pulmonary vessels [88]. Isoprenaline inhalation may also improve FEV without affecting Pa,o_2 [79].

Woolcock and Read [112] have pointed out that a few patients claim considerable subjective relief during treatment with corticosteroid drugs, in spite of little demonstrable improvement in FEV. They found that these patients might initially have an FRC, or even an RV, which was greater than the TLC recorded after recovery. Conducting their breathing at almost maximal lung inflation, as was necessary to obtain any tidal volume at all, must have greatly increased the work of inspiration and sense of dyspnoea because of the fully stretched elastic tissue of the lung. As the patients recovered, breathing occurred in a more and more deflated position, as witnessed by the decreasing FRC, with subjective improvement in spite, at first, of an unaltered FEV.

CLINICAL MANIFESTATIONS

ASTHMATIC ATTACKS

The classical attack of asthma is relatively sudden in onset. The main symptom is that of breathlessness. The patient has difficulty in forcing the air out of his lungs and the effort usually results in *wheeze* audible to himself and others. In a very severe attack the respiratory obstruction may be so extreme that there is no audible wheeze. In a bad attack there may also be some inspiratory difficulty, though this is usually much less obvious. Dean Swift, who was an asthmatic, is said to have remarked that if he could once get the air out of his lungs he would take good care never to let it in again! Occasionally the larynx is involved and there is *stridor*, though this is rare; when it occurs a local cause should be excluded by laryngoscopy and bronchoscopy.

The *duration* of the attack is very variable.

Of course the patient often cuts it short by the use of an inhaler or other therapy. It may last half an hour or an hour or it may go on for several days, or even weeks.

In the earlier stages most asthmatics have periods when they are completely free of symptoms and can indulge in quite violent exercise without distress, though children are often wheezy on exercise between attacks. In many severe or long-standing asthmatics some evidence of respiratory obstruction can be found, either by physical examination or by physiological testing, even at times when the patient says that he is quite free from symptoms. This respiratory obstruction may still be reversible by the use of adrenaline or other drugs. Presumably the patient has forgotten what it is like to be completely normal and regards himself as free from symptoms by contrast to the distress which he suffers during exacerbations.

There is every possible variety in the *frequency* and *duration* of asthmatic attacks. Some patients will have a single attack once or twice a year, lasting for only a few minutes, others will be in a state of chronic respiratory distress, with recurrent severe exacerbations lasting for weeks at a time.

Although dyspnoea and wheeze are the principal symptoms of asthma, *cough* is a frequent accompaniment. In those whose attacks of asthma coincide with a respiratory infection cough is usually a prominent symptom and the sputum may be purulent or mucopurulent. In some patients *paroxysmal cough* is almost as prominent a symptom as the dyspnoea and is relieved by the same measures. The cough may be due to irritation from impacted mucus in the lower respiratory tract and may be relieved by coughing up a little viscid mucus or even *plugs* or bronchial casts. The coughing up of plugs and bronchial casts is particularly associated with hypersensitivity to *Aspergillus fumigatus* (see Asthmatic Pulmonary Eosinophilia, p. 429).

PRECIPITATING FACTORS

A careful history is especially important in a patient with asthma and will often reveal important precipitating factors. The possibility of any of the following precipitating factors should be considered in all cases:

(1) *Allergens.* Ogilvie [78] found allergic factors in 35% of 1000 asthmatics in Britain, Rackemann and Edwards [83] in 40% of 688 children in the U.S.A. These should be particularly sought in patients in whom the asthma first began in childhood or young adult life. *Food allergens* are more often responsible in children than in adults. The relationship to common foods will often not be obvious from the history but may have to be revealed by skin testing or, more reliably, by actual dietary trial. Asthma tending to come on at a particular season of the year may be related to the *pollens* which are found at that period or to *fungi* or their *spores*, some of which also have a seasonal prevalence. Hypersensitivity to *Aspergillus fumigatus* is commonest in the middle aged and is often characterized by a particular clinical picture, including recurrent pulmonary shadows on the x-ray, eosinophilia and the coughing up of bronchial plugs (p. 429). On the other hand some patients are hypersensitive to the spores of *Aspergillus* and respond to them with simple asthmatic attacks [80]. A history of contact with pets, especially *birds*, *cats* and *dogs*, or with *horses*, should be sought in every case as allergy to animal dander is relatively common. In the housewife exacerbations during periods of springcleaning or intensive housework will often be suggestive of allergy to *housedust*, although sometimes these exacerbations seem to be nonspecific and merely due to dust in general. Attacks at night may be associated with an allergic reaction to *feathers* in pillow or eiderdown or to housedust, although often it is not possible to prove any definite association.

(2) *Infection.* In taking the history from a patient with asthma there is frequently an obvious association between upper respiratory infections and attacks of asthma. These attacks usually last several days or a week or more and are accompanied by cough and sputum. As already mentioned, no specific allergy to an infectious agent has yet been convincingly demonstrated in such patients and the proof of the association depends on a careful history. Asthma may also predispose to infection. Infection is often an important precipitating factor in *young children* [76] and in those, especially women, who first become asthmatic in *middle age*. The reduction of respiratory infections by the use of prophylactic antibiotics may result in a sharp decrease in the number of attacks of asthma, though not uncommonly the infection is merely a complication of the asthma. Naturally such patients tend to have more asthma in the winter than in the summer, in contrast to those whose asthma is precipitated by pollen allergy.

(3) *Psychological factors.* These have already been discussed (p. 398). It is doubtful whether asthma is ever caused directly by psychological stress alone but there is little doubt that such distress exacerbates asthma in many patients. It is seldom that a patient will make spontaneous suggestions about the sources of mental stress. The physician will therefore have to enquire tactfully and carefully. *In the child* the overanxious mother is often blamed, although it would be difficult for any mother not to be anxious when she sees her child in the acute distress of an asthmatic attack. The physician must beware of blaming the mother for his own inability to prevent the child's attacks! Nevertheless the child is often capable, however unconsciously, of exploiting his parents' anxiety, or indeed he may be infected by it, so that the whole family situation must be carefully assessed. It is astonishing how successfully asthma may be relieved by removing the child from home. Although one cannot be certain that this success is not due to separating the child from some specific allergen, it seems more likely that one is breaking a vicious circle of asthma and anxiety. On the other hand childhood infection has been found to be commoner in poor homes with inefficient maternal care [76].

In older patients the cause of trouble may be the relationship with another member of the family or a work situation. The adolescent with an ambitious father may be being driven too hard for his capabilities, the dependent wife may be unconsciously using her asthma to monopolize her husband's attention. Unfortunately it is often easier to identify these situations than to remedy them, but explanation alone may help and the attempt is well worth making.

(4) *Nonspecific factors.* The asthmatic with hypersensitive bronchi will often respond with an asthmatic attack, or an increase in respiratory obstruction, to a wide range of stimuli. Hard exercise or going out of the house into cold air in the winter will often result in increased respiratory obstruction. Dusty or foggy conditions usually make asthmatics worse. Many asthmatics give up smoking because they find it aggravates their symptoms. These factors have been discussed on p. 400.

PHYSICAL SIGNS

The basic manifestation of asthma is obstruction of the bronchi, particularly on expiration. Because of the narrowing of the bronchi complete expiration is difficult; the *lungs* are therefore often *overinflated*. During an attack physical signs may be suggestive of emphysema, namely a barrel-shaped chest, increased resonance and decreased liver and cardiac dullness. Between attacks, or after reversal of respiratory obstruction with corticosteroids, these physical signs may disappear, indicating that they were due to hyperinflation of the lungs rather than to true emphysema. Longstanding overinflation may lead to 'pigeon chest' deformity, though even this may be reversed if the asthma is effectively dealt with.

Wheeze is usually audible and *expiratory rhonchi* are audible all over the chest in a severe attack. In less severe attacks there may be only a few scattered rhonchi. In very severe attacks the extreme bronchial narrowing may result in a silent chest without rhonchi. Between attacks no rhonchi may be heard, although frequently they may be detected on forced expiration. There are sometimes inspiratory as well as expiratory rhonchi. Occasionally the larynx appears also to take part in the spasm and *stridor* may be audible, often expiratory and sometimes inspiratory also.

Because of the marked expiratory effort the intrathoracic pressure is often above atmospheric on expiration so that the *jugular venous pressure* may be raised on expiration and fall to normal or below normal on inspiration. This immediately distinguishes the findings from those in cardiac failure.

If the patient has a prolonged severe asthmatic attack, lasting more than 24 hours, he is often said to be in *status asthmaticus*. The patient is then in great distress, both from the acute discomfort of breathing, from the physical effort required to maintain it and from exhaustion. He is often unable to maintain adequate oxygenation of the blood and becomes *cyanosed*, although retention of CO_2 is a late phenomenon. He may develop peripheral vascular collapse and lowering of the blood pressure, presumably because the raised intrathoracic pressure interferes with the venous return to the heart. *Dehydration*, due to loss of fluid from hyperventilation, may also contribute. *Cor pulmonale* only occurs very late when the situation is desperate. *Tachycardia* is a danger sign; a pulse of 120 or above calls for urgent measures.

CLINICAL TYPES

CHILDREN

Two main types of asthma occur in children. In the *eczema-asthma type* there is often a family history of asthma. The child has infantile eczema and later develops asthma. In infancy there may be a demonstrable allergy to food but more often to inhalants. This type comprises a minority of asthma in children but the proportion of demonstrably allergic asthma has been as high as 40% in some series. More frequent is the *infective type*, commoner in boys, in which attacks are precipitated by respiratory infection, though there may be wheezing on exercise between the infective exacerbations. This form of asthma usually ceases to trouble the child as he grows older and the prognosis is therefore good [48, 64, 76 & 78].

YOUNG ADULTS

In young adults demonstrable allergy is often

found. The asthma is often paroxysmal and intermittent, though sometimes chronic. If the asthma persists the range of precipitating causes may increase. Psychological factors are not uncommon.

ONSET IN MIDDLE AGED OR ELDERLY

As already mentioned, a late onset of asthma is much commoner in women (p. 394). Infection is often the initiating and exacerbating factor, though wheeze is often chronic with only occasional periods of relative freedom. There is frequently eosinophilia in the blood or sputum. Without treatment this type of asthma often pursued a steadily downhill course and mortality was high. With the use of antibiotics and corticosteroids the prognosis is now very much better, though the recent increase in British mortality is causing concern (p. 394). There is sometimes difficulty in differentiating the condition from chronic bronchitis. In some it is relatively arbitrary which label is chosen. When the wheeze is out of proportion to the cough and when respiratory obstruction can be largely reversed, either spontaneously or by drugs, the condition will be called asthma. There is usually an infective precipitating factor and there may or may not be eosinophilia in the sputum or blood.

In all these age groups the asthma is often intermittent at its onset but may later become chronic. A chronic course is more likely the older the patient at the time of onset [78]. Chronic asthma carries an appreciably worse prognosis than the recurrent acute form [78]. A chronic course is often associated with complicating infection and bronchitis.

ASTHMATIC PULMONARY EOSINOPHILIA [24 & 80]

This condition is characterized by lung shadowing, often recurrent, sometimes accompanied by fever and eosinophilia in the blood and often in the sputum. Asthmatic attacks may precede or accompany the incident of radiological infiltration. Rarely there may be no asthma during the time when the lung shadowing is present, although asthma is present at other times. Patients frequently cough up plugs of mucus, often brownish in colour, or even bronchial casts. Bronchiectasis may be demonstrated at the sites of recurrent radiological infiltration. A number of these patients have been shown to be hypersensitive to *Aspergillus fumigatus* on skin or inhalation testing [80]. Fragments of mycelium may be found in the bronchial casts. The fungus however is usually difficult to isolate from the sputum. The condition is more fully discussed on p. 429.

CARCINOID TUMOUR

Asthmatic symptoms are not uncommon in patients with carcinoid tumour. This tumour usually occurs in the ileum, occasionally in the lung (p. 554) or elsewhere. The clinical condition is characterized by recurrent diarrhoea, peculiar flushing attacks and sometimes by asthma. The pathogenesis of the asthma is discussed on p. 402.

POLYARTERITIS NODOSA

The type of polyarteritis nodosa in which there is lung involvement is often initiated by asthmatic symptoms and sinusitis. In this type there is usually a marked blood eosinophilia. Polyarteritis nodosa should be suspected if asthmatic symptoms are accompanied by haematuria, peripheral neuritis, muscle nodules or other evidence of diffuse disease, or if there is high and persistent increase in the erythrocyte sedimentation rate (p. 438).

RADIOLOGY

Radiology is not very important in asthma. In chronic asthma or during an attack the chest film may show evidence of hyperinflation, as witnessed by a low diaphragm and, in the lateral view, an increased area of transradiancy above and in front of the heart. The heart may be long and narrow and the peripheral vessels not well seen. The difference from the normal chest is even more obvious if the film is taken in expiration, when the rise in the diaphragm and the decrease in transradiancy are often much less than normal. Fluoroscopy will reveal similar changes.

Nevertheless, the hyperinflation of the lungs is usually obvious enough clinically and the main point of the x-ray is to exclude the presence of other conditions or complications, especially pneumothorax. Secondary infection will, of course, sometimes result in a pneumonic shadow, and impacted mucus may cause segmental collapse [76]. Recurrent segmental opacities, or localized homogeneous shadows with a less clear segmental distribution, are characteristic of asthmatic pulmonary eosinophilia (p. 429). X-ray of the sinuses often reveals thickened mucosa, especially in allergic asthma, but we see little point in exposing the patient to the radiation involved in sinus radiography unless there is a suggestion of secondary sinus infection; even then the condition may be obvious enough clinically.

INVESTIGATIONS

HISTORY

The history is particularly important in asthma. As already mentioned, this may give important information as to precipitating factors, allergic, infectious or psychological.

TESTS FOR HYPERSENSITIVITY

The value of skin tests [82] is much contested by those interested in asthma. Enthusiastic allergists will be prepared to carry out tests with very large numbers of allergens and are impressed with their value. The range of potential allergens is of course almost infinite. There is bound to be some selection. On the other hand others assert that skin testing adds little to a carefully taken history. Many clinicians, if they carry out skin tests at all, will be content with utilizing extracts of pollens, animal dander or hair, fungi, house dust, feathers, etc., obtainable from commercial firms, and are guided by clues in the history. In testing for sensitivity to animals, reaction is more likely to dander than to fur or feathers [82]. Testing to aspergillin, extracted from *Aspergillus fumigatus*, is particularly important in middle aged asthmatics, especially those with episodes characterized by fleeting lung shadows in the x-ray. Skin tests are much less reliable in testing for food allergy, unless the clinical reaction to food is an immediate one. Skin tests can occasionally give rise to very severe reactions and it is wise to have a syringe charged with adrenaline available. Prick or scratch tests are much safer than intradermal injection and give fewer nonspecific reactions. The prick test is to be preferred.

A positive reaction shows an urticarial weal and an erythematous flare, maximal in 10–20 min and fading within 1–$1\frac{1}{2}$ hours. There is usually itching which may be helpful in interpreting a doubtful test. A positive test must be correlated with the clinical history. Reactions are relatively common in normal individuals with a positive family history, though a proportion of these will develop clinical allergy later. A negative reaction does not exclude clinical hypersensitivity, especially in the case of house dust. This may be because the specific allergen is not always included in the test material. There is recent evidence to suggest that the most important element in house dust is a mite of the *Dermatophagoides* species, which lives on human skin peelings and is commoner in damp houses and in damp years [103]. Antihistamine drugs and recently administered bronchodilator drugs may suppress the reaction, though corticosteroid drugs have little if any effect. There is no convincing or consistent evidence that skin testing with bacterial extracts or whole bacteria is of value in asthma [82 & 92], though a delayed reaction after intradermal injection (20 mm weal at 24 hours) has been claimed to accord with intrabronchial testing and clinical evidence [58].

It is claimed that hypersensitivity to such inhalants as house dust and moulds is best demonstrated by *inhalation tests*, assessing the results by serial measurement of VC. It certainly seems rational to employ the allergen by the route through which it usually reaches the bronchi but this does require some elaboration of apparatus [18, 60, 70, & 71] and a severe attack of asthma may be induced. Sometimes this severe attack is delayed for as long as 24 hours [70] and appropriate remedies must be available to the patient. The method may be used to demonstrate the success of hyposensitization, at least in pollen asthma [18 & 71]. Inhalation tests have been claimed [58] to be superior to intradermal or prick tests in demonstrating hypersensitivity to bacteria, especially *H. influenzae*, though there is closer correlation with 24-hour reading (late reaction) of intradermal tests. It is probably better to carry out inhalation tests in hospital. Because only one allergen can be tested at a time, because of the difficulty in assessing dosage and because of the danger of inducing a severe attack, this method of testing is not popular.

RESPIRATORY FUNCTION TESTS

The most valuable tests to carry out are the FEV and the FVC which give an objective measure of the severity of airways obstruction and are useful for following progress and assessing response to treatment. The Peak Expiratory Flow Rate (PEFR) may also be used. The best test for reversibility is to measure FEV 10 minutes after the inhalation of 1 ml 2% isoprenaline from a Wright nebulizer over 2 minutes, or 20 minutes after 0·5 ml of 1/1000 adrenaline subcutaneously. In chronic bronchitis the degree of reversibility is usually much less than in asthma. Atropine sulphate 0·6 mg given subcutaneously, with repeat of FEV testing 20 minutes later, usually improves FEV in chronic bronchitis to a similar extent as does adrenaline or isoprenaline, but gives lower readings in asthma [25] unless the patient is receiving corticosteroid drugs. In the latter case the response may be similar in asthma and bronchitis. As already mentioned (p. 403) the response to adrenaline or isoprenaline in asthma usually amounts to an improvement of FEV of at least 20% and sometimes as much as 100%.

In the hospital assessment of a new case of asthma, or as an aid to the differentiation from chronic bronchitis in a difficult case, our own routine is to give a week's course of prednisolone 40 mg daily with daily measurement of FEV and FVC. If psychological factors seem to be important placebo tablets may be given initially and, if there is a doubt about response, again substituted later in the course. A graph of the FEV data when the patient is receiving prednisolone or placebo usually makes it clear whether there is a genuine response to the corticosteroid. An impressive response suggests that the case should be classed as asthma rather than bronchitis. Sometimes response is unconvincing after a week, though it may be suggestive, and a second week's test may be necessary. If response is slow, improvement in FVC may be the first evidence of a corticosteroid effect. In slow or doubtful responders, especially if there is subjective improvement, it may be that serial FRC estimation may show an improvement preceding that in FVC or FEV, as reported by Woolcock and Read [112] (p. 404).

The very low levels of Pa,O_2, and the raised Pa,CO_2 and respiratory acidosis, which may occur in severe asthma, have only recently been appreciated. It seems desirable that these should be monitored in patients in severe *status asthmaticus* (p. 419).

BLOOD EOSINOPHILIA

In assessing a new case of asthma, or in differentiating asthma from chronic bronchitis, examination of the blood for eosinophils is useful. The blood eosinophilia is usually in the region of 500–800 per mm³, occasionally higher, but may be absent or intermittent. In a tropical area, or in a patient from a tropical area, a count of over 20% suggests tropical pulmonary eosinophilia (p. 432), especially if there is paroxysmal cough. In a temperate zone such a count, particularly if accompanied by a persistently high erythrocyte sedimentation rate, suggests the possibility of polyarteritis nodosa but may sometimes occur in severe cases of simple asthma.

SPUTUM

The majority of the cells in the sputum are often eosinophils, sometimes even when it appears macroscopically purulent. Curschmann's spirals, elongated spiral casts of the smaller bronchi, are a classical finding. Naylor [77] has again drawn attention to the compact clusters of epithelial cells which are found in large quantities almost exclusively in the sputum of asthmatics. Brownish plugs, or elongated or even branching casts, are seen particularly in asthmatic pulmonary eosinophilia, often associated with hypersensitivity to *Aspergillus fumigatus* (p. 429). Silver staining may reveal fragments of mycelium in the casts, though the amount of fungus is usually small and repeated cultures may be necessary to identify it. Culture for both bacteria and fungi should be routine. It must be remembered that *A. fumigatus* is a common contaminant, both of patients and of culture media, between October and April; the significance of a positive culture must be confirmed by skin testing.

DIAGNOSIS

The most important differential diagnosis in asthma is from acute or chronic bronchitis causing wheeze. Difficulty arises mainly in children and occasionally in the middle aged and elderly. As has been pointed out, the difference is partly semantic, the conditions tending to fade into one another. In children, in particular, the exact diagnostic term which is used for recurrent wheezing precipitated by infection is largely arbitrary. A diagnosis of 'bronchitis' is often less alarming to parents than if the child is labelled asthmatic. In the middle aged and elderly the term used may also be somewhat arbitrary but it is reasonable to call the condition asthma if the history reveals that the airways obstruction is sometimes absent or if it can be shown to be reversible to an important degree (p. 409). A careful history is therefore one of the most important factors in making a diagnosis of asthma and should reveal the paroxysmal nature of the attacks and periods of relative freedom from symptoms, at least in the initial stages. The history is also an essential factor in giving clues to possible precipitating causes. The presence of a blood eosinophilia or of eosinophils in the sputum favours the diagnosis. The occasional difficulties have been emphasized here, but in the great majority of cases the diagnosis is clearcut.

'Cardiac asthma', a term which is now fortunately going out of fashion, is usually easily differentiated by the accompanying cardiovascular findings and the presence of pulmonary oedema.

Once a diagnosis of asthma has been made the next step is to identify the precipitating or predisposing factors. The importance of the history has already been emphasized. Skin (p. 408) or bronchial sensitivity testing (p. 408), and occasionally elimination diets, may be used to confirm or supplement conclusions drawn from the history.

COMPLICATIONS [30]

THORACIC DEFORMITY

In the very young child with chronic asthma the sternum may be drawn inwards or there may be Harrison's sulcus. Older children tend to develop a pigeon chest or the same type of 'barrel' chest as adults. Fortunately even gross deformities may reverse to a surprising degree if the chronic asthma is relieved by corticosteroid drugs.

EFFECT ON GROWTH

The depression of growth rate in children by the use of long term corticosteroids will be discussed in the section on treatment (p. 418) but it is important to remember that asthma itself may have considerable retarding effect on growth as was well documented before the introduction of corticosteroid drugs [23].

RIB FRACTURES

These are seen from time to time and are attributed to cough. They tend to occur in an oblique line on the ribs corresponding to the interdigitations of the *serratus anterior* and external abdominal oblique muscles whose opposing action puts a strain on the ribs during coughing. In patients on long term treatment with corticosteroid drugs the demineralization of the bones may contribute to fractures (p. 417).

POSTOPERATIVE RESPIRATORY COMPLICATIONS

With appropriate preoperative care, and the use of corticosteroids when necessary, asthmatics usually tolerate surgical operations well. The postoperative complication rate was only slightly higher than that of the general population, even before the corticosteroid drugs became available [50]. Pneumonia or an acute asthmatic attack in the postoperative period are the major risks and, as in other respiratory conditions, are more common after upper abdominal operations.

PNEUMONIA AND ATELECTASIS

Segmental pneumonic or atelectatic shadows may be found in the x-ray of the chest during exacerbations, especially if these are due to infection. They are relatively common in children [76], less so in adults. However, in the group of conditions known as 'asthmatic pulmonary eosinophilia' (p. 429) recurrent pneumonic shadows may be accompanied by a blood eosinophilia and the coughing up of bronchial casts; about 50% of these cases are associated with hypersensitivity to *Aspergillus fumigatus*. In asthmatic pulmonary eosinophilia secondary *bronchiectasis* may occur in the parts of the lung which are affected by the recurrent pneumonic processes.

BRONCHITIS

Bronchial infection is a common complication of chronic asthma, less so of the acute paroxysmal type. It is associated with a much poorer prognosis [78].

SPONTANEOUS PNEUMOTHORAX

Spontaneous pneumothorax is comparatively rare but does occur from time to time. It is wise to x-ray the chest of any asthmatic patient with sudden severe dyspnoea as it is almost impossible to make a clinical diagnosis of spontaneous pneumothorax in the presence of severe asthma; failure to relieve an undiagnosed pneumothorax may result in death.

INTERSTITIAL PULMONARY OR MEDIASTINAL EMPHYSEMA

These complications may occasionally occur, and are sometimes associated with subcutaneous emphysema. They may be asymptomatic and only detected on the x-ray or may give rise to pain, cyanosis and collapse (p. 440).

CARDIAC COMPLICATIONS

Right ventricular hypertrophy is said to be present in most patients at autopsy [30]. There are not many reports of pulmonary artery pressure recordings during an attack of severe asthma, but increase in pressure has been noted on occasion [5]. The factors are presumably intrapulmonary pressure affecting small vessels and possibly vasospasm resulting from hypoxaemia. The electrocardiogram may sometimes show a *cor pulmonale* pattern but overt cardiac failure usually occurs only in very severe and prolonged *status asthmaticus*.

TREATMENT

It must be admitted that the treatment of asthma is largely palliative. At present we have no way of altering permanently and reliably the fundamental abnormality. It is true that some patients while under treatment cease to have asthma. In fact the great majority of asthmatic children lose their asthma as they get older and it is important to emphasize this to anxious parents [48, 64, 76 & 78]. A proportion of patients who first develop asthma in adult life cease to have attacks later. Sometimes patients may be free of disease for many years and develop attacks again in later life. Although the patient, and sometimes the doctor, often attributes the cessation of attacks to the treatment being used at the time, this is in fact unlikely, owing to the variety of treatments employed and their inability to repeat the success in the majority of other patients. One has the impression that in an occasional middle aged woman, in whom asthma follows a severe acute attack of bronchitis, it is possible to reverse the abnormal reaction of the bronchi by suppressing the hyperreactivity by corticosteroids for a number of months and using preventive chemotherapy to avoid further infectious insults. Some of these patients can later be weaned from therapy without recurrence of asthma, but it is difficult to be completely certain that this is the result of treatment.

In spite of our therapeutic inefficiency in dealing with the fundamental abnormality in asthma, a very great deal can be done to improve the patient's well-being and allow him to lead a normal life. In most patients the corticosteroids are capable of dealing with the worst horrors of the disease and saving a number of lives. As in most of the chronic diseases, the more trouble the physician takes the better the results. The very fact that he is available and interested helps to remove the anxiety which so often aggravates the disease.

THE TREATMENT OF PRECIPITATING FACTORS

ALLERGENS

As already indicated, it is important to take a very careful history with a view to identifying relevant allergens. It is comparatively seldom that skin tests give additional information but it is nevertheless wise to carry them out as a routine, concentrating on allergens that may be relevant in the particular case. If a specific allergen can be identified, then it is often possible to avoid it or at least reduce exposure. This is particularly true of food allergens and animal dander. The former can sometimes be identified by keeping a food diary and recording also attacks of asthma; elimination diets are sometimes required. When attacks occur particularly at night it is often helpful to advise radical changes in the patient's bedroom. These are designed to avoid accumulation of dust. Feather pillows and eiderdowns are banned. Carpets and mats are removed and the furniture reduced to a minimum. The bedroom is 'springcleaned' daily, a vacuum cleaner being used to remove all dust, including that behind and on top of cupboards, etc. If a vacuum cleaner is not available then a damp mop may be used instead. Dusting should also be carried out with a damp cloth to prevent dust rising into the air and being inhaled. Before this is done the bed should be made and covered. The pillow should be enclosed in plastic material to reduce the inhalation of dust from the usual linen cover. In some cases the adoption of this routine produces dramatic results.

The value of *desensitization*, or more correctly 'hyposensitization', is controversial.

Some allergists assert that, if testing is sufficiently detailed and extensive, specific allergens can frequently be found and desensitization to these is very valuable. On the whole these claims have not been supported by carefully controlled trials and in asthma the palliative effect of any form of placebo is well known. Almost any new treatment is effective for a time. Frankland et al. [43] obtained improvement in 50% of patients with carbol-saline. Most physicians feel that desensitization is only effective in a few cases where a very narrow range of allergens is involved, especially in the case of pollen allergy. In these it may sometimes be quite helpful. The literature has been critically reviewed by Citron [19].

Standardization of pollen extracts

The basic unit is the *Noon Unit*, named after one of the pioneers of the procedure. It equals 1 ml of a dilution of $1:10^6$; or approximately 1 millionth of a gramme of pollen. In the U.S.A. protein nitrogen standardization is routine and 1 Noon Unit is equal to 0·6 Protein Nitrogen Unit.

Formerly aqueous solutions were used but desensitization requires many and frequent injections. Attempts have recently been made to give 'slow-release' injections in which the allergen is injected in a depôt material from which it gradually diffuses out. Two forms of depôt have been used, an oily emulsion or a relatively insoluble complex, pyridine-extracted alum-precipitated extracts [19].

Desensitization with *aqueous solutions* is carried out by subcutaneous injection using ascending doses of the allergen. Allergen solutions both for testing and for desensitization can be obtained from commercial firms; full instructions are included. Pollen desensitization is usually done before the pollen season and has to be repeated annually. Starting in February with an injection of 20 Noon Units this may be increased by 20 units up to 200 and then by 15% at each injection. A final dose of 18,000 Noon Units may give as good a result as 100,000 [19] but the right dosage must depend on the individual patient and his reactions. It may be found that if a patient is successfully desensitized in 3 succeeding seasons he may not require it the 4th year [81]. Injections may actually provoke an attack so that close supervision and adjustment of dosage is necessary.

There is little reliable evidence to support the value of desensitization to allergens other than pollen and house dust. The results in the latter are variable, perhaps because of incomplete antigens. If the evidence for a mite allergen as the main component in house dust sensitivity (p. 398) proves correct, better desensitizing solutions may become available. However in the presence of definite sensitivity to an allergen which cannot be avoided, desensitization may justifiably be attempted.

Depôt desensitization with pollen extracts

Pearson [81] reported a cooperative trial in over 1000 patients, using an oily emulsion. Successive doses of 750 and 7500 Noon Units at intervals of 1 month gave better results than desensitization with aqueous solutions or than a single depôt injection of 750 units. Severe general anaphylactic reactions occurred, usually 2–4 hours later, in 0·7%, but these were less frequent than with aqueous solutions. Local reactions were common. An antihistamine drug was given at the time of injection and 4 hours later and reserve tablets of antihistamine and isoprenaline were also provided. Using a similar technique McAllen et al. [71] showed good clinical results in 75% of cases after 1 year and in 80% after 2 years' treatment, with marked improvement in tested bronchial tolerance. Depôt injections are therefore worth further trial, though the local reactions, and the occasional severe general reactions, merit caution and careful supervision.

Desensitization by inhalation

It has been suggested that desensitization by inhalation may be more successful, especially in the case of hypersensitivity to house dust [70]. The inhalation is increased by 30% at intervals of 4–7 days, with slower increase if there are reactions. It is said that desensitization to allergens other than pollen require repeating every 6 months, or even more often.

INFECTION

As already indicated, there is no clear evidence of a connection between any specific infecting agent and exacerbations of asthma, but in many patients, especially in children and those whose asthma comes on first in middle age, there is often clear historical connection between exacerbations of asthma and infection. The infection may precipitate asthma merely by causing inflammation of the bronchial mucous membrane. Although carefully controlled trials have not been carried out, experience suggests that the use of prophylactic tetracycline is of considerable value in these patients, especially when combined with corticosteroid drugs. If it is possible to keep the bronchi at rest for a number of months, reducing their hyperirritability by prednisolone and decreasing the likelihood of lower respiratory infections by preventive tetracycline, exacerbations of asthma are often much less frequent. Sometimes the patient can later be weaned from both drugs or need take them only during the winter. It is not easy to generalize about this type of case, but when the asthma has its first onset in middle age and is precipitated by respiratory infection it is well worth while, after controlling the acute exacerbation with corticosteroid drugs, to initiate preventive treatment with tetracycline in a dose of 0·5 g twice daily. At the same time corticosteroid drugs, for instance prednisolone in a dose of 2·5–5 mg twice daily, may be given for several months. It is desirable to keep the dose of prednisolone at 10 mg daily or below to minimize the chances of side effects. If the patient remains free from asthma for a number of months it may be possible to wean him from both drugs preferably in the summer months. If the initial attacks have been severe it may be wise to renew the treatment during the following winter and if the patient can be kept reasonably clear for 18 months or more it is well worth while trying without the drugs. Some patients with severe asthma may require to continue tetracycline throughout the year and may require long term corticosteroid treatment with higher doses in exacerbations (see below).

Controlled trials of stock or autogenous

vaccines in infective asthma have failed to show any beneficial effect [19 & 43].

PSYCHOLOGICAL FACTORS

As mentioned above, psychological influences are more often aggravating than initiating factors in asthma. They should be carefully sought in every case and may not be at all obvious on the surface. Children frequently seem to benefit physically by separation from home, if they go to a boarding school or a special institute at which asthmatics are taught. It is doubtful, however, whether young children are benefited psychologically by separation from their mother; in fact the contrary is probably the case and separation should only be advocated if the physical disability is very severe indeed. Nevertheless it is wise to explain to the mother that the child may, however unconsciously, use his asthma to get his own way with his parents. As far as possible the parents should attempt to take a matter of fact attitude towards the child's disability and conceal their understandable anxiety or distress. The doctor must realise that this is easier said than done.

In older children and adults psychological factors are more easily identified than remedied. Sometimes one finds that a boy of mediocre capacity is being driven too hard by an over-ambitious father; explanation and reorientation to a less ambitious programme may be surprisingly successful. Possible marital difficulties should always be investigated. These may sometimes be quite indirect. For instance, it may sometimes be found that a child's asthma is worse just before the time of his mother's period. On questioning she may admit that she is particularly irritable at this time and the irritability may be associated with anxiety about further pregnancy. Advice about contraception may do much to allay the anxiety and break the vicious circle. It is often helpful for the physician to work in close cooperation with the psychiatrist.

The value of *hypnosis* in asthma is uncertain. There has been a recent revival of interest in this method of therapy. It must be remembered that the asthmatic is always subject to suggestion and that hypnosis is a particularly valuable form of suggestion. The value of hypnosis has yet to be conclusively demonstrated by carefully controlled trials, though encouraging results have been claimed [73]. In severe asthma hypnosis may have to be used as cautiously as sedation (p. 416). We have known at least one patient die following its use.

SYMPTOMATIC TREATMENT

BRONCHODILATOR DRUGS [51]

Bronchodilator, or antispasmodic, drugs are the bread and butter of the treatment of asthma, both in dealing with the acute attack and for the long term relief of bronchial obstruction. Large numbers of such preparations are on the market, most of them mixtures of a few basic types of bronchodilator. There is in fact some evidence [51] that mixtures do potentiate the effect as do small doses of sedative such as phenobarbitone. For the rapid relief of an acute, but not very severe, attack the most convenient method is the use of an inhaler [38]. The most effective drug is 2% *isoprenaline*; 1% is somewhat less effective. Relief of bronchospasm is said to be prolonged by combining isoprenaline with atropine methonitrate, as in Isoprenaline Compound Spray BPC. Pocket pressurized inhalers are now available commercially and are widely used. They are highly effective in dealing with mild asthma or preparing the patient for unusual exertion but have very little effect in a severe asthmatic attack. There is the added danger that the patient may, contrary to instructions, continue to inhale in the hope of obtaining relief. Absorption, without relief of bronchospasm, can lead to hyperirritability of the heart (probably potentiated by hypoxaemia), ventricular fibrillation and death [56]. The combination of adrenaline and isoprenaline is particularly dangerous.

Orciprenaline is said to give a greater initial response and a longer duration of relief than 1% isoprenaline [40]. In more severe cases in hospital it is sometimes useful to give 0·5% isoprenaline with an intermittent positive pressure machine, such as the Bennett.

For a severe attack *adrenaline* 1/1000 0·2–

0·5 ml may be given subcutaneously and repeated as necessary, though it is dangerous to give more than 2 ml within 5–10 minutes. Large doses should not be given if the patient has recently received isoprenaline owing to the possiblity of dangerous combined action on the heart. Patients who have frequent severe attacks may be taught self-administration of adrenaline. There is a great deal of evidence that adrenaline rapidly relieves airways obstruction in most patients, though not always in very severe cases. Nevertheless, it has recently been shown that the hypoxaemia may not be relieved, presumably owing to the persistence of disturbed ventilation–perfusion relationships [87]. This may not matter in patients in a less severe attack in which the Pa,o_2 is over 70 mm Hg and in whom therefore there is no major unsaturation of haemoglobin, but it is important to bear in mind in very severe attacks in which the Pa,o_2 may be very much lower and in whom hypoxaemia may even be life-threatening. *Intravenous aminophylline* 0·25–0·5 g in 10–20 ml, given slowly over 2–10 minutes, is often highly effective in relieving airways obstruction, though there is some variation between patients. Rees et al. [88] confirmed that airways obstruction was usually relieved but the effect on Pa,o_2 was unpredictable. In some patients the existing hypoxaemia was worsened, possibly due to dilatation of pulmonary vessels. On the other hand aminophylline reduces the work of breathing and probably carries less risk for the cardiac muscle in a patient who may have received adrenaline or isoprenaline within the immediately preceding period.

In the treatment of *chronic asthma* or mild attacks oral preparations are convenient. Patients vary in their response to, and tolerance of, the different drugs. The most suitable for the individual should be found by trial and should be given as frequently and in as large doses as are necessary to obtain maximal relief. *Ephedrine* 15–60 or even 90 mg orally may be given up to 5 times daily, though palpitation or difficulty with micturition may prevent its use in some patients. Certain patients are kept awake by it and in these the last dose should not be later than

6 p.m. Tolerance to ephedrine may develop, resulting in loss of its antispasmodic action, sometimes even after a week's use. It is restored by stopping the drug for a few days. *Isoprenaline* 10–20 mg sublingually may be given 5 times daily or before any particular effort. It acts quickly though it may cause palpitations in some patients and care must be taken not to exceed the dose, owing to the risk of cardiac arrythmia. Orciprenaline 20 mg is an analogue which is effective when swallowed.

There is conflicting evidence as to the value of the *theophylline* group of drugs when given by the mouth. There are probably individual differences. The most effective is stated to be choline theophyllinate 100–400 mg 5 times daily. Nausea is sometimes a problem. Aminophylline Suppositories (BPC) are more effective but may cause proctitis if used more than twice a day.

Two drugs, *promethazine hydrochloride* and *deptropine*, with antihistamine and atropine-like effects, have a minor part to play in the treatment of asthma. The soporific effect of promethazine hydrochloride, together with its other properties, often reduces the frequency and severity of night attacks. There is a good deal of variation in the degree of sedation induced. The correct dose for an adult usually lies between 20 and 50 mg, the aim being to achieve the maximum effect in reducing night asthma without the patient being too sleepy in the morning. Although promethazine is of value for its sedative effect, in general antihistamine drugs are disappointing in asthma, the histamine factor being a relatively unimportant one in man [33]. Deptropine 1 mg orally 12 hourly is of value mainly in patients already receiving corticosteroid drugs; it has relatively little effect in others and atropine-like side effects may be troublesome [67]. Although it is ineffective when given alone by inhalation, a dose of 0·2 mg given by inhalation in combination with isoprenaline has been shown to potentiate and prolong the effect of the isoprenaline in the same way as does atropine methonitrate [66].

Antagonists to SRS-A (p. 401) might be more valuable than antihistamine drugs. One of these, *homochlorcyclizine*, which also has antiacetylcholine and anti-5-HT actions and is a mild sedative and bronchodilator, has been reported on enthusiastically [42], but has not yet come into general use.

Alcohol has often been thought clinically to relieve asthma and has been shown objectively to do so [34]. An evening whisky or brandy may therefore be useful in individuals who are not thought to be at risk of becoming addicts. Other *sedatives* in severe asthma have to be used with caution. Any depression of the respiratory centre may be lethal; morphia should never be given and even barbiturates are dangerous, though phenobarbitone in small doses may potentiate the action of bronchodilators and is safe enough in mild asthma. The use of promethazine hydrochloride has already been mentioned. Chloral and its derivatives may be employed in less severe cases.

CORTICOSTEROID DRUGS

In the great majority of asthmatics corticosteroid drugs are highly effective but their free use is limited by side effects. They should not be given lightly but on the other hand a patient should not be left in misery or exposed to mortal risk by undue apprehensions about possible side effects. The use of corticosteroid drugs is mandatory in a severe and prolonged attack (*status asthmaticus*: see below). In the patient who has occasional but relatively severe attacks the episodic use of corticosteroid drugs is quite justified; only moderate doses need be given for a relatively short time and undesirable side effects are minimal. It is more difficult to decide whether these drugs should be used in a patient with chronic asthma. One must accept that, once this form of treatment has been started on a long term basis, it will often have to go on indefinitely. Quite frequently the patient may be well controlled by small doses to begin with but may require larger doses later. As undesirable side effects mainly occur in patients on prolonged treatment the decision to initiate this must be carefully considered in each case. In our view long term corticosteroid treatment should not be undertaken until a corticosteroid drug has been demonstrated by objective tests to reverse the airways obstruction. Severe chronic asthma causes such misery, and interferes to such a very great degree with work and living, that the use of corticosteroid drugs is almost always justified. The physician's aim should be to obtain the optimal relief with the minimal dose and frequent readjustment of dose is usually necessary.

There is not a great deal to choose between the different forms of corticosteroid drug. It is best for the physician to use one particular drug and become thoroughly familiar with it. Prednisolone or prednisone are very suitable forms, as 1 mg tablets are available and these allow the precise control of dosage and the slow reduction which are often necessary and desirable.

For the patient who has an *occasional relatively severe attack*, not rapidly relieved by adrenaline or aminophylline, an initial dose of prednisolone 10 mg may be given, followed by 5 mg 4 times daily for 48 hours. If the attack is then relieved the dose may be reduced by 5 mg every 3rd day. In very severe attacks requiring admission to hospital we usually give higher doses (p. 419).

Before deciding to give *long term corticosteroid treatment* it is desirable to make sure, by serial measurement of FEV, that the bronchial obstruction is indeed reversed by prednisolone. In patients in hospital we usually carry this out by giving 10 mg prednisolone 4 times daily for a week with daily estimation of FEV. It is useful to know how long the effect will last. To avoid emotional factors influencing the result we often substitute dummy tablets at the end of the week to determine how long it is before the FEV deteriorates. If deterioration does not occur for several days the patient may be suitable for intermittent therapy. If there is any doubt about the response, several days of prednisolone treatment may be alternated with periods on placebo tablets. A chart of the FEV readings usually makes clear whether there has been a genuine response.

There is some suggestion that the frequency of side effects, such as hypercorticism, peripheral oedema and spontaneous fracture, is lower in patients on regimens of *intermittent treatment* than in those receiving prednisolone daily, although it is not quite certain whether this may not have been due to these patients having a lower overall mean dose [104]. The particular intermittent regimen may be chosen according to the time it takes for the FEV to deteriorate after treatment is stopped. Walsh and Grant [104] have used 20 mg on 3 consecutive days per week, 17·5 mg on 2 days in 4, or a similar dose on alternate days. On the whole, results were better in the patients who were found suitable for treatment 3 days per week or for 2 days in 4 than in those requiring treatment on alternate days, but this may have reflected the lesser severity of the asthma rather than the superiority of the treatment.

In patients on daily long term treatment it is highly desirable, if at all possible, to keep the daily dose of prednisolone to 10 mg or below. Side effects are relatively uncommon if this dose can be maintained. The dose will nearly always have to be varied from time to time, the physician aiming to keeping it at the lowest possible level which will enable the patient to lead a normal life. It will often have to be increased during infections or exacerbations. In most cases an increase to 15 or 20 mg for a few days is sufficient. Oxytetracycline 0·25–0·5 g 4 times daily should also be given during respiratory infection. In a very few patients the physician is forced to keep the dose above 10 mg for prolonged periods, in which case side effects are much more likely.

Side effects of corticosteroid treatment

Moon face is relatively common in those on the higher doses. Facial plethora, acne, striae, hirsutism, purpura and occasionally hypertension may be seen. Peripheral oedema is sometimes a nuisance and may even require treatment with a diuretic. The most important complication of long term therapy is osteoporosis which may lead to compression fracture of the spine or other fractures after relatively minor trauma [85 & 104]. This is due to decalcification. It seems reasonable therefore to treat long term patients with oral calcium and we find that 'Calcium (Sandoz)' 1 tablet 3 times a day is acceptable. There is,

however, no unequivocal evidence that this prevents or delays the osteoporosis. Anabolic steroid drugs have been given with the same object. Again there is no definite evidence of their value; in addition they may produce side effects and they are very expensive. We do not use them. Although peptic ulceration and its complications are frequently quoted as a complication of corticosteroid therapy, there is no real evidence that they are more common in these patients than in the general population. A few patients do complain of dyspepsia after oral prednisolone. In our experience this can always be removed by giving enteric-coated prednisolone tablets. Diabetes mellitus occasionally occurs in patients on larger doses. Tuberculosis is also a known risk and it is well to x-ray the chest of all asthmatics before starting treatment and at least at yearly intervals. A report of cataract following corticosteroid therapy [35] should be borne in mind although the risk would appear to be slight.

Patients on long term corticosteroids tolerate operation well, the dose being increased to cover the operation and the immediate postoperative period [85]. Oral administration may not be easy and cortisone acetate, 50 mg intramuscularly, may be given 6 hourly. These patients usually tolerate pregnancy well. It is often possible to reduce the dose of corticosteroids in the latter half of pregnancy. An increased dose may have to be given over the actual labour period. There is nothing to suggest that there is an increase in the complications of pregnancy or that the corticosteroid drugs adversely affect the foetus [105].

Patients on long term corticosteroids are, of course, liable to adrenal failure if exposed to undue stress, and require added doses in severe infections, after trauma or to cover operations. It is advisable that the patient should always carry a 'steroid card' giving details of the dosage and the address and telephone number of the relevant doctor.

Corticosteroid drugs in children

The main disadvantage of long term corticosteroid drugs in children is the effect on growth. Fortunately the majority of children only have an occasional severe attack. In these the drugs are quite justifiable for a brief period to treat an attack. Long term corticosteroids should be avoided if possible in children with mild chronic asthma but may be essential in a child with severe chronic asthma. The asthma may itself, of course, interfere with growth (p. 410). There is recent evidence [47] that corticotrophin does not have the same adverse effect on growth and that children whose treatment is changed from oral corticosteroids to corticotrophin begin to grow. Unfortunately corticotrophin has to be given by deep intramuscular injection (10–80 units in a single dose daily). It is claimed that children can become quite used to this, as in the case of diabetic children. It is not yet known whether a combination of oral corticosteroids and intermittent injections of corticotrophin would be equally effective in stimulating growth without requiring such frequent injections.

Corticosteroids by inhalation

Corticosteroids have been given by inhalation and it has been claimed that this allows reduction of oral steroids [29]. However, up to 16 inhalations a day may be necessary, there is some absorption from the respiratory and alimentary tract and infective complications have been reported [29]. We do not consider this method of treatment is of practical value.

BREATHING EXERCISES

It has been claimed that breathing exercises which concentrate on teaching the patient controlled inspiration, utilizing the diaphragm and abdominal muscles, have been demonstrated in a controlled trial to be superior to those in which controlled expiration was emphasized [8]. However, a very important part of the procedure is teaching the patient to relax and giving him confidence. If a patient is persuaded that breathing exercises may help to abort an attack, the effect of the suggestion itself, apart from any technical details of the exercises undertaken, may in fact enable him to do so. Very much depends on the personality of the physiotherapist. Details of

suitable exercises may be found in a publication by the Asthma Research Council [3].

SURGERY

Glomectomy, or the excision of one of the carotid bodies, was introduced in 1942 on the hypothesis that asthma partly resulted from an imbalance in the autonomic nervous system. It has been widely practised in certain parts of the world but it is very difficult to know how far any improvement obtained is due to suggestion. A controlled trial has recently been reported [26] in which the results in a group who had true glomectomy were compared with those in a group who had a sham operation. There was a small, but statistically significant, advantage in respiratory function tested 6 weeks after the operation in those who had the true glomectomy; but by 6 months there was no significant difference from the controls. This operation cannot therefore be recommended.

Vagotomy, by denervation of one or both lungs (which also involves sympathectomy) has been carried out for asthma at least since 1923. The results have been reported with varying degrees of surgical optimism [6] but, as far as we know, there have been no carefully controlled trials so that an objective assessment is virtually impossible. Unilateral resection of the autonomic supply to one of the lungs is said to give as good results as bilateral [6] which could indicate that the successes have been mainly due to suggestion. It is said that patients have subsequent difficulty in clearing secretions from the operated lung. With the availability of corticosteroids the popularity of operation has declined. We have never recommended it to our own patients.

STATUS ASTHMATICUS

This term has been used to describe a severe attack of asthma which has continued for more than 24 hours. Such a patient is not only in great distress but also at risk of dying from respiratory failure or exhaustion. Sometimes death occurs suddenly and unexpectedly in a patient who had not appeared to be desperately ill. Because of the severe distress, because of the risk of dying and because of the latent period of 6–12 hours before corticosteroid drugs take effect, all such patients should receive corticosteroids immediately. Most require transfer to hospital. The latter is essential if the patient has a tachycardia of 120 per minute or greater, if he is cyanosed, or if he is becoming exhausted. The dose of *corticosteroids* should depend on the state of the patient. If he is not too ill prednisolone 15 mg may be given immediately, followed by 10 mg 6 hourly for the first 2 days. If he is very severely ill massive doses may be given, such as prednisolone 100 mg by the mouth with or without 1000 mg of hydrocortisone given by intravenous drip over the first 12 hours [55]. With massive doses of prednisolone secondary infection is a real risk and the patient is best isolated with barrier nursing. There is no convincing evidence that hydrocortisone intravenously accelerates the speed of response. Prednisolone may be given by intramuscular injection if necessary.

The major problem is to try to obtain some relief for the patient during the latent period until the corticosteroid drugs take effect. *Adrenaline* can be given subcutaneously at once, but if the patient has previously received isoprenaline and adrenaline it is safer to give intravenous *aminophylline*. Another alternative is to give 0·5% *isoprenaline aerosol* by *intermittent positive pressure ventilation*, for instance with the Bennett respirator, but here again the risk of cardiac arrythmias must be remembered. It is a wise precaution to monitor the ECG [55]. Aminophylline may be repeated as necessary.

In a severe case it is useful to sample the Pa,o_2, Pa,co_2 and pH of the arterial blood by means of an indwelling catheter. Patients with hypoxaemia will require *oxygen*, which should be well saturated with water vapour and will usually have to be carefully controlled, especially if there is any rise in Pa,co_2. The patient is frequently dehydrated and the mucus in his bronchi inspissated. Oral fluids should be given in large amounts, as this helps to liquefy the bronchial secretions. Intravenous fluids are also helpful. In very severe and prolonged attacks with consequent acidosis (p. 47) an intravenous drip of sodium bicarbonate may be indicated. 90 mEq (100 ml of 0·3 M solution) is given intravenously over 5 min and repeated at 5–10 min intervals until the arterial pH has returned to near normal value or the clinical condition has improved.

With these procedures the great majority of cases of *status asthmaticus* are satisfactorily relieved. In a few cases it may be necessary to proceed to *intermittent positive pressure* respiration (IPPR). The 5 main indications for this are tachycardia of 140 per min or above, a Pa,co_2 of 60 mm Hg or above, a Pa,o_2 less than 40 mm Hg, a pH of less than 7·3 or exhaustion of the patient. IPPR is usually only necessary for a relatively short time so that endobronchial intubation is preferable to tracheostomy [1]. Although sedation must be carefully avoided when the patient is desperately fighting to maintain his own respiration, once this has been taken over by the machine intravenous morphine can be given up to a dose of 30–45 mg and morphine repeated as necessary [74]. Some now prefer phenoperidine or scoline as less likely to give rise to vomiting. Very high positive pressures are usually required. Conscious patients will require general anaesthesia and relaxants for the intubation.

If adequate doses of corticosteroid drugs have been administered, positive pressure ventilation may only be required for 12–24 hours though patients have been kept on this form of ventilation for as long as 6 days [1].

The question of *bronchial lavage* is controversial. It is known that in these patients the bronchi are filled with inspissated mucus. Broom [13] reports success by washing out the bronchi of intubated patients with trypsin in physiological saline. Thompson et al. [101] have carried out the same procedure by bronchoscopy under deep general anaesthesia, washing out the bronchi with 800–1500 ml of saline solution, 25–30% of which is returned. Ambiavagar and Sherwood Jones [1] find lavage through an endotracheal tube, with positive pressure respiration, more effective than lavage at bronchoscopy. They pour 10 ml of sterile, isotonic saline, warmed to body temperature, down the endotracheal tube and subsequently clear the trachea and main bronchi by mechanical suction. After a further 5 minutes of assisted ventilation they repeat the procedure. Spasms of coughing are often induced which assist the clearance. They may repeat the procedure for an hour or so.

Experience seems to vary with this method of treatment. It may well be that those who have most experience of it have the greatest success and that failure may be due to inadequate anaesthesia or to inadequate lavage. Its place in the treatment of *status asthmaticus* cannot yet be said to be definitely established.

As has been mentioned (p. 411), it is wise in all cases of *status asthmaticus* to take an x-ray of the chest to exclude *pneumothorax*. This should also be done if there is any sudden deterioration. *Cardiac arrest* may sometimes occur. Owing to the inflation of the lungs external cardiac massage is not satisfactory. If electrical stimulation is not available or is unsuccessful open cardiac massage may be required, though this is a desperate measure.

With these measures it is nearly always possible to salvage patients with *status asthmaticus* once they reach hospital. Assisted respiration is seldom necessary. But it is essential to get the patient quickly to skilled care. Many still die at home or in the ambulance on their way to hospital, because their peril has been realised too late.

CONCLUSION

Finally, as in all medicine, but particularly in asthma, the personality and enthusiasm of the doctor may have an important effect on the disease by the encouragement and self-confidence conveyed to the patient. Any new remedy may be temporarily effective. To prove its efficacy double-blind controlled trials are essential. The new remedy must be compared to previous remedies without either doctor or patient being able to identify which treatment the individual is receiving. Such a technique is essential for scientific assessment. For ordinary clinical handling of the patient, when the main objective is to improve symptoms, the doctor should use his personality to the full.

PROGNOSIS

The trends in asthma mortality in Britain have been outlined on p. 395. The initial fall in mortality after the introduction of corticosteroids has been mentioned and also the more recent rise, the cause of the latter being uncertain (p. 396). In a 20 year follow-up of a large group of asthmatics in Norway, mainly treated before the introduction of corticosteroids, Westlund and Hougen [106] found that the mortality in males was about twice that of the general population and in females slightly above that figure. In a follow-up of 1000 asthmatics of all ages in the North of England, with a mean observation period of about 11 years, Ogilvie [78] found an overall mortality from asthma or its complications of 7%, the figure being slightly higher in males than females.

There is a big difference in prognosis according to whether asthma first comes on in childhood or adult life. As already mentioned (p. 406), the prognosis for childhood asthma or 'wheezy chest' is remarkably good. In one 20 year follow up of a large group of child asthmatics Rackeman and Edwards [83] found a mortality of less than 1% and Dees [27], in a 14 year follow-up, found a mortality of about 1%. 71% of Rackeman and Edwards' cases were free from asthma at follow-up, though 21% had some other symptom such as hay fever. 29% had residual asthmatic symptoms but these were only troublesome in 11%. Goodall [53] found that only 5 out of 384 children with 'wheezy chests', seen in a group practice, were still wheezing at the age of 15. Fry [48] found that in general practice 80 out of 126 such children had only a single attack. After 10 years' observation only 13% of a group still had wheezing attacks and in only 3% were these sufficient to cause absence from school. Of 98 asthmatics with attacks beginning before the age of 15 years, 95% were free from asthma within 10 years. These last 2 series were probably diluted by children with slight attacks of wheezy bronchitis, but in more overt and severe asthma Dees [27] found that 44% of children were free from symptoms by the age of 14, 36%

had only mild attacks after that age and only 20% had severe episodes. Ogilvie [78] found that 60% of patients first seen with asthma before the age of 16 were in good health at follow-up. The prognosis is probably less good in children with infantile eczema followed by asthma. In a 10 year follow-up of a small group of such children Burrows and Penman [14] found that 80% still had chest symptoms; but most of these children would not yet have reached puberty, so the prognosis might be better than these figures suggest.

Apart from the better prognosis in patients whose asthma started in childhood, Ogilvie [78] found that the outlook was very much better, both for survival and for improvement in symptoms, in patients with intermittent as compared to those with continuous asthma. Only 2% of those with intermittent asthma had died compared to 9% of those with continuous. The condition at follow-up was poor in only 10% of those with intermittent asthma compared to 25% of continuous. The follow-up condition was good, with complete freedom from symptoms for 2 years or only very mild attacks, in 65% of those with intermittent asthma compared to 37% of those with continuous. He found that complicating bronchitis has an important adverse effect on prognosis. Bronchitis was very much commoner in those with continuous asthma. Although it was difficult to be quite certain about the clinical facts, he thought it likely that almost all the deaths had occurred in this group. The follow-up condition was poor in only 1% of those without bronchitis, but in 30% of those with it.

Although the majority of the patients in the series quoted were treated, during most of their period of observation, at a time when corticosteroid drugs were not available, it is likely that these would mainly have had an effect in modifying symptoms and perhaps in avoiding some deaths. In a group followed up at the present time there would no doubt be some change in emphasis and some variation in individuals, but it is probable that the overall pattern would not be radically different.

REFERENCES

[1] AMBIAVAGAR M. & SHERWOOD JONES E. (1967) Resuscitation of the moribund asthmatic. Use of intermittent positive pressure ventilation, bronchial lavage and intravenous infusions. *Anaesthesia* 22, 375.

[2] ARBORELIUS M.Jr., EKWALL B., JERNÉRUS R., LUNDIN G. & SUANBERG L. (1962) Unilateral provoked bronchial asthma in man. *J. clin. Invest.* 41, 1236.

[3] ASTHMA RESEARCH COUNCIL (1939) *Physical Exercises for Asthma*, 3rd Edition. London.

[4] AUGUSTIN R. (1966) Transmission of maternal immunity. Letter in *Lancet* ii, 1312.

[5] BATES D.V. & CHRISTIE R.V. (1964) *Respiratory Function in Disease. An Introduction to the Integrated Study of the Lung*. Philadelphia, Saunders.

[6] BELCHER J.R. (1961) The surgical treatment of asthma. *Br. J. Dis. Chest* 55, 77.

[7] BOHROD M.G. (1958) Pathologic manifestations of allergic and related mechanisms in diseases of the lungs. *Int. Arch. Allergy* 13, 39.

[8] BOLTON J.H., GANDEVIA B. & ROSS MURIEL (1956) The rationale of breathing exercises in asthma with results of a controlled clinical trial. *Med. J. Austr.* 2, 675.

[9] BOUHUYS A., JÖNSSON R., LICHTNECKERT S., LINDELL S.-E., LUNDGREN C., LUNDIN G. & RINGQUIST T.R. (1960) Effects of histamine on pulmonary ventilation in man. *Clin. Sci.* 19, 79.

[10] BRISTOW V.G. (1962) Aetiology of asthma—allergic and infective factors. *Bull. postgrad. Committee in Medicine, University of Sydney* 18, 50.

[11] BROCKLEHURST W.E. (1962) Slow reacting substance and related compounds. In *Progress in Allergy*, No. 6. Ed. Kallós P. and Waksman, B.H. Basel, Karger.

[12] BROCKLEHURST W.E. (1963) Pharmacological mediators of hypersensitivity reactions. In *Clinical Aspects of Immunology*. Ed. Gell P.G.H. and Coombs R.R.A. Oxford, Blackwell Scientific Publications.

[13] BROOM B. (1960) Intermittent positive pressure respiration and therapeutic bronchial lavage in intractable status asthmaticus. *Lancet* i, 899.

[14] BURROWS D. & PENMAN R.W.B. (1960) Prognosis of eczema–asthma syndrome. *Br. med. J.* ii, 825.

[15] CAMPBELL E.J.M., MARTIN H.B. & RILEY R.L. (1957) Mechanisms of airway obstruction. *Bull. Johns Hopkins Hosp.* 101, 329.

[16] CARDELL B.S. & PEARSON R.S.B. (1959) Death in asthmatics. *Thorax* 14, 341.

[17] CHOBOT R., UVITSKY I.H. & DUNDY H. (1951) The relationship of the etiologic factors in asthma in infants and children. *J. Allergy* 22, 106.

[18] CITRON K.M., FRANKLAND A.W. & SINCLAIR J.D. (1958) Inhalation tests of bronchial hypersensitivity in pollen asthma. *Thorax* 13, 229.

[19] CITRON K.M. (1966) Injection treatment for desensitization in asthma, hay fever and allergic rhinitis. *Br. J. Dis. Chest* 60, 1.

[20] CODE C.F., HURN MARGARET M. & MITCHELL R.G. (1964) Histamine in human disease. *Mayo Clin. P.* 39, 715.

[21] COHEN M.B. & ABRAM L.E. (1948) Growth patterns of allergic children. A statistical study using the grid technique. *J. Allergy* 19, 165.

[22] COOMBS R.R.A. & GELL P.G.H. (1963) Diagnostic methods in serology and immunopathology. In *Clinical Aspects of Immunology*. Ed. Gell P.G.H. and Coombs R.R.A. Oxford, Blackwell Scientific Publications.

[23] COOMBS R.R.A., HUNTER A., JONAS W.E., BENNICH H., JOHANSSON S.G.O. & PANZANI R. (1968) Detection of IgE (IgND) specific antibody (probably reagin) to castor-bean allergen by the red-cell-linked antigen–antiglobulin reaction. *Lancet* i, 1115.

[24] CROFTON J.W., LIVINGSTONE J.L., OSWALD N.C. & ROBERTS A.T.M. (1952) Pulmonary eosinophilia. *Thorax* 7, 1.

[25] CROMPTON G.K. (1968) A comparison of responses to bronchodilator drugs in chronic bronchitis and chronic asthma. *Thorax* 23, 46.

[26] CURRAN W.S., OSER J.F., LONGFIELD A.N., BRODERICK E.G. & CULVAHOUSE B.M. (1966) Glomectomy for severe bronchial asthma. A double-blind study. *Am. Rev. resp. Dis.* 93, 84.

[27] DEES SUSAN C. (1957) Development and course of asthma in children. *Am. J. Dis. Child.* 93, 228.

[28] DEKKER E. & GROEN J. (1956) Reproducible psychogenic attacks of asthma: a laboratory study. *J. Psychosom. Res.* 1, 58.

[29] DENNIS M. & ITKIN I.H. (1964) Effectiveness and complications of aerosol dexamethasone phosphate in severe asthma. *J. Allergy* 35, 70.

[30] DERBES V.J., WEAVER N.K. & COTTON A.L. (1951) Complications of bronchial asthma. *Am. J. med. Sci.* 222, 88.

[31] DOLL R., SPEIZER F., HEAF P. & STRANG L. (1967) Increased deaths from asthma. Letter in *Br. med. J.* i, 756.

[32] DOUGLAS A., SIMPSON D., MERCHANT SYLVIA, CROMPTON G. & CROFTON J. (1966) The measurement of endomural bronchial (or 'squeeze') pressures in bronchitis and asthma. *Am. Rev. resp. Dis.* 93, 693.

[33] EDITORIAL (1961) Drug treatment in asthma. *Lancet* i, 654.

[34] EDITORIAL (1963) Alcohol and asthma. *Lancet* ii, 1211.

[35] EDITORIAL (1963) Corticosteroid cataract. *Br. med. J.* i, 1628.

[36] EDITORIAL (1965) Adrenal function and asthma. *Lancet* i, 853.

[37] EDITORIAL (1966) Local asthmas. *Lancet* i, 1360.

[38] EDITORIAL (1966) Aerosol bronchodilators. *Lancet* i, 307.

[39] EDITORIAL (1968) Reagin and IgE. *Lancet* i, 1131.

[40] EDWARDS G. (1964) Orciprenaline in treatment of airways obstruction in chronic bronchitis. *Br. med. J.* i, 1015.

[41] FELARCA ALLISON B. & ITKIN I.H. (1966) Studies with the quantitative-inhalation challenge technique. I. Curve of dose response to acetyl-beta-methylcholine in patients with asthma of known and unknown origin, hay fever subjects and nonatopic volunteers. *J. Allergy* 37, 223.

[42] FISHERMAN E.W., FEINBERG S.M., FEINBERG A.R. & PRUZANSKY J.J. (1960) Homochlorcyclizine: an antiallergic drug with multiple clinical properties. *J. Allergy* 31, 232.

[43] FRANKLAND A.W., HUGHES W.H. & GORRILL R.H. (1955) Autogenous bacterial vaccines in treatment of asthma. *Br. med. J.* ii, 941.

[44] FRANKLAND A.W. (1961) Microbic flora and therapy with bacterial vaccines in chronic bronchitis with secondary asthma. *Folia allergol.* 8, 200.

[45] FRANKLAND A.W. (1963) The pathogenesis of asthma, hay fever and atopic diseases. In *Clinical Aspects of Immunology*, Ed. Gell P.G.H. and Coombs R.R.A. Oxford, Blackwell Scientific Publications.

[46] FRIEDEWALD V.E. (1952) Is skin testing in allergic patients worth the effort? *J. Allergy* 23, 420.

[47] FRIEDMAN M. & STRANG L.B. (1966) Effect of longterm corticosteroids and corticotrophin on the growth of children. *Lancet* ii, 568.

[48] FRY J. (1961) 'Acute wheezy chests': clinical patterns and natural history. *Br. med. J.* i, 227.

[49] FRY J. (1962) On Respiratory diseases. In *Studies on Medical and Population Subjects, No. 14—Morbidity Statistics from General Practice: Volume III (Disease in General Practice)*. Research Committee of the College of General Practitioners. London, H.M. Stationery Office.

[50] GAARDE F.W., PRICKMAN L.E. & RASZKOWSKI H.J. (1942) Is the asthmatic patient a good surgical risk? *J. Am. med. Ass.* 120, 431.

[51] GANDEVIA B. (1962) Management of asthma-bronchodilators. *Bull. postgrad. Committee in Medicine, Univ. Sydney* 18, 77.

[52] GLYNN A.A. & MICHAELS L. (1960) Bronchial biopsy in chronic bronchitis and asthma. *Thorax* 15, 142.

[53] GOODALL J.F. (1958) The natural history of common respiratory infection in children and some principles in its management. III.

Wheezy children. *J. Coll. Gen. Practitioners* **1**, 51.

[54] GRAHAM P.J., RUTTER M.L., YULE W. & PLESS I.B. (1967) Childhood asthma: a psychosomatic disorder? Some epidemiological considerations. *Br. J. prev. soc. Med.* **21**, 78.

[55] GRANT I.W.B. (1966) Treatment of status asthmaticus. *Lancet* **i**, 363.

[56] GREENBERG M.J. & PINES A. (1967) Pressurized aerosols in asthma. *Br. med. J.* **i**, 563.

[57] HAFEZ F.F. & CROMPTON G.K. (1968) The forced expiratory volume after hyperventilation in bronchitis and asthma. *Br. J. Dis. Chest* **62**, 41.

[58] HAJOS MARY-KATHARINE (1960) A comparative study of skin test and bronchial tests with bacterial solutions in infective bronchial asthma. *Acta allerg. Kbh.* **15**, 517.

[59] HERXHEIMER H. (1949) Antihistamines in bronchial asthma. *Br. med. J.* **ii**, 901.

[60] HERXHEIMER H. (1951) Induced asthma in man. *Lancet* **i**, 1337.

[61] HERXHEIMER H. (1951) Bronchial obstruction induced by allergens, histamine and acetyl-beta-methylcholine chloride. *Internat. Arch. Allergy* **2**, 27.

[62] HERXHEIMER H., HYDE H.A. & WILLIAMS D.A. (1966) Allergic asthma caused by fungal spores. *Lancet* **i**, 572.

[63] HIDDLESTONE H.J.H. (1964) Bronchial asthma and pregnancy. *N.Z. med. J.* **63**, 521.

[64] INKLEY S.R. & O'SEASOHN R.D. (1967) A study of illness in a group of Cleveland families. Ventilatory function in young adults a decade after repeated wheezing in childhood. *Am. Rev. resp. Dis.* **96**, 408.

[65] JOHANSSON S.G.O. (1967) Raised levels of a new immunoglobulin class (IgND) in asthma. *Lancet* **ii**, 951.

[66] KENNEDY M.C.S. (1965) 'Bronchodilator' action of deptropine citrate with and without isoprenaline by inhalation. *Br. med. J.* **ii**, 916.

[67] LECKIE W.J.H. & HORNE N.W. (1965) Preliminary assessment of deptropine dihydrogen citrate in chronic airways obstruction. *Thorax* **20**, 317.

[68] LEIGH D. & MARLEY E. (1967) *Bronchial Asthma: a Genetic, Population and Psychiatric Study*. Oxford, Pergamon Press.

[69] LOGAN W.P.D. & CUSHION A.A. (1958) *Studies on Medical and Population Subjects, No. 14—Morbidity Statistics from General Practice: Volume I. (General)*. London, H.M. Stationery Office.

[70] MCALLEN MONICA K. (1961) Bronchial sensitivity testing in asthma. An assessment of the effect of hyposensitization in house dust and pollen-sensitive asthmatic subjects. *Thorax* **16**, 30.

[71] MCALLEN MONICA K., HEAF P.J.D. & MCINROY P. (1967) Depôt grass-pollen injections

in asthma: effect of repeated treatment on clinical response and measured bronchial sensitivity. *Br. med. J.* **i**, 22.

[72] MCNEILL R.S., NAIRN JEAN R., MILLAR J.S. & INGRAM C.G. (1966) Exercise-induced asthma. *Quart. J. Med.* **35**, 55.

[73] MAHER-LOUGHNAN G.P., MACDONALD N., MASON A.A. & FRY L. (1962) Controlled trial of hypnosis in the symptomatic treatment of asthma. *Br. med. J.* **ii**, 371.

[74] MARCHARD P. & VAN HASSELT H. (1966) Last-resort treatment of status asthmaticus. *Lancet* **i**, 227.

[75] MESSER J.W., PETERS G.A. & BENNETT W.A. (1960) Causes of death and pathologic findings in 304 cases of bronchial asthma. *Dis. Chest* **38**, 616.

[76] MILLER F.J.W., COURT S.D.M., WALTON W.S. & KNOX E.G. (1960) *Growing up in Newcastle-upon-Tyne*. London, Oxford University Press.

[77] NAYLOR B. (1962) The shedding of the mucosa of the bronchial tree in asthma. *Thorax* **17**, 69.

[78] OGILVIE A.G. (1962) Asthma: a study in prognosis of 1000 patients. *Thorax* **17**, 183.

[79] PALMER K.N.V. & DIAMENT M.L. (1967) Spirometry and blood gas tensions in bronchial asthma and chronic bronchitis. *Lancet* **ii**, 383.

[80] PARISH W.E. & PEPYS J. (1963) Allergic reactions in the lung. In *Clinical Aspects of Immunology*. Ed. Gell P.G.H. and Coombs R.R.A. Oxford, Blackwell Scientific Publications.

[81] PEARSON R.S.B. (1965) Depôt injections in the treatment of hay fever and pollen asthma. *Br. med. J.* **ii**, 1148.

[82] PEPYS J. (1963) Skin tests in diagnosis. In *Clinical Aspects of Immunology*. Ed. Gell P.G.H. and Coombs R.R.A. Oxford, Blackwell Scientific Publications.

[83] RACKEMANN F.M. & EDWARDS MARY C. (1952) Asthma in children. A follow up study of 688 patients after an interval of twenty years. *New Engl. J. Med.* **246**, 815, 858.

[84] RATNER B. & SILBERMAN D.E. (1953) Critical analysis of the hereditary concept of allergy. *J. Allergy* **24**, 371.

[85] REES H.A. & WILLIAMS D.A. (1962) Long term steroid therapy in chronic intractable asthma. A study of 317 adult asthmatics on continuous steroid therapy for an average period of 2½ years. *Br. med. J.* **i**, 1575.

[86] REES L. (1967) Aetiological factors in asthma. *Hospital Medicine* **1**, 1101.

[87] REES H.A., MILLAR J.S. & DONALD K.W. (1967) Adrenaline in bronchial asthma. *Lancet* **ii**, 1164.

[88] REES H.A., BORTHWICK R.C., MILLAR J.S. & DONALD K.W. (1967) Aminophylline in bronchial asthma. *Lancet* **ii**, 1167.

[89] ROBERTSON C.K. & SINCLAIR K. (1954) Fatal bronchial asthma. A review of 18 cases. *Br. med. J.* i, 187.

[90] SCHILD H.O. HAWKINS D.P., MONGAR J.L. & HERXHEIMER H. (1951) Reactions of isolated human asthmatic lung and bronchial tissue to a specific antigen. *Lancet* ii, 376.

[91] SCHWARTZ M. (1952) Heredity in bronchial asthma. *Acta allerg. Kbh.* 5, Suppl. 2.

[92] SIMON S.W. & RINARD L.A. (1961) Bacterial antigen complexes (Hoffmann). An evaluation of skin test specificity versus patient reaction. *Ann. Allergy* 19, 877.

[93] SPEIZER F.E., DOLL R. & HEAF P. (1968) Observations on recent increase in mortality from asthma. *Br. med. J.* i, 335.

[94] SPEIZER F.E., DOLL R., HEAF P. & STRANG L.B. (1968) Investigation into use of drugs preceding death from asthma. *Br. med. J.* i, 339.

[95] SPENCER H. (1962) *Pathology of the Lung.* Pergamon Press, Oxford, p. 570.

[96] STANWORTH D.R. (1963) Reagins. *Br. med. Bull.* 19, 235.

[97] SWINEFORD O.Jr., JOHNSON E.R.Jr., COOK H.M.Jr. & OCHOTA L. (1962) Infectious asthma. An analysis of the asthmagrams of 100 cases and a critical review. *Ann. Allergy* 20, 155.

[98] SWINEFORD O.Jr. (1962) The asthma problem. A critical analysis. *Ann. intern. Med.* 57, 144.

[99] TAI E. & READ J. (1967) Response of blood gas tensions to aminophylline and isoprenaline in patients with asthma. *Thorax* 22, 543.

[100] TERR ABBA I. & BENTZ JOAN D. (1965) Skin-sensitizing antibodies in serum sickness. *J. Allerg.* 36, 433.

[101] THOMPSON H.T., PRYOR W.J. & HILL JACQUE-LINE (1966) Bronchial lavage in the treatment of obstructive lung disease. *Thorax* 21, 557.

[102] TIFFENEAU R. (1958) L'hyperexitabilité des terminaisons sensitives pulmonaires de l'asthmatique. Mesure. Caractères. Causes. Son rôle en tant que facteur asthmogène réflexe. *Presse méd.* 66, 1250.

[103] VOORHORST R., SPIEKSMA-BOEZEMAN M.I.A. & SPIEKSMA F. Th.M. (1964) Is a mite (Dermatophagoides sp.) the producer of house dust allergen? *Allerg. Asthma (Leipzig)* 10, 329.

[104] WALSH SADIE D. & GRANT I.W.B. (1966) Corticosteroids in treatment of chronic asthma. *Br. med. J.* ii, 796.

[105] WALSH SADIE D. & CLARK F.R. (1967) Pregnancy in patients on longterm corticosteroid therapy. *Scot. med. J.* 12, 302.

[106] WESTLUND K. & HOUGEN ANNE (1956) Prognosis in bronchial asthma. *J. chron. Dis.* 3, 34.

[107] WIENER A.S. (1948) Rh factor in immunological reactions. *Ann. Allergy* 6, 293.

[108] WILLIAMS ELSIE O. & WILLIAMS G.E.O. (1949) Natural history of asthma. A review of 300 cases. *Br. med. J.* i, 897.

[109] WILLIAMS D.A., LEWIS-FANING E., REES L., JACOBS J. & THOMAS A. (1958) Assessment of the relative importance of the allergic, infective and psychological factors in asthma. *Acta allerg.* 12, 376.

[110] WILLIAMS D.A. (1959) Definition, prevalence, predisposing and contributory factors. In *International Textbook of Allergy.* Ed. Jamar J.M. Oxford, Blackwell Scientific Publications.

[111] WILLIAMS D.A. & LEOPOLD J.G. (1959) Death from bronchial asthma. *Acta Allerg., Kbh.* 14, 83.

[112] WOOLCOCK ANN J. & READ J. (1965) Improvement in bronchial asthma not reflected in Forced Expiratory Volume. *Lancet* ii, 1323.

CHAPTER 25

Pulmonary Eosinophilia, Polyarteritis Nodosa and Wegener's Granulomatosis

DEFINITION OF PULMONARY EOSINOPHILIA

This term was originally coined [7] as a general one for a group of conditions in which, at one time or another, lung shadows were observed radiologically and were accompanied by a blood eosinophilia. Well-defined diseases, such as hydatid disease and Hodgkin's disease, were excluded. Subsequent to the original review [7] some of the subgroups of pulmonary eosinophilia have become better defined. For instance it seems relatively certain that tropical pulmonary eosinophilia (p. 432) is associated with a filarial infestation of some kind. Nevertheless it is still convenient to keep the term 'pulmonary eosinophilia' for the group as a whole.

In some publications this group of conditions has been referred to as 'Löffler's syndrome' but in fact the syndrome described by Löffler [30 & 31] corresponds only to one subgroup of pulmonary eosinophilia, that of 'simple pulmonary eosinophilia'. Some American publications refer to the group as the 'PIE' syndrome (pulmonary infiltration associated with blood eosinophilia) [11]. The subgroup of asthmatic pulmonary eosinophilia in which the bronchi may be blocked by inspissated mucus has sometimes been described as 'mucoid impaction of the bronchi' [20 & 23]; we doubt if this is a useful distinction.

The exact significance of the eosinophils in this group of conditions is as uncertain as the significance and function of eosinophils themselves. There is some evidence that eosinophils may remove histamine by engulfing granules containing it and may possess an antihistaminic action [6]. Increased blood histamine, associated with eosinophilia, has been shown in asthma, parasitism and tropical pulmonary eosinophilia [6] and increased histamine excretion in a case of simple pulmonary eosinophilia [13].

CLASSIFICATION

Pulmonary eosinophilia includes cases varying from a brief simple illness which may pass almost unnoticed by the patient to the severe and fatal manifestations of polyarteritis nodosa and Wegener's granulomatosis. A convenient classification is as follows:

(1) Simple pulmonary eosinophilia (Löffler's syndrome).
(2) Prolonged pulmonary eosinophilia.
(3) Asthmatic pulmonary eosinophilia.
(4) Tropical pulmonary eosinophilia.
(5) Polyarteritis nodosa and Wegener's granulomatosis.

It seems probable that in simple and in prolonged pulmonary eosinophilia there is a hypersensitivity reaction which is mainly confined to the alveoli. In asthmatic pulmonary eosinophilia and in tropical pulmonary eosinophilia the bronchi are also involved. In polyarteritis nodosa and Wegener's granulomatosis the blood vessels are mainly affected. In prolonged and in asthmatic pulmonary eosinophilia other organs may very occasionally be involved without necessarily the lethal implications of polyarteritis nodosa or Wegener's granulomatosis.

The chief characteristics of the different types of pulmonary eosinophilia are summarized in table 25.1.

TABLE 25.1

Characteristics of Different Types of Pulmonary Eosinophilia

Group	Severity of symptoms	White blood count	Eosinophils (%)	Other organs involved	Duration of illness	Fatal outcome
1. Simple pulmonary eosinophilia (Löffler's syndrome)	Slight	High normal	Usually under 20	Rarely	Under 1 month	Never
2. Prolonged pulmonary eosinophilia	Slight or moderate	High or very high	Usually over 20	Rarely	2–6 months or longer	Never
3. Asthmatic pulmonary eosinophilia	Slight, moderate or severe	Normal, sometimes high or very high	Occasionally over 20	Sometimes	Varies, often 3–4 months, may be years	Sometimes
4. Tropical pulmonary eosinophilia	Moderate or severe	High or very high	Usually over 20	Seldom	Months or or years	Never
5. Polyarteritis nodosa	Usually severe	Usually high or very high	Sometimes over 20	Always	Varies, usually months	Usually

SIMPLE PULMONARY EOSINOPHILIA [7, 30 & 31] (Löffler's Syndrome)

DEFINITION

Simple pulmonary eosinophilia is character-ized by transient shadows in the chest x-ray and by a blood eosinophilia which is usually relatively slight. Symptoms are mild and may even be absent. The illness usually lasts less than 2 weeks and always less than a month.

AETIOLOGY

Simple pulmonary eosinophilia has been described in many countries. It is probably due to a transient allergic reaction in the alveoli. A large number of allergens have been incriminated. The commonest in the cases originally described was *Ascaris lumbricoides*. *Ascaris* contains a number of substances which are powerfully allergenic. Skin tests may be positive and the condition has been repro-duced in volunteers [7]. Other worms have also been associated with the condition, such as *Ancylostomum braziliense*, *Trichuris tri-*

chiura, Taenia saginata and *Distomum hepa-ticum*. The syndrome has also occurred with a number of drugs. One of the more important of these is para-aminosalicylic acid (PAS); if x-rays of the chest are taken during febrile or dermatological hypersensitive reactions to this drug transient pulmonary infiltrations may be seen [48]. Other drugs which have been associated are aspirin, penicillin, nitro-furantoin and sulphonamides [15]. Among miscellaneous allergens are pollens (such as that of the privet, *Ligustrum vulgare*, and lily of the valley, *Convallaria majalis*), and there is an alleged association with smoke inhala-tion, poison ivy sensitivity and contact with nickel [7 & 15]. Other cases have been doubt-fully attributed to amoebiasis or hypersensi-tivity to tuberculin [7]. An increased urinary excretion of histamine has been described in one case hypersensitive to privet [13]; we know of no others in which this has been investigated. It is of interest that high levels of immunoglobulin E (IgND), the immunoglobulin associated with the reagins of allergic reactions, has been found in children in Ethiopia with a high rate of infestation by *Ascaris lumbricoides* [25].

PATHOLOGY

Occasional biopsies, or autopsies in patients dying from other conditions, have yielded some information about the pathology. The lesions in the lungs consist of irregular bronchopneumonic foci which microscopically represent small areas of alveolar exudate with many eosinophils. Foreign body giant cells are present in some cases. Although there is usually little evidence of vascular damage, in 2 cases there were perivascular collections of leucocytes and small thromboses [7].

CLINICAL FEATURES

A number of the original cases were found only on routine fluoroscopy and had no symptoms. When symptoms are present, cough is the commonest. It is usually slight but may be severe. There is often no sputum; when present it may be lemon yellow and occasionally blood-stained and often contains eosinophils. Other symptoms which have been described include malaise, headache, upper respiratory catarrh, hay fever, night sweats, substernal or unilateral chest pain, as well as other allergic conditions such as angioneurotic oedema and cheiropompholyx. There is often no fever; when present it is usually relatively low and settles to normal in a few days. Occasionally high fever has been recorded. Frequently there are no abnormal physical signs in the chest, but there may be slight impairment of percussion note, diminished breath sounds or a few crepitations.

Symptoms and physical signs usually disappear in a few days, almost always within a fortnight.

RADIOLOGY

The radiographic shadows are usually fan-shaped, fairly homogeneous and with indefinite borders. They may be unilateral or bilateral and may disappear in one part of the lung to appear in another. They may be small or may occupy most of the lung field. Occasionally the shadows are nodular or rounded. In most cases they disappear in 6–12 days and, by definition, always within a month.

INVESTIGATIONS AND DIAGNOSIS

The white blood count is usually normal or high normal with a relatively low eosinophilia. Higher counts, sometimes over 20,000 per mm^3 with 25% or more of eosinophils, have been recorded. Efforts should be made to identify the possible allergen and stools should be examined for parasites. The pulmonary migration of ascaris larvae, and hence the manifestations of simple pulmonary eosinophilia, occurs usually within 2 weeks of infection. The worms only become adult in 2 months and it is after that that eggs can be found in the stools. In consequence it is wise to re-examine the stools 2–3 months after the onset of symptoms.

The diagnostic problem will arise from the abnormal x-ray shadow. The main differential diagnosis is from pneumonia, infarct or tuberculosis. The transient nature of the shadow will exclude tuberculosis. Recurrent radiographic shadows in the lung are more often due to pulmonary infarcts than to pulmonary eosinophilia but the latter diagnosis will of course be suggested if there is a blood eosinophilia. Mild pneumonia can only be differentiated from pulmonary eosinophilia by the absence of eosinophilia.

TREATMENT

As the condition is so mild usually no specific therapy is required. Any infestation may of course need treatment. If the manifestations were prolonged or severe corticosteroid drugs might be justifiable.

PROLONGED PULMONARY EOSINOPHILIA

DEFINITION

There are a small number of cases which differ from simple pulmonary eosinophilia mainly in the longer duration of the illness and of the radiographic abnormalities. An arbitrary dividing line of 1 month may be accepted for differentiating prolonged from simple pulmonary eosinophilia.

AETIOLOGY

These cases are comparatively rare. Linde-smith [29] found 61 in the literature, but a few of these seem to have been eosinophil granuloma (p. 573). They have been reported from a number of different countries and in different races. Though described both in the old and in children, the disease is commonest in the third decade. In some patients there is a personal or family history of allergic conditions. Various worms, drugs, moulds or meats have been alleged as responsible agents in individual cases. *Brucella abortus* was blamed in 2 cases and coccidioidomycosis in another two.

PATHOLOGY

It seems likely that there is an eosinophil pneumonia, but we have not found any convincing pathological reports in the literature.

FUNCTIONAL ABNORMALITY

The limited evidence indicates that findings suggesting a restrictive lesion are present in at least some cases [29].

CLINICAL FEATURES

In reported cases there has been considerable variation in severity. High fever is relatively common but the patient may appear much less ill than the temperature chart would lead one to suspect. The fever frequently lasts for a month or more and may continue for several months. Some cases have no cough, but in most there is some, often nonproductive but sometimes with sputum containing eosinophils. Haemoptysis has also been recorded. By definition none of these cases has asthmatic symptoms. Crepitations are the commonest physical finding. Lesions in *other organs* have occasionally been recorded, such as angioneurotic oedema, focal necrosis of the liver, sinusitis, eosinophilic pleural effusions and local necrosis of skin [7]. Enlargement of liver and spleen has been reported [29].

RADIOLOGY

In reported cases there has been considerable variation in the appearances, ranging from indefinite localized mottling to a relatively homogeneous shadow occupying most of the lung field. Miliary mottling has been described [29]. The edges of the shadows are often indefinite and there may not be a clear association with anatomical segments. The shadows are usually more pronounced in the upper than the lower zones and in most cases are bilateral at some stage. The shadows often appear successively, one resolving to be replaced by others on the same or the opposite side. Occasionally one individual shadow persists throughout the illness.

INVESTIGATIONS

The degree of the eosinophilia tends to be higher than in simple pulmonary eosinophilia, the total white count usually being over 10,000 per mm^3 and the eosinophilia over 10%. Counts as high as 72% of 117,000 have been recorded. Other investigations should be similar to those described for simple pulmonary eosinophilia.

DIAGNOSIS

The differential diagnosis is similar to that of simple pulmonary eosinophilia, though the more prolonged course may raise problems of pulmonary tuberculosis, which will be excluded by the changing form of the lung shadows, the eosinophilia and the absence of tubercle bacilli. Occasionally a bronchial carcinoma will have to be excluded.

TREATMENT

Once the diagnosis is established, and if there are important symptoms, it is justifiable to give corticosteroid drugs. The response is usually good [11 & 32]. It should be sufficient to give prednisolone 5 mg 4 times daily until the pulmonary shadows have faded and then slowly to reduce the dose over several weeks, using serial x-rays and blood counts to detect any relapse. The drugs may be stopped after

4–6 weeks but thereafter the patient should be followed carefully as relapse may occur and need further treatment. Prolonged follow-up is necessary in case the initial diagnosis was incorrect.

PROGNOSIS

The illness usually lasts for 2–6 months, though some recover in 6 weeks and others not for more than a year [29]. One patient still had a cough, persistent radiographic shadows and eosinophilia 14 months after the onset of the illness, though without fever and continuing to work as a housewife [7]. Recovery is usually complete although relapses have been recorded in a few cases.

ASTHMATIC PULMONARY EOSINOPHILIA

DEFINITION

Asthmatic pulmonary eosinophilia is a condition characterized by asthmatic symptoms, recurrent shadows in the chest radiograph and blood eosinophilia. The coughing up of inspissated mucus in the form of pellets or casts is relatively common.

AETIOLOGY

This is much the commonest type of pulmonary eosinophilia and the geographical distribution is world wide. It is usually seen in the 4th or 5th decade of life but occasionally in young adults. The incidence in women is more than twice that in men. About half the cases are associated with hypersensitivity to *Aspergillus fumigatus*, which may be demonstrated by skin tests (p. 408). The organism may be cultured, though often with difficulty, from the sputum, and fragments of mycelium may be identified in the bronchial plugs or casts [38]. In other cases skin tests to pollens, dust or animal products have been positive. Hypersensitivity to various drugs has been blamed in some cases [3 & 7]. Asthma, eosinophilia and pulmonary shadows have also been recorded in established cases of filariasis and schistosomiasis (p. 366). Sometimes no potential allergen can be identified.

PATHOLOGY [7]

A few patients have come to autopsy or have had a resection in the belief that the pulmonary shadow might represent a carcinoma. Examination has shown areas of alveolar and interstitial exudate containing numerous eosinophils, sometimes also neutrophils, lymphocytes and plasma cells. In some cases there were granulomata containing giant cells. In most there was infiltration of the bronchial lumen, and sometimes the walls, with eosinophils. In several cases there were areas of arteritis, sometimes with actual necrosis.

FUNCTIONAL ABNORMALITY

The predominant functional abnormality is airways obstruction due to the accompanying asthma.

CLINICAL FEATURES

There is considerable variation in the severity and type of the clinical features. Most patients in this group have first developed asthma in the 4th or 5th decade though sometimes with a history of asthmatic symptoms in childhood. There is often a family history of allergic conditions. The attacks are usually characterized by *cough*, which may be paroxysmal and result in the coughing up of small *plugs* or *bronchial casts* which are often brownish and may contain eosinophils and portions of aspergillus mycelium. There may be accompanying *fever*. Sometimes the fever and tightness in the chest persist until the plugs are coughed up, after which they both subside. Sometimes the symptoms are much less obvious and the lung shadows are found only at routine x-ray of an asthmatic patient. The attacks may recur over weeks, months or years with variable intervals but may cease spontaneously. In many cases the lung infiltrations are merely incidents in chronic or recurrent asthma but in some patients the asthma is only present during the attacks and in others it may be absent during the attacks though occurring in the intervening period.

Fever is not always present but when it is it may be quite high. Often it will last for less than 10 days but some patients may have recurrent bouts of fever lasting more than a month. In a number of cases in the literature *other organs* have been involved, without overt evidence of polyarteritis nodosa although probably towards this end of the spectrum. These complications include pleural effusion, purpura, paralyses, adhesive pericarditis, ascites, polyarthritis, pericardial effusion, urticaria, large hilar glands, encephalitis and hepatomegaly [7]. Evidence of multisystem involvement always raises a suspicion of polyarteritis nodosa and, if possible, biopsy must be done to exclude this. However, there is no doubt that some cases with proved involvement of other organs have apparently recovered, which would seem to exclude polyarteritis nodosa.

Two conditions which have sometimes been given other names seem likely to be related to asthmatic pulmonary eosinophilia. In *mucoid impaction of the bronchus* [20 & 23] there are areas of collapse and bronchiectasis characterized by blocking of bronchi with inspissated mucus. There is local eosinophil infiltration in at least some of the cases. In *plastic bronchitis* [26] recurrent attacks of bronchitis or asthma are accompanied by lobar collapse due to the blocking of major bronchi with thick mucus, which may also contain fibrin,

pus cells and blood. Thick, whitish branching bronchial casts may be coughed up. At least some of the cases have had an eosinophilia and have been associated with *Aspergillus fumigatus*. We have seen a case in which collapse of a complete lung was associated with blockage of the bronchial tree by masses of aspergillus to which the patient was also hypersensitive.

RADIOLOGY

Characteristically there are recurrent abnormal shadows, one shadow clearing to be replaced by others. They are often bilateral and are commoner in the upper zones. They vary from quite small patches to extensive and explosive looking appearances occupying much of the lung field. They are often not well-defined by anatomical segments or lobes. Usually the shadows are relatively homogeneous, though sometimes there is mottling and occasionally they are bizarre, resembling plaits of hair or 'clouds of smoke rising after an explosion in the region of the hilum and drifting up against the chest wall peripherally' [7]. It is common to find bronchiectasis in the area of the recurrent shadows and this has been confirmed pathologically in patients who, for one reason or another, have had areas of lung resected [7, 20 & 23].

INVESTIGATIONS

BLOOD COUNT

Although the earlier cases described often had high white counts and high eosinophilia, in ordinary clinical practice it is very common to encounter this syndrome with the relatively low eosinophilia which is usual in asthmatics. Occasionally the total white count is over 20,000 per mm^3 and eosinophil counts as high as 82% of 70,000 have been recorded [7].

SKIN TESTS

It is now well established that about half the cases are hypersensitive to *Aspergillus fumigatus*, a fungus which is relatively common in Britain, mainly between October and April [38]. Prick tests with aspergillin derived from fungus show an immediate positive reaction in such cases. In a small proportion the weal resolves completely, to be followed by a second nodular reaction, appearing after 3–7 hours and beginning to resolve after 24 hours. In the milder of these delayed reactions biopsy shows lymphocyte infiltration; in the more vigorous, eosinophils predominate. The appearance and disappearance of the delayed reaction is more rapid than that of a tuberculin test performed at the same time, but, like the tuberculin reaction and in contrast to the immediate weal reaction, the delayed reaction is inhibited by corticosteroid drugs [37]. Skin tests to other allergens may also be positive in some patients, including some of those positive to aspergillin.

BRONCHIAL TESTS WITH ASPERGILLIN EXTRACTS (p. 408)

Bronchial tests are often positive but may cause severe reactions.

PRECIPITINS FOR A. FUMIGATUS

These are usually present in the blood serum [38].

SPUTUM

The condition is basically a hypersensitivity; aspergillus may not be readily cultured from the sputum and repeated attempts may be necessary. With appropriate staining scraps of mycelium may be identified in the sputum, plugs or casts. Eosinophils are often present in large numbers in the sputum.

DIAGNOSIS

The radiological appearances often closely resemble pulmonary tuberculosis. The possibility of asthmatic pulmonary eosinophilia must always be borne in mind in a patient with asthma and apparent tuberculosis. The varying nature of the shadows and the blood eosinophilia make differentiation simple. Recurrent shadows must also be differentiated from pulmonary infarcts and large local consolidations from carcinoma of the bronchus. The clinician familiar with the syndrome should have no difficulty.

TREATMENT

The individual attack usually responds to routine treatment for asthma, often including corticosteroid drugs, with or without the addition of antibiotics. We have the impression that secondary infection is sometimes important. Whether prolonged treatment with corticosteroid drugs is necessary depends on the pattern of the attacks and the severity of the asthma. Response is very variable. Some patients respond quite dramatically and can be kept free from attacks with small doses of prednisolone or remain free for long periods, or indefinitely, with no treatment. Others, particularly when there is much lung damage, respond relatively poorly. We have the impression that natamycin inhalations (e.g. 2·5 mg given in 4 ml of normal saline by a Wright's nebulizer) are of definite value. In hospital they can be administered 4 times a day, after an initial 1 ml inhalation to check for hypersensitivity. This can sometimes be arranged at home but requires an oxygen or compressed air cylinder. It may be found more convenient for the patient to come up to hospital 2 or 3 times a week for follow-up treatment. Sometimes long term tetracycline drugs must be given to prevent recurrent secondary infection (p. 431).

Unfortunately desensitization to aspergillin is unsatisfactory. Patients are liable to have severe, and sometimes dangerous, reactions without obvious clinical benefit.

PROGNOSIS

The prognosis of this condition is very variable. Many patients have had asthma for years and return to their chronic state after the acute illness has subsided. Most of the acute attacks last less than a month, often only a few days, though they may recur. Recurrent attacks over weeks, months or sometimes years, are not uncommon. Some recover completely and remain symptom free indefinitely. Death may occur but this is related primarily to the asthma rather than to the pulmonary eosinophilia.

TROPICAL PULMONARY EOSINOPHILIA

DEFINITION

The name 'tropical eosinophilia' was originally given by Weingarten [16] to a condition characterized by severe spasmodic bronchitis, leucocytosis, a very high eosinophilia and a dramatic response to treatment with organic arsenicals. If the condition is to be included within the spectrum of pulmonary eosinophilia it is perhaps convenient to refer to it as 'tropical pulmonary eosinophilia'. Mottled bilateral shadowing may be seen on the chest x-ray. Previously Frimodt-Möller and Barton [17] had noted this radiological appearance, associated with a high eosinophilia, in patients admitted to a tuberculosis sanatorium in India and had coined the term 'eosinophil lung', for what was clearly the same condition; this term is now little used.

AETIOLOGY

Large numbers of cases have been published from the Indian subcontinent where it is commonest in the northwest. Many cases have also been reported from Ceylon, Burma, Malaysia and Indonesia. There are reports from many parts of tropical Africa and some from South America and the Southern Pacific [24]. Investigations over recent years leave little doubt that the condition is related in some way to filarial infestation although the exact relationship is still uncertain. The strongest evidence is that the very great majority of patients with this disease have complement-fixing antibodies for filaria in their blood serum and that the titre diminishes after cure [8, 9 & 10]. The condition responds dramatically to antifilarial treatment. By examining numerous sections Webb et al. [45] have demonstrated microfilariae in the lung, liver and lymph nodes of typical cases. Microfilariae can virtually never be demonstrated in the blood, though there are a few reported cases with typical human filarial infestation and symptoms suggestive of tropical pulmonary eosinophilia [24]. It has been suggested that the disease may represent an allergic response to filaria normally affecting animals and conveyed to man by mosquitoes. It has also been suggested, on the basis of some limited experimental work on volunteers, that an individual may be initially sensitized by any form of filarial infestation. The first infestation causes no symptoms but later infestation may then result in tropical pulmonary eosinophilia which develops as a result of a hypersensitivity reaction [24]. The exact pathogenesis still remains uncertain.

A small proportion of patients do not have complement-fixing antibodies though these are not always typical cases. Biopsies by Udwadia and Joshi [42] in 26 patients revealed microfilaria in only one, though the search may not have been so intensive as in the studies of Webb et al. [45]. It may be that the host reaction is also important; in Malaya the condition is very much commoner in patients of Indian origin than in Malayans or Chinese, though the prevalence of filariasis is similar in all 3 races.

An increased amount of histamine has been found in the blood of patients with tropical pulmonary eosinophilia, possibly a reflexion of the possible histamine–antagonistic rôle of the eosinophils, though the correlation coefficients are not impressive [6].

PATHOLOGY

Information regarding the pathology of this condition has been derived from postmortem studies in patients dying with arsenical encephalopathy and, more recently, from biopsies [9, 42, 43 & 45]. *Macroscopically* the lungs contain palish scattered nodules. *Microscopically* the alveoli in the affected areas are filled with eosinophils, neutrophil polymorphs and large macrophages. There are focal granulomata, often containing very large multinucleated giant cells among which lies necrotic eosinophilic material possibly representing degenerated parasites. The granulomata may be in relation to the terminal bronchioles; these may also show infiltration with eosinophils and shedding of the mucous membrane. In longstanding cases there is an increasing amount of fibrosis. In some areas there may be alveolar necrosis with the formation of eosinophil abscesses. The liver may also contain similar nodules, with eosinophil infiltrations and granulomata, though sometimes there are only lymphocytes. The lymph nodes may show hyperplasia with eosinophil infiltration but may be normal.

FUNCTIONAL ABNORMALITY

Patients with wheeze will have evidence of airways obstruction. Udwadia [42a] found a restrictive ventilatory lesion in most cases and impairment of diffusion in those with long-standing disease.

CLINICAL FEATURES

The disease appears to be commoner in the young than the old and there is little evidence of a seasonal incidence. The onset is often insidious with *cough*, which may be dry or with scanty mucoid sputum. The cough is often paroxysmal and distressing. The patient is also frequently *wheezy*. Cough and wheeze may occur in the early morning and closely resemble bronchial asthma or, perhaps more frequently, wheezy bronchitis. About a third of the patients run a moderate *fever*. Some may have vague *pain in the chest* and *haemoptysis* may occur. The patient may have a series of mild attacks at variable intervals, but these may become longer and more severe. In chronic cases which have not been diagnosed and treated *cor pulmonale* may develop.

The most obvious *physical signs* are those of wheeze, together with scattered crepitations and rhonchi in the chest. The liver may be enlarged, especially in children, as may the spleen [24 & 47].

RADIOLOGY

The typical appearance is of bilateral indefinite mottling, fairly uniformly distributed in both lung fields. The individual shadows are 2–5 mm in diameter. Occasionally mottled shadows become confluent to produce a pneumonic appearance. Increased striations in the lung fields are also described. Rarely pleural effusion and cavitation have been reported. Rab et al. [39] have described complicating bronchiectasis. A proportion of patients, varying in different series, have no radiographic abnormality when seen, although this may of course have been present previously.

INVESTIGATIONS

BLOOD COUNT

The crucial investigation is the eosinophil count. There is nearly always an absolute eosinophil count of more than 2000 per mm^3: at least it has been found that patients with a count above this level virtually always respond to diethylcarbamazine [35]. The total white count is almost always above 15,000 per mm^3 and may be as high as 90,000 with 20–90% of eosinophils. There is not necessarily a correlation between the severity of symptoms and the degree of eosinophilia [24]. Red blood cell count, haemoglobin or sedimentation rate have no diagnostic value.

FILARIAL COMPLEMENT FIXATION TEST

As already mentioned, this is positive in almost every case with typical clinical findings and an absolute eosinophil count of more than 2000 per mm^3. The titre may range from 1 in 5 to 1 in 320; the higher the titre the greater the diagnostic significance [24].

MICROFILARIAE IN THE BLOOD

These are normally absent though occasional cases of classical filariasis have had clinical features suggesting tropical eosinophilia [24].

SPUTUM EXAMINATION

The sputum may contain eosinophils. In appropriate cases it should be examined for tubercle bacilli.

STOOL EXAMINATION

Since many helminths can produce eosinophilia, sometimes with pulmonary symptoms, search of the stool for parasites or ova is important.

OTHER SEROLOGICAL TESTS

Raised cold agglutinins have been found in some series, as have positive Wassermann and Kahn tests [24]. About half the patients have raised gamma globulin with diminution of the albumin fraction of the serum proteins.

ELECTROCARDIOGRAM

Mild changes, such as first degree heart block, peaked P or abnormal T waves have been reported but are said to revert to normal after treatment [27].

DIAGNOSIS

If the possibility is borne in mind the diagnosis is not difficult. The typical clinical and radiological findings, combined with the high eosinophilia and a positive complement fixation test for filaria, are virtually conclusive. It is of course very easy to mistake the condition for asthma or bronchitis if no blood count is done, especially as the chest x-ray may be normal. Fever, malaise, cough and bilateral radiological changes may suggest tuberculosis, but the appropriate investigations will clarify the diagnosis. Other causes of eosinophilia, in particular intestinal infestation, should be excluded. Polyarteritis nodosa may occasionally give rise to similar miliary mottlings in the chest x-ray accompanied by an eosinophilia, but there is likely to be evidence of lesions in other organs. The same is true of Wegener's granulomatosis.

TREATMENT

The antifilarial drug, diethylcarbamazine, is undoubtedly the best to use for treatment. A controlled trial has shown its superiority over organic arsenicals, which were formerly used, and it is free from the dangerous risk of arsenical encephalopathy [2]. A daily total of 6–8 mg/kg should be given orally in 3 doses. There is usually dramatic relief of symptoms in a few days though the eosinophilia may take 7–10 days to return to normal, sometimes longer. Treatment may be continued for 10–14 days or until the eosinophil count has become normal. Sometimes it has to be continued for 3–4 weeks. In the rare case in which there is no response to diethylcarbamazine the diagnosis should be reconsidered. If it is still thought to be correct organic arsenic should be tried. Diethylaminoacetarsol (acetylarsan) is said to be safer than other organic arsenicals. It is given as bi-weekly intramuscular injections of 0·75 g for 4–5 weeks. It is suggested that the first 2 doses should be smaller in case there are any side reactions. The patient should be kept under close supervision during the course of treatment with arsenic and the urine should be examined for albumin before each injection. If there is albuminuria the injection should be omitted [24].

PROGNOSIS

It is thought that spontaneous recovery sometimes occurs and is more frequent after bacterial infection. Untreated cases may persist for months or years, with recurrences and remissions. It seems that some very chronic cases, even if finally diagnosed and treated, may be left with residual fibrosis and lung damage [42a]. Some claim that 5–10% of cases are resistant to diethylcarbamazine and that some of these respond to organic arsenicals but it may be that the resistant cases have been incorrectly diagnosed. Successfully treated cases may sometimes relapse, perhaps due to reinfestation, but appear to respond to further treatment.

POLYARTERITIS NODOSA (Synonym: Periarteritis nodosa)

DEFINITION

Polyarteritis nodosa well illustrates the thesis that classification of clinical phenomena under disease names is only an approximation. Polyarteritis nodosa is a rare disease characterized pathologically by foci of necrotizing arteritis which, sooner or later, affect many organs in the body. In about a third of patients the lung is involved. Blood eosinophilia is very much commoner in pulmonary cases. In Rose and Spencer's large series [40] it occurred in 54% of those with lung involvement and in none of those without. Necrotizing lesions not demonstrably related to arteries are also commoner in these patients and are often infiltrated with eosinophils. Many patients with lung involvement have asthma. Sometimes necrotizing lesions of the lungs and upper respiratory tract predominate in the early stages (Wegener's granulomatosis). Sooner or later other organs are involved, especially the kidneys. The ultimate prognosis is bad. When there is lung involvement and blood eosinophilia the disease comes within the definition of pulmonary eosinophilia of which, on present evidence, it may only be an extreme form. We have already noted that, in the less serious types of pulmonary eosinophilia, other organs may be affected and there may be vascular lesions; polyarteritis nodosa may differ only in the extent and severity of the arterial and necrotizing lesions.

Although polyarteritis, with lung lesions but without eosinophilia, should strictly speaking be excluded from this section, it is convenient to include here all lung manifestations of the disease. Wegener's granulomatosis should provisionally be regarded as a subgroup of polyarteritis nodosa.

Polyarteritis nodosa shades out into other forms of angiitis (see below) as well as into the more benign forms of pulmonary eosinophilia. It is possible that even the fatal outcome, which was formerly regarded as an essential feature of polyarteritis nodosa, may be prevented in some cases by corticosteroid therapy.

AETIOLOGY

Although in polyarteritis nodosa as a whole there is a predominance of males, the sexes tend to be more equal in the third or so of cases who have lung involvement [40]. The incidence increases with age, though it has been described in young adults and adolescents, and is maximal in the 6th decade [40]. It is a rare disease. Crude annual mortality in 1951–59 inclusive in New York City was 0·15 per 100,000 for males and 0·12 for females. It is between a third and a quarter the mortality from systemic lupus erythematosus [33].

The cause is uncertain. Parish and Pepys [37] point out that the disease has features in common with serum sickness, asthma, the milder forms of pulmonary eosinophilia and ulcerating lesions in the upper respiratory tract without lung involvement. Necrotizing arteritis is also found in a number of other diseases such as rheumatoid disease, rheumatic fever, systemic lupus erythematosus, polymyositis, dermatomyositis, temporal arteritis and Henoch-Schönlein purpura [1].

A possible relationship to potential allergens, such as horse serum or drugs, has been considered. In Rose and Spencer's large series [40] about a quarter of the patients had had various drugs, most often sulphonamides, shortly before the onset of the disease. Several patients had also had the thiouracil group of drugs for thyrotoxicosis. A number had had repeated courses of the same drug. However, there was little evidence of drug sensitivity in these patients and it has been suggested that drug induced angiitis usually affects the smaller arteries, arterioles and veins, whereas polyarteritis nodosa usually affects the larger arteries [1]—though in fact the smaller vessels may be involved in the pulmonary form. A number of patients have had evidence of preceding haemolytic streptococcal infection, or of preceding rheumatic fever or rheumatic heart disease which might have been related to streptococcal infection [40]. Indeed the sulphonamides, which were given shortly before the onset of polyarteritis nodosa in some cases, were often administered for streptococcal infection. A few cases have developed the disease after having been given horse serum for therapeutic purposes, but sometimes this was part of the treatment of a condition which might already have been the early stages of polyarteritis nodosa. Some of these patients had serum sickness, but this again may in fact have been part of the polyarteritis.

15—R.D.

Rose and Spencer [40] have reviewed the production of arteritis in experimental animals. This has been initiated by horse serum, by various drugs and by streptococci, but there is a good deal of species difference and neither the pathological picture nor the overall disease closely mimics polyarteritis nodosa. These authors find the experimental evidence unconvincing as a pointer to the aetiology of the disease. Similarly Alarcón-Segovia and Brown [1] have reviewed the evidence that polyarteritis nodosa might be a disease of autoimmunity and have found it at present insufficient to support this view.

It still seems possible that the disease is some sort of hypersensitivity reaction, perhaps to a variety of allergens, and it is just possible that conditions with different aetiology are included within the group. But it has to be admitted that, at the present time, there is no firm evidence in favour of any individual theory of causation.

In 25% of Rose and Spencer's series [40] the patient had a preceding chronic respiratory illness, with chronic cough, established bronchiectasis or suppurative otitis media, which had usually existed for many years. The exact relationship of this to the pathogenesis of the disease remains uncertain.

Although some have had the impression that the frequency of polyarteritis nodosa, which is in any case a rare disease, is increasing, Symmers [41] in a survey of hospital autopsies over many years, has found a decrease in the number of cases of polyarteritis nodosa, with the exception of Wegener's granulomatosis. He suspects the decrease might be due to the decreasing use of sulphonamides. On the other hand there have been increasing numbers of Wegener's granulomatosis, which he considers might represent a complication of antibiotic treatment.

PATHOLOGY

We are here concerned mainly with the lung manifestations of the disease. The following account is based on Rose and Spencer's series [40]. *Macroscopically* 3 types of lesions may be found in the lung:

(1) Necrotic and caseous areas, which may resemble tuberculosis and vary from minute tubercle-like foci to massive destruction of a whole lobe. Sometimes they are nodular and cavitated. The nodules may be scattered throughout the lungs and are grey or yellow in colour. The necrotic lesions may give rise to areas of intra-alveolar haemorrhage which may be responsible for some of the transient soft shadows sometimes seen radiologically [12]. In some cases the larynx and trachea are extensively ulcerated.

(2) Infarcts, which may be visible macroscopically but sometimes are only microscopic.

(3) Bronchiectasis, which may be related to the nodular or fibrocaseous lesions but may occur independently. As already mentioned, there is evidence that in some cases the bronchiectasis precedes by many years the onset of polyarteritis nodosa.

Microscopically the tuberculosis-like lesions consist of necrosis surrounded by giant cells (Langhans or foreign body), lymphocytes, plasma cells and often neutrophils. Histiocytes and eosinophils are scanty in the region of the necrotic foci, though in those with high eosinophilia at death there may be diffuse and focal eosinophil infiltration. In the pulmonary arteries and veins there is often much proliferation of intimal connective tissue and infiltration with neutrophils and eosinophils. The media, particularly of the arteries, often show fibrinoid change, sometimes with giant cells. Fibrinoid change may also occur in the capillaries. It is mostly small arteries which are involved, both in the lungs and elsewhere. This is in some contrast to patients with polyarteritis but without lung involvement in whom it is mainly the larger arteries which are affected and who tend not to have necrotic lesions apart from vascular necrosis. The bronchial arteries may also be involved. The usual microscopic changes will be present in pulmonary infarcts, if present, and in areas of bronchiectasis.

In the *other organs* there are, in patients with lung involvement, often granulomatous necrotizing lesions as well as polyarteritis. In patients without lung involvement the lesions are usually confined to the vessels. In the kidney there is often glomerulitis as well as the other 2 types of lesion.

FUNCTIONAL ABNORMALITY

Although we have found little in the way of direct records, presumably those with asthma will have airways obstruction. In cases with extensive lung infiltration there may be evidence of a restrictive type of lesion if this is not overshadowed by airways obstruction. Serial measurement of FEV or PEFR may be useful in following progress in a patient with asthma under treatment with corticosteroids, but the measurement of ESR, haemoglobin and eosinophils, and serial chest radiography, will be of more value in assessing the progress of the underlying disease.

CLINICAL FEATURES

We are here concerned only with those patients who have lung involvement. This occurs in about a third of all cases of polyarteritis nodosa [40]. In Rose and Spencer's series [40] all those who were shown pathologically or radiologically to have the lung affected had an *initial respiratory illness*. Manifestations elsewhere followed in most cases within a year but in some were delayed, in one patient even for as long as 7 years. This latent period was longer in those who had *asthma*, in whom the manifestations of systemic illness were delayed for more than a year in 67%, compared with only 17% in those who did not have asthma. The onset of asthma is often preceded, for varying periods, by a productive *cough* and this cough tends to persist throughout the illness. The asthma is usually chronic and severe but remissions of up to 18 months have been recorded in some patients [40]. In most cases with asthma there is a high *blood eosinophilia*. Other patients have *chronic bronchitis* with cough, wheeze, rhonchi and coarse crepitations.

The serious nature of the illness may be suspected, even before the onset of obvious manifestations in other organs, because of the accompanying *weight loss* and *general weakness*. Incidents of *pneumonia* are comparatively common, with cough, blood-stained sputum and pleuritic pain. In the chest there are usually local medium or fine crepitations. The pneumonic incidents are sometimes transient (perhaps some of these are really infarcts) but sometimes progressive in which case they probably represent necrotic lesions. There is no response to antibiotics. Some of the lesions may break down with abscess formation. The *sputum* is often abundant and purulent and may contain eosinophils. Haemolytic streptococci are found in about a quarter of the cases [40]. Occasionally there may be pleural effusion, which is lymphocytic or seropurulent. *Clubbing* may occur. *Death* may result from respiratory failure, haemoptysis or rupture of an abscess.

Other *general manifestations* consist of fever, weakness and loss of weight. Later in the disease many bizarre manifestations may occur in different organs, producing strange clinical pictures. Evidence of involvement of the *urinary tract* should lead to a suspicion of the diagnosis. Renal involvement may present like acute glomerulonephritis, usually with persistent albuminuria and macroscopic haematuria, and this is often followed by hypertension. Haematuria and dysuria may occur due to vasculitis in the bladder. *Alimentary* manifestations may include bloody diarrhoea, abdominal cramps, perforation of stomach or duodenum, or even steatorrhoea [5]. Involvement of *cranial nerves, mononeuritis multiplex, polyneuritis* or *polymyositis* may occur. *Joint involvement* is relatively common and may present like rheumatic fever or rheumatoid arthritis. In the *heart* myocardial infarction, coronary insufficiency, cardiac failure due to hypertension, and acute pericarditis may all occur. There may be nodules in the *skin* or subcutaneous tissue, which are often tender and are due to arterial lesions. Various skin eruptions, including purpura and even gangrene, may occur. *Glossitis*, usually ulcerative, may be found in some cases. Symptoms related to the *nose* and *ears* may be present, especially in those with Wegener's granulomatosis. The most common are nasal obstruction and catarrh; these may be due to simple rhinitis or to ulcerating granulomatous lesions [21 & 40].

RADIOLOGY

In the chest film a pneumonic type of consolidation is the commonest finding [40]. The shadows may be ill-defined and transgress anatomical boundaries. They may disappear and reappear over periods of 2–12 weeks; some of these may represent intra-alveolar haemorrhage [12], others pulmonary infarcts. In certain patients there may be shadows resembling miliary tuberculosis or round homogeneous shadows which may cavitate. In some cases the radiological appearances closely resemble tuberculosis. Pleural effusion may occur.

INVESTIGATIONS

A leucocytosis is common. In Rose and Spencer's series [40] 54% of all those with lung lesions had *eosinophilia* of some degree, though there was considerable fluctuation in the amount. Those with asthma tend to have particularly high eosinophilia; it was greater than 5000 per mm^3 in half of Rose and Spencer's cases. The *erythrocyte sedimentation rate* (ESR) is usually very high. Consistent with this is a high *plasma globulin*, mainly the gamma component. It seems that *antinuclear factor* (ANF) is present in at least some cases but there is insufficient evidence so far to know in what proportion [22]. *LE cells* may sometimes be found.

The crucial investigation is to prove the diagnosis by *biopsy*. The classical tissue to biopsy has been muscle but blind biopsy is rarely helpful [18]. It has been found that electromyography is a valuable tool in selecting an appropriate muscle [18]. Renal biopsy may also be useful in those with renal manifestations.

DIAGNOSIS

This may be difficult before the onset of the systemic disease. It may sometimes be sus-

pected in a patient with asthma who has a persistently high ESR, especially if this is accompanied by a high eosinophilia. In cases without asthma a persistently high ESR with obscure pulmonary lesions might lead to a suspicion of polyarteritis nodosa or lupus erythematosus. Tuberculosis, multiple lung abscesses and carcinoma may enter into the differential diagnosis. The onset of renal lesions should always lead to a suspicion of the disease, as should widespread or obscure manifestations in other organs. Fortunately polyarteritis nodosa is a relatively rare disease and is suspected more often than it is proved.

TREATMENT AND PROGNOSIS

The only effective treatment consists of corticosteroid drugs. Patients often need large doses, such as 40–60 mg of prednisolone daily. It is thought best to aim at complete suppression of symptoms and a normal ESR. When this has been achieved the dose should be gradually reduced to a maintenance one which will keep the manifestations under control. With such regimens patients in the British Medical Research Council series [34] showed an improvement in survival over the first 12 months, compared to those not treated with corticosteroids. In a more recent series from the Mayo Clinic [18] there were 130 patients followed from 1946 to 1962. The 5-year survival in 110 patients who received corticosteroids was 48% compared with 13% in those who did not. The presence of hypertension or renal disease before the start of treatment was associated with a worse prognosis. Both these manifestations developed less frequently in those who had received treatment early. There was no difference in prognosis between those with and without pulmonary involvement. Most patients had to continue long term corticosteroids to avoid relapse but side effects of the steroids did not prove of major importance.

Without treatment the course of the disease in most patients consists of exacerbations and partial remissions. In Rose and Spencer's series [40] 70% of those beginning with a respiratory illness were dead within a year but there was 1 survivor for 13 years. After the onset of the systemic disease 65% were dead within 3 months but 1 survived for more than 7 years. Death was most often due to lung complications, but renal and cardiac deaths were frequent.

WEGENER'S GRANULOMATOSIS [16, 19, 28, 36 & 44]

It seems reasonable to regard this as a variant of polyarteritis nodosa. This appears to have been the view of Wegener [46] who described 3 patients in their 30s who suffered from a relatively brief fatal illness characterized by a septic type of fever, severe ulcerating granulomatous lesions of the upper respiratory tract and renal involvement. Two of the patients had macroscopic cavitating necrotic lesions of the lungs; the third had at least microscopic arterial changes. He described the characteristic lesions of polyarteritis nodosa in all 3 cases.

Wegener's granulomatosis occurs equally in both sexes and is most common in the 4th and 5th decades. As already mentioned, Symmers [41] suggests that this variant is becoming more common and that it may be related to hypersensitivity to antibiotics, but the true causation is as uncertain as in polyarteritis nodosa in general. The *pathology* does not differ importantly from that already described for polyarteritis nodosa. Carrington and Liebow [4] state that the vasculitis mainly affects the small arteries, arterioles, small veins, venules and probably the capillaries. The pulmonary vessels are always involved.

Clinically the onset is often insidious with nonspecific symptoms of infection in some part of the respiratory tract. In about two-thirds there is persistent, purulent rhinorrhoea and nasal obstruction with crusting, antral pain and epistaxis. Occasionally there is otorrhoea, deafness or ulceration of the gums. The lung symptoms consist of chronic cough, haemoptysis or pleurisy. There is often marked constitutional upset with fever, which may be of the swinging septic type, malaise and weakness. Leak and Clein [28] state that the upper respiratory tract is spared in about a third of cases.

The upper respiratory tract lesions may lead to ulceration of the nasal cartilage or caseous destruction. Later there may be con-junctivitis, exophthalmos, sore mouth or dysphagia with ulceration of fauces, pharynx or larynx. The skin of the face is seldom affected. Sooner or later the disease becomes generalized, with involvement of the kidneys and other organs, similar to that occurring in other forms of polyarteritis nodosa. Eosinophilia occurs in at least some cases.

Radiologically, in more than 50% of cases the chest x-ray shows dense circular opacities which may be very large, often cavitate and may be solitary or multiple. In a few cases there are miliary densities, bronchopneumonia or pleural effusion [14].

Without *corticosteroid treatment* deterioration is usually rapid. Cases on an average die within 5 months and some may die as soon as 4 weeks after the onset, but occasional cases have remained alive as long as 4 years.

Carrington and Liebow [4] have described a more benign form with longer survival, though only 6 of their 16 patients had been followed more than 2 years and a number had already died. However, 2 were well and off corticosteroid drugs at the time of reporting and one was clinically well though still with a raised sedimentation rate. One patient was still surviving 13 years after the onset and $6\frac{1}{2}$ years after starting corticosteroid drugs, which were still being maintained at the time of reporting. Fred et al. [16] reviewed the reports of 38 cases treated with corticosteroids, in 22 of which it was possible to evaluate the results. All of these showed varying degrees of improvement, sometimes only temporary. Lesions in the kidney were less favourably affected. These authors state that the lesions in the lungs may sometimes undergo spontaneous regression.

Corticosteroid drugs should be given in the same way as already suggested for pulmonary polyarteritis nodosa (p. 438). In the initial stages, if the lesions are localized, Walton [44] has suggested the use of radiotherapy and this seems to have been effective in some cases.

REFERENCES

[1] ALARCÓN-SEGOVIA D. & BROWN A.L. (1964) Classification and etiologic aspects of necrotizing angiitides: an analytic approach to a confused subject with a critical review of the evidence for hypersensitivity in polyarteritis nodosa. *Proc. Staff Meet. Mayo Clin.* **39**, 205.

[2] BAKER S.J., RAJAN K.T. & DEVADATTA S. (1959) Treatment of tropical eosinophilia. A controlled trial. *Lancet* **ii**, 144.

[3] BELL R.J.M. (1964) Pulmonary infiltration with eosinophils caused by chlorpropamide. *Lancet* **i**, 1249.

[4] CARRINGTON C.B. & LIEBOW A.A. (1966) Limited forms of angiitis and granulomatosis of Wegener's type. *Am. J. Med.* **41**, 497.

[5] CARRON D.B. & DOUGLAS A.P. (1965) Steatorrhoea in vascular insufficiency of the small intestine. Five cases of polyarteritis nodosa and allied disorders. *Quart. J. Med. N.S.* **34**, 331.

[6] CODE C.F., HURN MARGARET M. & MITCHELL R.G. (1964) Histamine in human disease. *Mayo Clin. P.* **39**, 715.

[7] CROFTON J.W., LIVINGSTONE J.L., OSWALD N.C. & ROBERTS A.T.M. (1952) Pulmonary eosinophilia. *Thorax*, **7**, 1.

[8] DANARAJ T.J. (1958) The treatment of eosinophilic lung (tropical eosinophilia) with diethylcarbamazine. *Quart. J. Med. N.S.* **27**, 243.

[9] DANARAJ T.J. (1959) Pathologic studies in eosinophilic lung (tropical eosinophilia) *Arch. Path.* **67**, 515.

[10] DANARAJ T.J., DA SILVA L.S. & SCHACHER J.F. (1959) The serological diagnosis of eosinophilic lung (tropical eosinophilia) and its etiological implications. *Am. J. trop. Med. Hyg.* **8**, 151.

[11] DIVERTIE M.B. & OLSEN A.M. (1960) Pulmonary infiltration associated with blood eosinophilia (PIE): a clinical study of Löffler's syndrome and of periarteritis nodosa with PIE syndrome. *Dis. Chest* **37**, 340.

[12] DIVERTIE M.B. & JOHNSON W.J. (1966) Pulmonary involvement in renal disease. *Med. Clin. N. Am.* **50**, 1055.

[13] DUNÉR H. & PERNOW B. (1956) The urinary excretion of histamine in a case of Loeffler's syndrome. *Acta med. scand.*, **156**, 313.

[14] FELSON B. & BRAUNSTEIN H. (1958) Noninfectious necrotising granulomatosis: Wegener's syndrome, lethal granuloma and allergic angiitis and granulomatosis. *Radiology* **70**, 326.

[15] FORD R.M. (1966) Transient pulmonary eosinophilia and asthma. A review of 20 cases occurring in 5702 asthma sufferers. *Am. Rev. resp. Dis.* **93**, 797.

[16] FRED H.L., LYNCH E.C., GREENBERG S.D. & GONZALES-ANGULO A. (1964) A patient with Wegener's granulomatosis exhibiting unusual clinical and morphologic features. *Am. J. Med.* **37**, 311.

[17] FRIMODT-MÖLLER C. & BARTON R.M. (1940) A pseudotuberculosis condition associated with eosinophilia. *Ind. med. Gaz.* **75**, 607.

[18] FROHNERT P.P. & SHEPS S.G. (1967) Long-term follow up study of periarteritis nodosa. *Am. J. Med.* **43**, 8.

[19] GILLANDERS L.A. & BRANWOOD A.W. (1965) Wegener's granulomatosis. *Scot. med. J.* **10**, 75.

[20] GREER A.E. (1957) Mucoid impaction of the bronchi. *Ann. intern. Med.* **46**, 506.

[21] HARVEY A.M. (1963) Polyarteritis. In *Cecil-Loeb Textbook of Medicine.* Ed. Beeson, P.B. and McDermott W., 11th Edition. Philadelphia, Saunders.

[22] HOLBOROW E.J. (1963) Systemic lupus erythematosus. In *Clinical Aspects of Immunology*, ed. Gell P.G.H. and Coombs R.R.A. Oxford, Blackwell Scientific Publications.

[23] HUTCHESON J.B., SHAW R.R., PAULSON D.D. & KEE J.L. (1960) Mucoid impaction of the bronchi. *Am. J. Clin. Path.* **33**, 427.

[24] ISLAM N. (1964) *Tropical Eosinophilia.* Chittagong, Anwara, Islam.

[25] JOHANSSON S.G.O., MELLBIN T. & VAHLQUIST B. (1968) Immunoglobulin levels in Ethiopian preschool children with special reference to high concentrations of immunoglobulin E (IgND). *Lancet* **i**, 1118.

[26] JOHNSON R.S. & SITA-LUMSDEN E.G. (1960) Plastic bronchitis. *Thorax* **15**, 325.

[27] JOHNY K.V. & ANANTHACHARI M.D. (1965) Cardiovascular changes in tropical eosinophilia. *Am. Ht. J.* **69**, 591.

[28] LEAK D. & CLEIN G.P. (1967) Acute Wegener's granulomatosis. *Thorax* **22**, 437.

[29] LINDESMITH L. (1964) Prolonged pulmonary infiltration with eosinophilia. *N. Carolina med. J.* **25**, 466.

[30] LÖFFLER W. (1932) Zur Differential-Diagnose der Lungeninfiltrierungen: über flüchtige Succedan-Infiltraten (mit Eosinophilie). *Beitr. Klin. Tuberk.* **79**, 368.

[31] LÖFFLER W. (1936) Die flüchtigen Lungeninfiltrate mit Eosinophilie. *Schweitz. med. Wschr.* **66**, 1069.

[32] MARK L. (1954) Loeffler's syndrome, with a report of 23 cases. *Dis. Chest* **25**, 128.

[33] MASI A.T. (1967) Population studies in rheumatic disease. *Ann. Rev. Med.* **18**, 185.

[34] MEDICAL RESEARCH COUNCIL (Collagen Diseases and Hypersensitivity Panel) (1960) Treatment of polyarteritis nodosa with cortisone. Results after 3 years. *Br. med. J.* **i**, 1399.

[35] NARANG R.K. & JAIN S.C. (1966) Oral diethyl-

carbamazine in tropical pulmonary eosinophilia. *Br. J. Dis. Chest* **60**, 93.

[36] NIELSEN K., CHRISTIANSEN I. & JENSEN E. (1967) Wegener's granulomatosis. A survey and 3 cases. *Acta med. scand.* **181**, 577.

[37] PARISH W.E. & PEPYS J. (1963) Allergic reactions in the lung. In *Clinical Aspects of Immunology*, ed. Gell P.G.H. and Coombs R.R.A. Oxford, Blackwell Scientific Publications.

[38] PEPYS J., RIDDELL R.W., CITRON K.W., CLAYTON Y.M. & SHORT E.I. (1959) Clinical and immunologic significance of *Aspergillus fumigatus* in the sputum. *Am. Rev. Tuberc.* **80**, 167.

[39] RAB S.M., SHAKUR S.A. & ALAM M. (1966) Complications and sequelae of tropical eosinophilia. *Br. J. Dis. Chest* **60**, 44.

[40] ROSE G.A. & SPENCER H. (1957) Polyarteritis nodosa. *Quart. J. Med. N.S.* **26**, 43.

[41] SYMMERS W.ST.C. (1962) The occurrence of angiitis and of other generalized diseases of connective tissues as a consequence of the administration of drugs. *Proc. roy. Soc. Med.* **55**, 20.

[42] UDWADIA F.E. & JOSHI V.V. (1964) A study of tropical eosinophilia. *Thorax* **19**, 548.

[42a] UDWADIA F. E. (1967) Tropical eosinophilia— A correlation of clinical, histopathologic and lung function studies. *Dis. Chest*, **52**, 531.

[43] VISWANATHAN R. (1947) Postmortem appearance in tropical eosinophilia. *Ind. med. Gaz.* **82**, 49.

[44] WALTON E.W. (1958) Giant cell granuloma of the respiratory tract (Wegener's granulomatosis). *Br. med. J.* **ii**, 265.

[45] WEBB J.K.G., JOB C.K. & GAULT E.W. (1960) Tropical eosinophilia. Demonstration of microfilariae in lung, liver and lymph nodes. *Lancet* **i**, 836.

[46] WEGENER F. (1936) Über generalisierte, septische Gefässer Krankungen. *Verh. dtsch. path. Ges.* **29**, 202.

[47] WEINGARTEN R.J. (1943) Tropical eosinophilia. *Lancet* **i**, 103.

[48] WOLD D.E. & ZAHN D.W. (1956) Allergic (Loeffler's) pneumonitis occurring during antituberculous chemotherapy: Report of 3 cases. *Am. Rev. Tuberc.* **74**, 445.

CHAPTER 26

Pneumothorax and Mediastinal Emphysema

DEFINITION, VARIETIES AND PATHOLOGY

The term pneumothorax always has the precise meaning of air in the *pleural cavity*. The normal pleural 'cavity' is a potential rather than an actual space for the visceral and parietal layers are held in contact by the cohesion of their moist surfaces. If the surfaces are separated by the introduction of air *via* a manometer needle the elastic retraction of the lung results in a negative pressure recording (p. 21). This is the force that draws air into the pleural cavity in pneumothorax. The hole through which air enters the cavity may be in the visceral or parietal pleura and may be the result of *disease*, chiefly lung disease, *traumatic injury* with or without penetrating wounds of the chest or the *deliberate introduction of air*. Corresponding to these 3 causative factors there are 3 principal types of pneumothorax—respectively *spontaneous, traumatic* and *artificial pneumothorax*.

Pneumothorax of whatever type may be *localized* when part of the pleural cavity has been obliterated by adhesions, or *generalized* when the whole cavity contains air. Furthermore, a pneumothorax is described as *open* when the air moves freely in and out of the pleural space during respiration, *closed* when no movement of air takes place, *valvular* when air enters during inspiration and is prevented from escaping during expiration. A valvular pneumothorax tends to enlarge progressively, and often rapidly, displacing the mediastinum, kinking the great veins, and causing increasing cardiac and respiratory embarrassment. At this stage it is usually termed a *tension pneumothorax* because of the rising pressure which builds up in the pleural cavity. If a pneumothorax is closed it means that the hole through which air entered has been sealed off. An open pneumothorax with a small hole will show fluctuations of intrapleural pressure during respiration, whereas if the hole is large and there is free communication with the bronchial system, e.g. in the presence of a substantial *bronchopleural fistula*, the intrapleural pressure changes are rapidly neutralized and the manometer records a practically constant reading at about normal atmospheric pressure.

SPONTANEOUS PNEUMOTHORAX

Spontaneous pneumothorax is by far the commonest form in clinical practice and is always secondary to pulmonary or pleural abnormality. This may be congenital or due to acute or chronic acquired disease.

AETIOLOGY

Usually the patient is a young adult male (M:F ratio 5–6:1) and the pneumothorax is due to the rupture of a pleural bleb, a bubble of air which has tracked between the layers of pleura from a minor defect in the wall of a subpleural alveolus [7 & 27]. In these patients the chief cause of alveolar wall leakage is probably a chance congenital defect in the elastica of the alveolar wall. The blebs are usually in the apical part of the lung and may be bilateral [4]. The 2 lungs are affected with equal frequency.

In patients over 40 spontaneous pneumothorax is most often due to chronic bronchitis and emphysema and the factors concerned are progressive destruction of alveolar walls and the high intrapulmonary pressures produced by coughing. When bullae are present as well as generalized emphysema it is usually from a bulla that the air escapes. When emphysema occurs without bullae, leaks may occur simultaneously from many sites on the delicate lung surface [8].

In children spontaneous pneumothorax may occur following rupture of congenital cysts derived from malformed terminal bronchioles [8 & 27]. These cysts often retain their connection with the bronchial system and develop a check valve mechanism at the bronchial opening which causes them to become distended with air and liable to rupture.

Rarer causes of spontaneous pneumothorax include bronchial asthma (p. 411), rupture of tension cysts in staphylococcal pneumonia (more commonly in children) (p. 122), rupture of caseating subpleural tuberculous lesions (p. 230) and cavities (p. 230), and rupture of tension cysts caused by partial obstruction of a terminal bronchus by carcinoma. Still rarer are the cases of spontaneous pneumothorax which follow rupture of subpleural cysts developing in the course of interstitial pulmonary fibrosis or honeycomb lung (p. 565) [37]. Spontaneous pneumothorax may occasionally occur as a complication of a number of occupational lung diseases including coalworker's pneumoconiosis (p. 478), silicosis (p. 479), berylliosis (p. 498) and particularly aluminosis (p. 492) and bauxite lung (p. 493). It is a rare complication of pulmonary sarcoidosis, occurring principally in the late fibrotic stage of the disease with associated bullous emphysema [44]. Spontaneous pneumothorax due to disease of the pleura but not of the lungs occurs occasionally when carcinoma of the oesophagus involves the pleura and establishes a fistulous connection between the oesophagus and the pleural cavity.

Escape of air through a weak area of the pleura may be initiated by marked variations in intrathoracic pressure such as may occur during ascent in an airplane to subatmospheric pressures [23] or due to too rapid decompression to atmospheric pressure of divers and caisson workers. Attention to appropriate pressurization will reduce these hazards considerably. Skin divers should be made fully aware of the dangers of surfacing with the glottis closed. Pilots who have to eject at high altitudes are also at special risk of developing a pneumothorax. Medical examination including a chest x-ray may help to exclude from exposure to these hazards those who have any pulmonary abnormality which might result in air trapping at increased intrathoracic pressures.

FUNCTIONAL ABNORMALITY

ACUTE PNEUMOTHORAX

As might be expected the functional abnormality produced by an acute pneumothorax depends on the general state of the lungs. The type and degree of parenchymal disease present determine the basic pattern of abnormality in any particular case and to this the effect of pneumothorax is added. In a patient with otherwise healthy lungs acute pneumothorax results in reduction in lung volumes and diffusing capacity to an extent comparable to the degree of lung collapse. With spontaneous re-expansion these indices of function return to normal values. A large pneumothorax (over 20% collapse) has been shown to cause immediate fall in arterial oxygen saturation [33, 41 & 50] in patients with relatively healthy lungs but because of progressive reduction of perfusion of the collapsed lung arterial oxygen saturation becomes normal within a few hours. In the patient with advanced chronic lung disease even a small pneumothorax can result in arterial oxygen unsaturation or worsen existing unsaturation. Treatment to expand the lung is an urgent necessity in these patients and the effects of whatever perfusion adjustment is possible have not been studied for obvious reasons.

Tachypnoea and hyperventilation with fall in arterial PCO_2 but normal arterial oxygen saturation occur after the experimental production of pneumothorax in the intact dog. In the vagotomized dog this compensatory mechanism does not operate and arterial unsaturation occurs. Anaesthesia also impairs the adaptation to an acute pneumothorax in dogs [25]. To what extent these observations can be applied to the understanding of adaptation in man is not known.

CHRONIC PNEUMOTHORAX

It is unusual for a chronic pneumothorax to be more than mild to moderate in degree since more than this will have demanded treatment to ensure re-expansion. The patient with chronic pneumothorax may have little respiratory discomfort on ordinary exertion but lung volume estimates will, of course, reflect the extent of lung collapse. Most studies of chronic pneumothorax have been made in patients with maintained artificial pneumothoraces [3, 14, 16, 36 & 38]. These have shown that the pleural changes and limitation of diaphragmatic movement secondary to long continued collapse can result in severe permanent impairment of function of the re-expanded lung. The pleural fibrosis imposes a restrictive ventilatory defect (fig. 16.1, p. 51) and there is some evidence that the ventilation of the normal lung is impaired, possibly by the rigidity of the affected side though by what mechanism is not known. Decortication can result in remarkable improvement of function [9, 11, 12, 39, 43 & 48] provided that the extent of the parenchymal disease is not great. Not only is ventilation improved but the freed lung is capable of re-establishing a normal circulation even although the blood flow in the bound down lung may have been minimal for many years.

CLINICAL FEATURES

Most of the patients with spontaneous pneumothorax under 40 years of age tend to be thin and underweight but these are not usual features in the over 40 group with bronchitis and emphysema. Pneumothorax due to rupture of a subpleural emphysematous bleb may follow some strenuous exertion but commonly there is no history of this. The onset is more or less sudden with unilateral *pleuritic pain* and *dyspnoea*. When the pneumothorax is relatively small it is common for the initial dyspnoea and discomfort to im-

prove after a few hours even although the x-ray shows no change in the degree of lung collapse. The degree of dyspnoea varies according to the size of the pneumothorax and according to whether the lungs are in a healthy condition or not. A pneumothorax of moderate size may cause little discomfort in an otherwise healthy young man whereas a reduction of lung volume by 10% or less may cause acute dyspnoea in an elderly patient with emphysema. *Cough* when present is usually short and unproductive (but many patients with pneumothorax also suffer from diseases which give rise to cough and sputum). The development of *tension pneumothorax* is associated with increasing anxiety, restlessness and respiratory distress to which may be added the weak, rapid pulse and cold, clammy skin of shock when increasing intrapleural pressure progressively impairs the venous return to the heart. Unless the condition is relieved death will occur from a combination of respiratory and cardiac failure.

Cyanosis is unusual in the younger patients except when severe tension pneumothorax is present, but in older patients with chronic bronchitis and emphysema cyanosis may occur even with a small pneumothorax. Fever, leucocytosis and raised ESR are not features of pneumothorax as such and if present are due to associated disease or to complications.

In a small number of cases mediastinal emphysema may accompany the pneumothorax (p. 449). Rarely pneumothorax may be present in both pleural cavities simultaneously.

In a few cases severe haemorrhage into the pleural space, usually from rupture of a pleural adhesion and involving arteries supplied at systemic pressure, will add the features of rapid blood loss to the clinical picture. More commonly any bleeding which occurs is slight.

In patients with *status asthmaticus* the development of pneumothorax may be suspected if the patient's condition appears to worsen despite treatment. It is extremely important to be aware of this complication (p. 411).

PHYSICAL SIGNS

The physical signs in the chest depend essentially on the degree of pulmonary collapse and whether or not there is an associated effusion. Small effusions generally mean that haemorrhage has occurred from a torn pleural adhesion. Larger effusions may occur in cases of tuberculosis and staphylococcal pneumonia. A small pneumothorax may not be detectable clinically.

The commonest physical sign is *diminution of breath sounds*. Unilateral *diminution of movement* associated with normal or even *hyper-resonance* on percussion may be present in variable degree. The vocal resonance is usually diminished. *Tracheal deviation* and *displacement of the apex beat* away from the affected side can be elicited if the pneumothorax is large. Bronchial breath sounds described as 'metallic' or 'amphoric' may rarely be heard. In *tension pneumothorax* distension of the chest wall on the affected side may be apparent on inspection; the physical signs include those of mediastinal displacement, and rising pulse and respiration rates indicate increasing cardiac and respiratory embarrassment. The much described 'coin test' in tension pneumothorax is of little practical value.

Right sided pneumothorax reduces the upper level of liver dullness and may actually depress the liver.

A small pneumothorax may occasionally give rise to a '*clicking sound*' (or 'crunching', 'grating' or 'crackling') which may be heard (sometimes by the patient himself), in time with the heart beat. It is often heard best in expiration and with the patient leaning to the left. A 'noisy' pneumothorax is usually small [45], often difficult to detect clinically and almost invariably left sided [47]. It may be due to sudden movement of air by the heart beat or the sudden contact and separation of the two layers of pleura. When the sign was first described by Hamman [21] it was regarded as diagnostic of mediastinal emphysema (p. 449) but it is now known to occur in pneumothorax without mediastinal emphysema.

An associated *effusion* will be clinically detectable only if moderate in size. The upper level of dullness is horizontal and moves when the patient's position is altered. The phenomenon of '*splashing*' may be elicited. 'Tinkling' sounds may sometimes be heard, particularly after coughing.

RADIOGRAPHIC APPEARANCES

The characteristic radiographic appearance in pneumothorax is the sharply defined lung edge separated from the bony cage by a clear zone devoid of lung markings. If the pneumothorax is very shallow these features may escape observation unless a radiograph is taken in full expiration. In major collapse the lung appears as a globular mass at the hilum the density proportional to the degree of collapse, and there may be mediastinal shift to the opposite side. A tension pneumothorax usually displaces the mediastinum to the opposite side. A major degree of collapse of one lung usually results in increased blood flow and congestion in the other with appearances which may simulate lobular pneumonia. Pleural effusion accompanying pneumothorax appears in the radiograph as an opacity with a horizontal upper edge. This may amount to no more than a blunting of the costophrenic angle.

DIFFERENTIAL DIAGNOSIS

In the typical case the sudden onset with chest pain and dyspnoea may simulate *myocardial infarction* or *pulmonary embolism* or *infarction* or occasionally *perforated peptic ulcer* but the correct diagnosis will usually be clear from the physical signs and the chest radiograph.

Obstructive emphysema and large emphysematous *bullae* or *congenital cysts* may be confused with pneumothorax on physical examination but can usually be distinguished by their radiographic appearances.

Diaphragmatic hernia with protrusion of stomach and colon through the hemidiaphragm (usually the left) may resemble basal pneumothorax on physical examination and even in radiographic appearances but can always be distinguished if barium studies are carried out. A history of injury, especially a crush or deceleration injury to the lower chest, either recent or in the past, may support a diagnosis of diaphragmatic hernia of traumatic origin but it should be remembered that developmental defects in the diaphragm may result in much the same radiographic appearances.

ARTIFICIAL PNEUMOTHORAX

Once a mainstay of treatment for the control of tuberculous lesions, therapeutic artificial pneumothorax has now been abandoned. A well recognized but unexplained accompaniment of maintained artificial pneumothorax was weight loss. This is still seen in cases of chronic spontaneous pneumothorax (p. 447). In modern medicine the principal use of artificial pneumothorax is as a diagnostic procedure for the differentiation of a peripheral pulmonary lesion from a lesion in the parietal pleura or chest wall.

TRAUMATIC PNEUMOTHORAX

Penetrating wounds of the chest, rib fractures and accidental puncture of the lung at pleural aspiration or biopsy are the common causes of traumatic pneumothorax. Rupture of a bronchus complicating closed chest injury [10 & 29] has become an increasingly common cause of traumatic pneumothorax in the past decade due to the increase in road accidents. Haemorrhage into the pleural space nearly always accompanies traumatic pneumothorax; the combined lesion is known as *haemopneumothorax*. Pyogenic infection of the pleural cavity is a common and important complication of traumatic pneumothorax, resulting in *pyopneumothorax* in which high fever and a polymorph leucocytosis are constant features.

TREATMENT OF PNEUMOTHORAX

The management of cases of uncomplicated spontaneous pneumothorax in young patients depends in the first place on the degree of pulmonary collapse which is present. A small pneumothorax (less than 20% collapse) usually causes little disability. Bed rest is not essential and although there should be some limitation of the patient's activities, nonmanual workers may be permitted to remain at work. The prognosis is uniformly excellent and reabsorption of the air occurs spontaneously, usually within a month. In most reported series, however, there has been more than a 50% collapse in two thirds of the cases. It has been calculated that reabsorption of air from a sealed off pneumothorax is 1·25% of the radiographic lung volume per day [26]. Thus a 50% collapse would take 40 days to expand spontaneously if no air leak persists. Most studies confirm the delay that conservative treatment entails, average times for expansion varying from 3 weeks to 3 months [24, 35 & 51]. The economic significances are obvious and compel consideration of measures to re-expand the lung rapidly. It must always be remembered that a patient continues to be in danger so long as the lung does not completely occupy the hemithorax.

When the pneumothorax is larger than about 20% and/or is accompanied by dyspnoea, air must be evacuated from the pleural cavity. This may be attempted by the use of a Foster-Carter type needle and a pneumothorax machine at the outset and this occasionally proves successful. Considerable care must be exercised to avoid tearing the expanding lung by the needle tip. Most clinicians, however, prefer as primary treatment the use of an intercostal catheter with underwater seal drainage to evacuate the air and promote a local irritative pleurisy. Under local anaesthesia a self retaining catheter of the Malecot type (size 22–28) stretched on an introducer is inserted through a cannula in the 4th or 5th intercostal space just behind the anterior axillary line, provided there are no adhesions to the chest wall in this site. With the catheter so placed any effusion which is present or may develop can be easily withdrawn simply by tipping the patient to the side. Lateral pleural adhesions and persistence of an apical pneumothorax may require insertion of the catheter in the anterior chest wall, usually in the second intercostal space. In the young female patient attention must be paid to cosmetic considerations when drainage tubes have to be inserted through the anterior chest wall. Re-expansion of the lung usually accompanies the escape of air through the catheter and underwater seal and attempts to hasten the process by forced suction are seldom necessary or effective. If the space persists it means that a broncho-pleural fistula has developed and no improvement can be hoped for from forced suction unless air can be sucked out of the cavity more quickly than it enters through the fistula. It is said that the only readily available instrument capable of this performance is the domestic vacuum cleaner!

The intercostal tube is usually left *in situ* for 24 hours after full re-expansion of the lung has been achieved; that is for a period of 3–4 days in most cases. It is well to remember that a tube in the chest can be very painful. The sooner it can be safely removed the better, but while it is in position analgesics should not be withheld and even morphine may be given provided that there are no contra-indications to its use such as severe bronchitis with emphysema. Should the intercostal catheter become blocked by fibrinous exudate it must be removed and replaced by another. It may happen that several catheters in succession are required before re-expansion of the lung and sufficient pleurodesis to prevent relapse have been achieved. If a persistent bronchopleural fistula prevents re-expansion thoracotomy should be carried out and the fistula closed. *Tension pneumothorax* may require emergency treatment by the insertion into the pleural space of a blunt ended, wide-bore needle connected to underwater drainage or to a finger cot slit so that it acts as a one way valve. As soon as possible the needle should be replaced by an intercostal catheter. Any significant degree of pleural effusion invites infection and it is important to aspirate the pleural space to dryness.

A device consisting of a plastic tube containing a one way valve has been introduced with the aim of allowing ambulation while evacuating the pleural space of air [28]. This has not yet received general acceptance. It is not recommended if there is more than a small amount of pleural fluid since the valve may become blocked before all the air has escaped. A suggested intermediate technique which still employs underwater seal is the use of a 12 or 14 FG Intracath which is much less painful than a Malecot catheter [34]. In an uncomplicated pneumothorax treated by intercostal catheter the patient is usually back to work in 1 week [42].

Thoracoscopy adds little of value to the management of pneumothorax.

RECURRENT AND CHRONIC PNEUMOTHORAX

About 20% of cases of spontaneous pneumothorax recur, most of them within a year. A few cases become chronic (i.e. persisting for 3 months or longer) because of the development of a persistent bronchopleural fistula. This occurs [7] (a) if adhesions prevent the lung from collapsing and so closing the fistula, (b) if the air leak is through a congenital cyst since epithelial tissue does not readily seal over, or (c) if, as mentioned previously, there are multiple leaks through the pleural membrane in generalized emphysema. A further reason for persistence of a pneumothorax is the development of a fibrinous peel over the visceral pleura. This is more likely to occur if there has been an associated effusion. The pleural peel may later calcify. Symptoms include dyspnoea, vague chest discomfort and weight loss.

Recurrent pneumothorax may be treated by the instillation of an irritant substance into the pleural cavity with the object of inducing a bland pleurisy and subsequent pleural adhesions. Several such chemical agents are available but the relative merits of each, and indeed the value of the method as a whole, are matters which are still debated. The use of silver nitrate to induce chemical pleurodesis has been abandoned because of the severe pain it causes. Poudrage with iodised talc is also a painful procedure, but nevertheless is regarded by some as the treatment of choice in recurrent pneumothorax [6]. The distribution of the talc over the pleural surfaces is carried out visually at thoracoscopy under general anaesthesia. Camphor in oil (10 ml of a 1% solution) injected into the space can be used instead of iodized talc and has the advantages of being virtually painless and requiring only local anaesthesia. Commonly the oil is inserted prior to attempting evacuation of the space by a pneumothorax machine, and is distributed evenly over the pleural surfaces by rolling the patient about on the affected side. The patient's own blood has sometimes been used in place of camphor in oil. In most cases, however, a first or second recurrence on the same side is treated by a further intercostal tube, chemical pleurodesis with camphor in oil being sometimes used in addition. Recurrence rates after an intercostal tube vary from 11 to 17% [40, 42 & 53] as opposed to 18–32% after conservative treatment [30, 35 & 42].

Certain major operative procedures may be required in the treatment of recurrent or chronic pneumothorax. *Pleurectomy* should be considered for patients in whom pneumothorax has recurred 3 times on the same side despite repeated tubes and attempts at chemical pleurodesis. The operation comprises stripping off the parietal pleura from the chest wall and the upper mediastinum so as to leave a raw surface to which the visceral pleura can adhere. The lower mediastinal and diaphragmatic parietal pleura is left intact. Recurrence after pleurectomy is rare. None occurred in the series reported by Ruckley and McCormack [42] and Andersen and Poulsen [1]. The impairment of ventilatory function after pleurectomy is remarkably slight [1 & 15]. When recurrence of pneumothorax is complicated by the development of a contralateral pneumothorax, pleurectomy is indicated on the side first affected with the minimum of delay. Rarely bilateral pleurectomy is necessary.

In chronic cases division of an adhesion may suffice; in other cases a rind of fibrin on the visceral pleura may have to be stripped off (*decortication*). Occasionally it may be possible to define the site of persistent leakage at operation whereupon it may be *sutured* or removed by *segmental resection*. These operative procedures usually require the patient to be in hospital for about a fortnight. In the patient with grossly impaired respiratory function from emphysema thoracotomy and pleurectomy, however desirable, may not be feasible and repeated intubation may be safer.

TREATMENT OF OTHER COMPLICATIONS

(1) *Severe bleeding* into the pleural space complicating traumatic pneumothorax or spontaneous pneumothorax with rupture of a pleural adhesion (haemopneumothorax) requires emergency thoracotomy to evacuate the clot and to secure the source of bleeding. Blood transfusion may be needed. Gaensler [15] found a reported mortality of 26% in severe intrapleural haemorrhage complicating pneumothorax.

(2) *Infection* of the pleural space with the development of empyema following traumatic pneumothorax or spontaneous pneumothorax (pyopneumothorax) associated with tuberculous or staphylococcal infection demands immediate aspiration of the effusion and the institution of appropriate chemotherapy (p. 446 and p. 272).

(3) *Atelectasis* may complicate any of the forms of spontaneous pneumothorax and may delay re-expansion. Physiotherapy may achieve the removal of viscid secretions but occasionally it may be necessary to resort to bronchoscopy.

(4) *Respiratory failure* may occur in patients whose respiratory reserve was impaired before the development of pneumothorax. Rapid re-expansion of the lung is the most important aspect of treatment. The other measures applicable are discussed in Chapter 18.

OTHER ASPECTS OF MANAGEMENT

Oxygen therapy is important in patients who are hypoxic from tension pneumothorax or chronic lung disease, the usual precautions being observed in the latter. Analgesia has already been mentioned. Complicating infection requires appropriate chemotherapy. In the rare situation where tuberculosis or bronchial carcinoma are thought to be aetiological possibilities, a tuberculin test, sputum culture, bronchoscopy and perhaps sputum cytology are indicated.

Chemotherapy with penicillin, tetracycline or ampicillin may be required if purulent sputum develops at any stage during treatment. Secretion retention resulting from painful coughing when a tube is *in situ* not infrequently leads to purulence of the sputum.

This is much more likely in the chronic bronchitic but may occur in patients with no associated chest disease.

Follow-up of cases of spontaneous pneumothorax should continue for 1 year with x-ray at 3 monthly intervals to ensure that no underlying pathology is missed. It is, however, exceedingly rare for any radiographic abnormality to develop (except for the 1 in 5 possibility of recurrence of pneumothorax) if the x-ray at the time of the initial incident was clear apart from the pneumothorax.

MEDIASTINAL EMPHYSEMA

DEFINITION

Air in the mediastinal tissues is referred to as mediastinal emphysema or pneumomediastinum.

AETIOLOGY AND PATHOGENESIS

The air enters the mediastinum directly from a *ruptured bronchus* or *oesophagus*, or indirectly either along the perivascular sheaths of the pulmonary vessels following *rupture of lung alveoli* [32], or through the retroperitoneal tissues in the rare case in which mediastinal emphysema follows *rupture of some part of the gastrointestinal tract* or perirenal insufflation.

Rupture of lung alveoli is usually precipitated by straining with the breath held in inspiration and may, therefore, occur in labour, or in any lung disease in which acute airways obstruction is combined with severe cough, e.g. bronchial asthma, bronchiolitis and whooping cough. So-called 'spontaneous mediastinal emphysema' probably follows unrecognized straining or coughing. The alveolar rupture which causes spontaneous pneumothorax may also cause mediastinal emphysema, especially if tension pneumothorax develops. Mediastinal emphysema occurring spontaneously with or without pneumothorax in the newborn may be due to rupture of alveoli or of congenital lung cysts. Enthusiastic efforts at resuscitation of an apneoic infant have sometimes resulted in

alveolar rupture followed by mediastinal emphysema and pneumothorax. Perforation of bronchi or of the oesophagus [17] is usually a complication of chest injury or local disease but sometimes it is an untoward sequel to endoscopic examination [2 & 49] and occasionally it follows the swallowing or inhalation of foreign bodies. Rupture of the oesophagus brought on by a bout of vomiting is probably due mainly to incoordinated oesophageal contraction and is characteristically associated with acute alcoholism. Spontaneous rupture of the oesophagus usually occurs in the lower 8 cms and results in a vertical tear on the left posterolateral wall [17] where the oesophagus is not supported by connective tissue.

The air in the mediastinum may escape upwards into the subcutaneous tissues of the neck and also, but much less commonly, downwards into the retroperitoneal tissues where it may result in intestinal pneumatosis. These extensions of emphysema are more likely to occur if the channel by which air entered the mediastinum remains open.

CLINICAL FEATURES

Since mediastinal emphysema is seldom a primary event the dominant clinical features are likely to be those of the condition to which it owes its origin, or of other complications which arise at the same time. Thus, two-thirds of the cases of ruptured bronchus give rise to *spontaneous pneumothorax* as well as *mediastinal emphysema*, and oesophageal rupture nearly always leads swiftly to *pleural effusion* and *empyema*, usually on the left side. Pleural effusion due to oesophageal rupture and the persistence of the pleuro-oesophageal fistula can be proved by giving the patient a marker substance (methylene blue) to swallow and noting its reappearance in the fluid drawn from the effusion.

Mediastinal emphysema *per se* is *virtually symptomless in most cases* because the air escapes freely into the subcutaneous tissues. Sometimes the patient may notice swelling and/or crepitus in the neck due to subcutaneous emphysema. When air accumulates in the mediastinal tissues, however, compression effects may give rise to *pain* sometimes indistinguishable from that of myocardial infarction, and to dyspnoea, cyanosis and hypotension. Physical signs in the classical case amount to subcutaneous emphysema, diminution or absence of cardiac dullness, distant heart sounds and coarse crepitant sounds over the mediastinum (Hamman's sign), sometimes best heard over the left sternal edge from the 3rd to the 6th intercostal spaces with the patient sitting up. These sounds are in time with the heart beat or, if present only in the upper sternal area, with respiration or with swallowing. Loud systolic 'crunching' or 'clicking' sounds may be heard over the precordium, especially if a pneumothorax (usually on the left) is also present. Hamman's sign [18, 19 & 20] is present in 50% of cases [52] and was once thought to be diagnostic of mediastinal emphysema. It may, however, be also present in left sided pneumothorax without mediastinal emphysema [46], in bullous emphysema of lingula, a dilated lower oesophagus, pneumoperitoneum with a high left diaphragm and gastric dilatation [52].

Fever may indicate the onset of mediastinitis.

RADIOGRAPHIC APPEARANCES

Air in the mediastinum is recognizable radiographically as an arc-shaped translucency scalloping the outline of the upper mediastinum, which is commonly widened, and air may outline the heart borders, usually the left [31]. A lateral film may show a substernal collection of air. Air may also be evident in the subcutaneous tissues of the neck. In a suspected case with none of these radiographic features a lateral view of the neck in the upright position may show air in the various fascial planes [5].

Pneumothorax of varying degree may also be seen in the radiograph in about one third of cases [22] and, if the mediastinal emphysema is due to oesophageal rupture, pleural effusion may be visible at an early stage.

DIAGNOSIS

The usual problem is to distinguish mediastinal emphysema from *myocardial infarction* and it will usually be decided on the basis of the physical signs and the radiographic appearances. The diagnosis is more difficult in cases with small air leaks although the ECG and the transaminase estimations may be helpful. It may be necessary to perform bronchoscopy and/or oesophagoscopy to determine the cause of the mediastinal emphysema.

TREATMENT

The cause of the mediastinal emphysema will often be the first consideration in treatment. If tension pneumothorax is present an intercostal catheter with underwater seal drainage must be inserted immediately (p. 447). Bronchial or oesophageal perforation due to an accident at endoscopy will usually be a minor injury requiring no special treatment but major perforations, particularly those due to trauma, usually require operative intervention. Pleural exudates must be drained at once (p. 448).

In spontaneous mediastinal emphysema the treatment varies from reassurance and mild analgesia to energetic measures directed towards anoxia and shock. In most cases spontaneous absorption of air occurs within a week. It has been suggested that incision of the superficial tissues just above the suprasternal notch may be made to relieve the effects of rapidly developing mediastinal emphysema associated with subcutaneous emphysema but in practice this is never necessary.

Subcutaneous and mediastinal emphysema have been shown to be improved by breathing 95% oxygen [13], replacing nitrogen by the rapidly absorbed oxygen, and it has been suggested that nonsurgical pneumomediastinum would probably respond to hyperbaric oxygen therapy [17] if the facilities were available.

REFERENCES

[1] ANDERSEN I. & POULSEN T. (1959) Surgical treatment of spontaneous pneumothorax. *Acta chir. scand.* **118**, 105.

[2] ANDERSON R.L. (1952) Rupture of the oesophagus. *J. thorac. Surg.* **24**, 369.

[3] AUTIO V. (1959) The reduction of respiratory function by parenchymal and pleural lesions. A bronchospirometric study of patients with unilateral involvement. *Acta tuberc. scand.* **37**, 112.

[4] BARANOFSKY I.D., WARDEN H.G., KAUFMAN J.L., WHATLEY J. & HAUNTER J.M. (1957) Bilateral therapy for unilateral spontaneous pneumothorax. *J. thorac. Surg.* **34**, 310.

[5] BARRETT N.R. (1952) In *Modern Trends of Gastroenterology.* Ed. Avery Jones F. 1st Edition, p. 224. London, Butterworths.

[6] BELCHER J.R. (1966) Spontaneous pneumothorax. *Br. med. J. Corresp.* **i**, 419.

[7] BREWER L.A., DOLLEY F.S. & EVANS B.H. (1950) The surgical management of chronic 'spontaneous' pneumothorax. *J. thorac. Surg.* **19**, 167.

[8] BROCK R.C. (1948) Recurrent and chronic spontaneous pneumothorax. *Thorax* **3**, 88.

[9] CARROLL D., McCLEMENT J., HIMMELSTEIN A. & COURNAND A. (1951) Pulmonary function following decortication of the lung. *Am. Rev. Tuberc.* **63**, 231.

[10] CHESTERMAN J.T. & SATSANGI P.N. (1966) Rupture of the trachea and bronchi by closed injury. *Thorax* **21**, 21.

[11] DARK J. & CHATTERJEE S.S. (1959) Pulmonary decortication. *Lancet* **ii**, 950.

[12] FALK A., PEARSON R.T. & MARTIN F.E. (1952) A bronchospirometric study of pulmonary function after decortication in pulmonary tuberculosis. *Am. Rev. Tuberc.* **66**, 509.

[13] FINE J., HERMANSON L. & FREHLING S. (1938) Further clinical experiences with 95% oxygen for the absorption of air from the body tissues. *Ann. Surg.* **107**, 1.

[14] FLEMING H.A. (1957) Pulmonary function before and after segmental resection and after 'ideal' pneumothorax treatment. *Br. med. J.* **i**, 485.

[15] GAENSLER E.A. (1956) Parietal pleurectomy for recurrent spontaneous pneumothorax. *Surg. Gynec. Obstet.* **102**, 293.

[16] GAENSLER E.A., WATSON T.R.Jr. & PATTON W.E. (1953) Bronchospirometry. VI. Results of 1089 examinations. *J. Lab. clin. Med.* **41**, 436.

[17] GRAY J.M. & HANSON GILLIAN C. (1966) Mediastinal emphysema: aetiology, diagnosis and treatment. *Thorax* **21**, 325.

[18] HAMMAN L. (1934) Remarks on the diagnosis of coronary occlusion. *Ann. intern. Med.* **8**, 417.

[19] HAMMAN L. (1937) Spontaneous interstitial emphysema of the lungs. *Trans. Ass. Am. Physns* **52**, 311.

[20] HAMMAN L. (1939a) Spontaneous mediastinal emphysema. *Bull. Johns Hopk. Hosp.* **64**, 1.

[21] HAMMAN L. (1939b) A note on the mechanism of spontaneous pneumothorax. *Ann. intern. Med.* **13**, 923.

[22] HAMMAN L. (1945) Mediastinal emphysema. *J. Am. med. Ass.* **128**, 1.

[23] HOLTER H.V. & HORWITZ O. (1945) Spontaneous pneumothorax produced by ascent in an airplane. *J. Am. med. Ass.* **127**, 519.

[24] HYDE L. (1963) Spontaneous pneumothorax. *Dis. Chest* **43**, 476.

[25] KILBURN K.H. (1963) Cardiorespiratory effects of large pneumothorax in conscious and anesthetized dogs. *J. appl. Physiol.* **18**, 279.

[26] KIRCHER L.T.Jr. & SWARTZEL R.L. (1954) Spontaneous pneumothorax and its treatment. *J. Am. med. Ass.* **155**, 24.

[27] KJAERGAARD H. (1932) Spontaneous pneumothorax in the apparently healthy. *Acta med. scand. Suppl.* **43**, 1.

[28] KNIGHT R.K. (1967) A pneumothorax valve. *Lancet* **i**, 190.

[29] LARIZADEH R. (1966) Rupture of the bronchus. *Thorax* **21**, 28.

[30] LINDSKOG G.E. & HALASZ N.A. (1957) Spontaneous pneumothorax: a consideration of pathogenesis and management with review of 72 hospitalized cases. *Arch. Surg.* **75**, 693.

[31] MACKLIN C.C. (1937) Pneumothorax with massive collapse from experimental local over-inflation of the lung substance. *Canad. med. Ass. J.* **36**, 414.

[32] MACKLIN M.T. & MACKLIN C.C. (1944) Malignant interstitial emphysema of the lungs and mediastinum as an important occult complication of many respiratory diseases and other conditions; an interpretation of the clinical literature in the light of laboratory experiment. *Medicine (Baltimore)* **23**, 281.

[33] MEAKINS J.C. & DAVIES H.W. (1925) *Respiratory Function in Disease.* Edinburgh, Oliver and Boyd.

[34] MORRIS M.D.R. (1966) Spontaneous pneumothorax. *Br. med. J. Corresp.* **i**, 420.

[35] MYERS J.A. (1954) Simple spontaneous pneumothorax. *Dis. Chest* **26**, 420.

[36] OSINSKA K., KOZIOROWSKI A. & BEDNARSKI Z. (1956) Zaburzenia oddychania w przebiegu odmy oplucnej. III. Fibrothorax poodmowy. (Respiratory disturbances during pneumothorax therapy. III. Fibrothorax as a sequel of pneumothorax therapy). *Gruzlica*, **24**, 269. (*Excerpta Med.* (*1957*) *XV* **10**, 206).

[37] OSWALD N. & PARKINSON T. (1949) Honeycomb lungs. *Quart. J. Med.* **18**, 1.

[38] PÄTIÄLÄ J. & KARVONEN M.J. (1954) Studies on pulmonary function after pneumothorax therapy. *Acta tuberc. scand.* **29**, 193.

[39] PETTY T.L., FILLEY G.F. & MITCHELL R.S. (1961) Objective functional improvement by decortication after 20 years of artificial pneumothorax for pulmonary tuberculosis: Report of a case and review of the literature. *Am. Rev. resp. Dis.* **84**, 572.

[40] REID J.M., STEVENSON J.G. & MCSWAN N. (1963) The management of spontaneous pneumothorax. *Scot. med. J.* **8**, 171.

[41] RICHARDS D.W.Jr., RILEY C.B. & HISCOCK M. (1932) Cardiac output following artificial pneumothorax in man. *Arch. intern. Med.* **49**, 994.

[42] RUCKLEY C.V. & MCCORMACK R.J.M. (1966) The management of spontaneous pneumothorax. *Thorax* **21**, 139.

[43] SAVAGE T. & FLEMING H.A. (1955) Decortication of the lung in tuberculous disease: a study of 43 cases. *Thorax* **10**, 293.

[44] SCADDING J.G. (1967) In *Sarcoidosis*, p. 136. London, Eyre and Spottiswoode.

[45] SCADDING J.G. & WOOD P.H. (1939) Systolic clicks due to left sided pneumothorax. *Lancet* ii, 1208.

[46] SCOTT J.T. (1957) Mediastinal emphysema and left pneumothorax. *Dis. Chest* **32**, 421.

[47] SEMPLE T. & LANCASTER W.M. (1961) Noisy pneumothorax—observations based on 24 cases. *Br. med. J.* i, 1343.

[48] SIEBENS A.A., STOREY C.F., NEWMAN M.M., KENT D.C. & STANDARD J.E. (1956) The physiological effects of fibrothorax and the functional results of surgical treatment. *J. thorac. Surg.* **32**, 53.

[49] SMITH C.C.K. & TANNER N.C. (1956) The complications of gastroscopy and oesophagoscopy. *Br. J. Surg.* **43**, 396.

[50] STEWART H.J. & BAILEY R.L.Jr. (1940) The effect of unilateral spontaneous pneumothorax on the circulation in man. *J. clin. Invest.* **19**, 321.

[51] STRADLING P. & POOLE G. (1966) Conservative management of spontaneous pneumothorax. *Thorax* **21**, 145.

[52] SULAVIK S. (1962) Mediastinal crunch (Hamman's sign). *GP. Kans. Cy.* **26**, 104.

[53] WOLCOTT M.W., SHAVER W.A. & JENNINGS W.D. (1963) Spontaneous pneumothorax. Management by tube, thoracotomy and suction. *Dis. Chest* **43**, 78.

CHAPTER 27

Pulmonary Thromboembolism

The term 'pulmonary thromboembolism' links in a single disease process thrombosis of peripheral veins, embolism of the pulmonary arteries and infarction of the lung parenchyma. Primary thrombosis of the pulmonary arteries and veins must also be included.

Pulmonary arterial embolism is much more common than primary pulmonary arterial thrombosis. Pulmonary embolism is, however, a common *cause* of pulmonary arterial thrombosis and lesions compounded of embolism and thrombosis are often indistinguishable from those due to thrombosis alone. Precision in diagnosis tends to be sacrificed to convenience in the sense that most cases are classified as thromboembolic phenomena unless there is strong evidence in favour of thrombosis being the initial feature.

Progress in the prevention and treatment of pulmonary embolism has been slow. Over a century has passed since Virchow described the pathology of venous thrombosis and the relation to pulmonary embolism and 50 years had to pass before Trendelenburg [79] first described pulmonary embolectomy. By 1930, 300 operations had been performed but only 7 successful cases reported. It was this experience which prompted more vigorous attempts at prevention and Homans in 1934 [32] attempted prevention of embolism from leg veins by ligation of the femoral vein. Five years later anticoagulants came into general clinical use and further research was directed towards prevention of thrombosis. More recently it has been appreciated that more precise methods are necessary for the diagnosis of pulmonary embolism for 2 reasons. First, repeated small pulmonary emboli may result in chronic heart disease and secondly advances in cardiac surgery have greatly reduced the risk of embolectomy when massive pulmonary embolism has occurred.

PULMONARY EMBOLISM

The term 'pulmonary embolism' has come to imply pulmonary artery blockage by thrombus of extrapulmonary origin. By far the commonest type of embolus is an intravascular thrombus arising in a peripheral vein. The thrombus consists mainly of layers of platelets, leucocytes and fibrin with relatively few entrapped red cells as opposed to an *in vitro* clot in which a loose fibrin mesh binds the cellular constituents in the proportions normally present in whole blood.

INCIDENCE AND PATHOGENESIS

Pulmonary embolism is found in 10–15% of postmortem examinations of adults (mainly middle aged and elderly) dying in hospital and in 3% it is the principal cause of death. In 30–40% of autopsies, including practically all cases of pulmonary embolism, leg vein thrombosis is found and is without doubt the source of the majority of emboli. The leg vein thrombosis is frequently bilateral although in life it may have been clinically detectable in one limb only or not at all.

A distinction has been made between thrombophlebitis and phlebothrombosis [52] which, theoretically, may have aetiological significances in the genesis of pulmonary embolism. As its name suggests thrombophlebitis is an inflammation of the vein wall (commonly femoral) which results in local thrombosis as a secondary phenomenon. The thrombus formed is usually firmly adherent to the wall of the vein and is, therefore, consequently less likely to become detached and to form an embolus. Clinically there is local tenderness and pain and swelling of the leg. The term 'phlebothrombosis' implies primary thrombus formation not affecting the vein wall importantly. By reason of this the thrombus may be easily dislodged to become an embolus. Phlebothrombosis may develop with no overt symptoms, which explains the incidence of unexpected venous thrombosis at autopsy [2, 34 & 65]. Both forms of venous thrombosis may result in embolism, however, and the clinician must regard each as potentially dangerous and treat accordingly.

CAUSES OF VASCULAR THROMBOSIS

Over a century ago Virchow enunciated the 3 factors responsible for vascular thrombosis. We know little more about the abnormalities that initiate thrombosis than Virchow did and his triad remains true today. Vascular thrombosis may occur (a) when the vessel walls are damaged, (b) when the blood flow is reduced below a certain critical level and (c) when there is increased coagulability of the blood. In individual cases one of these may be dominant but commonly they interlink. Of the 3 the present view is that, in most cases, damage to the endothelium appears to be the most important factor.

DAMAGE TO THE VESSEL WALL

The veins involved in thrombosis are usually those of the lower part of the body (legs and pelvis). It has been shown that the veins of the soleus muscle are more liable to thrombosis than those of the gastrocnemius [24 & 34] and it is thought that this difference may be due to greater physical trauma by the relatively greater venous pump action of the soleus muscle. Pathological studies of phlebothrombosis in human subjects [43 & 53] and in experimental animals [50] have usually failed to show any initial damage to the vessel wall but it must be remembered that changes in the vessel wall which are important for the development of thrombosis may not be detectable by ordinary histological methods. For example wetability of the endothelium and subsequent platelet adhesiveness, which

are important factors in the initial development of intravascular thrombosis [50], have been shown experimentally to become effective before any histological change in endothelium is evident. Presumably the damage results from hypoxia.

It is possible that the intima of the leg veins may be damaged by poor oxygenation in patients who are in bed since the veins are compressed and relatively empty [21].

Damage to the endothelium is sufficient of itself to cause thrombosis even when the blood flow is good.

REDUCTION IN BLOOD FLOW

Simple stagnation of blood in a healthy vein results in very slow clotting [81] and sometimes thrombin is so rapidly inactivated by antithrombins that no clot forms [45]. Stagnation of blood *per se*, therefore, may not be sufficient to explain leg vein thrombosis. It may, however, in conjunction with the other factors determine the onset and the site of thrombus formation.

Studies of the blood flow in leg veins with radioactive indicators have shown that blood takes about 18 seconds to pass from the foot to the groin in young normal subjects when the legs are horizontal [88]. It has also been shown that radio-opaque medium may be held up in the valve pockets of the deep leg veins for half an hour or more [31 & 42], and postoperatively the flow of blood in the leg generally [43 & 65] and the calf veins [4] is usually diminished, becoming most marked between the 13th and the 15th day after operation [38 & 69]. The importance of diaphragmatic movement in the maintenance of a good venous return from the legs was stressed by Lister [39] who believed that impairment of this mechanism contributed to the high incidence of pulmonary embolism after upper abdominal surgery. It has been shown, however, that there is no clear relationship between reduction in diaphragmatic movement and venous flow in the limbs [20].

INCREASED COAGULABILITY OF THE BLOOD

It has been shown that increased coagulability

of the blood combined with reduction in venous blood flow can result in thrombosis even though the endothelium is intact [7, 19, 46, 76 & 82]. Bed rest and meals with a high fat content both increase the blood coagulability [22].

After operation there are changes in the coagulability of the blood which have been attributed to changes in prothrombin [74], factor V, factor VII, fibrinogen and thromboplastin [15 & 84]. There is an increased resistance to the action of heparin in evidence by the 1st or 2nd day postoperatively and maximal by the 6th day [15, 26 & 33]. These changes in blood coagulability are more marked in older people and are greater the more extensive the operation [15 & 23]. The platelet count and platelet adhesiveness increase postoperatively and postpartum, reaching a maximum around the 10th day [8 & 87]. When thrombosis does occur the platelet count has been reported to decrease and it has been suggested that this is because adhesive platelets are deposited onto the thrombus [50 & 66]. This decrease in platelets has, however, been disputed by other workers [40].

VENOUS THROMBOSIS

The prime cause of leg vein thrombosis is venous stasis from rest in bed. Contributory factors abound, for rest in bed is frequently accompanied by other conditions which predispose to venous stasis, such as *immobility* due to old age, obesity or muscular weakness, *restricted respiratory movement* after abdominal operations, and *congestive cardiac failure*. Whether venous stasis initiates thrombosis or merely favours its propagation is not clear. It is thought that venous stasis may initiate thrombosis by interfering with the nutrition of endothelial cells. Foci of altered endothelium could give rise to minute thrombotic lesions, such as have been found in postmortem material, and these in turn could promote thrombosis on a larger scale. Advancing age, debilitating disease, and a host of other factors doubtless play their part in determining the susceptibility of endothelial cells to the effects of venous stasis in different individuals. For example when typhoid, tuberculosis and pneumonia were more serious diseases, venous thrombosis was a fairly common complication [80]. The large, deeply seated veins of the calf are the more prone to thrombosis. In these vessels venous stasis is at its worst when failure of the valvular mechanism leads to overdistension. For the same reason varicose veins carry an increased risk of thrombosis.

The *site* at which the initial venous thrombosis begins is not necessarily the site from which an embolus, particularly a large pulmonary embolus, originates. For example thrombosis of the foot veins may be followed by thrombosis of the deep calf veins and later the femoral or iliac veins [65] from which the thick, long, coiled thrombi causing death fairly certainly arise. Sevitt and Gallagher [65] have given the order of frequency of leg vein thrombosis as follows:

(1) deep veins of calf (67%);
(2) posterior tibial (54%);
(3) common femoral (48%);
(4) profunda femoris (43%);
(5) popliteal (33%);
(6) external iliac (26%).

Thrombosis of the leg veins in apparently healthy people with no known predisposing causes is probably more common than is appreciated [17]. The danger of pulmonary embolism in this 'idiopathic' form is just as great as that when thrombosis complicates an overt medical or surgical condition. Slight premonitory symptoms such as faintness and tiredness may be indications to begin what may be life-saving treatment.

Increase in thromboplastic activity and in the number and adhesiveness of *platelets*, occurring after operation and parturition, are generally held to predispose to thrombosis and embolism but other factors are always present as well.

The suggestion that oral contraceptives may increase the incidence of venous thrombosis and pulmonary embolism has led to many investigations. The current view is that expressed in the British Medical Research Council Report in 1967 [48]. Although it is a preliminary communication the Report states 'there can be no reasonable doubt that some types of thromboembolic disorder are associated with the use of oral contraceptives'. It must be emphasized that the positive findings apply only to venous thrombosis and pulmonary embolism. Increase in cerebrovascular thrombosis has not been proved and increase in coronary thrombosis appears to have been excluded. These findings must be considered in the appropriate context, principally the increased risk of thromboembolism complicating the unwanted pregnancy which might occur if oral contraception were not used. The Report indicates that oral contraceptives increase the risk of venous thrombosis 3 times while pregnancy increases it 6 times. The balance would, therefore, appear to have been redressed in favour of oral contraceptives. The compromise situation which practitioners have to face is that the use of oral contraceptives must at present be regarded as an interim measure until safer means become available. A particularly difficult decision concerns the patient with a previous history of thromboembolism complicating pregnancy who now requires some form of contraception; with our present knowledge alternative measures to the oral method are likely to be safer.

Pulmonary embolism occasionally follows thrombosis in veins other than the leg. The chief factor in these cases appears to be damage to the vein wall by trauma or sepsis though the victim may be a patient in bed, predisposed to thrombosis in various ways. Typical examples are *pelvic vein thrombosis* following parturition, pelvic operations and pelvic sepsis, and *internal jugular vein thrombosis* in association with operations on the head and neck or middle ear disease. Other cases depend less on local damage and more on general disorders predisposing to thrombosis, e.g. *primary polycythaemia*.

In most instances, therefore, the thrombosis and embolism make their appearance in the course of a clinically evident disease. The converse, with thrombosis as the first manifestation of disease, is less common but perhaps more interesting. A good example is the thromboplastin-liberating *carcinoma of pancreas* which is usually unsuspected until peripheral vein thrombosis occurs. Thromboplastin production is an occasional but ill-understood property of carcinomas in general. A study by Spencer [70] of 125 cases of carcinoma of the pancreas revealed thrombosis in over half of the cases. Venous thrombosis and pulmonary embolism have been found to be $2\frac{1}{2}$ times more common in patients with carcinoma in various sites [1] than in patients without malignant disease. The migrating thrombophlebitis which is the commonest form of venous thrombosis associated with malignant disease usually affects superficial veins and is not a common cause of pulmonary embolism. Removal of the tumour may sometimes halt the tendency to thrombosis [86].

It is rare for pulmonary embolism to occur in *children* and the sites of origin of thrombi vary from those in adults. In the *neonate* thrombi mostly arise from the hepatic and renal veins; in *older children* the cerebral sinuses and veins of the nasopharynx provide the greater number of emboli [9, 14, 29, 35 & 41]. It is usual for venous thrombosis in children and consequent pulmonary embolism to occur only in children who are ill [9 & 35] and the high mortality rate reflects the severity of the primary condition.

A *previous history of venous thrombosis* or embolism carries with it an increased liability to a further attack when conditions favour the development of venous thrombosis. Series have been reported giving incidences varying from 20% [55] to 44% [1] of venous thrombosis or embolism in patients with previous episodes of these conditions. De Takats and Jesser [75] reported that patients who survive one attack of pulmonary embolism have a 40% chance of a second episode and a 12% chance of a third.

The incidence of venous thrombosis and, therefore, of pulmonary embolism is much lower in Asian and African races than in Europeans [18, 71 & 77]. The reason for this is not precisely known but there are certainly racial differences in fibrinolytic activity [18,

49 & 71]. Diet does not appear to be the reason for the disparity in this instance but it is interesting that the incidence of pulmonary embolism was low in European countries during the Second World War, presumably due to the lower standard of nutrition.

There is no significant difference between male and female in the incidence of venous thrombosis or pulmonary embolism [51 & 78] when such obvious predisposing factors as pregnancy are taken into account.

OTHER SOURCES OF VASCULAR THROMBI

Some mural thrombi in the *heart* can give rise to pulmonary embolism; for example those which occur in association with atrial fibrillation, on the interventricular septum when it is included in an infarct and on diseased and damaged pulmonary and tricuspid valves. The sluggish circulation associated with congestive cardiac failure may also predispose to peripheral venous thrombosis and its consequences in these instances.

EMBOLI OF EXTRAVASCULAR ORIGIN

Pulmonary embolism due to nonthrombotic emboli, that is emboli of extravascular origin, is uncommon. *Fat embolism* probably occurs after most long bone fractures but is seldom evident clinically. Pulmonary oil embolism may rarely follow hysterosalpingography [27]. *Air embolism* has a particular medico-legal interest because of its occurrence during illicit attempts at procuring abortion. *Amniotic fluid*, normal *trophoblast* and fragments of *chorionepithelioma* may be carried via the uterine veins from the uterus to the lung. Other extravascular emboli include fragments of *tumour* which have invaded large veins, *Schistosoma ova* and emboli of human manufacture such as intravenous catheters and the like. In fat and air embolism small emboli may pass through the pulmonary capillaries and become impacted in the brain and other organs. Larger emboli may reach the systemic circulation via a patent *foramen ovale*, which is said to be present in 20–25% of otherwise normal subjects [12].

PATHOLOGICAL CHANGES DUE TO EMBOLISM

Thrombotic emboli are generally small and multiple and lodge in the distal branches of the pulmonary arteries at the periphery of the lungs, usually in the lower lobes, the right more often than the left. Animal studies have shown that small thrombotic emboli are quickly absorbed and that embolism is only serious when a great many small thrombi reach the lung simultaneously, or when large emboli block major vessels. A large thrombotic embolus is naturally more likely to prove fatal if the pulmonary circulation is already embarrassed by the presence of numerous small unabsorbed thrombi.

Evidence of recurrent embolism is often found in human cases at autopsy. Embolic blockage of major vessels (often bilateral owing to fragmentation of the embolus) is accompanied by small, healing, peripheral embolic lesions which are the result of earlier symptomless embolism. Impacted emboli cause local stasis and endothelial damage followed by thrombosis, which in the larger vessels may extend some distance proximally. Subsequently the thrombus is absorbed and recanalized, but the intima may be left thickened and the lumen diminished. If enough vessels are involved in this way pulmonary hypertension develops followed by right ventricular hypertrophy and right heart failure. Infarction of lung parenchyma does not necessarily follow embolic blockage, even of large arteries, as the circulation may be maintained by freely anastomosing branches of adjacent pulmonary arteries and by contributions from the bronchial arteries. If the venous return is impeded, as in left ventricular failure, infarction is much more likely to occur.

FUNCTIONAL ABNORMALITY

The effects of pulmonary embolism on function depend on the number and size of the emboli. A small single embolus may have no appreciable effect. A large embolus may cause fatal obstruction of the pulmonary circulation. Since patients with pulmonary embolism or infarction are too ill for extensive investigation there is a dearth of precise information regarding the pathophysiology of these conditions. There is also the complicating factor that the diseases which predispose to pulmonary thromboembolism may influence the results of lung function studies. No single test, or combination of tests, is diagnostic of pulmonary embolism.

Patients with pulmonary embolism may show *arterial hypoxaemia* as the only detectable abnormality. More often there is *hyperventilation* so that the Pa,co_2 as well as the Pa,o_2 is lowered. It seems clear that venoarterial shunting is mainly responsible for the hypoxaemia since oxygen breathing cannot achieve full oxygen saturation [57]. It has been shown by Robin and his colleagues [56 & 57] that ventilation is not immediately reduced after impaction of thrombus has reduced the circulation. Normally the partial pressure of CO_2 in alveolar gas (PA,co_2) is the same as that of arterial blood (Pa,co_2). If, however, some alveoli are not perfused they will contain very little CO_2 since they receive no CO_2 in gas exchange and what is present is simply that rebreathed from the dead space of the airways at the beginning of inspiration. An endtidal sample of gas will contain a mixture of normal alveolar gas and gas with a low CO_2 content from underperfused alveoli. This will mean an endtidal CO_2 pressure lower than the arterial CO_2 pressure and the difference is a measure of the volume of unperfused lung (dead space effect). Certainly experimental embolization in animals results in an $(a-A)Pco_2$ difference which can be used to estimate the volume of affected lung [37, 64 & 72]. The value of this test in clinical practice is limited, however, since the mutual adjusting of ventilation and perfusion which occurs when infarction develops soon removes the $(a-A)Pco_2$ difference. Also $(a-A)Pco_2$ difference may be found in chronic bronchitis which may coexist so that unless the difference is known before embolization occurs it is of little value; $(a-A)Pco_2$ difference may even occur in normal people if respiration is not deep enough.

In experimental pulmonary embolism the *diffusing capacity* is often lowered (6) and this in conjunction with increase in the physiological dead space, though not diagnostic of pulmonary arterial obstruction from embolism, makes the latter a reasonable presumption provided there is no other disease affecting the pulmonary arterial system. For example the fibrosis of sarcoidosis may be associated with obliterative arteriolitis which can result in similar abnormalities in lung function.

Studies by Duner, Pernow and Rigner [11] showed that complete recovery of cardiac and pulmonary function was possible within 3 months in patients whose cardiopulmonary function prior to a single episode of pulmonary embolism was normal. This is in keeping with the experimental evidence that autologous blood clot in dogs may completely disappear [47 & 59]. In contrast repeated microembolism may produce permanent changes in lung function.

Patients with *recurrent pulmonary microembolism* usually show no significant changes in the static lung volumes, and pulmonary compliance and airway resistance are normal. Gas distribution is normal. The diffusing capacity has been usually reported as near normal at rest; exercise has been reported to have variable effect. The dominant finding is the very marked hyperpnoea in relation to O_2 uptake on exercise. This results in a reduction in Pa,co_2. The Pa,o_2 may also be reduced because of ventilation–perfusion imbalance. The clinical picture may closely simulate hysterical overventilation but in the latter there is, of course, no associated pulmonary hypertension nor is there increased dead space. In 3 patients studied by Ehrner and his colleagues [13] the $\dot{V}o_2/\dot{V}E$ ratio on exercise was 2·04, 1·06 and 2·34% compared with the average normal value of about 4·8% [10]. Undoubtedly this is mainly responsible for the effort dyspnoea which is the commonest symptom of the condition. The mechanism is, however, not understood. It has been suggested that it occurs as a result of stimulation of ventilation from abnormal receptor impulses from the hypertensive pulmonary circulation [53]. The rôles of hypoxaemia and stretch reflexes from vessels are not known.

Chronic obstruction of one main pulmonary artery may be confirmed by broncho-spirometry (p. 48) [60 & 83]. Oxygen uptake by the affected lung would be greatly reduced whereas the ventilation in that lung would be little affected.

CLINICAL FEATURES

Thromboembolic disease of the pulmonary circulation may result in 3 more or less distinct clinical pictures. The first occurs characteristically after a major surgical operation and is due to obstruction of a main pulmonary artery by thrombus arising most commonly in the deep veins of the leg ('*massive pulmonary embolism*'). The second type, found commonly in patients with cardiac disease results in *pulmonary infarction*. In the third type, recurrent showers of small emboli lodge in the peripheral branches of the pulmonary artery, resulting in progressive reduction of the pulmonary vascular bed and consequent pulmonary hypertension ('*obliterative pulmonary hypertension*'). The first type is often dramatically fatal; the second usually presents as an acute illness, with all possible grades of severity; the third may not produce any immediate clinical symptoms and may only be suspected when the features of pulmonary hypertension become evident.

The distinction between the 3 clinical pictures may not be precise nor may the pathological effects be so compartmented as indicated above. Thus pathological and perhaps clinically evident infarction may occur in massive pulmonary embolism and sometimes in recurrent microembolism.

MASSIVE PULMONARY EMBOLISM

The classical description of an elderly, possibly obese, patient around the 10th postoperative day calling for a bed pan and expiring suddenly, or dying while in the act of defaecation, is well known. The precise cause of death in massive pulmonary embolism is not fully understood. Sudden reduction in blood flow must certainly be a major factor in bringing about cardiac arrest and may be the only one. The part played by reflex vagal action is still uncertain. It is known that defaecation commonly occurs in experimental embolism in dogs but before applying this observation to the disease in man it should be remembered that defaecation itself gives rise to violent fluctuations in venous pressure which could have the effect of dislodging a peripheral vein thrombus. The same mechanism may be at work in those cases in which massive pulmonary embolism follows immediately after the exertion of getting out of bed.

If the embolism is not immediately fatal the patient becomes suddenly *shocked* and experiences *central chest pain* due to failure of coronary blood flow. Distressing *dyspnoea*, *faintness* and acute *apprehension* soon follow associated with *cyanosis, tachycardia, profuse sweating* and *collapse*. If the patient survives, the features of *right heart strain* may appear in the ECG and *congestive cardiac failure* may rapidly develop. At this stage it may be recalled that the patient had previously suffered from varicose veins or thrombophlebitis, or had signs of deep vein thrombosis. In retrospect the 'flick of fever' which might have occurred earlier in the week could have been due to a small premonitory episode of pulmonary embolism.

In patients who survive massive pulmonary embolism characteristic changes may sometimes be seen in the *chest radiograph*. Bilateral hilar enlargement indicates obstruction of both pulmonary arteries while obstruction of a single pulmonary artery is shown by unilateral pulmonary artery dilatation, too rarely associated with an area of recognizable ischaemia of the lung for this to be of clinical value. Radiographic evidence is less likely to be obtained with the lesser degrees of embolism.

Radioscanning of the lung fields after the intravenous injection of macroaggregated human serum albumin (p. 49) is another method of detecting pulmonary embolism. 0·5 ml of a 2% suspension of human serum albumin, labelled with ^{131}I and aggregated into particles of 10–50 μ diameter, is injected intravenously. The particles become impacted in the pulmonary arterioles and capillaries according to the blood flow. Scanning with a scintillation counter will show which areas have no radioactivity and are, therefore, receiving no blood flow. The amount of aggregated albumin used is too small to cause any untoward effect by arterial blockage and since nearly all of the ^{131}I is excreted within a month there is no likelihood of long term effects from radioactivity. It is important to interpret the scan in conjunction with the chest radiograph since lesions such as pneumonia or pleural effusion may also show areas of absent radioactivity. Though safer than pulmonary angiography involving cardiac catheterization the technique is less discriminative. It also requires that the patient, who may be acutely ill, is kept still for 15–20 min and this is not always possible. Nor is the rather sophisticated apparatus widely available. *Pulmonary angiography* is a more precise method of confirming the diagnosis but is not often considered necessary. Adequate pulmonary angiography may be obtained by the simplified and relatively safe technique of rapid intravenous injection of radio-opaque contrast medium into a peripheral vein [85].

The intravenous radio-Xenon technique (p. 49) may be applied in pulmonary embolism but can only detect lack of perfusion due to obstruction affecting at least one lobe. Smaller embolization cannot be recognized by this method.

DIFFERENTIAL DIAGNOSIS

It may be very difficult initially to distinguish massive pulmonary embolism from *myocardial infarction*. The early symptoms of shock and central chest pain are common to both conditions and the chest pain in pulmonary embolism is actually due to myocardial ischaemia. Serum transaminase estimation and the ECG may be helpful in excluding myocardial damage but should they indicate that myocardial damage is present the diagnosis of massive pulmonary embolism is not thereby excluded, for myocardial infarction frequently complicates pulmonary embolism. The ECG is the less valuable of the two as it is notoriously variable in the early stages of pulmonary embolism. Fortunately in practice precise distinction between the two is not an urgent necessity as the first stages in treatment are the same. *Spontaneous pneumothorax* can be excluded from the diagnosis by the physical signs and the radiographic appearances.

The collapse and pain in *dissecting aortic aneurysm* may closely simulate myocardial infarction. The signs depend on the site of dissection and the degree of obstruction of the aorta and its branches.

Shock associated with injury or following operation may resemble the effects of embolism, as does bacteraemic shock following septicaemia (e.g. complicating urinary infection). In each case the venous pressure is low and this is shown in collapsed peripheral veins with a low jugular venous pressure.

Major pulmonary collapse usually occurs within 24–28 hours after operation whereas pulmonary embolism more commonly is later, at the end of the first week after operation or during the second week [36]. In massive collapse the physical signs are usually characteristic and the chest radiograph establishes the diagnosis.

PULMONARY INFARCTION

The great majority of cases of pulmonary infarction due to pulmonary embolism occur in *middle aged or elderly patients* with leg vein thrombosis due to rest in bed, associated with the other conditions already mentioned. In younger patients *pregnancy* and *parturition* associated with thrombosis in pelvic or leg veins provide the bulk of the cases. Other causes are *rheumatic heart disease* with atrial fibrillation giving rise to thrombosis in the right atrium, and *congenital defects* of the heart affecting the tricuspid and pulmonary valves and the interatrial and interventricular septa. In the rare examples of pulmonary infarction in apparently normal people it will usually be found that a predisposition to peripheral vein thrombosis exists in the form of one or other of the ordinary local and general causes of thrombosis.

PATHOLOGY OF PULMONARY INFARCTION

The vascularity and laxity of lung tissue allow intense engorgement to occur in the infarcted area followed by considerable haemorrhage from rupture of the over-distended and subsequently necrotic capillaries. Granulation tissue repair proceeding from the periphery gradually encroaches upon and absorbs the necrotic central part of the infarct which is finally replaced by a fibrous scar pigmented with haemosiderin and much smaller than the original infarct. Bronchioles in the infarcted area sometimes survive because of their independent blood supply and may remain as bronchiectatic cavities in or near the scar. Bacterial infection of an infarct may occur if the causative embolus is itself infected, but an infarct especially in the necrotic stage is liable to chance infection from the bronchi and the blood stream. The effect of infection is to transform an infarct into an abscess (p. 160). Since infarcts are generally caused by blockage of small pulmonary arteries they tend to involve the pleura and to be accompanied by pleurisy, pleural effusion and pleural adhesions. Only about 10% of pulmonary infarcts are in the upper lobes [28, 44 & 67]. The disparity of blood flow between the apex and the base of the lung in the upright (p. 37) or semi-upright position (in which most patients are nursed) is generally held to be the most likely explanation for the greater liability of the lower lobes.

CLINICAL FEATURES

Pulmonary infarction is the great dissembler in respiratory medicine and there is no single clinical or radiographic manifestation which cannot be found in most other forms of respiratory disease. Pleural involvement in pulmonary infarction is almost invariable and hence *pleuritic pain* is very common. *Pleural effusion* often develops and in some cases may be the only radiographic abnormality. *Haemoptysis*, a 'classical' feature of pulmonary infarction, occurs in only about 50% of cases and a source of embolism is clinically detectable in only about 60% [44]. There may be marked *leucocytosis* (as high as 20,000 per mm^3) in uncomplicated infarction. Cough and sputum, apart from haemoptysis, are not frequent unless respiratory disease due to other factors is also present. *Dyspnoea* is variable and linked with the degree of pleuritic pain. *Pyrexia* is usually low grade (99–100°F for 3–7 days) although occasionally temperatures of 102°F or higher may be recorded in the first 48 hours. *Tachycardia* above 100 per minute is found in the majority of cases, usually out of proportion to the degree of pyrexia. Cyanosis is not found unless the infarction is extensive or accompanied by cardiac failure. Icterus is unlikely except in patients with longstanding congestive cardiac failure and some degree of liver damage ('cardiac cirrhosis').

Infection of a pulmonary infarct may be reflected in rapid worsening of the clinical state and the development of features suggesting lung abscess or empyema—persistent fever, increased tachycardia, malaise, sweating and a rising leucocyte count above the usual upper figure of 20,000 per mm^3 for uncomplicated infarction. *Staphylococcus pyogenes* is one of the most dangerous bacterial invaders and if it has been acquired in hospital it is likely to prove resistant to the commonly employed antibiotics.

The *physical signs* in the chest in pulmonary infarction are due to 3 factors—pleurisy, elevation of the diaphragm and consolidation, although all 3 are not necessarily present or equally marked in every case. *Pleural friction* may be detected not only in the area corresponding to the radiographic changes but also on the opposite side since pulmonary embolism is often bilateral. Evidence of bilateral incidents should at once suggest a diagnosis of embolic infarction. Tenderness and hyperaesthesia of the chest wall may accompany severe pleurisy. Signs suggestive of *pleural effusion* may be present but can be misleading as they are not infrequently due to an elevated hemidiaphragm. *Consolidation* only occasionally gives rise to the classical signs, but its presence is suggested by diminished air entry with a few coarse crepitations, which are the commonest physical signs found during the first 36 hours.

RADIOGRAPHIC FEATURES

There are 4 principal types of radiographic abnormality in pulmonary infarction:

(1) *Pleural opacities*—effusion (p. 268) or thickening.

(2) *Pulmonary opacities*—homogeneous or patchy, resembling the consolidation of pneumonia or bronchopneumonia, or rarely rounded and well demarcated.

(3) *Horizontal linear opacities*—nonsegmental in distribution, usually situated peripherally at the bases and due possibly to pleural thickening or minute areas of peripheral pulmonary atelectasis (PLATE 27.1).

(4) *Elevation of a hemidiaphragm* with limited movement or, occasionally, paradoxical movement from true paralysis.

An infected pulmonary infarct may have the radiographic appearance of an abscess.

The oft-quoted 'wedge shaped' opacity is quite uncommon. Often the radiographic manifestations of pulmonary infarction are bilateral. When unilateral the right side is more commonly involved than the left. The radiographic appearances are nonspecific but horizontal linear opacities, especially if bilateral, strongly support the clinical diagnosis of pulmonary infarction. The radiographic changes often alter quite rapidly, particularly the linear shadows, and new opacities may develop from further infarction. To repeat the chest radiograph at short intervals is, therefore, a useful aid to diagnosis in difficult cases.

DIFFERENTIAL DIAGNOSIS

The differential diagnosis of pulmonary infarction includes *pneumonia* (p. 133) including aspiration types, say from megaoesophagus, *postoperative atelectasis* (p. 462), *pulmonary tuberculosis* (p. 228), *lung abscess* (p. 159), *bronchogenic carcinoma* (p. 517), *spontaneous pneumothorax* (p. 445), *dry pleurisy* (p. 264) and various types of *pleural effusion* (p. 267). *Pulmonary eosinophilia* is a rare alternative (p. 427). In some cases it is difficult or impossible to exclude pneumonia and treatment for both conditions must be given initially.

In *postoperative atelectasis* pleuritic pain is not usually prominent. Cough is usually present and the chest may sound rattling. There may be a clear history of increasing difficulty in coughing up secretions. The radiographic opacity in postoperative atelectasis has a strictly segmental or lobar distribution.

Serial estimations of various tissue products have been suggested as probable indicators of pulmonary infarction, e.g. lactic dehydrogenase, alanine and aspartate aminotransferase, alkaline phosphates, serum bilirubin and thymol turbidity. In a comparative study [63] it has been shown that no single one of these or any combination of them can be relied upon for diagnosis.

Constant awareness of the susceptibility of certain groups of patients to pulmonary infarction will increase the frequency of early diagnosis. The development of unexplained pyrexia, dyspnoea or chest pain in an older person, particularly when confined to bed, or in the postoperative or postpartum patient, should arouse suspicion of pulmonary embolism and careful examination should be made for evidence of *preceding phlebothrombosis* or *thrombophlebitis*. Not uncommonly the peripheral venous thrombosis may only become clinically evident *after* the development of pulmonary infarction. Infarction can sometimes be remarkably silent, particularly when obscured by the features of existing cardiac failure. Sometimes it may be suspected from the development of tachycardia or *cardiac arrhythmia* such as auricular fibrillation [68].

It cannot be overstressed that the 'classical' clinical features of pulmonary infarction— sudden pleuritic pain, haemoptysis, calf tenderness and conclusive radiographic evidence of pulmonary consolidation—are rarely all present in the individual case. Probably of no other clinical condition can it be more truly said that the practice of medicine is a matter of probabilities. It may be vitally important that the doctor constantly keeps infarction on the probability list. Even then pulmonary infarction may be unrecognized because it is 'silent' and it is probable that about one half of all cases are not diagnosed. Recurrent bilateral pulmonary incidents, either pain or radiographic abnormality, are strongly suggestive of the diagnosis.

RECURRENT OBSTRUCTIVE PULMONARY THROMBOEMBOLISM (OBLITERATIVE PULMONARY HYPERTENSION)

Thromboembolic pulmonary vascular disease confined to the small vessels sometimes obstructs the blood flow sufficiently to cause pulmonary hypertension [25]. In severe cases the characteristic clinical picture of progressive pulmonary hypertension develops. The patients complain of *dyspnoea* and *weakness on exertion, effort syncope* and *anginal pain.* The *physical signs* of the condition include a tapping apex beat, a left parasternal heave due to right ventricular hypertrophy, a loud pulmonary second sound which is narrowly split or single, and an ejection click after the first heart sound and progressive cardiac enlargement. The systemic blood pressure is usually normal and cardiac murmurs are variable or absent. There may be incidents compatible with pulmonary infarction or venous thrombosis. Overt *heart failure* occurs late in the disease and its first manifestations are venous distension and congestive hepatomegaly. Peripheral oedema or ascites may develop subsequently and cyanosis, if it appears at all, is also a later feature.

Typical ECG findings are tall, peaked P waves, an increased R wave in V_1 and T wave inversion in the right and central precordial leads.

The radiographic features on the plain x-ray are very variable but usually show cardiomegaly, dilatation of the main pulmonary artery and its proximal branches with diminished vascular markings in the peripheral lung fields [16, 30, 62 & 83]. In cases with a clear history of pulmonary infarction *pulmonary angiography* generally shows obstruction of the larger arteries. In patients without a history of pulmonary infarction and with no apparent source of embolism angiography often shows large main pulmonary arteries which are not obviously obstructed. The pulmonary vascular markings may be within

normal limits but in the more severe cases a general loss of vascularity is apparent, and the small branches appear to be attenuated and do not reach to the periphery of the lungs [30, 62 & 83]. In both types of case, as pulmonary hypertension increases, enlargement of the main pulmonary arteries, of the right ventricle and sometimes also of the right atrium, become apparent. It should be remembered that pulmonary angiography carries an appreciable risk if the pulmonary arterial pressure is high and the cardiac output low.

The importance of recognizing thromboembolic pulmonary hypertension lies in the fact that it is potentially treatable. Unfortunately pulmonary hypertension does not usually appear until about two thirds of the pulmonary vascular bed has been obliterated and this militates against early diagnosis. It is important to remember the possibility of thromboembolism in pregnancy or the puerperium because, if overlooked, it may progress to serious obliterative pulmonary hypertension. The rare occurrence of embolism by trophoblast can be excluded by tests for chorionic gonadotrophin in the urine. The diagnosis of 'primary' pulmonary hypertension should never be made in a patient who is or recently, has been, pregnant. Patients with pulmonary hypertension suspected to be due to recurrent pulmonary embolism require prolonged anticoagulant treatment and this should always be given unless there are prohibitive contra-indications.

PULMONARY VASCULAR THROMBOSIS

It has already been mentioned that *pulmonary artery thrombosis* is a common complication of pulmonary embolism, especially in the sense of thrombosis spreading proximally from the site of embolic blockage to involve larger pulmonary arteries. The converse process also occurs, thrombus in a large artery releasing embolic fragments to block the distal branches and the two sites being subsequently united by thrombosis. It is a truism that in most cases it is difficult to say where thrombosis ends and embolism begins. Nevertheless true primary thrombosis does sometimes occur. In the large pulmonary arteries the commonest cause of this rare condition is probably *atheroma* in *pulmonary hypertension* such as occurs in mitral stenosis. *Chronic bronchitis* is the most frequent association with pulmonary arterial thrombosis which may also complicate *thoracic operations* and *cardiac failure* and has been described in association with *pulmonary tuberculosis* and *pneumoconiosis*. It is probable that pulmonary artery thrombosis is under-diagnosed. Both pulmonary arteries are usually involved, but if the condition is unilateral, the right is more often affected than the left. The clinical features are increasing dyspnoea, fatigue and right heart failure and not infrequently the clinical picture has been erroneously attributed to chronic bronchitis alone when the patient has been known to suffer from this. Thrombosis in medium-sized or small pulmonary arteries occurs in the same circumstances and is also found in conditions of reduced pulmonary inflow, for example *congenital pulmonary stenosis* and *Fallot's tetralogy*.

Thrombosis of pulmonary arteries reduces the pulmonary vein blood flow and predisposes to *pulmonary vein thrombosis* and also to infarction, the latter seldom occurring if the venous flow is normal. Pulmonary vein thrombosis is also caused by many local conditions which damage or obstruct the veins. *Bronchial carcinoma* and *pulmonary tuberculosis* are familiar examples. *Polycythaemia*, primary or compensatory, and other *blood diseases predisposing to thrombosis* provide other examples of pulmonary vein thrombosis. *Injury* to pulmonary veins at *chest operations* is an additional but very occasional cause of pulmonary vein thrombosis which may lead to areas of infarction and later give rise to bronchopleural fistula and empyema [61].

TREATMENT OF PULMONARY THROMBOEMBOLISM

PREVENTION

Prevention is directed towards those patients at greatest risk—the old and obese, the patient with cardiac disease, the postpartum and postoperative patient. Continued ambulation of elderly people afflicted with minor illnesses should be encouraged. Early ambulation is theoretically advisable in postoperative and postpartum patients, although there is no clear evidence that this has reduced the incidence of postoperative phlebothrombosis. During operation the raising of the legs slightly above the horizontal will assist venous drainage [42] and the use of suitable padding may prevent pressure on leg muscles and contusion which may initiate thrombosis [49]. Attention to the bowel in patients with known phlebothrombosis is important to prevent straining at stool. Dehydration should be avoided and cardiac failure treated. Intravenous infusions should never be given *via* the saphenous veins for fear of initiating venous thrombosis.

Patients confined to bed should be examined frequently for the development of evidence of phlebothrombosis—increased warmth of the limb, tenderness over deep calf veins where a thrombosed vessel may be palpable, dilatation of superficial veins crossing the anterior aspect of the tibia and, in the developed case, pitting oedema. Homans' sign should be relegated to the archives. This manoeuvre is an excellent way to detach a loosely held calf vein thrombus and fatal pulmonary embolism has been encountered following its use.

Anticoagulant therapy should be begun immediately on suspicion of the development of deep venous thrombosis unless there are strong contra-indications. The use of phenindione as a prophylactic in surgical patients particularly susceptible to venous thrombosis and pulmonary embolism has been proved by controlled trial to be safe and practicable and to reduce markedly the incidence of thromboembolic phenomena [65]. In the series of hip fractures treated by pinning reported by Sevitt and Gallagher phenindione was begun on admission and did not cause any problem from haemorrhage at operation or subsequently. Full antithrombotic protection cannot, however, be separated from the risk of increased haemorrhage though in general the advantages outweigh the disadvantages. Heparin has the advantage over phenindione that overdosage is relatively unimportant since the drug is rapidly excreted and its effect is rapidly reversed by protamine sulphate. It also decreases platelet adhesiveness [50] and has been shown to be more effective than the coumarol derivatives in preventing extension of a developed thrombus [5]. Anticoagulants in myocardial infarction minimize the risk of thromboembolic complications.

Enthusiasm has waned for ligation of limb veins as a prophylactic measure. Thrombi are not uncommonly bilateral at postmortem even though clinically evident on one side only, and ligation at inferior vena cava level would be necessary to meet this problem. Inferior vena caval ligation is commonly associated with persisting leg oedema and should never be undertaken lightly. Ligature of the common iliac veins avoids the complication of residual oedema by allowing collateral circulation through the pelvic veins but both veins may require to be ligated to give effective prophylaxis against pulmonary embolism. Recurrent embolism from pelvic vein thrombosis requires ligation of the inferior vena cava.

TREATMENT OF MASSIVE PULMONARY EMBOLISM

The recognition of major pulmonary embolism is a medical emergency because the sooner treatment is begun the more effective it is. *Intravenous heparin* may be life-saving and at the moment is the first line of treatment. Fibrinolytic agents have not, so far, proved of value in this disorder. *Emergency embolectomy* is becoming increasingly a practical procedure with the use of hypothermia or cardiopulmonary bypass. At least 30% of patients who die with massive pulmonary embolism survive more than 2 hours and so are potential candidates for embolectomy [60, 73 & 75]. Pulmonary angiography is a useful aid to diagnosis for the surgeon who is considering embolectomy. Pulmonary scanning for radioactivity after the intravenous injection of radioactive albumin is at present being evaluated as a means of detecting pulmonary embolism (p. 459).

Some physiologists hold the view that reflex or chemical vasoconstriction and bronchoconstriction contribute importantly to the immediate clinical effects of pulmonary embolism but there is insufficient evidence at present to support the use of vasodilator or bronchodilator substances such as papaverine or atropine, or antagonists to tissue products, such as histamine, serotonin or bradykinin, which may be released at the time of embolism.

Morphine or *pethidine* is invaluable for the relief of pain and apprehension. *Oxygen* should be given freely and the usual measures for acute circulatory failure employed.

TREATMENT OF PULMONARY INFARCTION

In those patients in whom the history, clinical findings and radiographic appearances do not allow a clear distinction between pneumonia and pulmonary infarction the only safe rule is to treat for both, heparin and phenindione (p. 464) being begun at once along with an oral antibiotic such as ampicillin. Intramuscular injections should be avoided because of the possibility of haematomata but this is only a relative contra-indication and the severity of the condition may warrant the parenteral use of antibiotics in the individual case. Heparinization is maintained for 48 hours and anticoagulant therapy continued thereafter with phenindione to complete a 3 week course, the prothrombin level being measured frequently. It is unusual for therapy to be necessary beyond this time although further embolization has been known very occasionally to occur during the treatment period despite satisfactory control of the prothrombin level. Should there be evidence of further thromboembolism the anticoagulant regime should be continued longer, and in the rare case it may prove necessary to institute long term anticoagulant therapy. The wisdom of giving anticoagulants in the face of haemoptysis may be questioned, but the common finding is that haemoptysis rapidly subsides after treatment is begun.

High concentrations of *oxygen* (over 40%) may be given with impunity in pulmonary embolism or infarction. *Morphine* or *pethidine* may require to be used for the associated pleuritic pain. Coincident antibiotic therapy is usually not employed unless there is suspicion of associated infection or doubt about the diagnosis. Provided that the clinical signs of deep venous thrombosis have subsided the patient may be allowed up after the tenth day. By this time the thrombus will have become firmly adherent to the vessel wall. Persistence of oedema or deep tenderness in the calf may compel a longer period of bed rest.

The effusion complicating pulmonary infarction is usually small to moderate in size and self-limiting. The fluid may be blood stained, but more commonly it is clear and yellow in colour. Aspiration is not often required and it is rare for more than a single withdrawal to be necessary unless the pulmonary infarction complicates mitral stenosis or other cardiac disease, in which case the effusion may be large and persistent (sometimes for many months) or recurrent.

TREATMENT OF OBSTRUCTIVE PULMONARY THROMBOEMBOLISM

In obliterative pulmonary hypertension due to microembolism or thrombosis of larger vessels treatment with anticoagulant drugs should be continued for at least a year.

REFERENCES

[1] BARKER N.W. & PRIESTLEY J.T. (1942) Postoperative thrombophlebitis and embolism. *Surgery* 12, 411.

[2] BELT T.H. (1934) Thrombosis and pulmonary embolism. *Am. J. Path.* 10, 129.

[3] BORGSTROM S., GELIN L.E. & ZEDERFELDT B. (1959) The formation of vein thrombi following tissue injury; an experimental study in rabbits. *Acta chir. scand. Suppl.* 247, 1.

[4] BROWSE N.L. (1962) Effect of surgery on resting calf blood flow. *Br. med. J.* i, 1714.

[5] CAREY L.C. & WILLIAMS R.D. (1960) Comparative effects of dicoumarol, tromexan and heparin on thrombus propagation. *Ann. Surg.* 152, 919.

[6] COLP C.R. & WILLIAMS M.H. (1962) Pulmonary function following pulmonary embolism. *Am. Rev. resp. Dis.* 85, 799.

[7] COPLEY A.L. & STEFKO P.L. (1947) Coagulation thrombi in segments of artery and vein in dogs and the genesis of thromboembolism. *Surg. Gynec. Obstet.* 84, 451

[8] DAWBARN R.Y., EARLAM F. & EVANS W.H. (1928) The relation of the blood platelets to thrombosis after operation and parturition. *J. Path. Bact.* 31, 833.

[9] DECAMP P.T., OCHSNER A. & DEBAKEY M.E. (1951) Thromboembolism in children; analysis of 35 cases. *Ann. Surg.* 133, 611.

[10] DONEVAN R.E., PALMER W.H., VARVIS C.J. & BATES D.V. (1959) Influence of age on pulmonary diffusing capacity. *J. appl. Physiol.* 14, 483.

[11] DUNER H., PERNOW B. & RIGNER K.G. (1960) The prognosis of pulmonary embolism. A medical and physiological follow up examination of patients treated at the Departments of Internal Medicine and Surgery, Karolinska Sjukhuset in 1952–58. *Acta med. scand.* 168, 381.

[12] EDWARDS J.E. (1960) Congenital malformations of the heart and great vessels. A. Malformations of the atrial septal complex. In *Pathology of the Heart*, ed. Gould S.E., p. 261. Springfield, Thomas.

[13] EHRNER L., GARLIND T. & LINDERHOLM J. (1959) Chronic cor pulmonale following thromboembolism. A. Clinical and pathophysiological study of 3 cases. *Acta med. scand.* 164, 279.

[14] EMERY J.L. (1962) Pulmonary embolism in children. *Arch. Dis. Childh.* 37, 591.

[15] FERUGLIO G., SANDBERG H. & BELLET S. (1960) Postoperative changes in blood coagulation in elderly patients. *Am. J. Cardiol.* 5, 477.

[16] FLEISCHNER F.G. (1950) Pulmonary embolism. *Canad. med. Ass. J.* 78, 653.

[17] FLEMING H.A. & BAILEY S.M. (1966) Massive pulmonary embolism in healthy people. *Br. med. J.* i, 1322.

[18] FRANZ R.C., KARK A.E. & HATHORN M. (1961) Postoperative thrombosis and plasma fibrinolytic activity. A comparative study in Africans, Indians and Whites. *Lancet* i, 195.

[19] FREIMAN D.G. & WESSLER S. (1957) Experimental studies in intravascular thrombosis and pulmonary embolism. *Am. J. Path.* 33, 579.

[20] FRIMANN-DAHL J. (1935) Diaphragmabewegungen und der postoperative Venenstrom. *Acta chir. scand. Suppl.* 36, 1.

[21] FRYKHOLM R. (1939) Om ventrombosens patogenes och mekaniska profylax. *Nord. Med.* 4, 3534.

[22] FULLERTON H.W. & McDONALD G.A. (1960) The recalcified plasma clotting time as a measure of blood coagulability. In *Thrombosis and Anticoagulant Therapy*, ed. Walker W. Dundee, University St. Andrews.

[23] GEETER R. DE & DUMONT A. (1955) La fibrinolyse et les modifications de quelques facteurs de la coagulation au cours des interventions de chirurgie thoracique. *Acta chir. Belg.* 54, 324.

[24] GIBBS N.M. (1959) The prophylaxis of pulmonary embolism. *Br. J. Surg.* **47**, 282.

[25] GOODWIN J.F., HARRISON C.V. & WILCKEN D.E.L. (1963) Obliterative pulmonary hypertension and thromboembolism. *Br. med. J.* **i**, 701, 777.

[26] GORMSEN J. & HAXHOLDT B.F. (1961) Operative and postoperative changes in blood coagulation. *Acta chir. scand.* **121**, 377.

[27] GRANT I.W.B., CALLAM W.D.A. & DAVIDSON J.K. (1957) Pulmonary oil embolism following hysterosalpingography. *J. Fac. Radiol.* **8**, 410.

[28] GSELL O. (1935) Der Hämorrhagische Lungeninfarkt und seine Komplikationen (Infarktpleuritis, Infarktpneumonie, Infarktkaverne usw.) *Dt. med. Wschr.* **61**, 1317, 1360.

[29] HAMBURGER R. (1920) Über Gefässthrombosen junger Kinder. *Jb. Kinderheilk. phys. Erzieh.* **91**, 439.

[30] HANELIN J. & EYLER W.R. (1951) Pulmonary artery thrombosis: roentgen manifestations. *Radiology* **56**, 689.

[31] HODGSON D.C. (1964) Venous stasis during surgery. *Anaesthesia,* **19**, 96.

[32] HOMANS J. (1934) Thrombosis of deep veins of the lower leg, causing pulmonary embolism. *New Engl. J. Med.* **211**, 993.

[33] HOMANS J. (1943) Pulmonary emboli due to quiet venous thrombosis and simulating cardiac and pulmonary disease. *New Engl. J. Med.* **229**, 309.

[34] HUNTER W.C., SNEEDEN V.D., ROBERTSON T.D. & SNYDER G.A.C. (1941) Thrombosis of deep veins of leg: clinical significance as exemplified in 351 autopsies. *Arch. intern. Med.* **68**, 1.

[35] HUTINEL V. (1877) *Contribution à l'étude des troubles de la circulation veineuse chez l'enfant et en particulier chez le nouveau-né.* Paris, Delahaye.

[36] JENKINS L.C. & GRAVES H.B. (1961) Anaesthesia and pulmonary embolism. *Canad. anesth. Soc. J.* **8**, 143.

[37] JULIAN D.G., TRAVIS D.M., ROBIN E.D. & CRUMP C.H. (1960) Effect of pulmonary artery occlusion upon end-tidal CO_2 tension. *J. appl. Physiol.* **15**, 87.

[38] KVALE W.F., SMITH L.A. & ALLEN E.V. (1940) Speed of blood flow in the arteries and in the veins of man. *Arch. Surg.* **40**, 344.

[39] LISTER W.A. (1927) A statistical investigation into the causation of pulmonary embolism following operation. *Lancet* **i**, 111.

[40] LOEWE L., LASSER R.P. & MORRISON M. (1950) The prediction of thromboembolism. *Angiology*, **1**, 64.

[41] McCLELLAND C.Q. & HUGHES J.P. (1950) Thrombosis of the renal vein in infants. *J. Pediat. (St. Louis)* **36**, 214.

[42] McLACHLIN A.D., McLACHLIN J.A., JORY T.A. & RAWLING E.G. (1960) Venous stasis in the lower extremities. *Ann. Surg.* **152**, 678.

[43] McLACHLIN J. & PATTERSON J.C. (1951) Some basic observations on venous thrombosis and pulmonary embolism. *Surg. Gynec. Obstet.* **93**, 1.

[44] MacLEOD J.G. & GRANT I.W.B. (1954) A clinical, radiographic and pathological study of pulmonary embolism. *Thorax* **9**, 71.

[45] MARIN H.M., LEMIEUX J. & MUELLER L. (1961) The coagulation of blood in isolated venous segments. *Surg. Gynec. Obstet.* **113**, 293.

[46] MARIN H.M. & STEFANINI M. (1960) Experimental production of phlebothrombosis. *Surg. Gynec. Obstet.* **100**, 263.

[47] MARSHALL R. (1962) Pulmonary embolism and thrombosis. *Postgrad. med. J.* **38**, 13.

[48] MEDICAL RESEARCH COUNCIL (1967) Risk of thromboembolic disease in women taking oral contraceptives. A preliminary communication by a subcommittee. *Br. med. J.* **ii**, 355.

[49] MERSKEY C., GORDON H. & LACKNER H. (1960) Blood coagulation and fibrinolysis in relation to coronary heart disease. A comparative study of normal white men, white men with overt coronary heart disease, and normal Bantu men. *Br. med. J.* **i**, 219.

[50] MOOLTEN S.E., VROMAN L., VROMAN G.G.S. & GOODMAN B. (1949) Rôle of blood platelets in thromboembolism. *Arch. intern. Med.* **84**, 667.

[51] MORRELL M.T., TRUELOVE S.C. & BARR A. (1963) Pulmonary embolism. *Br. med. J.* **ii**, 830.

[52] OCHSNER A. & DeBAKEY M. (1939) Thrombophlebitis and phlebothrombosis. *Sth. Surg.* **8**, 269.

[53] PAPP O.A. (1962) Control of respiration: rôle of the pressure in the atria and pulmonary artery. Thesis for Diploma in Internal Medicine, McGill University, Montreal.

[54] PATTERSON J.C. & McLACHLIN J. (1954) Precipitating factors in venous thrombosis. *Surg. Gynec. Obstet.* **98**, 96.

[55] PHEAR D. (1960) Pulmonary embolism. A study of late prognosis. *Lancet* **ii**, 832.

[56] ROBIN E.D., JULIAN D.G., TRAVIS D.M. & CRUMP C.H. (1959) A physiologic approach to the diagnosis of acute pulmonary embolism. *New Engl. J. Med.* **260**, 586.

[57] ROBIN E.D., FORKNER C.E, BROMBERG P.A., CROTEAU J.R. & TRAVIS D.M. (1960) Alveolar gas exchange in clinical pulmonary embolism. *New Engl. J. Med.* **262**, 283.

[58] ROSENBERG D.M.L., PEARCE C. & McNULTY J. (1964) Surgical treatment of pulmonary embolism. *J. thorac. cardiovasc. Surg.* **47**, 1.

[59] SABISTON D.C.Jr., MARSHALL R., DUNNILL M.S. & ALLISON P.R. (1962) Experimental pulmonary embolism: Description of a method utilizing large venous thrombi. *Surgery* **52**, 9.

[60] SADOUL P., FAIVRE G., GILGENKRANTL J.M., CHERRIER F. & SAUNIER C. (1962) Étude de la fonction respiratoire dans le cœur pulmonaire

16—R.D.

chronique post-embolique. *J. fr. Méd. Chir. thorac.* **16**, 433.

[61] SALYER J.M. & HARRISON H.N. (1958) Pulmonary infarction complicating segmental resection. *J. thorac. Surg.* **36**, 818.

[62] SCHAUBLE J.F., ANLYAN W.G., DEATON H.L., DeLAUGHTER G.D., BAYLIN G.J. & LYNN J.A. (1960) A study of recurrent pulmonary embolism. *Arch. Surg.* **80**, 105.

[63] SCHONELL M.E., CROMPTON G.K., FORSHALL J.M. & WHITBY L.G. (1966) Failure to differentiate pulmonary infarction from pneumonia by biochemical tests. *Br. med. J.* **i**, 1146.

[64] SEVERINGHAUS J.W. & STUPFEL M. (1957) Alveolar dead space as an index of distribution of blood flow in pulmonary capillaries. *J. appl. Physiol.* **10**, 335.

[65] SEVITT S. & GALLAGHER N. (1961) Venous thrombosis and pulmonary embolism. *Br. J. Surg.* **48**, 475.

[66] SHARNOFF J.G., BAGG J.F., BREEN S.R., ROGLIANO A.G., WALSH A.R. & SCARDINO V. (1960) The possible indication of postoperative thromboembolism by platelet counts and blood coagulation studies in the patient undergoing extensive surgery. *Surg. Gynec. Obstet.* **111**, 469.

[67] SHORT D.S. (1951) A radiological study of pulmonary infarction. *Quart. J. Med.* **20**, 233.

[68] SHORT D.S. (1952) A survey of pulmonary embolism in a general hospital. *Br. med. J.* **i**, 790.

[69] SMITH L.A. & ALLEN E.V. (1940) Circulation time from foot to carotid sinus and from arm to carotid sinus of man. II. Effects of operation and of administration of thyroid gland; postoperative phlebitis and pulmonary embolism. *Arch. Surg.* **41**, 1377.

[70] SPENCER H. (1962) *Pathology of the Lung.* Oxford, Pergamon Press.

[71] SRIVASTAVA S.C. (1964) Absence of pulmonary embolism in Asians. *Br. med. J.* **i**, 772.

[72] STEIN M., FORKNER C.E., ROBIN E.D. & WESSLER S. (1961) Gas exchange after autologous pulmonary embolism in dogs. *J. appl. Physiol.* **16**, 488.

[73] STONEY W.S., JACOBS J.K. & COLLINS H.A. (1963) Pulmonary embolism and embolectomy. *Surg. Gynec. Obstet.* **116**, 292.

[74] STRAUSS L., BAY M.W. & KATZ A.D. (1957) Prothrombin time during the postoperative period. *Am. J. Surg.* **93**, 95.

[75] TAKATS G. DE & JESSER J.H. (1940) Pulmonary embolism: suggestions for its diagnosis, prevention and management. *J. Am. med. Ass.* **114**, 1415.

[76] THOMAS D.P. (1964) Some factors influencing the size of pulmonary emboli. *Lancet* **ii**, 924.

[77] TINCKLER L.F. (1964) Absence of pulmonary embolism in Asians? Letter in *Br. med. J.* **i**, 502.

[78] TORACK R.M. (1958) The incidence and etiology of pulmonary infarction in the absence of congestive heart failure. *Arch. Path.* **65**, 574.

[79] TRENDELENBERG F. (1907) Ueber die Operative Behandlung der Embolie der Lungenarterie. *Zentbl. Chir.* **44**, 1402.

[80] WELCH W.H. (1899) Thrombosis, p. 155; Embolism, p. 228. In *A System of Medicine*, Vol. 6, ed. Allbutt T.C. London, Macmillan.

[81] WESSLER S. & CONNELLY M.T. (1952) Studies of intravascular coagulation. I. Coagulation changes in isolated venous segments. *J. clin. Invest.* **31**, 1011.

[82] WESSLER S., REINER L., FREIMAN D.G., REIMER S.M. & LERTZMAN M. (1959) Serum-induced thrombosis. Studies of its induction and evolution under controlled conditions *in vivo*. *Circulation* **20**, 864.

[83] WILHELMSEN L., SELANDER S., SODERHOLM B., PAULIN S., VARNAUSKAS E. & WERKO L. (1963) Recurrent pulmonary embolism. *Medicine* **42**, 335.

[84] WILLE P. (1960) Die postoperativen Veränderungen im Gerinnungssystem und ihre Bedeutung für die Früherkennung der Thrombose. *Folia haemat.* **4**, 335.

[85] WILLIAMS J.R., WILCOX W.S., ANDREWS G.J. and BURNS R.R. (1963) Angiography in pulmonary embolism. *J. Am. med. Ass.* **184**, 473.

[86] WOMACK W.S. & CASTELLANO C.J. (1952) Migratory thrombophlebitis associated with ovarian carcinoma. *Am. J. Obstet. Gynec.* **63**, 467.

[87] WRIGHT H.P. (1942) Changes in adhesiveness of blood platelets following parturition and surgical operations. *J. Path. Bact.* **54**, 461.

[88] WRIGHT H.P. & OSBORN S.B. (1952) Effect of posture on venous velocity, measured with ^{24}NaCl. *Br. Heart J.* **14**, 325.

CHAPTER 28

Occupational Lung Disease

DEFINITION

Damage to the lungs caused by dusts (pneumoconiosis) or fumes or noxious substances inhaled by workers in certain specific occupations is known as 'occupational lung disease'. Since public money is paid in compensation to those who contract occupational lung disease the criteria for diagnosis are subject to statutory regulations. Distinctive signs or symptoms, characteristic radiographic changes and abnormalities in tests of respiratory function—each or all of these, or any combination of them, may be utilized in the diagnosis and in the assessment of disability.

In the first quarter of this century occupational lung disease was practically synonymous with silicosis. Since then improved radiology, extensive pathological studies, animal experiments, pulmonary function studies and modern epidemiological techniques have widened the field enormously. A great many varieties of occupational lung disease are already recognized by law in Britain and the number is still growing. The commonest are coalworkers' pneumoconiosis, silicosis and asbestosis (table 28.1).

AETIOLOGY

One of the hazards of our technological society is the production by industrial processes of a vast number of substances which are capable of causing respiratory disorders, ranging from minor ailments to chronic disabling diseases. Fortunately, however, the danger is so well recognized that control measures are often applied virtually *pari passu* with the introduction of any new volatile substance or dust which is judged to be potentially dangerous to the lungs. Nevertheless, with the present rapid expansion of industry, particularly in its chemical branches, there will inevitably be introduced an increasing number of respirable substances whose dangerous properties are not at first suspected. Some will escape detection because their ill effects are recognizable only after a long interval, an example being the belated discovery of the relationship of asbestos inhalation to pleural mesothelioma (p. 484).

Dust particles even if chemically inert will cause some harm by their mere presence in the lungs. Lungs clogged with dust inevitably lose something of their ability to expand and contract freely and with the minimum expenditure of energy, and it is on this ability that their functional efficiency depends. The fact that some workers are symptom free and show no very obvious impairment of respiratory function (e.g. early coalworkers' pneumoconiosis) should not condone a complacent attitude to prevention in any dusty occupation.

Apart from mechanical effects due to dust retention in the lungs, noxious substances responsible for occupational lung disease may exert their influence by:

(1) irritation of the air passages (e.g. chlorine, ammonia, sulphur dioxide) commonly associated with secondary infection;

(2) toxicity (e.g. mercury vapour);

(3) the ability to stimulate local fibrosis (e.g. silica);

(4) provoking allergic responses in the lungs (e.g. animal hair, furs, feathers and certain chemicals such as diazomethane); or

(5) by causing granulomatous inflammatory lesions in the lung parenchyma (e.g. beryllium, and the products of mouldy hay, p. 498 and p. 506).

In general the effects produced by inhaling these substances depend upon the concentration in the inspired air, the duration of

TABLE 28.1
Commoner Pneumoconioses

Disease	Cause	Sources of dust	Pathological effects
Baritosis	Barium sulphate	Mining of barium salts	Nil. X-ray changes only
Siderosis	Iron oxide	Welding	Nil. X-ray changes only
Stannosis	Tin oxide	Smelting	Nil. X-ray changes only
Kaolinosis	Hydrated aluminium silicate, etc.	China clay	Simple pneumoconiosis (rarely PMF)
Aluminosis	Stamped aluminium	Explosives, paints	Nodular fibrosis, emphysematous bullae, pneumothorax
Coalworkers' pneumoconiosis	Coal dust	Mining	Simple and complicated pneumoconiosis
Silicosis	Silica	Mining, quarrying, fettling, etc.	Simple and complicated pneumoconiosis
Talcosis	Hydrated magnesium silicate	Rubber industry, etc.	Pulmonary fibrosis
Berylliosis	Beryllium compounds	Atomic reactors, aero engines, electronic equipment, etc.	Granuloma formation, diffuse interstitial fibrosis
Asbestosis	Asbestos	Mining, lagging materials, brake linings, etc.	Pulmonary fibrosis, pleural calcification, bronchial carcinoma, pleural and peritoneal mesothelioma

exposure and, where dusts are concerned, the size of the dust particles. Individual susceptibility is an additional and important factor but one which cannot as yet be assessed. If a substance produces acute irritation of the respiratory tract the onset of symptoms follows immediately after exposure. With non-irritant substances there will be an interval before symptoms appear, depending for its length on the particular pathological process which is involved. An example of the first type is toluene di-isocyanate which is used as a 'foaming' agent in the plastics industry. As soon as the vapour is inhaled the effects of respiratory irritation become apparent with the onset of cough, tightness in the chest, dyspnoea and wheezing. Berylliosis (p. 498) is an example of the delayed onset type of occupational lung disease. Slowly developing granulomatous lesions in the lung give rise to respiratory symptoms 10 years or more after the first exposure to beryllium dust. The exposure need be relatively transient and it may not be remembered by the patient unless he is specifically questioned about it.

To the specific clinical pictures produced by the prolonged inhalation of dusts and fumes may be added chronic bronchitis since it is possible that industrial exposure may pre-dispose to bronchitis without producing radiographic or other signs to distinguish it from bronchitis of nonindustrial origin.

PULMONARY FUNCTION TESTS AND THE PNEUMOCONIOSES

The International Labour Organization Report of a Meeting of Experts [193] stresses the place of pulmonary function tests in prophylaxis, diagnosis, assessment and clinical management of respiratory impairment due to the pneumoconioses. The tests used should be standardized and made available on a worldwide scale so that comparisons can be made of the normal values for pulmonary function and of the effects of pneumoconioses in the different countries. Assistance in the form of grants and survey teams is recommended for the economically developing countries whenever necessary. The need for correlating respiratory impairment, dust exposure and lung pathology is stressed and recommendations are made for studies of patients in the different stages of the pneumoconioses and comparisons with nonindustrial control groups. Postmortem studies relating pathology to dust exposure will continue to play a valuable part in the understanding of any related pulmonary dysfunction. Pulmonary function tests should not only be used to assess functional disability. They should be an important part of pre-employment examination and periodic testing can play an important prophylactic rôle in certain occupations.

TYPES OF OCCUPATIONAL LUNG DISEASE

There are 4 principal types.

1. DUE TO MINERAL DUST

The effect on the lungs varies within a wide range from the mildest lesions caused by the inert, nonreactive dusts of iron, barium, antimony and tin to the most severe, caused by the highly fibrogenic dusts of silica, talc and asbestos. Lesions caused by coal dust, kaolin (China clay) and diatomaceous earth (used in ceramics) are of intermediate severity.

2. DUE TO ORGANIC DUSTS

The products of mouldy hay (farmer's lung), cotton dust (byssinosis), sugar cane dust (bagassosis) and the dust from maple bark (maple bark stripper's lung) are examples of organic dusts which can result in pneumoconiosis.

3. DUE TO GASES AND FUMES

Included in this group are the effects of exposure to ammonia, chlorine, phosgene, sulphur dioxide and trioxide, the oxides of nitrogen and the fumes of various metals. (The list of substances capable of causing irritation or chemical inflammation of the respiratory tract is lengthy and the reader is referred to larger works for more complete descriptions.)

4. PULMONARY AND PLEURAL MALIGNANCY

The development of cancer of the lung may be directly related to inhaled industrial products (p. 484). Pleural mesothelioma may result from asbestos inhalation (p. 484).

EPIDEMIOLOGY OF PNEUMOCONIOSIS IN BRITAIN

Long before any legislation regarding industrial hazards had been formulated a number of forms of occupational lung disease had been recognized and given colloquial designation. Among these were 'potters' rot', 'knife grinders' asthma' and 'masons' phthisis'. In the early part of the 18th century an increased incidence of lung disease was recorded among pottery workers in Staffordshire when finely ground flint was introduced into the manufacturing process. About the same time there were reports of black lungs seen at postmortem examination of coal miners in Fife and the Lothians and this condition was called anthracosis. In the first half of the 19th century it was observed that coal miners in some coal fields were more liable to suffer from chest trouble than in others and the part played by working with stone was appreciated early. The hazard of silicosis was highlighted at the beginning of this century by reports of 'miners' phthisis' among workers in the South African gold mines. The result was that, for a time, attention was focused on those industries in which silica in its various forms was used. There was a false sense of security about occupational disease in coal mining until about 1920 when reports from the South Wales coal field began to appear. Modern research in coalworkers' pneumoconiosis may be said to have developed from this time.

Although it is undergoing marked contraction the major industry in Britain is still coal mining and it is not surprising that the largest number of cases of pneumoconiosis is in coal miners. In 1964, 1213 cases of coalworkers' pneumoconiosis were certified as opposed to 435 cases in other industries. The other industries contributing the largest number of cases were asbestos handling 83, pottery 65, iron foundry works 54 and shale splitting 47. In the 5 years preceding 1964 there had been a fall in coalworkers' pneumoconiosis from 5·3 per 1000 wage earners to 2·4. This improvement undoubtedly reflected the efficacy of preventive measures. The rate of coalworkers' pneumoconiosis varies considerably from area to area (7·5 per 1000 in South Wales in 1964 to 0·2 per 1000 in Northumberland). This disparity is due to several factors including the method of coal production, the dust content of the pit and the 'rank' of the coal. Methods of dust suppression and efficient ventilation, often best in those mines in which gas is a recognized hazard, undoubtedly influence the incidence of pneumoconiosis. Studies in the 1940's concluded that the incidence of pneumoconiosis was somehow related to the hardness or rank of the coal [79 & 114]. Thus the disease was commoner in the anthracite (hard, high rank) than in the bituminous or steam coal (soft, low rank) pits. This situation did not obtain in the years 1951–55 [161] and it is possible that the higher incidence was related to the previously poorer ventilation in the anthracite mines compared with the others.

Pneumoconiosis is often due to the inhalation of several different noxious agents at the same time and the components of the mixture may vary in different sections of the same industry (e.g. coal mining, arc welding, etc.).

DEPOSITION AND RETENTION OF DUSTS IN THE LUNG

The mechanisms by which dust particles are trapped in the lung were first evaluated in 1935 by Findeisen [77] who constructed a model based on Newtonian principles, with the concept of inertia, Stokes' law concerning the rate of fall of small particles and the diffusion theory based on Brownian motion. Most particles carried into the bronchial tree on inhalation deposit on the walls above the level of the respiratory bronchioles. Inhaled particles with a diameter over 20 μ or so collide with the bronchial walls or settle on the walls by gravitation. Particles of unit density cannot enter alveoli if they are more than about 10 μ in diameter. In the range 2–10 μ some reach the alveoli and some deposit on the walls higher up. Particles between 0·1 and 2 μ in diameter nearly all reach the alveoli. Most of those below 0·1 μ settle on the bronchial epithelium by a process of diffusion. Deposition is least in the 0·4–0·5 μ range and up to 80% of particles in this size may be breathed out again.

Deposition of fine particles tends to be greatest in the lower halves of the upper lobes, the upper halves of the lower lobes and the middle lobe [212]. Faulds [70] attributed this distribution to drainage of mucus with entrapped dust particles into these parts of the lung during sleep. Particles larger than about 30 μ in diameter are carried to the lower lobes in the axial air stream, e.g. asbestos, talc.

The subsequent fate of inhaled particles of less than 10 μ diameter is described in the section on coalworkers' pneumoconiosis.

COALWORKERS' PNEUMOCONIOSIS

DEFINITION

The form of pneumoconiosis resulting from prolonged inhalation of coal dust.

PATHOGENESIS AND PATHOLOGY

The coal dust particles in the lesions of coalworkers' pneumoconiosis are mostly about 5 μ diameter. Being small enough to be carried into the alveoli during inspiration, but too large to remain suspended, they are deposited on the alveolar walls to which they adhere.

Eventually they become dislodged by respiratory movements or engulfed by alveolar wall phagocytes which are dislodged in their turn and the free dust particles and the dust laden phagocytes gradually move out of the alveoli into the bronchioles to be excreted in the sputum. The clearing mechanism is slower in alveoli with fixed attachments which restrict their movements. These alveoli, namely those attached to and opening into respiratory bronchioles and those attached to the pleura, interlobular septa and blood vessels, become clogged with coal dust and dust laden macrophages. Permanent fibrotic lesions develop after death of the macrophages has provided the protein and lipoid rich matrix needed for reticulin fibril production.

Some of the coal dust in the alveoli is cleared by the lymphatic route after entering the alveolar wall tissues in some manner not yet understood. Blocking of lymphatics leads to coal pigmentation and fibrosis in the interstitial tissues adjacent to the clogged alveoli, along the lymphatics and in the hilar lymph nodes. Fibrosis in the interlobular septa and alveoli at the periphery of the lobules leads to compensatory dilatation of the more mobile alveoli in the centre of the lobules (hence centrilobular emphysema).

The process outlined above accounts for the appearance of the lung in *simple coalworkers' pneumoconiosis*: coal impregnated nodular and diffuse fibrosis outlines the pleura and the lung lobules, the parenchyma of which has a spongier texture than usual because of compensatory emphysema.

Pulmonary fibrosis in pneumoconiosis does not occur through the direct action of dusts or their dissolution products. For fibrosis to occur dusts must be absorbed by macrophages. Subsequent degeneration of the cells liberates toxic substances which cause inflammation and fibrosis. Fibrosis, therefore, stems essentially from a lesion of the phagocytic cells.

Heppleston [119] by an ingenious technique demonstrated that dust in the lung is capable of active migration. He first produced a pneumoconiosis in animals with coal dust and when this was established exposed the animals to haematite. He found that the black and red dusts soon became intimately mixed. Even the apparently immutable classical fibrotic nodule of silicosis could become permeated by other dusts inhaled at a later date. This dynamic situation is presumably explained, in part at least, by the lung phagocytes.

A miner inhaling 1000 particles per ml of size 0·5–5 μ (rather higher than present approved conditions) might inhale 150 g of dust per year of which 1·5–15 g might be deposited in the alveoli and 0·5 g permanently retained. Airborne coal dust contains a little free silica (mean value less than 2% in South Wales)

and previously this was regarded as the cause of the pathological process. Were this the case the pure dust lesion of coalworkers should resemble the silicotic lesion but this is not so. There is, therefore, much to support the view that the simple dust lesion of coalworkers is a nonspecific reaction to the larger fraction of the dust which contains no free silica and that the contribution from free silica is slight and nonspecific [117]. That free silica is not necessary for the development of the lesion in simple coalworkers' pneumoconiosis is supported by a number of reports of pneumoconiosis due to carbon (e.g. workers with carbon black, graphite or carbon electrodes) in which the lesions produced were identical with those in coalworkers.

High concentrations of silica in coal dust do, however, alter the pathological picture. A mixture of coal and quartz produces more fibrosis in the lungs than the sum of each alone. In rats an intratracheal injection of 2 mg of quartz produces no fibrosis and 100 mg of coal results only in minimal amounts of reticulin. 98 mg of coal and 2 mg of quartz, however, results in some degree of fibrosis. The assumption from this is that the lungs can deal with 2 mg of quartz in the rat, probably by moving it on to the hilar glands, but the clogging effect of coal dust impedes the removal of quartz from the lung parenchyma so that it can then cause lung fibrosis [139].

All forms of pneumoconiosis due to dust particles of 1–10 μ size have the same mode of development and the same type and distribution of lesions, such differences as occur being due to the special properties of the dust particles concerned.

Simple coalworkers' pneumoconiosis being essentially due to the physical 'silting up' of coal dust in the lung will progress only as long as excessive amounts of coal dust continue to be inhaled. It does, however, predispose to a progressive form of pneumoconiosis known as *complicated pneumoconiosis* which is characterized by the lesions of *progressive massive fibrosis* (PMF).

PROGRESSIVE MASSIVE FIBROSIS

The lesions, which are almost invariably situated in the upper lobes, are rounded fibrotic masses several centimetres in diameter, sometimes with necrotic central cavities. Pneumoconiosis of the ordinary type is always present elsewhere in the lungs, but there is no relationship between the degree of pneumoconiosis and the development of PMF. The pneumoconiosis need not be due to coal dust; PMF occurs in several other dust diseases as well (e.g. the pneumoconioses due to haematite, kaolin or graphite) and is particularly common in silicosis. For PMF to develop in simple pneumoconiosis of whatever type the 'silting up' process already described must be supplemented by the action of some fibrosis-inducing factor which is independent of further dust inhalation. It is no longer believed that this factor is tuberculous infection. Miners with PMF do not show the symptoms of clinical tuberculosis and only rarely can tubercle bacilli be isolated from the sputum. Even in postmortem material it is rare to show evidence of tuberculosis in the lungs. The Medical Research Council's Epidemiological Research Unit tested the hypothesis that PMF of coalworkers was due in part to tuberculosis infection by studying the tuberculin sensitivity of a random sample of 1250 miners and ex-miners in South Wales. It was found that there was no difference in the tuberculin reaction to 5 TU between miners and ex-miners with PMF and men with either no pneumoconiosis or simple pneumoconious [113]. These findings confirmed the results of a previous study by Hart and Aslett [114]. Hendriks and Bleiker in Holland found similar results in Dutch miners. They showed that there was a well marked correlation between tuberculin hypersensitivity and age but no correlation with category of pneumoconiosis. There did not appear to be any difference in hypersensitivity between miners having PMF and men of the same age who had never worked underground [115]. Rogan has reported the failure of antituberculosis chemotherapy to influence PMF in coalminers [221].

Whatever the promoting factor for the development of PMF, it is thought that an enhanced immune reaction occurs followed by the deposition of immune globulin in the pneumoconiotic lungs. The globulins form a matrix suitable for fibrous tissue development but favouring the production of collagen rather than reticulin fibrils—an important difference from the fibrosis of ordinary coalworkers' pneumoconiosis. The evidence for immune mechanism activity in cases of PMF is discussed in the section on Silicosis (p. 480). Although the details of the process are still far from clear it is accepted that the PMF in coalworkers' pneumoconiosis is fundamentally the same pathological process. Coalworkers' pneumoconiosis does, however, provide an example of PMF-like lesions in which the participation of the immune mechanism can scarcely be doubted. These lesions, first described by Caplan (1953) [38] occur in patients with *rheumatoid arthritis and coalworkers' pneumoconiosis*, and consist of rounded, fibrotic nodules 0·5–5 cm in diameter situated at the periphery of the lung but without predilection for any particular lobe. On microscopic examination they show an arrangment of concentric layers of collagenous fibrous tissue exactly as in the PMF lesions but the necrotic central area, instead of being of a piece with the collagen as in PMF, is separated from it by a zone of palisaded histiocytes which is a typically rheumatoid histological picture. The Caplan lesions may precede, accompany or follow the clinical evidence of rheumatoid arthritis but they are clearly inseparable from it and hence owe their existence, in part at least, to the obscure immunity disturbance which is the fundamental basis of rheumatoid disease.

The lesions in 'rheumatoid pneumoconiosis' characteristically tend to appear in crops, fresh lesions developing at intervals of a few months, and they develop more rapidly than the PMF lesions in patients without rheumatoid arthritis. The course of rheumatoid nodules in the lung varies. Some remain quiescent, others may calcify and still others undergo necrosis. Necrotic material may be coughed up to leave one or more thin-walled cavities which may contract or even disappear radiologically. In many cases the Caplan lesions become incorporated in large areas of fibrosis indistinguishable radiologically from PMF. At autopsy the latter can be shown to be an aggregation of multiple nodules. Rarely a pleural effusion may complicate the picture.

The Caplan syndrome is not confined to coalworkers' pneumoconiosis. Examples of the Caplan lesion have also been reported in workers exposed to a variety of other dusts in potteries, sand blasting and brass and iron foundries. It may also occur rarely in asbestosis (p. 486).

Chemical studies have shown that the lungs in PMF may contain 40–50 g of dust. Over 80% of this is coal, 10–15% is mixed rock material and 2–3% quartz [30]. In a study of the lungs of 18 coalworkers with PMF Nagelschmidt and his colleagues [190] showed that the dust concentration in PMF lesions was on an average twice as high as in the rest of the lung but the quartz content was not significantly different. They felt that this was additional proof against the silica theory of PMF.

Cochrane and Miall [46] found an attack rate of PMF of about 1% per year in South Wales; elsewhere in the country the prevalence is lower.

COMPLICATIONS OF PMF

The spreading fibrosis at the periphery of PMF lesions implicates bronchi, arterioles, veins and lymphatics. Stenosis, dilatation and distortion of bronchi predispose to chronic bronchitis and bronchiectasis; fibrosis of blood vessels leads to intimal hyperplasia and favours ischaemic necrosis in the lesions, thrombosis particularly of pulmonary veins and, at a later stage of the disease, the development of pulmonary hypertension and *cor pulmonale*. Lymphatic obstruction by fibrosis hinders drainage and favours further coal dust retention and fibrosis.

X-RAY APPEARANCES

The x-ray appearances in the pneumoconioses depend on the quantity of dust retained in the lungs and its radiodensity. For example much larger quantities of coal dust are required than iron oxide to give similar x-ray appearances. In coalworkers' pneumoconiosis the earliest radiographic indication of dust retention in the lungs is likely to occur when the patient is symptom free and while the prognosis is still relatively good. The routine radiographic screening of coalworkers is designed to detect these early changes.

Simple coalworkers' pneumoconiosis is characterized radiographically by minute opacities diffusely scattered throughout both lung fields. The opacities are punctiform (up to 1·5 mm), micronodular or miliary (diameter between 1·5 and 3 mm) or nodular (between 3 and 10 mm diameter). The micronodular type of opacity occurs most frequently. The severity of the disease is classified radiographically under 3 headings as follows:

Category 1

A small number of opacities in an area equivalent to at least 2 anterior rib spaces and at the most not greater than one third of the 2 lung fields.

Category 2

Opacities more numerous and diffuse than in Category 1 and distributed over most of the lung fields.

Category 3

Very numerous profuse opacities covering the whole or nearly the whole of the lung fields.

In Category 1 simple pneumoconiosis the risk of developing complicated pneumoconiosis is extremely small [44]. The chances of PMF developing increase from about 1% for Category 1 to 30% or more for Category 3 [43]. Periodic x-ray examination is, therefore, one of the important preventive measures in the control of the disease. A miner with diagnosable pneumoconiosis is eligible for Industrial Injuries Benefit. Most commonly Category 2 simple pneumoconiosis (the stage at which a liability to PMF exists) must be present before a claim for compensation can be accepted (p. 478).

The more detailed International Labour Office classification proposed in Geneva in 1958 is shown in table 28.2. Small opacities are designated p, m or n according to size. Complicated pneumoconiosis is graded by the total area of the lesions into categories A, B and C. Increasing category correlates roughly with disability for any given age.

Progressive massive fibrosis may present as single or multiple opacities in the upper lobes, usually peripherally situated and frequently irregular in outline. The lesions progress even when all further contact with dust is avoided. Cavitation may occur in the PMF lesion. The nature of the PMF lesion is suggested by the background of simple pneumoconiosis.

The Caplan lesions (p. 474) may be associated with only very slight evidence of simple pneumoconiosis in the lung as a whole and the rounded peripheral lesions may be mistaken for metastatic neoplasia.

The later stages of advanced coalworkers' pneumoconiosis may terminate in *cor pulmonale* with x-ray evidence of dilated pulmonary arteries and cardiomegaly.

FUNCTIONAL ABNORMALITY

In a majority of miners coal dust can be demonstrated in the lungs on pathological examination even though there has been little or no demonstrable abnormality of pulmonary function as estimated by the commonly used tests. As has already been stated this does not mean that the accumulation of coal dust in the lungs is not harmful; it simply means that the standard pulmonary function tests cannot detect abnormality. The most commonly applied test has been the Forced Expiratory Volume which, of course, may be influenced by chronic bronchitis or asthma. Smoking is common among miners and abnormalities in FEV may be due to this rather than the pneumoconiosis [148].

In contrast to simple coalworkers' pneumoconiosis when it is the rule to find relatively normal indices of lung function the complicated form with PMF always shows abnormalities of lung function and these are more or less distinctive. Cochrane and Higgins [45] found that the area of the shadows of PMF commonly exceeded 20 cm^2 before disability was appreciable. The fact that PMF lesions occupy space in the lung and reduce the effective volume of tissue for gas exchange, the associated compensatory emphysema and the distortion of bronchi all contribute to functional abnormality. The changes in lung function are principally those of a space occupying lesion and, as the patient becomes older and recurrent infections are more frequent, chronic bronchitis with emphysema becomes superimposed leading to severe ventilatory defect with irreversible obstructive airways disease and finally arterial undersaturation, CO_2 retention and *cor pulmonale*. The FEV is reduced. The RV may be normal or increased resulting in an increased RV/TLC ratio. This does not necessarily mean the presence of emphysema since the TLC is reduced by the space occupying lesion of progressive massive fibrosis. Gas distribution is impaired but not so severely as is seen commonly in emphysema. Diffusing capacity is also reduced, but this is not marked until there is significant associated emphysema. The alveolar–arterial Po_2 difference has been shown to increase progressively as the radiological category increases [25]. When the patient is breathing air the exercise ventilation is normal or slightly increased in the earlier stages; later the ability to exercise is much reduced and at this stage the exercise ventilation may be reduced by oxygen therapy and the use of portable oxygen may be justified.

CLINICAL FEATURES

The diagnosis of pneumoconiosis should be suspected in a man who has worked in the mines for several years and who complains of increasing breathlessness on exertion. It is common for the patient to have associated chronic bronchitis and to be a cigarette smoker. The question of coalworkers' pneumoconiosis *per se* predisposing to chronic bronchitis has not yet been satisfactorily answered. In the absence of bronchitis the dyspnoea is usually unaccompanied by cough except in the later stages when cough is nearly

TABLE 28.2

International Classification of Persistent Radiological Opacities in the Lung Fields Provoked by the Inhalation of Mineral Dusts.* (*Geneva, 1958*)

Type of opacity	No pneumo-coniosis	Suspect	Pneumoconiosis									
			Linear opacities	Small opacities						Large opacities		
Qualitative features	O	Z	L	p		m		n		A	B	C
Quantitative features				1 2 3		1 2 3		1 2 3				
Additional symbols	(co)/ (cp)	(cv)	(di)	(em)		(hi)		(pl)		(px)		(tb)

* Including coal and carbon dusts.

DEFINITIONS AND COMMENTS

The object of the classification is to codify the radiological appearances of the pneumoconioses in a simple, easily reproducible way. It is intended to describe the radiographic appearances of the persistent opacities associated with pneumoconiosis, not to define pathological entities, nor to take into account the question of working capacity.

Where there is an appreciable difference in the appearance of the two lungs, the two appearances may be described separately, beginning with the right lung.

No pneumo-moconiosis	O	No radiographic evidence of pneumoconiosis

Suspect opacities	Z	Increased lung markings

Pneumoconiosis

Linear opacities	L	Numerous linear or reticular opacities, the lung pattern being normal, accentuated or obscured

The following types are defined according to the greatest diameter of the predominant opacities.

The categorization depends on the extent and the profusion of the opacities.

Small opacities[1]

p — Punctiform opacities. Size up to 1·5 mm

m — Micronodular or miliary opacities. Greatest diameter between 1·5 and 3 mm.

n — Nodular opacities. Size between 3 and 10 mm.

Category 1: A small number of opacities in an area equivalent to at least 2 anterior rib spaces and at the most not greater than one third of the 2 lung fields.

Category 2: Opacities more numerous and diffuse than in category 1 and distributed over most of the lung fields.

Category 3: Very numerous profuse opacities covering the whole or nearly the whole of the lung fields.

Large opacities[2]

A — An opacity having a longest diameter of between 1 and 5 cm, or several opacities each greater than 1 cm, the sum of whose longest diameters does not exceed 5 cm.

B — One or more opacities, larger or more numerous than those in category A, whose combined area does not exceed one third of one lung field.

C — One or more large opacities, whose combined area exceeds one third of one lung field.

Additional symbols

Recommended additional symbols[3]

(co) — abnormalities of the cardiac outline. To be replaced by (cp): *cor pulmonale*, if this condition is strongly suspected.

(cv) — cavity.

(di) — significant distortion of the intrathoracic organs.

(em) — marked emphysema.

(hi) — marked abnormalities of the hilar shadows.

(pl) — significant pleural abnormalities.

(px) — pneumothorax.

(tb) — opacities suggestive of active tuberculosis.

[1] The choice of order of the symbols is left to the convenience of the physician.
[2] The background of small opacities should be specified as far as possible.
[3] The use of these symbols is optional.

always present particularly in the morning on rising. The sputum when present is usually mucoid but infective exacerbations are common and, when bronchiectasis coexists, purulent sputum is the rule. When PMF lesions cavitate the sputum becomes jet black (melanoptysis). This, though alarming, is not of serious importance and is not necessarily associated with the development of tuberculosis. The sputum should, however, be examined repeatedly for tubercle bacilli if this feature occurs. Recurrent haemoptysis is common in PMF but it is unusual for bleeding to be severe. Again, it does not necessarily mean that tuberculosis is present.

Chest pain is common and may be due to various causes:

(1) intercostal myalgia which, if present, should be treated by local heat or infiltration of local anaesthetic;

(2) pleurisy;

(3) ischaemic heart disease or pulmonary hypertension giving a constricting type of retrosternal pain;

(4) pneumothorax in which the chest pain is associated with increased breathlessness.

The physical findings in the chest are not diagnostic of pneumoconiosis as such and any of the features of bronchitis, emphysema or *cor pulmonale* may be present.

There is no evidence to suggest that carcinoma of the lung is more common in patients with coalworkers' pneumoconiosis than in matched controls. There is, of course, the difficulty in diagnosis caused by the similarity between progressive massive fibrosis and bronchial neoplasm which may have led to confusion in early studies. When carcinoma of the lung does occur in patients with coalworkers' pneumoconiosis there is no appreciable overall difference in survival rates between miners and nonminers [97]. But, within the group of miners, Goldman [97] showed that survival rate of lung cancer tended to increase with rise in radiographic category of simple pneumoconiosis and suggested that this might be due to a retardation of spread of neoplasm in miners' lungs by the coal dust.

DIFFERENTIAL DIAGNOSIS

The radiographic appearances in conjunction with the history of occupational exposure usually suggests the diagnosis. The development of PMF may be difficult to differentiate from bronchial carcinoma or tuberculosis. Previous chest radiographs tracing the slow development of the lesion on a background of simple pneumoconiosis will frequently be helpful. Occasionally an absolute diagnosis cannot be made from carcinoma without recourse to thoracotomy if pulmonary function permits. The Mantoux test, tomography and bacteriological examination of the sputum may help to exclude an active tuberculous lesion. In patients with pneumoconiosis a certain diagnosis of active tuberculosis requires nothing less than the finding of tubercle bacilli in the sputum. Radiographic differentiation is not possible.

MANAGEMENT

There is no specific treatment for the condition and the most important aspect of management is prevention. In its essentials this implies effective dust suppression, the early recognition of dust retention by routine radiography and, when necessary, the provision of alternative employment in surroundings with low dust concentration to prevent progress of the disease.

If, through the development of respiratory symptoms or as a result of the discovery of a radiographic abnormality, a miner is suspected of having pneumoconiosis he may claim benefit under the National Insurance Industrial Injuries Act. In the first place his case must be reviewed by a Pneumoconiosis Panel who determine if diagnosable pneumoconiosis is present on the basis of radiographic appearances and the industrial history. If the disease is confirmed, disability is then determined on a percentage basis. The assessments are in the range of 1–100% by increments of 10. Any disablement award is in addition to sickness benefit allowable under the National Insurance Acts. There are also other supplementary benefits for particular cases. Certification of pneumoconiosis does not necessarily mean that further work underground is forbidden. Indeed, in most instances, the man can continue work in 'approved dust conditions' underground. The idea of men registered as having pneumoconiosis continuing to work underground may seem strange until it is appreciated that over 60% of those presently receiving compensation for coalworkers' pneumoconiosis have their disability assessed at 10% or less.

When the sputum is positive for tubercle bacilli bacteriological cure can be achieved by appropriate chemotherapy although radiographic improvement is usually disappointing [207]. In these cases bacteriological conversion can be achieved by chemotherapy just as quickly as in cases of tuberculosis without industrial disease [207]. Rarely anonymous mycobacteria have complicated PMF, raising difficulties because of primary resistance of many of these organisms to the antituberculosis drugs. The management of bronchial infection, generalized airways obstruction and *cor pulmonale* are discussed elsewhere.

SUPERVISION OF COALWORKERS' PNEUMOCONIOSIS CASES AT WORK

When a miner is certified as having pneumoconiosis the Pneumoconiosis Medical Panel make recommendations as to his employment and, if the worker agrees, the Management are informed of these. The Pneumoconiosis Medical Panel may advise work in dust free conditions on the surface or, as in most cases, in approved conditions underground. Men coming within this scheme are kept under regular supervision by Area Medical Officers who review not only the man but his place of employment with the help of the Coal Board's Scientific Department where random samples of dust are analysed. It is the aim of the National Coal Board to achieve 'approved dust conditions' generally. These conditions have special application in relation to the employment of pneumoconiosis cases. The following standards have been agreed in Britain:

(1) stone drifts and scourings (all Divisions): not more than 250 p.p. cm^3;

(2) all other locations:

(a) in all Divisions (except South Western Division): not more than 700 p.p. cm^3;

(b) in South Western Division (except anthracite collieries): not more than 500 p.p. cm^3;

(c) in anthracite collieries (South Western Division): not more than 400 p.p. cm^3.

All the standards refer to particles in the size range 1–5 μ.

When a Medical Panel decides that a claimant has pneumoconiosis a letter of advice is sent telling him whether or not he can safely continue at his work and, if so, under what conditions. This is most important in relation to cases with PMF. The claimant is free to decide for himself and can seek any further advice he wishes from his family doctor or trade union. His decision whether to continue at work or not does not affect his disability pension.

The Pneumoconiosis Medical Panel may also 'suspend a man from work in the process'. This is not common and is usually used when there is coincident pulmonary tuberculosis requiring treatment.

SILICOSIS

DEFINITION

The form of pneumoconiosis resulting from inhalation of dust containing silica particles 1–10 μ in diameter.

PATHOGENESIS

The earth's crust is composed mainly of silica and silicates. Their dusts are, therefore, encountered to a varying degree in mining and in the handling of quartz-containing stone where this involves dust production, e.g. stone trimming, granite crushing, etc. Also a large number of industrial processes involve the use of finely divided silica (table 28.3) which may be inhaled.

The distribution of silica particles in the lung and the initial production of lesions by

TABLE 28.3

Principal Industries Associated with Silica

(1) Mining of gold, tin, copper, mica, graphite

(2) Quarrying of granite, sandstone and slate

(3) Stone dressing

(4) Metal casting and sandblasting

(5) Pottery and ceramics

(6) Manufacture and trimming of refractory bricks used in furnaces

(7) Boiler scaling

(8) Some forms of enamelling

(9) Variably encountered in rubber and paint industries

the 'silting up' process is the same in silicosis as in coalworkers' pneumoconiosis. The further progress of the disease is modified, however, by effects due to the silica particles themselves and is characterized by more abundant fibrosis which is also denser and more collagenous than that of coalworkers' pneumoconiosis. A man can retain 30 g of coal dust in the lungs and still be reasonably healthy but one tenth of this amount of quartz would be fatal.

The strongly fibrogenic properties of the silica particles have been explained in several different ways. The original *solubility theory* which attributed all the effects of silica dust to liberation of silicic acid is no longer considered valid and extensions of the theory [120 & 125] according to which silicic acid takes the place of mucopolysaccharides in the bonding of proteins to form collagen, while acceptable up to a point, are not regarded as a complete explanation. At present 2 biological theories which are not mutually exclusive hold the field. The *antigen theory* interprets the reaction to silica as an immunity reaction. This is supported by the increased production of plasma cells and the high levels of serum globulin in patients with silicosis [259] and by the fact that the fibrous tissue in the silicosis lesions contains large amounts of

alpha and beta globulins and lipoid. The theory embraces a part of the extended solubility theory in so far as the antigen responsible for the reaction is held to be a compound of silica and body protein. The laying down of fibrous tissue is comparable to the deposition of amyloid at foci of chronic infection. In fact, the silicosis fibrous tissue closely resembles amyloid in its chemical composition [203].

The *phospholipid theory* of fibrosis emphasizes the part played by the tissue phagocytes. Experimental evidence seems to confirm that fibrogenesis is dependent on some substance liberated from dead macrophages. In experimental silicosis Fallon [69] showed that death of silica laden macrophages resulted in the formation of phospholipids which were fibrogenic. Silicates (e.g. mica, sericite, etc.) cause less damage to phagocytes, less phospholipid production and consequently less fibrosis.

The biological theories provide a better understanding of the way in which tuberculous infection stimulates the fibrogenic effects of silicosis. It is suggested that the addition of dead tubercle bacilli to the protein and lipoid material derived from dead macrophages acts in the manner of a 'Freund's Adjuvant' to 'boost', as it were, the immunity response to the silica-protein antigen [261]. This concept may be a possible basis for the PMF in other forms of pneumoconiosis, in which, however, the nature of the antigen is much more obscure.

PATHOLOGY

The lung in silicosis has the same general appearance as in coalworkers' pneumoconiosis except that the lesions are larger and more fibrotic and greyish black rather than inky black. The same features apply to PMF when it develops in silicotic lungs. Microscopically the silicotic lesions are made up of concentric layers of collagen containing silica particles as well as trapped carbon. The excessive fibrosis, like that of PMF in coalworkers' pneumoconiosis, involves bronchi, blood vessels and lymphatics. Silicosis specifically predisposes to pulmonary tuberculosis

(p. 183) and positive cultures are more likely to be obtained from the necrotic material in the larger nodules than in coalworkers' pneumoconiosis. As in coal dust pneumoconiosis the classical histological features of tuberculous granulation tissue are seldom seen. Pleural thickening and adhesions are common in the silicotic lung.

FUNCTIONAL ABNORMALITY

In general, abnormalities of pulmonary function have not been so well documented in silicosis as in coalworkers' pneumoconiosis. Relatively normal function may be present in about 15–20% of patients with the radiographic appearances of simple silicosis [15 & 224]. Impairment in exercise diffusing capacity appears to be important in some early cases but how frequently this occurs is not known. When the condition has been present for some time the pathological process results in a combination of restrictive (due to fibrosis) and obstructive (due to secondary emphysema) patterns of disability, one of which may predominate. Thus there may be reduced FRC and RV and relatively normal air flow, or the features associated with obstructive airways disease (p. 51) with decreased air flow. Diffusing capacity may be reduced with either pattern, though for different reasons. In early cases arterial oxygen unsaturation may be detectable with heavy exercise [15 & 223].

The functional abnormality associated with the development of PMF has not been studied sufficiently to allow patterns of abnormality to be defined. Obviously $\dot{V}/\dot{Q}$ abnormalities must be severe. In the later stages of the disease the features of chronic hypoxia and CO_2 retention are present.

X-RAY APPEARANCES

In *simple silicosis* diffuse miliary or nodular lesions are found throughout both lung fields although they are usually more marked in the upper and middle zones. In the *complicated form* the lesions of massive fibrosis appear as dense shadows, which may be cavitated, on a background of nodulation and may cause gross distortion of the surrounding tissues. Associated bronchitis, emphysema, tuberculosis and *cor pulmonale* may modify the radiographic appearances.

The hilar shadows may be enlarged. 'Egg shell' calcification of the hilar lymph glands is a distinctive feature of silicosis.

CLINICAL FEATURES

Symptoms do not usually appear until after several years of exposure to the dust but an *acute form* with symptoms appearing within a few months of exposure used to be encountered in workers engaged in the manufacture of abrasive soaps before the hazard of silicosis was fully appreciated [180]. A mixture of silica dust and alkali was thought to be responsible for this particular manifestation. The dominant clinical feature was dyspnoea and it was accompanied by cyanosis, fever and grave systemic upset, passing into cachexia and often leading to death within a few weeks. The replacement of millstone grit by carborundum has virtually abolished the acute form of silicosis.

The *chronic form* of the disease usually presents with slowly progressive dyspnoea on exertion to which is added unproductive cough and recurrent bouts of bronchitis. Haemoptysis occasionally occurs. The development of silico-tuberculosis is marked by deterioration in general condition, worsening of dyspnoea, increase in cough and sputum, pyrexia and loss of weight. Haemoptysis is more likely at this stage. Tubercle bacilli may be found in the sputum. The tuberculous lesions in the silicotic lung are so chronic and indurative that the demonstration of tubercle bacilli is often the only way in which the infection can be recognized.

Silicosis is not associated with an increased incidence of lung cancer [89 & 127]. The physical signs vary with the stage of the disease, the degree of associated bronchitis and emphysema and the amount of associated pleural thickening. In the late stages the features of *cor pulmonale* and congestive cardiac failure may be present.

DIAGNOSIS

The patient's occupation will usually suggest the possibility of exposure to dust. In the simple form the diffuse lesion may have to be distinguished from the many other causes of diffuse miliary or nodular opacities, including sarcoidosis (p. 371), haemosiderosis (p. 596), miliary tuberculosis (p. 207), etc. Investigations should always include bacteriological examination of the sputum for tubercle bacilli.

MANAGEMENT OF SILICOSIS

There is no specific treatment for the primary condition. The treatment of the associated conditions is dealt with elsewhere.

Since silicosis continues to progress even after exposure to dust has ceased it is vital to diagnose the condition at the earliest possible stage and to remove the patient from all further contact with the offending dust.

The disease is notifiable and compensation is covered by the National Health Industrial Injuries Act.

ASBESTOSIS

DEFINITION

The form of pneumoconiosis due to inhalation of asbestos dust.

THE NATURE AND USES OF ASBESTOS

Asbestos is a mixture of silicates of iron, magnesium, nickel, calcium and aluminium which has the unique property of occurring naturally as a fibre. Commercial asbestos consists of compact bunches of extremely fine crystalline filaments lying parallel to each other. The length of each filament may vary from a few millimetres to several centimetres. The manufacture of asbestos involves crushing rock to yield fibres and amorphous powder. Both the mining and manufacture of asbestos result in much dust. Small particles of an average length of 50 μ and a diameter of about 0·5 μ are mainly responsible for the harmful effects of asbestos inhalation.

The consumption of asbestos has increased 8-fold in the last 30 years and 1000-fold in the last 60 years. Although the diffuse crippling fibrosis due to pulmonary asbestosis was recognized as early as 1906 and precautionary measures were introduced officially from 1931 onwards the incidence of asbestosis has shown a steady increase. This is due to the fact that there are no known substitutes for some of its uses.

Asbestos (its name means 'indestructible') has many properties which make it indispensable in modern industry. These include its strength, fire resistance and acid and alkali resistance. Fireproof clothing, fire resistant bulkheads, brake and clutch linings, asbestos cement, tiles, paints, tyres, roofing felts, flooring compounds, pipe lagging and electric wire insulation are only some of the uses to which this valuable mineral is put. It is reported that there are at least 1000 different uses for asbestos [116]. Against this background of the rapidly increasing use of asbestos must be examined the hazards to health of those who have to deal with it. In contrast to coal mining which has a decreasing incidence of pneumoconiosis those industries in which asbestos is employed are providing increasing numbers of cases of asbestosis. The latter is, however, still numerically much less a problem than coalworkers' pneumoconiosis in Britain. Over the years 1959–64 the number of cases of coalminers' pneumoconiosis fell from 3523 to 1213 whereas the number of cases of asbestosis rose from 37 to 83.

Apart from the tremendous increase in the use of the substance a possible explanation for the lack of correlation between the effects of preventive measures (said to cost 7% of the wage bill) and the incidence of asbestosis is the fact that asbestos is being used more and more in industries which are not directly subject to statutory regulations. Disquieting evidence is now appearing that even the ordinary town dweller may be exposed to the risk of asbestos inhalation from atmospheric pollution. The persistence of asbestos, once inhaled and retained in the lungs, is of considerable importance with regard to potential disability in later life.

TYPES OF ASBESTOS

There are 4 main types of asbestos fibre, each with its particular properties. The most important in terms of amount used is *chrysotile* or serpentine asbestos, a hydrated magnesium silicate containing small amounts of iron and aluminium. It varies in colour from white to greyish green and is the softest of the forms of asbestos fibres. Its principal use is in heat and alkali resistant textiles. Chrysotile is mainly found among igneous rock containing high concentrations of ferromagnesium silicates. The chief sources are Canada, the U.S.S.R., South Africa and Rhodesia. *Anthophyllite* is a less important magnesium-containing, white asbestos found in Finland and Italy and used for coating welding rods. Like all the forms of asbestos it is potentially dangerous and pleural calcification (p. 485) has been reported following its use.

Amosite, which comes only from the Transvaal and is brown in colour, differs from chrysotile in containing more silica, a larger percentage of iron and much less magnesium. The fibres are extremely long, sometimes as much as 30 cm, but they have a low tensile strength and are brittle. Its principal use is in heat insulation. *Crocidolite* or blue asbestos also contains iron and has the important property of marked resistance to acids, making it extremely useful in pipe packings in the chemical industry. It is also remarkably strong and it has been stated that only especially hardened steel wire is stronger. Crocidolite comes mainly from the North West Cape; small amounts are also mined in North West Australia. It has been shown that amosite and crocidolite contain traces of 3:4 benzpyrene. Crocidolite contains roughly 3 times more than amosite (3 μg per 100 g for crocidolite as opposed to 1 μg per 100 g for amosite).

Two other forms of asbestos are *tremolite* and *actinolite*. Both contain calcium and a trace of iron and may also contain 3:4 benzpyrene. Their industrial use is limited and on this account they are less important as occupational hazards. Tremolite is used in filters and actinolite is sometimes used to strengthen paper.

The yearly production in 1000 tons of the various types of asbestos in 1962 was as follows: chrysotile 1700, crocidolite 132, amosite 75 and anthophyllite 11. From the point of view of occupational hazard, therefore, the most important of all the forms of asbestos is chrysotile. In the crude form the fibres may be up to 2 cm long but only a few microns in diameter. Being fragile and rigid they snap cleanly across the transverse diameter but they may also cleave in the plane of the long axis making a needle-like particle.

PATHOGENESIS

The needle shaped asbestos particles being about 50 μ long are too large to be distributed uniformly through the lung and tend to follow the axial bronchi into the lower lobes. Some are arrested in the smaller air passages, others reach the alveoli. How particles of this size can enter alveoli was a puzzle to earlier workers and at one time it was suggested that fibres gained access to the lungs by different means from that of other dusts. Timbrell [252] in a series of studies of the factors affecting deposition and retention of fibrous dusts has shown that the falling speed (the most important parameter influencing the entry of particles into the lungs) is predominantly determined by the diameter and not the length. Long, thin fibres (with a diameter less than 3.5 μ) have a slow falling speed and stand a good chance of escaping deposition onto the airways and so of penetrating far into the lung. The more symmetrical the fibre the greater the chance of its penetrating deeply. Quantitative inhalation experiments in animals, using asbestos, have recently been reported [173 & 266]. These have shown that chrysotile is less fibrogenic than amosite or crocidolite, probably due to the more rapid elimination of chrysotile from the lungs. Why this should be so is not known but it may be related to solubility. It has for some time been known that the lungs of patients with severe asbestosis often contain very little detectable mineral compared with other forms of pneumoconiosis [10 & 189]. This may be explained by the ability of the body to eliminate chrysotile.

The mechanism by which fibrosis is produced is still uncertain. The solubility and auto-immune theories with their various extensions have been proposed as alternatives to the original theory of physical irritation but these have not found support in recent work [264]. Asbestos is less toxic to phagocytes in tissue culture than quartz and it has been suggested that fibrogenesis is due to a direct stimulus to the fibroblasts.

When an asbestos needle is broken transversely magnesium hydroxide is formed at the free end which gives an alkaline reaction. A series of chemical reactions at the ends and along the sides of the needle result in the so-called 'asbestos body'. The asbestos fibres become coated with a film of proteinous material which is thickened over the sharp ends giving them a characteristic bulbous appearance. These are about 3μ thick and 70μ long. The naked needle of asbestos which may be found in the lung is smaller, averaging 15μ in length and 0.5μ in diameter. The asbestos body is less fragile and less rigid than the naked needle suggesting that some physicochemical change has occurred. Experimentally the asbestos body has been simulated by coating a needle with egg albumin. With the passage of time the needle in the centre of an asbestos body loses its definition and finally disappears, probably going into solution. The longer the patient survives after inhalation of asbestos the smaller the asbestos needles appear to be. The asbestos body itself alters with age and finally leaves only a collection of dark granules which are probably iron oxide. It is possible that the protein envelope of the asbestos body reduces the harmful effects of asbestos since it has been shown in guinea pigs that asbestos bodies provoke no reaction whereas inhaled asbestos dust results in pulmonary fibrosis [263].

The importance of the asbestos body in the pathogenesis of pulmonary fibrosis is not known. Whether or not asbestos bodies are important in the development of fibrosis they are certainly of considerable importance in the epidemiological field and provide an index of the degree of exposure to asbestos [163].

Because of their size and durability asbestos particles remain *in situ* for a long time and the physical irritation theory implies that the sharp ends of the particles continue to inflict injury on the alveolar wall which results in hyperplasia of the alveolar lining epithelium and fibrosis in the interstitial tissue. The alveoli are eventually obliterated by the fibrous tissue in which the asbestos particles are left incarcerated. The sharp fibres are capable of reaching the pleura and provoking dense adhesions, and may even penetrate the diaphragm and cause reactive peritoneal fibrosis.

ASBESTOS EXPOSURE AND MALIGNANCY

BRONCHIAL CARCINOMA

A possible association between asbestosis and bronchial carcinoma had been suggested as early as 1934 but final proof was not established until 1955 when Doll reported a mortality study of men working with asbestos in the textile industry [58]. 15 cases of bronchial carcinoma were found in 105 autopsies of asbestosis. Subsequent studies have confirmed the association [143]. The percentage of male cases of asbestosis with complicating lung cancer in Britain has risen from 19·7 in the decade 1931–40 to 54·5 in the years 1961–64. It is not yet clear whether the increased rate of bronchial carcinoma is always accompanied by the clinical picture of pulmonary asbestosis. There is some evidence [158 & 235] that an excess mortality from bronchial carcinoma may occur in workers exposed to asbestos who do not have clinically detectable asbestosis.

DIFFUSE MESOTHELIOMA OF PLEURA AND PERITONEUM

In recent years evidence has accumulated from many parts of the world that asbestos inhalation is aetiologically related to the development of diffuse mesothelioma of the pleura. Cases have been reported from South Africa [265 & 267], Germany [142], Britain [121, 177, 178 & 195] and the United States [235]. Present evidence suggests that crocidolite, the blue asbestos mined in South Africa, appears to be particularly carcinogenic but it cannot be concluded that this is the only type of asbestos fibre which results in tumour formation. Peritoneal tumours related to asbestos exposure have also been recorded [65, 121 & 135].

Certain types of asbestos have been found to contain oils, waxes and other organic matter. Also asbestos fibres can absorb hydrocarbons from sacks in which it is transported. Trace amounts of elements such as nickel and chromium, which are known to have an association with pulmonary neoplasia, may also be found in some types of fibre. The presence of 3:4 benzpyrene in crocidolite and amosite has already been mentioned. The possible rôle of these substances in the development of tumours after exposure to asbestos is not yet known.

All available evidence suggests that the hazard from asbestos is much more serious and widespread than was commonly appreciated. Contact with asbestos need be very slight for pleural or pulmonary malignancy to occur and may amount only to living near a factory or handling the dusty clothes of an asbestos worker. It is difficult to assess the present hazard of asbestos exposure with regard to tumour formation since the latent period from first exposure to the development of tumour is up to 40 years.

PLEURAL PLAQUES

The marked irritation of asbestos fibres in the pleura may lead to pleural plaques which may calcify [95, 96 & 122]. Plaques are usually bilateral, are most prominent in the lower halves of the pleura and tend to follow the lines of the ribs. They consist of laminated, hyaline collagen and commonly show a variable degree of calcification. Radiographic detection depends on their size and the amount of associated calcification. Only 15% are detectable in life. Single plaques are more frequently found on the diaphragmatic surfaces. In a study of 56 patients with a history of asbestos exposure in whom pleural plaques were present at autopsy asbestos bodies were found in the lungs of all 56. These comprised 16 who had clinical asbestosis, 8 cases in which only histological evidence of asbestosis was found but also 32 who showed no pulmonary lesion [121]. It is not surprising, therefore, that pleural calcification due to asbestos commonly occurs without radiographic evidence of pulmonary asbestosis. Histological evidence of pulmonary asbestosis is, however, nearly always found when calcified pleural plaques are present. The calcification is uneven or speckled with irregular outlines which have been likened to those of a holly leaf [121]. There is some evidence from Finland that nonindustrial exposure to asbestos may result quite commonly in focal pleural calcification [140].

The development of pleural plaques and their detection appear to be related to the degree of exposure. Radiographically undetectable plaques are small, have little or no calcification, are usually not associated with histological asbestosis and asbestos bodies are scanty in the lungs. There may be no historical confirmation of exposure to asbestos. Conversely those plaques which are easily detected because of their size or calcium content are usually associated with histological (though, as stated above, not often radiographic) pulmonary asbestosis and a history of asbestos exposure is the rule.

The relationship of mesothelial tumours and pleural plaques is not clear. In Finland where plaques are common mesothelial tumours are rare. In the Transvaal area no mesothelial tumours have yet been reported but plaques are common. In parts of South Africa where the incidence of mesothelial tumours is high the incidence of plaques is also high. This is only one of the many problems concerning asbestos exposure and public health. Proposals for further study are summarized in the Report and Recommendations of the Working Group on Asbestos and Cancer to the Geographical Pathology

Committee of the International Union against Cancer [213].

PATHOLOGY

The appearance of the lung in asbestosis reflects the operation of the pathogenic processes outlined above. The lesions, mainly in the lower lobes, are diffuse, greyish fibrotic consolidations covered by thickened pleura which is anchored to the chest wall by fibrous adhesions. Fibrosis in the lung occurs in relation to the sites where asbestos fibres lodge. The primary site of lodgement of asbestos fibres is in the alveoli arising directly from the respiratory bronchioles. The fibres along with dust particles and alveolar macrophages accumulate in the alveoli and are subsequently entrapped there by a network of reticulin fibres which develop following the disintegration of some of the macrophages. The reticulin is in time replaced by thicker fibres and the alveoli are finally obliterated by fibrous tissue. The primary lesion, therefore, is essentially an adding on of material from within the lumen of the respiratory bronchioles and not initially an interstitial fibrosis [264]. Fibrosis later spreads down to affect the terminal air sacs and alveoli so that finally individual lesions link up to form a widespread fine fibrotic network in the lung. Asbestos bodies may be found within the alveoli or in the fibrotic lesions. The lesions may be confined to the lower lobes. If the fibrosis is patchy in distribution cystic changes may occur in the relatively normal lung giving a honeycomb appearance [118]. In the more severe cases where all the lung is involved fibrosis is frequently more marked at the bases. When apical fibrosis has been an important feature there has usually been a history of exposure to mixed dusts containing silica.

Rheumatoid pneumoconiosis in association with asbestosis is rare; there are only 3 reports of this in the world literature [170, 215 & 249].

Two important complications may also be evident in the lung. These are tuberculous lesions at the apices of the upper lobes and malignant disease in the fibrotic lower lobes or in the pleura. The tendency to tuberculosis may be nonspecific, but the development of malignant disease is clearly influenced by the presence of asbestosis. Long continued hyperplasia of the alveolar epithelial cells and of the pleural serosal cells may be the factors responsible, respectively, for the development of bronchial carcinoma (p. 484) and of pleural mesothelioma (p. 484). Mesothelioma of the peritoneum may also occur. The latent period before malignant disease develops is often very long and the exposure to asbestos and the degree of asbestosis present may both be very slight. These factors can be attributed to the indestructibility of asbestos which ensures that the reactive hyperplasia will be continued for a very long time.

Merewether [162] reported that of 232 deaths associated with asbestos exposure over a 25 year period in Britain 160 were due to asbestosis, 72 (31%) were complicated by tuberculosis and 31 (13·2%) had associated lung or pleural malignancy. In contrast only 1·32% of 6884 patients with silicosis had intrathoracic malignancy as a complication.

FUNCTIONAL ABNORMALITY

The most important single parameter of respiratory function affected in asbestosis is the diffusing capacity which may be reduced even before there is x-ray evidence of the disease. Presumably at this stage the reduction in diffusing capacity is due to the alveolar lesion before it has progressed to diffuse fibrosis. Later a progressive restrictive lesion develops with reduction in TLC and VC and further decrease in diffusing capacity [5, 19, 147, 251 & 275] with consistently raised alveolar–arterial oxygen difference [278]. The arterial oxygen saturation is reduced on exercise. Marked $\dot{V}/\dot{Q}$ abnormality has been demonstrated [210]. The lowered diffusing capacity may, therefore, be due to pathological changes in the alveolar wall, reduction in lung volume or $\dot{V}/\dot{Q}$ abnormality, each playing a variable part according to the stage of the disease [13].

As would be expected from the nature of the

pathological process pulmonary compliance is markedly reduced [147].

X-RAY APPEARANCES

Disability does not necessarily match the x-ray appearances which may be slight at the time the patient first complains. The abnormality is mostly in the lower two-thirds of the lung fields and varies from very fine mottling to marked streaky fibrosis to which is commonly added a shaggy appearance of the outlines of the heart and diaphragm due to pleural adhesions. Plaques of calcification may be visible in the pleura, and tuberculosis, emphysema and heart failure, when present, will add their distinctive features.

There is considerable observer error in the interpretation of the early radiographic changes in asbestosis [274].

CLINICAL FEATURES

An asbestos worker with significant pulmonary damage, as shown by an impaired diffusing capacity, may have no symptoms and no x-ray abnormality. When symptoms develop these are due to the progressive diffuse fibrosis and include increasing shortness of breath on exertion and later cough, weakness, cyanosis, weight loss and finger clubbing. Bilateral basal crepitations may sometimes be due to bronchiectasis but more commonly are simply features of the fibrosis.

Emphysema, bronchiectasis, tuberculosis, bronchial carcinoma and pleural pathology, which may result in effusion, may modify the clinical features in the individual case. Tuberculosis is not so frequent a complication of asbestosis as of silicosis but in the past approximately one-third of the cases of asbestosis died of active tuberculosis.

DIAGNOSIS

The diagnosis of asbestosis in a patient with a history of exposure and suggestive clinical and radiographic features may be confirmed by the findings of asbestos bodies in the sputum. These are, however, an indication of exposure rather than disease. They may occur in the sputum as early as 2 months after first exposure but may not appear for 20 years. They are golden yellow structures with bulbous ends and each consists of a core of asbestos fibre with a covering of proteinous material impregnated by granules of haemosiderin. Asbestos bodies may also be found within the alveoli or in the fibrotic lesions at autopsy.

Tests of respiratory function may help in doubtful cases. The characteristic findings are a 'stiff lung' pattern of ventilatory abnormality and an impaired diffusing capacity.

The differential diagnosis of asbestosis includes severe generalized emphysema (p. 311), bronchiectasis (p. 352), diffuse interstitial pulmonary fibrosis (p. 565), honeycomb lung (p. 571), sarcoidosis (p. 382) and the collagen disorders.

MANAGEMENT

In the early case corticosteroid therapy may be worth a trial but evidence for the efficacy of this treatment is lacking. Any response is monitored by serial chest radiographs and, when possible, tests of ventilation and diffusing capacity. In the developed case only the complications can be treated.

As in silicosis, and for the same reason, the patient should be removed from exposure to the dust as soon as the diagnosis has been made.

CONTROL OF THE ASBESTOS HAZARD

In the Rock Carling Memorial Lecture in June 1967 Doll noted that malignant mesothelioma could be associated with very small exposures to asbestos and advocated a system of control by licence of the import of what is probably the most dangerous form of asbestos in regard to carcinogenesis, namely crocidolite. As has been mentioned previously none of the forms of asbestos can be clearly absolved from an association with intrathoracic malignancy and legislation will require to take note of this [94, 194 & 236]. The British Asbestos Industry in May 1967 announced measures to protect those who worked with or handled asbestos. These included proposals that asbestos fibres should be shipped in dustproof bags and that crocidolite should only be handled mechanically. The Draft Asbestos Regulations [59] which are intended to supersede the 1931 Regulations have already been circulated although it will probably be a long time before the regulations become law. The Draft Regulations may be too stringent to be practical in industry and may raise reasonable objections from those who are concerned with general atmospheric pollution and the particular hazard of asbestos. For example one of the requirements for equipment dealing with asbestos is that 'it produces an exhaust draught which prevents the escape into the air of any work place of dust consisting of or containing asbestos'. While ideal these provisions are unlikely to be possible in industry. Perhaps a more realistic approach would be to specify a maximum allowable concentration with penalties if this is exceeded. Also premises handling asbestos in the future are recommended to have 'a fixed vacuum cleaning equipment which has ducts . . . (and) is so designed that no dust consisting of or containing asbestos can escape or be discharged

. . . into the air of any work place'. The concern here relates to the possibility of discharge of asbestos dust into the general atmosphere with all the consequences of this. Fairly certainly discussion of the draft Regulations will take account of these problems and result in improvements before the Regulations pass into law.

A further aspect of the asbestos hazard is the accidental exposure both in industrial and nonindustrial situations due to the handling of materials which may contain asbestos unknown to the handler. It would seem reasonable to insist that asbestos-containing materials should be clearly marked so that adequate precautions can be taken. It is, of course, possible that the dangers of dealing with asbestos under good conditions may be overrated by workers' representatives. This might deny the use of a most valuable industrial commodity which in certain circumstances may save more lives than it can endanger. Industry is alive to the problem of asbestos and the new Asbestos Regulations will go far to ensure that all reasonable practical measures are taken to protect those who have to handle it.

PNEUMOCONIOSIS FROM OTHER SILICATE DUSTS

Fibrosis of the lungs may also result from exposure to the dusts of mica [74 & 239], sericite [129], sillimanite [133 & 165], kaolin (China clay) [104 & 165], mineral talc [155 & 159] and diatomaceous earth [34, 225 & 260]. The effects produced by these substances are usually less serious than those of silica or asbestos. Sericite and sillimanite are mined along with small amounts of quartz which may be the more important constituent of the dusts [229].

Talc is interesting in that it also produces an asbestos-like body which may appear in the sputum. A common contaminant of talc is tremolite which may be the main fibrogenic

agent in some cases. Malignant changes have not so far been reported in the talcotic lung and tuberculosis appears to be much less frequent than in asbestosis.

Kaolin pneumoconiosis is an example of an industrial disease which has resulted from a change in industrial processing. Although kaolin has been used in Britain since 1750 it was not until 1920 that kaolinosis became an important occupational disease when a dry process replaced a wet process which previously suppressed the dust. Massive fibrosis may occur in kaolin pneumoconiosis and necrotic changes with cavitation have been reported [244].

ACUTE LUNG IRRITANTS

Very many potentially dangerous gases and fumes may be encountered in modern industry. Data regarding their effects on lung

structure and function are often incomplete and this is particularly the case for exposure to low concentrations over long periods. The effects of prolonged exposure to noxious gases and fumes may not be recognized until permanent lung damage has occurred since the symptoms and signs are not specific and x-ray changes are not usually marked or distinctive. Tests of pulmonary function are likely to play an important preventive rôle in this context and detailed studies are urgently needed.

In general the initial effect of inhaled gases and fumes is a chemical inflammation of the alveoli and terminal air passages which usually results in pulmonary oedema. Secondary infection may follow.

IRRITANT GASES

AMMONIA, CHLORINE, PHOSGENE, SULPHUR DIOXIDE AND TRIOXIDE

Inhalation of these very irritant gases results in acute pulmonary oedema. With the exception of phosgene (chlorine carbonyl) the effects of irritation are immediate resulting in watering of the eyes, sneezing and coughing. After inhalation of phosgene or other carbonyls (nickel or iron) there is characteristically a latent period of several hours (up to 24) before pulmonary oedema occurs and there may have been very little initial irritation of the upper respiratory tract. A patient with a history of phosgene exposure should, therefore, be kept under observation overnight.

FUNCTIONAL ABNORMALITY

Although there are few reports in the literature there is little doubt that inhalation of the irritant gases can cause permanent lung damage with considerable impairment of function [26 & 149]. Gassing with chlorine and phosgene in the 1914–18 War was commonly followed by chronic bronchitis and the association seemed clear though it was not officially accepted. It has been shown that inhalation of low concentrations of sulphur dioxide increases airway resistance in man [81] and it is probable that all the irritant gases have this effect. The increasing problem of atmospheric pollution underlines the need for studies of the effect of inhalation of low concentrations of irritant gases over many years.

TREATMENT

The treatment of acute exposure to the irritant gases includes immediate removal of the patient to a safe area, removal of contaminated clothing, oxygen therapy and the general measures for shock. Secondary bacterial infection may require treatment with penicillin.

OXIDES OF NITROGEN

There are five oxides of nitrogen; two (NO_2 and N_2O_4) are important in industrial pulmonary disease, a third (N_2O_5) possibly so. These highly irritant gases may be accidentally inhaled in widely diverse industries. These include farming where nitrogen dioxide may be formed from decomposing corn in silage preparation ('silo filler's disease'), mining where nitro explosives are detonated in confined spaces and the chemical industry in its many branches which entail the use of nitric acid. The increasing use of nitrocellulose and plastics has brought the potential danger from nitrogen oxides into the domestic sphere since the slow combustion of these materials results in the production of a mixture of gases containing oxides of nitrogen in dangerous concentrations, particularly if the supply of oxygen is limited, e.g. in cupboards, etc. It is important to remember that x-ray films are made of nitrocellulose. This was the source of the toxic concentrations of nitrogen oxides in the Cleveland Clinic disaster in 1929 [192 & 256]. Nitrogen dioxide is one of the hazards of arc welding, particularly since the introduction of electrodes covered with heavy cellulose (p. 495). Oxyacetylene welding in restricted, unventilated spaces can oxidize atmospheric nitrogen to the dioxide.

PATHOLOGY

The initial pathological changes are those of extensive congestion and oedema affecting all parts of the lungs. Recovery from the acute episode may be followed by the development of an obliterative bronchiolitis which may progress to death some weeks later [152] or may heal with fibrosis [175]. Sometimes a progressive interstitial pulmonary fibrosis is superimposed [145].

FUNCTIONAL ABNORMALITY

As would be expected from the variety of pathological change the pattern of disturbed pulmonary function varies from case to case. Reduction of vital capacity, decreased air flow and increased airway resistance, uneven gas distribution and a lowered value for CO transfer factor may all occur in varying degrees. Exercise has been shown to lower the Pa,O_2 in some patients [149].

Abnormalities in air flow due to obliterative bronchiolitis may persist after all radiographic changes have resolved [14]. Abnormal values for CO transfer factor may persist for weeks or months [149].

It seems probable that chronic lung damage may result from inhalation of the nitrogen oxides but the problem has not been sufficiently studied from the point of view of pulmonary function to allow a clear statement on this. Certainly many patients whose symptoms have disappeared may finally have normal ventilatory function. As indicated above, however, many parameters of lung function may require to be studied before a complete picture of any residual functional abnormality is obtained in any particular case.

CLINICAL FEATURES

Nitrogen dioxide is not very irritating to the upper respiratory tract so that the victim may continue to inhale the gas for some time. Commonly there is a latent period of some hours before symptoms develop [192]. The patient may then become acutely ill with fever, nausea, cough, cyanosis and progressively worsening dyspnoea. Diffuse crepitations are usually heard. Death may occur in the acute stage from pulmonary oedema. Those who survive may go on to develop the features of severe generalized bronchiolitis which may prove fatal from a combination of respiratory failure and infection. Recovery from this stage may be complete although, as mentioned above, abnormality of some as-pects of pulmonary function may persist for several months.

RADIOLOGY

In the acute stage the x-ray shows changes compatible with patchy pulmonary oedema or bronchopneumonia. In those patients who make a symptomatic recovery there is usually no x-ray evidence of residual lung damage.

PREVENTION AND TREATMENT

Constant vigilance is necessary in those industries in which the nitrogen oxides are a potential hazard. Adequate ventilation in the working area is vitally important. The preventive rôle of repeated pulmonary function studies has already been mentioned.

Treatment of the acute pulmonary oedema stage consists essentially of the giving of high concentrations of oxygen, corticosteroid therapy and prophylactic penicillin. These measures are also indicated in the stage of obliterative bronchiolitis which may proceed to respiratory failure (p. 337) and may require assisted respiration.

OZONE

This powerful lung irritant is met with as an industrial hazard principally in argon shielded welding when it is usually mixed with the oxides of nitrogen. Ozone is used for bleaching flour and as a deodorant for organic effluents in factories. It may sometimes reach concentrations in which it may cause irritation of the respiratory tract in high flying aircraft [282]. It is an important air pollutant in Los Angeles [205] where the sunny climate effects a photochemical change in the nitrogen oxides and carbonyl compounds from automobile exhaust fumes to give compounds of the peracetyl nitrite type and ozone. Thus the air in Los Angeles takes on both irritant and oxidizing properties leading to irritation of the mucosa of the eyes, throat and bronchi.

The effects of acute exposure to concentrations as low as 9 parts per million can produce acute pulmonary oedema. The very low concentration of about 0.6 p.p.m. breathed for

2 hours has been reported as causing a 20% fall in the steady state diffusing capacity in normal subjects, with little change in vital capacity or air flow [283].

Adequate ventilation in arc welders' shops is an important preventive measure. Treatment of the patient with acute ozone poisoning is similar to that for acute poisoning with nitrogen oxides.

TOLUENE DI-ISOCYANATE

This toxic irritant is widely used in the manufacture of plastic foam and the clinical effects of acute exposure are now well documented [254]. The clinical picture is one of bronchitis with bronchospasm. Rhonchi are heard diffusely throughout the lungs. The x-ray shows no abnormality. It appears that there is a sensitizing process so that further exposure results in increasingly severe symptoms [284]. Tests of pulmonary function do not appear to have been undertaken in any of the cases reported.

CADMIUM

Cadmium has become increasingly important in industry. It is now used in the manufacture of copper alloys and of alkaline electric accumulators and in electroplating particularly in the motor industry. A more recent but increasingly important use is as a neutron absorber in reactor control rods. Welders may be exposed to high concentrations of the readily volatilized cadmium oxide when cutting scrap metal containing cadmium or when welding steel previously plated with cadmium anticorrosive. Acute and chronic effects of cadmium on the lungs are recognized.

PATHOLOGY

Acute exposure causes a severe reaction affecting mainly the alveoli and terminal air passages which become filled with protein-rich exudate. The alveolar epithelium is swollen and shows cellular proliferation and metaplasia; the lining cells desquamate. Bilateral cortical necrosis with widespread tubular degeneration and glomerular in-farction has been reported in acute cadmium poisoning [18].

Chronic inhalation results in a diffuse, severe pulmonary emphysema [21, 146 & 241]. Fibrosis is not a significant feature except around the blood vessels. The presence of cadmium in the lung can be confirmed by spectrographic analysis.

FUNCTIONAL ABNORMALITY

In cases of chronic exposure the pattern of disturbed pulmonary function is that of severe airways obstruction with moderate emphysema [134].

CLINICAL FEATURES

Acute exposure to the fumes of cadmium oxide usually causes no immediate symptoms so that no preventive action may be taken and exposure becomes cumulative. After about 8 hours or so some irritation of the throat may be noticed and this is followed by malaise, shivering, cough, headache and increasing dyspnoea. Central chest pain, headache and dizziness are variable features. The severe chemical pneumonia carries a high mortality, said to be about 16% [244]. The first few days of the illness appear to be the most important with regard to prognosis and if the patient survives beyond the first week recovery may be expected.

Chronic cadmium poisoning, which usually develops insidiously at least 2 years after exposure starts or may occasionally become evident some time after exposure ceases, results in chronic cough with increasing dyspnoea, progressive weight loss and weakness. Proteinuria due to toxic nephritis is common [240]. Death may occur from *cor pulmonale* and congestive cardiac failure, or from renal failure.

RADIOLOGY

The x-ray in acute exposure shows diffuse, pneumonic lesions and in chronic cadmium poisoning the x-ray appearances are compatible with generalized emphysema (p. 318).

PREVENTION AND TREATMENT

The importance of good ventilation in the

working area cannot be overstressed. The permissible quantity of cadmium in the atmosphere should not exceed 1 mg per 10 m³ of air. The value of serial pulmonary function studies in workers at risk from cadmium fumes is obvious. Recognition of chronic cadmium poisoning should imply immediate withdrawal from the industry. Treatment of the acute condition is along the lines described for poisoning with nitrogen oxide and ozone.

VANADIUM

Vanadium is used to harden steel and is a constituent of fossil fuel oil. Its toxic oxides (principally the pentoxide) may be encountered in the steel industry and when the soot or ash of fuel oil is inhaled [29 & 31] giving a combination of upper and lower respiratory tract irritation [61 & 248]. The effects of exposure are immediate and are principally cough, wheezing, dyspnoea, blockage of the nose and smarting of the eyes [150]. Sometimes nausea and vomiting occur after heavy exposures and the tongue may develop a greenish coating which can last for some weeks. Usually recovery is spontaneous in 2–3 days but sometimes the illness is prolonged by superimposed secondary bacterial infection. Recurrent exposure may result in chronic bronchitis.

Handlers of vanadium pentoxide may develop cough, shortness of breath and haemoptysis. Some of these show generalized reticulation [281] in the chest x-ray through deposition of vanadium.

OSMIUM

The highly volatile tetroxide of osmium is an acute lung irritant and severe exposure results in bronchiolitis or bronchopneumonia which may prove fatal [32 & 209]. Workers who have lesser degrees of exposure may develop cough and sputum but repeated contact does not apparently predispose to chronic respiratory disease [188].

MANGANESE PNEUMONIA

Acute pneumonia is common in those exposed to dust containing a high concentration of manganese or its salts [151 & 172]. Manganese fumes are sometimes responsible. Recurrent pneumonia often occurs and death is not infrequent. The condition has been reproduced experimentally.

PLATINUM ASTHMA

Inhalation of the complex salts of platinum during refining processes results in a clinical picture characterized by sneezing, rhinorrhoea, tightness of the chest, wheeze and dyspnoea [124]. Usually the symptoms subside very rapidly after exposure ceases at the end of a shift and within an hour the patient is well again. Sometimes a bronchitis-like picture is superimposed.

Prevention depends on adequate exhaust ventilation.

PRINTER'S ASTHMA

Exposure to gum acacia and tragacanth in alcohol solution can result in asthmatic symptoms which usually develop some hours later and can last for a few weeks [80]. The hazard principally affects workers in the printing trade.

A number of other industrial products (fumes and dusts) may act as acute lung irritants but these are more conveniently discussed under other headings.

THE METALS

ALUMINIUM

ALUMINOSIS

Following the demonstration by Kettle [138] that silica coated with iron oxide did not cause pulmonary fibrosis in animals, studies were made with aluminium dust [54 & 90] which showed that this also gave a measure of protection from silicosis. For a time there was a vogue for the use of aluminium dust as a modifying factor in industries in which silicosis was a hazard. The practice gradually ceased after an extensive controlled study by Kennedy [137] in 1956 had shown no important differences in the behaviour of pottery workers treated or untreated with aluminium dust.

Aluminosis is another example of an industrial hazard occurring through a change in manufacturing technique. Commercial aluminium consists of granules made from the molten metal or thin flakes stamped from the cold metal. The granules being covered by a film of oxide are inert, but the stamped flakes can react with water to produce aluminium hydroxide and hydrogen [49 & 50]. In the stamping process lubricants are added to assist the separation of the particles, the commonest being stearine and paraffin. Stearine completely covers the flake and acts like an oxide film but a paraffin covering is lost when shaken up with water so that the flake is exposed and can then react with water. Aluminium lung only occurs with stamped powders and was first reported when the German Armed Forces needed a stearine-free aluminium for explosives. Although stearine-free aluminium was still being made in Germany in 1956 [8] it has since been abandoned.

PATHOLOGY

Aluminium particles are taken up by phagocytes and soon reach the interstitial tissues where fibrosis occurs resulting in progressive dyspnoea.

FUNCTIONAL ABNORMALITY

Functional changes in aluminosis have been reported as showing a restrictive ventilatory disorder with reduced values for diffusing capacity and a varying degree of obstructive airways disease [131, 169 & 187].

CLINICAL FEATURES

The symptoms, which include cough, poor appetite, loss of weight and progressive shortness of breath, may occur as early as 3 months after first exposure but usually take longer [98, 99, 100, 101, 102 & 103]. In the more acute forms of the disease pneumothorax is a frequent complication.

Instances have been recorded in recent years of diffuse pulmonary fibrosis in workers in the fireworks industry in Britain and Sweden [2, 132, 168, 169 & 247]. In these cases fine aluminium dust was undoubtedly the fibrogenic agent.

PREVENTION AND TREATMENT

The use of alternatives to stamped aluminium powders would abolish aluminosis. When a worker has developed symptoms or signs of the disease he should be advised to leave the industry since the effect of recurrent exposure is cumulative.

BAUXITE LUNG
(Shaver's Disease, Corundum Smelters' Lung)

This condition was first recognized during the the 1939–45 War and was described by Shaver [238] and later by Riddell [217]. Alumina abrasives are manufactured by a process in which finely ground bauxite, iron and coke are fused by an electric arc using carbon electrodes. When a new batch of material is fed into the furnaces dense white fumes are given off which may be inhaled. The fumes contain about 7% silica, corundum (Al_2O_3), ferric oxide, traces of titanium and other constituents.

PATHOLOGY

The initial effect of inhaling the fumes is an alveolar oedema which is followed by fibrous thickening of the alveolar walls and the interlobular septa. It is thought that the total bauxite fume acts as a chemical irritant giving first the alveolar and intraseptal oedema and later an interstitial fibrosis with associated emphysema [280]. This is supported by the fact that chemical and spectrographic analysis of bauxite lung shows that all the elements of bauxite fumes are present in much the same proportions as in the fumes themselves.

FUNCTIONAL ABNORMALITY

Studies of pulmonary function have been reported in only very few cases. These have shown a range from complete normality to a combination of obstructive and restrictive patterns of ventilatory abnormality with impairment of diffusing capacity [131 & 169].

CLINICAL FEATURES

Symptoms may occur as early as 3 months after exposure and consist of cough with mucoid sputum, shortness of breath, cyanosis and substernal pain. Pneumothorax may sometimes be a complication.

RADIOLOGY

The *x-ray* shows reticular shadowing with perhaps denser focal shadows, bullae and atelectasis [218].

PREVENTION AND TREATMENT

Awareness by the worker of the danger of bauxite fumes will lead to efforts to avoid the hazard. A patient with the developed disease should immediately be removed from further exposure.

HARD METAL DISEASE

Tungsten carbide is almost as hard as diamond and is known as 'hard metal'. Its main use is in the making of the cutting edges of tools by bonding tungsten carbide with cobalt and soldering this to the tip of the tool. Sometimes other carbides—titanium, vanadium or tantalum—are incorporated in hard metal tips. The tip is finally shaped by grinding on diamond and carborundum (silicon carbide) wheels. A valuable feature of hard metal tips is that they become sharper as the temperature rises. The dusts in the hard metal workers' environment may, therefore, contain the carbides of tungsten, titanium, vanadium, and silicon and also aluminium oxide and diamond. Present evidence suggests that only silicon carbide and cobalt are potentially harmful. Cobalt has been shown to cause increase in serum globulin, polycythaemia and lung changes in animals [231 & 232].

There has been a rapid expansion of the hard metal industry since its beginning in Germany in the 1914–18 War. The manufacturing processes are dusty and inhalation of the dust may result in symptoms and pathological changes in the lung [11]. The incidence in exposed workers appears to be low but the true incidence is not known.

PATHOLOGY

One fatal case reported by Bech and his colleagues [11] showed a diffuse interstitial pulmonary fibrosis, peribronchial and perivascular fibrosis, and hyperplasia and metaplasia of the bronchial epithelium. It is interesting that an anaplastic carcinoma of the right lower lobe was also present.

FUNCTIONAL ABNORMALITY

Usually the features of mild obstructive airways disease are present (p. 51).

RADIOLOGY

Typical appearances include increase in linear markings, micronodular opacities particularly in the mid and lower zones and enlargement of the hilar shadows. The x-ray changes may regress after removal from exposure.

CLINICAL FEATURES

The symptoms of cough, dyspnoea and tightness in the chest characteristically have a sudden onset after durations of exposure varying from 2 to as long as 22 years, and in the earlier stages usually become evident towards the end of the working shift. The sudden onset after a variable duration of exposure has suggested that a hypersensitivity reaction may be involved. After many years the clinical picture resembles chronic bronchitis.

Serum globulins may sometimes be increased and there may be polycythaemia.

PREVENTION AND TREATMENT

The usual measures to suppress dust should be applied vigorously in the many industries in which hard metal is a known hazard. If there is clinical, radiographic or functional evidence of hard metal pneumoconiosis the question of removal from the industry must be considered.

SIDEROTIC LUNG DISEASE

This term includes 3 principal entities due to the inhalation of iron oxide, either in relatively pure form or more commonly mixed with dusts or fumes. These are silver polishers' lung, arc welders' lung and haematite miners' lung. Iron oxide itself is inert but pulmonary fibrosis may occur when it is inhaled along with silica particles or fumes of metallic oxides and silicates.

SILVER POLISHERS' LUNG

Rouge, an iron oxide powder, is used in the final stages of manufacture of silverware. Inhalation of this may be associated with cough and reddish sputum. No pulmonary fibrosis has been described in this condition [7] although the x-ray shows a generalized fine stippling [185].

Pathological examination of the lung shows 3 kinds of pigment—iron oxide and haemosiderin in phagocytes present in the alveoli and in subpleural and perivascular aggregations, and silver impregnating the elastic laminae of the pulmonary vessels and the alveolar walls.

ARC WELDING

Modern arc welding is a most complex affair so far as industrial hazard is concerned. Since most of the materials used are capable of being transformed into a gas or fume at the high temperature employed in modern welding there is a great variety of potentially respirable substances in the welder's environment [66, 153 & 160]. It is obvious that the danger is greater in confined spaces such as the hulls of ships and that all the hazards of welding can be minimized by adequate ventilation. Not only does high temperature welding vaporize the components involved but it also causes direct oxidations, both of the metals used and the oxygen and nitrogen in the atmosphere. Surface oxidation of metals which occurs more readily with higher temperatures tends to prevent the fusion on which the success of the weld depends. Hence a number of anti-oxidation techniques have been introduced. The latest development is to encase the arc in a sheath of inert gas, usually argon. When a metal is covered by paint [245], paint primer or plastic, or is galvanized or brought straight from the degreasing tank a great variety of fumes and gases is produced by the heat of welding. Bare electrodes have now been replaced by covered ones, the covering consisting of either heavy cellulose or a mixture of iron, titanium and manganese oxides, together with various silicates and carbonates. It will be seen, therefore, that the hazards of welding depend on the following:

(1) The metal used.
(2) The oxygen and nitrogen in the atmosphere.
(3) The surface coating of the electrodes.
(4) The surface coating of the metal.
(5) The temperature used in the welding process.
(6) The duration of the welding process.
(7) The ventilation and size of the welding shop.

Either the metal itself or its oxide may vaporize or fume. In steel welding iron oxide (Fe_2O_3) is produced and may be inhaled. This is taken up by macrophages and deposited in the perivascular and subpleural alveoli. The Prussian Blue reaction is negative when applied to the laden macrophages but becomes positive when chemical change within the cell converts iron oxide to haemosiderin. In most cases the presence of pure iron oxide (*siderosis*) has not resulted in reticulin or collagen fibre formation. When fibrosis has occurred it has usually been attributable to silica. The x-ray in siderosis shows generalized reticular and nodular shadows caused by deposits of iron oxide in the lung. If exposure ceases the x-ray abnormalities of siderosis tend to clear slowly over a period of years [57]. Pneumoconiotic siderosis has been regarded as benign and certainly there are usually no related symptoms and no disturbance in pulmonary function [76 & 171]. As mentioned previously, however, any foreign substance in the lung cannot be entirely harmless and there is the further concern that iron may be a carcinogen. Turner and Grace [255] found a higher incidence of cancer of all sites in iron and steel workers compared with control groups. Bonser, Faulds and Stewart [22] recorded an incidence of 8·85% of bronchial carcinoma in 192 autopsies on haematite miners compared with 1·85% in controls. Also Campbell [35] found support for the carcinogenic effect of iron in animal experiments. It is interesting that sarcomata can be produced by the intramuscular injection of ferric hydroxide–dextran complex into rats [214] whereas comparable injections of saccharated iron oxide appear to be harmless. There is no evidence at present to suggest that the siderosis produced by arc welding predisposes to lung cancer. It is possible that only certain physical forms of iron and its oxides are carcinogenic or that an iron–silica mixture (as in haematite) is necessary for malignancy to occur.

'*Metal fume fever*' is another hazard of the arc welder. This is caused by inhaling the oxidation products of various metals, principally zinc and copper, and is a transient acute febrile illness lasting a few hours to 2 days or so, sometimes complicated by secondary bacterial pneumonia. Beryllium–copper alloy (p. 498) and aluminium (p. 492) may also fume. So far beryllium has never been reported at more than half the maximum allowable concentration. There is no information regarding the concentrations of aluminium fumes during welding.

The temperature and photochemical conditions of modern welding result in the oxygen and the nitrogen of the atmosphere becoming oxidized to *ozone* [82] and *nitrogen dioxide* [56] respectively. The cellulose of the electrode coating is a further source of nitrogen oxides.

Trichlorethylene may cover the metal as it comes from the degreasing tank or may exist as a general pollutant in the working area. This substance is broken down by heat to form *phosgene* ($COCl_2$) (p. 489).

The coating of electrodes may also contain silica, asbestos and calcium fluoride but so far no cases of silicosis, asbestosis or fluorosis

have been reported in association with welding.

If the metal to be welded is painted, toxic effects from *lead* may be encountered. More commonly nowadays, however, paints based on zinc oxide are used, which can result in metal fume fever. Galvanized metals (i.e. iron coated with metallic zinc to prevent corrosion) are another source of zinc fumes. When metals have *cadmium* coatings the fumes of this can result in emphysema (p. 491). Some paint primers contain plastics which break down under heat to give a mixture of fumes and gases including phosgene. Vinyl coating had to be given up because of the production of *hydrogen chloride*, and polyethylene tetrafluoride ('teflon') is also proving disappointing because of the production of irritating *fluorides*.

The welder, then, is at risk from siderosis, acute pulmonary irritation and also chronic bronchitis and emphysema. Surveys have shown that as many as 60% of welders have symptoms of chronic bronchitis and 30% have signs of this [30].

HAEMATITE MINERS' LUNG

In Britain haematite has been mined in Cumberland since Roman times. Other sources are Belgium, Sweden, Canada and the U.S.A. In Cumberland haematite is mined in 2 areas some 30 miles apart which are entirely different geologically. In Whitehaven haematite ore is found in hard rock containing 10% silica, whereas around Millom it is found in a soft clay. Haematite miners' lung results from the associated silica dust (siderosilicosis) and in Britain it is almost entirely confined to Whitehaven. Iron oxide, like coal dust, has been thought to modify the effects of silica on the lung [88]. The silting-up process, as described in coalworkers' pneumoconiosis, occurs and finally results in similar types of lesions of which 3 forms are described—the diffuse, the nodular and the massive fibrosis varieties.

The *diffuse lesion* affects the whole lung which is brick red in colour and shows generalized fibrosis with centrilobular emphysema around collections of dust. The x-ray shows a generalized reticulation.

The *nodular variety* shows reddish-black silicotic nodules up to 1 cm in diameter on a background of brick red lung. The nodules may undergo necrosis. Pleural adhesions are common.

Massive fibrosis resembles that described in coalworkers' pneumoconiosis and silicosis, being mainly in the upper lobes, involving bronchi and pulmonary vessels and liable to ischaemic necrosis. In all the forms of haematite miners' lung the hilar lymph glands contain carbon and haematite which give them a mottled brick red and black appearance.

Pulmonary tuberculosis is as common in haematite miners' lung as in silicosis. An increased incidence of bronchial carcinoma in haematite miners is possible [70]. Since the pathological process so closely resembles coalworkers' pneumoconiosis which has no increased incidence of lung cancer it is possible that iron oxide when inhaled in company with silica may be carcinogenic.

The symptoms of haematite miners' lung are similar to those of coalworkers' pneumoconiosis. The sputum, however, instead of being coal black is brick red.

There has been no comprehensive study of the *functional abnormality* in haematite miners' lung but it seems probable that diffusing capacity will be reduced in the developed case. Ventilatory abnormality will depend on the severity of the pathological process and the degree of associated emphysema.

IRON IN OTHER INDUSTRIES

There is a large number of other industries in which iron or iron oxide may be inhaled either in relatively pure form or mixed with varying amounts of silica. In the first group are makers of electrolytic iron oxide, workers in iron and steel rolling mills, iron turners and steel grinders. The x-ray appearances of siderosis become apparent after long periods of exposure (10–25 years). There is no related functional disability.

Ochre miners and millers handle varieties of limonite (hydrated ferric oxides) contaminated with clays which are used to manufacture colours. Siennas, umbers, Venetian red and raddle are other iron-containing earths. These substances are mixed with free silica which varies from 2 to 35%. The workers in these industries may show varying degrees of silicosis combined with siderosis. In most cases the silicotic component has been slight and usually there is no clinical disability although the chest x-ray shows generalized reticulation and nodulation [41 & 258].

Foundry workers, particularly cleaners of steel castings, and fettlers (dressers or chippers) have a greater chance of exposure to silica, resulting in pulmonary fibrosis which in general varies with the amount of free silica in the dust [186]. Boiler scalers may also develop silicosiderosis [106, 107 & 108].

STANNOSIS

The inhalation of fumes or dust of tin dioxide (SnO_2) results after some years in quite a dramatic radiographic appearance but this is not associated with symptoms or signs, or with other features that can be ascribed to pneumoconiosis [219 & 220]. The dust which occurs in deposits around septa, vessels and bronchioles and beneath the pleura is relatively harmless and does not lead to fibrosis [244] or centrilobular emphysema to any extent and does not cause bronchitis. Pulmonary function tests, therefore, show no abnormality [92]. The x-ray appearances consist of widespread mottling with a highly radio-opaque material. Dust laden lymphatics may be clearly seen at the mediastinal reflection around the heart and the aorta, at the diaphragm, in the fissures and in the horizontal Kerley lines at the bases. The density of the opacity of any inhaled material depends mainly on the atomic weight and since that of tin is 118 it shows very readily and appears as dense as lipiodol.

OTHER NONFIBROGENIC RADIO-OPAQUE DUSTS

The dusts of emery (a mixture of magnetite, Fe_3O_4, and corundum, Al_2O_3), antimony and barium are similar to tin in that they produce dense reticular and nodular opacities through-out the lung [4, 78, 183, 196, 197, 198 & 199] with no symptoms or functional abnormality unless the dusts are mixed with lung irritants or fibrogenic agents. The opacities produced by these dusts do not coalesce. Since the atomic weight determines the radiodensity the most opaque shadows are found in *baritosis*. Removal of the worker from exposure may result in gradual radiographic improvement.

BERYLLIOSIS

Beryllium–copper alloy has many uses in industry because of its high tensile strength and its resistance to metal fatigue, high tem-perature and corrosion. Being in addition nonmagnetic with high electrical conductivity and not liable to spark it is used extensively in aircraft engines, electrical devices and the like. Its low atomic weight and transparency to x-rays make it ideal for x-ray tube windows. Beryllium is also an important component of atomic reactors in which it is used as a moderator to slow down and reflect neutrons without wastefully absorbing them. Weber and Engelhardt [268] in 1933 reported res-piratory symptoms among workers extracting beryllium from its principal ore beryl which is a beryllium aluminium silicate. Beryl itself does not apparently cause disease but metal-lic beryllium, its simple salts and the complex silicates of beryllium can all cause beryllium disease. In 1935 Fabrioni [68] exposed guinea pigs to the fumes of beryllium carbonate and produced lung lesions which he called 'berylliosis'. Then Gelman [91] recorded severe pneumonitis in Russian workers exposed to fumes in the extraction of beryl-lium from its fluorides. This illness occurred in 2 phases. An immediate reaction resembling metal fume fever and thought to be due to beryllium fumes was followed 4 days later by a severe bronchiolitis which Gelman attri-buted to fluorine. Beryllium poisoning was reported in Germany during the 1939–45 War [164 & 279] but after 1943 the widest experience of the harmful effects of beryllium was obtained in the United States where industrial epidemics led to the initiation in 1952 of a Beryllium Case Registry at the Massachusetts General Hospital. Over 600 cases were registered in the first five years. This explosive increase in incidence of beryl-lium disease reflected the many purposes which were found for this industrially highly desirable substance. For some years beryllium was used along with zinc, magnesium and manganese silicates to coat the inside of fluorescent light tubes and it was the occur-rence of beryllium disease in workers in this industry which highlighted the hazard of working with the metal or living in close proximity to factories manufacturing or using beryllium products. The problem in Britain was never important numerically and most cases occurred in the strip lighting in-dustry. After 1948 the use of beryllium in fluorescent lighting was abolished.

PATHOGENESIS

Since beryllium enters the body via the lungs and the pulmonary effects of beryllium disease dominate the clinical picture berylliosis is commonly designated a pneumoconiosis but essentially it is a systemic poisoning affecting many organs. The precise mode of action of beryllium in producing disease is not known. Several facts favour a hypersensitivity reac-tion. Only a small percentage of those at risk (0·4–2·0%) actually develop the disease. There may be a long latent period (10 years or more). Only about half of the cases of berylliosis have an excess of beryllium in the lungs or urine. In chronic berylliosis a skin patch test (p. 501) suggests a specific reaction along antigen–antibody lines [242]. Finally it has been shown [3] that beryllium ions can become attached to protein molecules to form a compound which could theoretically be antigenic.

Beryllium is extremely active biologically, particularly at an acid pH. Traces of the metal beneath the skin of a worker or an experi-mental animal produce a granuloma followed by fibrosis. Beryllium successfully competes with magnesium so that amounts less than 1 millionth of a mole will inhibit plasma alkaline phosphatase. It is known that beryllium has a marked effect on many intracellular enzymes in very low concentrations but at the moment these remain isolated facts only and have not been built into any theory of pathogenesis [30].

Beryllium is known to produce osteogenic sarcoma in dogs and there is some evidence that it is carcinogenic in the rat and some other animals. No beryllium-induced cancer has ever been reported in humans and it may be that the lung fibrosis which it causes proceeds at a pace which precludes any carcinogenic effect becoming apparent in man.

Exposure to beryllium can result in a variety of skin changes, including papulovesicular eruptions, ulcers and subcutaneous granulomata [130], and its inhalation may cause acute and chronic lung disease.

ACUTE BERYLLIOSIS

This is essentially a chemical pneumonia developing within a few weeks of the first exposure to beryllium and manifested by the development of dyspnoea and cyanosis with loss of weight and a radiographic appearance of diffuse miliary mottling. Most of the acute cases have been in workers in ore extraction plants following heavy exposure to a mixture of the oxides, sulphates and fluorides of beryllium. Fulminating cases may be fatal but these are uncommon and most acute cases recover although the x-ray changes may take several months to clear. Only about 1 in 10 cases of acute berylliosis later develop the chronic disease [250]. *Pathologically* the gross appearance of the lungs is that of severe pulmonary oedema. Microscopically the alveoli are filled with fibrin, red cells and a few polymorphs, the alveolar walls are infiltrated with lymphocytes and plasma cells and protein deposition on the alveolar wall gives the appearance of hyaline membrane. The bronchi show evidence of only mild irritation. Recovery from this phase is characterized by the appearance of phagocytes and lymphocytes in the alveoli, epithelialization of the alveolar walls and organization of the intra-alveolar exudate resulting in diffuse fibrosis.

There has been no comprehensive study of the *functional abnormality* in acute berylliosis

17—R.D.

but one would predict a restrictive ventilatory abnormality and an important diffusing defect as the main features.

The *treatment* of acute berylliosis is essentially the use of corticosteroid therapy in high dosage and oxygen in high concentrations.

CHRONIC BERYLLIOSIS

Chronic pulmonary berylliosis is a sarcoid-like granulomatous inflammation with fibrosis affecting all parts of the lungs. Most of the cases in the literature occurred in the United States in the period 1943–55 when beryllium was used extensively for fluorescent strip lighting. The first description of the disease was by Hardy and Tabershaw in 1946 [111] and following this the incidence of recognized chronic berylliosis increased to the extent that the condition became the subject of a Saranac Symposium in 1950 [262]. The number of cases reported in Britain has been small, only 11 in all [1, 132, 176, 222, 230, 242, 243 & 277]. Nine of these were exposed to beryllium phosphors in fluorescent lighting and 2 to beryllium–copper alloys. Exposure need only be brief for chronic pulmonary berylliosis to occur and the fact that there may be a latent period of as long as 10 years or more tends to obscure the memory of exposure. The degree of exposure may be so slight as to escape notice. A housewife whose husband is exposed to beryllium at his work may acquire berylliosis through inhaling the dust from his clothes as she brushes them. 'Neighbourhood cases' of berylliosis occurring in residents living near a factory using beryllium have been described [42 & 62] but it is possible that some of these were due to contact with workers whose clothes were contaminated.

The evidence from the Massachusetts Registry suggests that women are more susceptible than men. It has also been shown that beryllium can cross the placental barrier since it can be detected in the urine of newborn infants of mothers suffering from beryllium disease.

PATHOLOGY

When the fumes or salts of beryllium are

inhaled the lungs bear the brunt of the disease but lesions are scattered throughout the body affecting liver, kidney, spleen and lymph glands. Skin lesions may occur from superficial contact.

The lungs are firm, greyish-white in appearance with generalized pleural thickening. Subpleural bullae may be seen. The cut lung shows focal and diffuse fibrosis with numerous cystic spaces. The hilar glands are enlarged.

Microscopically there is a diffuse, chronic, noncaseating interstitial granulomatosis. In the early case follicles of epithelioid cells with a variable rim of lymphocytes and a few plasma cells occur in discrete foci throughout the interstitial tissue of the lung and involve the alveolar wall. At a later stage Langhan's type giant cells develop by fusion of epithelioid cells and inclusion bodies of the types found in sarcoidosis may occur (p. 378). With the passage of time reticulin develops in the granulomata which finally become areas of dense, hyaline collagen. Compensatory emphysema may occur but this may be limited by the pathological change in the alveoli whose walls become thickened, sometimes obliterating the alveolar space. Thick-walled alveolar cystic spaces are present diffusely among the grossly disorganized lung tissue. Patent alveoli may show a cuboidal type of epithelium. Pathologically the appearances are indistinguishable from chronic sarcoidosis but differentiation may be made by chemical analysis in tissue biopsies or at postmortem examination, since beryllium does not occur in normal tissues even in trace amounts.

The pathological changes in the hilar glands are similar to those in the lung, the granulomatous reaction giving way to a progressive fibrosis.

Chronic berylliosis may be complicated by *cor pulmonale* and cardiac failure.

FUNCTIONAL ABNORMALITY

Since the pulmonary pathology in chronic pulmonary berylliosis so closely resembles that in chronic sarcoidosis (p. 378) it is not surprising that the functional changes produced by each of these diseases is very similar.

Typically the changes are those of restrictive parenchymal disease, with hyperventilation and hypoxaemia on exercise and reduction in the diffusing capacity of the lung [51 & 86] and usually in the static lung compliance. In only a few cases can complicating emphysema be detected physiologically by reduced ventilatory capacity and increased residual volume. Some cases, however, have shown a significant degree of superimposed chronic obstructive airways disease [75, 86 & 136].

RADIOLOGY

The radiographic appearances depend on the stage of the disease. A diffuse fine granularity distributed uniformly throughout both lungs occurs early to be followed by definite micronodulation, reticular patterns and larger nodules (0·5–1 cm). The hilar shadows become enlarged, with indistinct margins. In the late stages the lungs appear shrunken with diffuse, sometimes irregular, fibrosis and increasing cardiomegaly may occur from *cor pulmonale* and congestive cardiac failure.

CLINICAL FEATURES

The dominant symptom in chronic berylliosis is progressive unremittent dyspnoea. Unproductive cough is the next most common symptom. Skin lesions resembling chronic skin sarcoids may occur. Delayed type hypersensitivities are depressed. A subacute stage of the process has been described in which chills and fever may occur. The clinical effects of chronic berylliosis may be delayed as long as 10–15 years after exposure although weight loss may be an earlier sign. Between the extremes of acute and chronic beryllium disease there is a whole spectrum of clinical pattern including those instances in which acute episodes subside only to progress later to chronic berylliosis even without further exposure. Recurrent infection and the effects of right heart failure add to the clinical picture. Spontaneous pneumothorax may occur. Finger clubbing was recorded in 5 of 45 cases by Hardy [109]. This is a much higher incidence than in sarcoidosis.

DIAGNOSIS

A combination of evidence is necessary for a diagnosis of berylliosis since no single factor can be more than suggestive. The clinical, functional [87] radiographic and histopathological features of beryllium disease closely resemble chronic sarcoidosis and similar abnormalities of serum protein and calcium metabolism [110] may be found in each. The difficulty is intensified by the fact that in each of these conditions biopsies of lung, lymph nodes, liver, skin, kidney or skeletal muscle may show identical histological pictures [60, 83 & 276]. Features found in some cases of sarcoidosis but not in berylliosis include uveitis, enlargement of salivary and lachrymal glands, widespread superficial lymphadenopathy and bone changes. For all practical purposes erythema nodosum does not occur in berylliosis nor does hilar and mediastinal adenopathy in the absence of lung changes. Progression to important disability is much more common in beryllium disease and the mortality is higher. Fortunately the management of both sarcoidosis and berylliosis is primarily concerned with the prevention of pulmonary fibrosis and its sequelae and the therapy is the same. A skin test specific for beryllium disease was devised by Curtis in 1951 [52]. The beryllium patch test, which indicates delayed type beryllium hypersensitivity, is performed with gauze moistened with 1% or 2% beryllium sulphate or nitrate. A positive reaction takes the form of an eczematous rash which develops in 2–3 days. Sneddon [242] biopsied the inflammatory reaction 3 weeks later and found the histological changes of a sarcoid-like granuloma. Curtis [53] showed that the Kveim test was negative in beryllium disease and James [126] showed that the beryllium patch test is negative in sarcoidosis. These 2 skin tests may, therefore, be helpful in distinguishing between the diseases although there have been doubts about the reliability and even the safety of the beryllium patch test since it may cause other than a local hypersensitivity response and worsening of lung lesions has been recorded following its use. A negative beryllium patch test does not exclude berylliosis.

The diagnosis of berylliosis depends on one or more of the following: a history of exposure, suggestive clinical and radiographic features, a positive skin test, and the detection of beryllium in the urine and affected tissues. Spectrographic analysis of biopsy of the liver or superficial lymphadenopathy may sometimes be helpful. Even a history of exposure plus the finding of beryllium in the urine or even in the lung may sometimes be misleading since these have been found in workers previously exposed to the hazard but who have died from other causes and whose lungs did not show any reaction to beryllium [257].

PROGNOSIS

The course of the disease is variable. Uncommonly radiographic abnormality may be the only evidence of disease. Most frequently chronic berylliosis results in mild symptoms which may remain unchanged for long periods or may be slowly progressive. A smaller group shows disabling, progressive disease characterized by dyspnoea, cough, weight loss, *cor pulmonale* and congestive cardiac failure and sometimes episodes of fever unrelated to complicating infection. Death in this group may occur after periods from 1 to 16 years. A mortality rate of 27% has been quoted by Hardy [109].

TREATMENT AND PREVENTION

Corticosteroid therapy should be begun whenever the condition is diagnosed and this may prove to be life-saving. As in sarcoidosis an intervening pregnancy has been known to produce a temporary relief in symptoms [176]. Presumably, as in sarcoidosis, this is due to a higher level of circulating cortisol during the later months of pregnancy. Treatment with corticosteroid may require to be indefinitely prolonged. Although improvement may be expected on this treatment if the pathology has not reached the immutable stage there is never full functional or radiographic recovery. Incidental infection, *cor pulmonale* or spontaneous pneumothorax will require their own specific measures.

It has been shown that the ammonium salt of aurintricarboxylic acid, a chelating agent, will protect mice against the effects of intravenous beryllium. This form of treatment, which theoretically might be useful in acute berylliosis, has not been used in human cases.

Prevention depends on a strict and effective level of control of beryllium in the working atmosphere. The U.S. Atomic Energy Commission and the American Industrial Hygiene Association have stated that maximum atmospheric concentration should not exceed 2 μg of beryllium per m³ of air [272] throughout an 8 hour day and this figure has also been adopted by the United Kingdom Atomic Energy Authority. Certainly acute berylliosis appears to be related to the concentration of beryllium in the atmosphere but individual susceptibility is important in chronic berylliosis. Much work would be needed to determine whether the chronic progressive form of berylliosis occurred only in those who are peculiarly at risk, immunologically or otherwise.

BYSSINOSIS

DEFINITION

Byssinosis is the industrial pulmonary disease caused by the inhalation of the dusts of cotton, flax or hemp.

TYPES OF VEGETABLE DUST DISEASE

There are 3 distinct clinical entities encountered in workers in flax, hemp and cotton mills. The first, often called *'mill fever'*, *'cotton fever'* or *'hemp fever'*, consists of fever and chills, nausea and vomiting lasting for a few days and occurring in workers first entering the industry or returning to it after a prolonged absence. The symptoms occur in a small proportion of the workers exposed, develop after about 6 hours of exposure and stop abruptly when exposure ceases. Tolerance appears to be acquired within a few days. These factors suggest an allergic type of response to the inhaled dust.

'Weaver's cough' tends to affect most of the workers in weaving sheds when mouldy cotton is being handled. This results in a illness resembling farmer's lung (p. 506) and the pathogenesis is similar.

Byssinosis proper is a chronic respiratory disease occurring in factory workers who have been employed for many years in cotton rooms, blowing rooms or card rooms. The nearer workers are to the carding engines the higher is the prevalence of disease [234]. Byssinosis is less prevalent in mills spinning fine cotton than in those where medium and coarse grades of fibre are used. The dust inhaled contains cotton fibres and foreign material. It is interesting that mill fever is uncommon in workers who have clinical byssinosis [233 & 271].

EPIDEMIOLOGY

The earlier view that the disease was limited to the Lancashire cotton towns suggested a combined effect of dust and general atmospheric pollution. Recognition that the condition is world-wide and that disabling disease can occur in the balmy, clean air of the Nile delta has convinced epidemiologists that cotton dust alone is responsible. Epidemiological studies have not been easy since the area in Britain with the highest incidence of byssinosis is also one where the risk of contracting chronic bronchitis from atmospheric pollution is considerable. In the years 1957–62 1500 Lancashire cotton workers received disability pensions for byssinosis.

CLINICAL FEATURES

The characteristic history of byssinosis is that the worker, after some years in the industry, becomes aware of chest tightness and wheeze after the weekend break—on Monday ('Monday fever') in European countries and on Saturday in Arab countries. Commonly the symptoms develop during the afternoon of the first day back at work and usually subside in the early evening. This situation may continue for several years without worsening and when the worker leaves the industry his symptoms cease. In some the condition progresses and chest tightness and breathlessness may persist on Tuesday, then on Wednesday and so on until there is constant dyspnoea on every working day and finally throughout the whole week. The features of chronic bronchitis may be superimposed at any stage and in time the eventual disability is indistinguishable from chronic bronchitis with asthmatic features and associated emphysema.

RADIOLOGY

There is no characteristic radiographic appearance. This is in contrast to most other forms of pneumoconiosis in which radiographic changes often precede functional disability by many years. In byssinosis the functional change is the earliest manifestation of the disease and it has been shown that even when symptoms have not been obtrusive the FEV falls with exposure to dust during the first day back at work after a break [182].

PATHOGENESIS AND PATHOLOGY

It has usually been postulated that the features of byssinosis represent a hypersensitivity or allergic reaction and in the pamphlet on 'Pneumoconiosis and Allied Occupational Chest Diseases' issued by the Ministry of Social Security in 1967, it is stated that 'The progress of the disease may be the result of repeated allergic reactions'. Schilling [233], however, found this concept difficult to reconcile with certain features of the disease. First, the symptoms in byssinosis have a delayed onset and improve as the week goes on. This clinical pattern has never been described in true asthma even when this has been due to industrial exposure, e.g. toluene diisocyanate. Further, in byssinosis a large proportion of those exposed may be affected whereas in true asthma only a small proportion of a total population develop the disease. Third, immediate-type hypersensitivity skin reactions have not been proved conclusively and what

work there is on this is conflicting [24, 28, 39, 40, 157, 166, 179 & 204].

The alternative explanation is that there is in the dust produced in the preparation of vegetable fibres a substance with a bronchoconstrictor effect which, for some reason as yet difficult to understand, becomes less effective with successive days during the working week. The causal agent is unknown but probably is contained in the leaves of the cotton plant. It has been shown that the dust from cotton mills contains substances which have a bronchoconstrictor action in animals and cause contraction of isolated human bronchial muscle.

When pathological studies have been possible these have usually shown only chronic bronchitis with varying degrees of emphysema [233].

FUNCTIONAL ABNORMALITY

The changes in lung function are those of obstructive airways disease. A decline in FEV has been shown in carding room workers throughout the first day at work after a weekend rest [93 & 182]. Increase in airways resistance and uneven distribution of inspired gas have paralleled these findings. Byssinosis is the example *par excellence* in which lung function tests corroborate the presence of industrial lung disease, since the radiographic appearances are usually normal.

Although the incidence of frank byssinosis is low in the hemp and sisal industries, a fall in FEV on Monday has been described without, however, symptoms of chest tightness [181].

PREVENTION AND TREATMENT

If a worker with the clinical features of byssinosis has demonstrable functional abnormality, even if this is only transient at the beginning of the week, he must be removed from the sections of the work with high dust concentrations and, if necessary, found work outside the industry. Much still remains to be known about the relationship between daily change in FEV from exposure to dust and eventual permanent disability. Routine medical checks may pick out those susceptible to the disease early on and so prevent the progressive pulmonary attrition which occurs in byssinosis. The most important preventive measure is, of course, the reduction to a minimum of cotton dust in the working atmosphere. In the developed case the treatment is the same as that of chronic bronchitis.

EXTRINSIC ALLERGIC ALVEOLITIS

The term 'extrinsic allergic alveolitis' has been applied to a growing number of conditions in which the inhalation of organic dusts results in hypersensitivity reactions at alveolar level, associated with the production of precipitins. In 1700 an Italian, Bernardino Ramazzini [206], described what is now the classical example of this group of diseases, namely farmer's lung. The condition occurred among 'sifters and measurers of grain' and we are told that the victims 'heaped a thousand curses on their calling'.

Two main forms of allergic response may occur in the lungs following the inhalation of organic dusts. In atopic individuals the bronchi may be affected, giving asthmatic symptoms mediated by nonprecipitating, reaginic antibody (Type I allergy). The second form of pulmonary allergic disease is that found in extrinsic allergic alveolitis which affects nonatopic persons after repeated exposure to the antigens concerned, is mediated by precipitating antibody (Type III allergy) and gives predominately alveolar reactions to dust particles small enough to reach the alveoli. Many organic dusts encountered at work, in the home or even as medical treatment cause extrinsic allergic alveolitis and at the moment 9 conditions are known certainly to belong to this group while a few others probably do, though the evidence is not as yet complete. The known examples include *farmer's lung* due to thermophilic actinomycetes [201], *bagassosis* [227] due to the inhalation of mouldy, overheated sugar cane bagasse, *maple bark stripper's lung* due to the fungus *Cryptostroma corticale* [64], *mushroom workers' lung* [27 & 226] in which thermophilic actinomycetes are suspect, *maltworkers' lung* due to the fungus *Aspergillus clavatus* [216], '*weaver's cough*' due to mouldy cotton, '*sequoiosis*' associated with inhalation of redwood sawdust [47], the lung disease due to the *grain weevil Sitophilus granarius* [154], *bird fancier's lung* due to antigens in avian excreta and serum, [6, 12, 23, 112, 191 & 211] and *pituitary snuff taker's lung* due to porcine and bovine posterior pituitary powder [156 & 202]. In each of these conditions precipitins have been found in the patients' serum against the relevant antigens. Other diseases with similar clinical features, but in which precipitins have either not yet been found or not identified with certainty, include *suberosis* due to cork dust, *paprika splitter's lung* [123], *smallpox handler's lung* [174] and a chronic lung disease found in New Guinea natives which has been attributed to the dust from thatched roofs [20]. '*Lycoperdonosis*', the respiratory disease caused by the excessive inhalation of puffball spores [246] in the folk-medicine treatment of epistaxis, may be an exotic example of extrinsic allergic alveolitis. 'Broken wind' or 'heaves' in horses is probably also in this category.

There is a common pattern of *clinical features* in extrinsic allergic alveolitis which contrasts strikingly with that of the asthmatic reaction in the atopic subject (table 28.4). Systemic symptoms are important and may consist of fever, chills, malaise, generalized aches and pains, followed by anorexia and loss of weight which may be marked. Symptoms and signs referable to the respiratory system are those of a dominantly alveolar reaction and consist of cough and dyspnoea. It is common for fine crepitations to be heard all over the lungs, principally at the bases, but this finding may not parallel the degree of dyspnoea. The *functional abnormality* is essentially a restrictive ventilatory disturbance which may not be marked, with impairment of gas transfer and decrease in lung compliance. Usually there is little evidence of

TABLE 28.4

Distinctions between Asthma and Extrinsic Allergic Alveolitis

	Asthma	*Extrinsic allergic alveolitis*
Individual predisposition	Important	Unimportant
Histology	Oedema and eosinophil infiltration of bronchial wall	Cellular infiltration of alveoli and interstitium, or epithelioid cell granuloma
Site	Bronchi	Alveoli and interstitium
Onset	Rapidly after exposure to allergen in allergic asthma	5–6 hours+ after exposure to relevant antigen
Systemic upset	Slight	Marked
Signs	Rhonchi	Crepitations
X-ray	Hyperinflation only (or nil)	Miliary mottling in acute stages (or nil)
Serology	No precipitins	Precipitins to relevant antigens
Eosinophilia	Common	Absent
Skin tests	Immediate type hypersensitivity reactions	May be Arthus type response after 3–4 hours
Physiology	Obstructive pattern of ventilatory abnormality	Restrictive pattern of ventilatory abnormality with marked diffusion defect

airways obstruction [201, 208 & 273] unless the patient has independent obstructive airways disease.

The *radiographic abnormality* in the acute stages is usually widely distributed micronodular shadowing. In the later stages the features are those of fibrosis with diffuse honeycombing which is most commonly marked in the upper lobes.

In the early stages the *pathology* of the lungs shows infiltration of the alveolar walls with polymorphs, lymphocytes and plasma cells [63] or epithelioid cell granulomata bearing a superficial resemblance to sarcoidosis and with variable fibrosis [9, & 55]. About one quarter of patients with farmer's lung also show the features of obliterative bronchiolitis [63]. Permanent lung damage due to interstitial fibrosis may occur after recurrent episodes.

At first it was believed that extrinsic allergic alveolitis only presented acutely but it is now recognized that subacute and chronic forms may occur [112 & 201]. The classical *acute form* presents with systemic and pulmonary symptoms 5–6 hours or more after exposure to the dust. The attack may subside rapidly but recurs on further exposure. Probably the more dangerous form is the type with an *insidious onset* since the association with the causal agent may not be appreciated. Thus medical advice may only be sought when irreversible fibrosis has occurred. It appears that the different modes of onset relate to the frequency and intensity of exposure to the dust. In both forms of the disease provocative inhalation tests induce classical acute symptoms after the usual interval [112].

The mainstay of *management* is avoidance of the offending antigens. The precipitin test may identify the specific antigen although the presence of precipitins can only be regarded as evidence of exposure. The clinical relevance of the immunological findings is confirmed by inhalation tests but in those conditions in which the significance of the serological tests has been established confirmatory inhalation tests are superfluous (e.g. farmer's lung). *Preventive measures* are obvious in certain of the industries. For example farmers can avoid exposure to farmer's lung hay antigen by taking thought about the preparation of stored hay, particularly the moisture content [105]. Those who work with mushrooms probably have greater problems in prophylaxis since very large numbers of spores of actinomycetes are produced [73]. The use of masks is of little practical value principally because the spores of thermophilic actinomycetes are extremely small, only about 1 μ in diameter [48]. It has been suggested [156] that a coarse grain preparation of posterior pituitary snuff with a particle diameter over 100 μ should be substituted for fine grain preparations which appear to be responsible for snuff taker's lung. In fact snuff is best avoided.

FARMER'S LUNG

DEFINITION

Farmer's lung is listed as prescribed occupational disease No. 43 under the British Industrial Injuries Act and is defined as: 'Pulmonary disease due to the inhalation of the dust of mouldy hay or of other mouldy vegetable produce, and characterized by symptoms and signs attributable to a reaction in the peripheral part of the bronchopulmonary system, and giving rise to a defect in gas exchange' [167].

The condition was described by Cadham in 1924 in Canada [33]. Campbell in 1932 [36 & 37] gave the first description in Britain of the disease occurring in farmworkers handling mouldy hay in Westmorland. The radiographic appearances and the earliest description of the pulmonary pathology in a fatal case were subjects of communications by Fawcitt in 1935 [71] and in 1938 [72]. The next major advance was the detailed description of the lung pathology from biopsy material by several authors [55, 85 & 253]. The findings of precipitins against antigens in mouldy hay reported by Pepys and his colleagues in 1961 and 1962 [201] and confirmed by Kobayashi et al. [141] represented a great advance in the understanding of the pathogenesis of the condition and stimulated interest in its incidence. This culminated in the recognition of farmer's lung as an occupational hazard in Britain and since 1965 a person contracting this disease has been entitled to Industrial Injuries Benefit.

The peak incidence of farmer's lung in Britain occurs from January to March when stored hay is being used for winter feeding. It is commoner in the wetter parts of the country and the incidence is higher after a wet summer when it is more difficult to dry the hay before storage. Good quality hay contains only about 16% of moisture and only a relatively small microflora will develop in this even after prolonged storage. But if hay is stored when too wet (moisture content greater than 29-34% water [76]), considerable heat (up to 60°C) may be produced and this encourages the growth of thermophilic micro-organisms, of which the actinomycetes have been shown to be the most important so far as the development of farmer's lung is concerned. The threshing of poor quality grain and the sweeping of barns also carry the risk of the inhalation of mouldy vegetable produce and can result in the clinical picture of farmer's lung. The speculative incidence in Britain may be as high as 1000 cases each year, of all grades of severity.

PATHOGENESIS

Combined studies by the British Medical Research Council's Clinical Immunology Research Group and the Rothamsted Experimental Station, led respectively by Dr. Pepys and Dr. Gregory, have defined what is termed farmer's lung hay (FLH) antigen complex, a group of antigens which appear in hay only after heating has occurred and of which the principal constituents are thermophilic actinomycetes. The richest sources of farmer's lung hay antigen are *Micropolyspora sp.* (*Thermopolyspora polyspora*) and to a lesser extent *Micromonospora* (*Thermoactinomyces*) *vulgaris* [200 & 201]. It has been calculated that a worker among mouldy hay may retain three quarters of a million of the spores of *Micropolyspora sp.* each minute [114]. The spores being only 1 μ in diameter can reach the alveoli where the main tissue reactions of the disease occur.

In 80% of patients with farmer's lung due to mouldy hay, precipitins can be demonstrated to FLH antigen; precipitins against other actinomycetes may be found in a further 2–3% [144 & 201]. When other dusts are responsible, such as those of barley and oats, 50% of patients have FLH precipitins. Clearly a number of other sources of antigen have still to be identified and all the features of farmer's lung may be present without a positive serological test. Thus a negative test does not exclude the diagnosis. Also 17–18% of exposed subjects who have no clinical features of farmer's lung may have precipitins to FLH antigen. The diagnosis, therefore, does not rest purely on a positive serological reaction and it is necessary to take into account both the clinical and the immunological findings [201].

Fog fever in cattle occurs after exposure to mouldy hay and 71% of the animals affected give FLH reactions on serological testing [128].

PATHOLOGY

The pathological appearances depend on the stage of the disease, all gradations being possible from an acute alveolar and interstitial reaction to a diffuse pulmonary fibrosis. The acute reaction is characterized by oedema and infiltration in the alveolar walls and interstitium of the lung by lymphocytes, plasma cells and neutrophils [63]. The pulmonary vessels may be involved in the process. Recurrent exposure leads to patchy areas of interstitial fibrosis and sometimes diffuse cystic changes.

Lung biopsy has sometimes shown a diffuse granulomatous lesion which affects the walls of the alveoli and the smaller bronchioles, the lung parenchyma generally, the interlobular septa and the subpleural tissues. The lumen of an affected bronchiole may be obliterated by inflammatory exudate. The granuloma consists of a collection of pale epithelioid cells with a rim of lymphocytes and plasma cells, and occasionally giant cells containing pale translucent fibres whose nature is unknown. When the larger bronchi have been examined bronchoscopically this has shown intense congestion [84].

Both *Micropolyspora sp.* [269] and *Micro-monospora vulgaris* [270] have been isolated from lung biopsy material of patients with farmer's lung.

FUNCTIONAL ABNORMALITY

The pattern of functional abnormality is that of restrictive lung disease of variable severity with striking impairment of diffusing capacity [55 & 208]. The changes include reduction in the static lung volumes, vital capacity, diffusing capacity and static compliance. The exercise ventilation is increased.

The functional abnormality is reversible in the earlier stages of the disease but repeated episodes may result in permanent lung damage and respiratory failure. Impairment of diffusing capacity can persist long after radiological clearing is complete [55, 228 & 273].

CLINICAL FEATURES AND RADIOLOGY

Two main groups are recognized: (a) acute and subacute and (b) chronic. The classical acute type presents with dyspnoea, shivering, fever and cough, occurring fairly suddenly some hours after exposure to mouldy hay. Wheeze is not a feature. The sputum is scanty and may rarely be bloodstained. Cyanosis may sometimes be marked even at rest. Crepitations are heard diffusely throughout the lungs. The chest x-ray may show no abnormality or may show a faint miliary mottling particularly in the middle and lower zones or, less commonly, patchy ill-defined opacities in these areas.

The symptoms and x-ray changes usually resolve spontaneously within 3–4 weeks but re-exposure will lead to recurrence of the development of a subacute phase in which clinical and radiographic resolution occurs more slowly. Some cases pass into the chronic phase and develop severe exertional dyspnoea and cough. The x-ray appearances in the chronic phase are nonspecific and consist usually of irregular opacities or diffuse honeycombing. Death is usually due to *cor pulmonale* with right-sided heart failure. Eosinophilia of the blood, sputum and tissues is not a feature of farmer's lung whereas it frequently occurs in asthma and pulmonary aspergillosis of the allergic type. There is no satisfactory skin test for farmer's lung.

DIFFERENTIAL DIAGNOSIS

Chronic bronchitis, emphysema, asthma (table 28.4), honeycomb lung, sarcoidosis and pulmonary aspergillosis may all have to be considered. The diagnosis of farmer's lung depends on the clinical history, clinical examination, x-ray appearances, lung function tests and serological tests. Of particular importance are the delayed onset of symptoms after exposure, the miliary type radiographic opacities, the marked diffusion abnormality and a positive precipitin test to FLH antigen.

PREVENTION AND TREATMENT

Adequate drying of hay, the use of open pit silage and forced ventilation in the working area are important preventive measures. Sensitized persons should be warned to avoid further exposure to mouldy hay. In a single man farm this may mean advising the patient to give up his work and seek other employment. As already stated the wearing of masks is of little value. Treatment of the acute and subacute case is by corticosteroids which sometimes have a dramatic effect.

The British Industrial Injuries Advisory Council has called for a publicity programme to draw attention to the hazards of handling mouldy vegetable produce.

WOOL SORTER'S DISEASE

Anthrax spores may be inhaled from animals' hides or wool to give a severe, often fatal illness due to pulmonary anthrax. The symptoms are cough, chest pain, fever and rapidly worsening dyspnoea, finally passing on to a septicaemic phase from which recovery is unusual. Strict control measures have eradicated the condition in Britain. The recommended treatment for a diagnosed case is antiserum and a combination of penicillin and sulphonamide [237].

HAIR SPRAYS

In 1958 attention was drawn to the possible association of the use of hair sprays and the development of pulmonary infiltration [16]. The initial cases of so-called 'thesaurosis' were identical with sarcoidosis in radiographic appearances and clinical course, and scalene node biopsy showed granulomatous change. Further cases studied with lung biopsy showed interstitial inflammatory change with fibrosis and hyperplasia of alveolar lining cells [17]. Chemical analysis failed to show polyvinyl compounds.

The existence of 'thesaurosis' is not proved beyond doubt and it is possible that the cases described were, in fact, due to sarcoidosis. In a survey of 505 hairdressers in Britain no cases were found [184].

Pulmonary function tests were not undertaken in any of the cases reported in the literature.

REFERENCES

[1] AGATE J.N. (1948) Delayed pneumonitis in a beryllium worker. *Lancet* ii, 530.

[2] AHLMARK A., BRUCE T. & NYSTROM A. (1960) *Silicosis and other pneumoconioses in Sweden.* Stockholm, Svenska Bokförlaget.

[3] ALDRIDGE W.N., BARNES J.M. & DENZ F.A. (1949) Experimental beryllium poisoning. *Br. J. exp. Path.* 30, 375.

[4] ARRIGONI A. (1933) La pneumoconiosis da bario (Osservazioni clinico-radiologiche experimentali). *Medna. Lav.* 24, 461.

[5] BADER M.E., BADER R.A. & SELIKOFF I.J. (1961) Pulmonary function in asbestosis of the lungs. An alveolar capillary block syndrome. *Am. J. Med.* 30, 235.

[6] BARBORIAK J.J., SOSMAN A.J. & REED C.E. (1965) Serological studies in pigeon breeders' disease. *J. Lab. clin. Med.* 65, 600.

[7] BARRIE H.J. & HARDING H.E. (1947) Argyrosiderosis of lungs in silver finishers. *Br. J. industr. Med.* 4, 225.

[8] BARTH G., FIRK W. & SCHEIDEMANDEL H. (1956) Die Aluminiumlunge; Verlaufsbeobach-

tungen und Neuerkrankungen in der Nach-kriegszeit. *Dt. med. Wschr.* **81**, 1115.

[9] BATES D.V. & CHRISTIE R.V. (1964) *Respiratory function in Disease.* London, Saunders.

[10] BEATTIE J. & KNOX J.F. (1961) In *Inhaled Particles and Vapours,* ed. Davies C.N. New York, Pergamon.

[11] BECH A.O., KIPLING M.D. & HEATHER J.C. (1962) Hard metal disease. *Br. J. industr. Med.* **19**, 239.

[12] BECKER W.B., LARSSON K. & KIPPS A. (1967) Serological studies in a case of pigeon breeder's lung. *S. Afr. med. J.* **41**, 194.

[13] BECKLAKE MARGARET R. (1965) Pneumoconiosis. In *Handbook of Physiology. Respiration* Ed. Fenn W.O. and Rahn H. Vol. 2, p. 1601 Washington, American Physiological Society.

[14] BECKLAKE MARGARET R., GOLDMAN H.I., BOSMAN A.R. & FREED C.C. (1957) The long term effects of exposure to nitrous fumes. *Am. Rev. Tuberc.* **76**, 398.

[15] BECKLAKE MARGARET R., DU PREEZ L. & LUTZ W. (1958) Lung function in silicosis of the Witwatersrand gold miner. *Am. Rev. Tuberc.* **77**, 400.

[16] BERGMAN M., FLANCE I.J. & BLUMENTHAL H.T. (1958) Thesaurosis following inhalation of hair sprays. A clinical and experimental study. *New Engl. J. Med.* **258**, 471.

[17] BERGMAN M., FLANCE I.J., CRUZ P.T., KLAM N., ARONSON P.R., JOSHI R.A. & BLUMENTHAL H.T. (1962) Thesaurosis due to inhalation of hair spray. Report of 12 new cases, including 3 autopsies. *New Engl. J. Med.* **266**, 750.

[18] BETON D.C., ANDREWS G.S., DAVIES H.J., HOWELLS L. & SMITH G.F. (1966) Acute cadmium fume poisoning: 5 cases with 1 death from renal necrosis. *Br. J. industr. Med.* **23**, 292.

[19] BJURE J., SÖDERHOLM B. & WIDIMSKY J. (1964) Cardiopulmonary function studies in workers dealing with asbestos and glass wool. *Thorax* **19**, 22.

[20] BLACKBURN C.R.B. (1966) Precipitins against extracts of thatched roofs in the sera of New Guinea natives with chronic lung disease. *Lancet* ii, 1396.

[21] BONNELL J.A., KAZANTZIS G. & KING E. (1959) A follow up of men exposed to cadmium oxide fume. *Br. J. industr. Med.* **16**, 135.

[22] BONSER G.M., FAULDS J.S. & STEWART M.J. (1955) Occupational cancer of the urinary bladder in dyestuffs operatives and of lung in asbestos textile workers and iron ore miners. *Am. J. clin. Path.* **25**, 126.

[23] BOYD G., DICK H.W., LORIMER A.R. & MORAN F. (1967) Bird breeder's lung. *Scot. med. J.* **12**, 69.

[24] BRAMWELL J.C. & ELLIS R. (1932) *Report of the Departmental Committee on Dust in Card-rooms in the Cotton Industry* H.M. Stationery Office.

[25] BRASSEUR L. (1963) *L'exploration fonctionnelle pulmonaire dans la pneumoconiose des houilleurs.* Brussels, Editions Arscia. Paris, Librairie Malone.

[26] BRILLE D., HATZFELD C. & LAURENT R. (1957) Emphysème pulmonaire après inhalation de vapeurs irritantes (Ammoniaque en particulier). *Arch. Mal. prof.* **18**, 320.

[27] BRINGHURST L.S., BYRNE R.N. & GERSHON-COHEN J. (1959) Respiratory disease of mushroom workers. *J. Am. med. Ass.* **171**, 15.

[28] BROWN A. (1932) (see [24]).

[29] BROWNE R.C. (1955) Vanadium poisoning from gas turbines. *Br. J. industr. Med.* **12**, 57.

[30] BROWNE R.C. (1966) *The Chemistry and Therapy of Industrial Pulmonary Diseases.* Springfield, Illinois, Thomas.

[31] BROWNE R.C. & STEEL J. (1963) The control of the vanadium hazard in catalytic oil-gas plants. *Ann. occup. Hyg.* **6**, 75.

[32] BRUNOT F.R. (1933) The toxicity of osmium tetroxide (Osmic acid). *J. ind. Hyg. Toxicol.* **15**, 136.

[33] CADHAM F.T. (1924) Asthma due to grain dusts. *J. Am. med. Ass.* **83**, 27.

[34] CAMPBELL A.H. & GLOYNE S.R. (1942) Cases of pneumoconiosis due to inhalation of Fuller's earth. *J. Path. Bact.* **61**, 375.

[35] CAMPBELL J.A. (1940) Effects of precipitated silica and of iron oxide on the incidence of primary lung tumours in mice. *Br. med. J.* ii, 275.

[36] CAMPBELL J.M. (1932) Acute symptoms following work with hay. *Br. med. J.* ii, 1143.

[37] CAMPBELL J.M. (1961) Farmer's lung again. *Br. med. J.* i, 727.

[38] CAPLAN A. (1953) Certain unusual radiological appearances in the chest of coalminers suffering from rheumatoid arthritis. *Thorax* **8**, 29.

[39] CAYTON H.E. FURNESS G. & MAITLAND H.B. (1952a) Studies on cotton dust in relation to byssinosis; skin tests for allergy with extracts of cotton dust. *Br. J. industr. Med.* **9**, 186.

[40] CAYTON H.E., FURNESS G., JACKSON D.S. & MAITLAND H.B. (1952b) Studies on cotton dust in relation to byssinosis; comparison of cotton dust and house dust by chemical and skin tests. *Br. J. industr. Med.* **9**, 303.

41] CHAMPEIX J. & MORCAN H.L. (1958) Observations récentes sur les pneumoconioses par terre d'ocre. *Arch. Mal. prof.* **19**, 564.

[42] CHESNER I.C. (1950) Chronic pulmonary granulomatosis in residents of a community near a beryllium plant: three autopsied cases. *Ann. intern. Med.* **32**, 1028.

[43] COCHRANE A.L. (1962) The attack rate of

progressive massive fibrosis. *Br. J. industr. Med.* **19**, 52.

[44] COCHRANE A.L. (1963) The international classification of the pneumoconioses. In *Industrial Pulmonary Disease. Br. J. Radiol.* **37**, 334.

[45] COCHRANE A.L. & HIGGINS I.T.T. (1961) Pulmonary ventilatory functions of coal-miners in various areas in relation to the x-ray category of pneumoconiosis. *Br. J. prev. Soc. Med.* **15**, 1.

[46] COCHRANE A.L. & MIALL W.E. (1956) Factors influencing the radiological attack rate of progressive massive fibrosis. *Br. med. J.* **i**, 1193.

[47] COHEN H.I., MERIGAN T.C., KOSEK J.C. & ELDRIDGE F. (1967) Sequoiosis: a granulomatous pneumonitis associated with redwood inhalation. *Am. J. Med.* **43**, 785.

[48] CORBAZ R., GREGORY P.H. & LACEY M.E. (1963) Thermophilic and mesophilic actinomycetes in mouldy hay. *J. gen. Microbiol.* **32**, 449.

[49] CORRIN G. (1963a) I. In vitro comparison of stamped aluminium powders containing different lubricating agents and a granular aluminium powder. *Br. J. industr. Med.* **20**, 264.

[50] CORRIN G. (1963b) II. Effect on the rat lung of intratracheal injections of stamped aluminium powders containing different lubricating agents and of a granular aluminium powder. *Br. J. industr. Med.* **20**, 268.

[51] CUGELL D.W., MARKS A., ELLICOTT M.F., BADGER T.L. & GAENSLER E.A. (1956) Carbon monoxide diffusing capacity during steady exercise. *Am. Rev. Tuberc.* **74**, 317.

[52] CURTIS G.H. (1951) Cutaneous hypersensitivity due to beryllium. *Arch. Derm.* **64**, 470.

[53] CURTIS G.H. (1959) The diagnosis of beryllium disease with special reference to the patch test. *Archs. ind. Hlth* **19**, 150.

[54] DENNY J.J., ROBSON W.D. & IRWIN D.A. (1939) Prevention of silicosis by metallic aluminium. *Canad. med. Ass. J.* **40**, 213.

[55] DICKIE H.A. & RANKIN J. (1958) Farmer's lung. An acute granulomatous interstitial pneumonitis occurring in agricultural workers. *J. Am. med. Ass.* **167**, 1069.

[56] DOIG A.T. & CHALLEN P.J.R. (1964) Respiratory hazards in welding. *Ann. occup. Hyg.* **7**, 223.

[57] DOIG A.T. & MCLAUGHLIN A.I.G. (1948) Clearing of x-ray shadows in welders' siderosis. *Lancet* **i**, 789.

[58] DOLL R. (1955) Mortality from lung cancer in asbestos workers. *Br. J. industr. Med.* **12**, 81.

[59] *Draft Statutory Instruments.* Factories: the Asbestos Regulations. Ministry of Labour (1966). Quoted in Editorial (1967) *Lancet*, **ii**, 1311.

[60] DUDLEY H.R. (1959) The pathologic changes of chronic beryllium disease. *Archs. ind. Hlth* **19**, 184.

[61] DUTTON W.F. (1911) Vanadiumism. *J. Am. med. Ass.* **56**, 1648.

[62] EISENBUD M., WANTA B.S., DUSTON C., STRADMAN L.T., HARRIS W.A. & WOLD B.S. (1949) Non-occupational berylliosis. *J. ind. Hyg. Toxicol.* **31**, 282.

[63] EMANUEL D.A., WENZEL F.J., BOWERMAN C.I. & LAWTON B.R. (1964) Farmer's lung: clinical, pathologic and immunologic study of twenty-four patients. *Am. J. Med.* **37**, 392.

[64] EMANUEL D.A., WENZEL F.J. & LAWTON B.R. (1966) Pneumonitis due to *Cryptostroma corticale* (Maple-bark disease) *New Engl. J. Med.* **274**, 1413.

[65] ENTICKNAP J.B. & SMITHER W.J. (1964) Peritoneal tumours in asbestosis. *Br. J. industr. Med.* **21**, 20.

[66] ENTWISTLE H. (1964) A casebook of welding accidents. *Ann. occup. Hyg.* **7**, 207.

[67] ENZER N. & SANDER O.A. (1938) Chronic lung changes in electric arc welders. *J. ind. Hyg. Toxicol.* **20**, 333.

[68] FABRIONI S.M. (1935) Patologia pulmonare da polveri di berillio. *Medna Lav.* **26**, 297.

[69] FALLON J.T. (1937) Specific tissue reaction to phospholipids; suggested explanation for similarity of lesions of silicosis and pulmonary tuberculosis. *Canad. med. Ass. J.* **36**, 223.

[70] FAULDS J.S. (1957) Haematite pneumoconiosis in Cumberland miners. *J. clin. Path.* **10**, 187.

[71] FAWCITT R. (1935) Fungoid conditions of the lung. *Br. J. Radiol.* **9**, 172, 354.

[72] FAWCITT R. (1938) Vol. I. Occupational diseases of the lung in agricultural workers. *Br. J. Radiol.* **11**, 378.

[73] FERGUS C.L. (1964) Thermophilic and thermotolerant moulds and actinomycetes of mushroom compost during peak heating. *Mycologia*, **56**, 267.

[74] FERGUSON T. (Quoted by Middleton E.L.) (1936) Industrial pulmonary disease due to inhalation of dust, with special reference to silicosis. *Lancet* **ii**, 59.

[75] FERRIS B.G.Jr., AFFELDT J.E., KRIETE H.A. & WHITTENBERGER J.L. (1951) Pulmonary function in patients with pulmonary disease treated with ACTH. *Archs. ind. Hyg.* **3**, 603.

[76] FESTENSTEIN G.N., LACEY J., SKINNER F.A., JENKINS P.A. & PEPYS J. (1965) Self heating of hay and grain in Dewar Flasks and the development of farmer's lung antigens. *J. gen. Microbiol.* **41**, 389.

[77] FINDEISEN W. (1935) Uber das Absetzen kleiner in der Luft suspendierter Teilchen in der Menschlichen Lunge bei der Atmung. *Pflügers Arch. ges. Physiol.* **236**, 367.

[78] FIORI E. (1926) Contributo alla clinica e alla

radiologia delle pneumoconiosi rare. *Osp. magg.* **3**, 78.

[79] FLETCHER C.M. (1948) Pneumoconiosis of coalminers. *Br. med. J.* **i**, 1015, 1065.

[80] FOWLER P.B.S. (1952) Printer's asthma. *Lancet* **ii**, 755.

[81] FRANK N.R., AMDUR M.O., WORCESTER J. & WHITTENBERGER J.L. (1962) Effects of acute controlled exposure to SO_2 on respiratory mechanics in healthy male adults. *J. appl. Physiol.* **17**, 252.

[82] FRANT R. (1963) Formation of ozone in gas-shielded welding. *Ann. occup. Hyg.* **6**, 113.

[83] FREIMAN D.G. (1959) Pathologic changes of beryllium disease. *Archs ind. Hlth* **19**, 188.

[84] FULLER C.J. (1953) Farmer's lung: a review of present knowledge. *Thorax* **8**, 59.

[85] FULLER C.J. (1958) In *Fungous Diseases and their Treatment*, ed. Riddell R.W. & Stewart G.T., p. 138. London, Butterworths.

[86] GAENSLER E.A., VERSTRAETEN J.M., WEIL W.B., CUGELL D.W., MARKS A., CADIGAN J.B.Jr., JONES R.H. & ELLICOTT M.F. (1959) Respiratory pathophysiology in chronic beryllium disease. Review of 30 cases with some observations after long term steroid therapy. *Arch. ind. Hlth* **19**, 132.

[87] GAENSLER E.A., VERSTRAETEN J.M., WEIL W.B., CUGELL D.W., MARKS A., CADIGAN J.B.Jr., JONES R.H. & ELLICOTT M.F. (1959) The differentiation of sarcoidosis and beryllium disease. *Arch. ind. Hlth* **19**, 160.

[88] GARDNER L.U. (1938) Reaction of the living body to different types of mineral dusts with or without complicating infection. *Min. Technol.* **929**, 1.

[89] GARDNER L.U. (1939) *Fourth Saranac Symposium on Silicosis*. Trudeau Sch. Tuberc., Saranac Lake, N.Y.

[90] GARDNER L.U., DWORSKI M. & DELAHANT A.B. (1944) Aluminium therapy in silicosis; experimental study. *J. ind. Hyg. Toxicol.* **26**, 211.

[91] GELMAN L. (1936) Poisoning by vapours of beryllium oxyfluoride. *J. ind. Hyg. Toxicol.* **18**, 371.

[92] GILSON J.C. (1960) The disturbance of pulmonary function in industrial pulmonary disease. In *A Symposium on Industrial Pulmonary Diseases*, ed. King, E.J. & Fletcher C.M. London, Churchill.

[93] GILSON J.C., SCOTT H., HOPWOOD B.E.C., ROACH S.A., McKERROW C.B. & SCHILLING R.S.F. (1962) Byssinosis: the acute effect on ventilatory capacity of dusts in cotton ginneries, cotton, sisal and jute mills. *Br. J. industr. Med.* **19**, 9.

[94] GILSON J.C. & WAGNER J.C. (1967) Asbestos in the lung. *Nature (Lond.)* **213**, 1170.

[95] GLOYNE S.R. (1933) Morbid anatomy and histology of asbestosis. *Tubercle (Lond.)* **14**, 445, 493, 550.

[96] GLOYNE S.R. (1938) In *Silicosis and Asbestosis*. Ed. Lanza A.J. London, Oxford University Press.

[97] GOLDMAN K.P. (1965) Prognosis of coalminers with carcinoma of the lung. *Thorax* **20**, 170.

[98] GORALEWSKI G. (1939) Klinische und tieres experimentelle Studien zur Frage der Aluminiumstaublunge. *Arch. Radiol.* **56**, 170.

[99] GORALEWSKI G. (1940) Zur Symptomatologie der Aluminiumstaublunge. *Arch. Gewerbepath. Gewerbehyg.* **10**, 384.

[100] GORALEWSKI G. (1941) Zur Klinik der Aluminiumlunge. *Arch. Gewerbepath. Gewerbehyg.* **11**, 106.

[101] GORALEWSKI G. (1943) Weitere Erfahrungen zum Krankheitsbild der Aluminiumlunge. *Dts. TuberkBl.* **17**, 3.

[102] GORALEWSKI G. (1947) The aluminium lung: a new industrial disease. *Z. ges. inn. Med.* **2**, 665.

[103] GORALEWSKI G. (1950) *Die Aluminiumlunge* (Arbeitsmedizin No. 26). Leipzig, Barth.

[104] GRANATA A. (1957) Kaolinosis. *Folia med. Napoli.* **40**, 329.

[105] GREGORY P.H., FESTENSTEIN G.N., LACEY M.E., SKINNER F.A., PEPYS J. & JENKINS P.A. (1964) Farmer's lung disease: the development of antigens in moulding hay. *J. gen. Microbiol.* **6**, 429.

[106] HARDING H.E. & MASSIE H.P. (1951) Pneumoconiosis in boiler scalers. *Br. J. industr. Med.* **8**, 256.

[107] HARDING H.E., TOD D.L.M. & McLAUGHLIN A.I.G. (1944) Disease of lungs in boiler scalers. *Br. J. industr. Med.* **1**, 247.

[108] HARDING H.E., TOD D.L.M. & McLAUGHLIN A.I.G. (1947) Pneumoconiosis in a boiler scaler. *Br. J. industr. Med.* **4**, 100.

[109] HARDY HARIET L. (1950) in *Pneumoconiosis*. Leroy U. Gardner Memorial Volume. Hoeber, New York.

[110] HARDY HARIET L. (1956) Differential diagnosis between beryllium poisoning and sarcoidosis. *Am. Rev. Tuberc.* **74**, 885.

[111] HARDY HARIET L. & TABERSHAW I.R. (1946) Delayed chemical pneumonitis occurring in workers exposed to beryllium compounds. *J. industr. Hyg.* **28**, 197.

[112] HARGREAVE F.E., PEPYS J., LONGBOTTOM J.L. & WRAITH D.G. (1966) Bird breeder's (Fancier's) lung. *Lancet* **i**, 445.

[113] HART J.R., COCHRANE A.L. & HIGGINS I.T.T. (1963) Tuberculin sensitivity in coalworkers pneumoconiosis. *Tubercle* **44**, 141.

[114] HART P.D'A. & ASLETT E.A. (1942) *Chronic pulmonary disease in South Wales coalminers*. Special Report Series. Medical Research Council. London. No. 243, 1.

[115] HENDRIKS CH.A.M. & BLEIKER M.A. (1964) Tuberculin sensitivity in coalminers with pneumoconiosis. *Tubercle* **45**, 379.

[116] HENDRY N.W. (1965) The geology, occurrences and major uses of asbestos. *Ann. N.Y. Acad. Sci.* **132**, 12.

[117] HEPPLESTON A.G. (1951) Coalworkers' pneumoconiosis; pathological and etiological considerations. *Arch. ind. Hyg.* **4**, 270.

[118] HEPPLESTON A.G. (1956) The pathology of honeycomb lung. *Thorax* **11**, 77.

[119] HEPPLESTON A.G. (1962) The disposal of dust in the lungs of silicotic rats. *Am. J. Path.* **40**, 493.

[120] HOLT P.F. (1957) *Pneumoconiosis*. London, Arnold.

[121] HOURIHANE D.O'B. (1964) The pathology of mesotheliomata and an analysis of their association with asbestos exposure. *Thorax* **19**, 268.

[122] HOURIHANE D.O'B., LESSOF L. & RICHARDSON P.C. (1966) Hyaline and calcified pleural plaques as an index of exposure to asbestos: a study of radiological and pathological features of 100 cases with a consideration of epidemiology. *Br. med. J.* **i**, 1069.

[123] HUNTER D. (1964) Paprika. In *The Diseases of Occupations*, p. 1021. London, English Universities Press Ltd.

[124] HUNTER D., MILTON R. & PERRY K.M.A. (1945) Asthma caused by the complex salts of platinum. *Br. J. industr. Med.* **2**, 92.

[125] JAGER R. (1954) Die Rolle der Ordnungszustände bei der Wechselwerkung zwischen Quarz und Organismus. In *Die Stablungenerkrankungen*, Vol. 2, p. 142, ed. Jötten K.W., Klosterkötter W. and Pfefferkorn G., Darmstadt, Steinkopff.

[126] JAMES D.G. (1959) Dermatological aspects of sarcoidosis. *Quart. J. Med.* **28**, 109.

[127] JAMES W.R.L. (1955) Primary lung cancer in South Wales coalworkers with pneumoconiosis. *Br. J. industr. Med.* **12**, 87.

[128] JENKINS P.A. & PEPYS J. (1965) Fog fever; precipitin (FLH) reactions to mouldy hay. *Vet. Rec.* **77**, 467.

[129] JONES W.R. (1933) Silicotic lungs: the minerals they contain. *J. Hyg. (Lond.)* **33**, 307.

[130] JONES-WILLIAMS W. & LAWRIE J.H. (1967) Skin granulomata from beryllium oxide. *Br. J. Surg.* **54**, 292.

[131] JORDAN J.W. (1961) Pulmonary fibrosis in a worker using an aluminium powder. *Br. J. industr. Med.* **18**, 21.

[132] JORDAN J.W. & DARKE C.S. (1958) Chronic beryllium poisoning. *Thorax* **13**, 69.

[133] JÖTTEN K.W. & EICKHOFF W. (1944) Lungenveränderurgen durch Sillimanstaub. Lung changes from sillimanite dust. *Arch. Gewerbepath. Gewerbehyg.* **12**, 223.

[134] KAZANTZIS G. (1956) Respiration function in men casting alloys: an assessment of respiratory function. *Br. J. industr. Med.* **13**, 30.

[135] KEAL E.E. (1960) Asbestosis and abdominal neoplasms. *Lancet* **ii**, 1211.

[136] KENNEDY B.J., PARE J.A.P., PUMP K.K., BECK J.C., JOHNSON L.G., EPSTEIN N.B., VENNING E.H. & BROWNE J.S.L. (1951) Effect of adrenocorticotrophic hormone (ACTH) on beryllium granulomatosis and silicosis. *Am. J. Med.* **10**, 134.

[137] KENNEDY M.C.S. (1956) Aluminium powder inhalations in the treatment of silicosis of pottery workers and pneumoconiosis of coalminers. *Br. J. industr. Med.* **13**, 85.

[138] KETTLE E.H. (1932) Interstitial reactions caused by various dusts and their influence on tuberculous infections. *J. Path. Bact.* **35**, 395.

[139] KING E.J. & HARRISON C.V. (1960) In *Industrial Pulmonary Disease*. London, Churchill.

[140] KIVILUOTO R. (1960) Pleural calcification as a roentgenologic sign of non-occupational endemic anthophyllite asbestosis. *Acta Radiol. (Stockh.) Suppl.* No. 194.

[141] KOBAYASHI M., STAHMANN M.A., RANKIN J. & DICKIE H.A. (1963) Antigens in mouldy hay as the cause of farmer's lung. *Proc. Soc. exp. Biol. (N.Y.)* **113**, 472,

[142] KÖNIG J. (1960) Über die Asbestose. *Arch. Gewerbepath. Gewerbehyg.* **18**, 159.

[143] KNOX J.F., DOLL R.S. & HILL I.D. (1965) Cohort analysis of changes in incidence of bronchial carcinoma in a textile asbestos factory. *Ann. N.Y. Acad. Sci.* **132**, 526.

[144] LACEY J. & LACEY M.E. (1964) Spore concentrations in the air of farm buildings. *Trans. Br. mycol. Soc.* **47**, 547.

[145] LA FLECHE L.R., BOIVIN C. & LEONARD C. (1961) Nitrogen dioxide: a respiratory irritant. *Canad. med. Ass. J.* **84**, 1438.

[146] LANE R.E. & CAMPBELL A.C.P. (1954) Fatal emphysema in two men making copper cadmium alloy. *Br. J. industr. Med.* **11**, 118.

[147] LEATHART G.L. (1960) Clinical, bronchographic, radiological and physiological observations in 10 cases of asbestosis. *Br. J. industr. Med.* **17**, 213.

[148] LEBOVITZ E., LEBOVITZ J.J. & SILVERMAN J.D. (1964) *Coalminers' pneumoconiosis*. Biochemical Clinics, Rubin H. Donelley Corporation. New York.

[149] LEPINE C. & SOUCY R. (1962) La bronchopneumopathie d'origine toxique. Évolution physio-pathologique. *Un. méd. Can.* **91**, 7.

[150] LEWIS C.E. (1959) The biological effects of vanadium exposure. II. The signs and symptoms of occupational vanadium exposure. *Archs ind. Hlth* **19**, 497.

[151] LLOYD-DAVIES T.A. & HARDING H.E. (1949) Manganese pneumonitis. Further clinical and

experimental observations. *Br. J. industr. Med.* **6**, 82.

[152] LOWRY T. & SCHUMAN L.M. (1956) Silo-filler's disease: a syndrome caused by nitrogen dioxide. *J. Am. med. Ass.* **162**, 153.

[153] LUCEY J.A. (1964) Survey of welding processes. *Ann. occup. Hyg.* **7**, 203.

[154] LUNN J.A. & HUGHES D.T.D. (1967) Pulmonary hypersensitivity to the grain weevil. *Br. J. industr. Med.* **24**, 158.

[155] LYONS H.A. (1953) Talc pneumoconiosis. *Milit. Surg.* **113**, 393.

[156] MAHON W.E., SCOTT D.J., ANSELL G., MANSON G.L. & FRASER R. (1967) Hypersensitivity to pituitary snuff with miliary shadowing of the lungs. *Thorax* **22**, 13.

[157] MAITLAND H.B., HEAP H. & MACDONALD A.D. (1932) (See [24]).

[158] MANCUSO T.F. & COULTER E.F. (1963) Methodology in industrial health studies. *Arch. environ. Hlth* **6**, 210.

[159] MANN B. & DEASY J.B. (1955) Talc pneumoconiosis in textile industry. *Br. med. J.* **ii**, 1460.

[160] MEICHAN F.W. (1960) Modern welding and health hazards. *Trans. Ass. ind. med. Offrs.* **10**, 39.

[161] MEIKLEJOHN A. (1960) In *Industrial Pulmonary Diseases in Great Britain* Ed. King E.J. and Fletcher C.M. London, Churchill.

[162] MEREWETHER E.R.A. (1955) Discussion. Recent advances in knowledge of the pathogenesis and pathology of the pneumoconioses. In *Proceedings, Third International Conference of Experts on Pneumoconiosis, Sydney, Australia 1950.* Geneva International Labour Office.

[163] MEURMAN L. (1966) Asbestos bodies and pleural plaques in a Finnish series of autopsy cases. *Acta. path. microbiol. scand. Suppl.* 181.

[164] MEYER J.E. (1942) Uber Berylliumerkrankungen der Lunge. *Beitr. Klin. Tuberk.* **98**, 388.

[165] MIDDLETON E.L. (1936) Industrial pulmonary disease due to inhalation of dust with special reference to silicosis. *Lancet* **ii**, 59.

[166] MINISTRY OF LABOUR AND NATIONAL SERVICE (1952) *A report on Dust in Card-rooms.* London, H.M. Stationery Office.

[167] MINISTRY OF SOCIAL SECURITY (1967) *Pneumoconiosis and Allied Occupational Chest Diseases.* H.M. Stationery Office.

[168] MITCHELL H. (1959) Pulmonary fibrosis in an aluminium worker. *Br. J. industr. Med.* **16**, 123.

[169] MITCHELL J., MANNING G.B., MOLYNEUX M. & LANE R.E. (1961) Pulmonary fibrosis in workers exposed to finely powdered aluminium. *Br. J. industr. Med.* **18**, 10.

[170] MORGAN W.K.C. (1964) Rheumatoid pneumoconiosis in association with asbestosis. *Thorax* **19**, 433.

[171] MORGAN W.K.C. & KERR A.D. (1963)

Pathologic and physiologic studies of welders' siderosis. *Ann. intern. Med.* **58**, 293.

[172] MORICHAU-BEAUCHANT G. (1964) Pneumonies manganiques. *J. fr. Med. Chir. thorac.* **18**, 301.

[173] MORRIS T.G., ROBERTS W.H., SILVERTON R.E., SKIDMORE J.W. & WAGNER J.C. (1966) *Proceedings of the Second National Symposium on Inhaled Particles and Vapours.* Cambridge, Pergamon Press.

[174] MORRIS-EVANS W.H. & FOREMAN H.M. (1963) Smallpox handler's lung. *Proc. roy. Soc. Med.* **56**, 274.

[175] McADAMS A.J.Jr. (1955) Bronchiolitis obliterans. *Am. J. Med.* **19**, 314.

[176] McCALLUM R.I., RANNIE I. & VERITY C. (1961) Chronic pulmonary berylliosis in a female chemist. *Br. J. industr. Med.* **18**, 133.

[177] McCAUGHEY W.T.E. (1958) Primary tumours of the pleura. *J. Path. Bact.* **76**, 517.

[178] McCAUGHEY W.T.E., WADE O.L. & ELMES P.C. (1962) Exposure to asbestos dust and diffuse pleural mesotheliomas. *Br. med. J.* **ii**, 397.

[179] MacDONALD A.D. & MAITLAND H.B. (1934) The examination of cotton, coir and esparto-grass dust for histamine. *J. Hyg. (Camb.)* **34**, 317.

[180] MacDONALD G., PIGGOT A.P., GILDER F.W., ARNALL F.A. & RUDGE E.A. (1930) Two cases of acute silicosis with suggested theory of causation. *Lancet* **ii**, 846.

[181] McKERROW C.B., GILSON J.C., SCHILLING R.S.F. & SKIDMORE J.W. (1965) Respiratory function and symptoms in rope makers. *Br. J. industr. Med.* **22**, 204.

[182] McKERROW C.B., McDERMOTT M., GILSON J.C. & SCHILLING R.S.F. (1958) Respiratory function during the day in cotton workers: a study in byssinosis. *Br. J. industr. Med.* **15**, 75.

[183] McLAUGHLIN A.I.G. (1960) Iron and other opaque dusts. In *Industrial Pulmonary Diseases* London, Churchill.

[184] McLAUGHLIN A.I.G., BIDSTRUP P.L. & KONSTAM M. (1963) Quoted in reference No. 2353 *Food Cosmet. Toxicol.* **i**, 171.

[185] McLAUGHLIN A.I.G., GROUT J.L.A. & BARRIE H.J. (1945) Iron oxide dust and lungs of silver finishers. *Lancet* **i**, 337.

[186] McLAUGHLIN A.I.G., JUPE M.H., LAWRIE W.B., PERRY K.M.A., SUTHERLAND C.L. & WOODS H. (1950) *Industrial Lung Disease of Iron and Steel Workers.* London, H.M. Stationery Office.

[187] McLAUGHLIN A.I.G., KAZANTZIS G., KING E., TEARE D., PORTER R.J. & OWEN R. (1962) Pulmonary fibrosis and encephalopathy associated with inhalation of aluminium dust. *Br. J. industr. Med.* **19**, 253.

[188] McLAUGHLIN A.I.G., MILLON R. & PERRY K.M.A. (1946) Toxic manifestations of osmium tetroxide. *Br. J. industr. Med.* **3**, 183.

[189] NAGELSCHMIDT G. (1965) Some observations of the dust content and composition in lungs with asbestosis, made during work on coal miners' pneumoconiosis. *Ann. N.Y. Acad. Sci.* **132**, 64.

[190] NAGELSCHMIDT G., RIVERS D., KING E.J. & TREVELLA W. (1963) Dust and collagen content of lungs of coalworkers with progressive massive fibrosis. *Br. J. industr. Med.* **20**, 181.

[191] NASH E.S., VOGELPOEL L. & BECKER W.B. (1967) Pigeon breeder's lung—a case report. *S. Afr. med. J.* **41**, 191.

[192] NICHOLS B.H. (1930) The clinical effects of the inhalation of nitrogen dioxide. *Am. J. Roentgenol.* **23**, 516.

[193] OCCUPATIONAL SAFETY AND HEALTH SERIES (1966) *Respiratory Function Tests in Pneumoconiosis*. No. 6. Geneva, International Labour Office.

[194] O'DONNELL W.M., MANN R.H. & CROSH J.L. (1966) Asbestos, an extrinsic factor in the pathogenesis of bronchogenic carcinoma and mesothelioma. *Cancer (N.Y.)* **19**, 1143.

[195] OWEN W.G. (1964) Diffuse mesothelioma and exposure to asbestos dust in the Merseyside area. *Br. med. J.* ii, 214.

[196] PANCHERI G. (1950) Su alcune forme di pneumoconiosi particolarmente studiate in Italia (Tio-pneumoconiosi e baritosi). *Medna Lav.* **41**, 73.

[197] PENDERGRASS E.P. (1938) *Lanza's silicosis and asbestosis*, p. 137. London, Oxford University Press.

[198] PENDERGRASS E.P. & GREENING R.R. (1953) Baritosis: report of case. *Archs ind. Hyg.* **7**, 44.

[199] PENDERGRASS E.P. & LEOPOLD S.S. (1945) Benign pneumoconiosis. *J. Am. med. Ass.* **127**, 701.

[200] PEPYS J. (1966) Pulmonary hypersensitivity disease due to inhaled organic antigens. *Postgrad. med. J.* **42**, 698.

[201] PEPYS J. & JENKINS P.A. (1965) Precipitin (FLH) tests in farmer's lung. *Thorax* **20**, 21.

[202] PEPYS J., JENKINS P.A., LACHMANN P.J. & MAHON W.E. (1966) An iatrogenic autoantibody: immunological responses to 'pituitary snuff' in patients with diabetes insipidus. *Clin. & exp. Immunol.* **1**, 377.

[203] PERNIS B. & PECCHIAI L. (1954) La composizione aminoacidica della sostanza ialina del nodulo silicotico. *Medna Lav.* **45**, 205.

[204] PRAUSNITZ C. (1936) *Investigations on respiratory dust disease in operatives in the cotton industry*. Special Report Series No. 212. London, Medical Research Council.

[205] *Proceedings of the National Conference of Air Pollution, Washington 1958* (1959) Public Health Service Publication No. 654. Washington, D.C., U.S. Department of Health, Education and Welfare.

[206] RAMAZZINI B. (1700) *De Mortis Artificium Diatriba*. (English translation: a treatise of the disease of tradesmen). London, 1705.

[207] RAMSAY J.H.R. & PINES A. (1959) Results of treatment of pneumoconiosis complicated by tuberculosis. *Br. med. J.* ii, 345.

[208] RANKIN J., JAESCHKE W.H., CALLIES Q.C. & DICKIE H.A. (1962) Farmer's lung. Physiopathologic features of the acute granulomatous pneumonitis of agricultural workers. *Ann. intern. Med.* **57**, 606.

[209] RAYMOND F. (1874) Empoisonnement par l'acide osmium. *Progr. méd. Paris* **2**, 373.

[210] READ J. & WILLIAMS R.S. (1959) Pulmonary ventilation. Blood flow relationships in interstitial disease of the lungs. *Am. J. Med.* **27**, 545.

[211] REED C.E., SOSMAN A.J. & BARBEE R.A. (1965) Pigeon breeder's lung. A newly observed interstitial pulmonary disease. *J. Am. med. Ass.* **193**, 261.

[212] REICHLE H.S. (1936) Bronchiogenic distribution of particulate matter: its site of predilection and the mechanism of transfer. *Am. J. Path.* **12**, 781.

[213] REPORT AND RECOMMENDATIONS OF THE WORKING GROUP ON ASBESTOS AND CANCER (1965) *Br. J. industr. Med.* **22**, 165.

[214] RICHMOND H.G. (1959) Induction of sarcoma in the rat by iron-dextran complex. *Br. med. J.* i, 947.

[215] RICKARDS A.G. & BARRETT G.M. (1958) Rheumatoid lung changes associated with asbestosis. *Thorax* **13**, 185.

[216] RIDDLE H.F.V. & GRANT I.W.B. (1967) Allergic alveolitis in a malt worker. Proceedings of the Thoracic Society. *Thorax* **22**, 478.

[217] RIDDELL A.R. (1948) Pulmonary changes encountered in employees engaged in manufacture of alumina abrasives; pathologic aspects. *Occup. Med.* **5**, 716.

[218] RIDDELL A.R. & SHAVER C.G. (1949) Pulmonary change in employees engaged in the manufacture of alumina abrasives. *Occup. Med.* **5**, 710.

[219] ROBERTSON A.J. (1964) The romance of tin. *Lancet* i, 1229.

[220] ROBERTSON A.J., RIVERS D., NAGELSCHMIDT G. & DUNCUMB P. (1961) Benign pneumoconiosis due to tin dioxide. *Lancet* i, 1089.

[221] ROGAN J.M. (1963) *Annual report for the year 1963*. Medical Service and Medical Research. London, National Coal Board.

[222] ROGERS W.N. (1957) Chronic beryllium poisoning in a beryllium worker. *Br. med. J.* i, 1030.

[223] ROSSIER P.H., BUHLMANN A.A. & LUCHSINGER P. (1955) Die Pathophysiologie der Atmung bei der Silikose und die Begutachtung der Arbeitsfähigkeit. *Dt. med. Wschr.* **80**, 608.

[224] ROSSIER P.H., BUHLMANN A.A. & WIESINGER K. (1960) (P.C. Luchsinger and K.M. Moser,

Editors and translators) *Respiration: Physiologic Principles and their Clinical Applications.* St. Louis, Mosby.

[225] SAKULA A. (1961) Pneumoconiosis due to Fuller's earth. *Thorax* **16**, 176.

[226] SAKULA A. (1967) Mushroom workers' lung. *Br. med. J.* **3**, 708.

[227] SALVAGGIO J.E., SEABURY J.H., BUECHNER H.A. & KUNDUR V.J. (1967) Pneumonitis due to *Cryptostroma corticale* (maple-bark disease). *J. Allergy* **39**, 106.

[228] SANDERS J.S. & MARTT J.M. (1963) Pulmonary function in 'farmer's lung' and related conditions. *Missouri Med.* **60**, 429.

[229] SAYERS R.R. (1937) *Third Saranac Symposium on Silicosis.* Trudeau Sch. Tuberc. Saranac Lake, N.Y.

[230] SCADDING J.G. (1967) Beryllium Disease. In *Sarcoidosis.* London, Eyre and Spottiswoode.

[231] SCHEPERS G.W.H. (1955) The biological action of particulate cobalt metal. *Arch. industr. Hlth* **12**, 127.

[232] SCHEPERS G.W.H. (1955) The biological action of tungsten carbide and cobalt. *Arch. industr. Hlth* **12**, 140.

[233] SCHILLING R.S.F. (1956) Byssinosis in cotton and other textile workers. *Lancet* ii, 261, 319.

[234] SCHILLING R.S.F. (1960) The epidemiology of byssinosis. In *Industrial Pulmonary Diseases*, ed. King E.J. and Fletcher C.M. London, Churchill.

[235] SELIKOFF I.J., CHURG J. & HAMMOND E.C. (1964) Asbestos exposure and neoplasia. *J. Am. med. Ass.* **188**, 22.

[236] SELIKOFF I.J., CHURG J. & HAMMOND E.C. (1965) Relation between exposure to asbestos and mesothelioma. *New Engl. J. Med.* **272**, 560.

[237] SHANAHAN R.H., GRIFFEN J.R. & VON AUERSPERG A.P. (1947) Anthrax meningitis: report of a case of internal anthrax with recovery. *Am. J. clin. Path.* **17**, 719.

[238] SHAVER C.G. (1948) Pulmonary changes encountered in employees engaged in manufacture of alumina abrasives: clinical and roentgenologic aspects. *Occup. Med.* **5**, 718.

[239] SMITH A.R. (1952) Pleural calcification resulting from exposure to certain dusts. *Am. J. Roentgenol.* **67**, 375.

[240] SMITH J.C. & KENCH J.E. (1957) Observations in urinary cadmium and protein excretion in men exposed to cadmium oxide dust and fume. *Br. J. industr. Med.* **14**, 240.

[241] SMITH J.P., SMITH J.C. & McCALL A.J. (1960) Chronic poisoning from cadmium fume. *J. Path. Bact.* **80**, 287.

[242] SNEDDON I.B. (1955) Berylliosis: a case report. *Br. med. J.* i, 1448.

[243] SNEDDON I.B. (1958) Beryllium disease. *Postgrad. med. J.* **34**, 262.

[244] SPENCER H. (1962) *Pathology of the Lung.* London, Pergamon Press, p. 850.

[245] STEEL J. (1964) Health hazards in the welding and cutting of paint-primed steel. *Ann. occup. Hyg.* **7**, 247.

[246] STRAND R.D., NEUHAUSER E.B.D. & SORNBERGER C.F. (1967) Lycoperdonosis. *New Engl. J. Med.* **277**, 89.

[247] SWENSSEN A., NORDENFELT O., FROSSMAN S., RUNDGREN K.D. & OHMAN H. (1962) Aluminium dust pneumoconiosis: a clinical study. *Arch. Gewerbepath. Gewerbehyg.* **19**, 131.

[248] SYMANSKI H. (1939) Gewerbliche Vanadinschadgunden, ihre Entstehung und Symptomatologie. *Arch. Gewerbliche Gewerbehyg.* **9**, 295.

[249] TELLESSON W.G. (1961) Rheumatoid pneumoconiosis (Caplan's syndrome) in an asbestos worker. *Thorax* **16**, 372.

[250] TEPPER L.B., HARDY HARIET L. & CHAMBERLIN R.I. (1961) *Toxicity of Beryllium Compounds.* Amsterdam, Elsevier.

[251] THOMSON M.D., McGRATH M.W., SMITHER W.J. & SHEPHERD J.M. (1961) Some anomalies in the measurement of pulmonary diffusion in asbestosis and chronic bronchitis with emphysema. *Clin. Sci.* **21**, 1.

[252] TIMBRELL V. (1965) The inhalation of fibrous dusts. *Ann. N.Y. Acad. Sci.* **132**, 255.

[253] TOTTEN R.S., REID D.H.S., DAVIS H.D. & MORAN T.J. (1958) Farmer's lung: report of two cases in which lung biopsies were performed. *Am. J. Med.* **25**, 803.

[254] TRENCHARD H.J. & HARRIS W.C. (1963) An outbreak of respiratory symptoms caused by toluene di-isocyanate. *Lancet* i, 404.

[255] TURNER H.M. & GRACE H.G. (1938) An investigation into cancer mortality among males in certain Sheffield trades. *J. Hyg. (Camb.)* **38**, 90.

[256] U.S. CHEMICAL WARFARE SERVICE (1929) *Proceedings of a board appointed for the purpose of investigating conditions incident to the disaster at the Cleveland Hospital Clinic, Cleveland, Ohio, on May 15th 1929.* Washington, D.C., U.S. Government Printing Office.

[257] VAN ORDSTRAND H.W. (1959) Diagnosis of beryllium disease. *Arch. ind. Hlth* **19**, 157.

[258] VERNHES A. & ROCHE D.H.R. (1955) Quelques considérations sur la silicose der travailleurs de l'ocre. *Presse méd.* **40**, 975.

[259] VIGLIANI E.C., BOSELLI A. & PECCHIAI L. (1950) Studi sulla componente emoplasmopatica della silicosi. *Medna Lav.* **41**, 33.

[260] VIGLIANI E.C. & MOTTURA G. (1948) Diatomaceous earth silicosis. *Br. J. industr. Med.* **5**, 148.

[261] VIGLIANI E.C. & PERNIS B. (1958) Immunological factors in the pathogenesis of the hyaline tissue of silicosis. *Br. J. industr. Med.* **15**, 8.

[262] VORWALD A.J. (1950) The beryllium problem:

the chronic or delayed disease: pathological aspects. *Sixth Saranac Symposium, Part III,* Ch. 11, p. 190. New York, Hoeber (Harper).

[263] VORWALD A.J., DURKAN T.M. & PRATT P.C. (1951) Experimental studies of asbestosis. *Arch. ind. Hyg.* **3**, 1.

[264] WAGNER J.C. (1965) The sequelae of exposure to asbestos dust. *Ann. N.Y. Acad. Sci.* **132**, 691.

[265] WAGNER J.C., MUNDAY D.E. & HARINGTON J.S. (1962) Histochemical demonstration of hyaluronic acid in pleural mesothelioma. *J. Path. Bact.* **84**, 73.

[266] WAGNER J.C. & SKIDMORE J.W. (1965) Asbestos dust deposition and retention in rats. *Ann. N.Y. Acad. Sci.* **132**, 77.

[267] WAGNER J.C., SLEGGS C.A. & MARCHAND P. (1960) Diffuse pleural mesothelioma and asbestos exposure in the north-western Cape Province. *Br. J. industr. Med.* **17**, 260.

[268] WEBER H.H. & ENGELHARDT W.E. (1933) Uber eine Apparatur zur Erzeugung niedriger Staubkonzentrationen von grosser Konstanz und eine Methode zur Mikrogravimetrischen Staubbestimmung. Anwendung bei der Untersuchung von Stauben aus der Berylliumgewinnung. *Zentbl. GewHyg. Unfallverhüt.* **10**, 41.

[269] WENZEL F.J., EMANUEL D.A. & LAWTON B.R. (1964) Isolation of the causative agent of 'farmer's lung'. *Ann. Allergy* **22**, 533.

[270] WENZEL F.J., EMANUEL D.A. & LAWTON B.R. (1967) Pneumonitis due to *Micromonospora vulgaris* (farmer's lung). *Am. Rev. resp. Dis.* **95**, 652.

[271] WERNER G.C.H. (1955) De la bronchiolite oedémateuse allergique. Essai statistique sur l'asthme des poussières textiles végétales. *Arch. Mal. prof.* **16**, 27.

[272] WILLIAMS C.R. (1959) Evaluation of exposure data in the Beryllium Registry. *Archs ind. Hlth.* **19**, 263.

[273] WILLIAMS J.V. (1963) Pulmonary function studies in patients with farmer's lung. *Thorax* **18**, 255.

[274] WILLIAMS R. & HUGH-JONES P. (1960) The radiological diagnosis of asbestosis. *Thorax* **15**, 103.

[275] WILLIAMS R. & HUGH-JONES P. (1960) The significance of lung function changes in asbestosis. *Thorax* **15**, 109.

[276] WILLIAMS W.J. (1958) A histological study of the lungs in 52 cases of chronic beryllium disease. *Br. J. industr. Med.* **15**, 84.

[277] WOOD C.H., BALL K.P. & TEARE N.D. (1958) A case of beryllium disease. *Br. J. industr. Med.* **15**, 209.

[278] WRIGHT G.W. (1955) Functional abnormalities of industrial pulmonary fibrosis. *Archs ind. Hlth* **11**, 196.

[279] WURM H. & RUGER H. (1942) Untersuchungen zur Frage der Berylliumstaubpneumonie. *Beitr. Klin. Tuberk.* **98**, 396.

[280] WYATT J.P. & RIDDELL A.C.R. (1949) The morphology of bauxite fume pneumoconiosis. *Am. J. Path.* **25**, 447.

[281] WYERS M. (1946) Some toxic effects of vanadium pentoxide. *Br. J. industr. Med.* **3**, 177.

[282] YOUNG W.A., SHAW D.B. & BATES D.V. (1962) Presence of ozone in aircraft flying at 35,000 feet. *Aerospace Med.* **33**, 311.

[283] YOUNG W.A. & SHAW D.B. (1963) Effect of low concentrations of ozone on pulmonary function. *Fed. Proc.* **22**, 396.

[284] ZAPP J.A. (1957) Hazards of isocyanates in polyurethane foam plastic production. *Archs ind. Hlth* **15**, 324.

CHAPTER 29

Tumours of the Lung

Bronchial carcinoma is by far the most important and common tumour of the lung. Other tumours are relatively rare. In the following list very rare tumours are placed in parenthesis.

CLASSIFICATION OF TUMOURS OF THE LUNG

OVERTLY MALIGNANT TUMOURS

(1) Carcinoma of the bronchus, p. 517.
(2) Alveolar cell carcinoma, p. 545. Synonyms: bronchiolar carcinoma, pulmonary adenomatosis.
(3) Pulmonary lymphomata. Synonym: reticuloses.

    (a) Hodgkin's disease, p. 552. Synonym: lymphadenoma.
    (b) Lymphosarcoma, p. 553.
    (c) Reticulum cell sarcoma, p. 553.
    (d) Leukaemias, p. 554.

TUMOURS WITH LESSER MALIGNANCY OR ONLY OCCASIONALLY OVERTLY MALIGNANT

(1) Bronchial adenoma

    (a) Carcinoid tumour, p. 554.
    (b) Cylindroma, p. 554.
    (c) (Mucoepidermoid tumour), p. 554.
    (d) (Mixed tumour), p. 554).

(2) (Myoblastoma), p. 561.

(3) (Neurofibroma and neurogenic sarcoma), p. 562.
(4) (Papilloma of trachea or bronchus), p. 562.
(5) (Plasmacytoma), p. 562.
(6) (Sarcoma), p. 562.
(7) Haemangiopericytoma, p. 562.

MALIGNANT CHANGE VERY RARE

(1) Hamartoma

    (a) Cartilaginous, p. 558.
    (b) (Fibroleiomyomatous), p. 559.

(2) (Chondroma of bronchus), p. 561.
(3) (Cystadenoma of bronchus), p. 561.
(4) (Fibroma), p. 561.
(5) (Myxoma), p. 561.
(6) (Lipoma), p. 561.

MALIGNANT CHANGE NOT DESCRIBED

(1) Pulmonary arteriovenous fistula, p. 559. Synonyms: pulmonary angioma, vascular hamartoma.
(2) (Histiocytoma), p. 561.

CARCINOMA OF THE BRONCHUS

DEFINITION

The term 'carcinoma of the bronchus' defines itself, but it should be pointed out that 'carcinoma of the lung' is sometimes used synonymously. The term of course does not apply to secondary carcinoma in lung or bronchus. Malignant change in adenoma of the bronchus (see p. 554) gives rise to a tumour which is usually more slowly progressive and should therefore be differentiated from carcinoma of the bronchus as such. Alveolar cell carcinoma (p. 545) and pleural mesothelioma (p. 484) should also be regarded as separate entities.

PREVALENCE AND MORTALITY

One of the most challenging aspects of the present medical scene in economically developed countries is the formidable rise in mortality from carcinoma of the bronchus over the last 30 years. This rise has been much greater in males than in females, probably owing to differences in smoking habits. All the evidence suggests that the rise is a genuine one and that little of it is due to better diagnosis [25]. Britain has the world's highest

In England and Wales the peak mortality in males has been moving towards the older age groups and was between 70 and 75 in 1963. There is evidence [113] that the increase has ceased in the younger age groups; there has been no increase in males under 60 since 1956. This is probably a 'saturation effect', the maximum influence of carcinogenetic

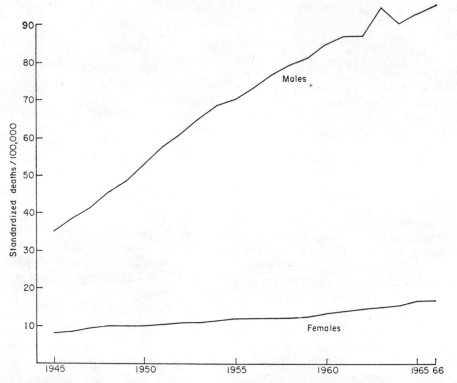

Fig. 29.1. Mortality from respiratory neoplasm in England and Wales. Males and females.

mortality for this disease and the death rate is still increasing rapidly. This unenviable distinction is probably due to the very high cigarette consumption in Britain and perhaps, to a lesser degree, to the pollution of the atmosphere.

The trends since 1945 for England and Wales are shown in fig. 29.1. Male mortality from the disease rose from 10 per 100,000 population in 1930 to 53 in 1950 and just under 100 (99·7) in 1966. The female rate in 1966 was 18 per 100,000. The Scottish rates for both sexes are a little higher still.

factors having been reached in these age groups. On the other hand in women, with their lower mortality from the disease, the rates continue to rise in all age groups and there is no evidence of 'saturation' having yet been reached.

Treatment for the disease is still relatively unsuccessful; therefore the attack rate is very similar to the mortality. In a major Mass Radiography campaign in Edinburgh in 1958, in which approximately 85% of the adult population were x-rayed, the prevalence for carcinoma of the bronchus in men over the

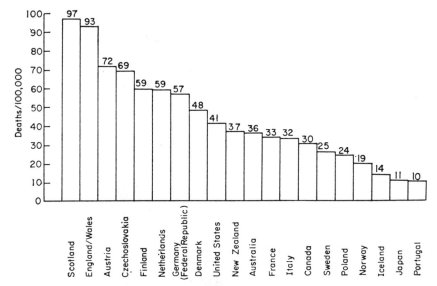

Fig. 29.2. International comparison of male death rates due to malignant neoplasm of trachea, bronchus and lung 1964.

age of 60 was 2·34 per 1000 examined compared to 3·4 for active pulmonary tuberculosis. At the present time the carcinoma figure would probably be appreciably higher and the tuberculosis figure lower. Other estimates from mass surveys include 1·3 per 1000 in London men over 45 [92], 2·8 per 1000 in Philadelphia men over 45 [13] and 0·4 per 1000 in Oslo men aged 50–69 [73].

Some international comparisons of male mortality from the disease are given in fig. 29.2. The grim precedence of Britain is obvious.

AETIOLOGY

All the available evidence incriminates the smoking of tobacco, especially of cigarettes, as the main cause of the great rise in mortality from bronchial carcinoma, probably with some small contribution from atmospheric pollution and a much smaller one from certain industrial processes. A very small proportion of bronchial carcinomata, especially adenocarcinomata, is probably unrelated to these causes. Some of the evidence for these statements will now be briefly reviewed.

SMOKING

RETROSPECTIVE STUDIES

The earliest evidence incriminating smoking was the classical study of Doll and Bradford Hill [37] in which the smoking habits of patients in hospital with carcinoma of the bronchus were compared with those of other patients, matched for age, sex and economic status. Among patients with carcinoma of the bronchus there were many fewer nonsmokers and many more heavy smokers than among the controls. This type of study has now been repeated in at least 29 different investigations in 9 different countries with similar results [2]. In general the degree of association increased with the amount smoked. Because of the interference of other factors there seems to be a complex, and not entirely straightforward, relationship between age, duration of smoking, amount smoked and risk of lung cancer [99].

The question of the effect of inhalation of cigarette smoke is also a complex one. Doll and Hill [37] found no apparent association between inhalation and lung cancer, though 4 subsequent investigations did find a significant association. It appears that inhalation may be an important factor with relatively low cigarette consumption but the difference between inhalers and noninhalers is lost at high levels of consumption [2]. A study in Venice [131], where there is no atmospheric pollution, confirmed the investigations carried out elsewhere.

highest for those who smoked cigarettes only. The risk for pipe smokers was appreciably higher than for nonsmokers but was a good deal less than for cigarette smokers. One encouraging finding was that the risk was less in those who had given up smoking, especially if they had done so for more than 10 years.

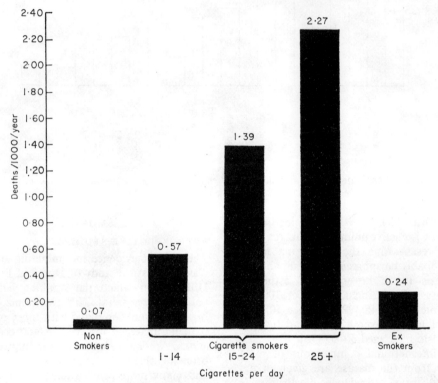

FIG. 29.3. Mortality from lung cancer in doctors related to previously recorded smoking habits (adapted from Doll and Hill 1964).

PROSPECTIVE STUDIES

Evidence which is even more convincing is provided by prospective studies of the association between smoking habits and the attack rate of carcinoma of the bronchus. For instance, in 1951 all male doctors over 35 in Britain were asked by Doll and Bradford Hill [42] to state their smoking habits and the proportion of these dying from carcinoma of the bronchus was determined during later years (fig. 29.3). It was found that the risk of dying from carcinoma of the bronchus increased with the amount smoked and was

About the same time a large scale prospective study was carried out in the United States [65] with similar results. Five other North American studies [2] were also confirmatory. For smokers of cigarettes only the ratio of mortality, compared to nonsmokers, varied from 4·9 to 20·2 in the 7 different studies, with a mean of 10·4. For those smoking more than 20 cigarettes a day the figure in Doll and Hill's study [42] reached 43·7. Pipe smoking showed a lower risk (ratio of 5·4). In the American studies cigar smoking showed no important association [2].

SEX RATIO

The sex ratio in the mortality from carcinoma of the bronchus is quite consistent with their smoking habits. In Britain male cigarette smoking principally began during the First World War and female during the Second. In spite of the fact that more women now smoke, the rate of tobacco consumption in males has risen even more steeply. Cohort studies, in which the male/female ratio for mortality from carcinoma of the bronchus was studied at all ages for those born in the same 10 year periods, have shown that the male/female ratio of deaths from carcinoma of the bronchus has been rising with each subsequent cohort, beginning with the cohorts who were aged between 20 and 40 in the 1914–18 war [30].

DIFFERENCES BETWEEN COUNTRIES AND GROUPS

Mortality from carcinoma of the bronchus in different countries is fairly closely related to the smoking habits in those countries 20 years previously [38]. Britain has the highest rate and one of the highest cigarette consumptions. The United States has a relatively low mortality considering its high cigarette consumption. Various studies have shown that this may be due to the fact that in the United States the average person leaves a very much larger cigarette stump than is the case in Britain and to the higher percentage of smokers in the older age groups in Britain [2]. On the other hand in Iceland both the cigarette consumption and the mortality rate for carcinoma of the bronchus are very low. Unfortunately cigarette consumption is now rising in Iceland and so is the mortality from carcinoma of the bronchus [45]. Rele [101] has compared in Bombay the mortality from carcinoma of the bronchus among Parsees, who are non-smokers, with that among non-Parsees. After age adjustment, in Parsees carcinoma of the bronchus in males is 3·2% of all cancer deaths compared with 13·2% in non-Parsees. Lemon et al. [82] found that the lung cancer mortality in male Seventh Day Adventists, who do not smoke, was only a third of

the expected; the deaths that did occur were in recent converts who had previously been heavy smokers.

EXPERIMENTAL EVIDENCE

It is difficult to mimic in animals the conditions of human smoking. So far there has been no convincing success in reproducing lung cancer experimentally, though the repeated direct application of cigarette smoke condensate to the bronchi of dogs has been reported to produce cancerous changes in a number of animals and an invasive carcinoma in one [105]. Tobacco tar painted on the skin of the ears of mice or rabbits induces cancer, but the success rate varies with the frequency and duration of painting [2]. Although cigarette smoke contains a number of known carcinogens, such as benzpyrene, the concentration of any one of these is thought to be much too small to account alone for the observed carcinogenic effect in man. A possible explanation for the discrepancy could be that cigarette smoke acts as a 'promoting factor' or 'cocarcinogen'. Painting an animal's skin with tobacco tar greatly increases the number of tumours produced by a weak dose of a true carcinogen [49]. It is also possible that cigarette smoking might act synergistically with carcinogens polluting the atmosphere (see below). It has recently been suggested that the radioactive substance ^{210} polonium, which is present in tobacco smoke in minute amounts and tends to accumulate in bronchial epithelium, might play a part [84]. The possible rôle of arsenic, present in American tobacco as a result of spraying of tobacco plants, has also been considered. The amount is minute but it might act as a promoting factor [48]. Prolonged oral treatment with arsenic, with chronic arsenic poisoning, has been associated with bronchial carcinoma in nonsmokers [104].

HISTOLOGICAL CHANGES

The double-blind controlled studies of Auerbach and his colleagues [3] together with related investigations [2] have established that certain changes in the bronchial mucosa are much commoner in cigarette smokers, with or without lung cancer, than in nonsmokers. The important changes are (a) loss of cilia, (b) basal cell hyperplasia and (c) appearance of atypical cells with irregular hyperchromatic nuclei. There is good reason to think that these changes are precancerous.

Kreyberg [78] pointed out that smoking appeared to be associated with squamous (epidermoid) bronchial carcinoma and with the anaplastic type (including the 'oat cell' variety) but not with adenocarcinoma, alveolar cell carcinoma or bronchial adenoma. Later studies [2 & 40] have confirmed this view.

ATMOSPHERIC POLLUTION

Both in Britain and in U.S.A. there is a clear increase in mortality in urban, as compared with rural regions, and with increasing degrees of urbanization (fig. 29.4), even allowing for differences in smoking habits [2]. Stocks [116] found in Lancashire that mortality was closely correlated with atmospheric pollution, not only in densely populated areas, where factors other than pollution might operate, but in less populous surrounding districts which received urban pollution in varying degrees. Later [117] he has correlated mortality with the atmospheric concentration of 5-hydrocarbons, especially 3:4 benzpyrene, a known carcinogen. Although his findings are true for north-west England such correlations have been less evident in other parts of Britain.

Evidence from South Africa [34 & 35] and New Zealand [46] has shown that mortality from carcinoma of the bronchus is higher in British immigrants than in the native born with similar smoking habits. The mortality rate in moderate or nonsmokers is much lower in rural South Africa than in rural England. It is suggested that the immigrants are affected by their earlier exposure to British atmospheric pollution.

Nevertheless, the evidence suggests that, whatever the actual carcinogenetic mechanism of smoking may be, it is a very much more important factor than atmospheric pollution. Not only is the correlation with smoking much closer, but bronchial cancer was a relative rarity, even in postmortem studies, at a time when atmospheric pollution in Britain was already high but the cigarette smoking habit had hardly begun [77].

INDUSTRIAL FACTORS [41]

There is known to be a higher mortality from carcinoma of the bronchus in certain industries, though of course this contributes only a small proportion of the total national mortality. The high attack rate in *pitchblende* miners in Czeckoslovakia has been known for many years and uranium miners in U.S.A. also have an excess mortality [126]. The exact factor is uncertain but is now thought to be probably the radioactivity to which the workers are exposed.

Higher mortalities from the disease have also been shown in workers dealing with *gas retorts* [43], *chromate* [11 & 74], *asbestos* and *nickel* [41, 47 & 74], *arsenic* [41 & 74] and in *haematite* workers in Cumberland [54]. Miners of *metal* other than uranium in the United States also have an excess mortality [125].

The association with *asbestos* has been established relatively recently [50 & 59]. Patients with asbestosis have a high attack rate and Doll [39] calculated the rate in British workers exposed to asbestos for more than 20 years to be 10 times that in the general population; similar figures have been found in the United States [107]. Mesothelioma of the pleura (p. 484) and peritoneum are also important risks of asbestos exposure, which is sometimes environmental rather than occupational. There is some evidence that dust control in the relevant occupations may be substantially lowering the risk [59].

The risk in *gas retort* workers seems to be a continuing one. *Nickel refining* gave rise to a relatively high rate of both nasal and lung cancer but a change of technique is claimed now to have eliminated the hazard [41]. The *chromate* risk is also in the manufacturing rather than the mining process and is similar in Britain and the United States [41]. The risk with *arsenic* has been in those manufacturing arsenical powder and in plant sprayers in Germany [74]. Doll [41] does not regard the risk in *haematite* workers as being yet conclusively proved; it was based mainly on autopsy figures. Although some occupations give rise both to a risk of lung cancer and of pneumoconiosis there does not seem to be a direct association between these conditions [41].

PETROL AND DIESEL FUMES [41]

Although fumes from internal combustion engines contain known carcinogens in certain conditions of engine running, it has not been possible to demonstrate any excess mortality from bronchial cancer in garage workers or others who are likely to be particularly exposed to the fumes. In any case diesel engines have not yet been generally used for long enough for an effect to have emerged, presuming an exposure of approximately 20 years to be necessary.

ASSOCIATION WITH OTHER DISEASES

It has been suggested that carcinomata tend to arise at sites of previous scarring [112], from tuberculosis [21 & 114] or other diseases. This is certainly so in individual cases, but its significance for the whole range of the disease is much less certain. In a follow-up based on abnormalities found in miniature films at mass x-ray, Brett [16] found no increase in attack rate of bronchial carcinoma in those who had had pneumonia, calcified tuberculous foci, pulmonary fibrosis or bronchiectasis, though his numbers were relatively small. Boucot *et al.* [14] found preceding evidence of fibrosis in 24% of men who developed lung cancers (mainly peripheral) but exactly the same prevalence of fibrosis in smoking controls; the figure for nonsmokers was distinctly lower. It must be remembered that, at least in males, both pulmonary tuberculosis and bronchial carcinoma are related to cigarette smoking. The same, of course, is true of the association between bronchial carcinoma and chronic bronchitis. Case and Lea [24] found that the attack rate of bronchial carcinoma was twice as high in chronic bronchitics as in controls but Doll [41] pointed out that this could have been due to the smoking association. Nevertheless a recent study in Holland

[123] suggested that the correlation was greater than could have been accounted for by smoking.

One may provisionally conclude that there is no unequivocal association between bronchial carcinoma and any previous disease, greater than could be accounted for by the common factor of smoking, but that such an association cannot yet be finally dismissed, at least in the case of scarring, tuberculosis and chronic bronchitis.

On the other hand a lower attack rate has been recorded among coal miners [76] which cannot be attributed to lower cigarette consumption [60]. It has been claimed that these workers have a higher survival rate after operation for carcinoma of the bronchus, perhaps because of the blocking of the lymphatic pathways through which spread and metastasis occur [1]. Goldman [61] found evidence of improved postoperative survival only in the higher grades of pneumoconiosis.

PATHOLOGY [108, 109 & 112]

PRECANCEROUS CHANGES

The increased prevalence of bronchial metaplasia and precancerous changes in the bronchi of smokers has already been mentioned (p. 521). These changes include not only basal cell hyperplasia and squamous cell metaplasia but also carcinoma *in situ*. The latter term is used to indicate small areas in which there are frequent mitoses and irregularity of cells but without actual invasion of adjacent tissues [3 & 112].

CLASSIFICATION

Most lung cancers, including squamous cell carcinomata and most of these of anaplastic type, probably arise from the bronchial epithelium. It is these types which are related to tobacco smoking [40 & 78]. The adenocarcinomata are probably derived from the mucous glands of the bronchial wall [108]. It is convenient to classify bronchial carcinomata histologically into 3 main types and a 4th group consisting of rare subtypes. The approximate frequency of each type given below is that found in a review by Nicholson *et al.* [93] and is reasonably representative of the findings of other workers. The differences between series often depend on definition. If a tumour contains any areas with differentiation into squamous cells some workers would class it under that category while others, if there is any evidence of anaplastic change, will class it with the latter.

(1) Squamous cell carcinoma: 56%.

(2) Anaplastic carcinoma, including oat cell carcinoma: 37%.

(3) Adenocarcinoma: 6%.

(4) Various subtypes, particularly alveolar cell carcinoma (p. 545): 1%.

SITE

In resected series about 50% of lung carcinomata are said to arise centrally, that is in, or proximal to, a segmental bronchus [128]. The remainder arise more peripherally. As central tumours are less often resectable they probably in fact constitute more than half of all lung cancers.

MACROSCOPIC APPEARANCES

Most central cancers appear as whitish or yellowish growths affecting the bronchial mucosa and invading the underlying wall. They grow around it and into the lumen which in due course becomes obstructed, with resultant collapse and infection of the distal lung. The tumour may completely fill the lumen and grow along the bronchial branches or within the actual wall. The surface of the growth is often ulcerated. Squamous cell carcinomata are said to spread mainly in the extracartilaginous part of the bronchial wall and to invade the adjacent lymph glands directly. A peripheral carcinoma appears as a nodule or an irregular mass. Particularly if it is an adenocarcinoma it may arise from a previous scar. Invasion of the surrounding lung tissue is usually visible macroscopically, in contradistinction to the more sharply defined edge of a secondary tumour. Squamous cell carcinoma is particularly liable to central necrosis with the formation of an irregular abscess cavity. A secondary abscess may also arise in infected lung tissue distal to the

carcinoma. Squamous cell carcinoma may occasionally arise in the walls of bronchiectatic or abscess cavities.

HISTOLOGY

(1) *Squamous cell carcinoma.* Four criteria are said to be necessary for the diagnosis of this type of carcinoma:

(a) the presence of intercellular bridges,

(b) definite cell nest formation,

(c) squamatization, and

(d) polarization or whorling arrangement of cells [112].

(2) *Anaplastic carcinoma.* It is convenient to group together the carcinomata with relatively undifferentiated histological appearances. In these the characteristic features of squamous cells are lost. The cell appearances may be classified as follows:

(a) Small round cell or oat cell carcinoma. The small round cells may superficially resemble lymphocytes. There is a high ratio between the nucleus and the cytoplasm. Occasionally the cells may seem to form vague tubes but lack the definite architecture of an adenocarcinoma. Mucus is never produced. The oat cell carcinomata are particularly rapidly fatal owing to early metastases with rapid invasion of mediastinal and more distant lymph glands. They are most often central but not uncommonly peripheral.

(b) Large cell and polygonal carcinoma. These cells are about the same size as in squamous cell carcinoma but have lost their characteristic appearance.

(c) Giant cell carcinoma. These are relatively rare. The cells are very variable and may be multinucleated resembling sarcomatous giant cells.

(3) *Adenocarcinoma.* Although these tumours occasionally arise from mucous glands in the larger bronchi the majority are peripheral. Unless picked up on mass radiography they may remain clinically silent until metastases have occurred. They may show acinar, capillary or solid alveolar form. All 3

forms may be seen in an individual tumour. They often produce mucus. Sometimes they grow continuously along the alveolar walls, using the lung as a basic stroma. Some of these may be difficult to differentiate from alveolar cell carcinoma.

(4) *Alveolar cell carcinoma* (see p. 545).

FUNCTIONAL ABNORMALITY

A peripheral carcinoma will have little effect on function beyond denying the patient the function of the volume of lung which the tumour occupies. Respiratory function will clearly be reduced if a segmental, lobar or main bronchus is partially or completely occluded. The ventilation of the relevant region of the lung will at first be impaired and later prevented. Investigation has shown that the pulmonary arterial flow through the affected area of lung rapidly diminishes so that there is no important shunt of unoxygenated blood [56].

Because of the association with cigarette smoking, patients with bronchial carcinoma often have chronic bronchitis in addition, with resultant airways obstruction. In considering a patient for operation it is important to assess the probable function of the residual lung. For this purpose the most useful investigations are FEV and blood gas studies, taken together with the clinical and radiological data. If the patient's FEV is more than 60% of the predicted value for his age and height he is unlikely to have severe postoperative dyspnoea. If it is below 40% the probability of postoperative death or later respiratory invalidism is high. Similarly an increase in Pa,co_2 is usually a contra-indication to operation.

Some patients with a carcinoma in a proximal bronchus appear to be more breathless than would be expected from objective tests, possibly a reflex effect from a rigid hilum. A patient with lymphatic carcinomatosis may show a diffusion defect in the early stages. Later he would be expected to have a restrictive lesion. Dyspnoea may also arise from weakness or paralysis of the diaphragm, usually due to the invasion of the phrenic nerve by tumour, occasionally to a complicating neuropathy.

CLINICAL FEATURES

The patient with carcinoma of the bronchus may be *symptom free* and first come to attention as a result of an abnormal shadow on a chest x-ray. More commonly he presents as a result of *respiratory symptoms*. These may have developed only recently or, more often, long standing mild symptoms of chronic bronchitis may have become more severe. Less often the presenting symptoms are those of *general disability*, tiredness, anorexia or loss of weight. Occasionally symptoms resulting from *metastases* first bring him to the doctor. For instance, the first symptoms may be those of a cerebral metastasis mimicking a primary brain tumour. More frequently the first symptoms may be due to *complications* of the tumour, such as pneumonia or pleural effusion or, more rarely, neuropathy or hypertrophic osteoarthropathy.

None of these symptoms is specific so that a patient in the appropriate age group who complains of any of them requires investigation, in particular x-ray of the chest, to exclude not only carcinoma of the bronchus but other diseases. The symptom groups will now be considered in more detail.

RADIOLOGICAL ABNORMALITY ONLY

The widespread use of miniature radiography, primarily with the object of detecting tuberculosis, has shown that carcinoma of the bronchus, particularly if originating peripherally in the lung, may give rise to an abnormal shadow on the x-ray before there are any clinical manifestations of the disease.

RESPIRATORY SYMPTOMS

The common respiratory symptoms of cough, sputum, haemoptysis, breathlessness or chest pain are also common initial symptoms of carcinoma of the bronchus. The patient is usually a smoker so that he may have had at least a morning *cough* for many years. Any patient with a morning cough should have his chest x-rayed and this is particularly important if there has been a recent increase in severity. There is nothing specific about the clinical appearance of the *sputum* in carcinoma of the bronchus. It may be mucoid or grey, or mucopurulent due to secondary infection. *Haemoptysis* usually brings the patient to the doctor and always calls for full investigation. Occasionally the haemoptysis is a moderate or large one but more commonly it consists of slight daily blood staining which, if continued over a number of days in a patient of carcinoma age, is always highly suspicious and should lead to bronchoscopy even if the chest x-ray appears normal.

Chest pain is often pleuritic, associated with secondary pneumonia or invasion of the pleura by the carcinoma. More continuous pain may occur due to invasion of the chest wall or to secondary deposits in the ribs. Some patients complain of deep chest pain perhaps associated with invasion of the mediastinum [115]. As with lymphadenoma and other neoplasms pain may very occasionally be aggravated by alcohol [18]. *Breathlessness*, which has already been discussed (p. 525), may be due to pulmonary collapse in a patient whose function is already impaired by chronic bronchitis. It may also be due to pleural effusion, to complicating pneumonia, to lymphatic invasion of the lung, to diaphragmatic paralysis or occasionally to neuropathy.

GENERAL SYMPTOMS

Sometimes the patient first complains of general symptoms such as *tiredness, anorexia* or *loss of weight*, though usually there are also respiratory symptoms. General symptoms without local symptoms often indicate widespread metastases.

SYMPTOMS FROM COMMON COMPLICATIONS

It is common for the patient first to present with *pneumonia* but on enquiry it can usually be determined that he has had symptoms for some time previously. The radiological appearances or the failure of the pneumonia to clear adequately after treatment should lead to bronchoscopy. The patient may present with a *pleural effusion* which may either be due to direct invasion of the pleura or secondary to a complicating pneumonia. In the first case there will usually be no pyrexia and the patient may merely present with dyspnoea or pleuritic pain. In the second case the effusion may clear with chemotherapy directed towards the pneumonia but the persistence of radiological shadows of the latter should lead to full investigation. Presentation with other complications will be considered below.

PHYSICAL SIGNS

Until a carcinoma has obstructed a large bronchus or produced metastases or complications there may be no abnormal physical signs in the chest. *Finger clubbing* is common. Its presence in a patient with a relatively recent history of respiratory symptoms should raise the possibility of carcinoma. If the history is suggestive of chronic bronchitis but finger clubbing is found on examination, a coexisting carcinoma needs to be excluded.

The commonest physical signs in the chest are those of *collapse*. Because the obstruction is often in a large bronchus auscultation reveals diminished breath sounds rather than bronchial breathing. There may be the physical signs of *complicating pneumonia, pleurisy* or *pleural effusion*. Invasion of the chest wall or rib metastases may cause *local tenderness*. Diminished breath sounds at a base may be due to *paralysis of the diaphragm* secondary to phrenic nerve involvement. The clinician must pay particular attention to the *scalene lymph glands* which often become involved. Axillary glands are usually affected only if the chest wall has been invaded. The abdomen should be palpated for possible *metastases in the liver*.

THORACIC INLET TUMOURS [69]

High apical tumours were at one time thought to be of a specific type and were called 'superior pulmonary sulcus' tumours, or 'Pancoast' tumours after the author who first drew attention to them and regarded them, incorrectly as it happened, as a specific type of growth. In fact their only peculiarity is their position and most are probably bronchial carcinoma with no particular histological predilection. *Pain* in the medial upper arm or shoulder is usually the first symptom. It often spreads down the ulnar side of the hand, and later to the front of the chest or between the scapulae if the mediastinum is invaded. The pain down the arm is due to invasion of the brachial plexus. C8, T1 and 2 roots are mainly affected with weakness of intrinsic muscles of the hand and paraesthesiae or sensory impairment in the medial hand and forearm. *Horner's syndrome*, due to invasion of the inferior cervical sympathetic ganglia, is common. The recurrent laryngeal nerve is sometimes involved, with resultant *hoarseness*. *Spinal cord* compression may occur, through invasion of the spinal canal. *Radiologically* one or more of the upper ribs may be eroded. Supraclavicular lymph nodes may be palpable.

RADIOLOGY

By the time the patient is first seen there is usually some abnormality to be found in the x-ray of the chest. Very occasionally the

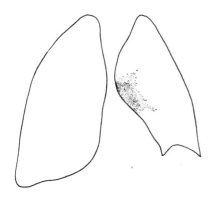

FIG. 29.4. Left hilar enlargement with phrenic paralysis.

patient first presents with haemoptysis due to a small tumour which produces *no x-ray changes*, the diagnosis being made by bronchoscopy. The most common appearance is *unilateral enlargement* of the *hilar shadow* (fig. 29.4). Gross abnormality is easy to detect but in a number of cases asymmetry of the hila

may be due to the patient being slightly turned to one side and the clinician is left in doubt. A further film or tomography may help but if symptoms are in any way suggestive it is safer to carry out a bronchoscopy. There is quite a high rate of observer error in assessing hilar shadows [111]; it is wiser to be over-suspicious rather than under-suspicious. It is worth noting that a tumour in the apex of a lower lobe may, in the postero-anterior film, simulate a hilar lesion. *Peripheral shadows* (figs. 29.5 and 29.6) are very variable in

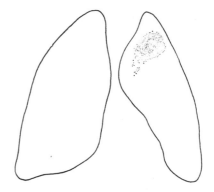

FIG. 29.5 Peripheral shadow

appearance. In a study of first radiographic manifestations in patients who were having an annual x-ray Boucot and her colleagues [14] found that the lesion might present as a nodule, a frank mass, a homogeneous irregular density or a small irregular non-homogeneous infiltrate. The margin of such shadows is usually not precisely defined. A hair-line edge makes malignant neoplasm less likely. There may be streaky shadows running out from the main mass into the surrounding lung, often better seen on the tomogram. This appearance is suggestive of neoplasm, but is sometimes due to fibrosis.

Cavitation may occur owing to necrosis. In this case the inner wall is often irregular with polypoid protuberances into the cavity (fig. 29.7). Although such an irregularity may be present in the early stages of a lung abscess the wall in this condition soon smoothes out. A persistent irregularity of the inner wall is suggestive of neoplasm, though occasionally

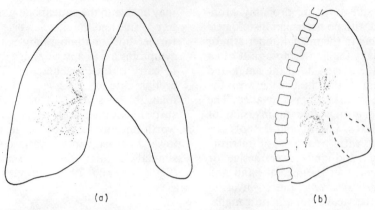

FIG. 29.6. Peripheral mass (adenocarcinoma) right lower lobe. (a) Postero-anterior view, (b) lateral view.

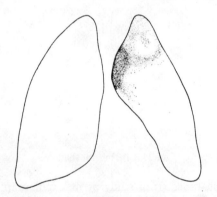

FIG. 29.7. Cavitated carcinoma left upper lobe. Note polypoid projection into cavity.

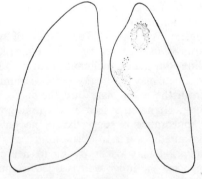

FIG. 29.8. Cavitated squamous carcinoma left upper lobe, resembling tuberculosis.

seen if there is a thick caseous lining in a tuberculous cavity. A carcinomatous cavity is not always thick-walled. On occasion a thin

wall is produced by almost total necrosis of the tumour (fig. 29.8). Sometimes a cavity represents a lung abscess distal to bronchial obstruction by the neoplasm (fig. 29.9).

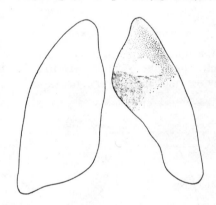

FIG. 29.9. Lung abscess with fluid level beyond hilar carcinoma.

Often the patient presents with symptoms due to *collapse* (figs. 29.10 and 29.11) or *consolidation* beyond the neoplasm. This may obscure the shadow of the tumour itself though sometimes some irregularity of the hilum may be detected. The tumour may also be obscured by a *complicating effusion*. The *mediastinum* may be broadened by deposits in the lymph glands. These, or the tumour itself, may invade the pericardium resulting in *pericardial effusion*. Sometimes broadening of the carina between the main bronchi may be visible in a penetrated film. Phrenic nerve

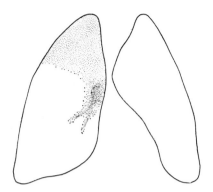

FIG. 29.10. Collapse right upper lobe due to carcinoma.

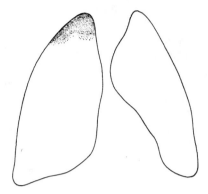

FIG. 29.12. Thoracic inlet tumour.

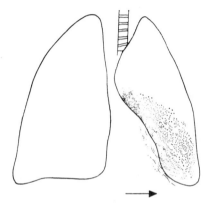

FIG. 29.11. Left hilar carcinoma with collapse left lower lobe and bronchopneumonia.

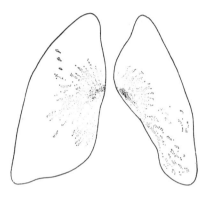

FIG. 29.13. Lymphatic carcinomatosis.

invasion may cause unilateral elevation of the diaphragm with *paradoxical movement* visible on fluoroscopy. If there is any question of a tumour being present the *bony cage* should be closely examined to ensure that all the ribs are intact. A missing portion of a rib, or a pathological fracture, may provide a clue to the diagnosis. Usually local pain gives an indication as to which part of the x-ray deserves particular attention.

A *thoracic inlet tumour* (p. 526) (fig. 29.12) produces a dense, irregular, somewhat crescentic shadow at the extreme apex, sometimes with invasion or destruction of one or more of the first 3 ribs. A tumour may invade the mediastinal glands and then spread along the lymphatics into both lungs. Radiographically this is seen as bilateral hilar enlargement with streaky shadows fanning out into both lung fields (*lymphatic carcinomatosis*, formerly known as lymphangitis carcinomatosa) (fig. 29.13). This appearance [66] may of course be caused by carcinoma originating elsewhere, e.g. stomach, pancreas or breast. Occasionally a tumour spreads via the pulmonary artery to both lungs so that there may be shadows both of the primary lesion and of rounded bilateral metastases.

COMPLICATIONS

Carcinoma of the bronchus may give rise to many complications. These may be grouped under 8 main headings:

(1) *mechanical* complications, such as collapse of a lobe or segment or obstruction of the superior vena cava;

(2) *inflammatory* complications such as pneumonia or lung abscess;

(3) *pleural* complications, either due to direct invasion of the pleura or to spread of inflammation from the underlying lung;

(4) *pericardial* and *cardiac* complications due to invasion by the tumour or secondarily from lymph glands;

(5) *metastases* in any part of the body;

(6) *neurological* complications;

    (a) invasion of phrenic nerve, left recurrent laryngeal nerve, brachial plexus or sympathetic;

    (b) metastatic deposits in the brain, simulating primary brain tumour;

    (c) neuropathies;

(7) *endocrine and metabolic* disorders, a rare but interesting group of conditions; and

(8) *hypertrophic osteoarthropathy.*

MECHANICAL COMPLICATIONS

These are common. The *collapse* of a segment, a lobe or a whole lung may be due to bronchial occlusion, either by an intrabronchial neoplasm or by pressure from outside. In a patient of carcinoma age any collapse which persists for more than a short time should be regarded as potentially due to neoplasm. *Superior vena caval obstruction* is usually due to compression or invasion by neoplastic tissue from the related lymph nodes, sometimes to direct invasion by a primary growth in the right upper lobe. The neck is enlarged and the neck veins distended. The patient may have noticed that he is having to take a larger size in collars. His face may be suffused and one or both arms may be oedematous. Distended venous collaterals may be observed on the anterior chest wall. Occasionally such patients complain of pain over the upper sternum, in the lower neck or in the face [115]. The *chest wall* may itself be invaded giving rise to local pain and tenderness and very occasionally to involvement of the intercostal nerves, resulting in paralysis and sensory loss.

INFLAMMATORY COMPLICATIONS

Pneumonia is a frequent complication of bronchial neoplasm, because bronchial occlusion or rigidity of the bronchus interferes with efficient drainage of the affected lung. Neoplasm must be excluded in any patient who has pneumonia which clears slowly radiologically. The pneumonia may be complicated by pleural effusion or empyema. An inflammatory effusion will usually clear with aspiration and chemotherapy of the underlying infection. On the other hand an effusion due to direct invasion of the pleura will re-accumulate after aspiration, and is quite often bloodstained. *Lung abscess* is not uncommon, either due to infection beyond the bronchial block or to necrosis of the neoplasm itself.

PLEURAL EFFUSION

Pleural effusion as already mentioned, is often due to direct invasion by the tumour. The effusion is frequently bloodstained and may contain malignant cells, though their identification in pleural fluid requires particular skill and experience (p. 280). The effusion is often large and tends to re-accumulate after aspiration. In Britain bronchial carcinoma is now the commonest cause of a pleural effusion persisting more than a month.

PERICARDIAL OR CARDIAC INVASION

Invasion may be directly by the tumour or secondarily from involved lymph glands, and may result in arrhythmias or pericardial effusion, often bloodstained.

METASTASES

Metastases may occur anywhere in the body. The commonest metastasis is to the *mediastinal* and *supraclavicular lymph glands*. The supraclavicular region should always be examined particularly carefully in any patient in whom a bronchial carcinoma may be present. Involvement of *axillary lymph glands* is usually secondary to chest wall invasion. The *liver* is often affected. *Lymphatic carcinomatosis* (p. 529) may occur and give rise to progressive dyspnoea, cough and repeated haemoptyses. *Bone metastases* usually cause pain and are locally tender, although occasionally they are painless. Metastases in or invasion of ribs are relatively common and are not always detectable radiographically. Metastases are common in the *brain*. They are said to be present in 30% of cases at death [15]; any patient presenting with an apparent primary brain tumour should have his chest x-rayed. Occasionally a patient is first seen with a *psychiatric disturbance* due to frontal lobe metastases. Mental disturbances may also be due to secondary neuropathy (p. 531). *Skin metastases* may occur; they usually consist of painless, somewhat flattened lesions.

NEUROLOGICAL COMPLICATIONS

Phrenic nerve paralysis, either due to invasion by the primary tumour or from secondary lymph glands in the hilum, is common and causes paralysis of the diaphragm. This is visible as a unilateral elevation on the x-ray and is confirmed by paradoxical movement seen on fluoroscopy. On the left side secondary glands in the hilum not uncommonly involve the *recurrent laryngeal nerve* as it hooks round the aorta, resulting in left-sided vocal cord paralysis and hoarseness. Much less commonly a thoracic inlet tumour may involve the right recurrent nerve. Thoracic inlet tumours (p. 526) often invade the *brachial plexus* and *cervical sympathetic chain*.

Certain other *neuropathic* and *myopathic* complications may occur. They are not related to metastasis and their pathogenesis is uncertain. They are not common in fully florid form, but if minor manifestations such as loss of limb reflexes are included they are said to be found in 12–15% of patients [29 & 75]. It is difficult to differentiate minor myopathic from minor neuropathic lesions as both may be characterized by muscle weakness and diminished tendon reflexes. The neuropathic lesions are associated with degenerative changes in the ganglion cells of the nervous system, the Purkinje cells of the dorsal root ganglia or the anterior horn cells of the spinal cord. There is a relative excess of these disorders in patients with oat cell carcinomata and in women [33]. The following main varieties have been described [15] though mixed forms are frequent.

(1) *Cerebellar degeneration* with ataxia, vertigo and dysarthria. Sometimes there is extrapyramidal tremor, pyramidal involvement, ptosis, ophthalmoplegia or bulbar palsy.

18—R.D.

(2) *Sensory neuropathy*. This often starts with numbness and sometimes pain in the face and limbs. It may gradually progress to loss of all forms of sensibility throughout the body, loss of reflexes and occasionally deafness.

(3) *Motor neuropathy*. There is progressive wasting, weakness and fasciculation. This has wrongly been called 'chronic progressive poliomyelitis'.

(4) *Polyneuritis* with mixed motor and sensory changes.

(5) *Mental abnormalities*. Progressive dementia, sometimes with depression, is the commonest manifestation. Confusion, stupor or emotional instability may occur [75].

(6) *Myopathy*. There are atrophic pareses, especially of the muscles of the limb girdles and the proximal limbs, often accompanied by a smooth red tongue.

(7) *Dermatomyositis* may complicate various forms of neoplasm, including bronchial carcinoma.

These syndromes tend to have an insidious onset and their manifestations may precede by months or even years symptoms directly due to the carcinoma. Their course is variable and is not necessarily directly related to the course of the original neoplasm. Remissions may occur, especially in the peripheral neuropathies and myopathies, but are not usually related to treatment of the neoplasm. In the neuropathies the cerebrospinal fluid may show a rise in lymphocytes and protein, and variable abnormality in the Lange test.

ENDOCRINE AND METABOLIC COMPLICATIONS [71 & 106]

These complications are comparatively rare in overt form but they usually arise late in the course of a bronchial carcinoma when the clinician is very properly considering the patient's comfort rather than the quirks of his clinical manifestations. It may be that these exotic syndromes are commoner than is thought. Occasionally they may arise earlier in the illness. Ross [106] mentions 2 patients with dilutional hyponatraemia first detected 2 and $2\frac{1}{2}$ years before death.

A very large variety of such complications

has been described. It is now considered that almost any tumour may produce almost any endocrine disturbance and there seems good evidence that at least the effective portion of the relevant hormone is produced by the tumour itself [52]. Occasionally more than one hormone is released. It has been suggested [52] that all normal cells, other than the reproductive cells, contain the same DNA and are basically totipotential. Specialization of cell lines may occur by the activation of repressor genes which inhibit activities not essential for that cell's special function. In the course of the chaotic mitoses of a tumour some of these repressor factors may be lost or inactivated releasing one or more processes of hormone production. All the hormones so far identified have been peptides, except for 5-HT and 5-HTP which are usually produced by carcinoid tumours (p. 554) but occasionally by bronchial carcinomata.

Some of the main manifestations will now be mentioned:

(1) *Cushing's syndrome.* Bilateral adrenocortical hyperplasia is probably the commonest endocrine manifestation of bronchial carcinoma, though it may also occur with tumours of the thymus, pancreas and ovary. Histologically the tumour is usually of the oat cell variety. The hyperplasia is due to the production of ACTH by the tumour. The stimulation of the adrenal cortex leads to very high plasma concentrations of cortisol. Nevertheless only a minority of patients with these levels of cortisol show the clinical features of Cushing's syndrome, possibly because they do not live long enough for the physical changes to develop. Oedema of the legs is common and diabetes may occur. The high level of cortisol may lead to the loss of large amounts of potassium in the urine and the development of hypokalaemic alkalosis. The loss may be so great that it is difficult to correct it with potassium supplements or spironolactone. If it is difficult to suppress the excess ACTH production by endocrine means plasma cortisol may be reduced by removal of the tumour or successful irradiation, though there may be recurrence if metastases develop.

(2) *Hypercalcaemia.* This is probably the second commonest manifestation and is usually associated with an oat cell carcinoma, though it may also occur with hypernephroma and other tumours. It seems to be due to the production of parathyroid-like hormone by the tumour, though it seems possible that not all cases are explicable in this way. Hypercalcaemia may, of course, also occur as the result of the release of calcium from bone by osteolytic metastases. The clinical manifestations are those of polyuria, thirst, constipation and mental confusion. Unlike the hypercalcaemia of parathyroidism hypercalcaemia secondary to bronchial carcinoma usually responds, at least initially, to cortisone [71]. It can also be abolished by removal or irradiation of the tumour.

(3) *Dilutional hyponatraemia.* An oat cell carcinoma may secrete antidiuretic hormone with retention of water, resulting in increased blood volume, decreased plasma sodium concentration, which may fall below 120 mEq/l, and low blood urea. In spite of the haemodilution the kidney continues to lose sodium. The condition is distinguished from Addison's disease by the absence of haemoconcentration and by the fact that the blood pressure is if anything elevated. By a mechanism which is uncertain some of these patients also have defective absorption by the proximal renal tubules of glucose, aminoacids and potassium. Patients with dilutional hyponatraemia are often drowsy and may be disorientated. Sometimes there is skin pigmentation. It is said that the plasma sodium concentration can be restored to normal, with improvement of the mental state, by giving fludrocortisone in a dose of 5 mg daily [106]. If there are renal tubular defects sodium and potassium supplements will be necessary.

(4) The *carcinoid syndrome*, if it is associated with a lung tumour, is more often due to an adenoma than a carcinoma but oat cell tumours are sometimes responsible. The syndrome is discussed on p. 554.

(5) *Hyperthyroidism.* This has occasionally been associated with carcinoma of the bronchus, although more often reported in trophoblastic tumours. The latter have been

shown to produce thyroid stimulating hormone.

(6) *Hypoglycaemia* has most often occurred in patients with liver carcinoma but has been reported with carcinoma of the bronchus and with mediastinal fibrosarcoma. There is some evidence that the tumour may produce either insulin or an insulin-like hormone.

(7) *Red cell aplasia.* This has been most often reported in association with thymoma but also as a complication of bronchial carcinoma [53]. The plasma contains a substance capable of depressing iron utilization in rabbits.

(8) *Gynaecomastia.* This may occasionally complicate bronchial carcinoma, especially in the presence of hypertrophic osteoarthropathy. The urinary oestrogen excretion has been shown to be high in patients with osteoarthropathy complicating carcinoma of the bronchus but the level is not closely related to the occurrence of gynaecomastia.

(9) *Adrenal metastases* often account for a rapid terminal deterioration in the patient's condition.

HYPERTROPHIC OSTEOARTHROPATHY [5 & 72]

The syndrome of hypertrophic osteoarthropathy includes periosteal and new bone formation, mainly in the long bones, and swelling and pain in the joints. In the great majority of cases, but not in all, gross finger clubbing is present. Sometimes there is flushing, blanching and profuse sweating, mainly in the hands and feet.

Hypertrophic osteoarthropathy is most often associated with carcinoma of the bronchus but may also occur with a fibroma of the pleura, pulmonary sepsis and most of the other potential causes of finger clubbing. It has even been recorded with aortic aneurysm. The *pathogenesis* is still uncertain. The blood flow to the affected limbs and bone is increased. It seems probable that the autonomic nervous system is involved as the condition may be abolished after resection of the vagus nerves. Even thoracotomy, without removal of the tumour, may sometimes be effective. The vasomotor instability which is

sometimes present also suggests an autonomic component. *Pathologically* there is periosteal new growth which results in irregular sheaths of new bone *radiologically* resembling elm bark. The bone is thereby widened and is initially denser than normal though ultimately the original cortex may be resorbed. The bones of the forearm and of the lower leg are primarily affected. In the bones of the hands 'collars' may form round the distal third of the metacarpals and the 1st and 2nd phalanges though the terminal phalanx usually shows no bony changes, apart from occasional osteoporosis, even in the presence of gross clubbing. *Microscopically* the earliest change is overgrowth of highly vascular connective tissue and lymphocyte infiltration. In the clubbed terminal phalanges there is oedema of the soft parts with proliferation of fibrous tissue and thickening of blood vessel walls. The synovium of the joints is infiltrated with round cells and there is often hydrarthrosis. Later there may be fibrinoid degeneration of cartilage. The skin and soft tissues of ankles, wrists, hands and feet show non-pitting swelling. There is usually moderate elevation of *serum alkaline phosphatase* and, for uncertain reasons, a rise in *serum phosphorus*. *Clinically* there is pain, which may be very severe, in the region of the wrists and ankles. Both the bone and the joints are tender and hot to the touch. In some cases there are bouts of profuse sweating, often confined to the hands and feet. Raynaud's phenomenon may alternate with periods of flushing. As already mentioned, *gynaecomastia* may accompany the condition. The manifestations usually disappear immediately and dramatically if the primary tumour can be dealt with. If it proves inoperable at thoracotomy local vagal resection is worth undertaking as this may relieve the symptoms. If radical treatment is not possible pain and swelling may respond rapidly to corticosteroid drugs.

DIAGNOSIS

The main tools in the diagnosis of bronchial carcinoma are radiology, bronchoscopy and cytology.

EARLY DIAGNOSIS

Theoretically *mass radiography* might be expected to detect cases in an early stage and so to improve prognosis, but results reported so far have been disappointing. McCormack [85] in a review of the results of 4 investigations, comprising 686 cases detected at mass radiography surveys found that the rate of resection was 45% compared to less than 30% in many routine series. The overall 5-year survival rate (3 years in one of the series) was only 15%, which was not a very impressive improvement on the 7% average in 7 other large series of routine cases. Nevertheless there is evidence that patients diagnosed in a presymptomatic stage have a better outlook [31].

Brett [17] has given preliminary results of a comparative trial in which 2 large groups of men over the age of 40 were x-rayed initially and after 3 years, one group having in addition 6 monthly films in the intermediate period. Although the '6 monthly' group had a higher resectability rate (65%) during the 3 year period than at the initial survey (51%) there was no difference in the provisional figures for mortality from bronchial carcinoma in the 2 groups during the 3 years. One must conclude that so far mass radiography has not proved an efficient method of improving the treatment of bronchial carcinoma by early diagnosis.

Mass sputum cytology would be a formidable undertaking and at present hardly practicable but the very sparse reports of the detection of lung cancer in this way in patients with normal x-ray [31] suggest that the outlook for successful resection might be better with this method of detection than with mass radiography. In one highly selected series only 1 of 15 patients had died of lung cancer, 9 being alive 4–8 years later [130].

PATIENTS WITH SYMPTOMS

Bronchial carcinoma must be considered in any patient of the relevant age group with respiratory symptoms which have lasted for more than 2 weeks, particularly if he is a smoker. Similarly, it must be considered in any chronic bronchitic who has had an exacerbation of symptoms. As has been indicated, the symptoms are nonspecific, the only suggestive one being repeated small haemoptyses. The presence of clubbing in a patient with a relatively short history is also suspicious. Unless there is evidence of metastases in palpable lymph glands or liver other physical signs are not diagnostic. *Radiologically*, unilateral enlargement of the hilar shadow is highly suspicious. A large irregular peripheral mass, or a lung cavity with irregular inner walls, are also suggestive but in many cases bronchial carcinoma is only one of the possible explanations for an abnormal shadow. The persistence of radiological evidence of collapse or pneumonia for more than 2 weeks always calls for investigation to exclude a carcinoma. By the time a patient develops symptoms there is nearly always a radiographic abnormality, though occasionally haemoptysis may lead to diagnosis by bronchoscopy or cytology in the presence of a normal x-ray.

If there is any doubt on clinical or radiological grounds the next step is to carry out *bronchoscopy* (p. 77). If the tumour is in a segmental bronchus or one of the larger bronchi a bronchoscopic abnormality is usually detectable and biopsy may confirm the diagnosis. If the tumour is not visible it may still be possible to obtain material for cytological diagnosis by bronchial washings. At bronchoscopy the relevant bronchus may be compressed from without or the tumour itself may be visible as a nodular area with or without bleeding and ulceration. The carina between the two main bronchi may be grossly broadened or invaded if there is a mass in the subcarinal lymph glands. The vocal cords are always inspected, and with particular attention if the patient is hoarse, in order to detect involvement of the recurrent laryngeal nerve.

Sputum cytology [31] is a valuable investigation in skilled hands. In one series positive results were obtained in 62% of 240 cases admitted to a surgical unit, compared with 31% positive results from bronchial biopsy [44]. Other series have given correct positive results in 46–88% of cases. False positives have mostly varied between nil and 5%, though figures as high as 13% and 24% have been reported [31]. The more specimens are examined the higher the positivity rate. Although small hilar tumours seem to be as often, or even more often, diagnosable cytologically as large, this is not true for peripheral tumours. In a review of various reported series Davies [31] found an average positivity rate of 50% for all peripheral tumours but the rate was higher for large tumours. The paraffin section method has been claimed to be superior to the more usual Papanicolaou smear [63]. Sputum cytology is particularly valuable when a bronchial neoplasm is suspected but bronchoscopy is negative. Cases have even been correctly diagnosed by cytology in the presence of a normal x-ray [31, 89 & 130]. Kuper and his colleagues [79] have described the use of soluble swabs for collecting material either directly from a tumour surface seen at bronchoscopy or from the bronchus draining a suspicious area. The swab can be subsequently dissolved and the cells concentrated by centrifugation.

Tetracycline is concentrated in necrotic tumour tissue and may be detected in sputum derived from tumours by the fact that it fluoresces in ultraviolet light. Burton and Cunliffe [20] have utilized this technique in the diagnosis of bronchial carcinoma. The patient is given 2 g of tetracycline a day in 4 divided doses for 2 consecutive days, the last dose being given 36 hours before the specimen is collected. In their hands it was found to be a more sensitive test than sputum cytology in proved malignant cases though the combined methods gave a detection rate as high as 84% with false positive results in about 5%. Hattori and his colleagues [67] have described a technique of passing a Métras bronchial catheter into the relevant segmental bronchus under vision, using the image intensifier. They insert a fine nylon brush, mounted on the end of a wire, deeply into the bronchus. The epithelium is brushed and smears made of the material obtained.

In cases in which there is a secondary pleural effusion *pleural biopsy* should be a routine. The examination of pleural fluid for *malignant cells* is particularly difficult but may be reliable in skilled hands. If pleural biopsy and bronchoscopy are negative, and it is thought possible on clinical grounds that the effusion may be due to pleural invasion by tumour, *thoracoscopy* may allow the diagnosis to be made by inspection and biopsy. If the x-ray shadow is peripheral but relatively superficial, diagnosis may sometimes be made by *needle biopsy* or biopsy by means of a *high speed drill*. *X-ray screening* should be carried out as a routine before thoracotomy or in any case where unilateral elevation of the diaphragm suggests the possibility of phrenic nerve involvement. A *barium swallow* should also be a routine in a suspicious case to exclude displacement of the oesophagus by secondary deposits in mediastinal lymph nodes.

An additional technique which may in due course prove of value is the determination of *local pulmonary arterial blood flow* by radioisotope scanning [97 & 127]. Human serum albumin labelled with radioactive iodine is injected intravenously in macroscopic particles which accumulate immediately in the lungs where their distribution can be displayed by automatic isotope scanning techniques. The concentration in various parts of the lungs is directly related to the pulmonary artery blood flow. Even when there is no collapse diminished blood flow may be found peripheral to a suspicious shadow. Such a diminution does not occur with secondary neoplasm. French workers [87] demonstrated diminished pulsation in pulmonary arterioles distal to bronchial carcinoma by means of photoelectric cinedensigraphy. The patient stands between the x-ray tube and a photoelectric cell which records the changes in density with pulsation of the pulmonary arterioles. Diminished pulsation is recorded peripheral to a bronchial carcinoma. This technique has not so far been widely adopted.

DIFFERENTIAL DIAGNOSIS

If a radiographic abnormality has been found the differential diagnosis is chiefly from an acute inflammatory lesion such as pneumonia or lung abscess, from tuberculosis, from benign tumour and occasionally from infarct. Slow clearing of an apparent pneumonia raises the possibility of either tuberculosis or neoplasm. If no tubercle bacilli are found in the sputum bronchoscopy will usually be indicated. Shadows of pulmonary infarct usually clear relatively rapidly but sometimes are sufficiently persistent to necessitate bronchoscopy or examination of the sputum for malignant cells. The solitary *cavitated shadow* may be due to neoplasm, tuberculosis or lung abscess. If the patient is ill and lung abscess is a possibility intensive chemotherapy should be initiated at once (p. 159). Thereafter investigations should be carried out to exclude the other two conditions. If tubercle bacilli are not present on direct smear tuberculosis is not excluded but bronchoscopy should be done. Indeed bronchoscopy is indicated in all cases of lung abscess in the relevant age group (p. 159) for the abscess may be occurring distal to a bronchus affected by a carcinoma. Tuberculosis and bronchial neoplasm are both common conditions and may coincide. In a doubtful case bronchoscopy should be carried out in spite of the finding of tubercle bacilli in the sputum.

A *rounded peripheral shadow* may pose a particularly difficult problem. Such a shadow may be due to a primary bronchial carcinoma but tuberculosis, benign tumour such as hamartoma, metastatic tumour and rarely hydatid cyst may give similar appearances. A well defined hair-line margin makes benign tumour or hydatid cyst more likely. Linear protrusions from the shadow into the surrounding lung are suggestive of primary carcinoma and are usually absent in metastatic tumour. Small satellite lesions suggest tuberculosis. The clinician should always enquire whether the patient has had any previous x-rays of his chest. If he has, these should be obtained even if they were recorded as negative. Knowing where the new lesion has appeared it is sometimes possible to detect a small abnormal shadow in the relevant area of a film taken several years previously. This would make tuberculosis a more likely diagnosis but it must be remembered that a neoplasm may start in an old scar. The presence of calcification in the lesion, which may sometimes be demonstrated on tomography if it is not obvious on the straight film, suggests tuberculosis or a benign neoplasm. The tuberculin test may also be relevant and sputum cytology may also be helpful. Nevertheless it is common not to be able to make a definite diagnosis. Even when the probabilities may be somewhat against a neoplasm the clinician frequently has to advise a thoracotomy because of the grim penalty of failing to operate on a carcinoma. When respiratory function forbids thoracotomy 'blind' radiotherapy may sometimes be indicated. If tuberculosis is a possible alternative diagnosis it is wise to carry out either thoracotomy or radiotherapy under cover of antituberculosis chemotherapy.

The differential diagnosis of malignant *pleural effusion* is considered on p. 269.

PREVENTION

SMOKING

Bronchial carcinoma is largely a preventable disease. On the basis of their studies in doctors Doll and Hill [42] calculated that nearly 90% of cases could be prevented if tobacco smoking were abolished. Indeed the effect of stopping smoking is fairly rapidly seen. Compared to a mortality rate of 1·28 per 1000 per year in those continuing smoking, the rate fell to 0·67 in exsmokers during the first 5 years, 0·49 during the 5th to the 9th year and 0·18 during the 10th to 19th year. During the 10 years of their enquiry the death rate for bronchial carcinoma in men aged 25 and over in England and Wales rose by 22%, whereas it fell by 7% in male doctors, who as a group had substantially reduced their smoking during this period.

We are far from discovering effective methods of reducing or abolishing this dangerous addiction. In Britain the public is now in general aware of the risks [26] and the percentage of smokers decreased between 1961 and 1965 from 57% to 54% [122]. The decrease, small though it was, occurred in males of all ages but only in the 16–19 age group in women. Nevertheless, though tobacco consumption decreased between 1961 and 1965 it rose in 1966. Advertising of cigarettes has been abolished on television and further restrictions may be imposed, but the amount spent on health education is very small compared to the vast sums still devoted to advertising tobacco and the enormous income the State derives from tobacco tax. No effective medical method has been found for curing the tobacco habit and social pressure is still the most important influence causing the exsmoker to start again [26]. Unfortunately the most important factor in preventing a child smoking is the possession of nonsmoking parents! There is a little evidence that social and intellectual pressures are beginning to decrease smoking among professional classes other than doctors and this may gradually affect other groups in the population but a much more rapid change is necessary if the present 'epidemic' of bronchial carcinoma is to be arrested. New methods must be constantly sought.

ATMOSPHERIC POLLUTION
Atmospheric pollution probably makes only a small contribution to the bronchial carcinoma problem, but control is highly desirable in the prevention of chronic bronchitis. Some success is being achieved [26] though there is still a long way to go.

OCCUPATIONAL FACTORS
Substantial progress has been made in reducing the risk in most industries in which there has been shown to be a lung cancer risk [41]. Unfortunately the success of the measures takes a long time to become apparent.

TREATMENT AND PROGNOSIS

The overall outlook for bronchial carcinoma is bad. In the large series from the Brompton and Royal Marsden Hospitals in London only 4% of cases survived 3 years after first attendance in the absence of surgical treatment or radiotherapy, and radical treatment was only

possible in a relatively small proportion [12]. The main hope of cure lies in surgery, though in a small but increasing proportion of cases success may be achieved by radiotherapy. At the present time the chemotherapy of bronchial carcinoma is only palliative. Radiographic and subjective improvement is obtained in some cases but there is no evidence that life is prolonged. Unfortunately in the great majority of patients all that can be done is to treat symptoms and to attempt to minimize the distress of the patient's last weeks or months.

SUMMARY OF MANAGEMENT
In this section a brief summary will be given of the management of a patient with bronchial carcinoma. More detailed consideration of the different facets of management will follow in subsequent sections.

Apart from anaplastic carcinoma, in which radiotherapy may be the treatment of choice (p. 542), the first consideration is whether the patient is suitable for *radical surgery*. Age, extensive invasion, distant metastases or poor respiratory function are frequent contra-indications to surgery (p. 539). In a patient considered for operation fluoroscopy and barium swallow are carried out to exclude phrenic paralysis or displacement of the oesophagus by carcinomatous mediastinal lymph glands. Respiratory function tests should include at least FEV and FVC and preferably Pa,co_2 estimation (p. 525). Lobectomy is the operation of choice if it is feasible (p. 539).

If surgery is not possible, suitability for *radical radiotherapy* must be considered as an alternative, though this also will be precluded if the tumour is very large or has given rise to distant metastases (p. 542). It is controversial whether poor lung function is a contra-indication (p. 542).

Unfortunately in many patients no radical treatment is possible. *Palliative radiotherapy* may be indicated to relieve symptoms due to pain, superior vena caval obstruction, serious haemoptysis, distressing cough or obstruction of a large bronchus (p. 543). *Chemotherapy* is less often used for these purposes but is the treatment of choice for malignant pleural effusion (p. 269). Secondary infection will frequently require antibiotic treatment.

In many cases only *symptomatic measures* are possible (p. 544). The physician has a particular responsibility to consider carefully what he will tell the patient and to minimize the *mental distress* of both the patient himself and of his close relatives (p. 544).

SURGERY

Surgery for carcinoma of the bronchus usually consists in the removal of a lobe or lung together with any apparently affected lymph glands. It is routine to remove those around the hilum. Some surgeons would also attempt to remove any affected mediastinal lymph nodes but it is virtually impossible to be sure of clearing all of these. Most do not operate if there is obvious mediastinal invasion or abandon the operation if it is revealed at thoracotomy. Others not only will attempt clearance of mediastinal lymph glands but are prepared to resect portions of the chest wall or pericardium [110]. As will be discussed below, there is a steadily diminishing success rate with increasing evidence of invasion. Many surgeons and physicians consider that if the chances of success are very low the patient's last months should not be made more miserable by the discomfort of a thoracotomy which may indeed shorten his life [94].

In spite of differences in policy by individual surgeons there are relatively little differences in the success rate between the various published surgical series, a selection of which is summarized in table 29.1.

It will be noted that in most series the 5 year survival rate lies between 20 and 33%, but that when the total of initial cases can be regarded as reasonably representative of the bronchial carcinoma problem in general the overall 5 year survival rate is only 3·5–9%. The proportion of patients submitted to

TABLE 29.1.

Five year Survival After Resection for Bronchial Carcinoma

Authors	No. of cases	% resected	Five year survival		
			% operative or early mortality	% of resected	% of all cases
Overholt *et al.* (1956)	733	37	12	21	
Gifford and Waddington (1957)	2156	21	22	28	4·5
Nicholson *et al.* (1957)	910	21		28	5·5
Bignall (1958)	1749	23		32	6
Ochsner *et al.* (1960)	875	41	16	15	6·5
Höst (1960)	903	23		37	9
Flavell (1962)	826	70	5·6	32·6	
Taylor *et al.* (1963)	2847	21		21	3·5
Clagett *et al.* (1964)	1401			33	
Goldman (1965)	746	33·5		22	
Belcher and Anderson (1965)	1134	79	10	26	
Bergh and Scherstén (1965)	219	82	16	26·5	

Table 29.1 showing percentage five year survival after resection for bronchial carcinoma, as given in a number of series. The series show evidence of varying degrees of selection. Those with a relatively low resection rate are in general more representative of unselected patients; for these series an overall survival rate, related to the total of original patients, has been calculated. In some of the series not all patients had been observed for 5 years or until death; the percentage 5 year survival relates only to the number of patients who had been so observed. The definition of deaths included in 'operative or early mortality' varies somewhat from series to series. It will be noted that there has been little change in survival rates in the last 10 years.

thoracotomy, and the proportion of thoracotomies in which resection is carried out, will vary partly with the policy of the surgeon but even more with the type of case which is referred to him. The variation in the percentage submitted to resection, as shown in table 29.1, is a reflection of these factors. The series in table 29.1 is given in chronological order of publication and it will be seen that there is no suggestion of improvement in success rate over the last 10 years. One could summarize the situation approximately by stating that only 20–25% of all cases are suitable for resection and that of these only a quarter to a third survive 5 years, giving an overall 5 year survival of approximately 5–8%.

TYPE OF OPERATION

Belcher [8] pointed out that the results of lobectomy for bronchial carcinoma were at least as good as, and often better than, the results of pneumonectomy. The better results are, of course, accounted for by the fact that the more restricted operation is only feasible in the more restricted lesions. In Belcher's report, which summarized the results of a number of London surgeons, the 2 year survival rate was 50%. It is claimed that lobectomy is possible in more than a third of cases and the operative mortality is less than half that of pneumonectomy, particularly in older patients [51]. A further advantage of lobectomy over pneumonectomy is the preservation of more functioning lung tissue, especially important in patients over the age of 50 [22]. As mentioned above only a proportion of surgeons will attempt a resection if the tumour is found to have invaded the mediastinum, the chest wall or the brachial plexus. The matter is discussed further below.

CONTRAINDICATIONS TO OPERATION

Nearly 80% of patients have to be denied operation mainly for one of the following reasons:

(1) *Advanced age.* There is a good deal of evidence that the immediate results of operation become less favourable with advancing age. For instance, Bergh and Schersténté [10] had an overall operative mortality of 19·5% in patients over the age of 60 compared to 11·5% under that age. For patients who had a pneumonectomy over the age of 60 the operative mortality was as high as 37·5%. Naturally the results are even worse in patients over the age of 70. Respiratory infection, pulmonary embolism and cardiac infarction are among the commoner causes of postoperative death.

(2) *Metastases.* Distant metastases in liver, brain or cervical lymph glands of course contra-indicate operation. A barium swallow should be carried out as a routine before operation. If the oesophagus is displaced by mediastinal glands operation is not worth undertaking. Paralysis of the left recurrent laryngeal nerve indicates mediastinal invasion and resection is usually not feasible. Phrenic nerve paralysis, as shown by paradoxical movement of the diaphragm, is usually due to invasion of the nerve in the mediastinum, making radical resection impossible, but occasionally a tumour below the level of the hilum may invade the phrenic nerve as it passes over the pericardium and it may be possible to excise the tumour with a portion of the pericardium.

(3) *Poor respiratory function.* Each case must be considered on its merits. It is very distressing for a patient to survive an extensive operation and have to live the rest of his life as a severe respiratory invalid. The use of function tests in assessing the patient for operation has been considered on p. 525.

(4) *Persistent pleural effusion.* A pleural effusion which recurs in spite of aspiration and is thought not to be due to secondary infection usually implies extensive pleural involvement. In such a case the tumour is almost always found at thoracotomy not to be resectable. Persistent pleural effusion should therefore be regarded as a contraindication to operation.

(5) *Extensive main bronchus involvement on the left.* A neoplasm which on the left side leaves less than 2 cm of the main bronchus uninvolved makes resection extremely difficult or impossible. For anatomical reasons

resection of the right main bronchus, and indeed part of the trachea, is technically feasible but because of the aorta this is much more difficult on the left.

(6) *Horner's syndrome*, or the *invasion* of *brachial plexus* or *chest wall* are regarded by most surgeons as contra-indications to operation. Invasion of the chest wall at the apex or medial to the angle of the ribs is usually an absolute contra-indication. Some surgeons may attempt resection, including part of the chest wall, if the invasion is elsewhere. The question of the treatment of the thoracic inlet tumours is discussed below.

(7) *Other serious diseases* may contra-indicate operation. The most common is, of course, severe chronic bronchitis impairing respiratory function. In the case of other diseases the whole clinical situation has to be assessed and the physician must decide whether the disturbance of an operation, and its uncertain outcome, are justified in the particular circumstance.

MEDIASTINOSCOPY

Although we have little personal experience of the use of mediastinoscopy [23] it seems a rational technique to apply in patients suspected of bronchial carcinoma; sometimes to assist in diagnosis, more often to decide whether thoracotomy is justifiable. The procedure causes relatively little disturbance to the patient and has the great advantage that, if mediastinal invasion is shown, he can be spared an unnecessary thoracotomy. Reynders [102] found that if unsuitable cases were excluded by this technique the resectability of carcinoma after thoracotomy rose to more than 90%; Bergh and Scherstén [10] were able to carry out resection in 80%. Nohl-Oser [94] found that only 9·7% of operated patients in whom the mediastinal lymph glands were involved survived 4 years and concluded that such patients should be spared the distress of a thoracotomy. Even the most radical surgeons would agree that by mediastinoscopy patients in whom the growth has spread outside the capsules of mediastinal lymph glands can be justifiably excluded from thoracotomy.

OTHER FACTORS AFFECTING THE RESULTS OF SURGERY

(1) *Delay in diagnosis.* In general one would expect that the earlier the diagnosis was made after the first manifestation the better would be the results of surgery. This is certainly suggested by some series. Overholt and Bougas [98] found that the average delay from the first manifestation to diagnosis was 6·7 months in their 5 year survivors compared with 11·2 months in the rest. Nevertheless sometimes such a delay is merely a manifestation of slow growth; a patient who is undergoing annual x-ray may have a small tumour missed one year to be picked up the next. This involves the paradox that a 'missed' tumour may have a better prognosis! There is certainly evidence from a number of series that patients who are diagnosed by routine radiography at a stage when they have no symptoms have a better prognosis. A 5 year survival rate of 75% has been reported for asymptomatic solitary nodules [28 & 32].

(2) *Site.* Although in some series better results have been reported for those with lesions in the upper lobes, in others the results have been better with lesions in the lower lobes. There is also some variation in the reports of the prognosis in peripheral lesions as compared with central. In view of these variations between different series it seems probable that site, as opposed to degree of invasion, has no important influence on the prognosis after surgery.

(3) *Histological type.* It is generally found that the outlook for squamous cell carcinoma after surgery is appreciably better than for anaplastic (including oat cell) and adenocarcinoma. The latter 2 types are much more likely to have metastasized by the time diagnosis is made. For instance, in Bergh and Scherstén's series [10] the 5 year survival rate for patients with squamous carcinoma after surgery was 33% as compared with 19% and 18% respectively for anaplastic and adenocarcinoma. As will be mentioned below, there is some evidence that radiotherapy may give better results than surgery in anaplastic carcinoma.

(4) *Lymph node involvement.* There is a

steady decrease in the survival rate after operation as successive groups of lymph glands are involved. If mediastinal lymph glands have been invaded the outlook is virtually hopeless, particularly if the growth has burst through the capsule of the gland and invaded the surrounding tissue.

(5) *Invasion of other tissues.* The survival rate is diminished with any evidence of pleural involvement or any evidence of crossing a fissure. Such an invasion facilitates access to lymphatics and leads to involvement of lymph nodes. The adverse significance of involvement of pericardium, phrenic nerve, recurrent laryngeal nerve, chest wall invasion, etc. has already been mentioned.

(6) *Invasion of blood vessels and evidence of tumour cells in the blood stream.* Collier et al. [28] found a sharp distinction in 5 year survival according to whether blood vessel invasion could be detected microscopically in the resected specimen. For those in whom there was evidence of such an invasion there were only 6% of 5 year survivals, whereas when there was no such evidence the survival rate was 75%. If there was blood vessel invasion the presence or absence of lymph gland invasion made little difference to the outlook. With no evidence of either blood vessel or lymph gland invasion the 5 year survival rate was as high as 83%. Both blood vessel invasion and lymph gland invasion were very much commoner in undifferentiated and adenocarcinomata than in the squamous type. Lymph gland invasion in those with no invasion of blood vessels reduced the 5-year survival rate from 76% to 50%. Others have found similar results [103]. In recent years techniques have been developed for detecting carcinoma cells in the blood. Hayata et al. [68] have obtained positive results in as many as 72 out of 160 cases. The highest frequency was found in arterial samples, especially those from the carotid artery. The blood findings were positive more often in central than in peripheral tumours; they were rare if the patient was symptom-free or with small peripheral tumours. Higher rates were found in those with haemoptysis, with lymphatic metastasis, with inoperable or with anaplastic

tumours. They point out that not all such tumour cells are viable but the association with other prognostic factors suggests that some of the cells may give rise to metastases [79]. Kuper and Bignall [79] demonstrated that at least some tumour cells obtained from pulmonary vein blood at operation are alive and have shown that the isolation of such cells is related to prognosis. All 5 of their patients with positive samples died within 2 years of operation, whereas 21 out of 30 with negative samples survived 2 years. As handling the tumour may encourage the release of such cells it is desirable that the surgeon should secure the pulmonary veins as early as possible in the operation.

RESPIRATORY CAPACITY AFTER OPERATION

The respiratory function after operation will depend on the function before operation, the contribution of the resected lung to the preoperative function and perhaps on any postoperative complications affecting the residual lung tissue. It is therefore not possible to generalize, but, as has already been pointed out, diminution in function will be less in those who have had a lobectomy than in those who have lost a whole lung and is likely to be more severe in older patients. Ogilvie and his colleagues [96] compared the function in a small group of patients who had had a pneumonectomy for carcinoma of the bronchus a year previously with that in a second small group who had had a pneumonectomy for the same reason 10 years before. All had some degree of breathlessness. As might be expected, there was a tendency for the 10 year group to have more severe dyspnoea and more evidence of bronchitis. None of the patients showed evidence of oxygen lack or carbon dioxide retention at rest but there was a diminution of ventilatory capacity, as reflected by VC, FEV and MVV, in the 10 year group. However, there was only a slight diminution, in the 10 year group, in the FEV expressed as a percentage of vital capacity, suggesting no major increase in airways obstruction. The diffusing capacity was at least as good as in the 1 year group but a number of the patients showed clinical and electrocardiographic evidence of *cor pulmonale*. These workers concluded that the reduction in ventilatory capacity after 10 years was due more to impaired mechanical efficiency of the thoracic cage than to progressive emphysematous or fibrotic changes within the lung itself. Of course 10 year survivors, considering the age at which pneumonectomy is carried out for carcinoma of the bronchus, must be a self-selected group and are not likely to be representative of the total sample. Many patients after operation show much more severe disability than might be suggested by the figures of Ogilvie and his colleagues [96].

RADIOTHERAPY

METHODS

The results of radical radiotherapy with orthovoltage x-ray apparatus were relatively poor, the reported 5 year survival rates varying from 1 to 4% [36] but with supervoltage x-rays it is possible to give a larger dose of radiation to deeply placed tumours with less damage to the skin and surrounding tissues and with less absorption and scatter by bone. Some of the machines allow treatment to be given in 2 or 3 minutes compared with 15 or 20 minutes with conventional apparatus.

RESULTS IN OPERABLE TUMOURS

It seems that surgery is still the treatment of choice for squamous carcinoma. Morrison *et al.* [90] carried out a controlled trial. In squamous carcinoma the 4 year survival rate with radiotherapy was only 6% compared to 30% for surgery; in anaplastic carcinoma there was no difference between the 2 treatments but the numbers were small. Subsequently a larger controlled trial has been carried out in patients with small cell or oat cell carcinoma [88]. Only clinically operable cases were admitted to the trial and treatment was randomized to resection or radiotherapy. Unfortunately the success rate in both groups was poor but at 24 months only 4% of the patients in the resected group survived compared to 10% of those treated by radiotherapy. The mean survival period in the radiotherapy series was significantly greater than that in the surgical. The results in this type of tumour are therefore very poor by any method of treatment but are marginally better with radiotherapy.

INOPERABLE TUMOURS

Megavoltage radiotherapy has also slightly improved the outlook for inoperable lesions. In Deeley and Singh's series [36] the overall 3 year survival rate was 8% and the 5-year survival rate 6%. The 3 year survival rate in squamous and adenocarcinoma was similar, 10% and 11% respectively, but in anaplastic and oat cell carcinoma was only 4%. In their series the hilum and mediastinum were included in the radiation field, whether or not there was clinical evidence of involvement. The results were somewhat better if the mediastinum was not involved, though the difference was not dramatic.

REACTIONS TO RADIOTHERAPY

Radical radiotherapy causes dysphagia, due to radiation damage to the oesophagus, in a high proportion of patients. This usually starts about the 3rd week of treatment, and occasionally necessitates its temporary cessation. Radiation also causes local reaction in the treated lung and there is often evidence of later fibrosis and shrinkage.

CONTRAINDICATIONS TO RADIATION

The presence of a large pleural effusion is regarded as a contraindication to radical radiotherapy. Extensive invasion of the mediastinum or chest wall, distant metastases, or a very large tumour (over 10 cm in diameter) will also preclude success. If there is evidence of acute infection this should be controlled before radiotherapy starts. If there is tuberculosis, definitely or potentially active, it is wise to carry out radiotherapy under the cover of antituberculosis drugs. With megavoltage radiotherapy lung function is said not to be impaired at the end of the course of radiotherapy but moderate functional disability has been found at the end of 1 year

[119]. Gillam *et al.* [58] investigated the influence of pre-existing chronic bronchitis on the tolerance of 161 bronchial carcinoma patients to radiotherapy, and on their health and survival after treatment. They found little evidence that the bronchitis influenced the results. There was no increased frequency of exacerbations of bronchitis after treatment; survival rate in patients with severe bronchitis was as good as that in those with mild bronchitis; and chronic bronchitis did not appear to contribute to any increased attack rate of radiation pneumonia or fibrosis. It must be added that some radiotherapists would not agree with this view and consider that many bronchitics are made worse by radiotherapy (J.G. Pearson: personal communication).

PALLIATIVE RADIOTHERAPY

Radiotherapy is often useful for palliation. Pain may be relieved, at least temporarily, in a high proportion of cases and haemoptysis with even greater success [36]. Cough can often be improved. Radiotherapy is of particular value in relieving superior vena caval obstruction. Szur and Bromley [120] found benefit in nearly 70% of cases and in 80% of these there was no later recurrence of the obstruction. Radiotherapy may also relieve obstruction of a main bronchus or of the trachea, but the treatment may lead to initial swelling of the lesion and increased obstruction so that it is best to give chemotherapy first followed by radiotherapy. The chemotherapy may produce initial shrinkage and does not result in reactionary swelling.

CHEMOTHERAPY

INDICATIONS

After a number of years' experience it is agreed by all workers that cytotoxic drugs do not prolong life, though they may shrink a tumour temporarily and are sometimes useful in palliation [4, 6 & 81]. It is generally agreed that anaplastic tumours respond best. Chemotherapy is of particular value in rapidly reaccumulating malignant pleural effusion. A single intrapleural dose may be sufficient to prevent recurrence. As already mentioned, cytotoxic drugs may be useful initial therapy where a large tumour is in danger of completely blocking the trachea or main bronchus, the chemotherapy being followed by radiotherapy after the tumour has shrunk sufficiently to give a good airway. Cytotoxic drugs are usually effective in relieving superior vena caval obstruction and may be used if radiotherapy is not available or if it has failed. Chemotherapy may sometimes relieve bone pain after radiotherapy has failed. It may also be useful for haemoptysis, although we would normally give radiotherapy first choice. Dyspnoea is sometimes improved and success has been reported in the treatment of endocrine dysfunctions secondary to a bronchial carcinoma [83].

METHODS

Several different drugs have been used but none has so far been shown to be superior to mustine (nitrogen mustard) or cyclophosphamide. The main side effects of these are nausea, loss of hair and bone marrow depression. In a comparative trial Barran *et al.* [4] found a higher improvement rate with cyclophosphamide but considered that they might not have pushed nitrogen mustard to the limit of tolerance. Cyclophosphamide has the advantage that follow-up treatment can be given orally. Intravenous therapy should be administered late in the evening. Bass's technique [6] minimizes nausea or vomiting after injection. He gives sodium amylobarbitone 0·2 g 2 hours before treatment and repeats this dose an hour before and at the time of injection. If the patient wakes during the night a further 0·2 g is given. A useful alternative is chlorpromazine 50–75 mg intramuscularly about 1 hour before the mustine injection; repetition of the chlorpromazine is often unnecessary. Mustine or cyclophosphamide is injected into the rubber tubing of a running saline drip. The drip is run very fast for 1 min after the injection to flush the drug out of the vein, and then allowed to run normally for a further 10 min after which it is taken down. With mustine on the whole it is less distressing for the patient to give a single dose of 0·4 mg/kg body weight. Alternatively this total dose can be divided into 3 and given on successive evenings. For *malignant pleural effusion* a single intrapleural injection of 20 mg of mustine in 100 ml may be administered after full aspiration of the fluid. This should be preceded by sedation as above.

Cyclophosphamide can similarly be given intravenously, but this is best done in divided doses of 100–400 mg daily to a total of not more than 7 g. As the drug depresses the bone marrow, daily white counts should be carried out and treatment stopped if the white blood cell count falls below 2000 per mm³. Some workers have followed up intravenous administration by oral treatment with 200 mg daily so long as the blood count showed no important granulopenia. This more prolonged treatment may be justified in dealing with certain symptoms, such as bone pain, but is less appropriate in dealing with haemoptysis or to obtain shrinkage of a tumour blocking a large bronchus. In general, as chemotherapy is palliative rather than curative, the minimum should be given which achieves the effect desired.

COMBINATIONS OF SURGERY, RADIOTHERAPY AND CHEMOTHERAPY

So far there is little evidence that combining different forms of treatment improves the survival rate. In a controlled trial Bromly and Szur [19] did not find that radiotherapy as a preliminary to surgery improved the results and there was a higher complication rate after operation. On the other hand Mallams *et al.* [86] reported 42 cases of *thoracic inlet tumour*, for obvious reasons a very difficult lesion to treat radically, to whom they gave preliminary irradiation with 'subcancerocidal doses' followed after 4 weeks by attempted total surgical resection. In order to avoid spread of the tumour they did not carry out any biopsy before operation. 33% of these cases were reported as living and well 2 years later. Poulsen [100] has reported a higher 12 month survival rate in patients receiving cyclophosphamide before and after operation than in those treated with surgery only. Combined forms of treatment require further exploration in carefully designed and

controlled trials [88]. At present one cannot say that any form of combined therapy has yet proved of unequivocal value.

OTHER PALLIATIVE TREATMENT

The palliative treatment of *superior vena caval obstruction, haemoptysis* and *obstruction of the trachea or a large bronchus* by radiotherapy, with or without chemotherapy, has been dealt with above. *Secondary infection* is common and can be treated by the same methods as are appropriate for primary pneumonia or lung abscess, though with a preference, in view of the poor outlook for the patient, for using oral drugs in order to save the discomfort of injections.

The patient's *mental state* will require particular attention. At an early stage the physician must decide what is to be told to him and his relatives. We have been increasingly convinced that there should be no standard procedure. The approach will depend on the stage of disease, the mental and emotional state of the patient and his relatives and their social background. There are occasions when, for social reasons and because of his own state of mind, the patient must be told the brutal truth but in our experience these circumstances are comparatively rare. Whatever their professions there are few patients who really desire to be deprived of hope. If the disease is advanced and death is unlikely to be long deferred a husband or wife will usually need to be told the full situation. If the patient is comparatively well and it is likely that he will last for quite a long time it may be more humane to withhold the full grimness of the situation and so make the last months of married life as free as possible from the searing distress of one of the partners knowing that the other will soon die. In these circumstances the family doctor will often be able to advise the best course and it is wise, if full information is withheld, that some other member of the family should be fully informed. It is impossible to generalize in these matters and it is our own practice to discuss with all the relevant people what decision should be taken in each individual case. In a hopeless situation the physician's primary duty is to minimize suffering, both physical and mental, and this may require as much care as the planning of curative treatment.

The patient is likely to have considerable anxiety as he may well suspect the diagnosis. Much can be done by tactful discussion but drugs can often be used to improve the sense of wellbeing and to damp down anxiety. Chlorpromazine in doses of 20–100 mg 4 times daily is useful for this purpose. Prednisolone in a dose of 30 mg daily may also improve the sense of wellbeing through its eutonic effect. Later an oral mixture containing morphine 15 mg and cocaine 10 mg, together with sugar and alcohol, is often successful in relieving pain and causing euphoria. The dose may be gradually increased. In the terminal stages morphia and hyoscine may be given.

ALVEOLAR CELL CARCINOMA (Bronchiolar Carcinoma, Pulmonary Adenomatosis) [70, 118 & 124]

DEFINITION

Alveolar cell carcinoma is a malignant tumour arising from either the alveolar, or possibly from the bronchiolar, epithelium. Characteristically it grows along, rather than invades, the alveolar walls, and is liable to manifest itself by multiple foci in one or both lungs.

AETIOLOGY AND PREVALENCE

This tumour comprises 1–2% of all malignant tumours of the lung [91]. It is said to be equally prevalent in both sexes and to occur in all races. It is commonest in patients between 50 and 70 years of age but has been recorded in a male as young as 16 [124]. There appears to be no relation to smoking or to any occupation. Similar tumours occur spontaneously in some strains of mice and can be induced with carcinogens. The disease jaagsiekte in sheep shows very similar pathological appearances but is almost certainly due to a virus or a mycoplasma. There is no rural bias in cases of alveolar cell carcinoma and jaagsiekte is virtually certainly an unrelated disease. One case has been reported in which thorotrast, containing thorium, had been given 16 years prior to death. A number of authors have emphasized the possible importance of previous pulmonary disease, either on the basis of history or pathological findings. Beaver et al. [7] obtained clinical evidence of previous pulmonary disease in 62% of 121 cases culled from the literature, and pathological evidence of old inflammation in 84%. Hewlett et al. [70] obtained a previous history of chest infections in 52% of cases and found pathological evidence of old inflammation in 47%. On the other hand Munnell and Kellar [91] describe the successful resection of 7 solitary lesions with no evidence of previous pulmonary disease in any. It seems that the tumour may sometimes arise in relation to old scar tissue or inflammation but this is by no means consistent.

PATHOLOGY

There has been considerable controversy as to whether this tumour arises from the alveolar or bronchiolar epithelium. The epithelium in fact forms a continuum so perhaps the matter is a little academic. At any rate the tumour tends to spread as a cuboidal or columnar 'epithelium' along the lining of the alveoli, with single or multiple rows of cells and often papillary formation which may completely fill the alveolus. The cytoplasm is usually finely granular with a vesicular nucleus in the base of the cell. Cilia are not common but do occur. Occasionally there is mucus formation [124]. Sometimes there is considerable fibrous tissue and scarring, or evidence of old inflammation. The bronchi are not usually obstructed. *Macroscopically* the tumour may be a solitary focus or there may be several nodules in close proximity with diffuse nodular formation occupying a segment, a lobe, a lung or both lungs. Sometimes the appearance may resemble pneumonia involving a segment or a lobe.

There is considerable controversy as to whether this tumour is multicentric in origin, as cases frequently present with diffuse nodulation but without evidence of metastases elsewhere. The success of surgery in solitary lesions has been adduced as an argument against a multicentric origin. Munnell and Keller [91] summarize 5 series, comprising 108 solitary lesions of alveolar carcinoma, with 69% of the patients living at various periods after surgery. They argue that if the lesions were multicentric in origin the recurrence rate would be much higher. Unless the solitary foci and multicentric tumours are 2 different types this argument appears compelling. Clagett *et al.* [27] do indeed consider that the solitary and diffuse types must be 2 different conditions because of the difference in outlook after resection. Reviewing a 10 year experience they say that among their patients with diffuse lesions at resection (presumably clinically confined to the lung tissue resected) there were no survivors. If, in fact, the disease is not multicentric presumably the diffuse foci arise by bronchial implantation of tumour.

Invasion of neighbouring tissue and lymph glands, and blood stream metastases, are less common than in the case of bronchial carcinoma though all these occur. Histologically the tumour closely resembles metastases from certain adenocarcinomata elsewhere and these must be carefully excluded.

CLINICAL FEATURES

The clinical features of the disease are very variable. A number of reported cases have been asymptomatic and have been detected at routine radiography. In some cases radiographic abnormalities have been present for a long period before diagnosis. Hewlett *et al.* [70] found radiographic abnormalities which had persisted for more than 2 years in 6 out of 39 cases; in 1 case abnormality had been present for over 8 years. In general the symtoms—cough, haemoptysis, chest pain, dyspnoea, anorexia, weight loss and malaise—are similar to those of bronchial carcinoma. As bronchial obstruction is unusual, secon-

dary infection is not an early manifestation. In late cases when there is diffuse tumour, often in both lungs, dyspnoea may be very severe. About 20% of cases are said to produce a large excess of mucus. Quantities as large as $1\frac{1}{2}$–4 l daily have occasionally been recorded [124].

RADIOLOGY (figs. 29.14 and 29.15)

The tumour is solitary in about one third of cases at the time of diagnosis. Sometimes more than one rounded shadow is visible in a local area. If inflammatory lesions can be

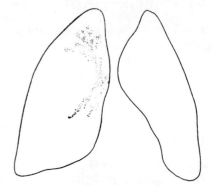

FIG. 29.14. Alveolar cell carcinoma of localized type.

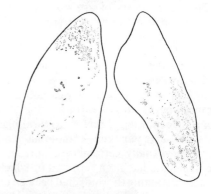

FIG. 29.15. Alveolar cell carcinoma of disseminated type.

excluded this might suggest an alveolar cell carcinoma. The shadows may be nodular and of very variable size and extent. They are often 5–10 mm in diameter and may be distributed over a localized area, throughout a lobe, throughout one lung or in both lungs, either diffusely or patchily. The appearances may closely resemble tuberculosis. Sometimes the shadows are confluent and mimic pneumonia, segmental, lobar or lobular. Occasionally the lesions are cavitated. Pleural effusion is not uncommon.

DIAGNOSIS

In the case of a solitary lesion the problem of diagnosis is similar to that of bronchial carcinoma (p. 517) and the correct diagnosis is usually only made after resection, or occasionally by cytology. Multifocal lesions present a much more difficult diagnostic problem. It is most important to bear the possibility of alveolar cell carcinoma in mind when faced with a difficult clinical and radiological problem. The initial impression is usually that the lesion is an inflammatory one but suspicion may be aroused by its failure to clear with chemotherapy directed towards an acute respiratory infection and the absence of supporting evidence for tuberculosis. Occasionally tuberculosis and alveolar cell carcinoma coexist. We have seen a patient in hospital for proved pulmonary tuberculosis who developed two new shadows in close proximity over a period of 6 weeks. As he was on effective chemotherapy it was thought that the lesions could not be tuberculous and the fact that there were two of them suggested the possibility of alveolar cell carcinoma. This proved to be correct when the lesions were resected.

As the larger bronchi are not normally invaded bronchoscopy is of little diagnostic value but a number of cases have been diagnosed by cytology. Lung biopsy, by needle, high speed drill or sometimes open thoracotomy, has a place. In a patient with marked bronchorrhoea electrophoresis is said to have shown a particular glycoprotein type not observed in bronchorrhoea due to other causes [124].

TREATMENT AND PROGNOSIS

In solitary lesions the prognosis after resection seems appreciably better than in the case of bronchial carcinoma. Munnell and Keller [91] described 7 such cases, all of which were living and well 1½–4 years later. As already mentioned, they summarized 5 series in which a total of 108 solitary lesions were resected and 69% of the patients were living after varying periods. Hewlett et al. [70] reported that 82% of their patients survived for more than 2 years after resection. On the other hand the prognosis for the diffuse lesions seems poor even when they are resectable. Clagett et al. [27] reported no survivors after 5 years. Nevertheless if the tumour is resectable this should certainly be attempted as it is the patient's only hope of cure. The tumour is said not to be susceptible to radiotherapy or chemotherapy [124].

In most cases with diffuse lesions the prognosis is poor and death follows relatively rapidly. On the other hand there are a few proved cases in which very long survival, even as long as 14 years, has occurred without specific treatment [124].

REFERENCES

[1] ABBEY SMITH R. (1959) Lung cancer in coal miners. Br. J. industr. Med. 16, 318.
[2] ADVISORY COMMITTEE TO THE SURGEON GENERAL OF THE PUBLIC HEALTH SERVICE (1964) Smoking and Health. Washington, U.S. Department of Health, Education and Welfare.
[3] AUERBACH O., STOUT A.P., HAMMOND E.C. & GARFINKEL L. (1961) Changes in bronchial epithelium in relation to cigarette smoking and in relation to lung cancer. New Engl. J. Med. 265, 253.
[4] BARRAN KATHARINE M., HELM W.H. & KING D.A. (1965) Bronchial carcinoma treated with nitrogen mustard and cyclophosphamide. Br. med. J ii, 685.
[5] BARTTER F.C. (1963) Hypertrophic osteoarthropathy. In Cecil-Loeb Textbook of Medicine, ed. Beeson P.B. and McDermott W. 11th Edition. Philadelphia, Saunders.
[6] BASS B.H. (1960) Nitrogen mustard in the palliation of lung cancer. Br. med. J. i, 617.
[7] BEAVER O.L. & SHAPIRO J.L. (1956) A consideration of chronic pulmonary parenchymal inflammation and alveolar cell carcinoma with regard to a possible etiologic relationship. Am. J. Med. 21, 879.
[8] BELCHER J.R. (1956) Lobectomy for bronchial carcinoma. Lancet i, 349.

[9] BELCHER J.R. & ANDERSON R. (1965) Surgical treatment of carcinoma of the bronchus. *Br. med. J.* i, 948.

[10] BERGH N.P. & SCHERSTÉN T. (1965) Bronchogenic carcinoma. A follow up study of a surgically treated series with special reference to the prognostic significance of lymph node metastases. *Acta chir. scand., Suppl.* 347.

[11] BIDSTRUP P.L. & CASE R.A.M. (1956) Carcinoma of the lung in workmen in the bichromates-producing industry in Great Britain. *Br. J. industr. Med.* 13, 260.

[12] BIGNALL J.R. (1958) Treatment and survival. In *Carcinoma of the Lung*, ed. Bignall J.R. Edinburgh, Livingstone.

[13] BOUCOT KATHARINE R., CARNAHAN W., COOPER D.A., NEALON T.Jr., OTTENBERG D.J. & THEODOS P.A. (1955) Philadelphia pulmonary neoplasm research project. Preliminary report. *J. Am. med. Ass.* 157, 440.

[14] BOUCOT K.R., COOPER D.A., WEISS W. & CARNAHAN W.J. (1964) Appearance of first roentgenographic abnormalities due to lung cancer. *J. Am. med. Ass.* 190, 1103.

[15] BRAIN LORD (1963) The neurological complications of neoplasms. *Lancet* i, 179.

[16] BRETT G.Z. (1963) Lung cancer and previous respiratory disease. *Tubercle, Lond.* 44, 285.

[17] BRETT G.Z. (1966) The presymptomatic diagnosis of lung cancer. *Proc. R. Soc. Med.* 59, 1208.

[18] BREWIN T.B. (1966) Alcohol intolerance in neoplastic disease. *Br. med. J.* ii, 437.

[19] BROMLEY L.L. & SZUR L. (1955) Combined radiotherapy and resection for carcinoma of the bronchus. Experiences with 60 patients. *Lancet* ii, 937.

[20] BURTON PATRICIA A. & CUNLIFFE W.J. (1966) A comparison of tetracycline fluorescence and exfoliative cytology in the detection of malignancy. *Lancet* i, 1002.

[21] CAMPBELL A.H. (1961) The association of lung cancer and tuberculosis. *Australas. Ann. Med.* 10, 129.

[22] CAPPELN C.Jr., EFSKIND L. & POPPE E. (1961) Bronchial carcinoma with special regard to the prognosis. *Acta path. microbiol. scand., Suppl.* 148, 23.

[23] CARLENS E. (1959) Mediastinoscopy: a method for inspection and tissue biopsy in the superior mediastinum. *Dis. Chest* 36, 343.

[24] CASE R.A.M. & LEA A.J. (1955) Mustard gas poisoning, chronic bronchitis and lung cancer, An investigation into the possibility that poisoning by mustard gas in the 1914–18 war might be a factor in the production of neoplasia. *Br. J. prev. soc. Med.* 9, 62.

[25] CASE R.A.M. (1958) The influence of improved diagnosis on the recorded death rates. In *Carcinoma of the Lung*, p. 21, ed. Bignall J.R. Edinburgh, Livingstone.

[26] CHIEF MEDICAL OFFICER, MINISTRY OF HEALTH (1967) *On the State of the Public Health.* London, H.M. Stationery Office.

[27] CLAGETT O.T., ALLEN T.H., PAYNE W.S. & WOOLNER L.B. (1964) The surgical treatment of pulmonary neoplasms: A 10 year experience. *J. thorac. cardiovasc. Surg.* 48, 391.

[28] COLLIER F.C., BLAKEMORE W.S., KYLE R.H. ENTERLINE H.T., KIRBY C.K. & JOHNSON J. (1957) Carcinoma of the lung: Factors which influence 5 year survival with special reference to blood vessel invasion. *Ann. Surg.* 146, 417.

[29] CROFT P.B. & WILKINSON MARCIA (1965) The incidence of carcinomatous neuromyopathy in patients with various types of carcinoma. *Brain* 88, 427.

[30] CROFTON EILEEN & CROFTON J. (1963) Influence of smoking on mortality from various diseases in Scotland and in England and Wales. An analysis by cohorts. *Br. med. J.* ii, 1161.

[31] DAVIES D.F. (1966) A review of detection methods for the early diagnosis of lung cancer. *J. chron. Dis.* 19, 819.

[32] DAVIS E.W., PEABODY J.W.Jr. & KATZ S. (1956) The solitary pulmonary nodule. *J. thorac. Surg.* 32, 728.

[33] DAYAN A.D., CROFT P.B. & WILKINSON MARCIA (1965) Association of carcinomatous neuromyopathy with different histological types of carcinoma of the lung. *Brain* 88, 435.

[34] DEAN G. (1959) Lung cancer among white South Africans. *Br. med. J.* ii, 852.

[35] DEAN G. (1961) Lung cancer among white South Africans. Report of a further study. *Br. med. J.* ii, 1599.

[36] DEELEY T.J. & SINGH S.P. (1967) Treatment of inoperable carcinoma of the bronchus by megavoltage x-rays. *Thorax* 22, 562.

[37] DOLL R. & HILL A.B. (1952) A study of the aetiology of carcinoma of the lung. *Br. med. J.* ii, 1271.

[38] DOLL R. (1955a) Etiology of lung cancer. *Advanc. Cancer Res.* 3, 1.

[39] DOLL R. (1955b) Mortality from lung cancer in asbestos workers. *Br. J. industr. Med.* 12, 81.

[40] DOLL R., HILL A.B. & KREYBERG L. (1957) The significance of cell type in relation to the aetiology of lung cancer. *Br. J. Cancer* 11, 43.

[41] DOLL R. (1958) Specific industrial causes. In *Carcinoma of the Lung*, ed. Bignall J.R. Edinburgh, Livingstone.

[42] DOLL R. & HILL A.B. (1964) Mortality in relation to smoking: 10 years' observation of British doctors. *Br. med. J.* i, 1399, 1460.

[43] DOLL R., FISHER R.E.W., GAMMON E.J., GUNN W., HUGHES G.O., TYRER F.H. & WILSON W. (1965) Mortality of gasworkers, with special reference to cancers of the lung and bladder, chronic bronchitis and pneumoconiosis. *Br. J. industr. Med.* 22, 1.

[44] DUGUID HELEN L. & HUISH D.W. (1963) Clinical evaluation of cytodiagnosis in bronchial carcinoma. *Br. med. J.* ii, 287.

[45] DUNGAL N. (1961) Lung cancer in Iceland. *Lancet* ii, 1350.

[46] EASTCOTT D.F. (1956) The epidemiology of lung cancer in New Zealand. *Lancet* i, 37.

[47] EDITORIAL (1957) Industrial lung cancer. *Lancet* i, 411.

[48] EDITORIAL (1961) Arsenic and lung cancer. *Br. med. J.* i, 115.

[49] EDITORIAL (1962) The cigarette as co-carcinogen. *Lancet* i, 85.

[50] EDITORIAL (1964) Asbestos and malignancy. *Br. med. J.* ii, 202.

[51] EDITORIAL (1965) Treatment of lung cancer. *Br. med. J.* ii, 604.

[52] EDITORIAL (1967) Hormones and histones? *Lancet* i, 86.

[53] ENTWISTLE C.C., FENTEM P.H. & JACOBS A. (1964) Red cell aplasia with carcinoma of the bronchus. *Br. med. J.* ii, 1504.

[54] FAULDS J.S. & STEWART M.J. (1956) Carcinoma of the lung in haematite miners. *J. Path. Bact.* 72, 353.

[55] FLAVELL G. (1962) Conservatism in surgical treatment of bronchial carcinoma. A review of 826 personal operations. *Br. med. J.* i, 284.

[56] GAULT JOAN H. & ROGAN MARY C. (1959) Lung function studies on bronchial carcinoma. *Scot. med. J.* 4, 35.

[57] GIFFORD J.H. & WADDINGTON J.K.B. (1957) Review of 464 cases of carcinoma of the lung treated by resection. *Br. med. J.* i, 723.

[58] GILLAM P.M.S., HEAF P.J.D., HOFFBRAND B.I. & HILTON GWEN (1964) Chronic bronchitis and radiotherapy of the lung. *Lancet* i, 1245.

[59] GILSON J.C. (1966) Health hazards of asbestos. Recent studies on its biological effects. *Trans. Soc. Occupational Med.* 16, 62.

[60] GOLDMAN K.P. (1965a) Mortality of coalminers from carcinoma of the lung. *Br. J. industr. Med.* 22, 72.

[61] GOLDMAN K.P. (1965b) Prognosis of coalminers with cancer of the lung. *Thorax* 20, 170.

[62] GOLDMAN K.P. (1965c) Histology of lung cancer in relation to prognosis. *Thorax* 20, 298.

[63] GRAY BRENDA (1964) Sputum cytodiagnosis in bronchial carcinoma. A comparative study of 2 methods. *Lancet* ii, 549.

[64] GRENVILLE-MATHERS R. & TRENCHARD H.J. (1964) Cytotoxic drugs in bronchial carcinoma. *Lancet* ii, 1200.

[65] HAMMOND E.I. & HORN D. (1958) Smoking and death rates—report on 44 months of follow up of 187,783 men. *J. Am. med. Ass.* 166, 1159, 1294.

[66] HAROLD J.T. (1952) Lymphangitis carcinomatosa of the lungs. *Quart. J. Med.* 45 (*N.S. 21*), 353.

[67] HATTORI S., MATSUDA M., SUGIYAMA T. & MATSUDA H. (1964) Cytological diagnosis of early lung cancer: Brushing method under x-ray television fluoroscopy. *Dis. Chest* 45, 129.

[68] HAYATA Y., MOTONOBU H., OHO K. & SHINOI K. (1964) Significance of carcinoma cells in the blood relative to surgery of pulmonary carcinoma. *Dis. Chest* 46, 51.

[69] HEPPER N.G.G., HERSKOVIC T., WITTEN D.M., MULDER D.W. & WOOLNER L.B. (1966) Thoracic inlet tumours. *Ann. intern. Med.* 64, 979.

[70] HEWLETT T.H., GOMEZ A.C., ARONSTAM E.M. & STEER A. (1964) Bronchiolar carcinoma of the lung. Review of 39 patients. *J. thorac. cardiovasc. Surg.* 48, 614.

[71] HOBBS C.B. & MILLER A.L. (1966) Review of endocrine syndromes associated with tumours of nonendocrine origin. *J. clin. Path.* 19, 119.

[72] HOLLING H.E., BRODEY R.S. & BOLAND H. CHRISTINE (1961) Pulmonary hypertrophic osteoarthropathy. *Lancet* ii, 1269.

[73] HÖST H. (1960) The value of periodic mass chest roentgenographic surveys in the detection of primary bronchial carcinoma in Norway. *Cancer* 13, 1167.

[74] HUEPER W.C. (1957) Environmental factors in the production of human cancer. In *Cancer*, Vol. I. Ed. Raven R.W. London, Butterworth.

[75] JERI R. (1963) *Las Manifestaciones Neurologicas del Carcinoma Broncogenica: Observaciones Clinico-Patologicas en una Serie Consecutiva de 383 Pacientes.* Lima. Quoted Editorial (1966) Neurological complications of lung cancer. *Lancet* i, 700.

[76] KENNAWAY E.L. & KENNAWAY M.N. (1953) Cancer of the lung in coalminers. *Br. J. Cancer* 7, 10.

[77] KENNAWAY E. & LINDSEY A.J. (1958) Some possible exogenous factors in the causation of lung cancer. *Br. med. Bull.* 14, 124.

[78] KREYBERG L. (1954) The significance of histological typing in the study of the epidemiology of primary epithelial lung tumours: A study of 466 cases. *Br. J. Cancer* 8, 199.

[79] KUPER S.W.A. & BIGNALL J.R. (1966) Survival after resection of bronchial carcinomas. Significance of tumour cells in the blood. *Lancet* i, 10.

[80] KUPER S.W.A., STRADLING P., DAVIS JANE & SHORTRIDGE DILYS (1966) The use of soluble swabs in exfoliative cytology of the bronchus and hollow viscera. *Lancet* ii, 680.

[81] LEES A.W. (1961) Tretamine compared with nitrogen mustard in the palliation of inoperable lung cancer. *Lancet* ii, 900.

[82] LEMON F.R., WALDEN R.T. & WOODS R.W. (1964) Cancer of the lung and mouth in Seventh-day Adventists: preliminary report on a population study. *Cancer (Philad.)* 17, 486.

[83] LINTON A.L. & HUTTON I. (1965) Hyponatraemia and bronchial carcinoma: Therapy with nitrogen mustard. *Br. med. J.* **ii**, 277.

[84] LITTLE J.B., RADFORD E.P.Jr., McCOMBS L. & HUNT VILMA R. (1965) Distribution of Polonium^{210} in pulmonary tissues of cigarette smokers. *New Engl. J. Med.* **273**, 1343.

[85] McCORMACK R.J.M. (1967) The results of surgical resection of bronchial carcinoma detected at mass radiography surveys. Personal communication (to be published).

[86] MALLAMS J.T., PAULSON D.L., COLLIER R.E. & SHAW R.R. (1964) Presurgical irradiation in bronchogenic carcinoma, superior sulcus type. *Radiology* **82**, 1050.

[87] MARCHAL M. & MARCHAL MARIE-THÉRÈSE (1951) Nouvelle méthode de ciné-densigraphie étalonné permettant le diagnostic differentiel du cancer du poumon. *C. r. Acad. Sci., Paris* **233**, 458.

[88] MEDICAL RESEARCH COUNCIL (1966) Comparative trial of surgery and radiotherapy for the primary treatment of small-celled or oat-celled carcinoma of the bronchus. *Lancet* **ii**, 979.

[89] MELAMED M.R., KOSS L.G. & CLIFFTON E.E. (1963) Roentgenologically occult lung cancer diagnosed by cytology. Report of 12 cases. *Cancer (Philad.)* **16**, 1537.

[90] MORRISON R., DEELEY T.J. & CLELAND W.P. (1963) The treatment of carcinoma of the bronchus. A clinical trial to compare surgery and supervoltage radiotherapy. *Lancet* **i**, 683.

[91] MUNNELL E.R. & KELLER D.F. (1966) Solitary bronchiolar (alveolar cell) carcinoma of the lung. *J. thorac. cardiovasc. Surg.* **52**, 261.

[92] NASH F., MORGAN M. & TOMKINS G. (1961) Detection of lung cancer. (Letter) *Lancet* **ii**, 46.

[93] NICHOLSON W.F., FOX M. & BRYCE A.G. (1957) Review of 910 cases of bronchial carcinoma with results of treatment. *Lancet* **i**, 296.

[94] NOHL-OSER H.C. (1966) Prognostic factors which may influence surgical management. In *Some Aspects of Carcinoma of the Bronchus and Other Malignant Diseases of the Lung.* Symposium, King Edward VII Hospital, Midhurst, U.K., p. 105.

[95] OCHSNER A., OCHSNER A.Jr., H'DOUBLER C. & BLALOCK J. (1960) Bronchogenic carcinoma *Dis. Chest.* **37**, 1.

[96] OGILVIE C., HARRIS L.H., MEECHAM J. & RYDER G. (1963) Ten years after pneumonectomy for carcinoma. *Br. med. J.* **i**, 1111.

[97] OKA S., SHIRAISHI K., ISAWA T., GOTO Y. & YASUDA T. (1967) Pulmonary diffusing capacity—its evaluation by scintillation scanning of the lungs in lung cancer. *Am. Rev. resp. Dis.* **95**, 239.

[98] OVERHOLT R.H. & BOUGAS J.A. (1956) Common factors in lung cancer survivors. *J. thorac. Surg.* **32**, 508.

[99] PIKE M.C. & DOLL R. (1965) Age at onset of lung cancer: Significance in relation to effect of smoking. *Lancet* **i**, 665.

[100] POULSEN O. (1963) Cytostatic treatment of lung cancer. *Acta chir. scand.* **125**, 498.

[101] RELE J.R. (1960) Demographic approach to the problem of the connexion between lung cancer and smoking. *Br. J. prev. soc. Med.* **14**, 181.

[102] REYNDERS H. (1964) Mediastinoscopy in bronchogenic carcinoma. *Dis. Chest* **45**, 606.

[103] RIENHOFF W.F., TALBERT J.L. & WOOD S. (1965) Bronchogenic carcinoma: A study of cases treated at Johns Hopkins Hospital from 1933 to 1958. *Ann. Surg.* **161**, 674.

[104] ROBSON A.O. & JELLIFFE A.M. (1963) Medicinal arsenic poisoning and lung cancer. *Br. med. J.* **ii**, 207.

[105] ROCKEY E.E., SPEER F.D., THOMPSON S.A., AHN K.J. & HIROSE T. (1962) Experimental study on effect of cigarette smoke condensate on bronchial mucosa. *J. Am. med. Ass.* **182**, 1094.

[106] ROSS E.J. (1965) Endocrine and metabolic consequences of carcinoma of the bronchus. *Proc. roy. Soc. Med.* **58**, 485.

[107] SELIKOFF I.J., CHURG J. & HAMMOND E.C. (1964) Asbestos exposure and neoplasm. *J. Am. med. Ass.* **188**, 22.

[108] SHINTON N.K. (1963a) The histological classification of lower respiratory tract tumours. *Br. J. Cancer* **17**, 213.

[109] SHINTON N.K. (1963b) Difference in biological characteristics of various histological types of lower respiratory tract tumours. *Br. J. Cancer* **17**, 222.

[110] SMITH R.A. (1963) Surgery in the treatment of locally advanced lung carcinoma. *Thorax* **18**, 21.

[111] SOMNER A.R. (1959) Observer disagreements in the interpretation of hilar shadows in chest radiographs. *Tubercle* **40**, 245.

[112] SPENCER H. (1962) *Pathology of the Lung.* Oxford, Pergamon Press.

[113] SPRINGETT V.H. (1966) The beginning of the end of the increase in mortality from carcinoma of the lung. *Thorax* **21**, 132.

[114] STEINITZ RUTH (1965) Pulmonary tuberculosis and carcinoma of the lung. A survey from two population based disease registers. *Am. Rev. resp. Dis.* **92**, 758.

[115] STEVENS A.E. (1963) Mediastinal pain in bronchial carcinoma. *Lancet* **i**, 1230.

[116] STOCKS P. (1959) Cancer and bronchitis mortality in relation to atmospheric deposit and smoke. *Br. med. J.* **i**, 74.

[117] STOCKS P. (1960) On the relations between atmospheric pollution in urban and rural

localities and mortality from cancer, bronchitis and pneumonia, with particular reference to 3:4 benzopyrene, beryllium, molybdenum, vanadium and arsenic. *Br. J. Cancer* **14**, 397.

[118] STOREY C.F., KNUDTSON K.P. & LAWRENCE B.J. (1953) Bronchiolar ('alveolar cell') carcinoma of the lung. *J. thorac. Surg.* **26**, 331.

[119] SUTTON M. (1960) The functional effect of pulmonary irradiation. *Br. med. J.* **ii**, 838.

[120] SZUR L. & BROMLEY L.L. (1956) Obstruction of the superior vena cava in carcinoma of bronchus. *Br. med. J.* **ii**, 1273.

[121] TAYLOR A.B., SHINTON N.K. & WATERHOUSE J.A.H. (1963) Histology of bronchial carcinoma in relation to prognosis. *Thorax* **18**, 178.

[122] TODD G.F. (1966) *Statistics of Smoking in the United Kingdom* Research Paper I, 4th Edition. London, Tobacco Research Council.

[123] VAN DER WAL ANNA M. (1964) *Chronic Non-Specific Lung Diseases (C.N.S.L.D.) as a Condition in the Pathogenesis of Lung Cancer.* M.D. Thesis. Groningen, Netherlands: N.V. Dijkstra.

[124] VIRÁGH Z. & WOODS J.R. (1962) Alveolar carcinoma of the lung. *Med. Thorac* **19**, 129.

[125] WAGONER J.K., MILLER R.W., LUNDIN F.E.Jr., FRAUMENI J.F. & HAIJ MARIAN E. (1963) Unusual cancer mortality among a group of underground metal miners. *New. Engl. J. Med.* **269**, 284.

[126] WAGONER J.K., ARCHER V.E., CARROLL B.E., HOLADAY D.A. & LAWRENCE P.A. (1964) Cancer mortality patterns among U.S. uranium miners and millers, 1950 through 1962. *J. Nat. Cancer Inst.* **32**, 787.

[127] WAGNER H.N.Jr., LOPEZ-MAJANO V., TOW D.E. & LANGAN J.K. (1965) Radioisotope scanning of lungs in early diagnosis of bronchogenic carcinoma. *Lancet* **i**, 344.

[128] WALTER J.B. & PRYCE D.M. (1955) The site of origin of lung cancer and its relation to histological type. *Thorax* **10**, 117.

[129] WANKA J. (1965) Alcohol-induced pain associated with adenocarcinoma of the bronchus. *Br. med. J.* **ii**, 87.

[130] WOOLNER L.B., ANDERSEN H.A. & BERNATZ P.E. (1960) 'Occult' carcinoma of the bronchus: a study of 15 cases of *in situ* or early invasive bronchogenic carcinoma. *Dis. Chest* **37**, 278.

[131] WYNDER E.L., FERRARI E. & FORTI E. (1961) Lung cancer in Venice. An epidemiological study. *Lancet* **ii**, 1347.

CHAPTER 30

Other Pulmonary Tumours

In this chapter the remaining pulmonary tumours will not be dealt with in the order given in the classification on p. 517 where they are grouped according to the degree of malignancy. Instead the more important tumours will be dealt with first. All the tumours described in this chapter are very much less common than carcinoma of the bronchus.

PULMONARY LYMPHOMATA
(Malignant Reticuloses)

HODGKIN'S DISEASE (Lymphadenoma)
PRIMARY HODGKIN'S DISEASE OF THE LUNG [30]

Hodgkin's disease may occasionally first arise in lymph glands related to the bronchi and may remain localized for months or even occasionally years.

PATHOLOGY
Macroscopically the tumour is a greyish yellow, fleshy, nodular or lobulated mass, often with small satellite lesions and occasionally with separate larger nodules in other lobes. The tumour often invades the bronchi. Lipoid pneumonia may occur in the adjacent lung. Microscopically the features are those of Hodgkin's disease anywhere.

CLINICAL FEATURES
As with Hodgkin's disease in general, patients tend to be younger than those with carcinoma of the bronchus. Some patients with this condition have no symptoms at the time of diagnosis, the lesion being detected at routine radiography. Cough, chest pain, fever and pruritus are the commonest symptoms. Haemoptysis sometimes occurs.

RADIOLOGY
The tumour is commonest in the upper lobes. There is nothing specific about it radiologically. Circumscribed shadows are seen, usually unilateral but occasionally bilateral. Air-containing bronchi may be visible as elongated translucencies in the opacity. Cavitation may occur.

DIAGNOSIS
By definition no lymphadenomatous glands are palpable elsewhere. Bronchoscopy is usually unrevealing but sometimes a positive biopsy has been obtained; most such cases are found to have mediastinal glandular involvement at thoracotomy. Indeed the majority are diagnosed at thoracotomy carried out when the shadows have failed to clear after repeated radiological observation, with or without chemotherapy. The diagnosis may be made by frozen section at operation.

TREATMENT
The recommended treatment is resection of the lesion with radiotherapy 3–4 weeks later.

PROGNOSIS
With the treatment mentioned there have been a number of 5-year survivals.

SECONDARY HODGKIN'S DISEASE OF THE LUNG [13, 15, 49 & 62]
The lung is said to be involved in Hodgkin's disease in about 40% of all cases. In about one fifth of these there is no evidence of mediastinal gland enlargement at autopsy [30].

PATHOLOGY AND RADIOLOGY
The pathological and radiological manifestations are varied but may be listed as follows:

(1) Hilar glandular enlargement with direct lung invasion (a) from the hilum with either fine or coarse streaking radiating into the lung,

or (b) direct invasion through the mediastinal pleura. This is the commonest appearance [62].

(2) Hilar glandular enlargement with intra- and peribronchial spread, which will give rise to coarse streaking radiating from the hilum on the x-ray.

(3) More or less lobar infiltrations which fairly frequently cavitate and may resemble tuberculosis.

(4) Fine or coarse unevenly disseminated nodules which tend to be well-defined at first but later irregular. They occasionally cavitate. The appearances often resemble tuberculosis, which may of course also complicate this disease. The apices tend to be spared in Hodgkin's disease.

(5) Confluent lobular foci with associated involvement of the mediastinal lymph glands.

(6) Disseminated rounded lesions resembling metastatic tumour.

(7) Miliary appearances. The shadows tend to be larger and vaguer than in miliary tuberculosis.

(8) Occasionally there is a unilateral hilar mass radiologically closely resembling a carcinoma of the bronchus.

(9) In addition to the above there is sometimes direct invasion of the ribs giving rise to an appearance like actinomycosis (p. 290). Pleural effusion may occur and may be of any type, serous, haemorrhagic, purulent or even chylous.

CLINICAL FEATURES

Cough and dyspnoea are the most common clinical features. Sometimes there may be chest pain or haemoptysis. Dyspnoea may be very severe if there is a large pleural effusion or diffuse infiltration causing the restrictive type of respiratory impairment.

DIAGNOSIS

Purely on radiological grounds it may be difficult to differentiate Hodgkin's disease involving the lung from tuberculosis, carcinoma or chronic pneumonia. If the mediastinal glands are enlarged in a patient of the relevant age group tuberculosis or chronic pneumonia are unlikely, though enlarged

mediastinal glands are sometimes seen in postprimary tuberculosis in non-Europeans. Enlargement of lymph glands elsewhere, or a palpable spleen, may give the clue or a gland biopsy may be carried out by mediastinoscopy if no glands are palpable elsewhere. Mediastinal lymph glands enlarged by Hodgkin's disease are likely to respond more rapidly to radiotherapy than those due to carcinoma.

TREATMENT

Treatment is that of Hodgkin's disease in general, that is radiotherapy or chemotherapy. Unfortunately intrapulmonary lesions are said to respond less well than those in the lymph glands [16, 46 & 62].

LYMPHOSARCOMA AND RETICULUM CELL SARCOMA
PRIMARY LYMPHOSARCOMA [46]

It is rare for lymphosarcoma to arise as a primary lesion in the lung but, like primary lymphosarcoma of the stomach, the lesion is more benign than lymphosarcoma arising in lymph glands. Most patients are over the age of 50 and there is a male predominance.

PATHOLOGY AND RADIOLOGY

Primary lymphosarcoma is rather commoner in the upper lobes than elsewhere. It may consist of a discrete rounded opacity on the x-ray or a massive homogeneous density with indefinite borders. The appearances are quite undiagnostic.

CLINICAL FEATURES

In more than 50% of reported cases patients were asymptomatic at diagnosis, the condition being picked up on routine x-ray. Cough, haemoptysis, weight loss, malaise and mild chest or shoulder pain are among the symptoms recorded. In some cases bronchial compression or a granular appearance of the mucosa has been seen at bronchoscopy and in a few the sputum has been positive for malignant cells.

DIAGNOSIS

Unless the diagnosis has been made by

bronchial biopsy or sputum cytology, or by biopsy of a metastatic gland, the nature of the lesion can usually only be established at thoracotomy or perhaps percutaneous lung biopsy. Most patients are operated on under the suspicion that the lesion is a carcinoma of the bronchus. If there are no metastases detectable the results of operation are surprisingly good, the prognosis with lobectomy being as good as that with pneumonectomy and better than in bronchial carcinoma.

SECONDARY INVOLVEMENT OF THE LUNG BY LYMPHOSARCOMA OR RETICULUM CELL SARCOMA

The lung or pleura is said to be involved in about 50% of such cases at autopsy, pleural deposits being more common than intrapulmonary metastases [55]. It is commonest in early middle age and in women. Clinically and radiologically the manifestations are the same as those of Hodgkin's disease [16]. The order of sensitivity to radiotherapy is said to be

(1) lymphosarcoma,
(2) Hodgkin's disease,
(3) reticulum cell sarcoma [49].

LEUKAEMIA [16, 22, 23, 49, 55 & 62]

PATHOLOGY AND RADIOLOGY

Mediastinal adenopathy, as part of generalized adenopathy, occurs in about 20% of cases of leukaemia. It is unusual to find mediastinal lymph gland enlargement without enlarged lymph glands elsewhere. In acute and chronic lymphatic leukaemia large mediastinal masses are common in the child; in adults often only the bronchopulmonary group are involved and the appearances may resemble sarcoidosis [49]. In myeloid leukaemia the adenopathy is minimal and late. In monocytic leukaemia there is frequently generalized lymphadenopathy which may include enlargement of the mediastinal nodes. Pulmonary shadows in the x-ray are most often not due directly to leukaemia but to complicating pneumonia, tuberculosis, infarction, abscess or fungal infection [22]. However, gross infiltration may occur, either localized or generalized. If the white blood count is greater than half a million per mm^3 the blood becomes viscous, the capillaries distended, the lung compliance decreased and diffuse streaky shadows may be obvious on the x-ray [55]. Pulmonary infiltrations are commoner in lymphatic than in myeloid leukamia. They may be unilateral or bilateral. There is seldom direct invasion of lung tissue from the mediastinal lymph glands, as occurs frequently in Hodgkin's disease. Linear, nodular, pneumonic or miliary shadows may be seen and pleural effusion is common. It is said that gross interstitial fibrosis can occur in the lung in cases where leukaemia has been complicated by myelofibrosis [55]. In cases complicated by *mycosis fungoides* x-ray of the chest may show a mediastinal mass and impressive lung infiltration of a lymphosarcomatous type [62].

CLINICAL FEATURES

In general the clinical features are those of leukaemia. Dyspnoea, cough and haemotysis may suggest pulmonary involvement, although, as mentioned above, the pulmonary symptoms are often due to complicating infections or infarcts.

TREATMENT

Treatment is that of the primary leukaemia.

BRONCHIAL ADENOMA

This term was originally applied to bronchial tumours which were thought to be benign but some of which have been shown subsequently to have malignant potentialities. The 2 major subgroups, *carcinoid tumours* and *cylindromata*, are now generally regarded as distinct tumours though, as they have many characteristics in common, they will be considered together here. Payne *et al.* [42] classify these tumours into 4 subgroups:

(1) Carcinoid tumours.
(2) Cylindromata (adenoid cystic and carcinoma).
(3) Mucoepidermoid tumours.
(4) Mixed tumours similar to the mixed tumours of salivary glands.

Approximately 90% of these tumours belong to the carcinoid group. Most of the rest are cylindromata and groups 3 and 4 are very rare.

FREQUENCY

Most series have been reported from surgical centres and, taken as a whole, have formed 1–6% of the numbers of bronchial carcinomata seen in the same period [20, 39, 54, 59, 60 & 66].

AGE AND SEX

Cases tend to be diagnosed at an earlier age than carcinoma of the bronchus. Mean ages in 2 series have been as low as 33 [54] and 28 [19]. In some earlier series it was suggested that there was a major female predominance [59] but later series have indicated that the excess in females, if there is any, is only slight.

PATHOLOGY

Although a *carcinoid* tumour sometimes presents as a pedunculated endobronchial mass of polyp (and this is the usual presentation of mucoepidermoid tumours), it is much more common for a carcinoid to form an 'iceberg' with a small intraluminal protuberance and a much larger mass outside the bronchus. Carcinoid tumours may occur in any of the large bronchi, 90% of them within bronchoscopic vision. There is a slight predilection for both lower lobes and for the right lung. They occasionally occur as peripheral tumours. *Cylindromata* tend to infiltrate the wall of the bronchus in a tubular fashion and often spread outside the wall, developing malignant characteristics. They most often occur in the large bronchi but may also affect the trachea where they are second in frequency only to carcinoma. Carcinoids are greyish-white or pink tumours and on section are often intersected with fibrous tissue. The endobronchial part of a cylindroma is often necrotic and on section may obviously contain mucus. Carcinoid tumours are said to be occasionally multicentric [39]. When a cylindroma is apparently multiple

this is said always to be due to metastases [42]. Mixed cell tumours behave like mixed cell tumours of the salivary glands.

Microscopically, carcinoid tumours consist of small, uniformly staining cells in solid clumps with trabeculae and pseudoacini [55]. Mitotic figures are rare. There is a vascular stroma which accounts for the tendency to bleed on biopsy; the stroma may degenerate to form hyaline tissue which may calcify or even form bone. Argentaffin staining cells have been demonstrated in some of these tumours [65]. The tumour surface is normally covered with intact bronchial epithelium, so that cytological examination of the sputum is usually unhelpful.

It has been suggested that carcinoid tumours are derived from vestigial bronchial buds, the tumour itself developing from outlying cells of neural origin [55]. It has been claimed that other congenital abnormalities have been found in these cases but Overholt *et al.* [39] found only one such abnormality among 60 patients.

Cylindromata consist of pleomorphic, darkly staining cells arranged in interlacing cylinders or tubes which may contain PAS-positive epithelial mucus. Occasionally the cells may be ciliated. They are probably derived from the bronchial glands [42]. There is usually more mitosis than in the carcinoids and these tumours are more likely to metastasize. There is often a loose collagenous stroma around the cells and this may become myxomatous and resemble cartilage. Cylindromata are particularly invasive locally. Both types of tumour may metastasize to the local lymph glands and occasionally to the liver and elsewhere. The *mucoepidermoid tumours* consist histologically of an 'intimate admixture of well differentiated mucous cells and benign-appearing squamous elements' [41]. The histology of the *mixed tumours* is similar to that of mixed tumours in the salivary glands [42].

All these tumours may give rise to secondary mechanical effects due to blocking of the bronchial lumen. The most common is collapse of a segment, lobe or lung, according to the position of the tumour. Occasionally there may be a check valve effect resulting in obstructive emphysema. Secondary infection beyond the blockage is common and may result in bronchiectasis, sometimes very gross (p. 347), suppurative pneumonia, lung abscess or empyema.

In a review of the literature McBurney *et al.* [33] concluded that about 10% of all bronchial adenomata gave rise to metastases; the incidence being 3 times higher in cylindromata than in carcinoid tumours. This may be an underestimate, as the published reports are unlikely to represent a complete follow-up.

CLINICAL FEATURES

Clinical manifestations may be due to (1) the tumour itself, (2) the mechanical effects of the tumour, (3) secondary infection, (4) metastases, or (5) general effects deriving from the products of the tumour (carcinoid tumours only).

(1) *Clinical manifestations of the tumour itself* consist mainly of cough and haemoptysis. Irritating *cough* is common. Recurrent small *haemoptyses* are a classical feature of bronchial adenoma, though they may not occur in more than 50% [59]. They are sometimes related to menstruation [19]. Haemoptysis may occasionally be severe. Bleeding is most often related to ulceration of the tumour but sometimes to infection beyond it.

(2) *Mechanical effects of the tumour.* Collapse may give rise to *breathlessness* which may also occasionally occur because of obstructive emphysema of a considerable portion of the lung. Collapse is sometimes intermittent. There may be *unilateral wheeze* owing to partial obstruction of the bronchus. This may occur without radiological abnormality. Unilateral 'asthma' should always suggest a mechanical obstruction of the bronchus. Cylindromata of the trachea, if they cannot be removed or dealt with by radiotherapy, may cause death by asphyxia. Occasionally a flapping polypoid tumour may result in a bizarre *click* synchronous with respiration [39].

(3) *Secondary infection* may result in *recurrent pneumonia* or the classical symptoms of *bronchiectasis, lung abscess* or *empyema. Finger clubbing* may be present if there is chronic infection [19].

(4) *Metastases.* The symptoms due to metastases are similar to those of metastases derived from other tumours except that metastases both from carcinoids and from cylindromata appear to be a good deal more slow growing and patients may even survive several years [66].

Because the majority of these tumours are not malignant, or do not become so for a number of years, symptoms have often been present for a very long period before the diagnosis is made. In published series a history of 5 or 10 years before diagnosis is common; one of the patients of Overholt *et al.* [39] had had symptoms as long as 45 years.

(5) *General effects* may consist of the carcinoid syndrome or endocrine effects.

THE CARCINOID SYNDROME

Rarely bronchial carcinoid tumours may give rise to the carcinoid syndrome, similar to that due to carcinoid of the intestine. This only occurred in 2% of a Mayo Clinic series [42]. In this syndrome there may be intermittent *cyanotic flushes*, usually of a patchy distribution. In some patients the flush is constant and may be accompanied by telangiectasia or purpura. *Abdominal cramps* and *diarrhoea* occur. There may be *oedema* of the face and arms as well as of the dependent parts. *Wheezing* and *dyspnoea* are common. In prolonged cases *valvular disease* of the right heart develops with pulmonary stenosis, tricuspid stenosis or incompetence. In a small number of cases *pellagra-like symptoms* are present and are probably due to the competition of the tumour for dietary tryptophan [29].

It was at first thought that the syndrome was due to the production of serotonin (5-hydroxytriptamine or 5HT). Later it was found that the tumour itself might produce a serotonin precursor, 5-hydroxytryptophan (5-HTP). Both could be estimated in the blood and were readily identified by their breakdown product in the urine, 5-hydroxyindole acetic acid (5-HIAA). Most cases who had the carcinoid syndrome had metastases.

This was thought to be due to the fact that both liver and lung contain monoamine oxidase which destroys serotonin. However, cases have been reported without metastases [29]. Later, cases were found in which there were high blood serotonin and high urinary 5-HIAA but without the carcinoid syndrome [45 & 64]. Oates *et al.* [38] have recently found evidence to suggest that, although serotonin may play some part in the reaction, the most important product may be a kinin related to bradykinin. They have shown that carcinoid tumours contain an enzyme kallikrein, which can probably be released from the tumour by adrenaline (accounting perhaps for the intermittent flushing). This enzyme catalyses the formation of the kinin peptide from a plasma protein substrate. The kinin appears to alter capillary permeability and may in this way be responsible for the fibrous overgrowth on the heart valve and also for bronchoconstriction.

ENDOCRINE ABNORMALITIES

At least 5 cases of Cushing's syndrome have been reported, in 1 of which the carcinoid syndrome also occurred. There have also been 4 cases of acromegaly and 3 of multiple endocrine adenomata [42].

RADIOLOGY

If there is no secondary mechanical effect or infection the chest x-ray may be normal, as may occur with a patient presenting with irritating nonproductive cough or with haemoptysis. There may be only partial deflation of a lobe, as shown by a change in the position of a fissure or a failure of part of a lung to lighten and darken normally on radioscopy. There may be obstructive emphysema. In a majority of patients the shadow of the tumour is obscured by collapse and other secondary effects in the lung, though Soutter *et al.* [54] were able to see some portion of the tumour in nearly 50%. Specks of ossification or calcification may occasionally be seen. More peripheral tumours have occurred in 10–50% of different series. These are sometimes circular but may be elongated, oval or slightly lobulated. Such a shadow may

be partly composed of a bronchus distended with mucus [52].

DIAGNOSIS

This diagnosis should be remembered in any patient with *recurrent haemoptyses*, especially if below the usual carcinoma age. Unilateral wheeze is also suggestive of bronchial obstruction and calls for bronchoscopy. Bronchial adenoma is one of the causes of *recurrent pneumonia*. Bronchoscopy will be indicated in any patient with persistent collapse of a lung or lobe. The tumour has been visible on bronchoscopy in about 90% of most series. Carcinoid tumours are particularly liable to bleed after biopsy. Cylindromata are said to be usually covered with necrotic material and also to bleed easily [41], while mucoepidermoid tumours tend to be clean; although there may be copious pus, they do not bleed easily on biopsy. Because the tumour is covered with intact bronchial epithelium exfoliative cytology is not usually helpful in the case of carcinoid though it has been positive in the case of cylindromata [41]. Ulceration of the tumour may make the interpretation of the biopsy difficult; a number of Zellos's cases [66] were misinterpreted as carcinoma until operation. As serotonin and 5-HTP may be produced by carcinoid tumours without the carcinoid syndrome it may be worth checking the urine for excess of 5-HIAA in any suspected case. The normal range is 2–9 mg/24 hours but in carcinoid tumours producing the relevant substances the figure may be within the range 40–2000 mg [29].

TREATMENT

The treatment of a bronchial adenoma is primarily surgical. As the tumour usually protrudes outside the bronchus endoscopic resection is unsatisfactory. It may be justifiable in some patients unfit for thoracotomy but will often have be repeated and is never curative. If the peripheral lung has not been severely damaged by infection sleeve resection of the involved bronchus may be feasible [59], but often severe damage beyond the bronchial block makes lobectomy, and sometimes even pneumonectomy, essential. Some success has been recorded with radiotherapy in cylindromata which were not resectable; this might apply in particular to cylindromata in the trachea. Vieta and Maier [63] report 6 patients surviving for more than 5 years with no recurrence and Zellos [66] reports 1 surviving more than 13 years. On the other hand these are very slow growing tumours and it is possible that radiotherapy did not make a major contribution to the survival.

Treatment of the carcinoid syndrome is unsatisfactory unless it is due to a resectable tumour. Antihistamine drugs have been used, usually with little success. Methyldopa has been reported as successful in cases secreting serotonin.

PROGNOSIS

If the tumour can be resected the prognosis is good. 75% of Thomas's cases [59] had survived 4–14 years after operation with only 1 recurrence. If there are lymph gland metastases locally, the glands should be removed as a number of such patients have survived for many years without recurrence [39 & 66]. Even with metastases elsewhere survival may be comparatively prolonged. Zellos [66] records one patient surviving with hepatic metastases for more than 3 years. On the other hand cylindromata are said to be 7 times as lethal as carcinoid tumours and recurrences 7 times more common [14]. Mucoepidermoid tumours do not usually invade surrounding tissue and do not metastasize, so that the prognosis after resection is good. The outlook is more doubtful in the invasive mixed tumours; local recurrence and malignant transformation may occur [42].

HAMARTOMA

DEFINITION

The term hamartoma is applied to tumours in which normal components of the organ are combined in a disorganized manner.

CAUSATION

Little is known of their causation. It might be thought that the anomaly is basically congenital but the lesions are rare in childhood and tend slowly to enlarge, which suggests that the components of the tumour are not subject to the normal control of growth.

CARTILAGINOUS HAMARTOMA

This term is applied to hamartomata of the lung in which cartilage predominates.

FREQUENCY AND AGE AND SEX DISTRIBUTION

The frequency is slightly less than that of carcinoid tumours of the lung. The tumours present most often in the 4th decade but an age range of 16–76 has been recorded [4]. There is probably little difference between the incidence in the two sexes; it has varied in different series.

PATHOLOGY

The tumour consists mainly of cartilage but may also contain epithelium, fibrous tissue and fat. It is most commonly peripheral but 3–5% occur within a bronchus [32]. Hamartomata grow slowly over months or years. They have varied in size from a few millimetres to filling the whole of one side of the thorax [32]. They occasionally become cystic due to necrosis [43] but an apparent cystic appearance on an x-ray is sometimes due to the transradiancy of contained areas of fat [10]. Calcification may occur within the tumour. Malignant change is apparently very rare [6] but Blair and McElvein [4] report carcinoma occurring in the same lobe some years later, possibly a coincidence, and another case in which an adenocarcinoma was found at resection in close proximity to the hamartoma. Bateson [3] records multiple cartilaginous tumours in a woman of 27.

CLINICAL FEATURES

The great majority of cases are picked up on routine x-ray. They are free from symptoms unless there is bronchial block in which case there may be secondary collapse or infection beyond the block with symptoms similar to those in bronchial adenoma (p. 556).

RADIOLOGY

The tumour usually shows as a circular shadow with a well-defined edge. It may be slightly lobulated and often contains a few spots of calcium visible on tomography. Rarely there may be a cystic appearance due to necrosis [43] or deposits of fat [10].

DIAGNOSIS

A rounded peripheral shadow with a well-defined hair-line edge suggests the possibility of a benign neoplasm. Carcinoid tumour is another possibility, as is hydatid cyst. Bronchial carcinoma, pulmonary metastasis and a tuberculous lesion will also come into the differential diagnosis (p. 525). If the tumour is peripheral bronchoscopy is unhelpful. Other investigations will include tomography, tuberculin testing and examination of the sputum for tubercle bacilli and malignant cells. In relevant areas the Casoni test for hydatid disease (p. 368) will be indicated. In many patients these tests prove unhelpful and, unless contra-indicated by age, other disease or poor lung function, a thoracotomy must be carried out. The rare endobronchial hamartomata do not necessarily show radiologically and may be obscured by the resulting collapse. The latter will call for bronchoscopy which usually reveals the diagnosis.

TREATMENT

It will be obvious that the treatment is surgical, provided that this is not contraindicated by age, poor respiratory function or other disease. The stony hardness of the lesion, as felt at thoracotomy, usually allows the surgeon to be confident of the diagnosis. It is then usually possible to remove the tumour without sacrificing lung tissue. It may be possible to remove an endobronchial hamartoma locally but if there is severe damage beyond the blocked bronchus the damaged lung will have to be resected.

PROGNOSIS

The prognosis after surgical removal is excellent. Recurrence is unlikely, but has been recorded [3]. If surgery is not carried out the rate of growth is usually slow but seems to be variable in individual cases. Malignant change may occur but is rare [6].

FIBROLEIOMYOMATOUS HAMARTOMA [8]

This type of hamartoma consists of localized or diffuse overgrowth of muscle, probably derived from small bronchi or bronchioles. The diffuse form may be associated with tuberous sclerosis, giving rise to one type of 'honeycomb lung' (p. 571); in this condition hamartoma may occur in other parts of the body [55]. The localized form is usually subpleural and gives rise to a limited shadow, not always well-defined, on the x-ray. Very rarely a fibroleiomyoma may be intrabronchial and form a greyish-red polypoid tumour giving rise to haemoptysis, infection and lung collapse [1 & 61]. Calcification may occur [55]. Histologically peripheral fibroleiomyomata must be differentiated from metastases from uterine fibroleiomyosarcoma, which may show little evidence of malignancy [55].

PULMONARY ARTERIOVENOUS FISTULA

(Pulmonary Angioma, Vascular Hamartoma, Pulmonary Arteriovenous Aneurysm)

DEFINITION AND PATHOLOGY

Strictly speaking this abnormality is a malformation rather than a tumour. It basically comprises a persistence of the short foetal capillary anastomoses between the arterial and venous sides of the pulmonary circulation. With the resultant lower resistance blood is deviated into the abnormality which therefore gradually dilates [55]. The lesions are said to be multiple in 20% of cases and bilateral in 10% [32]. Occasionally the supplying vessel is systemic, derived from the thoracic aorta, internal mammary, intercostal or even coronary artery. There are sometimes accompanying pulmonary venous abnormalities [24]. The condition is said to be associated with hereditary haemorrhagic telangiectasis in 50–60% of cases [7 & 55]. Conversely, about 6% of patients with the latter have pulmonary arteriovenous fistulae

[27]. Although any part of the lung may be affected, the lesion is commoner in the lower lobes. Vascular abnormalities are occasionally found in other organs, including cerebral arteriovenous fistula [7].

FUNCTIONAL ABNORMALITY

There may be a major shunt of unoxygenated blood from the right to the left side of the heart through the anastomosis. In that case there is diminution of Pa,O_2 while the Pa,CO_2 may be normal or decreased. The circulation time is said to be normal [7]. There is no increase in blood volume and, because there is no increased resistance, nor is there usually any hypertrophy of the heart. However, 3 cases have recently been described with raised pulmonary arterial pressure, the pathogenesis of which was uncertain [48].

FREQUENCY

This is a rare tumour. Le Roux [32] reported 8 cases seen in 10 years in a thoracic surgical unit which served a population of $1\frac{1}{2}$ million; during the same period 3000 cases of bronchial carcinoma and 40 of bronchial adenoma were seen. The lesions have been described in newborn infants but clinical presentation is usually in the 3rd decade or later, probably because the anastomoses gradually enlarge over the years. There is no particular sex or race bias.

CLINICAL FEATURES

The lesion or lesions may be *asymptomatic* and only found on routine x-ray. On the other hand if there is a major shunt from the right to the left heart there will be *cyanosis*, *polycythaemia* and *clubbing*. *Dyspnoea* may occur but is usually less than would be expected from the degree of the cyanosis. A vascular *murmur* may be heard over the lesion in about 50% of cases [18]. It may be audible throughout the cycle with systolic accentuation, or it may only be heard in systole. It is usually most noticeable on full inspiration and may only be heard if the patient is asked to take a full inspiration and then hold it. *Epistaxis* is commoner than haemoptysis and

is present in about 25%. *Telangiectasis* may be found elsewhere, in particular on the tongue, but often widely on the skin. Vascular abnormalities may occasionally be found in other organs [7]. *Haemothorax* has been recorded from rupture into the pleura. *Cerebral symptoms* may occur. Headache, vertigo, syncope, paresis, paraesthesiae, dysphagia and speech difficulties may be related to cerebral hypoxia or polycythaemia [18] but may sometimes be due to secondary *brain abscess*. The latter may be due to infected emboli reaching the systemic circulation through the fistula or, very occasionally, to *bacterial endangitis* of the lesion itself which may of course also result in infected emboli reaching other parts of the systemic circulation [55]. Cerebral symptoms due to air embolus have also been recorded. In a suspected case a personal or family history of bleeding, especially epistaxis, should be sought.

RADIOLOGY

The lesion usually shows as a rounded or lobulated opacity in the middle or lower zone of the lung fields. This may sometimes be seen to be multiple; more often multiple lesions, if they exist, are seen only on angiography. The enlargement of the supplying vessels between the lesion and the hilum can often be seen either on the PA or the lateral view. Sometimes these are visible only on tomography. Calcification may occur. Pulsation of the tumour is not usually detectable at fluoroscopy [58]. In a proportion, but by no means in all, the shadow may be seen to decrease in size with the Valsalva manoeuvre and to increase with the Mueller. A pulmonary angiogram should always be carried out before operation in order to ensure that the lesion is single or, if there are multiple lesions, to ensure that there are not too many for resection. Unfortunately after operation lesions which have previously been unsuspected may subsequently enlarge and cause symptoms.

TREATMENT

The treatment is surgical. It is usually possible to peel the enlarged vessels out of the lung without sacrificing pulmonary tissue. This is particularly important as it may, in subsequent years, be necessary to reoperate on lesions which develop later [32]. Occasionally segmental resection may be necessary.

PROGNOSIS

Without resection the mortality has been said to be as high as 50% in lesions presenting with symptoms [36]. After resection the prognosis is usually good but the development of further lesions may necessitate subsequent operation. In some patients the lesions are too numerous to justify operation.

RARE PULMONARY TUMOURS

There are a number of very rare pulmonary tumours. When these are intrabronchial they may give rise to haemoptysis and symptoms of bronchial obstruction similar to those of bronchial adenoma. When they are entirely outside the bronchus they are frequently diagnosed only on routine radiography though, if very large, they may give rise to cough or dyspnoea. In most cases a diagnosis can only be made if a bronchial biopsy is possible or at thoracotomy. Intrabronchial lesions may not be visible radiologically, or may be obscured by pulmonary collapse. A peripheral lesion usually presents radiologically as a rounded shadow which could well be a carcinoma. In the following paragraphs clinical and radiological features will not receive further comment unless they differ from the foregoing account.

CHONDROMA OF BRONCHUS

A purely cartilaginous tumour may arise from bronchial cartilage. It differs from an intrabronchial chondromatous hamartoma (p. 558) by the absence of other abnormal tissues [55]. Its clinical presentation is similar.

CYSTADENOMA OF BRONCHUS

These tumours arise from bronchial glands and differ from the cylindromatous type of adenoma in that there is no degeneration of the stroma and that they are confined within the cartilaginous layer of the bronchus [55].

FIBROMA AND MYXOMA [31, 35 & 55]

These are localized well-defined tumours which may occur in the lung substance or in the bronchial wall and give rise to a well-defined opacity on the x-ray. They may calcify or undergo myxomatous change. In myxoma there is mucoid change surrounding cells resembling fibroblasts.

HISTIOCYTOMA

This tumour has also been called a plasmacytoma (mistakenly according to Spencer [55]) or sclerosing haemangioma. It is usually spherical and well-circumscribed, yellow or grey in colour, and occasionally cavitates or calcifies [55]. It usually lies within the lung substance but may involve a bronchus [2]. Microscopically the appearance is variable. Plasma cells and spindle cells are characteristic, with variable numbers of lymphocytes and blood vessels. The tumour has been described at ages varying from 3 to 55. Malignant change apparently does not occur and it is possible that the lesion is a granuloma rather than a tumour.

LIPOMA

Pulmonary lipomata are very rare. They are commonest in the left main and lobar bronchi, forming smooth-walled polyps [34, 43, 55 & 56]. At least one has been described in the trachea [53]. Nearly all have occurred in males. Peripheral pulmonary lipomata are even rarer [50 & 55].

MYOBLASTOMA OF THE BRONCHUS

This very rare tumour occurs in the larger bronchi and presents as a sessile or polypoid growth [5 & 44]. It may extend outside the bronchus. Microscopically there are 3 types of cell: large granular and foamy cells with small dark nuclei, sometimes in syncytial masses; long fusiform cells; and cells with an eosinophilic cytoplasm and oval dark nuclei [44 & 55]. The age range at presentation has been 30–50 and metastases are said not to occur.

NEUROFIBROMA AND NEUROGENIC SARCOMA [9, 37 & 55]

Neurogenic tumours of the lung may be benign or malignant and have been reported between the ages of $2\frac{1}{2}$ and 57 with a slight preponderance in males. They are very much rarer than neurogenic tumours in the paravertebral gutter (p. 605). They may be multiple and are sometimes associated with generalized neurofibromatosis (von Recklinghausen's-disease). They are lobulated and well-encapsulated tumours, even when malignant, and may calcify. They may occur anywhere in the lung. Like other lung sarcomata they tend to remain localized.

PAPILLOMA OF TRACHEA OR BRONCHUS

Although papilloma of the larynx is the commonest benign tumour of the larynx in children [21], single or multiple papillomata of the trachea or bronchi are very rare. They may occur in children or young adults. Microscopically they consist of a connective tissue core covered with squamous epithelium. The papilloma may spread from the bronchus to adjoining alveoli. An inflammatory origin has been suggested [47, 55 & 57].

PLASMACYTOMA

Pulmonary deposits may occasionally be associated with multiple myeloma. Non-skeletal deposits have been called plasmacytomata. Myeloma may even more rarely present as a solitary intrapulmonary tumour without evidence of generalized myelomatosis [26]. Most reported cases seem to have originated in a rib or vertebra. If the lesion is solitary surgery or radiotherapy is indicated.

SARCOMA [12]

Sarcoma of the lung is very rare. Iverson [28] found only 16 cases in the literature between 1900 and 1950. Most probably arise in the bronchial walls but some in the lung parenchyma. They may originate from fibrous tissue, unstriped muscle, cartilage or undifferentiated primitive connective tissue cells. Those arising from nerves have already been considered above. Distant metastases are rarer than with sarcomata elsewhere but local invasion may occur. The tumours often remain localized for long periods. Thompson [60] and Iverson [28] report survivors a number of years after resection. Shaw et al. [51] also report good results in the case of *leiomyosarcomata*. *Rhabdomyosarcomata* have been described [11] and tend to invade the pulmonary veins and bronchi with polypoid formation. *Primary lymphosarcoma* is probably the commonest form of primary lung sarcoma [25 & 40]. Primary lymphosarcomata originate outside the bronchus and may remain localized to the lung for many months so that the outlook is good for resection [25 & 46]. They have been described at ages between 34 and 75 with an equal incidence in the two sexes. Radiotherapy has been successful if surgery is not possible or if there is recurrence after surgery.

PRIMARY THORACIC HAEMANGIOPERICYTOMA

Feldman and Seaman [17] reviewed 19 reported cases of this tumour. Of these 14 arose in the mediastinum, 4 in the lung and 1 in the pleura. Macroscopically the tumours often appear encapsulated and are yellow or tan-coloured, though very vascular when resected. The size has varied from a few centimetres to a tumour filling half the thorax. The growth rate has also varied; in many the tumour has grown importantly in a matter of months, but in one it was known to have been present for 60 years. Microscopically a proliferation of capillaries is surrounded by the tumour cell, the 'pericyte', a modified smooth muscle cell. Some are locally malignant and may later produce metastases by blood or lymph stream; death may occur within a year, but a number of patients have survived many years after resection. Other tumours appear benign. One case of pulmonary osteoarthropathy is recorded. X-ray shows a well-demarcated mass even in the malignant cases; it is seldom possible to see pulsation on fluoroscopy. The tumours should be treated by resection if feasible but they are also radiosensitive.

REFERENCES

[1] AAKHUS T. & MYLIUS E.A. (1962) Leiomyoma of the lung. *Acta chir. scand.* **124**, 372.

[2] BATES T. & HULL O.H. (1958) Histiocytoma of the bronchus. Report of a case in a 6 year old child. *Am. J. Dis. Child.* **95**, 53.

[3] BATESON E.M. (1967) Cartilage containing tumours of the lung: relationship between the purely cartilaginous type (chondroma) and the mixed type (so called hamartoma): an unusual case of multiple tumours. *Thorax* **22**, 256.

[4] BLAIR T.C. & McELVEIN R.B. (1963) Hamartoma of the lung. A clinical study of 25 cases. *Dis. Chest* **44**, 296.

[5] CAMPBELL D.C., SMITH E.P., HOOD R.H., DOMINY D.E. & DOOLEY B.N. (1964) Benign granular cell myoblastoma of the bronchus. *Dis. Chest* **46**, 729.

[6] CAVIN E., MASTERS J.H. & MOODY J. (1958) Hamartoma of the lung. *J. thorac Surg.* **35**, 816.

[7] CHANDLER D. (1965) Pulmonary and cerebral arteriovenous fistula with Osler's disease. *Arch. int. Med.* **116**, 277.

[8] CRASTNOPOL P. & FRANKLIN W.D. (1957) Fibroleiomyoma of the lung. *Ann. Surg.* **145**, 128.

[9] DIVELEY W. & DANIEL R.A. (1951) Primary solitary neurogenic tumours of the lung. *J. thorac. Surg.* **21**, 194.

[10] DOPPMAN J. & WILSON G. (1965) Cystic pulmonary hamartoma. *Br. J. Radiol.* **38**, 629.

[11] DRENNAN J.M. & McCORMACK R.J.M. (1960) Primary rhabdomyosarcoma of the lung. *J. Path. Bact.* **79**, 147.

[12] DYSON B.C. & TRENTALANCE A.E. (1964) Resection of primary pulmonary sarcoma. Review of literature and report of a case associated with pulmonary asbestosis. *J. thorac. cardiovasc. Surg.* **47**, 577.

[13] ELLMAN P. & BOWDLER A.J. (1960) Pulmonary manifestations of Hodgkin's disease. *Br. J. Dis. Chest* **54**, 59.

[14] ENTERLINE H.T. & SCHOENBERG H.W. (1954) Carcinoma (cyclindromatous type) of trachea and bronchi and bronchial adenoma: a comparative study. *Cancer* **7**, 663.

[15] FALCONER E.H. & LEONARD M.E. (1936) Hodgkin's disease of the lung. *Am. J. med. Sci.* **191**, 780.

[16] FALCONER E.H. & LEONARD M.E. (1938) Pulmonary involvement in lymphosarcoma and lymphatic leukaemia. *Am. J. med. Sci.* **195**, 294.

[17] FELDMAN FRIEDA & SEAMAN W.B. (1964) Primary thoracic haemangiopericytoma. *Radiology* **82**, 998.

[18] FOLEY R.E. & BOYD D.P. (1961) Pulmonary arteriovenous aneurysms. *Surg. Clin. N. Am.* **41**, 801.

[19] FOSTER-CARTER A.F. (1941) Bronchial adenoma. *Quart J. Med.* **10**, 139.

[20] GIBBON J.H.Jr. & NEALON T.F.Jr. (1962) Neoplasms of the lungs and trachea. In *Surgery of the Chest*, ed. Gibbon J.H.Jr. Philadelphia, Saunders.

[21] GORRELL D.S. (1952) Laryngeal papillomata in children. *Canad. med. Ass. J.* **67**, 425.

[22] GREEN R.A. & NICHOLS W.J. (1959) Pulmonary involvement in leukaemia. *Am. Rev. resp. Dis.* **80**, 833.

[23] GREEN R.A., NICHOLS W.J. & KING E.J. (1959) Alveolar capillary block due to leukemic infiltration of the lung. *Am. Rev. resp. Dis.* **80**, 895.

[24] GRISHMAN A., POPPEL M.H., SIMPSON R.S. & SUSSMAN M.L. (1949) The roentgenographic and angiocardiographic aspects of (1) aberrant insertion of pulmonary veins associated with interatrial septal defect and (2) congenital arteriovenous aneurysm of the lung. *Am. J. Roentgenol.* **62**, 500.

[25] HAVARD C.W.H., NICHOLS J.B. & STANSFELD A.G. (1962) Primary lymphosarcoma of the lung. *Thorax* **17**, 190.

[26] HERSKOVIC T., ANDERSEN H.A. & BAYRD E.D. (1965) Intrathoracic plasmacytomas. Presentation of 21 cases and review of the literature. *Dis. Chest* **47**, 1.

[27] HODGSON C.H., BURCHELL H.B., GOOD C.A. & CLAGETT O.T. (1959) Hereditary hemorrhagic telangiectasis and pulmonary arteriovenous fistula. Survey of a large family. *New Engl. J. Med.* **261**, 625.

[28] IVERSON L. (1954) Bronchopulmonary sarcoma. *J. thorac. Surg.* **27**, 130.

[29] JOSEPH M. & TAYLOR R.R. (1960) Argentaffinoma of the lung with carcinoid syndrome. *Br. med. J.* **ii**, 568.

[30] KERN W.H., CREPEAU A.G. & JONES J.C. (1961) Primary Hodgkin's disease of the lung. Report of 4 cases and review of the literature. *Cancer, Philadelphia* **14**, 1151.

[31] KOVARIK J.L. & ASHE S.M.P. (1963) Intrapulmonary fibroma. *Am. Rev. resp. Dis.* **88**, 539.

[32] LE ROUX B.T. (1964) Pulmonary 'hamartoma' *Thorax* **19**, 236.

[33] McBURNEY R.P., KIRKLIN J.W. & WOOLNER L.B. (1953) Metastasizing bronchial adenomas. *Surg. Gyn. Obstet.* **96**, 482.

[34] McCALL R.E. & HARRISON W. (1955) Intrabronchial lipoma. A case report. *J. thorac. Surg.* **29**, 317.

[35] MAYO P. (1965) Fibroma of the lung. Report of a case. *Dis. Chest* **47**, 338.

[36] MURI J.W. (1955) Arteriovenous aneurysm of the lung. *Am. J. Surg.* **89**, 265.

[37] NEILSON D.B. (1958) Primary intrapulmonary neurogenic sarcoma. *J. Path. Bact.* **76**, 419.

[38] OATES J.A., MELMON K., SJOEDSMA A., GILLESPIE L. & MASON D.T. (1964) Release of a kinin peptide in the carcinoid syndrome. *Lancet* **i**, 514.

19—R.D.

[39] OVERHOLT R.H., BOUGAS J.A. & MORSE D.P. (1957) Bronchial adenoma: a study of 60 patients with resections. *Am. Rev. Tuberc.* **75**, 865.

[40] PAPAIOANNOU A.N. & WATSON W.L. (1965) Primary lymphoma of the lung. An appraisal of its natural history and a comparison with other localized lymphomas. *J. thorac. cardiovasc. Surg.* **49**, 373.

[41] PAYNE W.S., ELLIS F.H.Jr., WOOLNER L.B. & MOERSCH H.J. (1959) The surgical treatment of cylindroma (adenoid cystic carcinoma) and mucoepidermoid tumours of the bronchus. *J. thorac. cardiovasc. Surg.* **38**, 709.

[42] PAYNE W.S., FONTANA R.S. & WOOLNER L.B. (1964) Bronchial tumours originating from mucous glands. Current classification and unusual manifestations. *Med. Clin. N. Am.* **48**, 945.

[43] PELEG H. & PAUSNER Y. (1965) Benign tumours of the lung. *Dis. Chest* **47**, 179.

[44] PETERSON P.A.Jr., SOULE E.H. & BERNATZ P.E. (1957) Benign granular cell myoblastoma of the bronchus. Report of 2 cases. *J. thorac. Surg.* **34**, 95.

[45] POLLARD A., GRAINGER R.G., FLEMING O. & MEACHIM G. (1962) An unusual case of metastasizing bronchial 'adenoma' associated with the carcinoid syndrome. *Lancet* **ii**, 1084.

[46] ROSE A.H. (1957) Primary lymphosarcoma of the lung. *J. thorac. Surg.* **33**, 254.

[47] SALEK J., PAZDERKA S. & ZAK F. (1958) Solitary bronchial polyps of inflammatory origin. *J. thorac. Surg.* **35**, 807.

[48] SAPRU R.P., HUTCHINSON D.C.S. & HALL J.I.: *Br. Heart J.*: to be published.

[49] SHANKS S.C. & KERLEY P. (1962) *A Textbook of X-ray Diagnosis by British Authors.* Vol. II, 3rd Edition. London, Lewis.

[50] SHAPIRO R. & CARTER M.G. (1954) Peripheral lipoma of the lung. Report of a case. *Am. Rev. Tuberc.* **69**, 1042.

[51] SHAW R.S., PAULSON D.L., KEE J.L. & LOVETT V.F. (1961) Primary pulmonary leiomyosarcomas. *J. thorac. cardiovasc. Surg.* **41**, 430.

[52] SIMON G. (1962) *Principles of Chest X-ray Diagnosis*, 2nd Edition. London, Butterworths.

[53] SMART J. (1953) Intrathoracic and intrabronchial lipomata. *Br. J. Tuberc.* **47**, 1.

[54] SOUTTER L., SNIFFEN R.C. & ROBBINS L.L. (1954) A clinical survey of adenomas of the trachea and bronchus in a general hospital. *J. thorac. Surg.* **21**, 412.

[55] SPENCER H. (1962) *Pathology of the Lung.* London, Pergamon Press.

[56] STAUB E.W., BARKER W.L. & LANGSTON H.T. (1965) Intrathoracic fatty tumours. *Dis. Chest* **47**, 308.

[57] STEIN A.A. & VOLK B.M. (1959) Papillomatosis of trachea and lungs. Report of a case. *Arch. Path., Chicago* **68**, 468.

[58] STEINBERG I. (1961) Diagnosis and surgical treatment of pulmonary arteriovenous fistula. Report of 3 new and review of 19 consecutive cases. *Surg. Clin. N. Am.* **41**, 523.

[59] THOMAS C.P. (1954) Benign tumours of the lung. *Lancet* **i**, 1.

[60] THOMPSON V.C. (1963) Tumours of the lung. In *Chest Diseases*, Vol. 2, ed. Perry K.M.A. and Sellors T.H. London, Butterworths.

[61] TURKINGSTON S.I., SCOTT G.A. & SMILEY T.B. (1950) Leiomyoma of the bronchus. *Thorax* **5**, 138.

[62] VIETA J.O. & CRAVER L.F. (1941) Intrathoracic manifestations of the lymphomatoid diseases. *Radiology* **37**, 138.

[63] VIETA J.O. & MAIER H.C. (1957) The treatment of adenoid cystic carcinoma (cylindroma) of the respiratory tract by surgery and radiation therapy. *Dis. Chest* **31**, 493.

[64] WARNER R.R.P., KIRSCHNER P.A. & WARNER GLORIA M. (1961) Serotonin production by bronchial adenomas without the carcinoid syndrome. *J. Am. med. Ass.* **178**, 1175.

[65] WILLIAMS E.D. & AZZOPARDI J.G. (1960) Tumours of the lung and the carcinoid syndrome. *Thorax* **15**, 30.

[66] ZELLOS S. (1962) Bronchial adenoma. *Thorax* **17**, 61.

CHAPTER 31

Diffuse Fibrosing Alveolitis and Honeycomb Lung

DIFFUSE FIBROSING ALVEOLITIS (Diffuse Interstitial Lung Disease,
Diffuse Interstitial Pulmonary Fibrosis, Hamman–Rich Syndrome)
[1, 15, 17, 39, 40, 42 & 49]

DEFINITION

This is a condition of unknown and possibly multiple causation characterized pathologically by a diffuse inflammatory process in the lung beyond the terminal bronchiole, having as its essential features:

(1) cellular thickening of the alveolar walls showing a tendency to fibrosis and

(2) the presence of large mononuclear cells, presumably of alveolar origin, within the alveolar spaces [41].

Clinically the chief feature is progressive and unremitting dyspnoea. Clubbing is common. The disease is often fatal, in the subacute form originally described by Hamman and Rich [17] usually within 6 months; in the commoner chronic form within a few years. Liebow et al. [28] differentiated 'desquamative interstitial pneumonia' as a separate condition in which desquamation of alveolar cells was a more prominent feature and which had a better prognosis, but Scadding and Hinson [41] regard this group as only one end of a continuous pathological and clinical spectrum. It is possible that diffuse fibrosing alveolitis is related to pulmonary fibrosis associated with collagen diseases such as rheumatoid arthritis (p. 578) and systemic sclerosis (p. 585), and to certain types of honeycomb lung (p. 571). The causes of these conditions also remain obscure. Diffuse lung fibrosis which is very similar both clinically and pathologically can be produced by certain drugs (p. 565).

AETIOLOGY AND PREVALENCE

Diffuse fibrosing alveolitis was at one time regarded as a rare disease but increasing numbers are being reported. More than 100 cases were reported between 1950 and 1962 [29]. The respiratory units in Edinburgh reported 42 cases in something under 10 years from a population between half and one million, but it is certain that not all cases came to their attention [44]. In one respiratory unit in Edinburgh this diagnosis was made in 45 patients over the 5 year period 1963–67.

AGE AND SEX

The disease has been reported at all ages from infancy to old age but the majority are middle aged or elderly. The mean age in Livingstone et al.'s 45 patients was 50 [29] but nearly half of Stack et al.'s 42 patients first developed symptoms in the 7th decade [44]. It seems that the sex representation is about equal; in some series males predominate, in others females. There appears to be no particular geographical distribution.

CAUSATION

The cause of this condition is uncertain. There are some known factors which cause diffuse lung disease closely resembling diffuse fibrosing alveolitis both clinically and pathologically. It is a matter of semantics whether these conditions should be included within the diagnosis. For instance, a very similar condition may be produced by hexamethonium, formmerly used to treat hypertension [35], and by busulphan used in chronic granulocytic leukaemia [24 & 35]. The reaction is perhaps a hypersensitivity phenomenon and responds rapidly to corticosteroid drugs. We have seen a similar case following chlorambucil. Poisoning with the weedkiller paraquat [12] may produce somewhat similar acute changes but is usually rapidly fatal. Closely related lung changes may occur in patients with overt rheumatoid arthritis [25 & 45] (p. 578), systemic sclerosis (p. 585) and Sjögren's syndrome (p. 580). Some patients may have arthralgia without overt rheumatoid arthritis [34]. These conditions are normally classified separately from diffuse fibrosing alveolitis but in a number of series without arthritic changes a rheumatoid factor has been found in up to 61% of cases [1, 30, 46 & 47], though more often the figure has been 20–30%. In some series (e.g. Stack et al. [44]) none was positive. Raised antistreptolysin titres were found in 3 out of 11 of the cases of Andér and Zettergren [1]. Whether patients with positive rheumatoid factor should be grouped as 'rheumatoid lung' or as diffuse fibrosing alveolitis is at present arbitrary.

The possibility that the lung abnormality might be an autoimmune reaction has been considered. Read [38] produced pulmonary fibrosis in rats by the intratracheal injection of anti-rat-lung serum, but no antibodies to lung have been found in patients when tests have been carried out [1, 44 & 47]. A rise in gamma globulins has been found in a few patients [42 & 44]. Mackay and Ritchie [30] found antinuclear factor (ANF) present in 41% of 17 cases and Turner-Warwick and Doniach in 28% of 34 cases but none was found in any of the 20 cases tested by Stack et al. Turner-Warwick [48] has described 8 cases with fibrosing alveolitis, chronic liver disease, non-organspecific autoantibodies and increase in immunoglobulins. It is possible that the variation between series reflects a variation in techniques of testing but any cryptic relationship to the collagen diseases must remain at present uncertain.

Histologically the findings resemble those in viral pneumonias in man and animals. The search for viral or other infective agents has not often been carried out in the early stages of the disease but the limited investigations so far reported have been negative [19 & 44].

There appears to be a genetic factor in at least some cases of diffuse fibrosing alveolitis. Hughes [21], in a review of the literature, found no less than 31 cases occurring in twins, siblings, and even in several generations of one family. Bonnani et al. [6] described a family with 8 proved cases and 3 suspected occurring in 3 out of 5 generations of a single family; one pair of identical twins had concordant disease. Inheritance was apparently an autosomal dominant trait. The condition was associated with a specific abnormal gamma globulin. A significant peripheral blood eosinophilia occurred in several of the cases. Donohue et al. [9] described 'interstitial pneumonitis' in infants in 2 families in which 1 or more adults had a condition apparently identical with diffuse fibrosing alveolitis. It is possible, of course, that there is merely a familial susceptibility to some external cause of the disease. A somewhat similar condition may be associated with tuberous sclerosis (p. 574), with neurofibromatosis [22] and with Sturge-Weber's disease [22], all of which are familial diseases.

PATHOLOGY

Scadding and Hinson [41] consider that there are 2 principal features of the disease,

(1) cellular thickening of the alveolar walls with a tendency to fibrosis and

(2) the presence of large mononuclear cells, presumably of alveolar origin, within the alveolar spaces.

The more prominent the second feature and the thinner the alveolar walls, the better they found the response to corticosteroid drugs. Cellular infiltration of the alveolar walls may consist of lymphocytes, plasma cells, mononuclear and giant cells, and eosinophil granulocytes, the nature and the proportion of cells varying in different cases. There may be haemosiderosis [19]. There is nearly always some evidence of fibrosis, at first with large thick fibroblasts, later with predominant collagen formation. In the later stages the lung architecture is so disrupted that it is difficult to be sure that the fibrosis is purely interstitial. In the early phase there may be fibrinous exudate in the alveoli and hyaline membrane formation. Later there may be hyperplasia of the bronchiolar epithelium to line the residual air spaces. Squamous metaplasia of bronchiolar and alveolar epithelium may occur [44]. One of our cases, who responded well to corticosteroid drugs, and remains well on a small dose 10 years later, had extensive deposits of bone [10].

Livingstone *et al.* [29] divided their cases pathologically into 5 grades, according to the amount of disruption of the lung architecture. *Grade I* is the mildest stage in which change is confined to the alveolar walls, the alveolar spaces being empty. In *Grade II* the architecture of the lung is still intact although the alveolar lumen is affected as well as the alveolar wall, the alveolar space usually being filled with fluid or cellular exudate. In *Grade III* the alveolar architecture is becoming blurred and perhaps lost altogether, though bronchioli may still be recognized. Staining for elastic fibres will show that the alveolar pattern is no longer intact. In *Grade IV* the normal lung structure is distorted by fibrosis, although remnants of bronchiolar epithelium and muscle may still be recognized. In *Grade V* the lung is converted to cystic spaces varying in diameter up to a centimetre or more. Grades IV and V often coexist. Within these grades there is often reduction in pulmonary artery filling and opening up of the anastomoses between the pulmonary and bronchial arteries. These authors also found an approximate correlation between radiographic appearances and the pathology of the biopsy specimens, fine and coarse mottling being commoner with Grades I and II, translucencies (honeycombing) being commoner in Grades IV and V.

Pulmonary muscular hyperplasia may occur in some patients. Such cases have been called 'bronchiolar emphysema' or 'muscular cirrhosis of the lung' [7, 14 & 49]. Most are probably variants of diffuse fibrosing alveolitis. Radiologically, honeycombing is common. Smooth muscle hyperplasia in the lung is a prominent histological feature of honeycomb lung associated with tuberous sclerosis (p. 574).

FUNCTIONAL ABNORMALITY
[4, 19 & 42]

The extensive interstitial changes in the lung lead to the classical restrictive lesion (p. 51), with decreased VC but a normal FEV/FVC ratio, indicating the absence of airways obstruction. TLC is usually lowered and RV normal or slightly increased. Reduction of diffusing capacity, by whatever method it is measured, is the earliest and most consistent change. The Pa,O_2 may at first be normal at rest but decreased on exercise, with accompanying hyperpnoea and often with lowering of Pa,CO_2 owing to over-ventilation of the more normal parts of the lung (p. 34). Minute ventilation at rest and on exercise may sometimes be increased without a fall in Pa,CO_2; this must be due to an increase in physiological dead space, which has been demonstrated in some cases. Later there is severe reduction of Pa,O_2. The oxygen extracted per unit of ventilation is greatly reduced.

The decreased Pa,O_2 may be partly due to shunting of blood through perfused but under-ventilated lung ($\dot{V}/\dot{Q}$ abnormality) and partly to the thickening of the alveolar membrane. On exercise an additional factor may be the increase in cardiac output through a decreased pulmonary vascular bed. This leads to increase in velocity of the blood in the capillaries, preventing complete saturation of end capillary blood and contributing to the decrease in Pa,O_2 [42]. The hypoxaemia will cause pulmonary vascular constriction and contribute to the rise in pulmonary artery pressure.

The extensive infiltration leads to decreased static and dynamic compliance of the lung, with greater transpulmonary pressure changes on breathing and consequent increase in the work of breathing. This may be the principal cause of the subjective sense of dyspnoea.

CLINICAL MANIFESTATIONS
[15, 17, 19, 29, 39, 40, 42 & 44]

Dyspnoea, usually progressive, is the outstanding characteristic of fibrosing alveolitis. In the rarer *subacute type*, originally described by Hamman and Rich [17], the condition may start as an apparent acute infection with pyrexia, cough and sometimes actual purulent sputum. There are bilateral diffuse crepitations in the chest and the illness is often initially regarded as a pneumonia, though there is no pleuritic pain. There may be a sensation of tightness in the chest. There is marked tachypnoea and cyanosis. Clubbing may develop rapidly. The clinical and radiological appearances often initially suggest pneumonia but the failure to improve on chemotherapy, the marked continued hyperpnoea, and perhaps the development of clubbing, in due course make it clear that the condition is not a simple pneumonia. The pyrexia may or may not subside but, in the absence of treatment, dyspnoea is progressive, cyanosis becomes more marked and the patient dies, usually within 6 months, of respiratory or cardiac failure. In our limited experience this type of patient may respond well to corticosteroid drugs.

The *chronic type* of diffuse fibrosing alveolitis is much more common. There is sometimes a relatively acute onset with an apparent respiratory infection, but more often the onset is insidious and there may be dyspnoea before there is any demonstrable radiological change. At first the patient is breathless only on exertion but later also at rest. Cyanosis also is at first present only on exercise but later may occur at rest. There is usually some cough but at first it is not a marked feature. Later in the disease there may be secondary infection with purulent sputum and more prominent cough. Finger clubbing is frequent but by no means always present. Hypertrophic pulmonary osteoarthropathy has been described [29]. Diffuse crepitations on auscultation of the chest are the main findings in the lungs. Rhonchi are absent unless there is considerable secondary infection. Mild haemoptysis is not uncommon. Later the signs of *cor pulmonale* develop.

Extrapulmonary manifestations may lead to a suspicion that the diffuse pulmonary disease does not conform to the narrow definition of idiopathic diffuse fibrosing alveolitis. Raynaud's phenomenon may suggest systemic sclerosis; joint changes may suggest rheumatoid disease. As already mentioned, the boundary between these conditions and diffuse fibrosing alveolitis is not clear cut.

INVESTIGATIONS

Apart from radiology and the physiological investigations which have already been outlined laboratory tests yield little of diagnostic importance. Occasional patients have a mild eosinophilia and polycythaemia may occur when the patient has chronic hypoxaemia. A few patients have a raised gamma globulin and these tend to have a high blood sedimentation rate. Antinuclear factor and rheumatoid factor should be measured in the serum and in certain series have been positive in a number of cases (p. 566). If the serum is positive for antinuclear factor a search should be made for LE cells, as lupus erythematosus may result in a similar clinical picture. The tuberculin test is usually unhelpful, though a strongly positive test might raise the question of pulmonary tuberculosis. The Kveim test is negative. A lung biopsy may be justifiable, at least in some cases (see below). The histology has already been outlined.

RADIOLOGY

In the early stages the x-ray can be normal in spite of symptoms of dyspnoea. In the subacute type the initial x-ray may resemble bronchopneumonia with extensive patchy shadows, confluent in places, and more extensive in the lower zones. In the commoner chronic type mottling is the most frequent appearance. When very fine it may show as confluent areas of low density consolidation similar to 'ground glass'. More often there is a fine mottling, with the individual shadows up to 2 mm, which later may become larger. Although widely diffused, the mottling is usually more marked in the lower zones. Later, when the mottling has become more coarse, translucencies appear, in most cases under 3 mm in size, mainly bounded by the mottling though sometimes with thin walls of their own [29]. This gives an appearance similar to 'honeycomb lung' though the cystic appearances are usually less well-defined. Larger translucencies, up to 5 mm or more, may occur but are less common. Like the other shadows they are more frequent at the base. Sometimes the shadows are reticular and occasionally there is obvious streaky fibrosis. Emphysematous bullae may be seen in the later stages. In many cases there is shrinking of the lungs with bilateral rise in the height of the diaphragmatic shadows. Shrinkage occurs particularly in the lower and middle lobes. It may result in marked unfolding of the aorta and kinking of the trachea. We have seen such a markedly unfolded aorta returning to normal as the lungs re-expanded under the influence of corticosteroid drugs. Sometimes predominant shrinkage of a particular lobe results in displacement of a fissure or shift of the mediastinum. As pulmonary artery pressure increases the pulmonary artery shadows may increase in size and later, with cardiac failure, the heart shadow enlarges also.

When the disease is advanced bronchograms may show lobar shrinkage and bronchial dilatation. In the late stages the distortion of lung architecture is reflected in bronchiolectasis and bronchial distortion [29]. We have seen one case in which there were, as well as coarse mottling and shrinkage of the lung, diffuse dense mottled shadows which in fact represented deposits of bone, some containing marrow cavities.

DIAGNOSIS

In the *subacute type* of the disease the main characteristics are the marked hyperpnoea and the bronchopneumonia-like shadows on the x-ray, perhaps with fever and perhaps with clubbing. Although the initial clinical impression is likely to be one of pneumonia, this will in due course be discarded when, over some weeks, the patient fails to respond to treatment. The development of clubbing will also indicate that the condition is not a pure pneumonia. The presence of bilateral crepitations with marked dyspnoea may initially suggest pulmonary oedema, but the absence of a cardiac cause and the failure to obtain response to diuretics will rule this out. If the x-ray appearances are appropriate, lymphatic carcinomatosis may have to be considered. This can give rise to clubbing and hyperpnoea, but there may be past or present evidence of malignant disease elsewhere. A rarer condition which may give rise to bronchopneumonia-like shadows is alveolar cell carcinoma. In both diseases bronchoscopy may be negative, but sputum cytology is sometimes diagnostic. As already mentioned, a condition closely resembling fibrosing alveolitis may develop as a response to drugs, in particular busulphan, chlorambucil and hexamethonium. It is possible that this list may later be extended. Enquiry may also be made for any history of having drunk the weedkiller paraquat by mistake. This leads to progressive and usually fatal lung damage, often after a latent period of a few days [12].

Tuberculosis and sarcoidosis seldom give such a degree of hyperpnoea in the presence of comparable radiological shadows, but of course the sputum should be checked as a routine for tubercle bacilli and a tuberculin test carried out; a Kveim test may be done. A rare disease which may give rise to a similar clinical picture is pulmonary alveolar proteinosis. This may be diagnosed either by finding PAS staining material in the sputum or by a lung biopsy. The appropriate extra-pulmonary manifestations, with a similar pulmonary picture, may suggest the possibility of rheumatoid lung (p. 578), systemic sclerosis (p. 585), disseminated lupus erythematosus or polyarteritis nodosa (p. 434). The blood should be investigated for rheumatoid factor, antinuclear factor and LE cells. The possibility of multiple pulmonary infarcts might also have to be considered but the shadows of infarcts appear successively and haemoptysis, pleuritic pain and a source of embolism would usually make such a diagnosis clear. If no evidence has been found to suggest one of the alternative diagnoses, lung biopsy, by thoracotomy or high speed drill, may be justified. If the patient is too ill, treatment may have to be initiated without a proved diagnosis.

In the *chronic type* of the disease in which the radiological shadows are nodular or reticular and there is no fever, pneumonia, pulmonary oedema, infarcts and pulmonary alveolar proteinosis would not enter into the differential diagnosis, but one would have to consider the other possibilities mentioned above. In fibrosing alveolitis there is much more dyspnoea, relative to the amount of radiographic change, than in sarcoidosis or tuberculosis, but it will often be necessary, in order to be certain, to carry out the tests already mentioned. Differentiation from the other possible conditions would be made as outlined in the previous paragraph. If any lymph glands are palpable in the neck a biopsy might be useful when tuberculosis, sarcoidosis or lymphatic carcinomatosis are possible alternatives. If none is palpable, in some cases it may be justifiable to do a mediastinoscopy in order to obtain a gland for biopsy.

The question of *lung biopsy* is often a difficult one. The patient may be old and very breathless. It may be felt that corticosteroid therapy, with or without antituberculosis drugs, is the only effective treatment for most of the treatable possibilities. There would be no effective treatment for lymphatic carcinomatosis, but even when that was considered likely it might be thought that corticosteroid drugs should be given with the slight hope that the condition might in fact turn out to be one of the other alternatives. On the other hand it is always unsatisfactory to be giving treatment, especially with potentially dangerous drugs, without a certain diagnosis. Lung biopsy with the high speed drill may be a satisfactory compromise in some patients, though it will not always give diagnostic information and postoperative pneumothorax, if it occurs, must be treated very promptly in an already dyspnoeic patient. We do not think that any general rule can be made as there is so much variation between patients. In each patient lung biopsy must be carefully considered and it must be decided whether the biopsy is in the interests of this particular individual. If an open biopsy is decided upon it is well to remove specimens both from a lung segment which is obviously affected by far advanced disease and from one affected by only slight disease. The far advanced part may show pure fibrosis and give little clue as to the actual diagnosis, while the slightly affected lung may, by being

in the earlier stages, provide a histological diagnosis.

TREATMENT

The only effective treatment is with corticosteroid drugs. There is little detail in the literature about the treatment of the rarer *subacute* type of disease, but in our limited experience the response is often favourable. In one of our patients gross clubbing disappeared within a month. The patient, from being virtually bedridden, was able to return to active work. He was kept well for approximately 18 months on a small maintenance dose and ultimately weaned without relapse. We have had other similar cases, in which the diagnosis was highly probable but not actually proved, who have responded very well. In the *chronic* type the results are very much more variable. Although dramatic improvement occurs in a small minority, and some improvement in a rather larger number, in many patients, especially the elderly and those in whom the condition has probably been present for a long time, the disease progresses ruthlessly in spite of corticosteroids. Livingstone *et al.* [29] found impressive improvement, with radiological clearing, in only 2 out of 31 patients, though an additional 5 showed moderate subjective improvement. 12 out of 31 of Stack *et al.*'s patients showed a significant response [44]. One may start with a dose of 5 mg of prednisolone 4 times daily, monitoring the response by radiological improvement and improvement in respiratory function tests, using in particular diffusing capacity, VC and Pa,o_2. Larger doses have not been found superior [44] but may be tried if there is no response. If improvement occurs within a few weeks the dosage should be gradually reduced over months to a maintenance dose which keeps the condition under control. Most patients will have to continue with a small dose, which may only have to be 5 mg daily, indefinitely, but it is worth while at intervals reducing the dose by 1 mg every few weeks to see whether it is possible to wean the patient completely.

Even if there is no response to initial

therapy with corticosteroid drugs it may be dangerous to take the patient off treatment suddenly. Severe deterioration has been recorded.

Other treatment is purely palliative. If the patient is severely disabled oxygen should be given in high concentration. In the later stages secondary infection may require treatment. Heart failure may be temporarily improved with diuretics and digitalis. Patients with fibrosing alveolitis do not retain CO_2 which might reduce the consciousness of dyspnoea. It is extremely important, therefore, to give appropriate sedation in the terminal stages.

PROGNOSIS

The duration of the illness has varied from 31 days to 15 years in different cases. In the absence of treatment most patients die in 2–4 years, though those with the rarer subacute type mostly die within 6 months [42].

We have seen apparent complete recovery of the subacute type, after weaning from corticosteroid drugs, and we have a patient well on a very small dose of steroids 10 years after being a complete respiratory invalid, though tending to relapse if taken off corticosteroid drugs. With treatment, as already mentioned, the prognosis is better in the more acute disease, in younger people and in those with less thickened alveolar walls on biopsy [41]. Livingstone et al. [29] found the prognosis somewhat better in those with finger clubbing than in those without. The presence of cyst formation or honeycombing on the chest x-ray is an unfavourable sign; such patients are less likely to respond to treatment [1, 29 & 31]. In a few, spontaneous arrest may occur.

Most patients die from respiratory or cardiac failure. A proportion have died from bronchial carcinoma, though the numbers are insufficient to be certain whether the risk of this disease is higher than in the general population [44].

HONEYCOMB LUNG

DEFINITION

This is a radiological term indicating the presence, often diffusely in both lungs, of cysts, usually 0·5–2 cm in diameter, relatively thick-walled and not filling with opaque material at bronchography. There is often nodulation or mottling in addition. This appearance may be congenital or may be produced by a number of different conditions. A localized form may be seen in a wide variety of diseases involving the alveolar septa, including sarcoidosis, berylliosis, asbestosis, systemic sclerosis, rheumatoid lung, tuberculosis and fibrosing alveolitis [37]. The term 'honeycomb lung' has usually been applied to conditions in which the honeycombing is diffuse in both lung fields. The main diseases in which this occurs are (1) some cases of diffuse fibrosing alveolitis, as already described (p. 567), (2) 'histiocytosis X' (Letterer-Siwe disease, Hand-Schüller-Christian disease and eosinophilic granuloma), (3) tuberous sclerosis, and, rarely, (4)

neurofibromatosis (Von Recklinghausen's disease).

PATHOGENESIS

A few cases may be congenital. Moffat [33], who also reviewed the literature on congenital cystic disease of the lung, described 9 cases, all under 18 months of age, some with localized but some with generalized cyst formation. In some of these cases the cysts were probably lymphatic (cystic hygroma), in some mainly septal and derived from pleural elements, but in others the cysts involved the terminal air passages as in honeycomb lung. Secondary infection had occurred in some patients, but the original lesions were almost certainly congenital. Several of the cases had died within a few days of birth; secondary infection and death from pneumonia complicated the disease in the older infants. It is possible that some cases of adult honeycomb lung may in fact be congenital in origin [36].

In acquired honeycomb lung the cysts are

bronchiolar dilatations with a well-defined wall made up of scar tissue or of a granulomatous process of varied aetiology [18]. Other bronchiolar lesions may be found, such as changes in direction and mode of division, amputations, and anastomoses between bronchioles and cysts belonging to anatomically independent airways [37]. The bullous appearances are probably due to multiple valvular distortions which allow the air in but not out of the cysts [37].

Diffuse fibrosing alveolitis has already been described (p. 565). An account of the other conditions mentioned now follows.

HISTIOCYTOSIS X
(Letterer-Siwe Disease,
Hand-Schüller-Christian Disease and
Eosinophilic Granuloma)

DEFINITION

Lichtenstein [27], in agreement with other workers, suggested that these 3 conditions could be put into a histological continuum, characterized by proliferation of histiocytes, and were probably different manifestations of the same unknown underlying process. He coined the term 'histiocytosis X' to emphasize our ignorance of the cause. The granulomatous lesions may occur in many different organs but often involve the lungs and bones. The condition is not familial or congenital. Although Letterer-Siwe disease has in the past usually been fatal there is a tendency to healing and recovery in the other 2 types.

PATHOLOGY [16, 26, 27, 37 & 43]

It has been suggested that the histological process may be divided into 4 stages, not rigidly demarcated and often overlapping in the different diseases [13].

(1) A proliferative phase with well marked increase of histiocytes and infiltration with eosinophilic granulocytes. This phase is 'lipoid free' and foam cells are absent.

(2) A granulomatous phase with increased vascularity and formation of fibrils. Cellular infiltration may still be marked and there may be giant cells and some lipoid phagocytosis.

(3) Xanthoma proper, with characteristic nests of xanthoma tissue and foam cells.

(4) A healed fibrotic phase, in which eosinophils are absent, and there may be little evidence of cellular infiltration.

In *Letterer-Siwe disease* the lungs are voluminous and filled with honeycomb cysts up to 1 cm in diameter. The walls of these consist of greyish-white tumour-like tissue. Microscopy shows marked histiocyte infiltration; the cytoplasm is often foamy and may contain lipoid. Eosinophils may occur and there are granulomatous deposits in bronchial walls, alveolar walls and in perivascular tissue. The lungs in *Hand-Schüller-Christian disease* may show granulomata, fibrosis and honeycombing with dots of orange-yellow lipid. Occasionally there is necrosis of the granulomata with cavity formation and bilateral hilar adenopathy may occur [3]. Microscopically, foamy histiocytes are characteristic and there may be some giant cells. Lipid, mainly of cholesterol type, is found in focal patches. Later there is increasing fibrosis, with collections of lymphocytes and a few plasma cells. In *eosinophilic granuloma* there are discrete greyish-white masses in the lung with honeycombing and diffuse miliary nodules. There may be polypoid granulomatous lesions in the bronchi and pleural plaques. Later there is increasing fibrosis. Microscopically, eosinophilic granulocytes are very prominent but histiocytes, giant cells, plasma cells, lymphocytes and a few neutrophils may occur. There may be some local haemorrhages and necrosis, and later foam cells may appear. In the final stages there is much fibrosis. Pulmonary artery walls may be infiltrated and this may give rise to pulmonary hypertension.

In Letterer-Siwe disease the skin, lymph nodes, bone, liver and spleen are frequently involved. The lung and bone are particularly affected in Hand-Schüller-Christian disease but lesions may occur in other organs. In eosinophilic granuloma bone lesions only may occur and are often solitary. It is being increasingly recognized that the lesions can be confined to the lung alone. Lesions in other organs are less common, though pituitary involvement may occur as in Hand-Schüller-Christian disease.

FUNCTIONAL ABNORMALITY

Letterer-Siwe disease is rapidly fatal. If investigated the functional abnormalities of the lung might well be similar to those of eosinophilic granuloma or fibrosing alveolitis but more severe. There may be little dyspnoea in Hand-Schüller-Christian disease, in spite of radiological changes. We know of no detailed functional investigations but these would probably show a milder form of restrictive lung disease. A few investigations in eosinophilic granuloma have been reported [20]. The abnormality is of the restrictive type, similar to that of diffuse fibrosing alveolitis (p. 567), but usually much less severe.

CLINICAL FEATURES AND RADIOLOGY

LETTERER-SIWE DISEASE

This is a usually fatal disease of infancy, occurring under the age of 3. It is of insidious onset and short duration. There may be fever, weakness, weight loss, and anaemia. Rashes, erythematous, papular or purpuric, sometimes even ulcerating, are common. Lymphadenopathy, hepatosplenomegaly and bone lesions may occur. There are often extensive cystic and granulomatous lesions in the lung and there may be secondary infection [2].

HAND-SCHÜLLER-CHRISTIAN DISEASE [2 & 3]

This disease usually begins in childhood, often under the age of 5, but first manifestations have been found as late as the 5th decade. The male/female ratio is approximately 3:2. The classical triad is of bone defects, exophthalmos and diabetes insipidus but the existence of all 3 in one patient is comparatively rare. The skull is usually involved and there may be soft tissue nodules over the punched out bone defects visible on the x-ray.

Other bones may be affected. The lesions may heal in weeks or persist for years. Gum lesions with loss of teeth are comparatively frequent. Otitis media is common and associated with bone lesions in the mastoid or petrous temporal bones. Exophthalmos may be unilateral or bilateral and is usually associated with orbital lesions. The bone lesions become sclerotic as they heal. 50% of patients have diabetes insipidus, and this may be the only manifestation. The skin is often involved, with isolated nodules or extensive eczematoid lesions. Pulmonary lesions occur in about one third of cases and show miliary or confluent shadows on the x-ray, sometimes with hilar adenopathy simulating sarcoidosis [3]. In children the pulmonary lesions may not give rise to symptoms and usually clear spontaneously, but in adults progressive fibrosis may occur. Honeycombing does not appear to be common. Defective growth is frequent. Enlargement of lymph glands, liver or spleen may occur.

EOSINOPHILIC GRANULOMA
[2, 5, 16, 20, 26 & 36]

Eosinophilic granuloma was originally recognized only as a disease of bone but it has been subsequently realized that about 20% of patients with multiple bone lesions have lung changes and that quite frequently it is the only organ affected. There may, however, be lesions elsewhere and diabetes insipidus is said to occur in 21% [20].

Dyspnoea and cough are the major respiratory symptoms but patients may be discovered at routine radiography when they have no symptoms at all. Rupture of a cyst may result in spontaneous pneumothorax which is a complication in about 30% of patients [20]. There are often no physical signs in the chest but crepitations may be audible in some patients. Clubbing occurs occasionally. There is usually no sputum unless secondary infection supervenes. Radiologically the characteristic appearance is of diffuse bilateral mottling with translucencies 5–20 mm in diameter, usually with fairly thick walls. After spontaneous improvement or treatment these walls may thin out so that the cysts show as fine bullae. The bone lesions are of the 'punched out' type but may later heal with sclerosis. Most cases have been diagnosed between the ages of 20 and 40 and the disease seems much commoner in males, but it can occur in children in whom its incidence may have been underrated.

Laboratory investigations are usually unhelpful. Blood eosinophilia is only occasionally seen but neutrophil leucocytosis is not uncommon. Sedimentation rate may or may not be raised. Eosinophils or fat laden histiocytes [26] are occasionally found in the sputum. Immunological and virological tests have so far been negative.

DIAGNOSIS

Diagnosis will be from the other conditions causing honeycombing which have already been mentioned. Lesions in bones or elsewhere may give a clue to the diagnosis of histiocytosis X but when eosinophilic granuloma is confined to the lung diagnosis can be made with certainty only by lung biopsy.

TREATMENT

Although eosinophilic granuloma, and probably Hand-Schüller-Christian disease, respond to radiotherapy [3], this treatment is only appropriate to localized lesions outside the lungs. There is increasing evidence that all types of histiocytosis X may respond to corticosteroid drugs [16 & 26]. Corticosteroid drugs should certainly be given to patients with Letterer-Siwe disease, which has a grim prognosis without treatment, and to patients with the other 2 types of disease if they have pulmonary symptoms or are deteriorating radiologically. The treatment is unlikely to be effective if the disease has already proceeded to fibrosis which may be irreversible. Corticosteroid drugs should be given along the same lines as already outlined for fibrosing alveolitis (p. 570). In the later stages symptomatic treatment may be necessary for *cor pulmonale*, infection or pneumothorax. Pneumothorax may be difficult to treat. It is often

recurrent and may be bilateral, so pleurectomy may be necessary.

PROGNOSIS

Letterer-Siwe disease was formerly always fatal but there are now some accounts of improvement, and perhaps permanent recovery, after treatment with corticosteroid drugs. Hand-Schüller-Christian disease and eosinophilic granuloma may recover spontaneously and survivals of at least 20 years have been recorded [26]. On the other hand without treatment eosinophilic granuloma may progress, with respiratory and cardiac failure or death from spontaneous pneumothorax. In children with Letterer-Siwe disease or Hand-Schüller-Christian disease death is more likely to occur if there is lung involvement and corticosteroid drugs will therefore be indicated. In these conditions, at least in children, the more widespread the visceral involvement the worse the prognosis [23].

TUBEROUS SCLEROSIS [8 & 11]

Pulmonary lesions with the clinical and functional characteristics of other forms of honeycombing may occur in patients with tuberous sclerosis. Histologically the lungs are characterized by hyperplasia of plain muscle as well as by fibrosis and much iron pigment. Lung symptoms usually develop in the third decade and death usually occurs within 5 years after development of symptoms. It seems unlikely that the lesions would respond to corticosteroid drugs but these might be worth trying.

Mental defect and epileptic fits, which are common manifestations of tuberous sclerosis, do not usually occur in those with lung manifestations. Extrapulmonary lesions may include adenoma sebaceum, subungual fibromata, retinal tumours, kidney tumours, rhabdomyomata of the heart and bone lesions. In the limb bones there may be nodular periosteal thickening and cyst formation visible on the x-ray and the skull radiograph may show increased density of the bone, either local or general, and 'cotton balls' due to calcification of the characteristic tuberous sclerotic lesions of the brain.

NEUROFIBROMATOSIS
(Von Recklinghausen's disease)

Honeycomb lung, with clinical and functional characteristics similar to those already outlined, may occasionally occur in this disease. The lung manifestations are sometimes closer to those of fibrosing alveolitis [32].

REFERENCES

[1] ANDÉR L. (1965) Idiopathic interstitial fibrosis of the lungs. I. Prognosis as indicated by radiological findings. *Acta med. scand.* **178,** 47.

[2] AVERY MARY E., McAFEE J.G. & GUILD HARRIET G. (1957) The course and prognosis of reticuloendotheliosis (eosinophilic granuloma, Schüller-Christian disease and Letterer-Siwe disease). A study of 40 cases. *Am. J. Med.* **22,** 636.

[3] AVIOLI L.V., LASERSOHN J.T. & LOPRESTI J.M. (1963) Histiocytosis X (Schüller-Christian disease). A clinico-pathological survey, review of 10 patients and the results of prednisone therapy. *Medicine* **42,** 119.

[4] BATES D.V. & CHRISTIE R.V. (1964) The Hamman-Rich syndrome. In *Respiratory Function in Disease. An Introduction to the Integrated Study of the Lung.* Philadelphia, Saunders.

[5] BICKERS J.N., BUECHNER H.A. & EKMAN P.J. (1962) Pulmonary eosinophilic granuloma. Its natural history and prognosis. *Am. Rev. resp. Dis.* **85,** 211.

[6] BONANNI P.P., FRYMOYER J.W. & JACOX R.F. (1965) A family study of idiopathic pulmonary fibrosis. A possible dysproteinemic and genetically determined disease. *Am. J. Med.* **39,** 411.

[7] DAVIES D., MACFARLANE A., DARKE C.S. & DODGE O.G. (1966) Muscular hyperplasia ('cirrhosis') of the lung and bronchial dilatations as features of chronic diffuse fibrosing alveolitis. *Thorax* **21,** 272.

[8] DAWSON J. (1954) Pulmonary tuberous sclerosis. *Quart J. Med. N.S.* **23,** 113.

[9] DONOHUE W.L., LASKI B., UCHIDA I. & MUNN J.D. (1959) Familial fibrocystic pulmonary dysplasia and its relation to the Hamman-Rich syndrome. *Pediatrics* **24,** 786.

[10] DOUGLAS A.C. (1960) Diffuse interstitial pulmonary fibrosis. Report of a case. *Br. J. Dis. Chest* **54,** 86.

[11] EDITORIAL (1954) Pulmonary tuberous sclerosis. *Lancet* **i,** 1175.

[12] EDITORIAL (1967) Poisoning from paraquat. *Br. med. J.* **iii,** 690.

[13] ENGELBRETH-HOLM J., TEILUM G. & CHRISTENSEN ERNA (1944) Eosinophil granuloma of bone—Schüller-Christian's disease. *Acta med. scand.* **118,** 292.

[14] FRAIMOW W. & CATHCART R.T. (1962) Clinical and physiological considerations in pulmonary muscular hyperplasia. *Ann. intern. Med.* **56,** 752.

[15] GRANT I.W.B., HILLIS B.R. & DAVIDSON J. (1956) Diffuse interstitial fibrosis of the lungs (Hamman-Rich syndrome) *Am. Rev. Tuberc.* **74,** 485.

[16] GRANT L.J. & GINSBURG JEAN (1955) Eosinophilic granuloma (honeycomb lung) with diabetes insipidus. *Lancet* **ii,** 529.

[17] HAMMAN L. & RICH A.R. (1944) Acute diffuse interstitial fibrosis of the lungs. *Bull. Johns Hopkins Hosp.* **74,** 177.

[18] HEPPLESTON A.G. (1956) The pathology of honeycomb lung. *Thorax* **11,** 77.

[19] HERBERT F.A., NAHMIAS BRIGITTE B., GAENSLER E.A. & MACMAHON H.E. (1962) Pathophysiology of interstitial pulmonary fibrosis. Report of 19 cases and follow up with corticosteroids. *Arch. intern. Med.* **110,** 628.

[20] HOFFMAN L., COHN J.E. & GAENSLER E.A. (1962) Respiratory abnormalities in eosinophilic granuloma of the lung. A long term study of 5 cases. *New Engl. J. Med.* **267,** 577.

[21] HUGHES E.W. (1964) Familial interstitial pulmonary fibrosis. *Thorax* **19,** 515.

[22] ISRAEL-ASSELAIN R., CHEBAT J., SORS CH., BASSET F. & LE ROLLAND A. (1965) Diffuse interstitial pulmonary fibrosis in a mother and son with von Recklinghausen's disease. *Thorax* **20,** 153.

[23] LAHEY M.E. (1962) Prognosis in reticuloendotheliosis in children. *J. Pediat.* **60,** 664.

[24] LEAKE ELEANOR, SMITH W.G. & WOODLIFF H.J. (1963) Diffuse interstitial pulmonary fibrosis after busulphan therapy. *Lancet* **ii,** 432.

[25] LEE F.T. & BRAIN A.T. (1962) Chronic diffuse interstitial fibrosis and rheumatoid arthritis. *Lancet* **ii,** 693.

[26] LEWIS J.G. (1964) Eosinophilic granuloma and its variants with special reference to lung involvement. A report of 12 patients. *Quart. J. Med., N.S.* **33,** 337.

[27] LICHTENSTEIN L. (1953) Histiocytosis X. Integration of eosinophilic granuloma of bone, Letterer-Siwe disease and Hand-Schüller-Christian disease as related manifestations of a single nosologic entity. *Arch. Path. (Chicago)* **56,** 84.

[28] LIEBOW A.A., STEER A. & BILLINGSLEY J.G. (1965) Desquamative interstitial pneumonia. *Am. J. Med.* **39,** 369.

[29] LIVINGSTONE J.L., LEWIS J.G., REID L. & JEFFERSON K.E. (1964) Diffuse interstitial pulmonary fibrosis. A clinical, radiological and pathological study based on 45 patients. *Quart. J. Med.* **33,** 71.

[30] MACKAY I.R. & RITCHIE B. (1965) Diffuse fibrosing alveolitis (diffuse interstitial fibrosis of the lungs): two cases with autoimmune features. *Thorax* **20,** 200.

[31] MALMBERG R., BERGLUND E. & ANDÉR L. (1965) Idiopathic interstitial fibrosis of the lungs. II. Reversibility of respiratory disturbances during steroid administration. *Acta med. scand.* **178**, 59.

[32] MASSARO D., KATZ S., MATTHEWS M.J. & HIGGINS G. (1965) Von Recklinghausen's neurofibromatosis associated with cystic lung disease. *Am. J. Med.* **38**, 233.

[33] MOFFAT A.D. (1960) Congenital cystic disease of the lungs and its classification. *J. Path. Bact.* **79**, 34.

[34] OGNIBENE, A.J. (1960) Systemic 'rheumatoid disease', with interstitial pulmonary fibrosis. A report of 2 cases. *Arch. intern. Med.* **105**, 762.

[35] OLINER H., SCHWARTZ R., RUBIO F.Jr. & DAMESHEK W. (1961) Interstitial pulmonary fibrosis following busulfan therapy. *Am. J. Med.* **31**, 134.

[36] OSWALD N. & PARKINSON T. (1949) Honeycomb lungs. *Quart. J. Med. N.S.* **18**, 1.

[37] PIMENTEL J.C. (1967) Tridimensional photographic reconstruction in a study of the pathogenesis of honeycomb lung. *Thorax* **22**, 444.

[38] READ J. (1958) The pathological changes produced by antilung serum. *J. Path. Bact.* **76**, 403.

[39] RUBIN E.H. & LUBLINER R. (1957) The Hamman–Rich syndrome: a review of the literature and an analysis of 15 cases. *Medicine* **36**, 397.

[40] SCADDING J.G. (1960) Chronic diffuse interstitial fibrosis of the lungs. *Br. med. J.* **i**, 443.

[41] SCADDING J.G. & HINSON K.F.W. (1967) Diffuse fibrosing alveolitis (diffuse interstitial fibrosis of the lungs) Correlation of histology at biopsy with prognosis. *Thorax* **22**, 291.

[42] SHERIDAN L.A., HARRISON E.G.Jr. & DIVERTIE M.B. (1964) Current status of idiopathic pulmonary fibrosis (Hamman-Rich syndrome). *Med. Clin. N. Am.* **48**, 993.

[43] SPENCER H. (1962) *Pathology of the Lung* (excluding Pulmonary Tuberculosis). London, Pergamon Press.

[44] STACK B.H.R., GRANT I.W.B., IRVINE W.J. & MOFFAT MARGARET A.J. (1965) Idiopathic diffuse interstitial lung disease. A review of 42 cases. *Am. Rev. resp. Dis.* **92**, 939.

[45] STRETTON T.B. & LEEMING J.T. (1964) Diffuse interstitial pulmonary fibrosis in patients with a positive sheep cell agglutination test. *Thorax* **19**, 79.

[46] TOMASI T.B.Jr., FUDENBERG H.H. & FINBY N. (1962) Possible relationship of rheumatoid factors and pulmonary disease. *Am. J. Med.* **33**, 243.

[47] TURNER-WARWICK MARGARET & DONIACH DEBORAH (1965) Autoantibody studies in interstitial pulmonary fibrosis. *Br. med. J.* **i**, 886.

[48] TURNER-WARWICK MARGARET (1968) Fibrosing alveolitis and chronic liver disease. *Quart. J. Med., N.S.* **37**, 133.

[49] ZISKIND M.M., WEILL H. & GEORGE R.B. (1967) Diffuse pulmonary diseases. *Am. J. med. Sci.* **254**, 117.

CHAPTER 32

Respiratory Manifestations of Systemic Diseases

RHEUMATIC FEVER. RHEUMATOID DISEASE. SJÖGREN'S SYNDROME. SYSTEMIC LUPUS ERYTHEMATOSUS. SYSTEMIC SCLEROSIS (GENERALIZED SCLERODERMA). DERMATOMYOSITIS. ERYTHEMA MULTIFORME EXUDATIVUM (STEVENS–JOHNSON SYNDROME).

(For Polyarteritis Nodosa see p. 434)

RHEUMATIC FEVER

RHEUMATIC PNEUMONIA

In addition to the well known respiratory complications of rheumatic fever or its sequelae—pulmonary oedema, pleural exudate (p. 274), congestive cardiac failure with pleural transudates, pulmonary infarction and pulmonary haemosiderosis—a specific pulmonary lesion which occurs in the course of acute rheumatic fever has been recognized and designated 'rheumatic pneumonia' [52]. Because of the absence of precise diagnostic criteria the frequency is uncertain. Probably it occurs more commonly than is appreciated. To what extent the use of corticosteroid drugs in the treatment of acute rheumatic fever has influenced the incidence of rheumatic pneumonia is not known.

PATHOGENESIS AND PATHOLOGY

Rheumatic pneumonia occurs during the active phase of rheumatic fever and is probably a hypersensitivity phenomenon. The pulmonary changes described resemble those found in patients with drug hypersensitivity and, experimentally, similar lesions have been observed in serum-sensitized rabbits [46]. The histological appearances are principally

(a) fibrinoid necrosis of the alveolar wall and interstitial mononuclear infiltration,

(b) protein exudation within the alveoli with the formation of a hyaline membrane, and

(c) hyaline thrombus formation and focal fibrinoid change in the smaller pulmonary arteries and the alveolar capillaries.

The presence of arterial and capillary damage, the interstitial cellular reaction and the nature of the alveolar exudate distinguish rheumatic pneumonia from uncomplicated left ventricular failure [52].

CLINICAL FEATURES

The symptoms of rheumatic pneumonia may develop at any time during an attack of rheumatic fever. Distressing cough, dyspnoea and pleuritic pain are common to most cases and fever, varying from low grade to hyperpyrexia and unresponsive to salicylates, is the rule. Cyanosis may develop. Haemoptysis may occur. The condition may be difficult to differentiate from pulmonary oedema or thromboembolism.

Physical signs in the lungs may suggest the presence of localized consolidation, or diffuse crepitations may be heard. The physical findings may be normal in the face of marked respiratory symptoms. Usually the features of carditis are evident and cardiac arrhythmia and pericarditis may also be present.

The laboratory findings are those of acute rheumatic fever.

RADIOGRAPHIC APPEARANCES

The radiographic appearances are not specific. Usually there are bilateral changes resembling pulmonary oedema and, less commonly, mottling or nodulation principally in the mid zones. Patchy confluence of lesions may occur. Frank consolidation is rare.

TREATMENT

When a diagnosis of rheumatic pneumonia is

made corticosteroid therapy is indicated in addition to salicylates.

RHEUMATOID DISEASE
[10, 24, 29, 37 & 53]

The following respiratory manifestations have been described in association with rheumatoid arthritis:

(1) Pleural adhesions, pleural thickening and pleural effusion, as discussed on p. 274. These are the commonest manifestations of rheumatoid disease in the respiratory system.

(2) Rheumatoid fibrosing alveolitis (diffuse interstitial rheumatoid disease of the lungs).

(3) Rheumatoid pneumoconiosis (Caplan's syndrome), described on p. 474.

(4) Lung nodules.

(5) Acute pulmonary infiltrations associated with pleuropericarditis.

(6) Pulmonary arterial obstruction with intimal hypertrophy and resultant pulmonary hypertension.

(7) Rheumatoid disease of the larynx.

(8) A higher incidence of respiratory infections.

There has in the past been some controversy as to whether the above conditions are truly manifestations of the rheumatoid process, rather than coincidental, but numerous series, some with controlled observations, now seem to have established that at least some of these conditions are definitely due to the rheumatoid process. The cause of the rheumatoid process is, of course, still unknown. It is virtually certain that rheumatoid pleurisy, rheumatoid fibrosing alveolitis, rheumatoid pneumoconiosis, rheumatoid lung nodules and rheumatoid laryngitis are definite entities. Rheumatoid pulmonary arterial disease [24] and acute pulmonary infiltration associated with pleuropericarditis [3] have been described in a smaller number of cases, but the latter at least is probably a definite entity. The higher incidence of respiratory infections has up to now been reported in only one series [57] but this was a large one and closely studied.

RHEUMATOID DIFFUSE FIBROSING ALVEOLITIS
(Rheumatoid Diffuse Interstitial Lung Disease)

DEFINITION AND PREVALENCE

This condition may be regarded as a variant of diffuse fibrosing alveolitis (p. 565). There is no absolute proof that fibrosing alveolitis, which in any case is uncommon, is more frequent in patients with rheumatoid disease. Nevertheless the fairly large number of cases which have now been reported in association with rheumatoid disease, and the histological evidence of specific rheumatoid features in the lungs, at least in some patients, makes it highly probable that rheumatoid fibrosing alveolitis is a definite entity. Up to 1965 Stack and Grant [53] were able to analyse 99 reported cases. Cruickshank [11] reported 6 cases among 100 autopsies of rheumatoid arthritis. Patterson et al. [45] found it in 1·1% of 702 patients. Doctor [14] suggested that if diffuse interstitial lung disease was associated with rheumatoid arthritis it should be called 'rheumatoid lung disease', but perhaps the term rheumatoid diffuse fibrosing alveolitis is better as there are other forms of rheumatoid lung disease.

In contradistinction to rheumatoid disease in general this condition is twice as common in males as in females. The average age of onset in 99 reported cases was 51 and only 6 were under the age of 40, 2 of these being associated with Still's disease in children [53].

PATHOLOGY

In a number of cases the initial granulomata, the increase in the lining cells of the alveoli and the later disorganization and honeycombing are similar to the pathological changes described in the idiopathic variety (p. 566) [14]. Nevertheless, in more than half the patients analysed by Edge [21] there was histological evidence suggesting rheumatoid disease. This consisted of gross collagen formation, hyaline and sometimes necrotic, with a tendency to peripheral palisading of fibroblasts [10].

FUNCTIONAL ABNORMALITY

Although in some patients with radiological changes there may be no respiratory symptoms and function tests may be normal [53], in most the changes are similar to those of diffuse fibrosing alveolitis of the idiopathic variety (p. 567).

CLINICAL AND RADIOLOGICAL MANIFESTATIONS

In most cases the lung manifestations appear after arthritis has developed but in about one sixth they may precede the arthritis [53]. There is no obvious relationship between the severity of the arthritis and the development of pulmonary changes, though patients with pulmonary disease tend to have anaemia and also a high erythrocyte sedimentation rate. There is no relationship to the height of the titre of serological tests for rheumatoid disease. A few patients have radiological changes but no symptoms. The main symptoms are dyspnoea and cough and are very similar to those in idiopathic fibrosing alveolitis (p. 567). Basal crepitations are common though perhaps less so than in the idiopathic variety. Clubbing is frequent, especially in the later stages. The appearances in the chest x-ray [37 & 56] are similar to those in the idiopathic variety except that pleural changes are commoner. In the lungs there are diffuse bilateral reticular, reticulonodular or cystic appearances which occasionally suggest true honeycombing.

TREATMENT

In reported cases only a small proportion have improved with corticosteroid drugs and most of these only temporarily and relatively slightly. Some clinicians even have the impression that the corticosteroid drugs may make the condition worse, especially after treatment is withdrawn. This may be partly a matter of the stage of the disease at which treatment is begun. In the rare acute fulminating cases corticosteroid drugs are well worth trying and in others it is difficult to avoid a trial if a patient is developing progressive symptoms of dyspnoea. Dosage may be similar to that recommended in systemic lupus erythematosus (p. 585).

PROGNOSIS

As already mentioned, the course is very variable. Some cases progress very rapidly to death from respiratory failure, others are arrested for long periods or even improve spontaneously. Most are said to progress slowly over many years [24]. No long term studies have yet given a true picture. It has been suggested, so far on limited evidence, that these patients have an undue tendency to develop bronchial carcinoma [53].

RHEUMATOID NODULES

Rheumatoid nodules in the lung are rare. Walker [56] found only 28 cases reported in the literature over a period of 12 years. 18 of these were in males aged between 40 and 74, with an average age of 55. The average age in females was 47. All had rheumatoid arthritis at the time of diagnosis.

Most cases have been diagnosed only at postmortem but in recent years a number of nodules have been removed surgically because of a provisional diagnosis of carcinoma of the bronchus. Radiologically the nodules are rounded or nodular and they may be single or multiple. There is no particularly common distribution in the lung but they are mostly subpleural. The size varies from minute up to 6 or 7 cm in diameter. The nodules may cavitate [1 & 44] or may fibrose and shrink [33, 37 & 56].

Many patients have no symptoms related to the nodules but cough and even haemoptysis has been recorded. Nodules have occurred in association with pleural effusion or rheumatoid fibrosing alveolitis [56]. Hart [29] described a nodule at the apex which caused pain by pressing on and eroding ribs and which was removed in the reasonable belief that it was a carcinoma.

Patients with rheumatoid nodules in the lungs are more likely to have rheumatoid disease elsewhere, especially subcutaneous nodules. They are also more likely to have anaemia and a high erythrocyte sedimentation rate.

As already mentioned, the nodules may increase in size, cavitate, remain stable or even shrink. Most of those which have become smaller had been treated with corticosteroid drugs. Response to treatment seems more likely than in the case of rheumatoid fibrosing alveolitis [37].

ACUTE PULMONARY INFILTRATIONS ASSOCIATED WITH PLEUROPERICARDITIS [3]

Beck and Hoffbrand [3] described 3 patients with rheumatoid arthritis who developed pleural effusion and pericarditis, with fever and dyspnoea but with little cough. In 2 there were lung shadows, in one patchy, in the other streaky, on the opposite side to the pleural effusion. In the third patient 'collapse-consolidation' was said to have underlain the pleural effusion. There was no evidence of secondary infection and the fever and abnormal shadows cleared only when corticosteroid drugs were given, in one patient leaving a persistent restrictive defect as shown by lung function studies. It is difficult to be certain that the lesions were not, for instance, pulmonary infarcts but the balance of evidence perhaps favours a rheumatoid origin.

RHEUMATOID ARTERITIS OF PULMONARY VESSELS

Very rarely patients with rheumatoid disease develop pulmonary hypertension without gross fibrosing alveolitis [27]. This has been shown to be due to intimal hypertrophy in the pulmonary arteries. These patients usually have Raynaud's phenomenon with similar histological changes in the digital arteries.

RHEUMATOID LARYNGITIS

Rheumatoid disease may affect the crico-arytenoid joints [29]. This may give rise to dyspnoea, stridor, hoarseness, inability to raise the voice and sometimes, as a result of secondary infection, to severe obstruction necessitating tracheostomy. There may be pain radiating to the ears, and a sensation of fullness of the throat on swallowing or speaking. Laryngoscopy may show oedema, redness and reduced mobility of the arytenoids and cords.

INCREASED INCIDENCE OF OTHER RESPIRATORY INFECTIONS

Walker [57] compared 516 patients with rheumatoid arthritis to a control group of 301 patients with degenerative joint disease. There was a highly significant excess of bronchiectasis in the patients with rheumatoid arthritis. The bronchiectasis had usually preceded the rheumatoid arthritis by many years and was thought possibly to have had some aetiological relationship to it. Both acute and chronic bronchitis were a good deal commoner in the patients with rheumatoid disease than in the controls but the patients with rheumatoid disease also smoked more heavily. A history of pneumonia was significantly commoner in the patients with rheumatoid arthritis, often preceding the arthritis, but this was usually associated with chronic bronchitis or bronchiectasis. There was no difference between the groups in radiological evidence of tuberculosis.

SJÖGREN'S SYNDROME
[7, 8, 13 & 55]

DEFINITION

Sjögen's syndrome is best regarded as a variant of rheumatoid disease characterized by (1) *keratoconjunctivitis sicca* due to lesions of the lachrymal glands, (2) *xerostomia* or dry mouth, due to damage to the salivary glands, which are often enlarged, and also damage to the mucous glands of the mouth, and (3) *rheumatoid arthritis*. The diagnosis may also be made when any 2 out of the 3 characteristics are present; rheumatoid arthritis is absent relatively frequently. The interrelationship of the various collagen diseases is indicated by the fact that Sjögren's syndrome may be associated with scleroderma, polymyositis, lupus erythematosus or polyarteritis nodosa [8]. *Other associated findings* may be hepatosplenomegaly, lymph gland enlargement, thyroid enlargement, acrodermatitis, purpura, achylia, pernicious anaemia, Raynaud's phenomenon and alopecia. *Rheumatoid factor* is almost always present in the blood serum, and often *antinuclear factor* and antibodies to various tissues [5]. The erythrocyte sedimentation rate is usually increased, as are the gamma globulins. Abnormal globulins such as cryoglobulin and C-reactive protein may also be present [13].

PATHOLOGY [51]

Pathologically the main finding is lymphocyte infiltration of the salivary and lachrymal glands, later leading to fibrosis and atrophy. The duct cells often proliferate and block the lumina. Plasma cells may also be present. The mucous glands of the trachea and bronchi may be affected, as well as those of the mouth, leading to a decrease of secretions. There may be bronchial wall infiltration with lymphocytes and plasma cells. This may also occur in the lungs. Pulmonary arteritis may also be present [7]. The infiltration may be followed by fibrosis which can be widespread. Nodules may occur in the lungs; these consist of densely cellular infiltration with lymphocytes, plasma cells, reticulum cells and occasional giant cells of the Langhans type, with a few neutrophils and eosinophils [6].

CLINICAL FEATURES

Pulmonary manifestations, somewhat similar to those of rheumatoid disease, may sometimes occur. Dry cough is relatively frequent, probably due to the decreased secretion in larynx, trachea and bronchi [7]. These patients, with their decreased secretion, are more liable to secondary infection and death is often due to pneumonia. Transient infiltrations and collapse can occur [7]. Recurrent pleurisy has often been reported and polyserositis in 3 patients [13]. Widespread pulmonary fibrosis is sometimes a manifestation and may give rise to dyspnoea [13]. Pneumothorax has also been recorded [25].

TREATMENT

The treatment of this condition is not very satisfactory. Artificial tears have been used to decrease the dryness of the eyes and the consequent secondary infection. It has been claimed that a combination of prednisolone and thyroid may be successful in improving the secretion even in patients with no evidence of hypothyroidism [13]. Corticosteroid drugs may also improve the joint symptoms. We have seen little account of their effect on any lung lesions but this might well be similar to that in systemic lupus erythematosus. Secondary infection would, of course, require treatment.

PROGNOSIS

Sjögren's syndrome is usually slowly progressive but relatively few deaths have been recorded. Most have been due to pneumonia.

SYSTEMIC LUPUS ERYTHEMATOSUS (SLE), Disseminated Lupus Erythematosus [15, 17 & 30]

Systemic lupus erythematosus (SLE) is a clinical syndrome of unknown cause or causes, characterized by multisystem involvement and multiple remissions and exacerbations. In the majority, diagnosis can be confirmed by finding LE cells in the blood, although the finding of LE cells alone, without the clinical characteristics, is not diagnostic [17]. It should be noted that LE cells may be found in patients with rheumatoid arthritis or lupoid hepatitis who never develop any disease elsewhere.

PREVALENCE AND MORTALITY [39]

Owing to a better awareness of the condition, to the value of the test for LE cells and probably to better survival with corticosteroid treatment, the prevalence of known disease is increasing. In Malmö, Sweden, the prevalence of known cases in 1955 was 2·9 per 100,000 population, increasing to 6·0 in 1961. Figures for East Manhattan, New York were very similar. On the other hand the mortality in New York city remained stable at 0·6 per 100,000 between 1955 and 1964, suggesting that the major contribution to the increased prevalence is better diagnosis.

The disease occurs mostly in young women

between the ages of 15 and 44, the ratio of females to males being roughly 3 to 1. The attack rate in males is fairly steady throughout life. The rate in negroes in the United States is 3–4 times that in whites.

AETIOLOGY

There is probably some genetic predisposition to the 'collagen diseases'. Relatives of patients with SLE have a higher incidence of SLE, rheumatoid disease and other collagen diseases in their families. Relatives without any clinical features of these diseases may have an increase in serum gamma globulins, or their serum may be positive for antinuclear or rheumatoid factor [16]. The cause of the disease remains uncertain. After review of all the evidence Dubois and Arterberry [16] do not find the popular autoimmune theory convincing. They consider that there may be a genetic predisposition, that a chronic viral infection, with or without some metabolic defect, may further predispose patients to the disease and that clinical manifestations may be triggered off by such factors as exposure to sun, drug reactions or other infections.

PATHOLOGY

The most specific histological feature is the presence of haematoxylin-stained bodies, but fibrinoid change is also frequently present [12]. Haematoxylin-stained bodies consist of ovoid or spindle-shaped bodies staining purplish-blue with haematoxylin, structureless and about the size of a red cell. They are probably derived from the nuclei of epithelial cells. The characteristic fibrinoid material consists of deeply eosinophil tissue, acellular, homogeneous and refractile. It occurs as fine threads, coarse fibres or agglomerated bands in loose connective tissue or in the walls of blood vessels. This change may be accompanied by mild inflammatory reaction with lymphocytes and plasma cells, sometimes also small numbers of neutrophils.

In the pleura the reaction consists of fibrinoid deposition, with haematoxylin-staining bodies in the active phase, later progressing to thick oedematous loose fibrous tissue. There has been little description of the patho-logical changes in the lung. Fibrinoid change in pulmonary vessels has only occasionally been described. The reaction in the more acute stage appears to consist of thickening of alveolar septa by infiltration of chronic inflammatory cells with mucinous oedema of alveolar walls. There may also be hyaline membrane formation, alveolar haemorrhage (sometimes extensive), focal necrosis of alveolar walls and focal organizing interstitial pneumonia. Focal atelectasis is common and may, with the interstitial inflammatory reaction and haemorrhage, account for the patchy pneumonia-like shadows seen on x-ray and of course for the appearance of linear atelectasis [34]. The cause of the atelectasis is uncertain but, in view of the hyaline membrane formation, it is possible that it is due to interference with the function of surfactant [34]. The fact that a number of patients have dyspnoea, in spite of the absence of radiological change other than high diaphragms with limited movement, suggests that widespread pathological changes, of the types outlined, may be occurring in areas of the lung too small to cast a radiographic shadow.

FUNCTIONAL ABNORMALITY
[17, 34 & 35]

Abnormality of respiratory function in SLE may be caused by

(1) pleural effusion or thickened pleura,

(2) pneumonic change, either directly due to SLE or due to secondary infection,

(3) interstitial lung disease and alveolar atelectasis, or

(4) cardiac or pericardial lesions.

Abnormalities of function due to pleural effusion (p. 29) or to secondary pneumonia (p. 118) are described elsewhere.

In recent years it has been appreciated that dyspnoea is a common complaint in SLE even in those without obvious pleural lesions, and often in patients whose only radiographic abnormality is that of high diaphragms which move sluggishly on fluoroscopy. Those who complain of dyspnoea and have a relatively normal chest x-ray often show evidence of a restrictive ventilatory defect with decrease in

VC, decreased lung compliance and often decreased TLC and IC. There is no evidence of airways obstruction. There may be minor degrees of $\dot{V}/\dot{Q}$ imbalance. These findings indicate that the lungs are small and stiff. It is not thought that this is due to pleural fibrosis because in some of the patients the pleural change is minimal radiographically and there may be dramatic improvement with corticosteroid drugs [34]. In those with dyspnoea but normal x-ray there may be no demonstrable diffusion defect, though this is often demonstrable when there is radiological change [17], and sometimes without it [35].

CLINICAL MANIFESTATIONS
[17, 30 & 34]

Clinical manifestations of SLE may occur in almost any organ. This disease, with poly-arteritis nodosa, is one that has to be suspected in any bizarre clinical picture with widespread organ involvement. The commonest initial presentation is *arthralgia* or *arthritis* of rheumatoid type, together with *skin lesions*, but *pulmonary manifestations* are common. The classical rash is that on the 'butterfly area' of the face on either side of the nose and may be erythematous, maculo-papular or, more rarely, discoid. There is *fever* in most cases and secondary infection, particularly pulmonary, is very common. *Pericarditis* and *pleurisy*, both often with *effusion*, are frequent (see below). There are often spontaneous *remissions* which last from a few months to several years.

Many *other manifestations* may occur. Among the more important are: weight loss, myalgia and myositis, subcutaneous nodules, myocarditis, endocarditis (including Libman–Sacks' atypical verrucous endocarditis), other skin lesions (including generalized discoid LE, photosensitivity, purpura, alopecia and Raynaud's phenomenon), hypertension, neurological lesions (hemiparesis and other central lesions, peripheral neuritis, psychoses, epilepsy), eye lesions (conjunctivitis, exudates or haemorrhages in the discs), renal lesions (resembling acute nephritis, chronic nephritis or the nephrotic syndrome), gastrointestinal manifestations (anorexia, nausea, vomiting, diarrhoea, abdominal pain, ascites), adeno-pathy (generalized or cervical), splenomegaly, hepatomegaly and blood abnormalities (anaemia, leucopenia, thrombocytopenia).

The main *pulmonary manifestations* are

(1) pleurisy, with or without effusion,
(2) various types of 'pneumonia' possibly directly due to LE,
(3) secondary pulmonary infections, including bacterial or viral pneumonia, lung abscess, tuberculosis or sometimes bizarre infections with fungi [30],
(4) dyspnoea without obvious pulmonary change on x-ray but with high diaphragms which move sluggishly on fluoroscopy and presumably due to radiologically cryptic interstitial lung infiltration and focal atelectasis.

These manifestations will now be discussed in more detail.

PLEURISY [17, 30 & 32]

Pleurisy, frequently bilateral, and not uncommonly with accompanying pericarditis, occurs in 42–60% of various reported series, with effusion in 16–55%. Pleurisy or effusion is sometimes the first manifestation. A history of recurrent pleuritic pain, unilateral or bilateral, is common. The pain usually lasts several days. The pleural effusion is usually small or moderate, seldom massive. The pleural fluid is straw coloured and cellular with a high percentage of mononuclear cells; LE cells may be present in the fluid if they are also present in the blood. The fluid is not usually haemorrhagic. Pleural effusions may clear spontaneously but respond well to corticosteroid treatment. There is often residual thickening visible on the x-ray. Some patients have recurrent attacks of cough, scanty sputum, dyspnoea and pleurisy, which respond dramatically to corticosteroid drugs [34].

PNEUMONIA

Pneumonia may be pyogenic or due to LE itself. There is frequently atelectasis, sometimes associated with bronchial blockage by mucus but sometimes without obvious cause.

It is perhaps due to an alteration in surfactant, as already mentioned. Different authors vary considerably in their estimate of what proportion of cases of pneumonia is due either directly to LE or to a bacterial or viral cause, but all agree that it is difficult to differentiate between the two groups. A consolidation persisting for weeks or months in a patient with SLE suggests a specific LE involvement. The type of pneumonia is very variable. The x-ray may show considerable consolidation, areas of atelectasis, sometimes with no obvious segmental distribution, or patchy irregular shadows in one or both lungs. If the lesions are small there may be no respiratory symptoms; if they are large there may be tachypnoea, dyspnoea and cyanosis with variable cough. There may be scattered fine or coarse crepitations. The LE type of pneumonia responds well to corticosteroid drugs.

DYSPNOEA WITHOUT OVERT PULMONARY CHANGE ON X-RAY

It is relatively common for patients to complain of dyspnoea without obvious radiographic change apart from high sluggish diaphragms on fluoroscopy [34]. The probable pathological basis and results of function testing have already been outlined (p. 582). The condition usually responds well to corticosteroid drugs. Overt diffuse *pulmonary fibrosis*, visible radiographically, is rare.

RADIOLOGY

There are no specific radiographic appearances. The presence of bilateral pleural effusions and pericardial effusion should suggest the possibility of SLE. The presence of obvious abnormality of the heart, whether due to pericarditis or to myocarditis, together with pleural and lung changes, should also suggest the diagnosis. Changes in the lung fields include the various types of pneumonic and atelectatic shadow already mentioned (p. 583). More rarely there may be pulmonary nodulation, diffuse micronodular infiltration, linear atelectasis, pulmonary oedema or, sometimes, persistent radiographic changes resembling pulmonary oedema but probably representing

LE lesions of the lung itself [17]. Appearances similar to those of fibrosing alveolitis seem to be rare, though one case is mentioned by Rubin and Lubliner [49] and we have seen several ourselves.

DIAGNOSIS [18]

In pulmonary disease SLE should enter into the differential diagnosis in a patient with recent repeated pulmonary infections or pleurisy who has had no previous respiratory trouble. Other causes of recurrent pneumonia, some of which are much more frequent, are discussed on p. 140. The presence of bilateral pleural effusion, especially if accompanied by pericardial effusion, should also give rise to a suspicion of SLE, though of course tuberculosis would be another contender in the differential diagnosis. The suspicion of SLE would be strengthened if there were skin lesions or appropriate lesions in other organs, though disseminated tuberculosis would also have to be considered. The search for *antinuclear factor* in the blood is a useful screening test, though this of course may be positive in other collagen diseases. The crucial criterion is the finding of *LE cells* in the blood on 2 or more occasions. As already mentioned, LE cells may occasionally be found in cases of rheumatoid arthritis or of 'lupoid hepatitis' who do not develop lesions elsewhere, but such patients will not of course have pulmonary involvement. In some patients with lupus erythematosus no LE cells may be found in spite of widespread suggestive lesions. The finding of typical skin lesions or of haematoxylin-staining bodies on *biopsy* is the only way in which the diagnosis can be established in such cases. One must remember that the group of conditions diagnosed as SLE merges into other diagnostic groups such as rheumatoid disease (p. 578), systemic sclerosis (p. 585), dermatomyositis (p. 587) and polyarteritis nodosa (p. 434).

TREATMENT AND PROGNOSIS [19, 20 & 40]

The avoidance of sunlight, ultraviolet light and heat are important in minimizing the initiation or exacerbation of the skin lesions, though these are not our concern in this book. In exacerbations rest is thought to be important. The pulmonary manifestations are merely incidents in the general disease. The outlook for exacerbations, and probably for long term prognosis, has been revolutionized by the introduction of the corticosteroid drugs. Without adequate treatment more than half the patients formerly died within 2 years. The evidence suggests that the prognosis is now much better; certainly many patients are living for at least 10 or 15 years, though often requiring repeated treatment [20].

The current tendency is to give very large doses of corticosteroid drugs in severe exacerbations, particularly if these involve the kidneys or the central nervous system, in order to avoid permanent and severe damage. Initial treatment may be with doses of prednisolone as high as 80 mg/day. If there is no response within 48 hours even higher doses may be given. Pulmonary and pleural lesions usually respond rapidly to smaller doses such as 20–40 mg/day. In a patient presenting with pneumonia it may be uncertain whether this is a bacterial pneumonia complicating SLE or an SLE phenomenon itself. It is best to initiate the necessary aetiological investigations and to treat as for bacterial pneumonia (p. 135), but to add a corticosteroid drug if there is failure to respond and if no infective agent is identified. If the patient is very severely ill it is wise to give both treatments initially. A dose of 40–60 mg of prednisolone daily is usually sufficient. After a response has been obtained this may be gradually reduced to 5–15 mg daily and continued for 6–12 months according to the circumstances, thereafter being reduced by 1 mg a week until the patient is off treatment. If there is any relapse the dose should again be raised. If relapse occurs it usually does so within 6 months of stopping treatment. Every patient has to be treated on an *ad hoc* basis, according to the clinical situation, both with respect to duration and to daily dosage.

SYSTEMIC SCLEROSIS
(Progressive Systemic Sclerosis, Generalized Scleroderma)

DEFINITION

Systemic sclerosis has been defined as 'a sclerotic and indurative process of the connective tissue which injures not only the cutis and subcutaneous tissue . . . but which can involve more or less precociously the connective tissue of any organ or system' [43]. This condition is undoubtedly related to certain others, such as dermatomyositis, systemic lupus erythematosus, rheumatoid disease and Sjögren's syndrome. Manifestations suggestive of one or other of these syndromes were found in 6% of a large series of cases of scleroderma at the Mayo Clinic [54].

PREVALENCE [39]

Systemic sclerosis is less common than systemic lupus erythematosus. It is 2 to 3 times commoner in females than in males. It occurs at all ages but is most frequently diagnosed between the ages of 30 and 50. In Baltimore, U.S.A., the mortality rate in white females has been quoted as 0·22 per 100,000 population, and 3 times higher in Negro females. The male rates were equal in both races.

AETIOLOGY

The cause of the condition is unknown. LE cells have occasionally been found [22 & 48]. The erythrocyte sedimentation rate is often raised and the albumin/globulin ratio may be reversed. Gammaglobulin has been found to be localized in the lesions of some cases [22]. Rheumatoid factor may be present in the blood serum and autoantibodies to intranuclear nucleoproteins have been demonstrated in a few cases [54].

PATHOLOGY

The essential pathological change is said to be the swelling and disintegration of collagen tissue, with cellular infiltration and fibrosis [36]. There may also be swelling of the intima of small vessels with fibrinoid necrosis and occlusion. When the lung is affected autopsy may show diffuse fibrosis of alveolar walls with obliteration of capillaries and alveolar spaces [36]. The process can also involve the bronchial walls and peribronchial tissue. Sometimes there is bronchiectasis. The pulmonary vessels may show endarteritis and sclerosis, which may result in pulmonary hypertension. Secondary infection, or spillover from the affected oesophagus, may give rise to acute inflammatory lesions.

FUNCTIONAL ABNORMALITY [9 & 36]

The lesions in the lung may not be visible on the x-ray; the patient may have dyspnoea and abnormal function tests with no obvious radiographic change. On the other hand, the patient may have no complaint in spite of radiographic abnormalities. The diffuse fibrosis gives rise to a restrictive ventilatory abnormality (p. 51). Diffusion defects are often demonstrable. In more severe cases the Pa,o_2 may be decreased, at least on exercise, and presumably also the Pa,co_2. In some cases the dyspnoea may be mainly due to involvement of chest wall or diaphragm by sclerosis, resulting in decrease of VC but no demonstrable diffusion defect.

CLINICAL FEATURES [23, 41 & 43]

SKIN LESIONS

Three types of skin lesion may occur in scleroderma:

(1) sclerotic lesions localized to small areas of the skin and usually resolving in months or years (morphoea),

(2) generalized scleroderma, widely affecting the trunk and limbs and often improving spontaneously; the skin is smooth, shiny and bound down to the deeper structure, and

(3) lesions mainly affecting the face, hands and feet.

It is the latter type of lesion which is usually associated with systemic sclerosis. The initial symptoms are often of pain in the fingers and Raynaud's phenomenon. Later there are atrophic changes in the fingers and toes, with ulceration and loss of tissue (acrosclerosis). The face becomes furrowed round the mouth.

There may be telangiectases of the face and hands and also pigmentation and calcinosis of the soft tissues. The hands may become fixed in semiflexion. Probably all these types of skin lesion are basically the same process.

CHANGES IN OTHER TISSUES

These include:

(1) dilatation and decrease in peristalsis of the *oesophagus*, often with an inefficient cardia resulting in dysphagia and heartburn;

(2) lesions of the *duodenum* and *colon* which may result in duodenal ileus and colonic diverticula, with symptoms of constipation or diarrhoea; there may be malabsorption and steatorrhoea;

(3) *cardiac* lesions, particularly fibrosis and sometimes adhesive pericarditis or pericardial effusion; more frequently cardiac lesions are secondary to hypertension resulting from kidney involvement [50];

(4) *renal* lesions, with multiple arterial occlusions, cortical infarcts and LE-like lesions of the glomeruli, resulting in hypertension and uraemia [47];

(5) lesions of *skeletal muscles*, which may consist of disuse atrophy, though sometimes of actual sclerosis;

(6) swelling of *joints* [4].

THE LUNGS [9, 23, 36, 41, 42 & 43]

Lung lesions may occur in between one third and one half of all patients who are radiologically examined. The main respiratory symptoms are dyspnoea and cough, sometimes with mucoid sputum. As already mentioned, dyspnoea may occur with no radiographic change. Alternatively, there may be x-ray evidence of pulmonary fibrosis but no dyspnoea. Pulmonary changes may precede those in the skin but more often follow them. As already mentioned, dyspnoea may sometimes be related to changes in the chest wall or diaphragm rather than the lungs. When dyspnoea is severe there may be cyanosis and there may also be basal crepitations. Secondary infection may occur, with purulent sputum and perhaps clinical and radiological evidence of pneumonia. Sometimes pneumonia is due to a spillover from the oesophagus. Although evidence of pleural thickening or effusion may be found at postmortem these are relatively seldom evident clinically or radiologically, and indeed may not be directly related to the systemic sclerosis. Pulmonary oedema may occur, most commonly due to systemic hypertension secondary to kidney lesions, but occasionally due to cardiac damage. Finger clubbing seems to be relatively uncommon.

RADIOLOGY [4, 41, 42 & 43]

Sometimes the x-ray shows only a mild local or regional fibrosis. More often there are generalized changes in both lower zones. These may be nodular initially but later streaky, and there may be honeycombing. Pleural changes have seldom been noted. Pneumonia-like shadows may be due to complicating pneumonia, to spillover from an affected oesophagus or perhaps occasionally, particularly when long continued, due to the disease itself. Bronchograms may or may not show evidence of bronchiectasis.

Although the fibrosis is classically in the middle and lower zones it may occasionally be apical and there may sometimes be difficulty in differentiating it from fibrosis due to tuberculosis.

DIAGNOSIS

The differential diagnosis is similar to that of fibrosing alveolitis of idiopathic type (p. 569). The diagnosis of systemic sclerosis can only be sustained if there are relevant lesions in other organs.

TREATMENT [4, 36 & 43]

As far as the lung lesions are concerned, the only possible specific treatment appears to be with corticosteroid drugs, though poorly substantiated claims have been made for various other forms of treatment. Even in the case of corticosteroid drugs the reports of success are variable, perhaps depending on the degree of irreversibility before treatment was initiated. Corticosteroid drugs have been unsuccessful in a number of cases but in others cortisone or prednisolone appear to have improved symptoms, respiratory function and x-ray appearances, though the drugs may have to be continued indefinitely. At the time of writing the evidence is far from conclusive. Prednisolone should be employed as for systemic lupus erythematosus (p. 584), using large doses if there are renal lesions as patients with these have a particularly bad prognosis.

PROGNOSIS

When the disease mainly affects the skin, joints and oesophagus it is characterized by periods of remission and exacerbation but when the heart, kidney and lungs are involved the disease is usually fairly rapidly progressive and, if untreated, results in death after several years' illness. Progress seems to be more rapid in women than in men [43]. In white residents in Baltimore, U.S.A., the average survival until death was 7 years, the average age at death being 56; in negroes the average survival was only 2 years and the average age at death 43. As already mentioned, it may be that the fatal outcome can be delayed, sometimes perhaps indefinitely, by the use of corticosteroid drugs, though in other patients treatment is unsuccessful.

DERMATOMYOSITIS

As already mentioned (p. 585), this condition is probably related to systemic sclerosis although a proportion of cases are associated with malignant disease. One might expect that some of these patients would have lung lesions similar to those occurring in systemic sclerosis. Bates and Christie [2] mention one such case of their own and state that there are others in the literature though they give no references. No mention of lung lesions is made in several full reviews of the condition [31 & 58]. We have had a patient who presented with a syndrome similar to the subacute type of fibrosing alveolitis (p. 567) whose condition responded to corticosteroid drugs but who later developed a polymyositis proved by biopsy.

ERYTHEMA MULTIFORME EXUDATIVUM

(Stevens–Johnson syndrome)

Erythema multiforme is a systemic disorder characterized by diffuse skin lesions due to focal vasculitis. The skin lesions include erythema, macules, papules, urticaria, purpura and bullae. All of these lesions may occur in a patient at the same time or crops of different lesions may develop in succession. The periphery of the body is mainly involved, with most of the lesions on the backs of the hands and feet, the shins and the genitalia. In severe cases the lips and throat are affected. Bullous eruptions on the lips and buccal mucosa develop into shallow ulcers which rapidly become secondarily infected.

Erythema multiforme appears to be commonly provoked by drugs such as aspirin, sulphonamides [28], hypnotics or antibiotics. Toxins of various kinds have sometimes appeared to be significant in triggering an attack. Often no precipitating cause is found. Individual hypersensitivity to the particular drug may be important as may the dosage and mode of excretion. Because of the association of Stevens–Johnson syndrome with long acting sulphonamides it has been recommended that these drugs should not be used in children [28].

When involvement of other organs is added to the skin manifestations of erythema multiforme the term *Stevens–Johnson Syndrome* is applied. Commonly a few days of symptoms of upper respiratory tract infection of influenza type precede the abrupt onset of the full clinical picture which is dominated initially by the skin lesions, conjunctivitis and fever. Cough, purulent sputum, retrosternal soreness and wheeze indicate establishment of secondary bacterial respiratory infection. Toxaemia develops in varying degrees. Carditis, arthritis and polyserositis may also occur. Associated haemolytic anaemia has been described.

Involvement of the lung parenchyma may not be suspected from physical examination but the chest radiograph may show one of a variety of appearances including diffuse miliary or nodular shadows, patchy areas of consolidation or a large pneumonic opacity.

The disease usually clears rapidly; occasional fatal cases have been due to overwhelming secondary infection.

Recent work has suggested that mycoplasmal infection (p. 131) is responsible for at least a proportion of the cases of Stevens–Johnson syndrome [26 & 38] and on this account tetracycline should be included in the treatment when this antibiotic can be excluded as a precipitating agent. It may be necessary to give other antibiotics for associated secondary infection. In severe cases corticosteroids given in high dosage may be lifesaving.

REFERENCES

[1] BASTEN A., CAMENS I. & SCHWARTZ C.J. (1966) Rheumatoid lung disease with report of a case. *Austr. Ann. Med.* **15**, 175.

[2] BATES D.V. & CHRISTIE R.V. (1964) *Respiratory Function in Disease. An Introduction to the Integrated Study of the Lung.* London, Saunders.

[3] BECK E.R. & HOFFBRAND B.I. (1966) Acute lung changes in rheumatoid arthritis. *Ann. rheum. Dis.* **25**, 459.

[4] BEIGELMAN P.M., GOLDNER F. & BAYLES T.B. (1953) Progressive systemic sclerosis (scleroderma) *New Engl. J. Med.* **249**, 45.

[5] BLOCH K.J. (1964) Serologic findings in Sjögren's syndrome. *Ann. intern. Med.* **61**, 518.

[6] BUCHANAN W.W. (1964) Case report. *Ann. intern. Med.* **61**, 510.

[7] BUCHER U.G. & REID LYNNE (1959) Sjögren's syndrome. Report of a fatal case with pulmonary and renal lesions. *Br. J. Dis. Chest* **53**, 237.

[8] BUNIM J.J., Moderator (1964) Clinical, pathologic and serologic studies in Sjögren's syndrome. Combined clinical staff conference at the National Institute of Health. *Ann. intern. Med.* **61**, 509.

[9] CATTERALL MARY & ROWELL N.R. (1963) Respiratory function in progressive systemic sclerosis. *Thorax* **18**, 10.

[10] CHRISTIE G.S. (1954) Pulmonary lesions in rheumatoid arthritis. *Austr. Ann. Med.* **3**, 49.

[11] CRUICKSHANK B. (1957) Rheumatoid arthritis and rheumatoid disease. *Proc. roy. Soc. Med.* **50**, 462.

[12] CRUICKSHANK B. (1966) The basic pattern of tissue damage and pathology of systemic lupus erythematosus. In DuBois E.L. (1966a) *op. cit.*

[13] DENKO C.W. (1960) The sicca syndrome

(Sjögren's syndrome). A study of 16 cases. *Arch. intern. Med.* **105**, 849.

[14] DOCTOR L. & SNIDER G.L. (1962) Diffuse interstitial pulmonary fibrosis associated with arthritis. With comments on the definition of rheumatoid lung disease. *Am. Rev. resp. Dis.*, **85**, 413.

[15] DUBOIS E.L. & TUFFANELLI D.L. (1964) Clinical manifestations of systemic lupus erythematosus. Computer analysis of 520 cases. *J. Am. med. Ass.* **190**, 105.

[16] DUBOIS E.L. & ARTERBERRY J.D. (1966) Etiology. In DUBOIS E.L. (1966a) *op. cit.*

[17] DUBOIS E.L. (1966a) The clinical picture of systemic lupus erythematosus. In *Lupus Erythematosus. A Review of the Current Status of Discoid and Systemic Lupus Erythematosus and their Variants*, ed. DUBOIS E.L. London, McGraw-Hill.

[18] DUBOIS E.L. (1966b) Differential diagnosis, criteria for diagnosis and classification of systemic lupus erythematosus. In DUBOIS E.L. (1966a) *op. cit.*

[19] DUBOIS E.L. (1966c) Management of discoid and systemic lupus erythematosus. In DUBOIS E.L. (1966a) *op. cit.*

[20] DUBOIS E.L. (1966d) Results of steroid therapy in systemic lupus erythematosus. In DUBOIS E.L. (1966a) *op. cit.*

[21] EDGE J.R. & RICKARDS A.G. (1957) Rheumatoid arthritis with lung lesions. *Thorax* **12**, 352.

[22] EDITORIAL (1962) Scleroderma and autoimmunity. *Lancet* **ii**, 767.

[23] EDITORIAL (1963) Pulmonary changes in systemic sclerosis. *Br. med. J.* **ii**, 196.

[24] EDITORIAL (1967) Rheumatoid lungs and rheumatoid piles. *Br. med. J.* **i**, 186.

[25] ELLMAN P., WEBER F.P. & GOODIER T.E.W. (1951) A contribution to the pathology of Sjögren's disease. *Quart. J. Med.*, N.S. **20**, 33.

[26] FEIZI T., MACLEAN H., SOMMERVILLE R.G. & SELWYN J.G. (1966) The rôle of mycoplasmas in human disease. *Proc. roy. Soc. Med.* **59**, 1109.

[27] GARDINER D.L., DUTHIE J.J.R., MACLEOD J. & ALLAN W.S.A. (1957) Pulmonary hypertension in rheumatoid arthritis. Report of a case with intimal sclerosis of the pulmonary and digital arteries. *Scot. med. J.* **2**, 183.

[28] HARRIS M.J., WISE G. & BEVERIDGE J. (1966) Stevens-Johnson Syndrome and sulphonamides. *Aust. paed. J.* **2**, 103.

[29] HART F.D. (1966) Complicated rheumatoid disease. *Br. med. J.* **ii**, 131.

[30] HARVEY A.M., SHULMAN L.E., TUMULTY A., CONLEY C.L. & SCHOENRICH EDYTH H. (1954) Systemic lupus erythematosus: Review of the literature and clinical analysis of 138 cases. *Medicine (Baltimore)* **33**, 291.

[31] HARVEY A.M. & SHULMAN L.E. (1960) Derma-

tomyositis. In *Arthritis and Allied Conditions—a Textbook of Rheumatology*, ed. Hollander J.L., 6th Edition. London, Kimpton.

[32] HASERICK J.R. (1966) Quoted DUBOIS E.L. (1966a) *op. cit.*

[33] HINDLE W. & YATES D.A.H. (1965) Pyopneumothorax complicating rheumatoid lung disease *Ann. rheum. Dis.* **24**, 57.

[34] HOFFBRAND B.I. & BECK E.R. (1965) 'Unexplained' dyspnoea and shrinking lungs in systemic lupus erythematosus. *Br. med. J.* **i**, 1273.

[35] HUANG C.-T., HENNIGAR G.R. & LYONS H.A. (1965) Pulmonary dysfunction in systemic lupus erythematosus. *New Engl. J. Med.* **272**, 288.

[36] HUGHES D.T.D. & LEE F.I. (1963) Lung function in patients with systemic sclerosis. *Thorax* **18**, 16.

[37] LOCKE G.B. (1963) Rheumatoid lung. *Clin. Radiol.* **14**, 43.

[38] LUDHAM G.B., BRIDGES J.B. & BENN F.C. (1964) Association of Stevens-Johnson Syndrome with antibody for *Mycoplasma pneumoniae*. *Lancet* **i**, 958.

[39] MASI A.T. (1967) Population studies in rheumatic disease. *Ann. Rev. Med.* **18**, 185.

[40] MEDICAL RESEARCH COUNCIL, COLLAGEN DISEASES AND HYPERSENSITIVITY PANEL (1961) Treatment of systemic lupus erythematosus with steroids. *Br. med. J.* **ii**, 915.

[41] MILLER R.D., FOWLER W.S. & HELMHOLZ F.H. (1959) Scleroderma of the lungs. *Proc. Mayo Clin.* **34**, 66.

[42] OPIE L.H. (1955) The pulmonary manifestations of generalized scleroderma (progressive systemic sclerosis). *Dis. Chest.* **28**, 665.

[43] ORABONA M.L. & ALBANO O. (1958) Progressive systemic sclerosis (or visceral scleroderma). Review of literature and report of cases. *Acta med. scand.* **160**, Suppl. 333.

[44] PANETTIERE F., CHANDLER B.F. & LIBCKE J.H. (1968) Pulmonary cavitation in rheumatoid disease. Review of the literature and an additional case. *Am. Rev. resp. Dis.* **97**, 89.

[45] PATTERSON C.D., HARVILLE W.E. & PIERCE J.A. (1965) Rheumatoid lung disease. *Ann. intern. Med.* **62**, 685.

[46] RICH A.R. & GREGORY J.E. (1943) On the anaphylactic nature of rheumatic pneumonitis. *Bull. Johns Hopkins Hosp.* **73**, 465.

[47] ROTTENBERG E.N., SLOCUMB C.H. & EDWARDS J.E. (1959) Cardiac and renal manifestations in progressive systemic sclerosis. *Proc. Mayo Clin.* **34**, 77.

[48] ROWELL N.R. (1962) Lupus erythematosus cells in systemic sclerosis. *Ann. rheum. Dis.* **21**, 70.

[49] RUBIN E.H. & LUBLINER R. (1957) The Hamman-Rich syndrome: review of the literature and analysis of 15 cases. *Medicine* **36**, 397.

[50] SACKNER M.A., HEINZ E.R. & STEINBERG A.J.

(1966) The heart in scleroderma. *Am. J. Cardiol.* **17**, 542.

[51] SOKOLOFF L. (1964) Pathologic changes in Sjögren's syndrome. *Ann. intern. Med.* **61**, 516.

[52] SPENCER H. (1962) *Pathology of the Lung.* London, Pergamon Press.

[53] STACK B.H.R. & GRANT I.W.B. (1965) Rheumatoid interstitial lung disease. *Br. J. Dis. Chest* **59**, 202.

[54] TUFFANELLI D.L. & WINKERMANN R.K. (1962) Scleroderma and its relationship to the 'collagenoses': Dermatomyositis, lupus erythematosus, rheumatoid arthritis and Sjögren's syndrome. *Am. J. med. Sci.* **243**, 133.

[55] VANSELOW N.A., DODSON V.N., ANGELL D.C. & DUFF I.F. (1963) A clinical study of Sjögren's syndrome. *Ann. intern. Med.* **58**, 124.

[56] WALKER W.C. (1966) *The Lungs in Rheumatoid Arthritis.* Edinburgh University, M.D. Thesis.

[57] WALKER W.C. (1967) Pulmonary infections and rheumatoid arthritis. *Quart. J. Med., N.S.* **36**, 239.

[58] WALTON J.N. & ADAMS R.D. (1958) *Polymyositis.* London, Livingstone.

CHAPTER 33

Hyaline Membrane Disease, Cystic Fibrosis, Idiopathic Pulmonary Haemosiderosis, Goodpasture's Syndrome.

HYALINE MEMBRANE DISEASE (Respiratory Distress Syndrome) [1 & 38]

DEFINITION

Hyaline membrane disease affects premature infants. It is characterized pathologically by a hyaline membrane lining the alveoli and clinically by respiratory distress which may be fatal. Full details should be sought in paediatric textbooks.

AETIOLOGY AND PREVALENCE

Hyaline membrane disease accounts for 30% of all neonatal deaths and 50–70% of deaths in premature infants. It is therefore an important disease. There is some evidence that it is associated with an abnormality of surfactant (p. 11), which in turn affects alveolar surface tension, but the basic cause is unknown.

PATHOLOGY

The characteristic membrane lining the alveoli consists of sloughed cell débris in a protein matrix and is more obvious the longer the child has survived. There are patchy areas of atelectasis and evidence of constriction of pulmonary arterioles, presumably caused by hypoxia. Macroscopically the lungs are purplish, dark, solid and liver-like.

FUNCTIONAL ABNORMALITY

As expected from the pathology the lungs show low compliance. Minute ventilation may be increased but alveolar ventilation is decreased with increased dead space/tidal volume ratio and ventilation/perfusion ($\dot{V}/\dot{Q}$) abnormalities. In the early stages Pa,O_2 may be only slightly lowered and so may Pa,CO_2. Later there is gross hypoxaemia with lowering of blood pH, though Pa,CO_2 is usually only slightly raised unless there is cerebral haemorrhage. Raised serum lactic acid, reflecting a metabolic acidosis due to inadequate oxygenation of muscle, may also develop. There may be systemic hypotension and a pulmonary-aortic shunt through the open ductus arteriosus, which is decreased by oxygen therapy. Severe hyperkalaemia may occur in infants with occult cerebral haemorrhage or who have become hypothermic.

CLINICAL CHARACTERISTICS AND RADIOLOGY

Grunting and distressed respiration, inspiratory retraction of sternum and costal margin, tachycardia and cyanosis are manifestations of the fully developed condition. Auscultation shows poor air entry but no crepitations. Oedema of the hands and feet is common. The x-ray of chest shows diffuse fine granularity throughout the lungs but no areas of local atelectasis.

In the early stages distress, cyanosis and tachycardia are relieved by oxygen. Less severely affected babies recover in a day or two; those with severe disease may die or continue dyspnoeic for many days or even weeks, though most who recover start to show improvement within 3–4 days. In those with oedema diuresis usually begins about this time. Jaundice is common between the 3rd and 7th day. Occult cerebral haemorrhage may be a complicating factor. Secondary pneumonia may occur.

TREATMENT

Treatment consists of full oxygenation, intravenous buffers, such as sodium bicarbonate, and careful protection from secondary infection. Digitalis is indicated if cardiac failure develops. Hyperkalaemia is treated with intravenous glucose and insulin. Intermittent positive pressure respiration may improve the outlook in very severe cases [32].

PROGNOSIS

The prognosis depends on the severity of the disease and the quality of medical care. If the initial capillary pH is 7·20 or below the mortality is 70–80% but has been reduced to 20% by intermittent positive pressure respiration [32]. Nearly all deaths occur within 72 hours of birth. In the remainder recovery is complete, with no residua.

CYSTIC FIBROSIS (Fibrocystic Disease of the Pancreas, Mucoviscidosis, Mucosis) [3, 5, 7, 33 & 35]

DEFINITION

Although originally described as a disease of the pancreas, it is now realized that cystic fibrosis is a hereditary disease affecting both mucus secreting and nonmucus secreting exocrine glands, with increased viscosity of mucus and a high sodium chloride content of sweat as major abnormalities [6]. Most of the clinical features are related to obstruction by viscid mucus; the lung, paranasal sinuses, pancreas, bile ducts, intestine, salivary glands and seminiferous tubules being particularly involved. Bronchial obstruction leads to secondary infection and lung damage which are prominent features in the great majority of cases and the commonest cause of death. Children are mainly affected, but increasing numbers of patients are now surviving into adult life.

PREVALENCE AND AETIOLOGY

Estimates of prevalence range from 1 in 500 to 1 in 3500 live births. Patients with mild symptoms may not be diagnosed in childhood and in one series nearly 50% of patients over the age of 17 were found to have been diagnosed after the age of 9 [35]. Cystic fibrosis is common in white Europeans and Americans but uncommon in negroes and orientals. The sexes are equally affected.

The disease is transmitted as a recessive gene. The patient is a homozygote and his healthy parents heterozygotes. It has been calculated that as many as 1 in 20 of the population may carry the recessive gene.

Until recently no method has been found of identifying the heterozygote, but it has now been reported that skin fibroblast cultures from heterozygotes, as well as from affected individuals, develop easily recognizable cytoplasmic intravesicular metachromasia [4A].

The exact nature of the underlying biochemical defect, if there is only one, is unknown. A recently published hypothesis [20] postulates that the basic defect is an inhibition of the movement of water and ions through the secretory cells of the affected glands. It is suggested that the defect is related to an abnormality of mucopolysaccharide in the extracellular space, either in the connective tissue proper or in the mucoid layer immediately outside the cell plasma membrane. At present this hypothesis is largely speculative.

PATHOLOGY

About 10% of patients present in infancy with *meconium ileus*. The obstruction is usually in the region of the terminal ileum and is due to the abnormal nature of the meconium. This is unduly viscid owing to the basic abnormality of secretion, and also contains a large amount of proteins owing to the absence of pancreatic enzymes. The presence of albumin is abnormal and it may also be found in siblings who later prove to have the disease [40]. The intestinal epithelium may be denuded and disorganized with evidence of viscid mucus secretion. In the earlier stages the *pancreas* shows dilatation of its ducts, with flattening of the epithelium and dilatation of acini to form cysts.

Later there is diffuse fibrosis with varying degrees of leucocyte infiltration. Later still the gland may show fat replacement with a few clusters of islet cells. Finally even the latter may be affected and diabetes can develop in patients who live sufficiently long. Changes in the *liver* are initially similar to those of the pancreas, with proliferation and dilatation of bile ducts and portal fibrosis which may result in multilobular cirrhosis, though this only develops in a small proportion. Jaundice is rare, although some liver function tests may be abnormal. As a result of cirrhosis hypersplenism occasionally occurs.

The basic abnormality in the *lungs* is the unusually viscid secretion of the mucous glands which leads to bronchial obstruction and secondary infection, resulting initially in purulent bronchitis and often later in widespread bronchiectasis due to damage of the bronchial walls. In addition there may be recurrent incidents of atelectasis, either of small areas of the lung or, especially in young children, of segments or lobes. These may become secondarily infected resulting in pneumonia or lung abscess. Recurrent infection results in progressive fibrosis and emphysema. There is no obvious histological abnormality of the mucous glands. The secretion of the mucous glands of the *paranasal sinuses* is also affected and chronic sinus infection is common.

Although the *sweat glands*, *salivary* and *parotid glands* produce an abnormal secretion they are histologically normal. The *lachrymal gland* secretions are normal.

It seems that biopsy is not a useful way of making the diagnosis, though it has been claimed that rectal biopsy shows a characteristic pattern of ciliated crypts packed with mucus which is sometimes lamellated. The crypt mouths may be gaping and goblet cells are often very prominent [31].

FUNCTIONAL ABNORMALITY

The main effect of the increased sodium chloride in the sweat is the heavy loss of sodium and chloride under hot conditions and the liability of infants and young children to develop consequent heat stroke. This, of course, occurs mainly in warm climates. The major damage is caused by the viscid nature of secreted mucus, leading to obstruction and resultant deficiency of pancreatic secretion and sometimes of bile. The diminished pancreatic secretion contributes to the failure to clear meconium from the intestine in some newborn infants, resulting in intestinal obstruction. Faecal impaction may occur in older children. The absence of pancreatic secretions also results in frequent large bowel movements and malabsorption. Occasionally the obstruction of the bile canaliculi is sufficient to cause jaundice.

Pulmonary function tests usually show decrease of VC in patients with radiological change. With recurrent or chronic bronchial infection, increase of airways resistance and decreased FEV are common. RV may be increased and there may be respiratory failure, with decreased Pa,o_2 and increased Pa,co_2, at first in exacerbations and later terminally [2 & 4].

CLINICAL FEATURES

RESPIRATORY SYMPTOMS

The disease should be suspected in any child with recurrent or chronic symptoms affecting the upper or lower respiratory tract. Respiratory symptoms affect virtually all patients who survive infancy. In most, symptoms begin in infancy but in a few they may develop later. Cough may be initially infrequent but is later persistent and often paroxysmal. Wheeze is common. As the disease progresses dyspnoea occurs and the cough becomes productive. There are recurrent episodes of acute respiratory infection, with pneumonia or purulent bronchitis, sometimes with collapse of a segment or lobe. The characteristic clinical features of bronchiectasis (p. 351) often develop and there may be finger clubbing. The child's general health is affected, with failure to grow and gain weight. Later there may be cyanosis and *cor pulmonale*. Chronic infection of the sinuses is common and there may be nasal polypi. The most common bacterial invader in the respiratory tract is *Staphylococcus pyogenes* but gram negative organisms, such as *Proteus*, *E. coli*, *K. pneumoniae* or *Pseudomonas*, may occur, particularly after the patient has received antibiotics.

GASTROINTESTINAL SYMPTOMS

Intestinal obstruction due to meconium ileus occurs in the newborn in about 10% of cases. Faecal impaction, intussusception and recurrent rectal prolapse may occur in older children. About 80% of patients develop symptoms suggesting pancreatic insufficiency or malabsorption. These include slow growth, failure to thrive, a good or huge appetite, frequent large foul stools and a protuberant abdomen.

HEPATIC SYMPTOMS

These are relatively uncommon. Sometimes there is jaundice. Later there may be evidence of cirrhosis of the liver which may be complicated by portal hypertension with or without hypersplenism.

HEAT STROKE

The loss of sodium and chloride in the sweat under hot conditions, together with excessive sweating, and loss of water, may result in circulatory collapse.

RADIOLOGY

Changes in the chest x-ray are variable, according to the stage of the disease and the severity of lung involvement. Scattered small areas of collapse or pneumonia may give a characteristic 'snowstorm' appearance in the x-ray but there may be lobar or segmental atelectasis, areas of pneumonia or the cavitated lesions of lung abscess. The lungs may become hyperinflated.

DIAGNOSIS

The most important factor in diagnosis is to suspect the possibility in any child, or indeed young adult, with chronic or recurrent respiratory infection, especially if there are also gastrointestinal symptoms of the relevant

type. All siblings of known patients should also be investigated. Much the most simple screening test, which is said to be 98% reliable in children, is the estimation of *sodium and chloride in the sweat*. The most frequent and painless method now employed is the pilocarpine iontophoresis method for stimulating local sweat production [15]. In cystic fibrosis the concentrations of both sodium and chloride are over 70 mEq/l in the sweat. This is very much less reliable in adults who may have values well above the diagnostic range although quite normal [24]. Factors affecting the level in adults are mentioned in the discussion of the alleged relationship of cystic fibrosis to chronic bronchitis (p. 310). Sweat levels are not altered in the heterozygote [35]. In patients with cystic fibrosis the high sweat sodium levels do not fall, as they do in normals, when given 9-α-fluorohydrocortisone or aldosterone. If the sweat sodium does not fall after aldosterone in a dose of 0·1 mg per kg has been given for several days the diagnosis is almost certain. This test may be of value in adolescents or adults in whom the absolute value of the sweat sodium is not diagnostic [12].

Sweat tests may be difficult in the newborn because of the difficulty of obtaining sweat, and in certain patients with dry skin. The sweat sodium can be measured by an expensive and elaborate technique in which a sodium sensitive electrode is placed directly on the skin [16]. In children and infants the analysis of nail clippings for raised sodium (and potassium) is said to be useful in early diagnosis if the sweat test gives a doubtful result [22].

Increase in viscosity and *decrease of trypsin* (and other pancreatic enzymes) in the duodenal aspirate was formerly used as an important diagnostic test. Duodenal aspiration is distressing to children and could well be omitted if the clinical features and sweat test make the diagnosis relatively certain. An indirect screening test for trypsin in the faeces, using gelatine film, might be substituted in order to avoid duodenal aspiration. When there is pancreatic insufficiency there is always an *increase of total free fatty acids* in the stool.

Patients may excrete as much as 30 g of fat per day.

PREVENTION

All unaffected siblings of children with the disease will be heterozygotes and should be warned about the risk of marrying any other known heterozygote. The family history, and perhaps now the skin fibroblast test (p. 592) may help to identify carriers of the gene. All children of known heterozygotes should have sweat tests as early as possible in infancy so that prophylactic measures can be taken before symptoms develop. Individuals who are known to have the trait should be given plenty of salt when in a warm climate or if they sweat excessively. Measles and whooping cough may be serious diseases in these children and vaccines should be given early. Dietary and pancreatic therapy should be begun as soon as the condition is diagnosed.

TREATMENT [3, 8, 28, 29 & 35]

It has been found very valuable to treat these patients at special centres where the staff can obtain experience of the disease and where it is easier to instruct parents in the care of the child and to maintain their morale. As far as possible the child should be treated as an outpatient, although admission to hospital may be necessary for emergencies.

Intestinal obstruction due to meconium ileus usually requires surgical treatment, often by ileostomy. In older children treatment is directed to maintaining nutrition, encouraging the drainage of the respiratory tract and controlling pulmonary infection. A high protein, high caloric *diet* is given, the amount of fat in the diet being adapted to the symptoms and the degree of pancreatic deficiency, as shown by the severity of steatorrhoea. The missing pancreatic enzymes are replaced by *pancreatin powder*, the dose of which is adjusted according to the severity of symptoms. *Additional salt* and fluid is given in hot weather to replace the sweat loss. *Additional vitamins* A, D and E are recommended [3]. Vitamin K should be given to small infants who are prone to hypoprothrombinaemia [35].

20—R.D.

Drainage of the bronchi is encouraged by postural drainage, breathing exercises and physical activity. Continuous *mist tent therapy* during sleep is said to give very impressive results in reducing the viscosity of sputum, reducing cough and decreasing secondary infection [29]. Special nebulizers are used employing compressed air; oxygen results in increased viscosity of secretions and damage to the bronchial mucosa. 10% propylene glycol is added to decrease the evaporation and disappearance of the water mist after inhalation. Nebulization aims at producing particles between 1 and 5 μ in diameter. The mist should be so dense that it is difficult to see the patient. Ultrasonic nebulizers have also been used [3]. If there is much wheeze 0·5% isoprenaline may be given by aerosol. Polymyxin and neomycin have been given by inhalation but should be used with caution. Neomycin inhalation can result in permanent deafness.

Antibiotic therapy should be based on the sensitivity of the invading organisms and may be given according to the principles outlined in Chapter 5. Its frequency and duration depend on the severity and chronicity of respiratory infection. Intensive and prolonged chemotherapy should be given for any exacerbation. Some authorities advise against giving continuous therapy, others recommend varying the chemotherapy every few weeks in order to reduce the chances of superinfection by resistant organisms.

PROGNOSIS

Before broad spectrum antibiotics became available the prognosis was poor and most children died before reaching 10 years of age. Death was usually due to respiratory infection. With the improvement of early diagnosis and the development of better methods of bronchial drainage and chemotherapy, the prognosis is now very much better. In 49 patients diagnosed early and having a full prophylactic régime no deaths and no deterioration in pulmonary function or pulmonary disease was found over an average follow-up period of $4\frac{1}{2}$ years. Another 49 patients already had severe pulmonary damage when first seen but in the entire group of 98 patients the mortality rate was only 2·5% per year and no death occurred under the age of 6 [8]. Shwachman [35] reported over 100 patients who had reached 17 years of age, many having completed a university course, 12 having married and 11 becoming mothers. To what age such patients will live is uncertain as the improvement in prognosis is so recent.

IDIOPATHIC PULMONARY HAEMOSIDEROSIS
[10, 11, 14, 19, 21, 30 & 37]

DEFINITION

Idiopathic pulmonary haemosiderosis is a rare disease of uncertain cause characterized by recurrent episodes of haemorrhage into the lung, haemoptysis and secondary iron deficiency anaemia. Most cases begin in childhood but some in adult life. The disease is often fatal though apparent complete recovery can occur. In certain cases a similar clinical picture is associated with acute or chronic nephritis (Goodpasture's syndrome) but there is some controversy as to whether these conditions are related.

AETIOLOGY AND PREVALENCE

This is a rare disease but Soergel and Sommers [37] were able to review 132 cases from the literature and from personal experience up to 1962. Most were aged between 1 and 7 at onset but about 15% were aged 16 or over when symptoms began. The sexes are equal in childhood but in adult life the disease is twice as common in men. The disease is not familial.

The accompanying iron deficiency anaemia is certainly due to loss of iron into the lung through haemorrhage, as has been shown by iron turnover studies [21]. The cause of the haemorrhages is uncertain. A possible developmental defect of the pulmonary elastic fibres is now thought not to be supported by the histological evidence [37] but it has been suggested that there is a primary abnormality of alveolar epithelial growth and function which may interfere with the mechanical stability of the alveolar capillaries [37]. If this is the case the origin of the epithelial abnormality is uncertain. It is fashionable to suggest that it may be due to some disturbance of immunological mechanisms. This might be supported by the presence of eosinophilia in about one eighth of cases, the aggregation of mast cells in the lung, an increase in plasma cells in the reticuloendothelial system and the presence of cold agglutinins in some cases [11]. It might also be supported by the occurrence in a few patients of lesions usually regarded as being associated with disturbance of immune mechanisms, such as rheumatoid arthritis or polyarthritis [36], myocarditis [21] and perhaps the nephritis in Goodpasture's syndrome (p. 598). Soergel and Sommer [37] found no evidence of autoantibodies to lung or kidney in any of 6 cases.

Heiner and his colleagues [18 & 19] found positive intradermal tests to cow's milk, and precipitins to cow's milk in the serum of some infants with proved or probable idiopathic pulmonary haemosiderosis, the symptoms disappearing on removal of cow's milk from the diet. But in other patients with proved pulmonary haemosiderosis the tests were negative.

One must conclude that the evidence at present available is insufficient to give a clear indication of the cause of the disease.

PATHOLOGY

Histologically there is degeneration, shedding and hyperplasia of alveolar epithelial cells and marked localized alveolar capillary dilatation [37]. There is infiltration with many haemosiderin-containing macrophages. One must remember that haemosiderin deposition is not specific to this disease. It can occur in haemolytic or aplastic anaemia, multiple blood transfusions, severe mitral stenosis or left ventricular failure and in bronchiectasis

[10]. It is also not uncommon in cases of fibrosing alveolitis or honeycomb lung. In remissions the haemosiderosis may not be a prominent feature. There may be varying degrees of diffuse pulmonary interstitial fibrosis; degeneration of the alveolar, interstitial and vascular elastic fibres; dilatation and moderate subendothelial sclerosis of pulmonary arteries and veins; and slight muscular hypertrophy of the bronchial arteries. These changes are regarded as secondary to the recurrent bleeding and are not always present [37]. *Macroscopically* gross pulmonary haemorrhages may be present in the more acute cases. In more chronic cases diffuse fibrosis may be obvious. The iron content of washed and dried lung tissue is from 5 to 2000 times greater than normal, the increase being roughly proportionate to the duration of the disease [11].

FUNCTIONAL ABNORMALITY

In acute incidents bronchial and alveolar flooding with blood will reduce the respiratory reserve to an extent which depends on the severity of the haemorrhage and how far it has been aspirated into different parts of the lung. In the more chronic cases dyspnoea is a feature, especially when fibrosis develops. The interstitial nature of the pathological process would lead one to expect a reduction in diffusing capacity, with hypoxaemia in spite of hyperventilation, and perhaps a reduction in Pa,co_2. These features were in fact found in 2 cases investigated by Bates and Christie [2].

CLINICAL AND RADIOLOGICAL FEATURES

Clinical and radiological features have been well summarized by Soergel and Sommers [37]. The intensity and duration of the pulmonary haemorrhages determine the clinical course. This is very variable. A frequent picture is one in which continuous, mild intrapulmonary bleeding results in a chronic nonproductive cough with tiredness, pallor and failure of the child to gain weight. The sputum may be intermittently bloodstained. An iron deficiency anaemia will be found and occult blood is occasionally present in the stools. In about one quarter of the patients there is generalized moderate lymphadenopathy. The chest x-ray may show transient, blotchy pulmonary shadows. After weeks or months the first severe bleeding occurs. There are small haemoptyses with prolonged coughing spells and there may be substernal or epigastric pain and tightness in the chest. There may be moderate pyrexia and anaemia becomes more severe. In the lungs there may be basal crepitations and dullness to percussion. In about 20% the liver and spleen become palpable. X-ray at this stage will show bilateral or unilateral, multiple patchy shadows, especially in the middle and lower zones. After 1–2 weeks the x-ray may clear and the patient improves with diminution of the anaemia.

These moderate bleeding episodes may continue for a long period and after several years the patient develops chronic mild breathlessness with continuing anaemia. At this stage there may be miliary nodulation in the lung film, most marked in the mid and lower zones, and sometimes an appearance of enlargement of mediastinal lymph nodes. About 25% of patients develop finger clubbing. Chronic *cor pulmonale* secondary to pulmonary fibrosis develops in only a small minority.

Massive pulmonary haemorrhage may occur at any time and most patients die in a severe bleeding episode. Occasional episodes of minor extrapulmonary bleeding have been recorded.

INVESTIGATIONS

Discovery of haemosiderin-containing macrophages in sputum or gastric washings is characteristic though such cells may also be found with other causes of lung bleeding. Hypochromic, microcytic anaemia is usual. Prothrombin, bleeding and clotting times are normal. Cold agglutinins may be present in some cases and blood eosinophilia in 20% [37]. Lung biopsy is sometimes justified.

TREATMENT

The iron deficiency anaemia responds to iron therapy. Repeated blood transfusions will be necessary for severe episodes of bleeding. Secondary infection is usually not a problem, even during bleeding episodes, causing a rise in temperature, and antibiotics are thought not to be necessary [37]. Some authors have had an impression that corticosteroid drugs were of value during the acute episodes, though most of these resolve spontaneously and it must be difficult to judge. It seems to be generally agreed that long term corticosteroid therapy does not alter the course or prognosis. Azathioprine has been thought to be effective in one case [38]. Splenectomy has been recommended but there is no good evidence that it influences the course of the disease.

PROGNOSIS

The course of the disease is very variable. Although it is often fatal a number of patients appear to recover and remain symptom free, at least for long periods. In an analysis of 68 patients Soergel and Sommers [37] found that 20 were dead after an average duration of the disease of 3·3 years; 17 still had active disease after an average duration of 5·5 years; 12 had relatively inactive disease but still with chronic symptoms, such as exertional dyspnoea and anaemia after an average duration of 5·4 years; 19 were apparently completely free from the disease and symptoms after an average duration of 4·5 years. They quote a 28 year old woman who died after an illness of only 9 days and a boy who was aged 6 at the onset and died of cor pulmonale 20 years later.

GOODPASTURE'S SYNDROME [9, 13, 23, 25, 26 & 34]
(Pulmonary Haemorrhage and Glomerular Nephritis)

DEFINITION

As already mentioned (p. 596), it is uncertain whether Goodpasture's syndrome should be regarded as a variant of idiopathic pulmonary haemosiderosis. Some of the patients, including the one originally described by Goodpasture [17], have probably been examples of polyarteritis nodosa (p. 434) but in most cases there is no evidence of arteritis and pulmonary haemorrhage is relatively unusual in polyarteritis nodosa. Goodpasture's syndrome differs from idiopathic pulmonary haemosiderosis in that it seems to be confined to individuals over 16 years of age and that the kidneys are involved as well as the lung. Massive pulmonary haemorrhage is said to be less common in Goodpasture's syndrome but intra-alveolar fibrin deposition more frequent. It is uncertain whether these differences are sufficient to warrant separate classification and the aetiology of both conditions is unknown.

AETIOLOGY AND PREVALENCE

Nearly 100 cases had been described up to 1965 [9]. In most, symptoms began between the ages of 18 and 35 and 75% were in males. The causation is unknown. Human gamma-globulin has been shown to be attached to the kidney glomeruli by fluorescent antibody techniques but this also occurs in glomerulonephritis associated with streptococci and no attachment to cells has been demonstrated in the lung [9]. In the majority of patients no evidence of infection with haemolytic streptococci, or of immune responses to streptococci, have been demonstrated, though these have been shown in an occasional case [25]. Duncan *et al.* [9] suggest that the condition may represent a primary viral infection of the lung and perhaps secondarily of the kidney, and that the glomerulonephritis may result from a reaction of antibody with antigen fixed to kidney cells. They admit that in the present state of knowledge this is pure speculation.

PATHOLOGY

The pathology of the kidney, by conventional methods, does not seem to differ from that of glomerulonephritis and may be acute or subacute according to the course of the disease, though a high incidence of necrotizing vasculitis has been reported [27]. On electron microscopy the lesions of the basement membrane are said to differ from those seen in acute streptococcal nephritis [9]. The lung lesions appear to be similar to those found in idiopathic pulmonary haemosiderosis, though severe haemorrhages are less common and, as already mentioned, in some cases there appears to be arteritis and necrotizing alveolitis [27], though it is possible that such patients should be classified with polyarteritis nodosa.

CLINICAL AND RADIOLOGICAL FEATURES

Lung haemorrhages, with clinical features similar to those of idiopathic haemosiderosis, but usually without severe bleeding incidents, commonly precede by a few weeks or months the onset of acute glomerulonephritis. The clinical features of the latter are similar to those of streptococcal glomerulonephritis except that hypertension is less frequent. The course of the disease is variable. The duration varies from less than a month to 12 years. Most patients die from renal failure rather than pulmonary haemorrhage or respiratory insufficiency. Others make an apparent complete recovery.

DIAGNOSIS

The main diagnosis will be from polyarteritis nodosa. Iron-containing macrophages in sputum or gastric washings may occur with any cause of lung bleeding. In some cases renal biopsy will be justifiable.

TREATMENT

What evidence is available suggests that corticosteroid drugs may be more effective in Goodpasture's syndrome than in idiopathic pulmonary haemosiderosis. In the review by Duncan and his colleagues [9], 9 of the 11 cases which 'recovered' received significant amounts of corticosteroid drugs at the stage when the renal manifestations were relatively mild. Treatment seems of little value once the renal disease is far advanced [9].

PROGNOSIS

Although most reported cases have been fatal, Duncan et al. [9] in their review reported 11 with apparent complete recovery and with up to 6 years of follow-up. Other recoveries have been subsequently reported [13 & 26]. The course in the fatal cases has been very variable. Some have died in a few weeks, others after a number of years, most within weeks or months. The outlook may be better in those who receive corticosteroid drugs while the renal lesions are relatively mild.

REFERENCES

[1] AVERY MARY E. (1964) Hyaline membrane disease. In *The Lung and its Disorders in the Newborn Infant*. Philadelphia, Saunders.
[2] BATES D.V. & CHRISTIE R.V. (1964) Fibrocystic disease of the pancreas (mucoviscidosis). In *Respiratory Function in Disease. An Introduction to the Integrated Study of the Lung*. Philadelphia, Saunders.
[3] COMMITTEE ON THERAPY OF THE AMERICAN THORACIC SOCIETY (1968) The treatment of cystic fibrosis. *Am. Rev. resp. Dis.* **97**, 730.
[4] COOK C.D., HELLIESEN P.J., KULCZYCKI L., BARRIE H., FRIEDLANDER L., AGATHON S., HARRIS G.B.C. & SHWACHMAN H. (1959) Studies of respiratory physiology in children. II. Lung volumes and mechanics of respiration in 64 patients with cystic fibrosis of the pancreas. *Pediatrics* **24**, 181.
[4A] DANES B.S. & BEARN A.G. (1968) A genetic cell marker in cystic fibrosis of the pancreas. *Lancet* i, 1061.
[5] DiSANT'AGNESE P.A. (1965a) Cystic fibrosis of the pancreas. *Am. J. Med.* **21**, 406.
[6] DiSANT'AGNESE P.A. (1956b) Fibrocystic disease of the pancreas. A generalized disease of exocrine glands. *J. Am. med. Ass.* **160**, 846.
[7] DiSANT'AGNESE P.A. & ANDERSEN DOROTHY H. (1959) Cystic fibrosis of the pancreas in young adults. *Ann. intern. Med.* **50**, 1321.
[8] DOERSHUK C.F., MATTHEWS L.W., TUCKER A.S. & SPECTOR S. (1965) Evaluation of a prophylactic and therapeutic program for patients with cystic fibrosis. *Pediatrics* **36**, 675.
[9] DUNCAN D.A., DRUMMOND K.N., MICHAEL A.F. & VERNIER R.L. (1965) Pulmonary hemorrhage and glomerulonephritis. Report of 6 cases and study of the renal lesion by the fluorescent antibody technique and electron microscopy. *Ann. intern. Med.* **62**, 920.

[10] EDITORIAL (1961) Idiopathic pulmonary haemosiderosis. *Br. med. J.* **i**, 1450.

[11] EDITORIAL (1963) Idiopathic pulmonary haemosiderosis. *Lancet* **i**, 979.

[12] EDITORIAL (1964) Early diagnosis of fibrocystic disease. *Lancet* **i**, 801.

[13] ELDER JANET L., KIRK G.M. & SMITH W.G. (1965) Idiopathic pulmonary haemosiderosis and the Goodpasture syndrome. *Br. med. J.* **ii**, 1152.

[14] ELLMAN P. (1960) Pulmonary haemosiderosis. *Proc. Roy. Soc. Med.* **53**, 333.

[15] GIBSON L.E. & COOKE R.E. (1959) A test for concentration of electrolytes in sweat in cystic fibrosis of the pancreas, utilizing pilocarpine by iontophoresis. *Pediatrics* **23**, 545.

[16] GOLDBLOOM R.B. & SEKELN P. (1963) Cystic fibrosis of the pancreas. Diagnosis by application of a sodium electrode to the skin. *New Engl. J. Med.* **269**, 1349.

[17] GOODPASTURE E.W. (1919) The significance of certain pulmonary lesions in relation to the etiology of influenza. *Am. J. med. Sci.* **158**, 863.

[18] HEINER D.C., SEARS J.W. & KNIKER W.T. (1962) Multiple precipitins to cow's milk in chronic respiratory disease. *Am. J. Dis. Child.* **103**, 634.

[19] HEINER D.C. (1967) Pulmonary hemosiderosis. In *Disorders of the Respiratory Tract in Children* ed. Kendig E.L.Jr. Philadelphia, Saunders.

[20] JOHANSEN PATRICIA G., ANDERSON CHARLOTTE M. & HADORN B. (1968) Cystic fibrosis of the pancreas. A generalized disturbance of water and electrolyte movement in exocrine tissues. *Lancet* **i**, 455.

[21] KENNEDY W.P.U., SHEARMAN D.J.C., DELAMORE I.W., SIMPSON J.D., BLACK J.W. & GRANT I.W.B. (1966) Idiopathic pulmonary haemosiderosis with myocarditis. Radioisotope studies in a patient treated with prednisone. *Thorax* **21**, 220.

[22] KOPITO L., KHAW K.T., TOWNLEY R.R.W. & SHWACHMAN H. (1965) Studies in cystic fibrosis. Analysis of nail clippings for sodium and potassium. *New Engl. J. Med.* **272**, 504.

[23] LLOYD-RUSBY N. & WILSON C. (1960) Lung purpura with nephritis. *Quart. J. Med., N.S.* **29**, 501.

[24] LOBECK C.C. & HUEBER DOROTHY (1962) Effect of age, sex, and cystic fibrosis on the sodium and potassium content of human sweat. *Pediatrics* **30**, 172.

[25] LUNDBERG G.D. (1963) Goodpasture's syndrome. Glomerulonephritis with pulmonary haemorrhage. *J. Am. med. Ass.* **184**, 915.

[26] MCCALL C.B., HARRIS T.R. & HATCH F.E. (1965) Nonfatal pulmonary haemorrhage and glomerulonephritis. *Am. Rev. resp. Dis.* **91**, 424.

[27] MCCAUGHEY W.T.E. & THOMAS BETTY J. (1962) Pulmonary hemorrhage and glomerulonephritis. The relation of pulmonary hemorrhage to certain types of glomerular lesions. *Am. J. clin. Path.* **38**, 577.

[28] MATTHEWS L.W., DOERSHUK C.F., WISE M., EDDY G., NUDELMAN H. & SPECTOR S. (1964) A therapeutic regimen for patients with cystic fibrosis. *J. Pediat.* **65**, 558.

[29] MATTHEWS L.W., DOERSHUK C.F. & SPECTOR S. (1967) Mist tent therapy of the obstructive pulmonary lesion of cystic fibrosis. *Pediatrics* **39**, 176.

[30] OGNIBENE A.J. & JOHNSON D.E. (1963) Idiopathic pulmonary hemosiderosis and related syndromes. *Am. J. Med.* **32**, 499.

[31] PARKINS R.A., EIDELMAN S., RUBIN C.E., DOBBINS W.O. & PHELPS P.C. (1963) The diagnosis of cystic fibrosis by rectal biopsy. *Lancet* **ii**, 851.

[32] REID D.H.S., TUNSTALL M.E. & MITCHELL R.G. (1967) A controlled trial of artificial respiration in the respiratory distress syndrome of the newborn. *Lancet* **i**, 532.

[33] ROSSI E. & STOLL E. eds. (1967) *Cystic Fibrosis. Physiology and Pathophysiology of Serous Secretion, Clinical Investigations and Therapy.* Proceedings of the 4th International Conference on Cystic Fibrosis of the Pancreas (mucoviscidosis). Basel, Karger.

[34] SALTZMAN P.W., WEST M. & CHOMET B. (1962) Pulmonary hemosiderosis and glomerulonephritis. *Ann. intern. Med.* **56**, 449.

[35] SHWACHMAN H. (1967) Cystic Fibrosis. In *Disorders of the Respiratory Tract in Children*, ed. Kendig E.L.Jr. Philadelphia, Saunders.

[36] SMITH B.S. (1966) Idiopathic pulmonary haemosiderosis and rheumatoid arthritis. *Br. med. J.* **i**, 1403.

[37] SOERGEL K.H. & SOMMERS S.C. (1962) Idiopathic pulmonary hemosiderosis and related syndromes. *Am. J. Med.* **32**, 499.

[38] STAHLMAN MILDRED T. (1967) Hyaline membrane disease. In *Disorders of the Respiratory Tract in Children*, ed. Kendig E.L.Jr. Philadelphia, Saunders.

[39] STEINER B. & NABRADY J. (1965) Immunoallergic lung purpura treated with azathioprine. *Lancet* **i**, 140.

[40] WISER W.C. & BEIER FRANCES R. (1964) Albumin in the meconium of infants with cystic fibrosis. A preliminary report. *Pediatrics* **33**, 115.

CHAPTER 34

Diseases of the Mediastinum

ANATOMY OF THE MEDIASTINUM

The mediastinum is the region between the pleural sacs. Bounded laterally by mediastinal pleura it extends from the thoracic inlet to the diaphragm and from the sternum to the spine. It is potentially mobile and normally maintained in the central position of the thorax by a balance between the pleural pressures on the two sides. Rarely fenestrations in the mediastinal pleura allow communication between the pleural sacs. In the infant and young child the mediastinum is highly mobile; in later life it becomes more rigid so that unilateral change in pleural pressure has proportionately less effect.

The mediastinum is divided by the anatomist into 4 compartments (fig. 34.1). The lower boundary of the superior mediastinum is a plane drawn between the lower borders of the manubrium and the 4th thoracic vertebra. This arbitrary dividing line is just below the aortic arch and just above the tracheal bifurcation. The anatomical boundaries of the other subdivisions are listed in table 34.1. Mediastinal space-occupying lesions may distort the anatomical boundaries so that a particular lesion usually confined to one compartment may occupy more than one. Lesions involving the small, crowded superior mediastinum are particularly liable to transgress the arbitrary limits. Certain structures are, however, normally common to more than one compartment, e.g. thymus extending from neck through superior mediastinum to anterior mediastinum; aorta and oesophagus are in both superior and posterior mediastinum. The anatomical division of the mediastinum has little clinical significance but the site of mediastinal lesions gives valuable information regarding the probabilities in diagnosis (table

TABLE 34.1
Subdivisions of Mediastinum (fig. 34.1)

Division	Anatomical boundaries	Normal contents
Superior (above pericardium)	Manubrium anteriorly, 1–4 thoracic vertebrae posteriorly	Aortic arch and its 3 branches, trachea, oesophagus, thoracic duct, superior vena cava and innominate veins, thymus (superior part), sympathetic nerves, phrenic nerves, left recurrent laryngeal nerve, lymph glands.
Anterior (in front of pericardium)	Body of sternum anteriorly, pericardium posteriorly.	Thymus (inferior part), fatty tissue, lymph glands.
Middle	Bounded by other 3 divisions	Pericardium and its contents, ascending aorta, main pulmonary artery, phrenic nerves.
Posterior	Pericardium and diaphragm anteriorly, lower 8 thoracic vertebrae posteriorly	Descending thoracic aorta and branches, oesophagus, sympathetic and vagus nerves, thoracic duct, lymph glands along aorta.

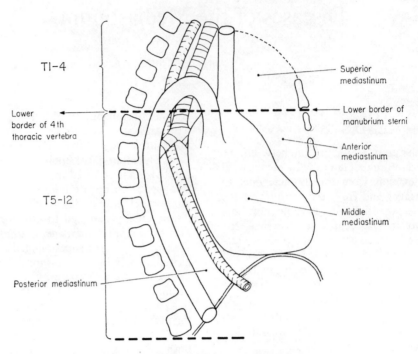

T1–4

Lower
border of 4th
thoracic vertebra

T5–12

Posterior mediastinum

Superior
mediastinum

Lower border of
manubrium sterni

Anterior
mediastinum

Middle
mediastinum

FIG. 34.1. Subdivisions of mediastinum.

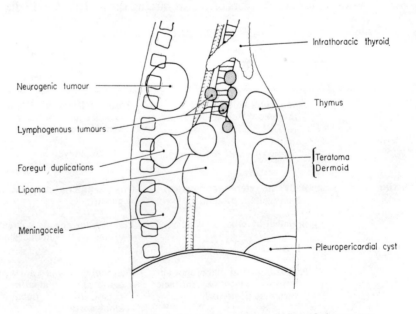

Neurogenic tumour

Lymphogenous tumours

Foregut duplications

Lipoma

Meningocele

Intrathoracic thyroid

Thymus

Teratoma
Dermoid

Pleuropericardial cyst

FIG. 34.2. Sites of mediastinal tumours and cysts in lateral chest x-ray.

Sites	Lesions
Superior	Thymic tumours
	Teratomata
	Cystic hygroma
	Haemangioma
	Mediastinal abscess
	Aortic aneurysm
	Intrathoracic thyroid
	Oesophageal lesions
	Lymphomata
	Lymphadenopathy (e.g. tuberculosis, sarcoidosis, leukaemia)
Anterior	Thymic enlargement, tumours and cysts
	Heterotopic thymus
	Teratomata
	Intrathoracic thyroid
	Heterotopic thyroid
	Pleuropericardial cyst
	Hernia through foramen of Morgagni
	Cystic hygroma
	Lymphomata
	Lymphadenopathy
Middle	Aortic aneurysm
	Anomalies of great vessels
	Cardiac tumours
	Bronchogenic cyst
	Lipoma
Posterior	Neurogenic tumours and cysts
	Gastroenteric and bronchogenic cysts
	Oesophageal lesions
	Hernia through foramen of Bochdalek
	Meningoceles
	Aortic aneurysm
	Posterior thyroid tumours

34.2 & fig. 34.2). Diagnosis can, however, rarely be certain and still more rarely is it possible to distinguish between malignant and benign lesions before the precise histology is known. As many as 1 in 5 mediastinal tumours or cysts may eventually undergo malignant change.

TYPES OF LESION AND THEIR GENERAL MANIFESTATIONS

Mediastinal lesions comprise a great variety of tumours and cysts. Most derive from developmental anomalies which are prone to occur since the area is embryologically very complex. Here the more caudal of the branchial arches develop; the lung bud develops from the primitive foregut and the latter itself differentiates; the heart and great vessels undergo the changes from foetal to adult state; the pleural and pericardial cavities are formed and the lower boundary of the mediastinum, the diaphragm, develops from the septum transversum. In addition the many adult tissues present in the mediastinum (table 34.1) may be subject to infective, degenerative or neoplastic change. Infections may also occur in the mediastinal tissues; mediastinal emphysema is described elsewhere (p. 449).

During embryological development the thymus, parathyroid and thyroid are intimately related and, since they migrate downwards from the primitive pharynx to different levels in the neck and mediastinum, heterotopic situations of the mature glands may result and occasionally there may be inclusion of part of one gland in the substance of another. The heterotopic gland may present as a mediastinal tumour.

Convention dictates that metastatic lesions, tumours invading the mediastinum from extramediastinal structures, tumours of the trachea, lesions of the oesophagus (e.g. megaoesophagus), and of the heart and great vessels (e.g. aortic aneurysm) are excluded from the classification of mediastinal lesions so far as description is concerned. Although they are mentioned in table 34.2 for completeness and must always be considered in differential diagnosis of mediastinal lesions, they will not be discussed further in any detail.

CLINICAL EFFECTS OF MEDIASTINAL TUMOURS AND CYSTS

Whether or not malignant change occurs, tumours and cysts of the mediastinum tend to enlarge and to compress adjacent structures. In general, cysts and simple tumours displace but do not interrupt the function of the longitudinal structures of the mediastinum. In contrast, malignant tumours and aortic aneurysm do interrupt function. This rule may not apply, of course, when cysts and simple tumours are in a confined space (e.g. thoracic inlet; 'dumb-bell' extensions of neurogenic tumours) when function of compressed structures may be interrupted. Cough and dyspnoea may be caused by pressure on bronchi and trachea, dysphagia by pressure on the oesophagus, distension of neck veins and the development of collateral circulation by venous obstruction and tachycardia by displacement of the heart limiting diastolic filling. Neurogenic tumours may give rise to pain which may be intercostal or more vaguely distributed in the chest, and those with 'dumb-bell' extensions into the vertebral canal may result in symptoms due to cord compression. Laryngeal nerve involvement may lead to hoarseness. Secondary infection of cysts may result in rupture of the contents into a bronchus. Sudden enlargement of cysts or tumours may occur from haemorrhage and, particularly in the case of retrosternal goitre, this complication can be fatal. Retrosternal goitres may also undergo toxic change with associated hyperthyroidism. Thymic tumours may be associated with myasthenia gravis though in less than a quarter of cases. Cysts derived from the foregut may show peptic ulceration when they contain gastric mucosa.

These potential effects, linked with the uncertainty of diagnosis and the ever present risk of malignant change, make a formidable case for surgical resection of most mediastinal tumours and cysts. Because of the increasing use of mass miniature radiography mediastinal lesions are as likely to be detected when clinically latent as when giving rise to symptoms.

INCIDENCE OF MEDIASTINAL CYSTS AND TUMOURS

This is difficult to assess with any accuracy since most reported series have been highly selected. Le Roux and Dodds [38] quote the Edinburgh experience over a 10 year period as follows: 105 patients with mediastinal cysts and tumours were treated in the Thoracic Surgical Unit. This figure is to be compared to the 3000 cases of bronchial carcinoma, 700 cases of oesophageal carcinoma and 40 cases of bronchial adenoma treated over the same period. A family doctor in Britain might, therefore, be expected to see on an average only one patient with a primary mediastinal cyst or tumour during his lifetime. Le Roux and Dodds also comment that while retrosternal thyroid is among the commoner mediastinal lesions, a thyroid which extends only a little into the thorax is likely to be dealt with by general surgeons thus making the reported incidence an underestimate in most thoracic centres. It was not included in the 105 cases mentioned above. These comprised 30 neural tumours, 21 teratomata, 20 pericardialcoelomic cysts, 17 thymic tumours or cysts, 14 cases of foregut duplication and 3 heterotopic mediastinal thyroids.

The combined series reported by Morrison in 1958 is the largest so far reported [44]. Neural tumours were the commonest (30·4%) followed by cystic lesions and teratomata, thymic tumours, lymphomata and a small number of rarer growths. Other series have confirmed the predominance of neurogenic tumours [50]. With the development of thoracic surgery in the postwar years thymic tumours have featured more prominently. Previously a precise diagnosis was not possible and many were undoubtedly classified as a form of reticulosis.

The increase in incidence of all forms of mediastinal tumours and cysts since the 1939–45 War is entirely due to the wider use of the routine chest x-ray, and their classification has been made possible by advances in anaesthesia and thoracic surgical technique which permit surgical removal and precise histological diagnosis.

X-RAY APPEARANCES OF MEDIASTINUM

The central mediastinal shadow in the standard PA film is bounded by the pericardium and the great vessels. Usually the air-filled trachea and sometimes the spine are also recognizable but the other normal contents of the mediastinum cannot usually be identified. For a mediastinal lesion to be detectable in the PA film it has to be sufficiently large to alter the normal mediastinal contour. Possible exceptions are: (a) mediastinal emphysema (p. 449) and (b) certain lesions such as hiatus hernia and neurogenic tumour, which may be seen through the cardiac shadow but give rise to no associated mediastinal enlargement. Because of the importance of precise anatomical localization the lateral and sometimes oblique views are particularly important in the assessment of mediastinal lesions; these may reveal lesions unsuspected in the PA film.

Generally speaking mediastinal lesions may be of any size, may be solid or cystic and some may be calcified. Hilar enlargement may be simulated by extension of a mediastinal mass to one or other side.

In the first month of life the mediastinum is proportionately wider than at any other period and may amount to two thirds of the transverse diameter of the chest. The thymus is variable in size and it is difficult to identify the pulmonary vessels and aorta distinctly. From 1 to 12 months the thymus usually shrinks but sometimes increases in size; the pulmonary vessels become proportionately larger and the heart size decreases. From 1 to 3 years the thymus progressively shrinks and the heart also becomes relatively smaller. From 4 years onwards the proportions of the various mediastinal shadows are the same as in the adult.

TECHNIQUES EMPLOYED IN DIAGNOSIS OF MEDIASTINAL LESIONS

Most of these are radiographic. Tomography may sometimes be useful in outlining the lesion more clearly and less frequently is necessary for demonstrating its precise location since the lateral film usually suffices. Barium swallow may give useful information by demonstrating displacement or narrowing of the oesophagus and the form this takes. Screening is particularly important when vascular lesions are suspected or the phrenic nerve involved. Lesions of the great vessels may be defined precisely by angiography. Pneumomediastinum is of particular value in outlining lymphadenopathy at the roots of the lungs but is rarely necessary.

Bronchoscopy is commonly valuable to confirm compression of the trachea and bronchi. Mediastinoscopy has greatly widened the scope of diagnostic procedures aimed at securing a precise diagnosis short of exploratory thoracotomy.

NEUROGENIC TUMOURS

The neurogenic group is the commonest of the mediastinal tumours. Since they arise from the paravertebral sympathetic nerve trunk and spinal nerves, these occur mainly in the paravertebral gutter and posterior mediastinum [4].

PATHOLOGY

There are 4 types of neurogenic tumour: neurilemmoma, neurofibroma, ganglioneuroma and neuroblastoma.

NEURILEMMOMA

This is derived from the sheath of Schwann of an intercostal nerve; very occasionally from the intrathoracic vagus [15]. It may lie partly in an intervertebral foramen, forming a 'dumb-bell' tumour which may compress the spinal cord. It is a well encapsulated, rounded, white, benign tumour and is often grouped clinically with the neurofibromata, though with differences from them. A neurilemmoma is formed of Schwann cells, long, slender and with elongated nuclei; palisading, whorls and eddies are usual. Reticulin fibres may be present. Nerve fibres are found only in the sheath. Neurilemmoma is much the commonest of the neurogenic tumours.

NEUROFIBROMA

This tumour may sometimes be associated with neurofibromatosis (von Recklinghausen's disease). It grows on an intercostal nerve. Malignant change can occur. It is really more a malformation than a tumour and contains all the elements which comprise the nerve trunk; sheath cells, axons and connective tissue. It may also protrude into an intervertebral foramen. Microscopically the structure is tangled and reticular, though also containing a variable amount of whorls and palisades derived from Schwann cells. With

special stains nerve fibrils can be seen. It is
the Schwann cells which may develop malignant sarcomatous form: the earliest change is
the presence of large, hyperchromatic nuclei.
Malignant change is commoner in patients
with neurofibromatosis.

GANGLIONEUROMA

This is a benign tumour arising from one of
the sympathetic ganglia. It is usually elongated and may overlie several rib spaces. Like
the first 2 types it may protrude into an intervertebral foramen to form a 'dumb-bell'
tumour [47]. It consists of nerve fibres and
varying numbers of large adult ganglion cells.
It is commoner in childhood but may occur
at any age. An adrenal ganglioneuroma [6]
grows from ectopic medullary adrenal tissue
and may be associated with the thoracic
sympathetic nerves. The tumour is grey in
colour and contains chromaffin tissue. It is
said that it may be associated with hypertension.

NEUROBLASTOMA

This is a malignant neoplasm of the sympathetic nervous system. It has been divided
into less differentiated (sympathicogonioma)
and more differentiated (sympathicoblastoma)
forms [47]. The less differentiated consists of
cells of about lymphocyte size with dense
hyperchromatic nuclei and a fibrillar stroma.
There may be pseudorosettes. The more
differentiated form has cells with a vesicular
nucleus and containing only a rim of cytoplasm; the cells are larger than in the first
type. Fibrillar stroma is also present; pseudorosettes are less common; there may be
occasional ganglion cells. Calcification may
occur in both types. These tumours are commoner in children.

CLINICAL FEATURES [1, 6 & 10]

Unless they cause pressure on the spinal cord
by protrusion through an intervertebral
foramen, as sometimes happens (the so-called
'dumb-bell' tumour), or become extremely
large, or undergo malignant change, most
neurogenic tumours are symptomless and

come to notice through routine radiography.
If the tumour is very large there may be local
pain, cough or dyspnoea; similar symptoms
may occur with smaller tumours after the
patient knows he has a radiographic abnormality. The commonest neurological complication is spinal compression from a 'dumb-
bell' tumour protruding through an intervertebral foramen but compression of the
brachial plexus, Horner's syndrome, phrenic
paralysis or laryngeal nerve paralysis have all
been occasionally recorded. Sometimes the
presence of other evidence of neurofibromata
such as 'café-au-lait' patches on the skin and
neurofibromata elsewhere, may give an additional clue to the diagnosis. In this case there
may be multiple lesions on the intercostal
nerves. Neurofibromata complicating neurofibromatosis are said to be particularly prone
to malignant change.

RADIOLOGY

Neurilemmomata and neurofibromata show
radiologically as rounded or oval, dense, well-
defined shadows, visible in the paravertebral
area and merging medially with the mediastinal shadow in the postero-anterior x-ray.
They are most often seen in the upper half of
the chest. In the lateral film they lie posteriorly
in the paravertebral gutter. Calcification is
occasionally seen [54]. The extreme posterior
position is characteristic and highly suggestive
of the diagnosis, although of course such
conditions as bronchial neoplasm may sometimes be seen in the extreme posterior part
of the lungs and cause confusion. The posterior ribs may be splayed apart by the
tumour. The ribs may be thinned out by
compression but are not irregularly eroded
unless there is malignant change. In the case
of 'dumb-bell' tumours the intervertebral
foramen may also be enlarged by compression
of the bone. Pedicles and bodies of neighbouring vertebrae may also be affected.

Neurogenic tumours of the vagus or sympathetic give rise to elongated shadows which
may stretch over several rib spaces. On the
posteroanterior film the lateral margin may
be well-defined but the medial tends to merge
with the mediastinal shadows and the mass

loses definition above and below. In the lateral film these tumours may be very difficult to define [10].

TREATMENT

Neurogenic tumours are best removed surgically because the diagnosis can never be completely certain, because later growth to a large size could make removal difficult, because neurofibromata carry the risk of malignant change and because the histological diagnosis usually cannot be made preoperatively. In the case of multiple neurofibromata associated with neurofibromatosis, multiple removal is impractical, but if a tumour enlarges, becomes painful or erodes a rib it should be removed.

PROGNOSIS

The prognosis after removal of neurilemmomata or neurofibromata is good. Only 2 out of 86 had recurred in one series [10] and these 2 were apparently cured by a second operation. Even those with malignant change may do well with operation, perhaps followed by radiotherapy. Naturally the less differentiated neuroblastomata are more likely to metastasize and consequently to have a poorer prognosis, but these tumours are very radiosensitive and have been apparently arrested by radiotherapy alone [1].

The rate of growth of unoperated neurilemmomata is very variable. They may grow slowly or remain static for years.

INTRATHORACIC THYROID

Although intrathoracic thyroid is nearly always an extension of a diseased cervical thyroid it is convenient to discuss this condition here since it is relatively common and must be considered in the differential diagnosis of tumours in the superior and anterior mediastinum. The lack of precise knowledge regarding the incidence of intrathoracic thyroid has already been mentioned; when it has been included in reported series it comprises 15–20% of the total. Heterotopic thyroid, which may be the patient's only functioning thyroid tissue, occurs relatively rarely and presents as an anterior mediastinal mass usually diagnosed only at thoracotomy. This differs from the commoner form of intrathoracic thyroid in having no vascular connections with a cervical thyroid although the blood supply may originate in the neck.

PATHOLOGY

DEVELOPMENTAL PATHOLOGY OF INTRATHORACIC THYROID

The thyroid develops from the endoderm of the primitive pharynx as a median outgrowth where the foramen caecum of the tongue is ultimately situated. The future thyroid first appears about the 4th embryonic week, is closely related to the aortic sac and grows downwards on the hollow thyroglossal duct, the proximal end of which persists as the foramen caecum. Aberrant thyroid tissue may, therefore, be found anywhere along the course of the thyroglossal duct from the base of the tongue through the superior and anterior mediastinum to the pericardium or even the heart [58]. Heterotopic mediastinal thyroid in the mediastinum, pericardium and heart results from developing thyroid tissue being pulled into the thorax during descent of the heart and great vessels. Usually it lies in the anterior mediastinum alongside the thymus. Whether or not it has connections with a normally situated cervical thyroid determines the blood supply which may be either from the neck or from local vessels.

MORBID ANATOMY

Most examples of intrathoracic thyroid are extensions of simple colloid goitres. These occur equally in male and female and are most commonly encountered in the middle aged and elderly. Toxic changes with the features of hyperthyroidism are uncommon; malignant change occurs more frequently.

Most commonly the intrathoracic goitre extends from the lower pole of a lateral lobe, the right more commonly than the left. It lies, therefore, anterior to the trachea in the superior part of the anterior mediastinum and immediately behind the sternum. In about

10% of cases the goitre arises from the posterolateral aspect of the gland and finally lies posterior to the trachea and posterolateral to the oesophagus which is progressively more displaced as the mass extends into the thorax. The factor principally determining the intrathoracic extension of a cervical goitre is the limitation to anterior and lateral enlargement imposed by the muscles of the neck. Once it has entered the thorax the line of least resistance is downwards.

Since the thyroid enlargement is usually asymmetrical it displaces the more mobile of the mediastinal structures, particularly the trachea and the oesophagus, to the opposite side.

CLINICAL FEATURES

The growth of the goitre is usually slow so that symptoms due to compression develop insidiously and many years may pass, and the patient reach a stage of serious disability due to dyspnoea, without the cause having been recognized. The trachea bears the brunt of the compression since the oesophagus is more mobile and is usually only displaced. Dysphagia is unusual with the commoner type of intrathoracic goitre. When the oesophagus is compressed, causing dysphagia, this is most often due to malignant change. Dyspnoea and stridor may occur from compression of the trachea which may result in erosion of the tracheal rings so that even after the mass has been removed the floppy trachea may lead to airway obstruction. Should the recurrent laryngeal nerve become stretched over the tumour, vocal cord paralysis with hoarseness may occasionally occur but is much more often a complication of operation. Obstruction of the great veins may result in engorgement of the neck veins, made worse when the patient lies down or when he bends.

Commonly the patient is in the over 50 age group and is frequently obese because of increasing limitation of exercise. The obesity often militates against early clinical and radiological diagnosis. As well as causing dyspnoea, tracheal pressure may result in an irritative cough. The tempo of events may be dramatically hastened by bleeding into a colloid intra-thoracic goitre. This may be an acute surgical emergency requiring immediate treatment for relief of dyspnoea. Usually a patient with an intrathoracic thyroid has a palpable thyroid in the neck. An intrathoracic extension has sometimes been missed at cervical thyroidectomy.

The chest x-ray shows an upper mediastinal rounded opacity in the PA film, usually situated anteriorly in the lateral view. Because of its asymmetry the mass is usually more prominent on one side than the other (more commonly on the right) and the diagnosis is suggested by the fact that the borders of the mass are ill-defined superiorly and continuous with the soft tissue shadows of the neck. The trachea is displaced and may be narrowed. Calcification may sometimes be seen in longstanding thyroid adenomata and cysts. Barium swallow shows movement of the thyroid mass on deglutition; in those few cases which are posterior to the trachea oesophageal displacement may be demonstrated. Radioactive iodine studies may be used to demonstrate functioning thyroid tissue in the mediastinum as well as a normal complement of thyroid tissue in the neck. Radioiodine may not be taken up in every case and previous iodine treatment invalidates the test. The clinician should not be put off by a negative result but a positive result is valuable evidence of intrathoracic thyroid tissue. Aortic aneurysm and thymic tumours may occasionally be mistaken for retrosternal goitre. Angiography may be indicated when aneurysm cannot be otherwise excluded.

Intrathoracic goitre may be affected by Hashimoto's disease. This is likely to result in severe compression symptoms such as occur with carcinomatous change. The finding of thyroid autoantibodies proves the diagnosis and since treatment with thyroxine is usually successful, surgery may be avoided.

TREATMENT

With the possible exception of Hashimoto's disease all intrathoracic goitres should be removed surgically. Heterotopic mediastinal thyroid tissue is nearly always diagnosed only at thoracotomy.

MEDIASTINAL PARATHYROID ADENOMA

A parathyroid adenoma may occasionally occur in the anterior mediastinum. Norris [46] recorded 17 cases out of a total of 322. Of these patients 8 showed skeletal changes only, 7 showed both skeletal changes and nephro-calcinosis or renal calculi, 1 had no bone lesions but had renal calculi and 1 was not associated with any evidence of hormonal activity. The incidence of the systemic effects of mediastinal parathyroid adenomata is much the same as when the adenoma is in the neck [53].

The histology of mediastinal parathyroid adenoma is the same as that found in the neck. Colloid-filled follicles, dense spherical nuclei and clear cytoplasm characteristic of parathyroid adenoma are intimately associated with remnants of the thymus.

The presence in the mediastinum has been explained by the proximity of the parathyroid and the anlage of the thymus in the 3rd pharyngeal pouch. Inclusion of the parathyroid in the larger thymus might result in its transfer to the anterior mediastinum. It has, however, been shown that the anlage of the thymus is multipotent and can produce parathyroid tissue under some circumstances. Thus a mediastinal parathyroid adenoma may arise in the thymus independently of the normal glands.

The diagnosis of mediastinal parathyroid adenoma has rarely been made preoperatively.

TERATOMATA

The teratomata are the second most common of the mediastinal tumours. In this section it is convenient to discuss dermoids and teratomata together although the pathologist may find it more satisfactory to classify these tumours as benign (e.g. benign epidermoid or dermoid cysts) and malignant (e.g. malignant teratomata and the rare choriocarcinoma [53]). Clinical descriptions of the lesions under a single heading are justified since they have a common origin and all the germinal layers are usually represented in each, though to a varying degree. Thus the dermoid contains largely tissues of ectodermal origin whereas all 3 are clearly discernible in the teratoma; the dermoid is usually cystic and the teratoma mainly solid; both occupy the anterior mediastinum as a rule and posterior mediastinal lesions of this type are rare [53].

The genesis of these lesions continues to be a matter of dispute. Perhaps the most acceptable is the view that the scene is set for embryogenic disorder when all the primitive layers come together in the fusion of the 3rd and 4th branchial arches in the mid line. From this fusion primitive cells may enter the anterior mediastinum along with the heart and great vessels with which they are in intimate contact. The embryogenic complexity in the mediastinum rivals that in the gonads and the area is second only to the gonads in the incidence of teratoid tumours. The reader is referred to the numerous reviews on the subject [2, 9, 14, 18, 24, 26, 28, 30, 37, 39, 40, 44, 48, 49, 50, 51 & 56].

PATHOLOGY

Dermoid cysts or so-called benign teratomata may be lobulated and multilocular. They have a dense fibrous capsule which is lined by stratified squamous epithelium. The capsule frequently contains remnants of the thymus [53]. Macroscopically the contents are milky or cheesy in consistence and may include such varied tissues as skin, hair, nervous tissues, sebaceous material, intestinal and bronchial epithelium, pancreatic tissue, teeth, bone (sometimes with marrow cavities and active haemopoietic tissue), cartilage and muscle. If muscle is present, most commonly it is of the smooth variety. Papillary intraluminal projections may be present and it is from the surface of these that hair frequently grows [53]. Microscopic examination confirms that mesodermal as well as ectodermal elements are present.

Malignant teratomata contain elements of all 3 germinal layers and may sometimes become very large. The variety of the contents is the same as in dermoid cysts but ectodermal derivatives such as skin or nervous tissue are less common [53]. Most of the epithelial components are of endodermal origin and poorly differentiated. The malignant component can frequently be identified as adenocarcinoma although the cells are usually markedly pleomorphic. The connective tissue stroma is loosely arranged. Foci of bone and cartilage are common but they are less mature than in dermoid cysts [53].

Choriocarcinoma is a variant of the malignant teratoma whose principal neoplastic elements are cells resembling those that cover the normal placental villi. It is rare and few cases have been reported [25 & 34]. A complete diagnosis must exclude a teratoma of the testis which may have metastasized to the mediastinum. Sometimes a primary testicular tumour which behaves in this manner is very small. The tumours are markedly haemorrhagic and friable. The pericardium is early infiltrated with tumour, and metastasis to the lungs is common. On microscopy the principal cells are small cuboidal trophoblasts and masses of syncytial cells with large nuclei and abundant cytoplasm. Commonly the syncytial cells surround thin-walled vascular spaces [53].

In addition to the signs and symptoms of other malignant teratomata in the anterior mediastinum the choriocarcinoma may result in gynaecomastia and testicular atrophy. Hormone assays have shown increased chorionic gonadotrophin in the urine and increase in oestrogen and pregnanediol levels.

CLINICAL FEATURES

In most cases these tumours are symptomless until complications occur. These are infection and malignant change. Infection transforms the lesion into an abscess which ruptures into a bronchus or into the pleura. Bronchial fistula may sometimes occur without overt infection and cases have been reported of the expectoration of the contents of the cyst, such as hair. But the most important complication is malignant change which may affect about 15–20% of all teratoid tumours. Malignant change occurs almost exclusively in males and the risk is much lower for dermoid cysts than for solid teratomata. Something like 30% of dermoid cysts become malignant; 70% of solid teratomata do so.

Pathognomic symptoms such as the coughing up of hairs are rare and teratomata are usually diagnosed from the radiographic appearance.

The dermoid cyst or malignant teratoma discovered as a consequence of symptoms usually presents because of pressure on the trachea with dyspnoea, cyanosis, substernal pain and cough, or the features of infection. Very large tumours may rarely compress the oesophagus and give rise to dysphagia. Pressure on the pulmonary artery may give rise to a systolic murmur which disappears when the tumour is removed. Pressure on the heart commonly results in palpitations.

RADIOLOGY

These tumours appear as dense homogeneous, uniform globular shadows which are sharply circumscribed in the anterior mediastinum. They often extend posteriorly and laterally and so may displace the lung. The clear margins of the tumour, extending to one or other side of the sternum, may be altered as a consequence of recurrent attacks of inflammation so that the edges become shaggy. Should a fistula develop, a fluid level may be seen. Teeth may be recognized in dermoids. Calcification is common in their walls but may also occur in many other mediastinal lesions. Among the more important conditions to be considered in differential diagnosis are thymic hyperplasia and tumours, substernal thyroids, lung cysts, fibromata and lipomata.

TREATMENT

Commonly the diagnosis is one of probability but there is never any doubt about treatment. Surgical exploration and removal is imperative and in those cases showing malignant change operation may be followed by irradiation. Technical difficulty in the removal of teratomata occurs only if malignant infiltration is present or if infection has previously occurred leading to dense adhesions.

PROGNOSIS

Even when an apparently satisfactory operation has been performed the presence of malignant change compels a guarded prognosis and the late development of metastases is not uncommon.

DISORDERS OF THE THYMUS

The precise function of the thymus gland is unknown but it is generally agreed that it plays a vital rôle, particularly in early life, in lymphopoiesis and in immunological activities. It is believed to be the site of origin of the lymphocytes responsible for most of the immunological activity of the body. The thymus is most active immunologically in the neonatal period; in later life other lymphoid organs take over this function. Within the thymus, stem cells from the bone marrow become immunologically competent. Also, a hormone is secreted by the thymic epithelial cells which makes lymphocytes elsewhere in the body capable of responding to antigenic stimulation. It has been suggested that all primary immune patterns originate in the thymus and that the cells involved in these migrate from the thymus to the lymph glands and spleen where they proliferate in response to immunological need.

The size of the thymus is relatively greatest at birth and thymic hyperplasia is a common finding in infancy and early childhood. Thymic tissue in the young is soft and gelatinous so that pressure symptoms from hyperplasia are unusual, although wheezing in infancy has sometimes been thought to be associated with a significantly enlarged thymus. In the young child the size and shape of an enlarged thymus varies greatly and is more prominent on expiration and when crying. It is a good rule to consider any suspicious mass in the superior and anterior mediastinum in a child under 2 years as being most likely to be due to thymic enlargement. The x-ray in thymic hyperplasia shows bilateral, globular widening of the upper mediastinal shadow, sometimes with steplike appearances to which the term 'sail shadow' has been given. Simple enlargement of the thymus has to be distinguished from thymic tumours, retrosternal thyroid, dermoid cysts, teratomata, lipomata, mediastinal lympha-denopathy and cystic hygroma. Diagnostic pneumomediastinum has sometimes been employed when the diagnosis has been in doubt.

When simple thymic enlargement seems the probable diagnosis no treatment is indicated since spontaneous regression may be expected over some months.

The fate of the thymus after infancy is interesting. There is rapid growth in the first 2 years of life, a more or less stationary situation until age 7, with again a phase of increase until puberty when it begins to regress. Throughout adult life there is progressive involutional change so that in the elderly the normal structure may only be represented by fatty tissue. To some extent, however, the facts that postmortem change is extremely rapid and that any prolonged wasting disease results in marked shrinkage of the thymus may have influenced anatomists and pathologists in their views regarding atrophy of the gland in the adult.

ANATOMY OF THE DEVELOPMENT OF THE THYMUS

The thymus has a right and left lobe closely bound together by fibrous tissue and is situated in the upper part of the anterior mediastinum immediately behind the sternum. It lies between the 2 pleural sacs, above the pericardium and overlapping it, and extends into the root of the neck. In the young child it is subdivided into lobules and follicles by fibrous septa. Cortical and medullary zones can be distinguished. The cortical zone is crowded with lymphocytes and has only sparse epithelial cells. The thymus is known to enlarge on occasion in thyrotoxicosis when lymphoid structures elsewhere apparently also increase. Thymic hyperplasia may also be a feature of systemic lupus erythematosus. The medullary zone contains more prominent epithelial cells grouped in places into the distinctive concentric corpuscles of Hassall. These corpuscles and the reticulum of branching cells which form the framework of the follicle are derived from both ectoderm and endoderm in its development from a pair of solid buds growing from the 3rd branchial arches at about the 6th week of embryonic life.

ABNORMALITIES OF THE THYMUS

Because of its embryological complexity it is not surprising that the thymus is a common site of tumours and cysts. Sometimes an accessory thymus may be left behind in the neck, more commonly near the lower parathyroid and only rarely near the upper parathyroid. Other abnormalities which may occur include hypoplasia, pathological involution, hyperplasia (often with germinal centres in the lymphoid follicles) and infiltrations. These may result from a variety of causes, some hormonal, some based on immunological deficiency and some due to autoimmune disease.

Several clinical syndromes have been related to pathological changes in the thymus. Myasthenia gravis is the most familiar example. Thyrotoxicosis and systemic lupus erythematosus have already been mentioned. Hypogammaglobulinaemia, myositis, myocarditis, acquired haemolytic anaemia and erythroblastic anaemia are others. A recent addition is an immunological deficiency disease of infants, known as hereditary lymphocytophthisis, in which thymic aplasia is associated with generalized lymphoid aplasia and hypogammaglobulinaemia.

CYSTS OF THE THYMUS

These are rare and are usually small and multiple and embedded in the gland. Uncommonly they may reach several centimetres in diameter and may then be attached to the gland by a broad pedicle. The larger cysts have a thin fibrous wall and are lined by flattened cells of epithelial or reticulum cell origin. The more common small cysts are lined by ciliated epithelium or by columnar, mucus-secreting cells which are thought to arise from a degenerated Hassall's corpuscle. Pathologists are not agreed whether these cysts represent postembryonal differentiation of the thymic reticulum or are derived from branchial pouch remnants [53]. From some studies in animals there is reason to believe

that at least some of the cysts develop after birth.

Most thymic cysts are asymptomatic. If large they may produce cough or chest pain. The chest x-ray shows the features of an enlarged thymus. Since diagnosis cannot be made from thymic tumour surgical removal is the treatment of choice.

TUMOURS OF THE THYMUS

Thymomata are usually believed to be the third most common of the mediastinal tumours though it must be remembered that their precise incidence is not known. The pathology of thymomata is so varied that although numerous attempts at classifications have been made none is entirely satisfactory [8]. The only safe rule regarding their management is that all should be considered malignant, and this in spite of the macroscopic or microscopic appearances.

PATHOLOGY

The tumours may be solid or cystic, with a well-defined margin or diffusely invasive, soft or with areas of calcification. Neither the presence of a capsule nor calcification infers that they are benign. It is a feature of thymic tumours that they are associated with dense fibrous tissue reaction in adjacent tissues but this does not prevent the tendency to erupt through these confines to involve structures beyond. Local invasion is, therefore, usually rapid with severe consequences. Metastases to distant organs are rare although involvement of mediastinal lymph glands is frequent. Infiltration of the pleura, lung and pericardium, and obstruction of the great veins, are commonly encountered.

In those cases of thymic enlargement (hypertrophy or thymoma) in adults which are associated with myasthenia gravis the disease often progresses rapidly and usually proves refractory to treatment. Thymic tumour is much more commonly associated with myasthenia than is simple hyperplasia.

The histology of thymic tumours is varied. Some resemble the normal gland and can be classified as adenomata; others are composed of reticulum cells with variable amounts of lymphocytes. Both of these types may be well-encapsulated by fibrous tissue. Other forms have been described as lymphosarcoma, myxosarcoma, carcinoma and spindle cell carcinoma according to the dominant histological features. Mitoses and giant cell formation are common; Hassall's corpuscles are uncommon in thymomata.

CLINICAL FEATURES

When the features of myasthenia are not present the lesion may be found only at routine radiography or because of pressure symptoms. The latter include stridor, wheezing, respiratory distress due to bronchial or tracheal compression and, occasionally, dysphagia due to oesophageal compression. When tracheal compression is marked the patient is usually hypoxic and cyanosed. Retrosternal pain may also be a feature. Superior vena caval obstruction may occur. Sometimes paroxysmal attacks of coughing and bronchospasm may result from pressure on the vagus.

RADIOLOGY

Every patient with myasthenia gravis should be suspected of having a thymoma and should be examined radiographically for this. A thymoma presents as an irregular tumour on one or other or both sides of the superior mediastinal shadow in the PA x-ray but may not be detectable except in lateral views when it appears as a rounded or elongated shadow in the anterior part of the upper mediastinum. The upper pole of a thymoma can usually be seen clearly in the PA film and this differentiates it from retrosternal goitre. About 10% of thymomata show calcification either on plain x-rays or on tomography. Thymoma associated with myasthenia can always be recognized in either PA or lateral x-rays and air insufflation is never necessary to demonstrate it.

TREATMENT

Whether myasthenia gravis is present or not, every thymoma should be treated surgically. In some centres radiotherapy is frequently given before surgical removal, principally as a therapeutic test. Irradiation always results in rapid shrinkage of the tumour. This does not, however, improve the results of surgical treatment since it is the lymphocytic elements which are mainly affected by radiotherapy and these are not the most important with regard to malignancy or the tendency to myasthenia; these appear to be mainly associated with thymic epithelial cells which are notoriously radioresistant even when megavoltage therapy is employed. Thymic tumours are found only in about 10–15% of cases presenting with myasthenia gravis but the incidence of myasthenia (at the time of presentation or later) in patients who present with a thymic tumour varies from 25 to 75% [38].

With regard to thymectomy for myasthenia gravis this is certainly indicated if a thymoma is present since these tumours are in any case commonly malignant. Myasthenia in association with malignant thymoma does, however, pursue a relentless course in most patients. Thymectomy in patients without a thymoma appears to have its best result in young women with generalized myasthenia of recent onset and in men with generalized weakness refractory to medical treatment. The localized or bulbar types of myasthenia have little tendency to affect the muscles diffusely and thymectomy is not indicated. Similarly when cholinergic drugs control the disease thymectomy is superfluous.

The reader is referred to the review by Simpson [55] whose findings are in agreement with most other workers in this field, and also to the review of operation cases by Holmes Sellors and his colleagues [27].

OTHER TUMOURS OF THE MEDIASTINUM

Apart from involvement of mediastinal glands by such conditions as lymphadenoma and leukaemia a number of other forms of neoplasia occur in the mediastinum. These include cavernous haemangioma (a rare benign tumour of the upper mediastinum), cystic hygroma (lymphangioma), lymphomatous tumours (lymphadenoma, lymphosarcoma, lymphoblastoma, reticulum cell sarcoma and giant follicular lymphoblastoma) and a great variety of tumours of mesenchymal origin (e.g. fibroma, lipoma and leiomyoma and their malignant counterparts).

LYMPHOMATOUS TUMOURS

Lymphadenoma and lymphosarcoma are the commonest forms of lymphatic tumours in the mediastinum. The two are difficult to distinguish clinically and even histologically. The mediastinal lesion is usually part of a generalized lymphatic involvement and since lymph glands are present in the superior and anterior mediastinum the disease may involve both of these. Consequently the enlarging mass blends with the cardiac outline. The cell is the mature, medium sized lymphocyte, later replaced by mononuclears, polymorphs with considerable numbers of eosinophils and multinucleated large hyperchromatic cells with basophilic cytoplasm, round or oval nuclei and prominent nucleoli. Mitoses may be recognizable.

Reticulum cell sarcoma has larger, paler, multinucleated cells with a reticular appearance.

The term *lymphoblastoma* is used to describe those lesions due to the more primitive lymphocytes.

Giant follicular lymphoblastoma is less common than the other forms of lymphomatous tumour. The histological findings are of immature lymphocytes compressing normal tissue.

All of these tumours may in time involve adjacent structures and bone marrow, and wider dissemination may occur. The x-ray shows a lobulated mass in the upper mediastinum, often bilateral. Malignant pericarditis may be due to lymphomatous tumours.

Other causes of multiple lymph gland enlargement around the trachea and main bronchi must be excluded. These include sarcoidosis, secondary malignant lymphadenopathy and primary pulmonary tuberculosis.

DIAGNOSIS AND TREATMENT

The primary lymphatic component may be suspected from the radiographic appearances, which are typical, or if there are palpable lymph nodes in the neck or elsewhere. A definite diagnosis can usually be made by scalene node biopsy or mediastinoscopy. The most effective treatment is x-radiation which results in rapid reduction in size of the tumour. Some cases respond to nitrogen mustard, methotrexate or chlorambucil. The prognosis, however, is poor with any form of treatment.

CYSTIC HYGROMA

Cystic hygroma is rare, commonly occurs in childhood and is usually associated with a hygroma of the neck. It is composed of a number of variable sized cysts, lined with epithelium and with walls which may contain smooth muscle and variable amounts of lymphocytes. They contain a clear or strawcoloured gelatinous fluid. Their derivation is thought to be from aberrant portions of pericardial or coelomic tissues. Pressure symptoms are uncommon and the lesion is usually found by noting a swelling in the neck due to extension of the lesion from the mediastinum. The x-ray shows a mass extending from the hilum to the jaw in which numerous cysts may be seen. The treatment is surgical removal as early as possible [19].

MENINGOCELES

Meningoceles in the posterior mediastinum are very rare. They are accompanied by a defect in the anterior aspect of the vertebral body and are usually on the right side. Signs and symptoms depend on the size, and such features as dysphagia, dyspnoea and cyanosis may all occur. Myelography demonstrates a connection with the spinal canal, screening usually shows pulsations and a bifid vertebra is a common accompaniment. Treatment is by excision.

CYSTS OF THE MEDIASTINUM

Cysts may arise in the mediastinum as congenital malformations of the pericardium, thymus (p. 612), tracheobronchial tree and gastrointestinal tract.

PLEUROPERICARDIAL CYSTS

These are usually adherent to the parietal pericardium, have a thin fibrous wall and are lined by flattened cells which may be mesothelial. It has been suggested that they may be due to failure of the primitive coelomic lacunae to fuse [35]. Other theories imply a sequestration of part of the pleuroperitoneal cavity by the developing diaphragm or the development from a persisting 'ventral parietal recess' of the pericardium. About 10% communicate with the pericardium.

The cysts, which may be up to 10 cm in diameter or more, are filled with a clear fluid and are situated anteriorly in the cardiophrenic angle, 70% of them on the right side. A colloquial designation is 'spring water cysts' because of their content. The fluid does not collect under tension except in the very rare complication of infection. Their incidence has been estimated as 1 per 100,000 of the population [36]. They are commonly first recognized at routine radiography and their benign nature may be confirmed if a previous chest x-ray taken some time before is available for comparison. Radiographically they present as a smooth, rounded opacity in the right cardiophrenic angle situated in the lateral chest radiograph in the sternodiaphragmatic angle. If there is no previous x-ray the insertion of a needle and aspiration of the characteristic fluid will confirm the diagnosis. Barium studies may be necessary to distinguish from a hernia through the foramen of Morgagni.

Infection only very rarely occurs and malignancy not at all. Since they are usually entirely symptomless the patient may be given an excellent prognosis although it is wise to continue follow-up to be certain that they are not increasing in size which would indicate excision, mainly on account of uncertainty about the nature of the lesion in this context.

INTRATHORACIC DUPLICATIONS OF THE FOREGUT

Foregut duplications are of two varieties and may result in the development of mediastinal cysts. The first form of duplication occurs fairly late in the development of the wall of the primitive foregut; the second develops much earlier as part of a more diffuse congenital abnormality called the split notochord syndrome.

Since the respiratory system develops as a bud from the ventral surface of the primitive foregut, duplications of the first type may be in the wall of the trachea, major bronchi or oesophagus. These are the so-called *bronchogenic* and *gastroenteric cysts* (sometimes called gastrogenous cysts). They appear to develop within the circular muscle coat of the parent respiratory or alimentary canal. They are lined by epithelium which is nearly always ciliated columnar in type but occasionally stratified squamous. If infection is a complication the type of epithelium may not be recognizable. Duplications which are part of the split notochord syndrome are usually associated with abnormalities of the vertebra and perhaps also of the spinal cord.

BRONCHOGENIC CYSTS

It is fairly certain that bronchogenic cysts occur more frequently than recorded series suggest. These have placed bronchogenic cysts between 5th [44] and 3rd [50] in order of frequency of mediastinal tumours and cysts.

Bronchogenic cysts are thin-walled and occur characteristically near the tracheal bifurcation [33]. They may be classified according to their location [41]:

(1) Paratracheal, when they are attached to the tracheal wall usually on the right side and just above the tracheal bifurcation.
(2) Carinal, when the cysts are attached at the level of the carina and often to the anterior oesophageal wall as well. These are probably the most serious and can give rise to tracheobronchial compression in early life.
(3) Hilar, when the cysts are attached to one of the main or lobar bronchi. Most bronchogenic cysts in older children or adults are in this group.

(4) Paraoesophageal, when the cysts are in intimate relationship with the oesophagus and may even be within its walls, separated entirely from the tracheobronchial tree.

PATHOLOGY

The wall is from 1 to 5 mm in thickness consisting of rather loose connective tissue containing bundles of smooth muscle. Mucous glands and cartilage may also be present. The epithelium has already been mentioned. In the paraoesophageal type of cyst the distinction from an oesophageal cyst depends on the finding of cartilage.

Infection is prone to occur with consequent rupture into a bronchus. The cyst may then contain pus, blood and air. An uninfected cyst usually contains a clear or milky, mucoid material with desquamated epithelial cells.

CLINICAL FEATURES

Bronchogenic cysts are frequently asymptomatic. Many are only discovered as incidental findings at routine radiography or even at autopsy. They are uncommon in childhood but have been known to produce signs of tracheobronchial obstruction. Because of their location on the posterior surface of the trachea or main bronchi they may extend upwards between the trachea and oesophagus and even laterally. Thus compression of the trachea, bronchi and the oesophagus may occur, the degree depending on the size of the cyst. Bronchogenic cysts becoming evident in childhood commonly result in poor feeding, dysphagia, noisy breathing and dyspnoea. When there is infection and fistulous connection with a bronchus haemoptysis, fever and purulent sputum may occur. These may result in chronic ill health with some similarities to bronchiectasis. Carcinoma has also been reported as a complication [42].

Radiographically the lesion is a smooth, round or oval homogeneous opacity most commonly in the superior or middle mediastinum, at or just anterior to the spine but not usually as far posteriorly as neurogenic tumours. Occasionally the presence of a fluid level indicates communication with the tracheobronchial tree. Calcification is not a feature. The barium swallow may show displacement of the oesophagus posteriorly.

Elective *treatment* is surgical removal.

GASTROENTERIC CYSTS

These are segments of the alimentary tract though they are completely or partially separated from it. They tend to produce symptoms early and most reported cases have been in infants under 1 year of age though examples in older people are not uncommon. The histological appearances are characterized by a mucosal lining resembling some part of the gut, usually the oesophagus or the stomach. They may secrete gastric juice so that ulceration may occur, particularly into the bronchi. Two types are recognized:

(1) Duplications. These are spherical or tubular cystic lesions in continuity with the alimentary canal and sharing a common blood supply. They may or may not have some communication. Muscular and mucosal layers are present in the wall and the fluid is that of the parent viscus. Oesophageal duplications are most commonly in the mid third of the posterior mediastinum on the right side. They may, on occasion, project into the hemithorax.

(2) Dorsal enteric remnants: These cysts have fibrous attachments to the spine and gut and may be located before, or rarely behind, the vertebrae.

As occurs with most other congenital abnormalities other malformations may coexist, such as cysts and diverticula elsewhere or spina bifida.

Treatment is by surgical removal which may be life-saving in infancy and is indicated at any age.

ACUTE MEDIASTINITIS

The commonest cause of acute mediastinitis is oesophageal perforation which may be traumatic or spontaneous. Among the traumatic causes are endoscopy and attempts to dilate or intubate oesophageal strictures (particularly carcinomata). Operations on the larynx, trachea and oesophagus or perforation of these by a foreign body are also among the commoner causes of acute mediastinitis. Spontaneous perforation is usually postemetic.

Suppurative lymphadenopathy secondary to infection of the lungs, oesophagus and pharynx may also lead to acute mediastinitis, as may rarely tuberculosis or osteomyelitis of the cervical or thoracic spine. Haematogenous infections and extension of subphrenic infection above the diaphragm are also rare causes. With the commoner aetiologies the posterior mediastinum is more likely to be affected by direct spread of infection along the tissue planes.

Clinical features include substernal pain, rigors, fever, dysphagia, neck pain, torticollis if the process descends from the neck, and, if the trachea is involved, a brassy cough and dyspnoea. The patient is usually toxaemic, cyanosed, restless and anxious. Tenderness may be elicited over the sternum. The white cell count may show a marked leucocytosis. Since most oesophageal perforations involve the mediastinal pleura, pleural effusion or pyopneumothorax, usually on the left side, rapidly develops. Mediastinal emphysema may be evident (p. 449). The chest x-ray shows widening of the upper mediastinal shadow by a dense shadow bulging outwards with a convex border. The lateral view may show displacement of the trachea and the oesophagus forward by a posterior abscess. The radiographic appearances of mediastinal emphysema and pleural effusion may be present.

The early use of antibiotic treatment may control the condition and prevent abscess formation. When an abscess has developed the treatment is primarily surgical. Surgical drainage is indicated when there is tracheal and oesophageal displacement as shown by the lateral x-ray, barium meal and perhaps bronchoscopy. Any complicating pyopneumothorax will, of course, require its own management.

CHRONIC FIBROUS MEDIASTINITIS
(Idiopathic mediastinal fibrosis)

As the name implies, chronic fibrous mediastinitis is a slowly progressive scarring of the mediastinal tissues. The mode of presentation and the severity of the illness vary with the extent of the process and with the structure or structures principally involved.

AETIOLOGY

The condition has been known for over a century [22]. The cases described in the earlier part of this century were thought to be either tuberculous or syphilitic in origin [31 & 32]. Bacteriological and histological examination of most cases, however, have excluded these possibilities. Knox [32] suggested a histological resemblance between keloids and the fibrosis of chronic fibrous mediastinitis and later workers have confirmed this [21 & 23]. There is, however, nothing in the past and family histories of reported cases which shows any tendency towards cutaneous keloid development. Allen [3] suggested the possibility of visceral keloid formation but this remains entirely theoretical. It was almost inevitable that autoimmunity would be included among recent theories, but there is no satisfactory evidence for this [12]. The less exotic theory of spread of infection via mediastinal lymph glands has been proposed but, again, receives little support from case histories [11]. The histology has suggested to several workers [5, 13 & 20], that mediastinal and retroperitoneal fibrosis are related and that these in turn have features in common with other fibrosing diseases such as fibrosing (Riedel's) thyroiditis, [5], pseudotumour of the orbit, Dupuytren's contracture of the palmar fascia and Peyronie's disease of the penis. More recently sclerosing cholangitis has been suggested as an addition to the list [7]. *Histoplasma capsulatum* infection has been proved in 4 reported cases [52]. Another possibility is a link with the retroperitoneal fibrosis known to occur after administration of Methysergide [16 & 59] though no such association has been demonstrated in mediastinal fibrosis.

Methysergide has been used, mainly in the United States, for the prevention of severe migraine. Although this is a very effective drug about 1 in 5 patients have side effects sufficient to warrant stopping its use. These include vertigo, unsteadiness, nausea and peripheral vasoconstriction. A more serious side effect may be heralded by aches in the loins, groins and thighs which, if the drug is continued, may be followed by recurrent fever, oliguria and dysuria due to retroperitoneal fibrosis compressing the ureters and leading to hydronephrosis. Stopping the drug results in progressive improvement and in some cases even in return of the pyelographic appearances to normal. Surgery alone has not been satisfactory treatment if the drug has been continued. Relapse has been recorded in some patients who have restarted the drug. About 150 cases of the condition have been reported so far [17]. 27 have been found in patients taking Methysergide in the past 3 years, making a fortuitous association unlikely. In addition cardiac murmurs and attacks of pleural friction and effusion have also been reported during Methysergide treatment, and lung biopsy in a few cases has shown perivascular and peribronchial fibrosis. Graham and his colleagues [17] warned that in patients treated with Methysergide the possibility of fibrosis other than in the retroperitoneal tissues should constantly be kept in mind.

Since mediastinal and retroperitoneal fibrosis were described long before the use of Methysergide clearly there must be other causes. Fibrosis, whether in the mediastinum, retroperitoneum, or elsewhere, may merely be an overresponse of fibrous tissue to a variety of stimuli. These stimuli may be infective, traumatic, toxic or immunological. In our present state of knowledge most cases of chronic mediastinal fibrosis remain firmly in the idiopathic category.

PATHOLOGY

Masses of fibrous tissue develop in the upper mediastinum. This is whitish, hard and fixed and usually infiltrates the connective tissues diffusely, appearing at thoracotomy as an indefinite plaque which has been likened to a pancake [5]. Less commonly it develops as a solid lump. It never invades the heart or lungs and its chief effect is on the superior vena cava and its tributaries which it compresses or even obliterates. The bronchi and large pulmonary vessels [45] may also be compressed by the encroaching fibrous tissue. Stricture of the pulmonary veins, trachea or main bronchi or oesophagus may also occur.

It is of interest to compare those patients in whom mediastinal and retroperitoneal fibrosis have been found in the same individual. The case described by Tubbs [57] was a male aged 25 with symptoms of superior vena caval obstruction for 4 years. Operation to relieve obstruction was unsuccessful and at autopsy there was stenosis and thrombosis of the inferior vena cava due to retroperitoneal fibrosis as well as mediastinal fibrosis. Inkley and Abbott [29] recorded the case of a man aged 59 who had a 9 years' history of recurrent haemoptysis and a broadening mediastinal shadow. Because of oesophageal varices portocaval anastomosis was performed and retroperitoneal fibrosis was found involving the portal vein and the hilus of the right kidney. At autopsy 9 days later the fibrosis in the mediastinum and retroperitoneum was found to be identical. Morgan and his colleagues [43] also described combined mediastinal and periureteric fibrosis and they make the point that the mediastinal and retroperitoneal lesions appear to have been anatomically separate, i.e. that the lesion is not a spreading process. They also stress the fact that the diagnosis of idiopathic fibrosis in one site should lead to continued observation to ensure that others are not involved. This infers follow-up for an indefinite number of years.

CLINICAL FEATURES

Chronic fibrosing mediastinitis may begin at any age but most commonly the diagnosis is made in the 4th decade; males and females are equally affected. Because of the indolent progress of the condition the symptoms are insidious at the beginning and are at first mild. The superior vena cava is mainly affected but the innominate and the azygos veins may also be included. All the veins of the head and neck, with the exception of the retinal veins, may become distended. The veins of the upper extremities may also be involved but to a lesser extent. Characteristically the face and neck begin to swell and this is particularly in evidence when the patient stoops or lies down. Later, swelling of the eyelids and subconjunctival oedema may be noted on rising in the morning. A feeling of fullness and pressure associated with headaches, breathlessness, giddiness and sometimes epistaxis may all occur and these are made worse by coughing, straining or exercise. The neck veins are dilated, and distended veins appear at the base of the neck. All of these features occur in the absence of fever or systemic upset and investigations may be unrewarding at this stage. As time passes collateral venous channels develop which allow many of the features to subside and the patient's condition may undergo slow improvement. In any case recognized early the immediate prognosis is, therefore, relatively good but the fibrosis is progressive and there is never full recovery. Stricture of the pulmonary veins, trachea, main bronchi or oesophagus may add their distinctive features.

RADIOLOGY

There is nothing characteristic about the x-ray appearances. Widening of the upper mediastinum is found in most cases, tomography may show tracheobronchial stricture and oesophageal stricture may be demonstrated by barium swallow. Angiography may show superior vena caval obstruction and the marked collateral circulation in the mediastinum. None of these procedures can give a diagnosis; differentiation from the more common alternative of malignant infiltration of the mediastinum can only be made by thoracotomy.

TREATMENT

Apart from those cases possibly associated with Methysergide in which the drug should obviously be stopped, treatment of idiopathic mediastinal fibrosis is essentially surgical and is aimed at relieving the pressure on the involved mediastinal structures. When the lesion is localized, removal is relatively easy; when it is diffuse, removal of the infiltrating mass may be difficult or impossible. Occasionally superior vena caval obstruction can be relieved by a bypass graft. Stricture of the oesophagus may require dilatation. Corticosteroid drugs have usually proved unhelpful.

With regard to the use of Methysergide it is recommended that treatment be interrupted for several months each year, high dosage avoided and the drug completely discontinued on suspicion of the development of any of the features of retroperitoneal or mediastinal fibrosis.

REFERENCES

[1] ACKERMAN L.V. & TAYLOR F.H. (1951) Neurogenous tumours within the thorax. A clinicopathological evaluation of 48 cases. *Cancer* 4, 669.
[2] ADLER R.H., TAHERI S.A. & WEINTRAUB D.H. (1960) Mediastinal teratoma in infancy. *J. thorac. Surg.* 39, 394.
[3] ALLEN A.C. (1954) *The Skin*, p. 176. St. Louis, Mosby.
[4] ANDERSON W. (1967) *Boyd's Pathology for the Surgeon*, 8th Edition. Philadelphia, Saunders.
[5] BARRETT N.R. (1958) Idiopathic mediastinal fibrosis. *Br. J. Surg.* 46, 207.
[6] BARRETT N.R. (1963) The chest wall. In *Chest Diseases*, ed. Perry K.M.A. and Sellors T.H. London, Butterworths.
[7] BARTHOLOMEW L.G., CAIN J.C., WOOLNER L.B., UTZ D.C. & FERRIS D.O. (1963) Sclerosing cholangitis; its possible association with Riedel's struma and fibrous mediastinitis. *New Engl. J. Med.* 269, 8.
[8] BERNATZ P.E., HARRISON E.G. & CLAGETT O.T. (1961) Thymoma: a clinico-pathologic study. *J. thorac. Surg.* 42, 424.
[9] BLADES B. (1946) Mediastinal tumours. *Ann. Surg.* 123, 749.
[10] CAREY L.S., ELLIS F.H.Jr., GOOD C.A. & WOOLNER L.B. (1960) Neurogenic tumours of the mediastinum, a clinico-pathologic study. *Am. J. Roentgenol* 84, 189.
[11] CHISHOLM E.R., HUTCH J.A. & BOLOMY A.A. (1954) Bilateral ureteral obstruction due to chronic inflammation of the fascia around the ureters. *J. Urol.* 72, 812.
[12] DeGENNES L., BRICARIE H., TOURNEUR R. & CURNOT L. (1960) Les rétrécissements peri-urinaires idiopathiques. *Lyon méd.* 203, 279.

[13] EDITORIAL (1962) Idiopathic mediastinal fibrosis *Br. med. J.* ii 720.

[14] ELLIS F.H.Jr. & DUSHANE J.W. (1956) Primary mediastinal cysts and neoplasms in infants and children. *Am. Rev. Tuberc.* **74**, 940.

[15] GAYOLA G. & WEIL P.H. (1965) Intrathoracic nerve sheath tumour of the vagus *J. thorac. cardiovasc. Surg.* **49**, 412.

[16] GRAHAM J.R. (1964) Methysergide for prevention of headache. Experience in 500 patients over 3 years. *New Engl. J. Med.* **270**, 267.

[17] GRAHAM J.R., SUBY H.I., LeCOMPTE P.R. & SADOWSKY N.L. (1966) Fibrotic disorders associated with Methysergide therapy for headache. *New Engl. J. Med.* **274**, 359.

[18] GROSS R.E. (1953) Cysts and primary tumours of the thorax. In *Surgery of Infancy and Childhood*, p. 762. Philadelphia, Saunders.

[19] GROSS R.E. & HURWITT E. (1948) Cervicomediastinal and mediastinal cystic hygroma. *Surg. Gynec. Obst.* **87**, 599.

[20] HACHE L., WOOLNER L.B. & BERNATZ P.E. (1962) Idiopathic fibrous mediastinitis. *Dis. Chest* **41**, 9.

[21] HACKETT E. (1958) Idiopathic retroperitoneal fibrosis: a condition involving the ureters, the aorta and the inferior vena cava. *Br. J. Surg.* **36**, 3.

[22] HALLET C.H. (1848) On the collateral circulation in cases of obliteration or obstruction of the venae cavae. *Edinburgh med. J.* **69**, 269.

[23] HAWK W.A. & HAZARD J.B. (1959) Sclerosing retroperitonitis and sclerosing mediastinitis. *Am. J. clin. Pathol.* **32**, 321.

[24] HENER G.J. & ANDRUS W. (1940) Surgery of mediastinal tumours. *Am. J. Surg.* **50**, 146.

[25] HIRSCH O., ROBBINS S.L. & HOUGHTON J.D. (1946) Mediastinal chorionepithelioma in a male. *Am. J. Pathol.* **22**, 833.

[26] HODGE J., APONTE G. & McLAUGHLIN E. (1959) Primary mediastinal tumours. *J. thorac. Surg.* **37**, 730.

[27] HOLMES SELLORS T., THACKRAY A.C. & THOMSON A.D. (1967) Tumours of the thymus: a review of 88 operation cases. *Thorax* **22**, 193.

[28] HOPE J.W. & KOOP C.E. (1959) Differential diagnosis of mediastinal masses. *Pediat. Clin. N. Am.* **6**, 379.

[29] INKLEY S.R. & ABBOTT G.R. (1961) Unilateral pulmonary arteriosclerosis. Unusual fibrous connective tissue growth associated: Review of literature and discussion of possible physiological mechanisms involved in these changes. *Arch. intern. Med.* **108**, 903.

[30] JOANNIDES M. & LANGSTON H. (1960) Mediastinal tumours and cysts in the adult. *Dis. Chest* **38**, 243.

[31] KEEFER C.S. (1938) Acute and chronic mediastinitis. *Arch. intern. Med.* **62**, 109.

[32] KNOX L.C. (1925) Chronic mediastinitis. *Am. J. med. Sci.* **169**, 807.

[33] LAIPPLY T.C. (1945) Cysts and cystic tumours of the mediastinum. *Arch. Pathol.* **39**, 153.

[34] LAIPPLY T.C. & SHIPLAY R.A. (1945) Extragenital choriocarcinoma in the male. *Am. J. Pathol.* **21**, 921.

[35] LAMBERT A.V.S. (1940) Aetiology of thin-walled thoracic cysts. *J. thorac. Surg.* **10**, 1.

[36] LE ROUX B.T. (1959) Pericardial coelomic cysts. *Thorax* **14**, 27.

[37] LE ROUX B.T. (1960) Mediastinal teratomata. *Thorax* **15**, 333.

[38] LE ROUX B.T. & DODDS T.C. (1964) *A Portfolio of Chest Radiographs*. London, Livingstone.

[39] LITTLE E.H. (1953) Congenital cysts and cystic tumours of the mediastinum. *South. med. J.* **46**, 742.

[40] LYONS H.A., CALVY G.L. & SAMMONS B.P. (1959) The diagnosis and classification of mediastinal masses I. *Ann. intern. Med.* **51**, 897.

[41] MAIER H.C. (1948) Bronchiogenic cysts of the mediastinum. *Ann. Surg.* **127**, 476.

[42] MOERSCH H.J. & CLAGETT O.T. (1947) Pulmonary cysts. *J. thorac. Surg.* **16**, 179.

[43] MORGAN A.C., LOUGHRIDGE LEVINA W. & CALNE R.Y. (1966) Combined mediastinal and retroperitoneal fibrosis. *Lancet* **i**, 67.

[44] MORRISON I.M. (1958) Tumours and cysts of the mediastinum. *Thorax* **13**, 294.

[45] NELSON W.P., LUNDBERG G.D. & DICKERSON R.B. (1965) Pulmonary artery obstruction and cor pulmonale due to chronic fibrous mediastinitis. *Am. J. Med.* **38**, 279.

[46] NORRIS E.H. (1947) The parathyroid adenoma. *Internat. Abstr. Surg.* **84**, 1.

[47] OBERMAN H.A. & ABELL M.R. (1960) Neurogenous neoplasms of the mediastinum. *Cancer* **13**, 882.

[48] PEABODY J.W., STRUG L.H. & RIVES J.D. (1954) Mediastinal tumours. *Arch. intern. Med.* **93**, 875.

[49] RICHARDS G.J. & REEVES R.J. (1958) Mediastinal tumours in children. *J. Dis. Child.* **95**, 284.

[50] RINGERTZ N. & LIDHOLM S.O. (1956) Mediastinal tumours and cysts. *J. thorac. Surg.* **31**, 458.

[51] SABISTON D.C.Jr. & SCOTT H.W.Jr. (1952) Primary neoplasms and cysts of the mediastinum. *Ann. Surg.* **136**, 777.

[52] SALYER J.M., HARRISON H.N., WINN D.F. & TAYLOR R.R. (1959) Chronic fibrous mediastinitis and superior vena caval obstruction due to histoplasmosis. *Dis. Chest* **35**, 364.

[53] SCHLUMBERGER H.G. (1951) Tumours of the mediastinum. In *Atlas of Tumour Pathology*. Washington, National Research Council.

[54] SHANKS S.C. & KERLEY P. (1962) *A Text-book of X-ray Diagnosis*, by British Authors, 3rd Edition. London Lewis.

[55] SIMPSON J.A. (1958) Evaluation of thymectomy in myasthenia gravis. *Brain* **81**, 112.

[56] SINGLETON E.B. & BILES E.W. (1956) Mediastinal tumours in children. *Texas J. Med.* **52**,
588.

[57] TUBBS O.S. (1946) Superior vena caval obstruction due to chronic mediastinitis. *Thorax* **1**,
247.

[58] WILLIS R.A. (1958) *The Borderland of Embryology and Pathology.* London, Butterworths.

[59] UTZ D.C., ROOKE E.D., SPITTELL J.A. &
BARTHOLOMEW N.L. (1966) Retroperitoneal
fibrosis in patients taking Methysergide. *J.
Am. med. Ass.* **191**, 983.

Diseases of the Chest Wall

THE RIBS

CONGENITAL DEFORMITIES AND ABNORMALITIES [15]

Bifid ribs are common, particularly in the upper 6 ribs. Their only importance is that, if the abnormality is not suspected on the x-ray, it may give rise to confusion in interpretation, the appearance being incorrectly attributed to a lesion in the lung. *Extra ribs, fused ribs* and *absence of ribs* may also occur. Again these are only of radiological importance. The only important clinical syndrome is that which arises from *cervical rib*, which may occur on one or both sides and is associated with the transverse process of the 7th cervical vertebra. Cervical ribs give rise to symptoms in about 10% of cases, but the symptoms are neurological or vascular and need not be enumerated in a book on respiratory disease.

Bone islands may occur in ribs. They are focal deposits of dense cortical bone, less than 1 cm in diameter, in areas normally occupied by cancellous bone. They sometimes have to be differentiated from osteosclerotic metastases, for instance from carcinoma of the prostate.

FRACTURES OF RIBS

TRAUMA

Major trauma of the chest wall is primarily of interest to surgeons and will not be discussed here. Lesser degrees of trauma may be forgotten by the patient or be sustained when he is under the influence of alcohol, anaesthetics or in coma, and may sometimes give rise to problems in differential diagnosis. A rib fracture should be suspected if there is local rib tenderness at the site of pain of recent onset or if pain occurs on 'springing' the ribs. Unless there is displacement the

fracture is often not visible on the x-ray in the acute stage and callus formation, visible radiologically, does not occur for several weeks. Sometimes the x-ray shows linear shadows 2–3 cm long underlying the fractured rib and possibly due to bruising of the lung [21]. Treatment with analgesics is usually all that is necessary, though occasionally it may be useful to infiltrate with local anaesthetic.

'FATIGUE' FRACTURES

These may occur in the first or second ribs, most commonly in young soldiers carrying heavy rucksacks or rifles. Often there is little pain but the fracture may result in fibrous union or a residual cyst [21].

COUGH FRACTURES

Cough fractures are relatively common and are presumably due to severe opposing muscular tension during cough. They may occur without specific predisposing factors but may also do so in calcium deficiency, associated for instance with corticosteroid osteoporosis or osteomalacia. They are seen most often in the region of the axillary line. There is a sudden onset of pain, which may resemble pleurisy but is usually worse on coughing than breathing. The local signs of fracture are those already outlined. Later there may be a tender lump. As with traumatic fracture, there may be no visible abnormality radiologically until callus appears. Treatment is similar to that outlined for traumatic fracture.

PATHOLOGICAL FRACTURE

Pathological fracture may occur with rib metastasis (p. 530) or osteolytic primary tumour of rib such as myeloma.

SLIPPING RIBS

Each of the upper 7 ribs has a joint between the cartilage and the sternum. This can be the site of painful osteoarthritis or clicking joints. Sometimes there is inefficient junction between the cartilage of the 8th or 9th rib and the costal margin resulting in a painful clicking with movement. This may be traumatic or may occur after pregnancy. The click may occasionally be striking on auscultation and may be induced by breathing or movement. We have not seen a case in which it has been necessary to excise the affected area, but this might be reasonable if it were really troublesome [3].

INFLAMMATORY LESIONS OF THE RIBS

OSTEOMYELITIS [3]

Osteomyelitis is relatively uncommon. It is most frequent in children but sometimes seen in adults. One of the upper 3 ribs is usually affected, most commonly the first. It is often post-traumatic. The suppuration may strip the periosteum from the rib and form a subperiosteal extrapleural abscess which may be large. Radiologically there may be no change in the appearance of the rib for 10 or 12 days. Initially there is nonspecific local destruction, with reactionary sclerosis in longstanding cases [15]. The extrapleural collection of pus may give rise to a puzzling local shadow in the chest x-ray, especially in a subacute case. Local osteomyelitis of a rib may be secondary to the drainage of an empyema with inflammation spreading from the drainage site into the bone. Sequestra may be formed. These may sometimes discharge into the empyema which persists until they are removed [3]. Typhoid osteitis or chondritis may occur years after an attack of typhoid and give rise to indolent inflammatory swelling in the bone. Radiologically there may be a translucent area resembling Brodie's abscess. It has been suggested that the lesion is best treated by intensive antibiotics, perhaps high doses of ampicillin, with excision of the affected area when it has become sterile [3].

SUPPURATIVE CHONDRITIS

Suppurative chondritis may occur after thoraco-abdominal operations when a cartilage is excised and the remnant becomes infected. This may give rise to a discharging sinus. The condition is treated by antibiotics and excision [3]. It is very rare.

TUBERCULOSIS OF THE RIB [15]

This is rare. Cold abscess of the chest wall usually arises from intercostal lymph nodes (p. 626). Rib lesions may cause local pain, swelling and sinus formation. Radiologically there is an initial small area of bone destruction which may progress to periosteal elevation and soft tissue swelling. There is usually no evidence of pulmonary tuberculosis; rib lesions with chronic pulmonary disease are more often due to actinomycosis (p. 290). Multiple lesions of the costovertebral portions of the ribs may accompany Pott's disease and paravertebral abscess formation. Tuberculosis very occasionally causes multiple cystic areas of destruction in the ribs or a localized destructive lesion at the costochondral junction. Tuberculosis of the sternum sometimes occurs.

BLASTOMYCOSIS, COCCIDIOIDOMYCOSIS, TORULOSIS, BRUCELLOSIS AND SPOROTRICHOSIS

These may rarely affect the ribs and produce changes similar to those of tuberculosis [15].

ACTINOMYCOSIS

Actinomycosis may spread from the lungs into the chest wall and ribs, producing destructive lesions with irregularity of the rib margins caused by periostitis.

SYPHILIS OF THE RIBS

Syphilis of rib is very rare and gives rise to irregular tender swelling of the rib. Radiologically there are irregular osteolytic lesions in the medulla with laminated periosteal reactions [15]; yaws may give a similar appearance. The diagnosis of syphilis will be made only by serology [3].

HYDATID CYSTS

Hydatid cysts may occur in ribs, with local expansion and cortical thinning [15].

COSTOCHONDRITIS
(Tietze's disease; thoracochondralgia)

This is a condition of obscure origin in which there is pain, swelling and tenderness of one or more of the 6 upper costal cartilages, though the sternoclavicular joint was also thought to be involved in one of Tietze's [24] original 4 cases. Some 200 cases have been described in the literature but there must be many unreported; we have seen a number in our own practice. There is no sex bias and it has been described at all ages between 11 and 80, with a large number of patients in early adult life [17]. Recorded *biopsies* have shown minimal or no abnormality [17] and there is no particular association with calcification of the cartilages. Although an overt history of trauma is unusual it may be that minor trauma is responsible, in view of the negative histological findings.

CLINICAL FEATURES [17, 20 & 24]

The chief complaint is pain, which may be exacerbated by coughing, wheezing or deep breathing. Occasionally there is swelling without pain. On examination a firm, fusiform swelling is found over one or more of the costal cartilages, most often one of the first 4. The swelling is usually tender, though there is no redness or heat. The tenderness usually disappears in 1–10 weeks; pain often lasts longer but gradually subsides. The swelling may decrease over months or may remain permanently; even in those regressing there is usually some residual swelling. There may be later recurrence.

Radiologically, as a rule there is no abnormality.

Diagnosis is not usually difficult. If there is no radiographic abnormality a tumour is unlikely. If there is no fluctuation, heat or redness of skin, and tenderness is not severe, an acute inflammatory lesion is unlikely, though we have once been deceived by the early stages of an unusual cold abscess of the mediastinum presenting anteriorly. A number of rare and exotic inflammatory lesions have been described in the costal cartilages, as already mentioned.

TREATMENT

Usually reassurance and a mild analgesic are all that are required. Salomon [20] obtained rapid improvement by the local injection of 15 mg of hydrocortisone, repeated in a few days. Partial or complete resection, leaving a cuff of perichondrium, has been performed in refractory cases [17] but we have never had to advise this.

VASCULAR DISEASES AFFECTING RIBS

Notching of the inferior rib borders by dilated intercostal arteries may occur in *coarctation of the aorta* but usually not before the age of 12. The 4th to the 8th ribs are most often affected. Notching occasionally occurs in other congenital vascular anomalies [15].

METABOLIC DISEASES AND TOXIC AGENTS AFFECTING THE RIBS

Lead lines, areas of increased bone density at the ends of the ribs, may be seen radiologically in *lead poisoning*; the wrist and knee may be x-rayed for confirmation. *Fluoridosis* may give rise to bony overgrowths at the sites of muscular insertions in the inferior margins of the ribs. There may also be thickening of the cortex. Rib fractures may occur in *osteoporosis* due to many causes, including old age, Cushing's disease and corticosteroid drugs. For a review of other metabolic conditions affecting the ribs see Gayler and Donner [15].

TUMOURS OF THE RIBS AND TUMOUR-LIKE ABNORMALITIES

Metastatic tumours are much more common than primary tumours of rib. Of the simple primary tumours chondroma, osteochondroma and fibrous dysplasia are the least rare; of the malignant primary tumours the commonest are chondrosarcoma, osteochondrosarcoma and myeloma. Pain and swelling are the principal clinical manifestations, the former suggesting malignant change. Cartilaginous tumours are particularly liable to become malignant and in them the presence or absence of malignancy may be difficult to judge histologically. Because of the difficulty in making a diagnosis, and because of the risk of malignancy, primary rib tumours should be removed surgically. More detailed comment follows.

Most types of tumour of bone, primary or metastatic, can affect the ribs. Some 'tumours', which may produce swelling of the ribs, are probably not strictly neoplastic, for instance fibrous dysplasia and eosinophil granuloma. In an analysis of 48 cases of 'tumours' of the ribs Barrett [2] found that 19 were chondromata, of which 8 were malignant; 14 were the solitary type of fibrous dysplasia; 6 were solitary osteochondromata; 4 were cases of rib tumour associated with generalized diaphysial aclasis; 3 were eosinophil granulomata without generalized skeletal involvement; 1 was an osteoclastoma and 1 a solitary myeloma. He also saw a number of sarcomata of the chest wall which might or might not have arisen from ribs.

CHONDROMA

These tumours probably arise from islands of cartilage in the rib substance. Surprisingly, they never arise from the costal cartilages. The island of cartilage expands to replace the normal bone and grows inwards or outwards or both. The tumour feels hard and fixed; it may be bossed and may have an overlying bursa. It occurs in both sexes and at all ages and is sometimes multiple. Radiologically the tumours are often lobulated and relatively opaque, frequently containing areas of calcification but without trabeculation. They may become malignant (*chondrosarcoma*) and a figure of 40% has been quoted. They are then more likely to cause pain. Owing to the risk of malignancy the tumour is best removed. In the late stages this may not be feasible but partial removal may be required to relieve pain.

The ribs may sometimes be involved in various cartilaginous abnormalities. For a review see Gayler and Donner [15].

OSTEOCHONDROMA [2]

This tumour may occur in any position on the rib other than, surprisingly, the costal cartilage. There may be a bursa over the surface of the tumour. There is often a bony base with a thick cartilaginous cap. If the tumour is rubbed it may be painful and there may be inflammation in the bursa. It is thought that these tumours usually stop growing when the growth of the rib ceases. Nevertheless, as it is difficult to be certain of the precise nature of the tumour, and as it will not be possible to exclude malignancy, it is best removed.

OSTEOMA

Osteoma is very rare. It shows radiologically as a fairly well demarcated area of very dense bone [15].

MULTIPLE EXOSTOSES (Diaphysial Aclasis)

Multiple chondromata may occur on the ribs in association with lesions in other bones. The exostoses may protrude into the chest cavity. Occasionally they may occur on the scapular border, when, on the posteroanterior x-ray, they will have to be differentiated from intrapulmonary tumours [2]. They may become malignant.

FIBROUS DYSPLASIA

Generalized fibrous dysplasia (Albright's syndrome) occurs as an obscure general disease of bone, involving endocrine and biochemical abnormalities [9 & 18]. This will not be further discussed here.

Localized (monostotic) fibrous dysplasia may occur in one or several ribs producing a localized mass and sometimes pain. There is no abnormality of blood chemistry and no general symptoms. Pathologically the lesion consists of vascularized fibrous tissue which may contain spicules of bone and cartilage. Radiologically it forms a mass which destroys the architecture of the bone. Between the edge of the bone and the mass is usually a rim of increased density, about 1 mm in width, which thins out over the outer part of the mass. Trabeculae may occur within the mass and there may be cyst formation and calcification, although this is usually not prominent. Because the diagnosis is usually uncertain the 'tumour' is best removed [2].

EOSINOPHIL GRANULOMA

This is a disease of uncertain causation. It is probably not a tumour. It may affect bone and lungs (p. 573) or be confined to either. The ribs are often involved if there are bone lesions. 80% of bone lesions are said to be solitary [15]. There may be no symptoms, or there may be pain and local tenderness. Rib lesions may be single, multiple or loculated and show radiologically as lytic lesions, sometimes with a slight marginal sclerosis, which tend to expand the bone. Pathological fractures may occur.

GAUCHER'S DISEASE

Gaucher's disease may also give rise to lytic areas in the ribs.

GIANT CELL TUMOURS

Giant cell tumours are often painful and produce a palpable mass. Radiologically the rib is expanded and translucent, with thinning of the cortex; trabeculae are usually seen crossing the translucent area [15].

HAEMANGIOMA

Haemangioma may occur, especially in the posterior shaft, and give rise to a similar radiological appearance to giant cell tumour [15].

EWING'S TUMOUR

Ewing's tumour occurs in ribs. About half the patients are under 30 years of age. There is usually local pain and a palpable tumour. Radiologically there may be irregular bone absorption with expansion of the rib and periosteal reaction but sometimes only a widening of the shaft with 'onion peel' periosteal reaction [15].

MULTIPLE MYELOMA

Multiple myeloma may show radiologically as multiple areas of bone destruction, sometimes 'punched out', sometimes ill-defined. Pathological fracture is common and there is sometimes a large soft tissue mass [15].

METASTASES

Metastases are common in the ribs, especially from lung, breast or kidney. There is usually local pain and tenderness, but they are sometimes painless. A lump may be felt. In the early stages there may be no radiological change; later there is rib destruction and pathological fracture may occur.

COLD ABSCESS OF THE CHEST WALL [3]

Cold abscess of the chest wall originates in tuberculosis of the intercostal lymph glands. There are 2 main groups of these, the first at the angle of the ribs from which the pus may track backwards with the posterior primary division of the intercostal nerve presenting near the erector spinae muscles or forwards with the anterior division to present in the lateral chest wall. In our experience the latter is the commoner. The abscess may also arise from lymph nodes in the region of the internal mammary artery and present near the intercostal cartilages. Cold abscess is usually relatively painless and often merely noticed by the patient as a swelling. It is of course fluctuant but may be mistaken for a lipoma. A number of our patients have been explored surgically with the latter in mind and pus, with or without tubercle bacilli, has been found on exploration. After aspiration of the pus these abscesses usually respond very well to chemotherapy.

GUMMA OF THE CHEST WALL [3]

This is now very rare and is described as arising in the anterior mediastinum and giving rise to a hard, fixed lump in the intercostal space which may later soften and form a punched out ulcer. Radiologically the lesion may resemble a tumour of the anterior mediastinum. The true nature may be suspected if a punched out ulcer has developed, or as a result of serology.

OTHER TUMOURS OF THE CHEST WALL

LIPOMA

This may originate in the muscles or the endothoracic fascia and form a swelling on the chest wall and, in the x-ray, a circumscribed peripheral shadow based on the wall. Because of the typical consistency of the lipoma diagnosis may be relatively easy clinically. The tumour is best excised. As already mentioned, it is sometimes confused with a cold abscess.

ANGIOMA

Angioma of the chest wall has been described [3] but is rare.

MYXOMA OF THE CHEST WALL [3]

This is a small, circumscribed tumour arising in the intercostal muscle layer which may be cystic and firm. X-ray may show an opacity based on the chest wall. These tumours are probably benign but may contain areas of degeneration similar to those in a sarcoma. They are best excised.

KYPHOSCOLIOSIS

AETIOLOGY

Kyphoscoliosis, or scoliosis without kyphosis, may be due to:

(1) congenital abnormality, with or without vertebral defects,

(2) vertebral disease, such as tuberculosis, rickets, osteomalacia or trauma,

(3) neuromuscular disease, such as poliomyelitis or Friedreich's ataxia,

(4) thoracic abnormality, such as thoracoplasty or destroyed lung with subsequent fibrosis,

(5) external causes, such as irradiation or 'frame' scoliosis, or

(6) it may be idiopathic, probably the commonest group [5 & 16].

We are here concerned only with the respiratory effects of kyphoscoliosis.

21—R.D.

PATHOLOGY AND FUNCTIONAL ABNORMALITY

Pathological investigation of the lungs indicates that severe kyphoscoliosis results in distortions of the lung outline with local dilatations and compressions of alveoli but no true emphysema unless there is superadded bronchitis. There is often terminal pneumonia or bronchopneumonia. The proximal pulmonary arteries are often dilated, with hypertrophy of the media. This is associated with pulmonary hypertension. There is no evidence of compression of vessels sufficient in itself to cause pulmonary hypertension [4 & 5].

Impairment of respiration, and pulmonary hypertension with eventual *cor pulmonale*, occur mainly in patients with severe scoliosis. Milder degrees may cause no obvious disability. Bergofsky *et al.* [5] found disability mainly in those over the age of 35 and with more than 100° of scoliosis. Brown and his colleagues [7] find that the position of the scoliosis is important; those with high dorsal curves of more than 90° are most likely to develop respiratory failure. It seems that the main factors are the reduction in lung volume, due to compression of the lung by the distorted chest wall, and the rigidity of the chest wall which increases with age. This rigidity results in increase in the work of breathing. The decreased lung volume and the rigid chest wall cause decrease in VC and tidal volume, with rapid shallow breathing and decreased alveolar ventilation, resulting in hypoxaemia and eventually in hypercapnia. There is evidence of $\dot{V}/\dot{Q}$ abnormalities with venous admixture through perfused but underventilated areas [8 & 23]. Pulmonary hypertension and later *cor pulmonale* result from decrease in the pulmonary vascular bed, due initially to lung compression and later to secondary contraction of pulmonary vessels caused by hypoxia and perhaps, during superinfections, by acidosis [25]. There is no evidence of vascular compression and cardiac murmurs are absent unless there is associated cardiac disease [14]. Dollery *et al.* [14] found, by ^{133}Xe studies, that in the upright position perfusion was even throughout the lung, in contrast to the predominantly basal perfusion in normal people. They attributed the even distribution of blood partly to the reduced height of the lungs in kyphoscoliosis, which reduced the hydrostatic pressure difference between apex and base, and partly to increased pulmonary artery pressure, which would facilitate apical perfusion. They point out that this even perfusion reduces the reserve of unperfused apical capillaries, which would normally take up the increased flow on exercise and thus keep down the pulmonary artery pressure. In those with kyphoscoliosis the normal reserve is absent and the increased flow on exercise would be likely to result in increased pulmonary artery pressure.

Decrease of FEV/FVC ratio, indicating airways obstruction, results only from complicating bronchitis which seems, understandably enough, commoner in British than in American series [5, 8, 10, 23 & 25]. There is some suggestion that respiratory disability develops more rapidly in kyphoscoliosis due to poliomyelitis, perhaps because of additional paralysis of muscles of respiration. Zorab [27] states that VC is the most convenient single measurement for following progress. In general he has found that, provided respiratory function tests give results above 50% of the predicted, the patient is well able to tolerate operation or parturition.

CLINICAL FEATURES

The main clinical features, apart from the orthopaedic and aesthetic results of the deformity, are dyspnoea on effort and, later, the symptoms and signs of *cor pulmonale* (p. 317). The latter is often precipitated by a respiratory infection. In Britain at least the condition may be complicated by chronic bronchitis, not necessarily directly related to the deformity but clearly likely to hasten respiratory and cardiac failure. The rate of progression will depend on the degree of deformity, the paralysis of muscles of respiration by poliomyelitis and the extent of complication by chronic bronchitis. It has been stated that the average age of death is 46 and that it is not uncommon for death to occur in the 3rd decade [4].

RADIOLOGY

Radiology will reveal details of the spinal deformity and may help in its elucidation, but it may also be helpful in assessing the respiratory disability. Fluoroscopy may reveal paralysis of the diaphragm in poliomyelitis. Good radiography may also show diminution in the pulmonary vasculature, localized or generalized. This is commoner in those with severe scoliosis, particularly in paralytic cases. It is almost always present in congenital cases, even when the curvature is relatively mild [27].

TREATMENT

In the young, correction of the deformity before the chest wall has become rigid is likely to benefit respiratory function. An increase in vital capacity of 50% within 6 months has been claimed in patients treated in plaster jackets [12]. Operative procedures seem unhelpful and may even worsen respiratory function [4]. The literature on the effect of treatment on respiratory function is somewhat conflicting and there is a need for further systematic and sophisticated study.

Any secondary infection should be vigorously treated and prophylactic measures appropriate to chronic bronchitis should be used if this is present (p. 319). *Cor pulmonale* should be treated by intensive therapy of the precipitating respiratory infection. Early tracheostomy, and intermittent positive pressure respiration, is of value to increase alveolar ventilation and to reduce the work of moving the rigid chest wall [5]. Diuretics and digitalis will also be appropriate. After recovery from the acute episode long term treatment should be similar to that used in chronic bronchitis (p. 320) but unfortunately at this stage the ultimate prognosis is poor.

PECTUS EXCAVATUM
(Pectus Recurvatum, Funnel Chest)

AETIOLOGY AND PATHOLOGY

This condition is probably due to fibrous replacement of the muscle of the anterior diaphragm which is normally attached to the lower part of the anterior chest wall and the xiphisternum. In the normal person the muscle in this region contracts on inspiration and the muscle attachments to the lower chest wall on either side of the xiphisternum and lower sternum prevent these being dragged backwards as the diaphragm descends. When this muscle is lacking the unopposed action of the posterior diaphragmatic muscle displaces the sternum and xiphisternum backwards as the diaphragm descends [11]. This movement occurs in newborn infants and in small children but later the sternum becomes fixed in the retracted position, with accompanying deformity of the costal cartilages. It is said that if the condition is diagnosed in newborn infants tenotomy of the strips of fibrous diaphragmatic tissue attached to the back of the sternum prevents the establishment of the deformity. In the fully developed condition the manubrium of the sternum is normal but the body is angled backwards with maximum recession at the xiphoid, below which the costal margin bends forwards. Sometimes the condition is asymmetrical with the sternum lying deeper on one side than the other.

There is said to be a hereditary tendency but no sex linkage. Pectus excavatum may be associated with kyphoscoliosis or other deformity. The condition was reported in 2·2% of boys and 2·5% of girls in a German series quoted by Reusch [19].

FUNCTIONAL ABNORMALITY

Although respiratory function tests often show only mild decrease in TLC, VC and FEV, in a few the disability may be much greater and *cor pulmonale* has been recorded [4]. Brown and Cook [6] claimed that MBC (and so presumably FEV) was improved by operation in 30% of cases.

CLINICAL FEATURES AND RADIOLOGY

In most cases the main symptom due to the deformity is the embarrassment caused to the patient by the deep vertical furrow in the chest. Chin [11] found some patients with severe symptoms of dyspnoea, praecordial

pain, palpitation, syncope on moderate exertion and repeated lung infections; two patients with severe deformity even had dysphagia. A second group had dyspnoea and recurrent bronchitis. These were usually children in whom the paradoxical movement of the lower sternum preceded fixation in the retracted position; there were often basal crepitations. Chin's cases were, of course, patients referred to a surgeon and therefore probably selected for disability. In the great majority the disability, if any, is only psychological, though this itself is not necessarily negligible.

In the posteroanterior x-ray the heart is often displaced to the left and the anterior ribs may show marked obliquity. The physician can often guess that this condition is present from the posteroanterior chest x-ray but of course it is obvious in the lateral film which shows the depressed sternum. The displacement of the heart often gives rise to systolic murmurs and sometimes thrills, with splitting of the heart sounds and the presence of a third heart sound. The electrocardiogram may show persistence of the juvenile pattern with T inversion in the right praecordial leads, incomplete right bundle branch block and right axis deviation. Because of cardiac rotation there may be inversion of P in V_1 and a QR pattern, reflecting the cavity potentials of the right atrium which has been rotated forwards against the chest wall [13]. All the electrical changes are probably due only to rotation and displacement of the heart. There are probably no haemodynamic abnormalities and the electrocardiographic abnormalities tend to reverse after surgery [19].

TREATMENT

In some cases surgical treatment may be desirable for aesthetic reasons but sometimes recurrent respiratory infections in childhood may suggest operation. It is usual to carry out wedge chondrotomies on the angulated costal cartilages, and an osteotomy between the manubrium and the sternum, the lower sternum being held forwards by a strut from rib front to rib front behind the sternum [3].

PIGEON CHEST
(Pectus Carinatum)

In this condition the sternum is prominent, forming an anterior ridge with the ribs falling steeply away on either side, sometimes actually with a vertical groove on each side of the sternum. In most cases it is probably secondary to childhood rickets and one has the impression that such patients have more frequent respiratory infections than others. This is probably merely a reflection of the fact that pigeon chest is more likely to occur in poorly nourished individuals who have had frequent childhood respiratory infections and poor general resistance. No treatment is necessary for the deformity as such.

HARRISON'S SULCUS

This mild deformity consists of a horizontal groove on each side of the chest, 2 or 3 rib spaces wide and lying a little above the costal margin. It probably is also due to respiratory infections in childhood, sometimes complicating rickets. No treatment is necessary.

ANKYLOSING SPONDYLITIS

FUNCTIONAL ABNORMALITY

Ankylosing spondylitis results in increasing fixation of the thoracic cage. The degree of fixation can be well estimated by merely measuring the chest expansion [26]. Zorab [26] found, in an investigation of 35 patients, that the limitation of chest wall expansion was usually well compensated by diaphragmatic movement. The thorax tended to be held at rest at a rather greater degree of inspiration than normal, perhaps in an unconscious attempt to obtain a relaxation of painful ligaments. As might be expected, RV and FRC were increased, though there was little decrease in VC until the thorax was severely affected. The FEV/FVC ratio remained normal, indicating an absence of airways obstruction. Diffusing capacity was normal but lung compliance variable. Others have found a decrease in chest wall compliance [22]. It seems that functional respiratory disability is

not an important complication of ankylosing spondylitis.

PREDISPOSITION TO RESPIRATORY DISEASES

Patients with ankylosing spondylitis do appear more liable to pulmonary tuberculosis. This accounted for more than 25% of 82 deaths among 2026 cases in the records of the British Ministry of Pensions and National Insurance [1]. Apart from the well known excess of leukaemic deaths in irradiated patients there was no obvious association with any other respiratory cause of death, though there were 5 deaths from pneumonia. In contrast, therefore, to severe kyphoscoliosis, patients with ankylosing spondylitis do *not* appear to be susceptible to *cor pulmonale*, probably because there is less interference with ventilation and pulmonary blood flow. Upper abdominal operations may be hazardous, as they interfere with the function of the diaphragm.

REFERENCES

[1] ABBATT J.D. & LEA A.J. (1956) The incidence of leukaemia in ankylosing spondylitis treated with x-rays. *Lancet* ii, 1317.

[2] BARRETT N.R. (1955) Primary tumours of rib. *Br. J. Surg.* 43, 113.

[3] BARRETT N.R. (1963) The chest wall. In *Chest Diseases*, ed. Perry K.M.A. and Sellors T.H. London, Butterworths.

[4] BATES D.V. & CHRISTIE R.V. (1964) *Respiratory Function in Disease*. Philadelphia, Saunders.

[5] BERGOFSKY E.H., TURINO G.M. & FISHMAN A.P. (1959) Cardiorespiratory failure in kyphoscoliosis. *Medicine* 38, 263.

[6] BROWN A.L. & COOK O. (1951) Cardiorespiratory studies in pre- and postoperative funnel chest (pectus excavatum). *Dis. Chest.* 20, 378.

[7] BROWN I.K. & OGILVIE C.M. (1968) Personal communication.

[8] BRUDERMAN I. & STEIN M. (1961) Physiologic evaluation and treatment of kyphoscoliotic patients. *Ann. intern. Med.* 55, 94.

[9] BUKER R.H. & MASHBURN J.D. (1965) Polyostotic fibrous dysplasia (Albright's Syndrome). A case report. *J. thorac. cardiovasc. Surg.* 49, 241.

[10] CARO C.G. & DUBOIS A.B. (1961) Pulmonary function in kyphoscoliosis. *Thorax* 16, 282.

[11] CHIN E.F. (1957) Surgery of funnel chest and congenital sternal prominence. *Br. J. Surg.* 44, 360.

[12] COTREL Y. Personal communication, quoted Editorial (1963) The lungs in kyphoscoliosis. *Lancet* **i**, 205.

[13] DE OLIVEIRA J.M., SAMBHI M.P. & ZIMMERMAN H.A. (1958) The electrocardiogram in pectus excavatum. *Br. Heart J.* **20**, 495.

[14] DOLLERY C.T., GILLAM P.M.S., HUGH-JONES P. & ZORAB P.A. (1965) Regional lung function in kyphoscoliosis. *Thorax* **20**, 175.

[15] GAYLER B.W. & DONNER M.W. (1967) Radiographic changes of the ribs. *Am. J. med. Sci* **253**, 586.

[16] JAMES J.I.P. (1967) *Scoliosis*. Edinburgh, Livingstone.

[17] KAYSER H.L. (1956) Tietze's Syndrome. A review of the literature. *Am. J. Med.* **21**, 982.

[18] PRITCHARD J.E. (1951) Fibrous dysplasia of the bones. *Am. J. med. Sci.* **222**, 313.

[19] REUSCH C.S. (1961) Hemodynamic studies in pectus excavatum. *Circulation* **24**, 1143.

[20] SALOMON M.I. (1958) Thoracochondralgia (Tietze's Syndrome). Report of 3 cases. *N.Y. St. J. Med.* **58**, 530.

[21] SHANKS S.C. & KERLEY P. (1962) *A Text-book of X-ray Diagnosis* by British Authors, 3rd Edition. London, Lewis.

[22] SHARP J.T., SWEANY S.K., HENRY J.P., PIETRAS R.J., MEADOWS W.R., AMARAL E. & RUBINSTEIN H.M. (1964) Lung and thoracic compliances in ankylosing spondylitis. *J. lab. clin. Med.* **63**, 254.

[23] SHAW D.B. & READ J. (1960) Hypoxia and thoracic scoliosis. *Br. med. J.* **ii**, 1486.

[24] TIETZE A. (1921) Ueber eine eigenartige Häufung von Fällen mit Dystrophie der Rippenknorpel. *Berl. klin. Wschr.* **58**, 829.

[25] TURINO G.M., GOLDRING ROBERTA M. & FISHMAN A.P. (1965) Cor pulmonale in musculoskeletal abnormalities of the thorax. *Bull. N.Y. Acad. Med.* **41**, 959.

[26] ZORAB P.A. (1962) The lungs in ankylosing spondylitis. *Quart. J. Med. (N.S.)* **31**, 267.

[27] ZORAB P.A. (1967) The medical aspects of scoliosis. In *Scoliosis* by James J.I.P. Edinburgh, Livingstone.

CHAPTER 36

Abnormalities and Diseases of the Diaphragm

The diaphragm is the most important muscle of respiration. It is rarely affected by intrinsic disease but, because of its complex embryological development, it is subject to a number of congenital abnormalities. Primary disorders of the diaphragm such as diaphragmatic hernia may present with symptoms suggestive of intrathoracic disease. Conversely x-ray abnormalities of the diaphragm may indicate disease in the chest or the abdomen.

ANATOMY AND DEVELOPMENT [15]

The arched musculotendinous division between the thorax and the abdomen has its origin in vertebral, costal and sternal attachments from which muscular fibres curve upwards and inwards from the periphery to be inserted into the fibrous sheet called the central tendon. The diaphragm is formed from the union of 4 main parts, ventral, dorsal, right and left lateral. At about the end of the 2nd month of foetal life they unite to form a fibrous sheet which is later largely converted to muscle. The largest contribution is the ventral part which is derived from the septum transversum, a large block of mesoderm lying immediately caudal to the pericardial cavity and chiefly derived from the 4th mesodermal somite. The dorsal part develops from the dorsal mesentery of the foregut. Folds of mesoderm from the lateral body walls (pleuroperitoneal folds) become the lateral segments which grow toward the mid line and unite with each other and with the dorsal component. The process of fusion is a complex affair and defects and areas of weakness may occur through which some of the abdominal contents may enter the thorax (fig. 36.1). Failure of the lateral folds to fuse with the dorsal segment, particularly on the left side, leaves the pleuroperitoneal opening unclosed (foramen of Bochdalek). The foramen of Morgagni lies between the muscle fibres which are inserted into the xiphoid process and the 7th costal cartilage. Fat or other abdominal contents may protrude through these foramina and appear in chest films as intrathoracic masses. Herniation occurs most commonly at the oesophageal hiatus (p. 636). The other normal openings in the diaphragm are for the passage of the inferior vena cava and the aorta. Herniation through either of these is rare.

Since the septum transversum is first found cephalic to the heart in the cervical region of the embryo it obtains its phrenic nerve supply locally and takes this with it as it migrates caudally. In man the phrenic nerve is usually stated as comprising components from C3 to C5 (principally C4, although there is some evidence that C6 may make a small contribution) [13]. The innervation of the diaphragm has been studied intensively [2, 6 & 24]. Scott [27] confirmed the presence of neural arcades noted by earlier workers and underlined the importance of the distribution of the phrenic nerves so that incisions in the diaphragm may be made in such a way as to cause the least damage to phrenic branches. He suggests that this might avoid much postoperative morbidity and even mortality, particularly in the aged, the debilitated or the acutely ill patient

NORMAL POSITION OF THE DIAPHRAGM

The right hemidiaphragm is normally higher than the left and the common explanation given for this is the underlying liver. However, studies of situs inversus have suggested that the position of the heart determines which is the lower of the two hemidiaphragms. X-ray studies of isolated dextrocardia and laevocardia by Carlson et al. [3] showed that the relative position of the hemidiaphragms

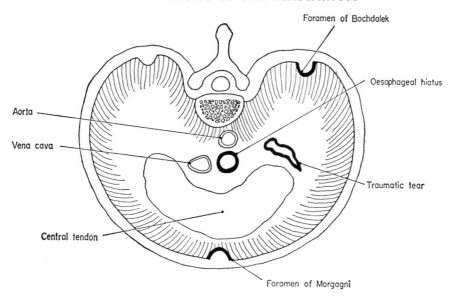

Foramen of Bochdalek

Oesophageal hiatus

Aorta

Vena cava

Traumatic tear

Central tendon

Foramen of Morgagni

FIG. 36.1. Diaphragm viewed from above, showing sites of possible herniation. Thick lines show commonest sites.

depends predominantly on depression of one side by the mass of the overlying heart rather than on elevation by the underlying liver. The relative position is, therefore, an unreliable guide to abdominal situs inversus. Of 17 patients with both heart and liver on the right side the right hemidiaphragm was lower than the left in 12, slightly higher than the left in 1 and the same height as the left in 4, 3 of whom had hearts near the midline. In each of 4 patients with both heart and liver on the left side the left hemidiaphragm was lower than the right.

Diaphragmatic movement may be assessed roughly by tidal percussion which has shown that tidal excursion can vary from 1·5 cm during quiet breathing to as much as 10 cm during deep breathing. In extreme expiration the level of the diaphragm may be as high as the 4th intercostal space anteriorly. The body position alters the level of the diaphragm (p. 634) and most workers believe that the reduction in total lung capacity when a normal subject lies supine, and which amounts to about 300 ml, is due to the upward displacement of the diaphragm by the abdominal viscera [17, 21 & 32].

DISPLACEMENTS OF THE DIAPHRAGM

Pathological displacement of the diaphragm can occur from a variety of conditions arising in the thorax or the abdomen. *Elevation* results from therapeutic or diagnostic pneumoperitoneum (affecting both hemidiaphragms); loss of lung volume (usually unilateral) after pulmonary resection, atelectasis, fibrosis of the lung or pleura; as a consequence of pulmonary infarction (which may be bilateral); or paralysis of the phrenic nerve, or eventration. Amoebic liver abscess is classically associated with a raised right hemidiaphragm. Subphrenic abscess may result in elevation of the diaphragm, usually on the right side. Increase in intra-abdominal pressure from obesity, pregnancy, large abdominal tumours or ascites will elevate the diaphragm bilaterally.

Dry pleurisy of any kind may result in elevation of a hemidiaphragm. Presumably in these cases the terminal filaments of the phrenic nerve are involved, or the nerve itself in its course over the pericardium.

Depression of the diaphragm occurs with large intrathoracic tumours, tension pneumothorax or massive pleural effusion. In each case only one side is usually involved. Hyper-inflation of the lungs such as occurs in severe bronchial asthma or diffuse pulmonary emphysema will result in bilateral depression and flattening.

FUNCTION AND FUNCTIONAL ABNORMALITY

In normal quiet breathing the diaphragm is responsible for 75% of the air inhaled and the intercostal muscles for 25%. Nevertheless total bilateral diaphragmatic paralysis is compatible with life because of partial compensation by the other muscles of respiration.

Contraction of the diaphragm pulls the central tendon downwards, increasing the length of the thoracic cavity and raising the abdominal pressure. In the normal subject contraction of the intercostal muscles results in upward and outward movement of the lower ribs. During descent of the diaphragm the peripheral attachments may be regarded mainly as fixed points which allow the muscle to carry out its function of ventilating the lungs. If, however, voluminous lungs due to emphysema result in the diaphragm being depressed and flattened there may be no 'slack' to be taken up. Contraction of the diaphragm on inspiration may then result in indrawing of the lower ribs, reducing the transverse and posteroanterior diameters of the lower thorax. This is particularly in evidence when bronchial infection increases airways resistance and the work of breathing, e.g. in croup (p. 95), or in an exacerbation of chronic bronchitis (p. 312).

When a patient is lying on his side the diaphragm is more elevated on the side of the dependent lung than on the upper side, presumably due to the effect of the abdominal contents. Pulmonary function studies have shown that the FRC is decreased, the fraction of the tidal volume increased, the deadspace reduced and the alveolar ventilation relatively increased in the dependent lung which also shows a much more rapid clearance of nitrogen than the upper lung [19, 20 & 30]. The proportional oxygen uptake of the dependent lung is also much greater [1]. Bates and Christie [1] stressed the practical importance

of these findings since patients are frequently nursed with the injured lung dependent. They make the point that since the dependent lung is responsible for a higher proportion of ventilation and oxygen uptake it is theoretically more sensible to nurse the patient with the more normal lung in the dependent position unless there are reasons which prevent this.

Thoracic movement becomes progressively restricted in ankylosing spondylitis (p. 630) and respiratory efficiency becomes more dependent on diaphragmatic movement which, fortunately, is usually very good. Any impairment of diaphragmatic movement will have serious consequences. Upper abdominal surgery is hazardous in these patients and can precipitate respiratory failure.

DIAPHRAGMATIC PARALYSIS

Once a common cause of this was therapeutic phrenic nerve crush or avulsion in the treatment of pulmonary tuberculosis. This is never practised nowadays. The most common cause of diaphragmatic paralysis is bronchogenic carcinoma. Involvement of the nerve by tumour above the level of the hilum excludes all possibility of surgical treatment. Sometimes when the lesion is demonstrated to be wholly below the level of the hilum, surgical treatment has been attempted with resection of the tumour, nerve and pericardium (p. 539).

Diaphragmatic paralysis may occur from involvement of the phrenic nerve at any point from its central connections to the periphery. A large number of causes have been described. These include poliomyelitis, herpes zoster, motor neurone disease, Huntington's chorea, haemorrhage into or tumours of the spinal cord, transverse myelitis, injuries or disease of the cervical vertebrae, diphtheria, lead poisoning, tetanus antitoxin [28], measles, typhoid or rheumatic fever, pulmonary infarction, mediastinitis [14] and pericarditis. It has also been recorded in association with pneumonia [8 & 12]. Pressure on the phrenic nerve from mediastinal masses or, rarely, from a large aortic aneurysm [26], has been described. When primary tuberculosis was more common in Britain, enlargement of the mediastinal and paratracheal lymph nodes sometimes involved a phrenic nerve. Trauma from neck wounds, birth injuries (stretching or tearing of a phrenic nerve from hyperextension of or pulling on the neck at delivery) and the radical removal of malignant tumours are other causes. Sometimes phrenic paralysis exists without satisfactory explanation [10].

Phrenic crush to elevate the diaphragm and reduce temporarily the size of the hemithorax was a routine procedure in most centres when lobectomy was performed for pulmonary tuberculosis. It is doubtful how useful this was and phrenic crush is no longer used as an adjunct to pulmonary resection for whatever cause.

FUNCTIONAL ABNORMALITY

In a subject otherwise normal, unilateral paralysis of the diaphragm reduces the ventilatory capacity by about 20% [29]. Svanberg showed that ventilation on the affected side was reduced to one quarter to one half the normal value and the oxygen uptake to one half to three quarters of normal [29]. Comroe *et al.* [7] commented on the orthopnoea in patients with bilateral diaphragmatic paralysis due to motor neuritis following tetanus antitoxin. McCredie and his colleagues later studied 3 patients with bilateral diaphragmatic paralysis [22]. In all cases the vital capacity was much reduced, particularly when the patient was supine, and the respiratory flow rates were also reduced. Airways resistance and diffusing capacity were normal in 2 out of 3 and in 2 there was arterial oxygen unsaturation when laid flat.

PATHOLOGY

Crushing of the phrenic nerve results in diaphragmatic paralysis which may last up to 6 months or be permanent. Trophic changes occur early and may be evident even after 3 days. Within a month a paralysed diaphragm shows reduction in thickness, deposition of fat and variable fibrosis. Presumably most or all of these are recoverable when the effects of crush diminish and normal diaphragmatic movement is re-established. In the nonrecoverable forms of diaphragmatic paralysis the changes are permanent.

CLINICAL AND RADIOGRAPHIC FEATURES

The features of the causative disease may be present. Otherwise unilateral paralysis rarely gives rise to symptoms (usually only transient gastric flatulence when the left side is involved) although bilateral paralysis may cause dyspnoea and, if complete, may sometimes require assisted respiration.

Apart from elevation, the plain film may show displacement of the heart to the opposite side. The diaphragm shows paradoxical movement on respiration. This is confirmed by fluoroscopy. When the patient is asked to sniff in, the paralysed diaphragm rises, reflecting the change in intra-abdominal pressure, whereas the intact diaphragm moves normally downwards.

MANAGEMENT

Further investigation and management will depend on the likely diagnosis. For example the presence of a pulmonary lesion near the hilum will indicate bronchoscopy and the other investigations for carcinoma. Differentiation from eventration may be difficult.

EVENTRATION OF THE DIAPHRAGM

Elevation and paradoxical movement may result from a condition, usually congenital but in some cases possibly a consequence of some unrecognized process involving the phrenic nerve, in which the hemidiaphragm is largely composed of fibrous tissue with only a few interspersed muscle fibres [18 & 23]. Males are rather more frequently affected than females and it is almost invariably left-sided. Usually there are no symptoms but sometimes the patient may complain of undue gastric flatulence. Eventration may be localized and when this is the case the right hemidiaphragm is more commonly affected, with the defect mainly in the anteromedial quadrant into which the liver bulges [31]. Localized eventration may closely resemble diaphragmatic herniation or pleuropericardial cyst in the plain x-ray.

Distinction from acquired phrenic paralysis depends on the absence of evidence of a cause for paralysis. An x-ray taken some time previously and showing similar appearances is of great importance in differentiating from the commonest cause of diaphragmatic paralysis, namely bronchial carcinoma.

Physical examination shows poor movement of the left hemithorax and tidal percussion shows a virtually immobile left hemidiaphragm. Fluoroscopy confirms the paradoxical movement. A barium meal will exclude the possibility of hiatus hernia.

Most cases do not require any treatment. Rarely plication or partial excision of the hemidiaphragm, sometimes with the insertion of tantalum mesh or a plastic prosthesis, has been undertaken because of the severity of associated dyspeptic symptoms [4]. When operation has been performed the phrenic nerve has usually been found to be normal in all respects.

DIAPHRAGMATIC HERNIA

The consideration of diaphragmatic hernia does not fall within the scope of this book. Herniation through the oesophageal hiatus is the commonest type but herniation may also occur through the foramen of Morgagni (between the costal and sternal slips of origin of the diaphragm), the foramen of Bochdalek (the pleuroperitoneal hiatus), through defects in the dome of the diaphragm or through a diaphragmatic rupture, the result of trauma.

Respiratory embarrassment may occur if the hernia is very large and is most commonly seen in the neonate with a Bochdalek hernia or in the patient with a ruptured diaphragm. Urgent surgical treatment is necessary in these patients.

The only other relevance of diaphragmatic hernia to the present discussion is that a hernia may present radiological features simulating pleuropulmonary disease. Thus a hiatus hernia may present in the chest film as a retrocardiac opacity containing a fluid

level and sometimes resembling a pulmonary or mediastinal cyst. The large hernia following diaphragmatic rupture may give a radiological picture that can be confused with a pneumothorax. Herniation through the foramen of Morgagni may be confused radiologically with a pleuropericardial cyst.

DUPLICATION OF THE DIAPHRAGM

An accessory diaphragm is a rare abnormality most commonly found above the right lower lobe [16]. Other intrathoracic anomalies may coexist, e.g. lobar hypoplasia, anomalous venous drainage. When associated with multiple abnormalities the child may not survive. The condition is usually discovered in the neonatal period when it may give rise to recurrent respiratory infection.

HICCUP, DIAPHRAGMATIC TONIC SPASM, TIC AND FLUTTER [11]

Sudden inspiratory spasm of the diaphragm with associated closure of the glottis (*hiccup*) is a familiar and harmless occasional symptom in the normal subject. It is usually precipitated by irritation of the diaphragm by gastric distension or inflammation due to rapid or excessive eating or drinking, and commonly it occurs repetitively for a short time. Long continued hiccup can, however, be a serious symptom and a manifestation of important disease.

Apart from the gastric and less common intestinal causes of hiccup, mediated through the phrenic nerve, peripheral causes of hiccup include pericarditis and mediastinitis. Hiccup of central neurological origin occurs most commonly in uraemia and epidemic encephalitis. Sometimes no satisfactory cause can be found for persisting hiccup and in a proportion of these cases it is difficult to avoid the conclusion that the symptom is psychological in origin.

Treatment depends on the cause and the severity. Everyone is aware of the homely remedies recommended for transient hiccup.

Perhaps many of these receive undeserved credit for stopping an attack.

Prolonged and distressing hiccup may compel the use of tranquillizing drugs (e.g. chlorpromazine) or, when these fail, the ultimate measure of phrenic paralysis by phrenic crush.

Tonic spasm may complicate rabies, tetanus and strychnine poisoning, and less commonly toxaemia of pregnancy, encephalitis and epilepsy. Acute dyspnoea is the dominant symptom, occurring in addition to the features of the primary illness. The patient is usually also aware of upper abdominal pain. Management may demand tracheostomy and assisted respiration.

The rapid contraction of the diaphragm (up to 100/min or more) known as *diaphragmatic tic* may be a feature of encephalitis but more commonly is a hysterical phenomenon. The increased frequency of respiratory movement may result in chest or abdominal pain resembling coronary occlusion and the increased excretion of CO_2 may result in tetany. When the rate is faster the term *diaphragmatic flutter* is used. Sometimes the condition affects only one hemidiaphragm. Phrenic paralysis by crush or injection of local anaesthetic is indicated when the condition persists.

SUBPHRENIC ABSCESS

This will not be dealt with here. Reference is made to the effects on the diaphragm and pleural space in the section on pleural effusion (p. 273). Very rarely the diaphragm may be weakened by infection, leading to diaphragmatic herniation.

TRICHINIASIS OF THE DIAPHRAGM

One of the few primary diseases of the diaphragm is trichiniasis. The larvae of the nematode *Trichinella spiralis* when ingested in undercooked pork, or much less commonly in bear meat, may be freed in the intestines where mating of male and female produce new larvae which can penetrate the intestinal wall and enter the blood stream. Their subsequent fate is variable. Some settle in organs where they die out, others in the diaphragm where they may remain alive for years, subsequently becoming encysted.

The phases of intestinal invasion and encystment are usually symptomless. Symptoms usually occur 1–2 weeks after ingestion. These include fever, oedema which may affect the face only or be more widespread, muscle aches, skin rashes, chest pain (usually attributed to involvement of the intercostal muscles and diaphragm), hiccup, cough and haemoptysis (due probably to parasites in the lung).

Eosinophilia is a fairly constant and early feature and the parasite may be recovered from the blood in the early stages. Other diagnostic procedures in a suspected case are muscle biopsy (after the 3rd week) and skin and precipitin tests with trichinella antigen.

The condition is usually self-limiting and no treatment is required or, indeed, is available. Prevention is the most important aspect of management of trichiniasis and the disease can be eradicated by making it widely known that the longer pork is cooked the safer it is.

CYSTS AND TUMOURS OF THE DIAPHRAGM

These are rare but are important since something like half of the reported diaphragmatic cysts and tumours are malignant [5].

Congenital cysts of mesothelial origin are related embryologically to pleuropericardial cysts and may develop within the substance of the diaphragm. These have a fibrous wall lined by a single layer of flattened epithelium [9 & 25].

Although the diaphragm is commonly involved by intrathoracic or intra-abdominal tumour, usually carcinoma, the commonest primary tumour is the sarcoma of which many varieties have been described. Next most frequent is the lipoma, but mesothelioma, fibroma, neurofibroma, chondroma, angiofibroma, haemangio-endothelioma and even endometrioma have all been described. The lesion may be discovered at routine radiography or on account of the development of pain of pleuritic type in the lower chest. Diagnostic pneumothorax or pneumoperitoneum may be necessary to define its relation to the diaphragm but most commonly the diagnosis is made at exploratory thoracotomy. When possible the tumour is excised with a wide area of surrounding diaphragm and subsequent closure of the diaphragm requires the use of other tissue such as fascia lata or some prosthetic material.

REFERENCES

[1] BATES D.V. & CHRISTIE R.V. (1964) *Respiratory Function in Disease*, pp. 100–102. Philadelphia, Saunders.

[2] BOTHA G.S.M. (1957) The anatomy of phrenic nerve termination and the motor innervation of the diaphragm. *Thorax* **12**, 50.

[3] CARLSON H.C., KINCAID O.W. & ONGLEY P.A. (1962) Position of the diaphragm. *Proc. Mayo Clin.* **37**, 25.

[4] CHRISTENSEN P. (1959) Eventration of the diaphragm. *Thorax* **14**, 311.

[5] CLAGETT O.T. & JOHNSON M.A. (1949) Tumours of the diaphragm. *Am. J. Surg.* **78**, 526.

[6] COLLIS J.L., STACHWELL L.M. & ABRAMS L.D. (1954) Nerve supply to the crura of the diaphragm. *Thorax* **9**, 22.

[7] COMROE J.H.Jr., WOOD F.C., KAY C.F. & SPOONT E.M. (1951) Motor neuritis after tetanus antitoxin with involvement of the muscles of respiration. *Am. J. Med.* **10**, 786.

[8] COUGH A.H.C. (1953) Paralysis of the diaphragm after pneumonia and of undetermined cause. *Thorax* **8**, 326.

[9] CRUICKSHANK G. & CRUICKSHANK D.B. (1951) Intradiaphragmatic mesothelial cysts. *Thorax* **6**, 145.

[10] DOUGLAS B.E. & CLAGETT O.T. (1960) The prognosis in idiopathic diaphragmatic paralysis. *Dis. Chest* **37**, 294.

[11] DRESSLER W. & KLEINFELD M. (1954) Tic of the respiratory muscles. Report of 3 cases and review of literature. *Am. J. Med.* **16**, 61.

[12] FREEDMAN B. (1950) Unilateral paralysis of diaphragm and larynx associated with inflammatory lung disease. *Thorax* **5**, 169.

[13] GOETZ O. (1925) Die effecktive Blockade des Nervus Phrenicus (Radikale Phrenicotomi). *Arch. Clin. Chir.* **135**, 595.

[14] GUPTA S.K. (1960) Spontaneous paralysis of the phrenic nerve with special reference to chronic pulmonary tuberculosis. *Br. J. Dis. Chest* **54**, 283.

[15] HAMILTON W.J., BOYD J.D. & MOSSMAN H.W. (1962) *Human Embryology*. Cambridge, Heffer.

[16] HASHIDA Y. & SHERMAN F.E. (1961) Accessory diaphragm associated with neonatal respiratory disease. *J. Pediat.* **59**, 529.

[17] LAGNEAU D., NAMUR M. & PETIT J.M. (1960) Influence de la position corporelle sur les values pulmonaires de l'homme normal. *Arch. Int. Physiol.* **68**, 596.

[18] LAXDALE O.E., MCDOUGALL H. & MELLIN G.W. (1954) Congenital eventration of the diaphragm. *New Engl. J. Med.* **250**, 401.

[19] LILLINGTON G.A., FOWLER W.S., MILLER R.D. & HELMHOLZ H.F.Jr. (1959) Nitrogen clearance rates of right and left lungs in different positions. *J. Clin. Invest.* **38**, 2026.

[20] MILLER R.D., FOWLER W.S. & HELMHOLZ H.F.Jr. (1956) Relative volume and ventilation of the two lungs with change to the lateral decubitus position. *J. lab. clin. Med.* **47**, 297.

[21] MILLS J.N. (1949) The influence upon the vital capacity of procedures calculated to alter the volume of blood in the lungs. *J. Physiol. (London)* **110**, 207.

[22] MCCREDIE M., LOVEJOY F.W.Jr. & KALTREIDER N.L. (1962) Pulmonary function in diaphragmatic paralysis. *Thorax* **17**, 213.

[23] NEUMAN H.W., ELLIS F.H.Jr. & ANDERSEN H.A. (1955) Eventration of the diaphragm. *Proc. Mayo Clin.* **30**, 310.

[24] PERERA H. & EDWARDS F.R. (1957) Intra-diaphragmatic course of the left phrenic nerve in relation to diaphragmatic incisions. *Lancet* **ii**, 75.

[25] ROBSON K. & COLLIS J.L. (1944) Tumours of the diaphragm with report of a diaphragmatic cyst. *Br. J. Tuberc.* **38**, 3.

[26] SANGUINETTI A.A. & GALZERANO D.A. (1943) Sindrome diafragmático por aneurisma de la aorta toráma. *Rev. Asoc. méd. argent.* **57**, 413.

[27] SCOTT R. (1965) Innervation of the diaphragm and its practical aspects in surgery. *Thorax* **20**, 357.

[28] SMITH H.P. & SMITH H.P.Jr. (1955) Phrenic paralysis due to serum neuritis. *Am. J. Med.* **19**, 808.

[29] SVANBERG L. (1956) Clinical value of analysis of lung function in some intrathoracic diseases. A spirometric, bronchospirometric and angio-pneumonographic investigation. *Acta chir. scand.* **111**, 169.

[30] SVANBERG L. (1957) Influence of posture on the lung volumes, ventilation and circulation in normals. A spirometric-bronchospirometric investigation. *Scand. J. clin. lab. Invest.* **9**, Suppl. 25.

[31] VOGEL A. & SMALL A. (1955) Partial eventration of the right diaphragm (congenital diaphragmatic herniation of the liver). *Ann. intern. Med.* **43**, 61.

[32] WADE O.L. & GILSON J.C. (1951) The effect of posture on diaphragmatic movement and vital capacity in normal subjects, with a note on spirometry as an aid in determining radiological chest volumes. *Thorax* **6**, 103.

CHAPTER 37

Some Rarer Pulmonary Diseases

BRONCHIOLITIS FIBROSA OBLITERANS, PULMONARY ALVEOLAR
PROTEINOSIS, PULMONARY ALVEOLAR MICROLITHIASIS,
AMYLOIDOSIS OF THE RESPIRATORY TRACT, TRACHEOBRONCHOMEGALY,
TRACHEO- AND BRONCHOPATHIA OSTEOPLASTICA, TRANSPLANT LUNG

BRONCHIOLITIS FIBROSA OBLITERANS [3]

This is primarily a pathological diagnosis characterized by a widespread obliterative process of the bronchioles. There is extensive damage to the bronchial walls and the lumina are partially or totally occluded by organizing bronchial exudate. It may be regarded as merely an extreme form of chronic severe bronchiolitis. It is very rare and most cases have been due to the inhalation of poison gases, either war gases or industrial gases such as oxides of nitrogen or chlorine. A few have been associated with severe infection, for instance following whooping cough or foreign body inhalation. In certain others the cause has been obscure.

The symptoms of cough, chest pain, dys-pnoea and haemoptysis are similar to those following poison gas inhalation (p. 489) or severe infective bronchiolitis and are very variable. As the diagnosis is a histological one most recorded cases have been fatal. The chest x-ray may show changes similar to those of miliary tuberculosis. In the idiopathic type x-ray changes have been recorded at a stage when the patient had no obvious respiratory symptoms.

Cases following poison gas or infection should be treated along the appropriate lines. If an idiopathic case were diagnosed by lung biopsy, trial of a combination of cortico-steroid drugs and antibiotics would be justi-fiable.

PULMONARY ALVEOLAR PROTEINOSIS [9 & 26]

DEFINITION

Pulmonary alveolar proteinosis is a rare disease of unknown origin usually character-ized by an initial febrile incident, followed after an interval by progressive dyspnoea associated with productive cough, low fever, chest pain and loss of weight. The radiological appear-ances are similar to those of pulmonary oedema. Histologically the alveoli contain a granular eosinophil material which is strongly positive to periodic acid/Schiff (PAS) stain.

AETIOLOGY

The disease is 3 times as common in men as in women. It usually occurs in young adults, though it has been described in 2 children aged $2\frac{1}{2}$ and 15 and in a man of 72. It has been reported from many parts of the world. The aetiology is unknown. A few cases have been exposed to various dusts but this seems likely to be coincidental. Two cases have been associated with *Cryptococcus neoformans* which produces somewhat similar changes in mice [6]. Nocardiosis has also been described in 7 cases [2 & 10] but these and other organ-isms which have been described from time to time are probably secondary invaders.

PATHOLOGY

Macroscopically the lungs contain firm, grey-white, nodular or diffuse masses, which micro-scopically consist of alveoli, bronchioles and bronchi stuffed with eosinophilic granular material staining with PAS. This material contains very large amounts of lipoid [26] but has also been said to contain large amounts of nucleic acids and amino acids without true protein [23]. The alveoli are often lined by epithelial cells and occasional foamy mono-nuclear cells containing lipoid. In frozen sections long, thin, birefringent crystals may be present which sometimes occur in the sputum and are said to be of diagnostic value [33]. Laminated calcified bodies may also occur. A few cases may have some interstitial fibrosis.

FUNCTIONAL ABNORMALITY
[5, 17 & 26]

The extent of the abnormality will depend on the amount of lung involved. The effect is similar to that of pneumonia and without airways obstruction. Decrease in VC and FRC, a low diffusing capacity, decreased Pa,O_2, especially on exercise, with normal Pa,CO_2, at least in the earlier stages, and normal MVV and FEV/VC ratios, have all been recorded and are what would be expected from the pathology.

CLINICAL FEATURES

There is often initial fever and sometimes later bouts. These are followed by progressive dyspnoea, usually with cough and white or yellow sputum. Chest pain and loss of weight are common. The initial illness is usually regarded as a pneumonia and it is only the later course which suggests the presence of some other condition. The physical signs are less than might be expected from the x-ray. There may be scattered fine crepitations. Cyanosis and clubbing may be present in the later stages.

RADIOLOGY

The x-ray shows diffuse perihilar shadows resembling pulmonary oedema. Changes in the radiological appearances are not always related to changes in the patient's symptoms. In fact, sometimes these are paradoxical, clinical improvement coinciding with radiological deterioration and vice versa [18].

INVESTIGATIONS

The sputum may contain PAS staining material and birefringent crystals. There may be leucocytosis and polycythaemia may occur in the later stages. However, various blood dyscrasias such as leucopenia, anaemia, an excess of platelets, eosinophilia and basophilia [15, 20 & 22] may occur. A raised serum lactic acid dehydrogenase occurs at least in some cases [24 & 25].

DIAGNOSIS

The radiological appearances are similar to those of pulmonary oedema which may be differentiated by the absence of a precipitating cardiac cause and failure to clear with diuretics. The fever will suggest pneumonia. It is only the persistent and recurrent symptoms, with the characteristic x-ray appearances resembling pulmonary oedema, which should suggest the possibility of the diagnosis. PAS staining material and birefringent crystals may be found in the sputum or may be obtained by bronchial washings [24]. Most cases have been diagnosed only at autopsy or at lung biopsy. In the latter this condition has to be diagnosed from *Pneumocystis* pneumonia, but the latter condition is almost confined to children and the causal organisms ought to be detectable histologically.

TREATMENT

In the early cases few treatments appeared to be satisfactory though some patients recovered, apparently spontaneously. Most patients have failed to respond to cortico-steroid drugs. Potassium iodide in a high dose (8 g daily) was possibly helpful in 2 cases. Oral chymotrypsin has also been reported successful in 1 case, although the recovery might have been coincidental [8]. However, increased success has recently been claimed for a technique by which the lung is repeatedly washed out either with heparin (7·5 units per ml of 0·5% buffered normal saline) or with 1% acetyl cysteine [25]. Recently a Carlens catheter, similar to that used for broncho-spirometry, has been employed to isolate and ventilate one lung while the other was washed out with large quantities of fluid. A number of recoveries have been reported following this treatment.

PROGNOSIS

About 20–25% of reported cases have died within 5 years but about 20% have recovered or greatly improved. The course is often progressive over a number of months, death being due to respiratory failure, occasionally to *cor pulmonale*. There is often secondary infection. It seems possible that the new technique of lung lavage may improve the recovery rate.

PULMONARY ALVEOLAR MICROLITHIASIS [28 & 31]

DEFINITION

Pulmonary alveolar microlithiasis is a disease, often familial, characterized by a radiographic appearance of very fine, sand-like mottling uniformly distributed through both lungs (plate 37.1). This mottling represents an extensive intra-alveolar deposit of calcium-containing bodies. Symptoms at the time of discovery are often minimal, in spite of extensive radiographic changes but later there is gradual progression to respiratory failure or *cor pulmonale*.

AETIOLOGY

The cause of the disease is quite uncertain. A number of cases have been exposed to dusts of various types but, in view of the diversity, it is doubtful whether this is significant. Some have claimed that the calcifications represent calcified fungi, but no fungi have ever been isolated and this seems improbable. There is no evidence of any upset of calcium metabolism or any deposit of calcium elsewhere but it has been suggested that the disease represents a local error of calcium metabolism [28]. Cases have been described at all ages between 6 and 72 but the majority are between 30 and 50 at the time of discovery. There is an equal distribution in the sexes. A familial incidence, with siblings affected, is common.

PATHOLOGY

The lungs are solid and may sink in water. Throughout them there are sand-like grains diffusely distributed but maximal at the bases.

The lung can be difficult to cut. Microscopically there are 'onion skin' bodies, resembling corpora amylacea, in 30–80% of alveoli and these bodies are usually densely calcified. There may or may not be interstitial fibrosis and cellular infiltration. There may be emphysematous blebs at the apices or the anterior margins of the lungs. There are usually no changes in the other organs.

FUNCTIONAL ABNORMALITY

Dyspnoea is the major complaint and will obviously be caused partly by the deletion of functioning lung tissue and partly by the rigidity of the lung. However, respiratory function tests are often normal or near normal even with extensive x-ray changes, though there are relatively few records of investigation. Decreased VC, diffusion defects and disturbed $\dot{V}/\dot{Q}$ ratio have all been reported.

CLINICAL FEATURES

These cases are often discovered by routine radiography at an asymptomatic stage when the patient may have no complaints in spite of dramatic x-ray changes. Later there is increasing dyspnoea, cough with a little sputum and, later still, cyanosis, polycythaemia and perhaps *cor pulmonale*. Death occurs from respiratory or cardiac failure. The patient may occasionally cough up calcified bodies. Spontaneous pneumothorax has been recorded. There are often no physical signs in the chest even in the presence of extensive x-ray changes, though later there may be crepitations and later still signs of *cor pulmonale*. Clubbing may be present.

TREATMENT

No satisfactory treatment has been reported. At least one failure with corticosteroid drugs has been recorded.

PROGNOSIS

The disease is probably slowly progressive. One case died 25 years after diagnosis, others deteriorated in 4 or 5 years or remained symptom free as long as 14 years.

AMYLOIDOSIS OF THE RESPIRATORY TRACT [11, 12, 14 & 29]

Amyloidosis is usually secondary to one of the well-recognized causes but primary amyloidosis, of unknown cause, may occur. *Primary amyloidosis* may be generalized or localized to a particular organ. In *secondary amyloidosis* the lung is said to be involved in 10% of cases [13], with deposits in the walls of the pulmonary arteries. Occasionally this may be the dominant clinical feature and cause death from respiratory insufficiency [11]. The lungs are said to be involved in 30% of cases of *generalized primary amyloidosis* which affects pulmonary arteries and alveolar walls, although the lesions elsewhere tend to dominate the clinical picture [30]. *Primary amyloidosis confined to the respiratory tract* is very rare but there are a number of cases in the literature. This condition will now be discussed.

PATHOLOGY

Primary amyloidosis confined to the lower respiratory tract occurs in 3 forms (1) multiple diffuse bronchial deposits (2) localized bronchial deposits and (3) single or multiple localized deposits in the lung parenchyma.

(1) Multiple bronchial deposits consist of numerous grey-white smooth nodules, up to 1 cm in diameter, in the trachea or larger bronchi. The entire wall may become diffusely infiltrated. Microscopically the epithelium remains intact, although there may be squamous metaplasia. Foci of calcification and giant cells may occur at the edge of the deposit. The larynx may be involved.

(2) Single localized bronchial deposits are much rarer. They occur in the larger lobar or segmental bronchi.

(3) Single or multiple parenchymatous deposits are usually subpleural. The amyloid staining may be atypical and the deposits may contain calcium, cartilage or even bone. Plasma cells, lymphocytes and giant cells may occur at the periphery of the lesion.

CLINICAL AND RADIOLOGICAL FEATURES

Patients usually present in their 6th or 7th decade and males predominate. The bronchial lesions come to notice by causing symptoms of obstruction, often with a history of many years before the diagnosis is made. Clinically and radiologically, therefore, they resemble bronchial adenoma or, if the history is short, bronchial carcinoma. Parenchymal lesions are often detected on routine radiography and are usually thought to be bronchial carcinoma or, if multiple, metastases. Multiple bronchial deposits may cause cough, wheeze and symptoms resulting from bronchial obstruction. The patient is often hoarse as a result of deposits in the larynx or trachea.

TREATMENT

Treatment, if it is possible, is surgical. Localized parenchymal lesions will usually be removed as possible carcinomata. Localized bronchial lesions, if the diagnosis has been made by biopsy, may be removed by sleeve resection, though lobectomy may prove necessary. If neither is possible endoscopic removal will be justified but may have to be repeated. Endoscopic removal is usually all that is possible in patients with multiple bronchial deposits.

PROGNOSIS

The lesions probably progress slowly over years. The prognosis after removal of localized solitary lesions of lung or bronchus appears to be good.

TRACHEOBRONCHOMEGALY [1 & 21]

Tracheobronchomegaly is a rare disease characterized by unusual width of the trachea and main bronchi and, because of the ineffectiveness of cough, often complicated by lower respiratory infection. It is probably congenital and inherited as an autosomal recessive; it has been recorded in association with Ehlers-Danlos syndrome. Most reported cases have been young adults but it has been found in children. There is an atrophy or congenital defect of the connective tissues of the trachea and main bronchi. The condition may be missed on the straight chest film but is obvious on the tracheobronchogram. There is gross variation in diameter of the trachea with respiration and there may be distortions and irregularities.

TRACHEO- AND BRONCHOPATHIA OSTEOPLASTICA
[4, 7, 16 & 32]

DEFINITION

Tracheo- or bronchopathia osteoplastica is a rare disease characterized by numerous cartilaginous and calcified plaques which project into the lumen of the trachea and large bronchi, occasionally also affecting the larynx.

PREVALENCE, AETIOLOGY AND PATHOLOGY

Some 144 cases had been reported in the world literature up to 1967 [32], mostly in middle aged and elderly men, but occasionally in women. The bony or cartilaginous bosses or plaques arise over the cartilages and are continuous with the perichondrium. They may be localized or diffuse and sometimes obstruct bronchi, though most have only been diagnosed at autopsy. They may arise as a metaplasia in association with the connective tissue cells which form the elastic fibres of the lamina propria of the trachea. The cause is unknown.

CLINICAL FEATURES

Most cases have only been diagnosed at autopsy in patients dying of other diseases, but a few have been diagnosed by the characteristic bronchoscopic appearances [19] Obstruction of a bronchus may give rise to pneumonia which may lead to bronchoscopy and thus to the diagnosis.

RADIOLOGY

Bronchial obstruction may lead to collapse and pneumonia. The conditions cannot be recognized on the straight x-ray but tomography of trachea or main bronchi may reveal the characteristic projecting nodules [4].

TREATMENT

Treatment is only necessary for complications, such as infection or collapse. If the collapsed lung is not severely damaged endoscopic removal or sleeve resection of the blocked bronchus might be justified.

TRANSPLANT LUNG [27]

Lung complications are common in patients who have received a kidney transplant. They are often associated with infection by unusual organisms, such as *P. carinii*, cytomegalic inclusion virus or fungi, presumably because of the reduction of the patient's immune mechanisms by large doses of corticosteroid drugs, and the efficiency of antibiotics in coping with the more usual infecting agents. A number of patients have been described who developed fever and dyspnoea at varying periods after transplant, sometimes simultaneously with a 'transplant rejection' episode, and in whom this was not thought to be due to infection. Some also had cough. Radiographically there might be no abnormality, or there might be miliary or pneumonia-like shadows. Lung function studies showed reduced Pa,O_2, and often reduced Pa,CO_2, and decrease in diffusing capacity. Most patients recovered, usually after an increase in corticosteroid dosage. It has been suggested that the condition is an immunological phenomenon and due to a similar antigen occurring in the patient's lung and in the transplanted kidney. This may be so, but it remains possible that these are merely episodes of lung infection from which the patient can make a spontaneous recovery.

REFERENCES

[1] AL-MALLAH Z. & QUANTOCK O.P. (1968) Tracheobronchomegaly. *Thorax* 23, 320.

[2] ANDRIOLE V.T., BALLAS M. & WILSON G.L. (1964) The association of nocardiosis with pulmonary alveolar proteinosis. A case study. *Ann. intern. Med.* 60, 266.

[3] BAAR H.S. & GALINDO J. (1966) Bronchiolitis fibrosa obliterans. *Thorax* 21, 209.

[4] BAIRD R.B. & MACARTNEY J.N. (1966) Tracheopathia osteoplastica. *Thorax* 21, 321.

[5] BATES D.V. & CHRISTIE R.V. (1964) *Respiratory Function in Disease. An Introduction to the Integrated Study of the Lung.* Philadelphia, Saunders.

[6] BERGMAN F. & LINELL F. (1961) Cryptococcosis as a cause of pulmonary alveolar proteniosis. *Acta path. microbiol. scand.* 53, 217.

[7] BOWEN D.A.L. (1959) Tracheopathia osteoplastica. *J. clin. Path.* 12, 435.

[8] BRODSKY I. & MAYCOCK R.L. (1961) Pulmonary alveolar proteinosis. Remission after therapy with trypsin and chymotrypsin. *New Engl. J. Med.* 265, 935.

[9] BRUN J., PERRIN-FAYOLLE M., TOMMASI M., QUENTIN R. & POZZETTO H. (1962) Protéinose alvéolaire mortelle associée à une fibrose pulmonaire (documentation anatomo-clinique). *Rev. lyon. Méd.* 11, 491.

[10] CARLSEN E.T., HILL R.B.Jr. & ROWLANDS D.T.Jr. (1964) Nocardiosis and pulmonary alveolar proteinosis. *Ann. intern. Med.* 60, 275.

[11] COTTON R.E. & JACKSON J.W. (1964) Localized amyloid 'tumours' of the lung simulating malignant neoplasms. *Thorax* 19, 97.

[12] CRAVER W.L. (1965) Solitary amyloid tumour of the lung. *J. thorac. cardiovasc. Surg.* 49, 860.

[13] DAHLIN D.C. (1949) Secondary amyloidosis. *Ann. intern. Med.* 31, 105.

[14] DOMM B.M., VASSALLO C.L., ADAMS C.L. (1965) Amyloid deposition localized to the lower respiratory tract. *Am. J. Med.* 38, 151.

[15] DOYLE A.P., BALCERZAK S.P., WELLS C.L. & CRITTENDEN J.O. (1963) Pulmonary alveolar proteinosis with hematologic disorders. *Arch. intern. Med.* 113, 940.

[16] EDITORIAL (1968) Rigid trachea. *Br. med. J.* ii, 4.

[17] FRAIMOW W., CATHCART R.T. & TAYLOR R.C. (1960) Physiologic and clinical aspects of pulmonary alveolar proteinosis. *Ann. intern. Med.* 52, 1177.

[18] HARRISON E.G.Jr., DIVERTIE M.B. & OLSEN A.M. (1960) Pulmonary alveolar proteinosis. Report of a case with a fatal outcome. *J. Am. med. Ass.* 173, 327.

[19] HUZLY A. (1960) *An Atlas of Bronchoscopy.* New York, Grune and Stratton.

[20] JONES C.C. (1960) Pulmonary alveolar proteinosis with unusual complicating infections. A report of 2 cases. *Am. J. Med.* 29, 713.

[21] KATZ I., LEVINE M. & HERMAN P. (1962) Tracheobronchomegaly. *Am. J. Roentg.* 88, 1084.

[22] LEVINSON B., JONES R.S., WINTROBE M.M. & CARTWRIGHT G.E. (1958) Thrombocythaemia and pulmonary intraalveolar coagulum in a young woman. *Blood* 13, 959.

[23] LULL G.F.Jr., BEYER J.C., MAIER J.G. & MORSS D.F.Jr. (1959) Pulmonary alveolar proteinosis: report of 2 cases. *Am. J. Roentg.* 82, 76.

[24] RAMIREZ-R J., NYKA W. & MCLAUGHLIN J. (1963) Pulmonary alveolar proteinosis. Diagnostic technics and observations. *New Engl. J. Med.* 268, 165.

[25] RAMIREZ-R. J. (1967) Pulmonary alveolar proteinosis. Treatment by massive bronchopulmonary lavage. *Arch. intern. Med.* 119, 147.

[26] ROSEN S.H., CASTLEMAN B. & LIEBOW A.A. (1958) Pulmonary alveolar proteinosis. *New Engl. J. Med.* 258, 1123.

[27] SLAPAK M., LEE H.M. & HUME D.M. (1968) Transplant lung—a new syndrome. *Br. med. J.* i, 80.

[28] SOSMAN M.C., DODD G.D., JONES W.D. & PILLMORE G.U. (1957) The familial occurrence of pulmonary alveolar microlithiasis. *Am. J. Roentg.* 77, 947.

[29] SPENCER H. (1962) *Pathology of the Lung.* London, Pergamon Press.

[30] SYMMERS W.ST.C. (1956) Primary amyloidosis. A review. *J. clin. Path.* 9, 187.

[31] VISWANATHAN R. (1962) Pulmonary alveolar microlithiasis. *Thorax* 17, 251.

[32] WAY S.P.B. (1967) Tracheopathia osteoplastica. *J. clin. Path.* 20, 814.

[33] WILLIAMS G.E.G., MEDLEY D.R.K. & BROWN R. (1960) Pulmonary alveolar proteinosis. *Lancet* i, 1385.

CHAPTER 38

Glanders and Melioidosis

GLANDERS

AETIOLOGY AND EPIDEMIOLOGY

Glanders is primarily a disease of horses, more rarely of mules and donkeys. It is due to a non-motile gram-negative bacillus (*Malleomyces mallei, Bacillus mallei, Pseudomonas mallei*, or *Loefflerella mallei*, among other names!). Even when the disease was common in horses it was rare in man. Since its virtual abolition in horses by a slaughter policy it is largely of historical interest. It mainly affected those who came into close contact with horses, but laboratory infections have been reported and the organism is a dangerous one to handle [4 & 14].

Infection could certainly occur through abrasions but in most cases the mode of infection was uncertain. The incubation period varied from a few days to weeks or months [2].

PATHOLOGY

The lesions mainly consisted of abscesses or granulomata, which might be found in many different organs, though the lungs were often affected. Histologically there was neutrophil infiltration but epithelioid and giant cells might occur [2].

CLINICAL FEATURES [2, 4 & 14]

In man the disease was either acute or chronic. It was often localized chiefly to the respiratory system, with severe prostration, fever, mucopurulent nasal discharge, cough and purulent sputum. A generalized eruption, at first papular and then pustular, was not uncommon. There were sometimes generalized abscesses, particularly in lungs, lymph glands, muscles and subcutaneous tissue. Pneumonia has been the main manifestation in laboratory infections [4]. Leucocytosis seems to have been unusual. Death usually occurred within 10 days.

The chronic disease affected the same organs and was characterized by remissions and exacerbations, sometimes with ultimate recovery.

There was some evidence that subclinical infection could occur and that the virulence of the organism varied [14].

DIAGNOSIS

Diagnosis can only be made with certainty by isolating the organism. The agglutination test appears to be unreliable [14], but, on the basis of laboratory experiment, the complement fixation test might be more sensitive [7].

TREATMENT

Sulphadiazine was successful in all of 6 accidental laboratory infections in man [4].

MELIOIDOSIS [1, 3, 6, 11 & 12]

AETIOLOGY AND EPIDEMIOLOGY

Melioidosis is a rare disease, occurring mainly in Burma, Malaysia, Viet-Nam, Thailand and Indonesia. A few cases have also been reported from Ceylon, Madagascar, the Caribbean region and Ecuador [10], as well as from Turkey [5], North Australia [11], the South Pacific, and even the U.S.A. [9]. Melioidosis is due to a motile gram negative bacillus, *Loefflerella whitmori* (*Pseudomonas pseudomallei, Bacillus whitmori, Pfeifferella whitmori*, etc.). Natural infections have been found in man, horse, cow, pig, sheep, goat, cat, dog, wallabies and several rodents [10], but it seems that the main source of human infection, perhaps through abrasions, is probably

645

from water or mud from which it cannot infrequently be isolated in the relevant countries [7]. It seems likely, on the basis of serum antibody surveys, that subclinical infections may not be uncommon [8] and that clinical disease is more likely in those already debilitated; most of the original cases described in Rangoon by Whitmore [13] were in morphia addicts.

PATHOLOGY

The lesions are basically abscesses, sometimes macroscopically resembling miliary tuberculosis, with granulomatous margins and filled with caseous pus. The exudate is initially neutrophil but giant cells may occur; epithelioid cells are rare [9]. The appearances are indistinguishable from glanders. Abscesses may be found in lungs, liver, spleen, kidney, lymph glands, bone, brain or other organs.

CLINICAL FEATURES AND RADIOLOGY

The course may be acute or chronic. The acute disease may be fulminant, often predominantly respiratory and resembling acute pneumonia or lung abscess, sometimes bilateral. There is often delirium and sometimes diarrhoea. The diarrhoea may resemble cholera. There may be a leucocytosis. The chronic form may closely resemble tuberculosis, both clinically and radiologically. There may be multiple subcutaneous abscesses in connective tissue, muscle or elsewhere, often with sinus formation.

DIAGNOSIS

Diagnosis is best made by culturing the organism from sputum or pus; blood culture is often positive in the acute form. The agglutination test is unreliable, since the patient may die before the titre has risen and also because positive titres may be found in healthy people [14]. In chronic cases it is possible that the complement fixation test may be of more value [7].

TREATMENT

The organism is usually sensitive to sulphadiazine [6 & 9] and to chloramphenicol [1 &

3]. Treatment should be intensive and prolonged, as the mortality without treatment is very high and relapse is not uncommon. Cases have been treated with chloramphenicol combined with novobiocin and kanamycin [1]. When time allows, laboratory sensitivity tests should be carried out to a wide variety of drugs. Bactericidal drugs, best given in combination, are to be preferred if the organism is sensitive to them *in vitro*. Even with chemotherapy the reported mortality is relatively high.

REFERENCES

[1] BAUMANN B.B. & MORITA E.T. (1967) Systemic melioidosis presenting as a myocardial infarct. *Ann. intern. Med.* **67**, 836.

[2] BERNSTEIN J. M. & CARLING E.R. (1909) Observations on human glanders, with a study of six cases and a discussion of the methods of diagnosis. *Br. med. J.* i, 319.

[3] COOPER E.B. (1967) Melioidosis. *J. Am. med. Ass.* **200**, 452.

[4] CRAVITZ L. & MILLER W.R. (1950) Immunologic studies with *Malleomyces mallei* and *Malleomyces pseudomallei*. II. Agglutination and complement fixation tests in man and animals. *J. infect. Dis.* **86**, 53.

[5] ERTUG C. (1961) Melioidosis. *Dis. Chest* **40**, 693.

[6] HARRIES E.J., LEWIS A.A.G., WARING J.W.B. & DOWLING E.J. (1948) Melioidosis treated with sulphonamides and penicillin. *Lancet* i, 363.

[7] NIGG CLARA & JOHNSTON MARGARET M. (1961) Complement fixation test in experimental clinical and subclinical melioidosis. *J. Bact.* **82**, 159.

[8] NIGG CLARA (1963) Serologic studies on subclinical melioidosis. *J. Immunol.* **91**, 18.

[9] PREVATT A.L. & HUNT J.S. (1957) Chronic systemic melioidosis. *Am. J. Med.* **23**, 810

[10] REDFEARN M.S., PALLERONI N.J. & STANIER R.V. (1966) A comparative study of *Pseudomonas pseudomallei* and *Bacillus mallei*. *J. gen. Microbiol.* **43**, 293.

[11] RIMINGTON R.A. (1962) Melioidosis in North Queensland. *Med. J. Aust.* **49**, 50.

[12] THIN R.N.T. (1968) *Melioidosis. A Report of Clinical Cases and of a Survey for Antibodies among Non-Indigenous Men living in an Endemic Area.* Edinburgh University, M.D. Thesis.

[13] WHITMORE A. (1913) An account of a glanders-like disease occurring in Rangoon. *J. Hyg.* **13**, 1.

[14] WILSON G.S. & MILES A.A. (1964) Glanders and melioidosis. In *Topley and Wilson's Principles of Bacteriology and Immunity*, 5th Edition, Vol. 2, p. 1711. London, Arnold.

CHAPTER 39

Paraquat Lung [4]

AETIOLOGY

Paraquat ('Gramoxone W') is a potent weed-killer. It also is highly toxic for animals and man, even in small doses. The lungs bear the brunt and death has usually been due to respiratory failure. Human cases have mostly resulted from the accidental drinking of paraquat from lemonade or other common household bottles in which it has been stored unlabelled and within easy access of young people.

The toxicity of paraquat for animals was demonstrated as early as 1966 [2]. Marked individual variation in response to paraquat was observed in animals of the same species. The most severe effects occurred when the chemical was given on an empty stomach. Ingestion is not necessary to produce pulmonary changes, which have been observed in man after subcutaneous injection of about 1 ml of a 20% solution.

It seems probable that the same varieties of effect occur in man as in experimental animals and the minimal lethal dose is not known. Death has been reported after a single mouthful [1 & 5].

PATHOLOGY

The basic lung lesion is a proliferative bronchiolitis and alveolitis; intra-alveolar hyaline membrane and fibrosis occur and are thought to be the consequence of intra-alveolar haemorrhage [3]. The histopathological features in man resemble those in experimental animals. The rôle of pulmonary surfactant is not yet known [4].

FUNCTIONAL ABNORMALITY

As expected from the pathological changes the dominant findings are impairment of CO transfer values, moderate airways obstruction and/or restrictive ventilatory abnormality. The few studies made early in the condition have to be interpreted in the light of the frequent inability of the patient to make maximum physical effort. Thus effort-dependent measurements such as the FVC or FEV_1 may not reflect the true state of affairs. The Tco is the most refined of the lung function tests available in this context and is a useful monitor of progress when blood gas studies are within normal limits, as we have found in a case studied personally. Severe lung damage will, of course, result in hypoxia and a low Pa,o_2.

CLINICAL AND RADIOGRAPHIC FEATURES

Ingestion results in painful lesions of the tongue, mouth and fauces and in painful oesophagitis and gastritis. Excretion is by the kidney which suffers in the process; albuminuria, haematuria and raised blood urea may occur. There may also be hepatic damage. Respiratory symptoms characteristically begin some days after ingestion and consist of progressive cyanosis and dyspnoea. Particularly when renal damage is severe, paraquat may continue to be detected in the urine for at least a week [4] unless haemodialysis is performed.

Radiographically the lungs initially show fine mottling which may coalesce to give the appearance of marked pulmonary oedema.

TREATMENT

Essential elements of treatment are scrupulous barrier nursing, prednisolone in high dosage to suppress tissue reaction, and repeated haemodialysis until no paraquat is being excreted by the urine. Lung transplantation (p. 649) is rational in severe cases. The recent case reported by Matthew *et al.* [4] demonstrated the feasibility of the procedure although the outcome in this particular case was fatal. Histopathological findings in the patient indicated that death was not due to tissue rejection but was most likely to be the consequence of paraquat poisoning of the transplant since the substance was still present in the blood at the time of operation.

REFERENCES

[1] BULLIVANT C.M. (1966) Accidental poisoning by paraquat: report of 2 cases in man. *Br. med. J.* i, 1272.

[2] CLARK D.G., McELLIGOTT T.F. & HURST E.W. (1966) The toxicity of paraquat. *Br. J. industr. Med.* 23, 126.

[3] MANKTELOW B.W. (1967) The loss of pulmonary surfactant in paraquat poisoning. *Br. J. exp. Path.* 48, 366.

[4] MATTHEW H., LOGAN A., WOODRUFF M.F.A. & HEARD B. (1968) Paraquat poisoning—Lung transplantation. *Br. med. J.* iii, 759.

[5] OREOPOULOS D.G., SOYANNWO M.A.O., SINNIAH R., FENTON S.S.A., McGEOWN M.F. & BRUCE J.H. (1968) Acute renal failure in case of paraquat poisoning. *Br. med. J.* i, 749.

CHAPTER 40

Lung Transplantation [1]

Lung transplantation was first performed experimentally in animals in 1951 by Juvenelle *et al.* [3] who reimplanted a separated lung. In 1963 a lung homograft in man [2] functioned for 18 days, the longest survival time so far recorded. Lung transplantation raises the same problems as in the case of other organs, the most important being immunological rejection. Unexpectedly the likelihood of rejection appears to bear no relation to the complexity of the tissue transplanted.

Apart from tissue rejection 2 other problems beset lung transplantation. The transplanted lung, unlike the heart, depends for its function on a poorly understood complex of voluntary, biochemical and autonomic control. The lung naturally has to be denervated and this results in a slow, deep type of ventilation. It has been suggested that the only method of dealing with this difficulty is to retain part of the host's lung to provide the 'drive' necessary for appropriate function of the graft. The second problem is the early development of a defect in gas transfer. This may improve with time but so far has never become normal. It is thought that the defect may be caused by pulmonary oedema due to obstruction of pulmonary venous drainage.

The purely surgical problem seems less difficult though it is suggested that implantation of the bronchial arteries into the aorta might improve the results.

The indications for lung transplantation are difficult to define. It would seem reasonable to consider it in younger patients affected by lung disease with a hopeless prognosis and preferably without infection. Paraquat poisoning is one such disease, provided the substance can be eliminated by haemodialysis before operation so as to avoid a toxic effect on the transplanted lung.

Lung transplantation is still in an experimental stage and so far no lasting success has been achieved. It should only be attempted in large centres where teams are specifically equipped for the highly technical procedures involved. It is still uncertain whether it will in fact prove to be a practicable and ethically justifiable method of treatment.

REFERENCES

[1] EDITORIAL (1968) Lung transplantation. *Br. med. J.* **iii**, 755.
[2] HARDY J.D., WEBB W.R., DALTON M.L. & WALKER G.R. (1963) Lung homotransplantation in man. *J. Am. med. Ass.* **186**, 1065.
[3] JUVENELLE A.A., CITRET C., WILES C.E.Jr. & STEWART J.D. (1951) Pneumonectomy with reimplantation of the lung in the dog for physiologic study. *J. thorac. Surg.* **21**, 111.

CHAPTER 41

The Investigation of Commoner Clinical Problems of the Respiratory System

THE INVESTIGATION OF HAEMOPTYSIS

The coughing up of blood is an alarming symptom which almost always brings the patient to the doctor. Even though in many cases no important cause is found, especially if the haemoptysis is a small one and is not repeated, all such cases do need investigation because haemoptysis may first draw attention to a serious underlying disease, in particular carcinoma or tuberculosis.

It is first of all important to make sure that the blood has really been coughed up, not vomited, and that it is not due to a nose bleed. Haemoptysis is usually easy to distinguish by the history. If the history is doubtful and the material is available it will be found that a haematemesis consists of changed brownish blood and is usually acid in reaction. Blood from an epistaxis may drop down the back of the pharynx and be coughed up, but, on questioning, the patient is usually aware of this and has blown blood down his nose as well.

If the condition is really a haemoptysis an assessment of the possible cause is influenced by

(1) the age of the patient,
(2) the amount of blood produced and
(3) whether there are acute symptoms, symptoms of chronic cough or no other symptoms at all.

If there are acute respiratory symptoms, such as fever, cough and chest pain of recent onset, *pneumonia* and *pulmonary infarct* are the first conditions to be considered, remembering that pneumonia may be secondary to a *bronchial carcinoma* or very occasionally to a *benign tumour* such as an adenoma of the bronchus. *Lung abscess* is a less frequent cause. Haemoptysis from pneumonia and infarct often merely consists of blood streaking of the sputum, though the sputum may be deeply bloodstained and sometimes mainly consists of blood.

If the cough has lasted for weeks or months *tuberculosis* as well as *bronchial carcinoma* will have to be considered. In most cases of *bronchiectasis* cough will date back to childhood and the haemoptysis consist of blood streaking of purulent sputum. Occasionally bronchiectasis is first manifested by severe haemoptysis, most often from the middle lobe and due to the erosion of an artery by a broncholith derived from old primary tuberculosis. *Repeated small haemoptyses*, occurring daily over a week or more, are highly suggestive of bronchial carcinoma (p. 526). Haemoptysis is occasionally due to a *vascular tumour* of the lung, respiratory tract or bronchi, sometimes associated with *hereditary haemorrhagic telangiectasia* and a personal or family history of nose bleeds (p. 559). Haemoptysis may also complicate a *foreign body* in the bronchus and blood streaking is not uncommon in *acute* or *chronic bronchitis*, though usually only as an isolated incident.

All patients who have coughed blood should have a *chest x-ray*. This may give an immediate indication of the probable diagnosis, for instance a hilar mass suggestive of a carcinoma or bilateral upper zone shadows suggestive of tuberculosis. Clinical and radiological evidence may be sufficient to suggest pneumonia or infarct, though the possibility of underlying carcinoma must not be forgotten and *bronchoscopy* must be undertaken if the haemoptysis is repeated, if it consists of more than a single incident of blood streaking, or if there are clinical symptoms consistent with possible carcinoma. In a younger person longstanding chronic cough, purulent sputum and localized crepitations may suggest bronchiectasis and bronchography should be undertaken if this diagnosis seems clinically possible. Occasionally severe or repeated haemoptysis may be due to quite localized *apical fibrosis* associated with healed tuberculosis, sometimes with demonstrable local bronchiectasis. Sputum cytology for malignant cells, sputum or laryngeal swabs for tubercle bacilli and the tuberculin test will all be appropriate investigations in clinical situations where carcinoma or tuberculosis are probabilities.

It must also be remembered that haemoptysis may complicate *mitral stenosis* or *left ventricular failure*, though these causes are usually fairly overt clinically. We have sometimes seen haemoptysis complicating *coronary thrombosis*, perhaps due to small accompanying pulmonary infarcts, usually not radiographically visible.

The problems of haemoptysis with diffuse pulmonary radiographic abnormality are dealt with on p. 654.

If no cause for the haemoptysis is found, and both chest x-ray and bronchoscopy show no abnormality, the patient should be reviewed with a further x-ray after 4–6 weeks and if necessary thereafter. A recurrence of haemoptysis may well be an indication to repeat the bronchoscopy. Bronchography may also be done at this stage if it has not been done already. It is wise to follow up a patient with unexplained haemoptysis for at least a year.

Unexplained haemoptysis is common. Johnston *et al.* [1] were unable to find a cause in 44% of 324 patients. Among the causes of haemoptysis chronic bronchitis or bronchiectasis accounted for 20% of the total and were more than 7 times as frequent as either bronchial carcinoma or active pulmonary tuberculosis. Patients with otherwise unexplained haemoptysis had a higher rate than controls of calcified primary tuberculous lesions visible in the chest film; expectoration of a broncholith or underlying bronchiectasis were excluded and the explanation of the haemoptysis was obscure. These authors doubt the value of follow-up if no explanation of the haemoptysis is found after full investigation. Only 2 of their patients, radiologically regarded as normal at the first attendance, developed lesions later, bronchial carcinoma and pulmonary tuberculosis respectively. Poole and Stradling [2], in a series of patients referred for radiography because of haemoptysis, found abnormalities in only 42%. The films were double read and in 281 cases, reported as normal, were repeated a month later; in only 1 patient was an abnormality discovered in the second film. A follow-up of 76 patients at 1 year suggested that in only 2 might there have developed later lesions possibly related to the haemoptysis.

Both these groups doubt the value of later follow-up, if initial investigation reveals no cause for the haemoptysis but both record a small percentage of patients in whom a later abnormality was, in fact, discovered. We consider, therefore, that follow-up should be carried out when adequate facilities are available, the interval between x-rays and the duration of follow-up varying according to the clinical circumstances.

ROUNDED SOLITARY LESION IN AN X-RAY OF THE CHEST

It is relatively common to find a single rounded shadow, perhaps 1·5–3 cm in diameter, in a routine chest x-ray, in a patient with no, or entirely nonspecific symptoms. The following are the main diagnoses to be considered:

(1) *bronchial carcinoma*,
(2) *metastasis* from a carcinoma elsewhere,
(3) *tuberculosis*, the so-called 'tuberculoma',
(4) *benign*, or relatively benign, tumour, and
(5) *hydatid cyst* (in a patient from certain countries or areas).

Occasionally (6) *pneumonia*, (7) *lung abscess* or (8) *infarct* may give rise to a rounded shadow in the postero-anterior x-ray, but the shadow is usually more than 3 cm in diameter, its edge is relatively ill-defined and a lateral film often indicates a segmental rather than a rounded outline. The first 5 possibilities are the most important to differentiate from one another.

When confronted with a rounded shadow of the type indicated, the clinician should immediately enquire whether the patient has ever had a previous chest x-ray. It is not uncommon, with the benefit of hindsight, to be able to find that the same shadow was present in a film taken perhaps 4 or 5 years previously. This makes carcinoma of any kind very unlikely and removes a good deal of the urgency from the situation. Tuberculosis and benign tumour remain possibilities.

The *margin* of the shadow should be carefully observed. A hairline edge, with a precisely defined border between the shadow and the surrounding lung, suggests the possibility of a benign tumour or a hydatid cyst rather than a carcinoma or a tuberculoma, though we have occasionally been deceived. A hydatid cyst, if unruptured, is usually completely *uniform in density*, though not always precisely round in outline. Complete uniformity in density with a precise edge makes hydatid an important possiblity to be considered. On the other hand if the cyst has ruptured there may be reaction in the surrounding lung and the edge will not be precisely defined. Moreover a crescent of air may be visible, within the shadow, where the endocyst is separated from the ectocyst (p. 367), an appearance which is only mimicked by an aspergilloma in an old tuberculous or other cavity (p. 287). A benign tumour may not be of uniform density. If *calcification* is not apparent on the straight film tomography may reveal it. Tomography may also show one or more translucencies suggestive of cavities, though these are more often due to less dense tissue rather than to air. Cavitation or calcification may also occur in a tuberculoma. The presence of surrounding mottling, the so-called 'satellite' lesions which are sometimes only revealed by tomography, is suggestive of tuberculosis. Both in tuberculosis and in carcinoma the edge of the lesion is not precisely defined and the lesion may not be entirely round.

So much for the radiographic appearance,

assessment of which may or may not limit the number of possibilities. The *tuberculin test* should be done; a strongly positive test makes tuberculosis more likely, though it does not prove it; a negative or only weakly positive test makes tuberculosis unlikely. The patient should be carefully examined for palpable *lymph nodes*, paying particular attention to the retroclavicular regions. If none is found, and if the radiological appearances and age of the patient are consistent with the possibility of carcinoma, a *mediastinoscopy* may be done to search for mediastinal lymph nodes, especially if the patient's respiratory function and general state would justify thoracotomy. A positive biopsy from a mediastinal lymph node would spare the patient an ineffective operation (p. 540). Routine *bronchoscopy* is normally unhelpful as the tumour is beyond the reach of vision, though occasionally the appearances may suggest invasion of subcarinal lymph glands. Some cytologists are willing to search washings taken at bronchoscopy for malignant cells; others consider that bronchoscopy may distort normal cells and give rise to false positives. *Cytological examination* of the sputum may be helpful and should be done. *Tubercle bacilli* are seldom seen in direct smear in such a patient, though they should be looked for; culture is not positive in time for the result to influence management.

There is often a question of how far one should go in trying to exclude a solitary metastasis from a carcinoma elsewhere. If there is no symptomatic lead we are usually satisfied with examining the faeces on at least 3 occasions for *occult blood*, looking for red cells in the urine and carrying out an *intravenous pyelogram*. In a woman the pelvis should be examined. In our experience a hypernephroma is the commonest primary neoplasm to be symptomatically cryptic and to give rise to rounded pulmonary lesions.

After all these investigations one is often still left uncertain about the diagnosis. In such a case the most dangerous lesion, as well as one of the most common, is a carcinoma of the bronchus and *thoracotomy* must be considered, if there are no contra-indications (p.

539). Fluoroscopy will be done to exclude diaphragmatic paralysis and barium swallow to exclude displacement of the oesophagus by mediastinal tumour. If there is any possibility of tuberculosis the thoracotomy should be carried out under cover of appropriate chemotherapy. At operation the surgeon may still be uncertain about the diagnosis. He may be assisted by examination of a frozen section or he may have to decide the extent of resection on purely clinical grounds.

If operation is contra-indicated it must be considered whether the patient should be given radiotherapy, in spite of the absence of proof of carcinoma. In fact the results of megavoltage radiotherapy in a carcinoma of the size being considered are relatively good (p. 542), especially when the tumour is of the well-defined squamous type. If the tuberculin test, or other evidence, makes tuberculosis also a possible diagnosis, antituberculosis chemotherapy should be given at the same time as radiotherapy and continued for 6 months to 1 year or more, according to the progress and the likelihood of the diagnosis.

THE INVESTIGATION OF A LUNG CAVITY

The commonest causes of a cavity in the lung, demonstrated in the chest x-ray, are *tuberculosis*, *lung abscess* or *bronchial carcinoma*. A cavity complicating a bronchial carcinoma may be caused by necrosis of the growth itself or by infective necrosis of the lung beyond a carcinomatous stenosis of the bronchus. Radiologically the inner wall of a cavity in a necrotic growth is often characteristically thick and persistently irregular, though irregularity may also occur in the initial stages of an abscess, as the slough separates, and occasionally in the thick caseous wall of a tuberculous cavity. Complete necrosis of a growth may sometimes give rise to a thin-walled cavity. Bilateral apical shadows with mottling or calcification favour tuberculosis, though abscesses due to *K. pneumoniae* (p. 122) or *actinomycosis* (p. 290) may give very similar appearances (except calcification). The presence of periostitis of the ribs favours actinomycosis (p. 290), though, of course, this disease is rare.

Rarer causes of lung cavities are (1) the breakdown of an area of progressive massive fibrosis in complicated pneumoconiosis (p. 474) or Caplan's syndrome (p. 474) and (2) the breakdown of a pulmonary rheumatoid mass (p. 579). In both the clinical context should make diagnosis simple, though complicating tuberculosis should be excluded by repeated sputum examination.

If the patient is *ill* and *febrile* when first seen lung abscess is an important possibility and rapid deterioration may occur if the physician unduly delays treatment pending diagnosis. The *sputum* should be sent at once for bacteriology, including anaerobic culture, and *treatment* with large doses of penicillin initiated (p. 159). But the diagnosis of lung abscess is only provisional at this stage. The sputum should be examined daily for tubercle bacilli and malignant cells should be sought. A tuberculin test should be initiated. A *white blood count* should be done. A high count favours lung abscess, though the abscess may, of course, be secondary to a bronchial carcinoma. *Bronchoscopy* can usually be deferred for a week or more pending the response to penicillin (or other antibiotic if suggested by the culture result) and the results of sputum examination. If no tubercle bacilli are found on direct smear, and the age and other circumstances make carcinoma a possibility, bronchoscopy should be carried out even if, as is usual, the temperature has responded to penicillin. If bacteria such as *K. pneumoniae* or staphylococci, resistant to penicillin, are cultured from the initial sputum there should be an appropriate change in chemotherapy (p. 159). If the white blood count is normal, the sputum negative for tubercle bacilli on direct smear, the bronchoscopy negative and if the *temperature persists* in spite of penicillin or the failure to demonstrate penicillin resistant pathogens, the diagnosis of tuberculosis may nevertheless have to be seriously considered; direct smear examination is sometimes negative even in the presence of extensive tuberculous cavitation. A strongly positive tuberculin test would favour the diagnosis, though in an ill patient the test may be less positive. By now the patient will probably have had penicillin for 10 days or so and a trial of *antituberculosis chemotherapy* may well be justified (p. 235).

Serial radiology will, of course, be helpful in confirming the response of a lung abscess to chemotherapy and in indicating bronchoscopy if the fever responds to penicillin but the x-ray does not. A *bronchial foreign body* may also account both for the development of a lung abscess and its failure to improve radiologically under penicillin.

Less common causes of fever and lung cavitation are the infection of an *emphysematous bulla* or cyst, characterized by a thin wall and a fluid level (p. 330), or of a *ruptured hydatid cyst*, in which case there is usually a crescentic air shadow in the upper part of the opacity and sometimes evidence of the collapsed endocyst protruding above the fluid level. In the latter case portions of endocyst may be coughed up and the *Casoni test* may be positive (p. 368). Occasionally it may be difficult to differentiate between a large posterior lung abscess and a *pyopneumothorax*. Marked dullness on percussion may indicate pleural fluid or the presence of an old empyema drainage scar may suggest the likelihood that an encysted empyema has ruptured into the lung. In a patient who has been to the tropics a basal cavity may suggest the possibility that an *amoebic liver abscess* has ruptured through the diaphragm, especially if the sputum contains the characteristic reddish-brown 'anchovy sauce'.

If the patient is *afebrile throughout*, it is unlikely that the cavity is due to a lung abscess. Tuberculosis or a necrotic carcinoma are more probable. Investigation should proceed along the lines already indicated but a cavitated peripheral tumour may not show bronchoscopic abnormality. If the sputum is negative for tubercle bacilli on smear, no malignant cells have been found and there is no evidence of metastases in lymph nodes or elsewhere, *thoracotomy* may have to be considered in the absence of other contra-indications (p. 539). A preliminary *mediastinoscopy* may be justified (p. 540). If tuberculosis remains a possibility thoracotomy should be carried out under cover of antituberculosis chemotherapy.

THE INVESTIGATION OF DIFFUSE RADIOGRAPHIC PULMONARY ABNORMALITY

From time to time, either as a result of a routine chest x-ray, or in the course of the investigation of symptoms, a patient is found to have abnormal shadows, mottled, nodular or reticular, throughout both lung fields. There are very large numbers of potential causes for these appearances. In the investigation of such a patient the most important evidence is usually provided by

(1) clinical data, such as occupational history and presence or absence of cough, dyspnoea, fever, pulmonary crepitations, finger clubbing or lesions elsewhere in the body,

(2) the result of the tuberculin test, particularly important in differentiating tuberculosis from sarcoidosis,

(3) direct smear and cultural examination for tubercle bacilli,

(4) the Kveim test for sarcoidosis (p. 379),

(5) biopsy of lymph node, liver, lung or other organ,

(6) therapeutic tests for tuberculosis, and occasionally the use of corticosteroid drugs.

Pulmonary function tests have little diagnostic value in such cases; they may show a limitation of pulmonary diffusion and ventilatory abnormality of the restrictive type, the degree of which may parallel the clinical evidence of dyspnoea.

THE PATIENT WITH FEVER

The first point to establish is whether the patient is *febrile* and ill. If he is febrile the investigation must be undertaken urgently but fortunately the number of possibilities is limited. The most important cause to exclude is *miliary tuberculosis* (p. 207). The major alternative is a diffuse *bronchopneumonia* (p. 123), though in this case the mottling is usually less well defined. Occasionally a patient with *allergic alveolitis* (p. 504) will present in this way. A patient with miliary tuberculosis may have a history of contact with tuberculosis and may have been unwell for some weeks; the onset in pneumonia is more acute. A patient with allergic alveolitis should have a history of exposure to mouldy hay, birds or one of the other recognized causes (p. 504), and usually presents little problem as long as the clinician bears the possibility in mind. Fine pulmonary crepitations may be heard in any of the 3 conditions, though perhaps less frequently in miliary tuberculosis unless this is very advanced. Choroidal tubercles should be sought since their presence is diagnostic of miliary disease (p. 209); an enlarged spleen or liver will also be suggestive. A positive direct smear sputum examination for tubercle bacilli will clinch the diagnosis, but it is often negative in miliary disease and one cannot afford to await the results of culture. A leucocytosis will favour bronchopneumonia, though occasionally occurring in miliary tuberculosis. A strongly positive tuberculin test suggests tuberculosis, but it is important to remember that the test may be negative or only weakly positive in miliary disease; in any case, if the patient is very ill, the initiation of treatment cannot await the result. Liver biopsy and search of bone marrow for tubercle bacilli (p. 210) may be justified in some cases.

All these investigations must be carried out at once, and in most cases the correct diagnosis becomes clear or at least probable. If it still remains in doubt the best course is to treat both for miliary tuberculosis and pneumonia and come to a conclusion on the basis of the rapidity with which the chest film clears—within weeks with pneumonia, within months with miliary tuberculosis—and on the final results of culture for tubercle bacilli. Sputum culture for nontuberculous organisms should also have been done, as well as blood culture and the taking of the first blood serum for viral antibody titres (p. 133). Mycoplasmal pneumonia may mimic miliary tuberculosis so it is as well to include tetracycline in the initial treatment.

Theoretically one might imagine that a patient with pulmonary sarcoidosis might sometimes present with fever. Oddly enough we have never seen one do so. When there is fever with sarcoidosis our experience is that the disease is never confined to the lung and clinical evidence of skin lesions, lesions of salivary glands, iridocyclitis, or splenomegaly will suggest the possibility of the diagnosis. The exception, of course, is a patient presenting with erythema nodosum but here the bilateral hilar lymph gland enlargement will suggest the diagnosis (p. 380).

In pulmonary alveolar proteinosis (p. 639) the shadows resemble those of lung oedema rather than miliary disease. The disease, in any case, is very rare. Polyarteritis nodosa (p. 434) is another rare cause.

THE PATIENT VIRTUALLY FREE FROM SYMPTOMS

A patient with extensive bilateral pulmonary lung shadows, yet well and virtually free from symptoms, is much more likely to be suffering from *sarcoidosis* than from any other disease. The diagnosis will have to be established by tuberculin test, biopsy (skin, liver, lymph gland or lung) or Kveim test, according to the circumstances (p. 385). A patient with such diffuse shadows due to tuberculosis will usually be ill, though tubercle bacilli should, of course, be sought in all cases. Patients with uncomplicated *pneumoconiosis* may also be symptom free but the diagnosis should be suggested by the occupational history. Very occasionally a patient with apparent diffuse fibrosis, perhaps as the result of 'burnt out' *diffuse interstitial lung disease (fibrosing alveolitis*, p. 565) may be free from symptoms and present only with radiological abnormality. In our experience such patients are usually elderly and lung biopsy is often not justifiable; the diagnosis will be made by observation and exclusion, and can then only be provisional. *Pulmonary alveolar microlithiasis* (p. 641), a very rare condition, may be discovered in a symptom free patient by routine radiography. The pinhead, fine, intensely white, diffuse shadows are pathognomonic and only simulated by the residua of the old type of oily lipiodol formerly used for bronchography, though lipiodol residua are usually localized rather than diffuse. Microlithiasis may also be found in the patient's siblings.

THE PATIENT WHO HAS SYMPTOMS BUT IS AFEBRILE

In such a patient the commonest symptoms are dyspnoea, cough, haemoptysis, malaise and loss of weight. If cough, malaise and loss of weight rather than dyspnoea are the most prominent symptoms one thinks particularly of *pulmonary tuberculosis* or *diffuse pulmonary metastases*. The x-ray appearance, the examination of the sputum for tubercle bacilli and malignant cells, evidence of a possible primary lesion elsewhere (remembering the thyroid as well as the breast, bronchus, kidney and gastrointestinal tract) may provide the answer. If it remains uncertain, lung biopsy may or may not be justified. If biopsy is not thought to be justified it is better to treat potentially treatable disease and give antituberculosis chemotherapy; regression or progression of symptoms, and x-ray changes, will usually clarify the situation within a few weeks. Leukaemic lung shadows will be diagnosed by blood examination; other lymphomata are virtually always diagnosable on clinical grounds by the time the lung has become involved (p. 552).

If dyspnoea is the most prominent symptom *diffuse interstitial lung disease* (*fibrosing alveolitis*, p. 565), *allergic alveolitis* (p. 504), *rheumatoid lung* (p. 578), *honeycomb lung* (p. 571), *haemosiderosis* (p. 596), *diffuse pulmonary metastases* (including *lymphatic carcinomatosis*, p. 529) and *diffuse pulmonary lymphomatoses* are among the important possibilities. When *pneumoconiosis* is severe enough to give rise to marked dyspnoea it has usually already become 'complicated' by progressive massive fibrosis which will be suggested by the radiographic appearance as well as by the occupational history (p. 474). Well-marked clubbing, in the absence of large quantities of purulent sputum, favours diffuse interstitial lung disease. In allergic alveolitis there should be an appropriate history of exposure (p. 504). In rheumatoid lung there is evidence of rheumatoid disease elsewhere. The patient with honeycomb lung shows the

typical fine radiographic cysts (p. 571) as well as mottling; he is often a young man and may have bone cysts if the abnormality is associated with eosinophil granuloma (p. 573), or mesodermal abnormalities if it is associated with tuberous sclerosis (p. 574). A patient with idiopathic pulmonary haemosiderosis will be young and will give a history of recurrent haemoptysis (p. 596); if it is secondary there will be clinical and radiographic evidence of mitral stenosis.

It is usually possible to find evidence of the primary tumour if metastases are suspected. There may be a history of previous mastectomy; lung metastases may occur many years later. There may be a history of some other operation for malignant disease. The thyroid should be examined, as lung secondaries from a thyroid carcinoma may be relatively chronic. Occult blood should be sought in the faeces and a barium series carried out if necessary. Bronchial carcinoma should always be remembered. In older men the prostate should also be investigated; it should be examined clinically and the serum acid phosphatase checked. Renal tumours may also be cryptic (p. 652). As already mentioned leukaemia is usually obvious from the blood count and other lymphomata nearly always give rise to suggestive clinical evidence by the time the lung is invaded.

The diagnosis, therefore, is often obvious, or highly suggestive, on purely clinical grounds or after fairly straightforward investigation. Other investigations for conditions such as tuberculosis and sarcoidosis can be carried out, when indicated, along the lines already mentioned. Only relatively seldom is lung biopsy necessary or justifiable, though sometimes biopsy with the high speed drill (p. 78) may be justified where a formal thoracotomy is thought too risky or too disturbing.

Occasionally, after full investigation short of lung biopsy, the clinician is left with tuberculosis, sarcoidosis, diffuse interstitial lung disease or diffuse metastases as possibilities in a patient whose age or general condition do not justify biopsy. If the relative chronicity makes it justifiable a Kveim test for sarcoidosis can be initiated and antituberculosis chemotherapy given. The Kveim test will be read after 6 weeks and the result of the sputum cultures for tubercle bacilli may be available by then; either may clinch the diagnosis. After 2 months or so a patient with tuberculosis should be improving under treatment. If he is not, or is deteriorating, corticosteroids, perhaps as prednisolone 5 mg 4 times daily, may be added, in case the condition is due to interstitial lung disease (which may or may not respond, p. 570) or sarcoidosis with a negative Kveim test (in which case, unless it is fibrotic or burnt out, there should be some radiological clearing within another 2 months). Ruthless progression in spite of these measures suggests malignant disease.

THE INVESTIGATION OF RECURRENT 'PNEUMONIC' SHADOWS IN THE X-RAY (p. 140), OF PLEURAL EFFUSION (p. 279) AND OF MEDIASTINAL LESIONS (p. 601)

These diagnostic problems are fully discussed in the relevant chapters, as indicated above.

REFERENCES

[1] JOHNSTON R.N., LOCKHART W., RITCHIE R.T. & SMITH D.H. (1960) Haemoptysis. *Br. med. J.* i, 592.

[2] POOLE G. & STRADLING P. (1964) Routine radiography for haemoptysis. *Br. med. J.* i, 341.

Author index

This index contains the names of all authors whose work is quoted in the text. References are given at the end of each chapter. The first figure after the name indicates the page on which the full reference appears; the figure in square brackets indicates the number of the reference on that page.

Subject index

Figures in bold type indicate a major reference or the most important reference under that heading. For references to authors see separate author index.

Asthma—(*contd.*)
  locusts and 397
  mast cells in 401
  mediastinal emphysema in 411, 449
  menstruation and **397**
  metaplasia, squamous and 402
  in the middle-aged 407
  migraine and 397
  mites and 398, 408
  morphia in treatment of 416
  mortality of **394**, 420
    by age 396
    Australia 396
    bronchodilator drugs and 396
    Canada 396
    corticosteroid drugs and 394
    Denmark 396
    England and Wales 394, 396
    Finland 396
    France 396
    Germany 396
    Ireland 396
    Italy 396
    Japan 396
    Netherlands 396
    New Zealand 394, 396
    Norway 396
    Scotland 394, 396
    Spain 396
    U.S.A. 396
  mucous glands in 396, 402
  mucous membrane in 396
  mucus in 396
  multiple factors in 399
  nasal polyposis and 398, 400
  neurosis and 398
  nitrogen washout in 403
  non-specific factors in 406
  orciprenaline in 414
    oral 415
  orris root and 398
  oxytetracycline in 417
  Pa,co_2 in 403, 409
  paint and 400
  Pa,o_2 in 403, 409
  pathogenesis of **396**
  pathology of **402**
  perfume and 400
  phenobarbitone in 414
  physical signs in **406**
  pigeon chest in 410
  placebos in 412
  platinum in **492**
  plugs in 404, 405, 407, 410
  pneumonia in 411
  pneumothorax in 408, 411
  pollen extracts in 412
  pollens and 398, 405
  polyarteritis nodosa and 407, 409, 435, 437

Asthma—(*contd.*)
  postoperative complications in 410
  precipitating factors in **404**
  pregnancy and **397**
  prevalence of **394**
  prevalence of, by age 394
    England and Wales 394
    men 394
    North America 394
    Northern Europe 394
    women 394
  printer's **492**
  prognosis in **420**
    in England 420
    in Norway 420
  promethazine hydrochloride in 415, 416
  psychogenic factors and 398
  psycho-social stress and 399
  psychological factors in **405**
    in treatment of **414**
  pulmonary artery pressure in 411
  radioactive xenon in 403
  radiology of **407**
  reagins in 400
  reflex factors in 400
  reversibility tests in 409
  rib fractures and 410
  sedatives in 416
  serotonin in 402
  serum sickness and 397
  shunt effect in 403
  sinuses in 408
  skin tests in 408
  slow reacting substance in 401
  smoke and 400
  sputum in **409**
  SRS-A in 401
  status asthmaticus (*see* Status asthmaticus)
  stimuli causing **397**
  stridor in 404, 406
  surgery in 418
  tachycardia in 406
  tetracycline in 413
  thoracic deformity in 410
  Tokyo-Yokohama and 400
  treatment of **411**
    adrenaline in 414
    alcohol in 416
    allergens and **412**
    aminophylline in 415
    aminophylline suppositories 415
    atropine methonitrate in 415
    barbiturates in 416
    breathing exercises in 418
    bronchodilator drugs in 414
    choline theophyllinate in 415

Asthma—(*contd.*)
    corticosteroid drugs in **416**
      intermittent 417
      long term 416
    deptropine in 415
    ephedrine in 415
    glomectomy in 418
    homochlorcyclizine, in 415
    infection and 413
    intermittent positive pressure in 414
    isoprenaline in 414
      oral 415
    morphia in 416
    orciprenaline in 414
      oral 415
    oxytetracycline in 417
    phenobarbitone in 414
    promethazine hydrochloride in 415, 416
    psychological factors in **414**
    sedatives in 416
    unilateral bronchospasm 403
    surgery in 418
    vagotomy in 418
  vaccines in 398, 414
  vagotomy in 418
  vasomotor rhinitis and 397
  ventilation/perfusion ($\dot{V}/\dot{Q}$) relationships in 403, 415
  ventricular fibrillation in 414
  wheat and 398
  work of breathing 403
  in young adults 406
Astrup interpolation micro method **45**
Atelectasis 11, 35
  in asthma 411
Atmospheric pollution, bronchial carcinoma in, *see* Carcinoma, bronchial, atmospheric pollution in
  chronic bronchitis and 305, **307**, 309, 316
  chronic bronchitis and, treatment of 320
  in Los Angeles 490
  prevention of 319
Atomic reactors 498
Atrium, pulmonary 10
Atropine, and effects of cigarette smoke 306
  goblet cells and 16
  methonitrate, in asthma 415
Attack rate, tuberculosis, *see* tuberculosis, attack rate
'Atypical' mycobacteria, *see* mycobacteria, 'atypical'
Auricle, dilated left 4
Auricular fibrillation, in pulmonary infarction 462